VISUAL AGNOSIAS
AND OTHER DISTURBANCES OF VISUAL PERCEPTION AND COGNITION

Vision and Visual Dysfunction

General Editor Professor John Cronly-Dillon

Dept of Optometry and Vision Sciences, UMIST, Manchester, UK

VISION AND VISUAL DYSFUNCTION
VOLUME 12

Visual Agnosias and Other Disturbances of Visual Perception and Cognition

Otto-Joachim Grüsser

Dept of Physiology
Freie Universität
Berlin, Germany

and

Theodor Landis

Dept of Neurology
University of Zurich
Switzerland

CRC Press, Inc.
Boca Raton   Ann Arbor   Boston

Published in the USA, its dependencies, and Canada by
CRC Press, Inc.
2000 Corporate Blvd., N.W.
Boca Raton, FL 33431, USA

Typeset in Monophoto Ehrhardt by August Filmsetting, Haydock, St Helens, UK
Printed and bound in Great Britain by William Clowes Limited, Beccles and London

Library of Congress Cataloging-in-Publication Data
Vision and visual dysfunction/edited by John Cronly-Dillon.
    p. cm.
  Includes index.
  ISBN 0–8493–7500–2 (set)
  1. Vision. 2. Vision disorders. I. Cronly-Dillon, J.
  [DNLM: 1. Vision. 2. Vision Disorders. WW 100 V831]
QP474.V44
612.8′4—dc20
DNLM/DLC
for Library of Congress   90–1881
                                                   CIP

Visual agnosias/O. Grüsser, T. Landis.
      p. cm.— (Vision and visual dysfunction; v.12)
  Includes index.
  ISBN 0–8493–7512–6
  1. Visual agnosia. I. Grüsser. Otto-Joachim. II. Landis, T.
  (Theodore) III. Series.
  [DNLM: 1. Agnosia–physiopathology. 2. Cognition. 3. Visual
  Perception. WW 100 V831 v.12]
QP474.V44 vol. 12
[RC394.V57]
612.8′4 s—dc20
[616.8]
DNLM/DLC
for Library of Congress   90–1889
                                                   CIP

Contents

Preface

Nearly three years ago, when we received the kind invitation from Professor Cronly-Dillon and the publishers to contribute a volume on *Visual Agnosias and Related Disorders* to *the Vision and Visual Dysfunction* series, we optimistically assumed that we would have enough leisure time together to discuss the content and problems of the twenty-three chapters extensively, to write, to read and mutually to correct our manuscripts. Since our days as medical students in the early 1950s and 1960s, we have both been interested in the physiology and pathophysiology of vision and have collected notes systematically on our observations in patients. While one of us (O.-J. G.), after finishing his training in neurology and psychiatry, continued his main research work in the field of experimental neurophysiology of the visual and vestibular system, the other (T. L.) performed his principal research as a clinician. T. L. had, however, the privilege of working in a centre of neurology in which, owing to the interest in research projects of its clinical director, Professor Günter Baumgartner, clinical studies were complemented by several experimental neurophysiological research laboratories in which the study of the visual, vestibular and oculomotor system was the main goal. Thus, when discussing and writing these chapters, we not only had common research interests and tested our hypotheses by investigating patients together at the Zurich Department of Neurology, but were also in close contact with research groups working in fields close to the topics of this book.

In the course of our work we finally realized that the time alotted by the deadlines set for publication was too short to elaborate on all the topics included in this volume with the thoroughness that we had originally planned. As a matter of fact, we ultimately found ourselves under serious pressure of time, but with the help of our native North American co-workers we hope to have written a readable and comprehensive text, introducing those interested in vision to the wide field of visual pathology.

Since visual agnosias and related disorders frequently affect not only human-specific higher brain functions but also those abilities depending essentially on cultural and educational background, we have included some chapters on normal, higher-order, visual brain functions, in which this broader, socio-cultural background is discussed. We also thought that a brief historical introduction including the time before the nineteenth century might be helpful in putting present-day knowledge into the framework of its historical development. Thus, we decided to write a chapter about the history of Western thought on higher brain functions and cognition, and we have also added short historical introductions to the individual chapters. This 'historicizing' attitude may not please all readers, since in modern neuroscience it has become rather fashionable to forget the work accomplished by preceding generations, where the length of a 'generation' seems to becoming shorter and shorter. Since the 'turnover' in clinical knowledge and observations in patients suffering from brain lesions is much slower than that in the more technical research fields of modern neuroscience, reading old literature was extremely helpful in clarifying symptoms, details of observations and theoretical concepts of visual agnosias.

In several volumes of this series extensive descriptions of the anatomy and neurophysiology of the peripheral and central visual systems are presented in great detail. Our coverage of these areas (Chapters 3–7) is not intended as a review of the research work in this field but rather to give the reader who is interested in visual agnosias and related disorders a basic knowledge of the 'normal' physiological mechanisms serving vision. In our opinion this knowledge is necessary for an understanding of the pathological symptoms and processes discussed in the following chapters as well as for the design of adequate tests used in agnosia research. Of necessity such an overview has to simplify some complicated facts and discard certain details important for research workers in a special field. Finally it also has to make a selection from the various opinions interpreting the research data. All readers who wish to learn more than a rough outline of the anatomy and physiology of the eye and the central visual system and who require more abundant information on the state of the art are referred to other volumes in this series. The selection for our material was based, of course, on our personal preference as well as on the arbitrary availability of research literature in our laboratories.

In order to maintain consistency with other volumes in

this series, some compromises on historical terminology became necessary: for example, we have used the spelling 'Purkinje' rather than the orthographically correct 'Purkyně'.

We would never have been able to finish the manuscript without the careful help of our co-workers. In Zurich: Ms S. Kirschner; in Berlin: Mrs J. Dames, Mrs B. Hauschild, Mr P. Holzner, Mrs M. Klingbeil, Mrs I. Knierim and Mrs U. Saykam. The collaboration of Mrs J. Dames, Mr Andrew Port and Mr Norman Cook in the English translation is also gratefully acknowledged. Mrs U. Krawczynski, Mr S. Müller and Mrs D. Starke are responsible for a major part of the graphic work. Since we preferred to redraw and combine many of the published figures instead of using the originals, this part of the work was particularly extensive.

Many of our friends and co-workers read parts of the manuscript and suggested inprovements and additions. For this assistance we wish to especially thank Professor G. Baumgartner (especially on Chapter 10), Dr P. Brugger and Dr Marianne Regard at the Department of Neurology, University of Zurich, and Dr S. Akbarian and Professor U. Grüsser-Cornehls at the Department of Physiology, Freie Universität Berlin. The work was begun while one of us (O.-J. G.) was supported by an Akademie-Stipendium of the Volkswagen Foundation. During the months of completing the last chapters and proofreading O.-J. G. held an F. C. Donders Professorship at the University of Utrecht. Thus, both institutions have contributed to the book, which is also gratefully acknowledged. The research work carried out in Zurich was supported by funds of the Swiss National Science Foundation (Schweizerischer Nationalfond, grants Nos. 3.876.-0.81; 3.884.-0.83; 3.821.-0.87), the Janggen-Poehn-Stiftung and the EMDO-Stiftung, while the experimental work mentioned in the text from the Berlin laboratory was financially supported in part by the Deutsche Forschungsgemeinschaft, Bonn-Bad Godesberg (grants Gr 161/18–38). The very low basic research support available at the Freie Universität Berlin was supplemented through additional financial assistance from the Freie Universität Berlin to the 'Forschungsprojektschwerpunkt Physiologie und Pathophysiologie des visuellen und vestibulären Systems', a research group at the Department of Physiology in Berlin.

Finally we must thank our families for tolerating repeated retreats from family life on long weekends and vacation, while working together in Zürich, Berlin or Utrecht.

O.-J. G.
T. L.
Berlin and Zurich
1991

In memoriam
Günter Baumgartner
1924–1991

1 Introduction

In the following 22 chapters, we shall attempt to review the higher-order perceptual and cognitive aspects of vision and its disturbances. We shall discuss the physiological mechanisms underlying these partly man-specific abilities in visual cognition. Since these abilities are not only rather complex but also highly adaptive, they considerably influenced the cultural development of mankind. Certain brain lesions affect cognitive visual functions, but the clinical symptoms of the different types of visual agnosias and other impairments of visual cognition vary considerably not only according to the site and size of the lesions, but also with the cultural and educational level the patient had acquired before the brain lesion.

The second chapter will deal with the history of Western thought on visual perception and cognition as well as on abnormal vision. We believe that even old-fashioned interpretations should not be forgotten, since they help us to understand the roots of modern ideas about brain function. The long historical development of Western scientific interest in visual perception and cognition led to ideas and models which, even when outdated, often have the same charm as peculiar old buildings or whimsical gardens designed by former generations. Such relics of past scientific work serve to remind us that our present models of scientific thought, if not forgotten in the future, could become a mere footnote to the scientific achievements of later generations. On the other hand, when discussing categories into which higher-level vision can be divided, we realize that our present thoughts do not differ essentially from the level reached by the great Arabic scientists of the tenth or eleventh centuries, or by Albertus Magnus during the thirteenth century.

Chapters 3–8 will deal with the principles of visual brain functions. By summarizing neuroanatomical, neurophysiological, psychophysical and neuropathological findings, we have tried to construct a gross framework of present-day knowledge in this field, which might be useful in order to understand some of the pathological conditions discussed extensively in Chapters 9–23.

Following the handbook tradition, we shall begin this chapter with some principal considerations on the main topic of this volume and try, by introducing some definitions, to clarify for the non-expert reader some basic concepts about visual agnosias. We will then discuss what modern neuroscience in collaboration with artificial intelligence can teach us about the general principles of visual perception of objects and space, will present some thoughts on ontogenetic development of higher visual brain functions and finally will discuss principles of the correlation between visual neuronal activity and visual perception.

Definition and Types of Visual Agnosias

Visual or optic agnosias are defects of associative or cognitive visual functions caused by circumscribed brain lesions (e.g. trauma, local ischaemia, tumour) or by diffuse (toxic, metabolic, infectious or degenerative) impairments of brain function, which affect higher-order visual centres or their connections through the white matter of the brain (Wilbrand, 1887; Pötzl, 1928; Kleist, 1934). The functions impaired in visual agnosia are normally considered to be present in adolescent and adult subjects. In brain-lesioned children, the symptoms and time course of visual agnosias differ from those in adults. This point will be treated only cursorily. Related to and sometimes accompanying visual agnosias are 'productive' pathological visual symptoms, such as phosphenes, visual hallucinations, visual pseudo-hallucinations and abnormal deformations of the visual percepts (e.g. dysmorphopsias and dysgnosias, which will be discussed in separate chapters). Also related to visual agnosias are congenital defects (genetic or intrauterine developmental), which lead to an impairment of visual cognitive functions. As a rule, these are followed by behavioural disturbances, as for example in juvenile autism, in which cerebral mechanisms related to averbal social communication are severely impaired, or by difficulties acquiring cultural cognitive functions, such as in congenital dyslexias. Such congenital defects of visual data processing will not be discussed in this volume, but rather in Volume 13 of this series.

The generation of clinical neurologists who investigated and treated patients suffering from brain-wounds received during the First World War became aware that two large groups of agnosias exist besides lesions in the primary visual cortex (area striata). Kleist (1934) summarized the observations of these neurologists, and discriminated visual object agnosias from visual space agnosias ('*Störung der Objektwahrnehmung*' – '*Störung der Raumwahrnehmung*'). He explained these two types of agnosias by pointing to the different brain regions that were affected: object agnosia appears when the occipito-temporal visual structures are affected, while spatial agnosias develop when the occipito-parietal system is affected. Thus Kleist realized that with regard to perception of the visual world, both an object-related cerebral 'what?' system and a space-related 'where?' system exist. One might add that considering visuo-motor aspects, i.e. the interaction between the visual world and the acting subject, frontal lobe structures are also involved ('where to?' system).

On the basis of present-day knowledge of the anatomy and physiology of the primate central visual system, one may classify the clinical symptoms appearing after lesions in the central visual system into the following general categories:

Visual Field Defects

These appear after lesions in the retina, the afferent visual pathways and the primary visual cortex (area 17 = area V1). As a rule, such central sensory defects are not included in the visual agnosias, but will nevertheless be briefly discussed in Chapter 9. The extent, quality (achromatic, chromatic) and binocular congruence of the visual field defects vary, depending on the site and the size of the lesion within the afferent or central visual system. Cortical blindness will be included in this category as an extreme case.

Perceptive Visual Agnosias

Caused by circumscribed lesions of visual centres in the peristriate regions of the brain located outside the primary visual cortex (area striata, area V1), these are impairments of elementary precognitive visual functions, such as movement perception, colour perception and stereoscopic depth perception. In some cases, these perceptive defects are found to be only in a portion of the binocular visual field (e.g. hemifield defects), i.e. these phenomena underlie the elementary rules of retinotopic mapping. Since brain lesions are rarely restricted to one or two functionally different cytoarchitectonic cortical areas, perceptive visual agnosias either are frequently 'masked' by higher-order deficits of visual cognition, or are accompanied by other neurological defects outside of the visual domain. We include 'local' changes in visual object perception as dysmorphopsias, macropsias or micropsia in the group of perceptive agnosias.

Apperceptive Visual Agnosias

These are caused by lesions in the occipito-temporal and occipito-parietal visual associative centres, and lead to impairment of visual shape or general visual space recognition. Frequently but not always, shape agnosias affect the whole field of vision or field of gaze, while spatial visual recognition defects may be restricted to one half of the extra-personal space (e.g. in unilateral visual 'hemineglect'). Diffuse lesions in the extended extrastriate visual cortical areas lead to global visual agnosia due to severe amblyopia, which is observed, for example, after recovery from cortical blindness caused by intoxication or bilateral cerebral ischaemia.

Associative Visual Agnosias

These lead to an impairment in the ability to recognize and comprehend certain distinct classes of visual signals and to recognize objects or visual surroundings despite their shape being comprehended. Although brain lesions leading to these agnosias might be lateralized, the defects are usually invariant with respect to the signal position in the visual fields. Face agnosia or 'pure' alexia are typical examples of this type of visual agnosia, which, as a rule, is not restricted to certain parts of the visual field or field of gaze.

General Agnosias

These are multimodal cognitive defects that can also affect the visual domain. These intellectual impairments are caused mainly by diffuse ischaemic, toxic or degenerative brain lesions affecting extensive parts of the cortex. In general agnosia, memory retrieval and the correct association of signals belonging to different modalities are impaired and the construction of a meaningful multimodal percept or object unity is no longer possible; it is frequently accompanied by spatial and temporal disorientation, as is the case in patients suffering from progressive states of Alzheimer's disease or extended viral meningoencephalitis.

Cortical Visuo-motor Defects

These may be caused by an interruption in the input–output coupling of visual percepts with gaze-motor, hand-motor or locomotor activity. Such defects appear after parietal and prefrontal cortical lesions. In turn, reduced visuo-motor abilities and impairment of spatially directed attention, especially with regard to gaze motor control, affect visual cognitive abilities, since normal visual perception is performed as a sequence of sampling gaze movements (eye saccades and/or head movements) across different parts of the visual space.

Productive Symptoms

Among these are phosphenes and hallucinations; they appear when parts of the brain undergo pathological stimulation. Such a state can be caused by lesions in other brain areas, leading to traumatic impairment of the metabolism of brain areas that are still working (e.g. collateral oedema in the area surrounding a lesion) or to a functional disinhibition of higher-order visual areas. The visual percepts evoked vary from such simple structures as the scintillating, 'fortification' phosphenes of 'classical' migraine to the complex, scenic hallucinations experienced by patients suffering from an alcoholic Korsakoff psychosis.

Physical and Cognitive 'Descriptors' of 'Natural' and 'Artificial' Visual Stimuli: A Converging Research Approach in the Neurosciences and in Artificial Intelligence

Vision is the ability of an organism or robot to detect by means of light part of its world, and to use these light signals for interaction with the world. In addition to suitable sense organs, the biological organism needs for this task a central nervous system, and the robot a programmable as well as adaptive signal processor and memory. Both systems operate according to algorithms, extracting from the abundant amount of visual information exactly or at least predominantly those components that are relevant for the selected task. Nets of nerve cells in the retina and the brain provide a symbolic representation of biologically relevant facts in our visual world. Their operation guarantees simultaneously that in normal function our visual world remains stable, even though the retinal image shifts every 0.18 to 1.2 seconds because of eye or head movements. Furthermore, the biological space (at least the grasping space and the near-distant action space) with the

coordinates left–right, above–below, forward–backward, is approximately perceived as Euclidean. Under normal conditions, locomotion within that space does not disturb the perceived constancy of the coordinates of the extrapersonal space.

One of the basic problems in understanding visual perception and the cognitive capacities of man is the search for the retinal and cerebral mechanisms which extract from the optical image, projected onto the retina, the behaviourally relevant information from a visual scene. The search for such descriptor functions can be approached in different ways:

1. Ideas leading to descriptor functions of image processing are derived from quantitative psychophysics data.

2. Intuitively meaningful reductive descriptor operations are invented in order to optimize image processing for machine vision. This approach is the one preferred by artificial intelligence (AI). The computational success of a selected set of descriptor operations acts, in turn, as a selection factor for further research.

3. When one records the activity of single neurones or of neuronal networks of the visual system, one has to apply an intuitively selected stimulus parameter again, since neurones in the visual brain frequently respond only to rather narrow visual 'features'. If a successful parameter is selected, optimal neuronal activation can be recorded. In order to evaluate the neuronal responses, computer-supported data processing is necessary. Meaningful or meaningless programs can again be applied to find the essential operations that the recorded neurone is performing. From the neurobiological data obtained using this method, general principles of neuronal signal processing are derived, which then can be compared with the descriptor functions selected by methods (1) or (2). Concepts deduced from correlations between psychophysical and neuronal data may be especially helpful in guiding the search for meaningful descriptors.

During the last three decades, the scientific approaches (1), (2) and (3) have provided partially overlapping results. This convergence has been optimistically interpreted as an indication that science is on a successful path (e.g. Marr, 1982).

Historical Observations: The Discovery of the Principles of Visual Data Processing

Before we deal in more detail with the remarkable progress that methods (1) and (2) have made, we shall first introduce the reader to the field by discussing the efforts of

Ernst Mach (1838–1916) to describe quantitatively the transformation of the retinal optical image (i) into a perceptual image (p). We shall designate these different levels the 'i-space' and the 'p-space'. To our knowledge, Mach was the first to discuss extensively the idea that the local light intensity distribution of the retinal image as well as its first and second spatial derivative are evaluated by the brain processes of visual perception. In his studies, he discovered that the perceived brightness distribution depends on spatial interaction between different points in the i-space. Furthermore, he emphasized the idea that the first spatial derivative of the intensity distribution leads to monocularly perceived 'local' depth cues: the perception of shapes and solid bodies is generated from shades of grey.

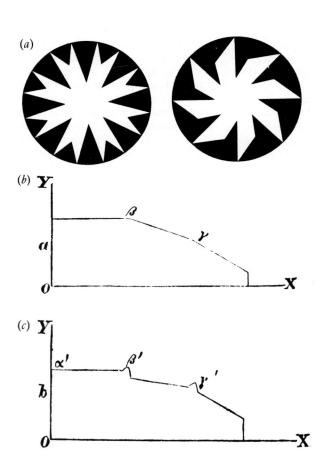

Mach was concerned primarily with the transformation of the signals in the i-space into neuronal signals that are represented in a retinotopic fashion in the retina or visual brain (p_r-space). Mach did not investigate in detail the next transformation from retinotopic coordinates to spatiotopic coordinates (egocentric coordinates, p_s-space). He tacitly assumed that, within certain limits, a linear transformation between retinotopic and spatiotopic coordinates is valid for the projection of the p_r-space into the p_s-space and argued that this transformation is controlled by an internal feedback of signals controlling gaze movement or gaze position. This principle of 'efference copy' mechanisms is further discussed on p. 6 (Mach, 1885).

Figure 1.1 illustrates the principal discoveries made by Mach in 1864 which prompted further thoughts on this matter. When the disc shown in Fig. 1.1(a) is rotated at sufficient speed above flicker fusion frequency, the effective average luminance distribution corresponds to Fig. 1.1(b) because of the temporal inertia of the visual process. What one perceives, however, is a brightness distribution as illustrated in Fig. 1.1(c). A bright band is seen whenever the spatial luminance profile produces a convex kink in the i-space. In the case of a black 'fan' on a white background (i.e. a 'negative' of Fig. 1.1(a)), the spatial luminance profile has two concave kinks and causes small dark bands in the p_r-space. Mach performed many experiments of this type, and produced illusionary bright or dark 'Mach bands'. In using stroboscopic illumination of simultaneously presented stripes of different shades of grey he found that the development of the simultaneous contrast mechanisms leading to Mach bands needs a certain time. Mach systematically varied the spatial luminance distribution (i), producing 'concave' or 'convex' one- or two-dimensional changes. He came to the general conclusion that at the perceptual level, the perceived brightness $B(x)$ is

$$B(x) = f(i) \pm f\left(\frac{\mathrm{d}^2 i}{\mathrm{d}x^2}\right) \qquad \text{[perceptual units]} \qquad (1.1)$$

For the description of the local transformation between light intensity (I) and perceived brightness (B) Mach applied Fechner's law (Fechner, 1860):

$$B = k \log\frac{I}{I_s} \qquad \text{[perceptual units]} \qquad (1.2)$$

where I_s represents a threshold value that depends on the average retinal light adaptation.

Mach described his findings on unidimensional spatial brightness distribution $B(x)$ to be a function of $i = f(x)$, the '*Lichtkurve*' of the unidimensional luminance distribution:

$$B(x) = a \log\left[\frac{i}{b} \pm \frac{k}{i}\left(\frac{\mathrm{d}^2 i}{\mathrm{d}x^2}\right)\right] \qquad \text{[perceptual units]} \qquad (1.3)$$

Fig. 1.1 *(a) When the discs shown are rotated at a sufficiently high speed above flicker fusion frequency, the time-averaged retinal luminance corresponds to three rings, as shown in (b). The perceived brightness, however, deviates as illustrated in (c). Brightness enhancement occurs at the kinks and the 'slope' of the shades of grey for the two outer rings deviates from the time-averaged luminance distribution (From Mach, 1865).*

with the constants a, b and k. Equation 1.3 can also be written as

$$B(x) = a \log \left[\frac{i}{b} \pm \frac{k}{i\rho_x} \right] \quad \text{[perceptual units]} \quad (1.4)$$

whereby ρ_x represents the spatial curvature of the '*(Licht-curve*'. For the two-dimensional case where $i = f(x, y)$ of a 'light plane' ('*Lichtfläche*'), equation 1.4 is transformed into

$$B(x,y) = a \log \left[\frac{i}{b} \pm \frac{k}{i}\left(\frac{1}{\rho_x} + \frac{1}{\rho_y} \right) \right] \quad \text{[perceptual units]} \quad (1.9)$$

Mach (1865, 1866a) emphasized with equations 1.3–1.5 that the second spatial derivative of the light distribution is somehow extracted by the neuronal network of the retina or the central visual system for recognition of the outlines of objects, an idea that resembles the 'primal sketch' of Marr and Hildreth (1980) discussed below.

Mach also found that although the first derivative of the spatial luminance distribution (i) is not essential in brightness perception, it contributes to the perceived depth and corporeality of solid objects. In the course of his studies, Mach (1866a) also discovered a phenomenon similar to what we now call the Craik–Cornsweet illusion: a border

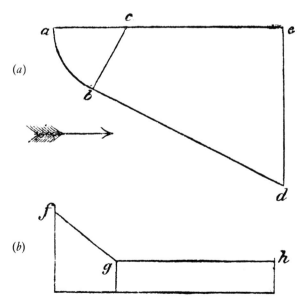

Fig. 1.2 *(a) Horizontal section through a three-dimensional quasi-cylindrical body. The surface a–b–d is illuminated by homogeneous light from the direction illustrated by the arrow. A spatial light distribution results as shown in (b). The distance f–g corresponds to a–b in (a). One can perceive a Mach band in g and simultaneously the corporeality of a–b–d–e (From Mach, 1866b).*

with a spatially asymmetric luminance profile dividing a homogeneous grey plane leads to a brightness step between the two half-fields which are actually of equal luminance. Mach concluded: 'The perceived brightness of a given point in the visual field [*Netzhautstelle*] depends on the luminance of a large area surrounding this point. The immediate neighbouring points have, of course, the strongest influence' (Mach, 1866a, p. 140). Mach attributed this phenomenon to the signal convergence that was discovered by histologists during his lifetime to be present in the human retina: about 100 rods were then assumed to converge onto a single retinal ganglion cell.

In the course of his studies concerned with varying the two-dimensional luminance distribution $i(x, y)$, Mach discovered that the values di/dx and di/dy determine the perceived depth of the surfaces. Firstly, he tested whether the law expressed by equation 1.3 or 1.5 is also valid for the perception of surfaces of solid shapes. One experiment confirming this is illustrated and explained in Fig. 1.2. He concluded: 'The eye reconstructs the shape of the plane illuminated from the light plane [*Lichtfläche*]. The result of this construction is not imagination, it is spatial sensation.'

The impression of three-dimensionality for solid shapes is thus generated by a spatial derivation from a two-dimensional 'light plane'. Depending on the shading, i.e. the di/dx curve relative to the illuminating gradient of the surrounding, one perceives either convex or concave surfaces. Mach assumed that each small area of the retina can develop its own 'depth' value, which essentially depends on the spatial first derivative relative to its immediate surrounding. In general, Mach concluded that by processing i, di/dx and d^2i/dx^2, 'the retina schematizes and caricatures' (Mach, 1868, 1906/1959, p. 217).

Mach's essential discoveries were the following:

1. The spatial light distribution within the visual field or within the retinal surface is respectively processed by retinal and cerebral neuronal mechanisms, whereby the spatial light distribution $i(x, y)$ on the retina as well as the first and second derivatives of this distribution constitute essential signals used for object recognition and spatial perception.

2. The first spatial derivative of the light distribution $i(x, y)$ determines the perceived monocular depth of an object ('corporeality', '*Körperlichkeit*'); the shading of the object's surface automatically generates a 3-D response at the p_r level.

3. The second spatial derivative of $i(x, y)$ is used in the perception of object contours, separating one object from another.

4. By performing psychophysical experiments, Mach obtained data supporting his theoretical approach aimed

at finding general laws of visual object and space recognition.

5. It should be noted that Mach's ideas were not appreciated by most vision physiologists, apart from the fact that some of his discoveries (e.g. the Mach bands along light–dark contrast borders) were often considered to be a curiosity of visual perception. Only in the present generation of 'computer vision' scientists were Mach's principles rediscovered and applied to vision research. This is usually done without giving credit to one of the leading physicists of his time, who worked at the universities of Graz, Prague and Vienna not only on problems of physics, but also on psychophysics, for he believed that a unitary approach to all phenomena experienced by man was necessary and important.

Eye Movements and Visual Perception

The average 'natural' visual stimulus consists of stationary structures as well as a few objects moving within the three-dimensional extra-personal space. Man moves his gaze across this space by eye saccades, slow-pursuit eye movements (when gazing at a moving object), head movements and/or body movements. Thus the percept of a stationary and coherent world is generated in the p_s-space by a set of successive images transformed from the i-space into the p_r-space images, which are shifted by every saccade with varying amplitudes across the retina. This fact leads us to the problem of perceived coherence and coordinate constancy of the visual percept.

To our knowledge, Johann Georg Steinbuch (1811) and Jan Evangelista Purkinje (1825a,b) were the first in the field of modern visual sciences to ask which cerebral mechanisms might guarantee the perceived stability of the extra-personal space, i.e. the transformation of the visual percept from the retinotopic p_r-space to the spatiotopic p_s-space, the objects of which are perceived to be independent of gaze position. Both scientists suggested the same answer, which had also been proposed by the Renaissance natural scientist and Jesuit Priest Franciscus Aquilonius (1613): the motor commands controlling eye, head or body movements are fed back within the central nervous system and are combined with the afferent visual signal flow in order to create the percept. This interaction must necessarily occur with opposite signs. Purkinje and later also Mach (1885/1906) believed that the motor movement signals controlling the gaze movements are simultaneously used by the central visual system to cancel the afferent visual movement signals caused by the shift of the retinal image that occurs with gaze movements. This model exactly corresponds to what modern neuroscientists today

refer to as the 'reafference principle' (von Holst and Mittelstaedt, 1950): the sensory input is continuously updated by an 'efference copy' of the motor commands moving the sense organs (cf. von Uexküll, 1928; historical review: Henn, 1969, 1971; Grüsser, 1986a). When the organism or a robot has 'solved' the question of the correlation between the 'retina-stable' visual field and the 'earth-stable' perceptual p_s-space by using such internal feedback mechanisms, other difficult theoretical problems still have to be addressed in order to describe human vision scientifically, i.e. by means of mathematical algorithms that can be matched to the findings of the neuroscientists.

Visual flow, which is generated on the two retinae when man moves through his environment, only recently became of interest again; in fact, the systematical investigations proposed by Gibson (1966) are still being performed. The visual flow in the i-space depends on the speed and direction of the observer's movement as well as on the fixation target selected. It is easiest to compute when a far distant visual target is fixated upon straight ahead at eye level (Koenderink and van Doorn, 1975; Koenderink, 1986). When one walks through familiar surroundings, the fixation point is continuously shifted across the extra-personal space by eye saccades every 0.3 to 1.2 seconds (average values). During the time in between the saccades, the head-in-space movements are compensated for by slow eye movements which keep the fixation point on the selected target. This mechanism is partly visual, partly vestibular (vestibulo–ocular reflex, VOR). In fact, with normal body movements composed of translatory and rotatory components, a rather complex input signal, which changes after each saccade, is generated on the retina. The relative change depends on the angle at which the fixation point is shifted by the saccade across the extra-personal space, the distance of the fixation point in and the visual structures of, the extra-personal space. In the natural conditions of a familiar environment, object and space recognition does not need more than the time of one or two fixation periods between goal-directed saccades. This time is also sufficient for the transfer of the visual percept from the retinotopic coordinates to the coordinates of the extra-personal space represented in the p_s-space. Except for rather complex objects, recognition of most objects in our environment does not need more than 0.5–0.8 seconds.

During fast saccades, which generally last 25 to 80 ms, retinal signals correspond to short 'grey intervals', since, because of the speed of the saccadic eye movements, the frequency of change in stimulation of retinal photoreceptors is above critical flicker fusion frequency (CFF), provided that the average spatial frequency of the visual surroundings is high enough. Under laboratory conditions, one can demonstrate that visual signals can also be sampled during fast saccades (Lamansky, 1869), and that only a very small decrease (if any) in visual sensibility ('saccadic inhibition') is induced by saccadic eye movements. As Lamansky demonstrated in 1869 while working at the Helmholtz laboratory in Heidelberg, one can construct stimuli, e.g. intermittent spots of light, for which effective visual signal uptake can be demonstrated during saccades. Lamansky used them to measure the angular speed of saccadic eye movements. Since the condition of intermittent illumination can be discarded under natural conditions for vision, however, only signal uptake during the fixation or pursuit periods between saccades must be considered for object and space perception. The retinal signals during a saccade are equivalent to short grey stimuli, which do not interrupt visual pattern perception (similar to eyeblinks). During and after each saccade, a recalibration of the spatial values of the retinal coordinates (p_r) in relation to the p_s-space occurs. The time course of this recalibration can be measured experimentally (Grüsser *et al.*, 1987). It is longer than the duration of a saccade (for details see Fig. 22.1). Some problems in temporo-spatial visual signal processing of the Lamansky type have been observed in people working with TV screens or computer monitors, most of which operate nowadays at a raster frequency below 70 Hz. At least 200 Hz are recommended for this artificial visual stimulus of our modern world in order to adequately approximate 'natural' stimulus conditions.

'Fixation periods' with respect to visual signal uptake are not only periods when the eye fixates on a target in a stationary visual world, but are also those intersaccadic periods during which the eye performs slow pursuit movements, keeping its optical axis as near as possible to the moving target, e.g. a bird flying across the extra-personal space. When one walks along an unknown and somewhat difficult path (e.g. in the mountains), the eyes usually fixate on a target located on the ground a few metres ahead. A predominantly vertical optokinetic gaze nystagmus is evoked as one walks. This keeps the fixated target stationary on the retina during the downward pursuit movements between the upward saccades. The shift in the visual image on each retina is then caused by two factors: the optokinetic eye movements and the visual flow, depending on the visual structure of the extra-personal space and on the translatory changes in head position during walking. These facts suggest that the 'natural' retinal stimulus patterns, from which visual information about the extra-personal space and the objects within it is extracted, are rather complex and also depend on the tuned interaction of visual signals with several other non-visual sensory modalities (somatosensory, vestibular) as well as with efference copy signals representing the motor commands for eye, head and body movements. It seems probable that the space and object constancy perceived under such conditions is contributed to by a short-

time memory for the gross spatial structure of the extra-personal space (e.g. Irwin *et al.*, 1990). We assume that space-related object perception requires a neuronal computation of spatial cross-correlograms between the 'neuronal images' sampled during successive fixation periods.

The Modern Search for Descriptor Functions of the Optic Image

Scientists working in visual psychophysics or in computer vision have become more and more interested in object recognition during the last twenty years. In their efforts, they have abandoned traditional visual psychophysics in which light spots, flicker stimuli, simple patterns related to simultaneous contrast, sinewave gratings or chequer-boards were used as typical stimuli, and have instead tried to analyse more complex stimulus patterns derived from simplified natural scenery. Their goal was to search for mathematically defined, i.e. computable descriptor functions for such stimulus patterns, and usually set aside the transfer of the reference frame from retinal coordinates to space coordinates. It was assumed that the retinal image (the *i*-space) is transformed into a multilayer representational process of the p_s-space, leading directly to classification of objects and to their visible relationship within a given scene. Whenever problems of binocular vision were investigated, two related *i*-space signals form the input signals for the descriptor functions.

We shall not discuss in our summary of these studies the simplification usually made when eye movements are not taken into consideration. We shall also not discuss the necessary remapping of retinal coordinates to extra-personal space coordinates which the organism performs during and after every gaze movement. Reviews of the rather complex efforts aimed at deriving meaningful descriptors for p_s-space percepts were published by Koenderink and van Doorn (1978, 1987, 1988), Treisman and Gelade (1980), Pylyshyn (1984), Callaghan (1984, 1989, 1990), Sutter *et al.* (1989), Duncan and Humphrey (1989), Biederman (1990), Yuille and Ullman (1990), Kosslyn (1990), Todd and Reichel (1989), Reichel and Todd (1990) and Watt (1990). In these and other studies, a hierarchy of filters that could possibly be used as descriptors for visual stimuli is discussed, with the goal of analysing precognitive and cognitive visual functions. Some of these descriptor functions were based on optical parameters, while others are descriptors of cognitive operations and were selected at least in part on an intuitive basis.

Visual objects in the extra-personal space have a certain position in space and relative to each other; they possess a distinct shape, size, distribution of surface colours, surface texture and 'internal' structure, which, along with the intensity and spectral composition of the illumination, determine the optical image, i.e. the input signal at any given moment of time. For the purpose of vision, the three-dimensional signal is transformed by the dioptric apparatus of the eye into a two-dimensional optical image on the retina, i.e. a spatio-temporal distribution of photons reaching the receptor surface of the retina, which determines the *i*-space. For every standard physical description of this image sufficiently precise to allow for the analysis of human vision, the image has to be parcelled down to not more than the diameter of a photoreceptor outer segment. The effect of photons absorbed into the outer segments of the photoreceptors generates the first level of the 'physiological' input signal. The activation of each photoreceptor depends on the 'local' spectral composition $C(r)$ of the light stimulus. The momentary excitation $E(r)$ of a photoreceptor, recorded in time bins of 20–50 ms, is a function of the convolution integral $C(r) * S(r) = i(r)$ divided by an adaptation factor which represents the average excitation $\bar{E}(r)$ of the surrounding photoreceptors. $S(r)$ is the spectral sensitivity of the absorbing visual pigment of the photoreceptor selected. $S(r)$ differs for rods and for the three different classes of cones. At a given time (t), the values $E(r, t)$ for all photoreceptors constitute the overall physiological input signal to the visual system.

These considerations lead to a 'physicalistic' point-by-point description of the optical image and of the action produced by photons in each photoreceptor outer segment. Such a description is an extremely tedious and redundant procedure. Simplification is possible for most of the experimental stimuli, however, as follows:

1. If black–white stimuli are used instead of chromatic stimuli, the average stimulus intensity $I(r)$ across the visible spectrum given at each photoreceptor can be considered to be an input signal when it is normalized relative to the spectral response curve of the photoreceptor and to the average stimulus luminance $I(r)_{surround}$ in the photoreceptor surroundings. Since average luminance variability in the natural environment remains mostly in a range below 1:100, the error is not very large when the overall retinal luminance I_{ret}, i.e. the general 'adaptation level' of the eye, is taken instead of $I(r)_{surround}$ for each photoreceptor.

The next step in the transformation of the physiological input signal is a compression of the intensity scale. Instead of Fechner's law (equation 1.2), this non-linear compression is more appropriately described by the following equation proposed by Hering (1874):

$$B(x) = aW/(W + S) \quad \text{[units of sensation]} \quad (1.6)$$

where W is the 'white value' and S the 'black-value' of a given local stimulus. One can transcribe equation 1.7 into

$$B(x) = a'I/(1 + kI) \quad \text{[units of sensation]} \quad (1.7)$$

where a' and k are constants and I is the stimulus intensity.

In principle, equations of type 1.7 are also valid for the relationship between the membrane potential changes in a single photoreceptor and stimulus intensity (Chapter 3). Hering's law describes at a psychophysical level the relationship between the brightness (B) and the stimulus intensity (I) for large, unstructured light spots. An S-shaped curve results when B is plotted as a function of log I. Equation 1.7 corresponds to the Michaelis–Menten kinetics in biochemistry. Although the afferent visual system compresses the signal related to general luminance within the visual field, it preserves in 'compressed' form the signal which is present at the receptor output level. This signal is still a highly redundant descriptor function of the retinal image.

2. The maximum information content present in an optical image can be estimated by expanding the analogy of a television screen across the whole visual field. A television screen composed of $(n \cdot m)$ pixels is a first-order descriptor for a visual input signal. It can produce many of the stimulus patterns on the retina, corresponding well to everyday vision when both movement of the observer through his extra-personal space and binocular disparities are discarded. For black-and-white stimuli, the stimulus luminance for each pixel has to be considered with a precision of 6 to 7 [bit], since less than $2^7 (= 128)$ shades of grey can be discriminated by the human observer. Because of the temporal frequency limits of our visual system, intermittent light stimuli extending beyond 100 Hz can be discarded when possible flicker perception is considered. Only values up to 8 Hz are relevant for Gestalt perception (cf. van de Grind *et al.*, 1973). The overall necessary information content of a visual pattern on a black-and-white TV screen with 512×512 pixels is therefore smaller than $(18 + 7) = 25$ [bit/frame]. Adequate simulation of the chromatic composition of a pixel for 'everyday' colour vision is obtained by three colour channels, for which an intensity variation of about 7 [bit] is sufficient. For chromatic visual patterns, the information content would thus increase by 14 [bit]; one would therefore end with a maximum necessary information content of less than 39 [bit/frame]. If we take a frequency limit of 50 or 60 Hz, i.e. the repetition frequency of a TV screen, the information flow for a stimulus on the screen is less than 2340 [bit s^{-1}].

Applying the TV screen model to the retina, the upper information content of the optical image in the *i*-space is scaled by the number of photoreceptors (about 125 million per retina) with no more than 7 bit in the intensity domain per receptor. Thus the information content of one image on the retina is about $7 + \text{ld } 1.25 + \text{ld } 10^8 = 33.88$ [bit]. Since flicker fusion frequency is below 60 Hz under natural stimulus conditions (under laboratory conditions, higher values can be reached, cf. van de Grind *et al.*, 1973), the maximum information capacity is less than 2032 [bit

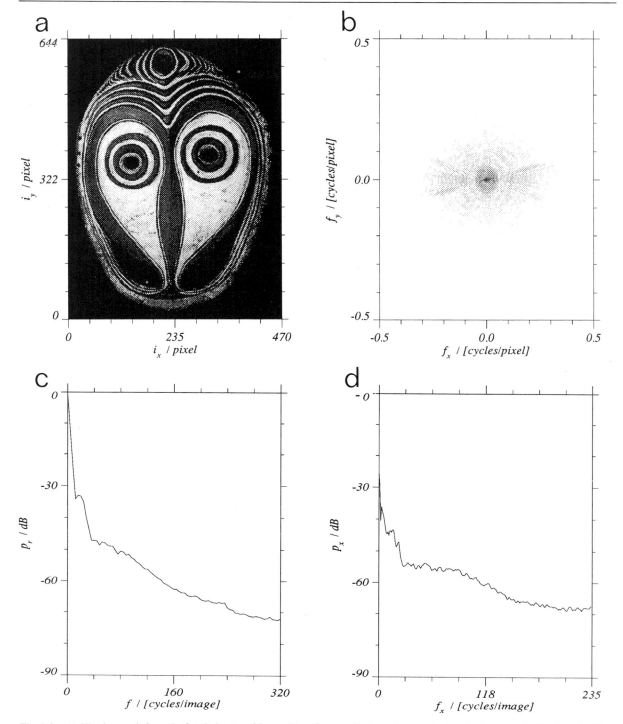

Fig. 1.3 *(a) Wooden mask from the Sepik district of Papua New Guinea. Such masks were fixed to the house roofs. Black-and-white reproduction of a computerized colour plate as published in Kussmaul (1982). In (b) the corresponding two-dimensional spatial frequency diagram is shown. In (c) the spatial frequency diagram was averaged along a rotating radius centred on (0,0) of (b). In (d) the spatial frequency distribution was averaged for the x-axis of (b). Computations by K. H. Dittberner and W. Seidler, Berlin.*

s^{-1}]. These values are upper estimates. In reality, of course, information content of an image and information capacity are very much lower. Futhermore, only a very small fraction of this information is really processed by the central visual system. Therefore, information rejection and information selection are the main tasks performed by the neuronal operations acting within the retina and the central visual system; the same is also true for computer vision.

3. Comparing different stimulus patterns quantitatively by means of the set of numbers corresponding to the three-dimension or five-dimension (chromatic stimuli) descriptors of a TV screen pattern is not a practical method, because a great deal of unnecessary, redundant information would enter the computation. The same is also true for a 'pixel analysis' of the physiological process. Vision and computer scientists are therefore searching for better descriptors in order to analyse the stimulus, hoping at the same time to understand operative parameters relevant for signal processing within the retina and the central visual system. It became popular during the last two decades to describe black-and-white stimulus patterns in a two-dimensional spatial frequency domain. Such a description, first suggested by Mach (1865), is certainly helpful when one is analysing a stimulus: it reduces, for example, the amount of information necessary to transmit an image by electronic devices across long distances. For the reconstruction of the real image from the spatial frequency spectrum, the phase spectrum has also to be preserved. Nowadays, computer programs have been developed that transform the set of pixel values by Fourier transformation into a two-dimensional spatial frequency and phase space. This transformation, which was applied to stimulus analysis by Caelli and Bevan (1982), for example, is illustrated in Fig. 1.3 for a 'simple' stimulus. A similar spatial frequency analysis can be performed for the chromatic components of a colour picture, of course, whereby a red, green and blue spatial frequency channel with adequate spectral sensitivity (as in a TV monitor) is used as a descriptor. Computing Fourier transforms of a visual signal is only one way to perform formal image analysis. Other transformations (i.e. sets of spatial filters), such as multiplying the image with Gabor functions or wavelets (second derivatives of Gaussian distribution of different widths), might lead to descriptor functions better adapted to the processes acting in the visual system.

4. Based on the idea of spatial frequency analysis first expressed by Mach (1866), simplified experimental designs were derived for the investigation of the visual system: spatial sinewave gratings or squarewave gratings. The latter contain, in addition to the basic sinewave frequency, higher harmonics which are relevant only up to the second or third order. Such a simplified stimulus either drifts across the stimulus field or is presented sta-

tionary and flickers with reversing maxima and minima. It was used in a large number of psychophysical and neurophysiological studies in which spatial frequency response characteristics were derived as functions describing the performance of a human observer or of single nerve cells in the peripheral or central visual system. As soon as the responses to complex stimulus patterns have to be explained, however, the success of this method is rather limited, since non-linear neuronal operations then become effective. An important hypothesis derived from psychophysical experiments with gratings was the observation that selective adaptation to a certain range of spatial frequencies occurs when the retina is stimulated by a grating with a certain frequency. From systematic studies using selective frequency adaptation, the following hypothesis was developed: 4 to 7 spatial frequency channels, which process the local stimulus pattern, exist for every part of the retina. This *ad hoc* hypothesis is widely accepted by vision scientists, some of whom assume 9 or 10 different spatial frequency channels.

5. Spatial frequency and phase analysis is a rather 'neutral' physicalistic approach used to describe visual stimulus patterns. It has produced meaningful results when elementary properties of visual sensation and perception

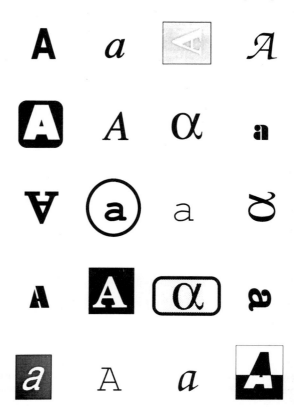

Fig. 1.4 *Different letters 'A'; for further explanation, see text.*

were analysed. It is seemingly irrelevant, however, when object perception, i.e. visual operation at a higher apperceptive or cognitive level, is considered. Figure 1.4, for example, depicts letters 'A' and 'a'. Everyone who has learned to read will recognize either letter regardless of its size (which varies with viewing distance), or whether it is written in upper or lower case, in the Greek or Latin alphabet, whether it is shaded, seen in outline or only in part, whether it is upright or upside down (then recognition takes more time), whether it is on the left or right side of the page, whether it is seen with the fovea or with parafoveal vision. From such observations, one can immediately conclude that the recognition of the letter is invariant over a wide range of signals representing different spatial frequency and phase information. Neuroscientists and scientists interested in computer vision have therefore searched for other methods that would allow them to parcellate a complex two-dimensional stimulus pattern, which would lead, in turn, to more adequate descriptors.

6. Marr and his co-workers (cf. Marr, 1982) proposed a formal subdivision of the low-level mechanisms of visual signal processing into three stages:

(*a*) The 'primal sketch', a reductive two-dimensional representation of the intensity distribution of an image (for human vision < 128 grey levels) formed by adequately chosen operations enhancing the edges in the image.

(*b*) The '2.5D sketch' summarizes the analysis of the primal sketch by using certain descriptor functions, and leads to a partial representation of the three-dimensional visual space. This level is perhaps comparable to the efforts of Renaissance artists to represent objects in their drawings correctly by using the technique of central perspective (e.g. Brunelleschi, Dürer, Fig. 1.5).

(*c*) The solid-model volumetric 3D representation of bodies in the scene (cf. Watt, 1988).

When one looks at a natural image, one realizes that the three components of intensity distributions are preserved in the primal sketch: on a large scale, the average brightness of the scene or of parts of the scene (intensity compressed according to equation 1.7), the first spatial derivative which is relevant for shading, shades and shadows, and the second spatial derivative leading to an enhancement of edges and contours (Mach, 1865, 1866a, b; cf. p. 4). Marr and his co-workers emphasized that the second spatial derivative dominates the primal sketch. This selection is certainly important for those interested in object recognition. Presumably because of neurophysiological data (Chapter 3), Marr and Hildreth (1980) preferred a convolution of the *i*-space into the p_r-space by means of a Laplacian operator $\nabla^2 G(r)$ of a two-dimensional Gaussian distribution $G(x, y)$ instead of applying a simple second-order spatial differentiation of the light distribution:

$$G(x,y) = e^{-\frac{x^2 + y^2}{2\pi\sigma^2}} \tag{1.8}$$

$$\nabla^2 G(r) = \frac{-1}{2\pi\sigma^4}\left(1 - \frac{r^2}{2\sigma^2}\right) e^{-\frac{r^2}{2\sigma^2}} \tag{1.9}$$

where *r* represents the radial distance from the origin, σ the standard deviation of the Gaussian (equation 1.8) and $\nabla^2 G(r)$ the Laplacian operator. Equation 1.9 is the circular symmetric 'Mexican-hat operator', which is very akin to

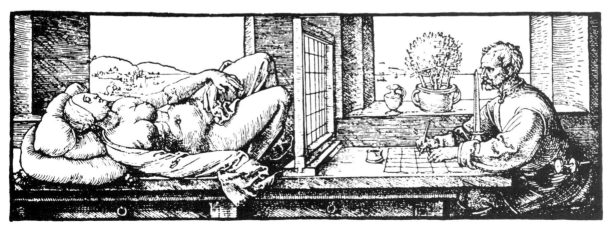

Fig. 1.5 *Illustration from Albrecht Dürer,* Underweysung der Messung *(1525, 1538). The technique of central perspective and correct outline drawing is illustrated in this woodcut of an artist drawing a recumbent woman. The artist uses a frame with a grid of parallel horizontal and vertical lines to look at the model. The paper on which the artist draws contains the same grid of squares to facilitate correct proportionality of the outline drawing and of central perspective, which depends on the distance of the artist and the object drawn from the screen.*

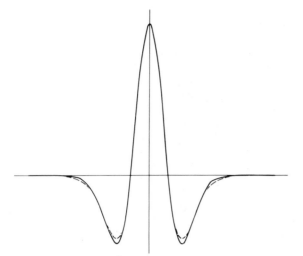

Fig. 1.6 *The function* $\nabla^2 G$ *(continuous line) may be approximated by the difference curves of two Gaussian distributions (DOG, dotted curve) when the ratio of the inhibitory and the excitatory space of the Gaussian distribution is about 1:1.6. (Reprinted by permission from D. Marr and E. Hildreth 1980.)*

the difference curve of an 'excitatory' and an 'inhibitory' two-dimensional Gaussian distribution (DOG) as illustrated in Fig. 1.6; this is a function also used as a reasonable representation of the concentric receptive fields of retinal ganglion cells (cf. Chapter 3).

Fig. 1.7 illustrates an example from Marr's book (1982). To determine the edges between the surfaces in the *i*-space, the zero crossings of the convolution of the image with $\nabla^2 G(r)$ are determined. Considerable efforts have been taken in order to derive from Marr's 'primal sketch' further meaningful steps that would lead to automatic object recognition in computer vision.

7. The recognition of edges, i.e. step changes in image intensity, is a first useful, elementary descriptor function, which is presumably realized in the retina and the afferent visual system for every region of the visual field by several simultaneously operating spatial frequency channels, as mentioned above. In addition to edge recognition in the primal sketch, of course, the information about the position of a certain edge within the image is also maintained. Other useful descriptor functions were proposed for further fractionating of the primal sketch: orientation of finite-length contours, blobs, i.e. closed edges, and L-type, X-type and T-type edge junctions which mark surface orientation discontinuity. T-junctions are frequently generated by unconnected 'occluding contours' of two objects. An 'occluding contour' is defined as the locus of all points where luminance changes abruptly (Watt, 1990). The general shape of occluding contours (convex,

concave), which may be determined by oriented small segments, refers to the shape of the respective body. The 'local spatial curvature of an edge' is another possible descriptor. Surfaces of natural objects are often characterized by shading, which is contained in the first derivative of the spatial intensity distribution (Fig. 1.2). Smoothly curved 3D surfaces are perceived from surface contours, whereby a large variety of continuous or broken contour patterns generate the 3D impression (Todd and Reichel, 1990).

8. Visual objects are also generated in a natural or artificial setting through differences in surface texture. Texture is determined by three elementary factors: the size of the particles, the shape of the particles and the spatial grouping of the particles. In recent years, considerable efforts have been made aimed at investigating texture effects on visual form perception. Hereby texture was frequently simplified in comparison with natural stimuli. Structural contrast phenomena between local signs and background textures and differences in the 'local' structure of the textures ('textones') lead to perception of simple shapes (e.g. Julesz, 1980, 1981; Beck, 1966a, b, 1972; Treisman, 1982; Nothdurft, 1985a, b; Bergen and Adelson, 1988). Texture along with the variable shading in the surface of an object, i.e. luminance gradients and shadows, are important descriptor operations that discriminate objects from their background. 'Local' shading and shades modify texture perception.

Coherent Movement Contributes to Object Recognition

Object motion contributes to a better separation of object and background if one of the two is moved separately or both are moved at different angular velocities or directions. For the retinal image, variable object movement occurs, for example, when one moves through a natural environment and perceives parallax shifts of the objects relative to each other. Shifts due to parallax contribute not only to depth perception but also to the separation of the different objects, since all points in the visual image of a certain object are shifted coherently according to simple translatory and circular motion when the observer moves. In a classic experiment, Wallach and O'Connell (1953) demonstrated that a shadow of a figure projected onto a tangent screen leads to quasi-three-dimensional object perception when rotated along an axis parallel to the screen. This effect is enhanced when the shadow consists only of characteristic contours and illustrates the perception of structure from coherent motion (e.g. Braunstein, 1976; Todd, 1982, 1984; Ullman, 1979; Hildreth, 1984; Yuille and Ullman, 1990). Johannson and his co-workers performed extensive studies on the generation of moving figures by placing a few dots of light at characteristic

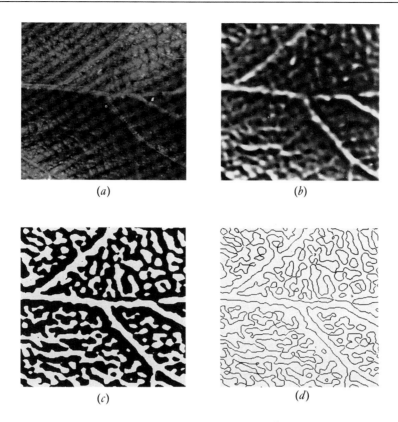

(a) *(b)*

(c) *(d)*

Fig. 1.7 *Examples of 'zero-crossing' detection using convolution of the figure with* $\nabla^2 G$. *The image (part of a leaf, a) is presented by* 320×320 *pixels. (b) shows the convolution of the image with* $\nabla^2 G$. *(c) depicts the positive values of (b) in white, the negative values in black. In (d) the zero-crossings of (b) are shown (from Marr, 1982, reproduced with permission).*

points on the figure (e.g. Johannson, 1975). The perception of three-dimensionality depends on the temporal integration of the displacement of the light spots within the sequence of several frames, indicating the existence of a short-time memory mechanism for the 3D operations in the p_s-space.

Colour Vision

The perception of colours depends predominantly on three components: the chromatic composition and intensity of the light illuminating the scene, the spectral reflectance of the surfaces of the objects in that scene and the spectral sensitivity of the three different types of cones in the retina. Minor contributions affecting colour and hue are caused by the spectral absorbance of the medium between the objects and the eye and by the spectral absorbance of the dioptric apparatus in the human eye or in the retinal pigments located outside the photoreceptor outer segments. As everyday experience teaches us, colour contributes considerably to object perception. This mech-

anism was presumably very important during pre-hominid evolution, since our primate ancestors depended heavily on a diet consisting of leaves and of colourful fruits collected from trees. In addition, the different shades of green, the main colour of the environment, had to be discriminated. It was recently claimed that colour mechanisms do not contribute to form vision, since contrast between colours of equal brightness is very weak (e.g. Livingstone and Hubel, 1988). It should be pointed out, however, that equal brightness colour contours rarely exist in a natural environment. Under natural illumination conditions, the colour constancy of the objects in our environment is rather well preserved, even when the spectral composition of the illuminating light changes, as is the case when one compares the light of an early, cloudy winter morning with that of a brilliant sunset evening in late summer. It was claimed (Land, 1977; Land and McCann, 1971) that the mechanisms of colour constancy operate so well that colour constancy is preserved over a very wide range of changes in chromatic composition of the illuminating light. A closer investigation indicates, however, that colour constancy is rather limited in a pattern composed of many patches having different chromatic compositions ('Mondrian pattern') (T. Caelli and O.-J. Grüsser, unpublished 1985). Quantitative psychophysics indicates that at least four 'physiological' levels of colour vision, all of which are also relevant for object recognition, exist:

1. trichromatic colour vision at the receptor level;
2. red–green, yellow–blue and black–white antagonistic colour vision in the afferent and central visual systems;
3. colour constancy mechanisms and categorization of different hues in colour-specific regions of the central visual system;
4. categorization of colours by behavioural categories and by naming.

For further remarks on colour perception, see Chapters 5 and 21.

Higher-level Vision

The ability to recognize objects from different shades of grey and colour as well as from contours or motion signals requires further steps which lead finally to a comparison between the percept and a representation of the object in visual memory. Object recognition is rather invariant relative to the intensity of the illuminating light, the three-dimensional aspect of the object, object size, whether or not the object is seen entirely or only in part (*pars-pro-toto* function), whether it is camouflaged by stimuli located in front of it or whether it is made less distinct by fog, etc. The set of signals provided by lower-level visual processes have to be combined before these invariant operations can be performed. Although it is unknown which operations are performed in the nervous system for this goal, models were developed in order to understand the processes allowing for object recognition. Biederman (1987, 1988, 1990) has suggested interesting ideas about 'recognition-by-components' (RBC), assuming that at the entry stage of 'higher-level vision processes' data from lower visual processes are combined to form 'geons', the combination of which constitute elementary raw shapes for objects. Assuming that the combination of the geons is easily changeable by simple mental operations, Biederman speculated that with 24 possible geons and objects composed of 2 or 3 geons in different spatial relations, one would yield a large amount of possible 2-geon objects (186,624) or 3-geon objects (about 1.4×10^9). Combination of geons could provide a basic structure for classifying 'real objects'. Other models of higher-level vision assume that a certain object or a distinct visual pattern is generated by selective feedback from a visual memory store 'downstream' to the perceptual visual centres, in which the signals from lower visual operations are processed. McClelland and Rumelhart (1981), for example, provided such a model in order to explain why letters are better recognized within a meaningful sequence, i.e. within words, than in a meaningless sequence, i.e. within a nonword.

Behavioural Dimensions in Visual Object Classification

Thanks to the combined efforts of computer vision and psychophysics, lower-level visual processes are nowadays much better understood than they were twenty years ago; on the other hand, higher-level visual processes still merit extensive study. At present, it is still helpful to follow Aristotle and his successors (Chapter 2) in searching in a more intuitive way for 'cognitive dimensions' or cognitive descriptors, by which the natural visual world can be adequately processed. In other words, one has to search for 'handy' stimulus categories in order to investigate higher-order visual functions in normal subjects and agnosic patients at a descriptor level far above the 'primal sketch'. Admittedly, the 'dimensions' of such apperceptive categories contain arbitrarily selected components, and their scientific 'success' also depends on whether or not the data obtained using stimuli classified according to such categories are accepted by the majority, or at least a significant number, of neuroscientists and neuropsychologists. Although Marr (1982) used the term 'modularity' to denote the perceptual categories, he did not substantiate their application (cf. also Fodor, 1983). In our opinion, a rather useful categorial division of visual objects was proposed by Konorski (1967). We shall present a modified version of Konorski's scheme, since we believe that the resulting categorization can be of use for clinical studies with agnosic patients.

Konorski (1967) thought that different gnostic areas are organized in the brain into separate 'gnostic units', i.e. category-selective neuronal networks, which create templates, i.e. operative filters, which process the visual input. One must necessarily assume that such gnostic units or neuronal templates are only partly innate, and that they are heavily modified by early life experiences. Konorski (1967) proposed the following nine categories within the visual stimulus domain:

1. small manipulable objects (keys, watches, dishes, etc.);
2. large objects that are in part manipulable (furniture, cars);
3. large non-manipulable objects (rocks, buildings, trees);

4. faces;
5. different classes of facial expressions;
6. animated objects (human figures, animals);
7. printed words, signs and symbols;
8. handwriting;
9. position of limbs.

For further studies on visual agnosia and visual object recognition, we propose a similar set of categories, but suggest that a polar organization be considered in addition to the several categorial 'strata' of signal processing. These functional categories form an *n*-dimensional categorical space in which all real objects can be represented. The following basic 'vectors' for classifying visual stimuli beyond the geometrical descriptors, which lead to the 2.5D-sketch of the visual image (Watt, 1990), seem to be suitable:

1. manipulable (small) – non-manipulable (large);
2. self-moving – stationary;
3. near (reachable) – far (unreachable);
4. physiognomic – verbal;
5. belonging to own body – not belonging to own body.

In a second set of categorical classifications, a 'cloud' in this five-dimensional space defined by (1) to (5) is further differentiated according to the following categories:

6. natural – man-made;
7. friendly (positive) – dangerous (negative);
8. edible – non-edible;
9. joyful – sad;
10. known (familiar) – unknown (unfamiliar).

In a third level of categorical classification, mainly physiognomic signs, facial expressions and gestures (body language) are further differentiated, i.e. the message conveyed by facial expression and gesture is specifically categorized. Another class of categories at this level is comprised of the visual signs used for visual verbal signal transmission ('reading' in the broadest sense). It should be pointed out that as a result of these categorial analyses, a given object or visual sign occupies part of a multi-dimensional descriptor space. The extension of this space ('cloud') is continuously modified by experience. A botanist differentiates between natural, small, stationary, and manipulable objects having little physiognomic expression, which are primarily useful, sometimes edible, and most frequently joyful, in the manifold Linnaean system of plants; a bird-watcher learns, on the other hand, to discriminate between small, self-moving, not too distant, manipulable objects having physiognomic characteristics, and eventually learns to recognize a large number of birds by sight.

For reading and other forms of learned purposeful

visual communication, a fourth level of categorization has to be assumed, which leads to the transmodal grapheme–phoneme correlation of all written language. Visual cognitive functions interact with speech-related auditory functions at this level.

Since all of these categorical dimensions heavily depend on learning, the effect of a brain lesion affecting cognitive visual performance depends not only on which operations are disturbed by the brain lesion, but also on the pre-lesion differentiation of these categorical dimensions that had occurred in the individual brain during a lifetime of learning.

Searching for the Neuronal Mechanisms of Visual Cognitive Functions: The Primate Model and Man-specific Visual Abilities

To explain the sometimes puzzling symptoms of visual agnosias, it is necessary to understand some basic principles related to the structure and function of the human visual system. It is also helpful to know the main properties of the adaptive mechanisms by which brain tissue and its neuronal organization respond to local lesions in the grey or white matter of the cerebral cortex. These mechanisms will be discussed in greater detail in Chapter 8. In order to understand the function of a highly complex neuronal structure, a basic understanding of anatomical connections, synaptic organization and neuronal network operations is necessary. Man shares a considerable part of his central visual system with other primates, since the essential developments in primate vision occurred during a phylogenetic period long before hominid evolution branched off from the primate ancestral stem about 8 to 10 million years ago. Therefore results from neurophysiological and neuroanatomical studies of the primate visual system are very helpful in order to understand better the neurobiology of human vision. Thanks to extensive research projects performed during the last 30 years on different species of primates, the neurosciences now possess a rather solid basic knowledge of the neuronal mechanisms by which visual signals are transformed from the *i*-space into the p_r-space and p_s-space. Of course, one has to be cautious when trying to 'explain' visual functions in man based on neurophysiological data obtained in anaesthetized and immobilized animals. More recent recordings performed with chronically implanted electrodes in awake, behaving animals, however, indicate that data obtained in anaesthetized and immobilized animals are at least in part applicable to the function of the awake brain. Since anatomical homologies can be demonstrated for the afferent visual system and for the primary visual cortex in man and other primates, and since microelectrode recordings from the human brain indicate that the same elementary principles are applicable in both man and monkeys, the use of animal research for the interpretation of human brain function is well justified. Thus the primate model of elementary visual brain function can serve to explain human visual performance. Research done on monkeys during the last thirty years has provided essential insight into the cellular mechanisms of data processing in the visual brain, and has thus helped to provide meaningful interpretations of the observations made by clinical neurologists in patients suffering from circumscribed brain lesions.

The phylogenetic separation of *Homo habilis* from the other hominid branch, the extinct australopithecines, occurred only about 2.5 million years ago (e.g. Tobias, 1985). Although a large variety of the properties of the human visual system can be understood by analysing neurophysiological and neuroanatomical data obtained in other primates, some *man-specific* functions do exist in the visual domain. These functions are based on brain structures that developed during the recent hominid phylogenesis from *Homo habilis* to *Homo erectus* and finally to *Homo sapiens sapiens* over the last 2 million years. Man-specific functions contribute to the following 'visual' cognitive abilities:

1. Some visual signals that are used for averbal primate social communication by facial expression and gestures are based on inborn genetic motor schemes and form the basis for generally understood 'universals' in human communication (Darwin, 1872; Eibl-Eibesfeldt, 1970; Ekman and Frièsen, 1975, 1978). Many averbal human social signals depend on learning, however. The meanings of characteristic facial expressions and gestures, i.e. of 'body language', are learned during childhood and adolescence. As a consequence, man possesses a much richer vocabulary for facial and gestural communication than all other primates. It seems likely that the perceptual mechanisms necessary for recognizing these averbal social signals, as well as the ability to identify faces and to understand facial expression and gestures, are developed in man considerably beyond the basic primate level.

2. The small-scale visual planning necessary for tool-making is only rudimentarily developed in apes (Köhler, 1917; Goodall, 1987). This ability of man considerably surpassed the level now reached by other apes over 2 million years ago, i.e. since *Homo habilis*. Visual conceptualization with regard to individual objects or the transformation of the extra-personal space is only rudimentarily developed in apes: it seems that we developed these abilities as specific signs of hominization when *Homo habilis* branched off from the australopithecines.

3. Visual arts and aesthetics, including axial or rotatory symmetry in stone tools and the use of colours, developed slowly at the level of late *Homo erectus* about 0.5 million years ago, and have included the ability to produce sculptures and wall paintings since Upper Palaeolithic times. At least since the Neolithic period, moving visual displays such as ritual dances, theatre performances, shadow theatre, etc., have been added to man's visual arts repertoire. During the last three generations, technically-produced, dynamic visual stimuli, such as movies and television performances, have considerably extended the man-specific visual world.

4. Large-scale spatial planning, necessary for architecture and the design of human living quarters, villages, cities, streets and bridges, i.e. man's entire environment, has its phylogenetic roots in the abilities possessed by late *Homo erectus* and *Homo praesapiens*, who built fairly large huts that served as temporary shelter about 0.2–0.3 million years ago (e.g. the Terra amata site in Nice). *Homo praesapiens* also modified the caves in which they were living.

5. Visual design of fashion, tattooing and man-made visual signs such as symbols of social rank or the visual symbols used for group identification, etc., are presumably of more recent, Neolithic origin. The use of red and yellow ochre to paint corpses and presumably living bodies as well dates back at least 100,000 years, however. At some Lower Palaeolithic sites (Terra amata in Nice, Becov in Czechoslovakia), different-coloured ochre pieces dating back about 250,000 years have also been found, which indicates the use of red and yellow paints by *Homo praesapiens* (Fridrich; 1975; Wreschner, 1985).

6. The development of visual symbols used for verbal communication, i.e. alphabetic, syllabic or ideographic script used for reading and writing, first began in Mesopotamia about 5300 years ago (e.g. Schmandt-Besserat, 1977; Nissen *et al.*, 1990, cf. Chapter 17). Man's ability to read and write probably depends on a phylogenetically much older, man-specific function, which we call 'visual *pars-pro-toto*-function' (Grüsser, 1988, cf. Chapter 17). This function is used, for example, in track reading by Neolithic hunters. The sign language used by deaf-mutes is a special category of visual 'reading' and 'writing', while Braille script demonstrates that the tactile domain can also serve as an instrument of non-auditory verbal communication. Related to reading and writing but certainly not any older is the use of visual symbols in calculus and geometry. For both script and numerical symbols, no palaeoanthropological findings exist to our knowledge from the periods before *Homo sapiens sapiens*. Precursors of this 'modern' visuo-motor ability in man did not occur earlier than the abstract signs and pictograms found on Upper Palaeolithic wall paintings originating 30,000 years ago or later; these are rather difficult to interpret (Földes-Papp, 1975; cf. Chapter 17).

These annotations suggest that a rather large part of man's visual and visual-constructive abilities are man-specific; they are based, of course, on retinal and 'simpler' cerebral mechanisms related to image processing, which man shares with other primates. Thus data obtained in animal experiments constitute an important foundation allowing for greater understanding of man's higher-order visual cognitive abilities. These data, however, are certainly not sufficient to explain man-specific functions. Only systematic studies of normal and impaired visual cognition, plus studies using normal subjects and patients volunteering for neuropsychological research programmes, will promote scientific advancement in this field. As already mentioned in the preceding section, efforts in connection with computer vision will certainly facilitate this goal. Nevertheless, many of the questions posed by visual agnosias still affect a level of visual cognition that surpasses the present knowledge of the experimental neurosciences, which is based on single unit recordings and on the descriptor functions successfully applied in computer vision.

Developmental Aspects of Visual Perception and Cognition

The visual system beyond area V1 is a complex analytical structure composed of many extrastriate 'visual association' and 'visual integration areas', extending considerably beyond the occipital lobe into the posterior parietal and the inferior temporal cortex. The activity in part of the visual association and integration regions is heavily dependent on motor action, general arousal and spatially directed or object-related attention. The function of these cortical regions is modified by learning and experience, i.e. by former interactions between the organism and its habitat. In addition to cognitive learning, however, the normal function of the higher visual cortical centres also depends on unconscious shaping and maturation of its signal-processing properties. During certain sensitive periods in childhood and adolescence external stimuli determine the future abilities of these cortical structures. As one knows from observations in adult illiterates, for example, man's ability to learn to read and write depends on age. Beyond adolescence it is a difficult task and usually yields rather meagre results. Since our ability to read and to write relies on man-specific brain regions which developed during the hominid evolution of the last 2 million years for other purposes (cf. Chapter 12), a high plasticity of the cortical functions involved in reading and writing seems to be a priori fairly probable. From everyday experience it is less clear whether we also learn to perceive three-dimensional objects instead of coloured spots, to estimate the distance

of objects from each other or the observer, or to judge the speed of a bird flying through our habitat. These abilities may be based essentially on innate mechanisms. Since we cannot perform goal-directed experiments to settle the 'nature vs. nurture' question in man, we have to rely on the few observations possible when 'nature' made such experiments spontaneously.

The philosophical discussion behind the question of whether our elementary abilities in colour, shape, form or movement perception are all dependent upon learning or whether these abilities are based predominantly on innate neuronal mechanisms has a considerable longevity: during the great days of Athenian philosophy idealistic Platonists and empiricist Aristotelians developed contradictory positions on this matter. These positions were rephrased repeatedly during the history of Western philosophy, as for example in the extended quarrel between the 'nominalistic' and 'realistic' scholastic philosophers. The clearest formulation of the problem regarding nature or nurture related to visual perception stems from the late seventeenth century, when the Irish lawyer and philosopher William Molyneux (1656–1698) wrote in a letter to John Locke (1632–1704) on 2 March 1693:

> *Suppose a man born blind, and now adult, and taught by his touch to distinguish between a cube and a sphere of the same metal, and, nighly of the same bigness, so as to tell, when he felt one and the other, which is the cube, which the sphere. Suppose then, the cube and sphere placed on a table, and the blind man to be made to see; quaere, whether by his sight, before he touched them, he could now distinguish and tell which is the globe, which the cube? To which the acute and judicious proposer answers: 'Not. For though he has obtained the experience of how a globe, how a cube, affect this touch; yet he has not yet obtained the experience, that what affects his touch so or so, must affect his sight so or so; or that a protuberant angle in the cube that pressed his hand unequally, shall appear to his eye as he does in the cube'. I agree with this thinking gentleman . . . in his answer to this his problem . . . .*
> (*Essay*, Chapter IX)

Locke replied to Molyneux that 'your ingenious problem will deserve to be published to the world' and therefore included Molyneux's letter in the second edition (1693) of his *Essay Concerning Human Understanding*. Evidently Locke held Molyneux's question for very important and predicted the outcome of his experiment:

> *I . . . am of opinion that the blind man, at first sight, would not be able with certainty to say which was the globe, which the cube, whilst he only saw them; though he could unerringly name them by his touch, and certainly distinguish them by the difference of their figures felt.*
> (*Essay*, Chapter IX)

George Berkeley (1685–1753) extended Molyneux's question to space perception. In his *Essay Towards a New Theory of Vision* he wrote that '. . . a man born blind, being made to see would at first have no idea of distance by sight; the sun and stars, the remotest objects as well as the nearer, would all seem to be in his eye, or rather in his mind' (section 41). In contrast to Locke and Berkeley, G. Leibniz (1646–1716) in his *New Essays Concerning Human Understanding* set forth the belief that Molyneux's man could distinguish 'by the principles of reason' between the globe and the cube. Nevertheless Leibniz admitted that the man seeing the globe and the cube for first time would be 'confused by the novelty' of these objects.

One generation later, an empirical test related to Molyneux's problem was published. In 1728 the London anatomist and surgeon William R. Cheselden (1688–1772), who also had a high reputation as an ophthalmic surgeon at St Thomas's Hospital (Cope, 1953), reported on a successful cataract operation performed in a 13- to 14-year-old young gentleman who had developed bilateral cataract very early in life. Cheselden reported that his patient, when seeing for the first time without a cloudy lens (but with of course a considerable hypermetropia), was able neither to recognize the objects well known to him by using sight (e.g. his cat) nor to estimate distances correctly. 'He thought all objects whatever touched his eyes.' He had great difficulty guiding his locomotor activities by vision. Concerning the early age of Cheselden's patient, it seems rather probable that, by learning, the young gentleman was soon able to use visual signals for his interaction with objects and space.

In the following generations, several cases similar to that of Cheselden were published (reviewed in Uhthoff, 1891, and Wilbrand, 1897). In some of the patients Molyneux's problems were investigated as he had recommended. One of such observations was made by J. C. A. Franz, a British physician, and published in 1841. He placed

at the distance of 3 feet, and on a level with the eye, a solid cube and a sphere, each of four inches in diameter . . . [in front of the patient]. *I now let him open his eye. After attentively examining these bodies, he said he saw a quadrangular and a circular figure, and after some consideration he pronounced the one a square and the other a disc. His eye being closed, the cube was taken away, and a disc of equal size substituted and placed next to the sphere. On again opening his eye he observed no difference in these objects but regarded them both as discs. The solid cube was now placed in a somewhat oblique position before the eye, and close beside it a figure cut out of pasteboard, representing a plane outline prospect of the cube when in this position. Both objects he took to be something like flat quadrates . . . .*

On the conclusion of these experiments I asked him to describe the sensations the objects had produced, whereupon he said that immediately upon opening his eye he had discovered a difference in the two objects, the cube and the sphere, placed before him, and perceived that they were not drawings; but that he had not been able to form from them the idea of a square and a disc, until he perceived a sensation of what he saw in the points of his fingers, as if he really touched the objects. When I gave the three bodies, the sphere, cube, and pyramid, into his hand, he was much surprised that he had not recognized them as such by sight as he was well acquainted with them by touch.

(*Philosophical Transactions*, communicated by Sir B. C. Brodie, London, 1841, I, 59–69)

Molyneux's question was extensively discussed in the philosophical literature of the eighteenth and nineteenth centuries, whereby the empiricist philosophers considered their position as proven by the empirical data obtained in these patients, who were indeed object-blind and whose behaviour was not unlike that of patient suffering from shape and object agnosia (cf. Chapter 11; for a historical discussion see Abbott, 1904; Davis, 1960).

In 1903 an interesting aspect in such a patient was reported by A. M. Ramsay, an ophthalmic surgeon in Glasgow. Abbott (1904) described this patient with additional details communicated to him by Dr Ramsay: a 30-year-old man, blind from birth due to bilateral cataracts, had been able prior to the cataract operation to tell day from night and could also locate a source of light. He worked in a garden and had learned to pluck flowers, arrange them in bunches and pack them in boxes. He distinguished the different flowers by touch or smell. The lenses of both eyes were extracted within 1 week:

For about 10 days after the operation the patient appeared quite dazed, and could not realize that he was seeing. From the outset he took a most intelligent interest in his own case and asked numerous questions of his fellow patients. The first thing he actually perceived was the face of the house-surgeon. He said, that at first he did not know what it was he saw, but that when Dr Stewart asked him to look down, the sense of hearing guided his eye straight to the point whence the sound came, and then regarding what he knew from having felt his own face he realized that this must be a mouth and that he must be looking at a face.

Dr Ramsey showed the patient a ball and a toy brick and asked him as Molyneux suggested whether he could tell the one from the other. The recognition task took the patient many minutes during which he moved his fingers 'nervously, trying to feel them in imagination', till he finally was able to discriminate the objects. Dr Ramsey also noted considerable differences in the visually guided locomotion of his patient on a horizontal plane as compared with stairs, where he had great difficulty estimating the height of the steps. Ramsey's patient, in contrast to Cheselden's boy, did not have the feeling that the objects touched his eyes.

In this century observations on such patients were summarized by von Senden (1932). Gregory and Wallace (1963) reported in detail on another case. Despite a great variability in the recognition abilities of such patients, it seems to be clear that in all of them elementary visual perception was impaired at least in part, and the conclusion one can draw is straightforward: the development of the elementary mechanisms used for form, object, space and spatial movement perception are seriously impaired by bilateral deprivation of vision. The outlines of the objects, however, are evidently perceived and the patients make intelligent use of kinaesthetic information by tracing these outlines for object recognition.

The effects of binocular deprivation on the development of pattern recognition in man led, of course, to the question of which physiological mechanisms could be responsible for these findings, which indicated that experience – but not necessarily conscious learning – plays an essential role in the development of elementary abilities for visual perception. Since several chapters of *Vision and Visual Dysfunction* are devoted to the development of the visual system, we will only briefly summarize the main aspects from this field which we believe important for the comprehension of the growth of man's higher visual cognitive abilities. The prenatal and postnatal development of the central visual system seems to follow *grosso modo* the Kielmeyer–Haeckel rule (the biogenetic law), i.e. the ontogenesis of an organism follows along programmes which can be understood as a schematic repetition of taxonomic systematics and phylogenesis.

The prenatal development of the primate visual system was studied by Rakic (1977): With an average time of gestation of 165 days in macaque monkeys, retinal ganglion cells develop on embryonic day 30 and lateral geniculate nucleus cells around day 36, while the different layers of the visual cortex appear between embryonic days 43 and 102. At birth the essential structural basis of the afferent visual system is laid out and the primate baby, as the human baby born at term, can direct his gaze towards his visual world, although the visual acuity in man and primates is very low during this early period of life (Fig. 1.8). The postnatal development of the central visual system is characterized by:

1. Development of axonal terminals, differentiation of nerve cell dendrites and dendritic spines and formation of axo–dendritic synapses in area V1.
2. Reduction in the number of nerve cells in the cortical grey matter, corresponding to the general rule that in many cortical areas an embryonic 'overproduction' of neurones had occurred.
3. Reduction of some transcortical connections. For example, the callosal connections of the visual cortices in the newborn animal (experiments in cats) cover a very large part of the cytoarchitectonic fields, while later in life these connections are to a varying extent restricted to the cerebral representations of the vertical meridian, where the two visual hemifields contact each other (Innocenti, 1981).

4. Axonal sprouting and myelinization of the axons are further important mechanisms shaping the function of the central visual areas.
5. A specification of synaptic connections develops under visual control. Hereby 'the timing of growth and interaction after birth can be seen as a natural continuation of a carefully orchestrated development programme that had largely been completed before the moment of birth' (Blakemore, 1988).
6. Growth and interaction of new neuronal connections within the central visual system are under the control of the visual input, but age of the organism is a crucial factor in the effectiveness of visual experience. Presumably the beginning and end of the 'sensitive periods' are defined by a genetic programme. During the sensitive periods 'genetically expected' input signals are required to maintain and reinforce cortical synaptic connections within area V1 and beyond. When sensory deprivation or sensory deformation of the 'adequate' visual signal patterns occur during a sensitive period, the 'carefully orchestrated development programme' breaks down and a morphological and physiological mismatch of visual neuronal interactions characterizes the function of area V1 and probably also of the higher visual cortices. Once the sensitive periods have passed, the plasticity of the visual cortices decreases rapidly and leaves little opportunity for repair of the functional defects which have developed (Blakemore *et al.*, 1978, 1981).

The development and the sensitive periods of the afferent visual system including area V1 are much better known than the corresponding developmental aspects of extrastriate visual association cortices or the visual integration areas of the parietal and temporal lobe. Visual acuity, for example, was measured in primates parallel to neurophysiological explorations of the developing afferent visual system. Figure 1.8 illustrates the limits of spatial resolution, as measured in cycles per degree using a grating pattern, in monkey babies at different ages. Early in life the spatial resolution is much better for the photoreceptor layer than for the LGN neurones and for neurones of area V1. As measured in behavioural studies (data included in Fig. 1.18), the monkey's behavioural visual resolution is lower during the first 80 days of life than the optimum visual resolution in single cortical neurones. Both values converge at a postnatal age of about 80 days and continue to improve up to the end of the first year of life. The differences existing between behavioural visual acuity and that of area V1 neurones indicate a delayed maturation of extrastriate cortical regions as compared to area V1. These extrastriate regions are necessary, however, for the animal to respond in the spatial resolution task.

Measurements of the development of visual acuity have also been performed in human infants, including preterm

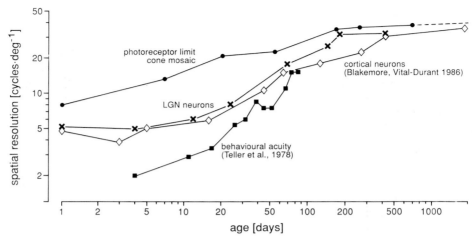

Fig. 1.8 *Development of the afferent visual system in monkeys. The spatial resolution limits were computed from the spatial density of the foveal cones, the responses of on-centre and off-centre neurones of the lateral geniculate nucleus (LGN, parvocellular layer) and the responses of area V1 foveal projection region nerve cells. Data were obtained at different postnatal ages (abscissa) and compared with behavioural findings on monkey visual acuity (Blakemore 1990; by permission of Macmillan Publishers).*

babies (Dobson *et al.*, 1979; Fantz *et al.*, 1975): visual acuity improves during the first years of life (Atkinson *et al.*, 1974; Mayer and Dobson, 1980). At birth acuity values reach about 0.6 cycle deg^{-1} on the average, then improve to about 6 cycles deg^{-1} at an age of 30 weeks and to about 10 cycles deg^{-1} towards the end of the first year (Kriazda *et al.*, 1980). Other studies, however, reported somewhat higher visual acuity values. Comparing these data with Fig. 1.8 one realizes that visual acuity is higher in monkeys of the same age (Teller *et al.*, 1978). Corresponding to the development of visual acuity, stereopsis also improves considerably during the early postnatal period. Between 15 and 30 weeks of life stereoacuity increases rapidly from values higher than 60 minutes of arc to values of less than 1 minute of arc. Stereoacuity only develops, however, when no congenital squint is present and monocular deprivation is absent.

Visual Deprivation

One can discriminate different levels of visual deprivation: monocular or binocular pattern deprivation as spontaneously occurs in congenital cataract, binocular fusion deprivation caused by congenital squint, binocular mismatch in the size of the retinal image caused by errors in the eye optical apparatus and absence of any visual structure when the animal grows up in 'empty' visual surroundings. The impact of monocular deprivation has been studied extensively by using monocular lid suture in cat and monkey. Early monocular deprivation leads to deprivation amblyopia accompanied by a shift in ocular dominance from the 'normal' left–right equilibrium to a

strong dominance of the seeing eye. Evidently, congenitally preformed synaptic contacts within area V1 binocular neurones are altered drastically. The efficiency of afferent LGN axon terminals in activating nerve cells of the primary visual cortex is changed. As a consequence the development of 'ocular dominance columns' (Chapter 4) is shifted considerably in favour of the seeing eye (Hubel and Wiesel, 1977a, b; LeVay *et al.*, 1980). The impact of monocular deprivation is especially serious during a sensitive period lasting several weeks postnatally in monkeys and extending in man most likely up to the second year of life. Vaegan and Taylor (1980) summarized the effect of unilateral cataract, predominantly of traumatic origin on the visual acuity of children and adolescents. They found that cataract occurring during the first four years of life and lasting at least several months led to a very low visual acuity (< 0.1, in many cases < 0.01[min of arc^{-1}]), while cataract occurring beyond an age of 8 years had little effect on visual acuity. Most of the patients of Vaegan and Taylor suffered from traumatic cataract. Naturally the time which had elapsed between development of cataract and ophthalmic surgery also played a role in the reduction in visual acuity.

Animal experiments concerning the effect of binocular deprivation on extrastriate visual functions are still fairly rare. For example, Hyvärinen reported on five laboratory-born stumptail macaques which underwent bilateral lid closure immediately after birth (Hyvärinen *et al.*, 1978; Hyvärinen, 1982a). The eyelids were opened bilaterally between 7 and 11 months. Except for a spontaneous irregular nystagmus developing several days after the opening of the eyes no particular irregularities of the eye themselves were observed. Nystagmus improved after a couple of weeks. The visual behaviour of the animals, however, remained grossly changed; all the monkeys were blind:

They bumped into obstacles, fell from tables and were unable to reach for food with their hand or mouth under visual guidance. Visual placing reactions were not developed by them although tactile placing was normal, and they never showed a teeth-chattering response to threatening facial expressions, although this innate response typical of a macaque monkey was readily evoked by threatening voices. In the colony they were uninfluenced by visual communication of the other monkeys although auditory signals and somatic contacts triggered normal behavioural patterns. Because of harassment by other monkeys caused by lack of comprehension of visual signals, these monkeys could not be kept with monkeys other than their mothers for any length of time.

(Hyvärinen, 1982a)

In one of the binocularly deprived monkeys, Hyvärinen and his colleagues performed microelectrode recordings from area 17 and area 19. They found few changes in the distribution of ocular dominance columns in both areas and reported that the deprived monkey's visual cortices did not differ functionally from normal animals. This was a somewhat surprising finding. Since most of the studies were done with multiple-unit recordings, however, Hyvärinen's conclusion should be taken with some reservation. He observed a slight change in the ocular dominance distribution in area 19 in favour of the contralateral eye and reported that the numbers of binocularly activated neurones diminished. Interestingly, an increase in somatic activation of the neurones located in the visual area 19 was observed in comparison with normal monkeys in which area 19 appeared entirely devoted to visual functions. Hyvärinen thought that this change was due to lack of foveation in the binocularly deprived animals, which used a 'manual fovea' instead of the eyes' fovea.

The most characteristic changes in neuronal activity were found in area 7 of binocularly deprived monkeys. The responses of area 7 neurones were studied in four binocularly deprived animals (Hyvärinen *et al.*, 1981a, b; Hyvärinen, 1982a) and the recording sites were area 7a and area 7b. A dramatic change in visually controlled neuronal responses as compared with normal animals of the same age was found and 'a great reduction in the proportion of cell groups activated by visual stimulation' was reported 'as a consequence of binocular deprivation' (Hyvärinen, 1982a). Very few visually driven cells gave weak responses to visual stimuli typically activating normal area 7 neurones. In normal animals studied with the same experimental techniques 24 per cent of the neurones recorded in area 7 responded to moving visual stim-

ulus patterns, in the binocularly deprived animals only 2 per cent. 'Bimodal' units, i.e. nerve cells responding to visual and somatic stimulation, are encountered in normal animals in about 30 per cent of the recordings. 'Bimodal' units were reduced in binocularly deprived animals to 1 per cent. To compensate for this effect, neurones responding to somatic (active or passive) stimulation alone increased from 43 per cent in normal animals to 88 per cent in the bilaterally deprived animals.

In one of the binocularly deprived animals the neurophysiological study was repeated after a lapse of 2 years following the opening of the eyes. This animal showed a very poor recovery of visually guided behavioural functions and, corresponding to this observation, the percentage of visually activated cells in area 7 had increased very little compared with the recordings done immediately after the eyelids were opened. In normal animals of this age about 54 per cent of area 7 neurones responded monomodally to visual or bimodally to visual and somatic stimuli. This value was reduced in the monkey to 3 per cent during the first recording session after the eyelids were opened and only recovered to a meagre 13 per cent after 2 years of normal visual sight.

Hyvärinen concluded that in area 7 the 'principle of competition' between 2 neuronal input classes (visual and somatosensory) led to the dramatic shift induced by binocular deprivation. He compared this shift from visual to somatosensory data processing in area 7 with the same 'principle of competition' which is evident in the case of monocular deprivation. In neurones of the primary visual cortex, a dominance of the seeing eye is then established, and once the sensitive period has passed, binocular vision, again possible through surgical intervention, can no longer change this dominance (cf. Hyvärinen *et al.*, 1978, 1981a, b; Hyvärinen and Hyvärinen, 1979).

Little is known from animal experiments about deprivation effects on higher-order visual integration cortices. From the work of Harlow and Harlow (1962) and their co-workers one knows that deprivation from social interaction leads to serious behavioural changes in baby and adolescent monkeys. We assume that the development of neuronal mechanisms in general, leading to specialized responses to visual submodalities such as oriented contours, chromatic contours, textures, stereoscopic depth vision, movement direction and evaluating parallax movements during locomotion, is genetically preprogrammed in rough outlines but requires a behavioural confirmation during the sensitive periods by sensory and sensorimotor signals, normally present in the habitat of the developing animal. Complete or partial visual deprivation leads to changes in neuronal data processing in area V1 and in the extrastriate visual association cortices, which ultimately produce symptoms very similar to the different types of visual agnosias discussed in this volume.

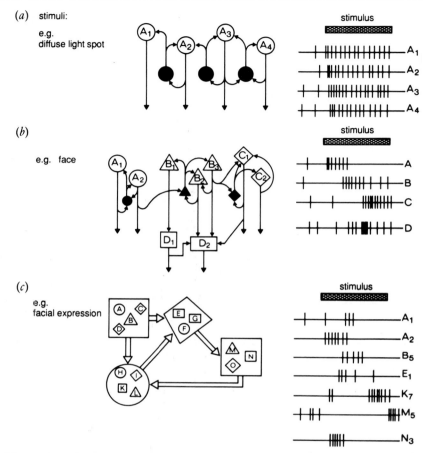

Fig. 1.9 *Scheme of the correlation between cerebral nerve cell activity and selected cases of visual stimuli. (a) The stimulus is a large-field white spot of light, which evokes uniform responses in on-centre neurones of the retina and the lateral geniculate nucleus and in layer 4 concentric receptive field nerve cells. A corresponding inhibition in off-centre neurones is recorded. The perceived brightness is linearly correlated with the neuronal impulse rate. (b) When a face photograph is selected as a stimulus, the neuronal activity in the 'face-responsive' region in the inferior temporal lobe of a monkey brain is changed in a complex manner, involving different neuronal classes specialized in part to respond to certain features characteristic of faces. (c) When facial expression is recognized in an individual real face, in addition to the responses shown in (b) extended nerve cell nets involving the occipital and the temporal lobe and some limbic structures are coactivated.*

Correlations between Brain Activity and Perceptual Phenomena: Some Elementary Thoughts

In the following chapters we will repeatedly claim that certain brain lesions lead to impairments of visual perception and cognition. Such a claim supposes a close correlation between brain neuronal activity and subjective experience. What are the arguments supporting the hypothesis of a close correlation between physiological mechanisms and subjective experience? Epistemological restrictions forbid the application of the category 'causality' when we are speaking about the correlation between

physiological and psychological events. As Immanuel Kant convincingly argued, the category of causality is not applicable for psychophysical correlations, since the phenomena of subjective experience are well defined regarding the time domain ('down' to the perceptual 'moment' lasting about 80 ms), while they are ill-defined regarding space. The perceptual 'ego' only has a rather vague spatial location. In contrast, one can describe physiological processes as events in time with a precision of 1 ms or less and in space with a precision in the micrometre-range or even down to the molecular level, when one studies the neuronal events at the level of single nerve cells or membrane channels. Kant argued in a postscript to Soemmerring's *Über das Organ der Seele* (1796)

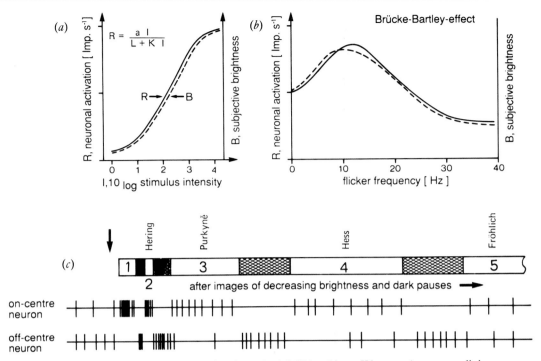

Fig. 1.10 *Examples of the simplest linear correlations found in retinal, LGN and layer IV area striata nerve cells between neuronal impulse rate and corresponding brightness and darkness pereception. (a) Neuronal activity and subjective brightness are similarly related to stimulus luminance. (b) The same is true for the perceived brightness enhancement in flicker stimuli (Brücke–Bartley effect; Grüsser and Creutzfeldt, 1957). (c) A bright, narrow slit moving rapidly across the visual field is seen followed by a sequence of bright and dark bands. These afterimages correspond to an oscillatory activity of on-centre and off-centre neurones in the afferent visual system as illustrated (Grüsser and Grützner,1958; Grüsser and Grüsser-Cornehls, 1962).*

that only the category of time is common to both phenomena, since the 'soul cannot define for itself any place whatsoever' ('... *nun kann die Seele ... sich schlechterdings keinen Ort bestimmen, weil sie sich zu diesem Behuf zum Gegenstand ihrer eigenen äusseren Anschauung machen und sich ausser sich selbst versetzen müsste; welches sich widerspricht'*).

The reader should take this caveat not as a case for dualism (e.g. Eccles, 1986) but as the epistemological limits of the monistic interpretation of brain functions which the authors support (e.g. Grüsser, 1956, 1965, 1990). The assumption of a close correlation between perceptual and physiological events is – as frequently observed for global hypotheses in science – mainly justified by its pragmatic success, and psychophysical monism or parallelism has, since Hering (1864/1920), Mach (1896) and Wundt (1896), been considered by many neuroscientists as a successful heuristic principle.

Modern neuroscience has to classify the correlation between perceptual or cognitive events on the one hand and brain cell activity on the other into different stages. This is schematically illustrated in Fig. 1.9(a): simple phenomena of visual perception such as subjective brightness or darkness, chromatic thresholds, short- or long-

lasting afterimages have their 1:1 correlate at the level of retinal ganglion cell activity. Despite sophisticated elaboration of the neuronal signals within the afferent or central visual system, elementary properties of visual data processing are preserved within the afferent visual signal flow and are represented in the activity of nerve cells in the primary visual cortex. For many phenomena of brightness and darkness perception a mutual prediction from neuronal activity to perception and back has been successfully established. Three examples illustrating the close correlation of single neurone activity and subjective brightness perception are depicted in Fig. 1.10. Once neuronal activity in the layer of retinal on-centre and off-centre ganglion cells had been established, certain phenomena of brightness and darkness perception were correctly predicted. As a matter of fact, we discovered some psychophysical effects only after we knew the corresponding behaviour of retinal ganglion cells or of nerve cells of the cat primary visual cortex having concentric or 'simple' receptive fields (e.g. the discovery of darkness enhancement in flickering patterns; Grüsser and Rabelo 1958).

As soon as elementary contour or shape perception comes into play, of course, one always has to consider carefully the spatially distributed activity within the visual

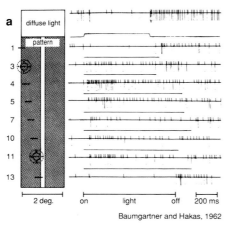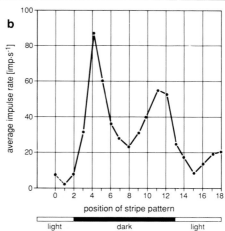

Baumgartner and Hakas, 1962

Fig. 1.11 *(a) Responses of a cortical off-centre neurone (cat encephale isolé preparation, area 17, presumably layer 4) evoked by a periodic vertical stripe pattern composed of small white and broad dark stripes. The RF centre of the neurone was placed at different positions relative to the light–dark stripe pattern as indicated. Note the border contrast activation. The horizontal bars indicate the diameter of the RF centre. (b) Same neurone and same stimulus pattern as in (a). The average impulse rate measured during the first 500 ms after stimulus onset is plotted as a function of the RF centre position relative to the stripe pattern. Note the enhancement of neuronal contrast activation when the RF centre was placed on the dark stripe near the light–dark border. Similar but less strong border contrast effects were found in retinal ganglion cells and LGN-neurones (from Baumgartner and Hakas, 1962, modified).*

neuronal networks. Baumgartner and Hakas (1960), for example, demonstrated that Mach's border contrast is easily explained when one looks at the spatial distribution of activity in the neuronal network of retinal on-centre and off- centre ganglion cells or area striata simple cells evoked by a light–dark border. Mach's border contrast is primarily caused by the centre–surround organization of these neurones (Fig. 1.11; Baumgartner, 1990). Large-field brightness contrast, however, and the generation of illusionary contours are not phenomena found in the neuronal activity of the afferent visual system, but require the activity of the neuronal network of area V2 (for details see Chapter 5).

Even more complex is the correlation between neuronal activity and the perception of certain visual shapes or structures like everyday objects or faces. As will be elaborated in Chapter 7, one has to know the temporo-spatial distribution of the activity of many neuronal classes in order to find a meaningful correlation between nerve cell activity and a defined perceptual phenomenon such as 'seeing a female face'. Neurones representing perceptual universals ('grandmother neurones', 'red-Volkswagen neurones') are inventions and do not exist in the real brain. This statement regarding the cerebral representation of perceptual wholes (or universals) is not a man-specific problem. Even for such elementary mechanisms as the prey-catching behaviour of frogs or toads, no 'bug detectors' exist (despite having been repeatedly claimed). A spatio-temporal complex sequence of activity of several neurone classes is correlated with the simple behavioural event 'frog catches fly' and the interdigitation of neuronal activity and motor acts changing the relation between frog

and prey is an essential component in the 'recognition' of a fly by a frog (for details see Grüsser and Grüsser-Cornehls, 1976).

Figure 1.8(b) illustrates schematically the complex interaction of different classes of neurones within a distinct neocortical area related to the recognition of a face. More complex, and involving extended spatial neuronal interactions and activity distributions across many brain areas, is the act of recognition related to the 'face of Margaret Thatcher', or, even more so, 'the faces of the authors of this volume after having completed the manuscript'. Recognizing such complex patterns requires (in the brain of our friends) a complex interaction of neuronal networks in widely spaced brain areas interconnected by thousands of transcortical axons. This is schematically illustrated in Fig. 1.8(c).

The consequences of this type of interpretation of brain activity are clear: as soon as visual recognition of more than elementary visual patterns is investigated, one is dealing with the time–space coordinated activity of extended brain regions and the claim of 'brain centres' for certain cognitive tasks can only mean that these 'centres' are composed of many important nerve cell nets, which are more involved than other brain regions in a certain perceptual task. Since every cortical nerve cell is connected with every other one through a chain not longer than 7–10 neurones, even very simple cognitive tasks change the activity level of large amounts of cortical regions. Whenever we speak in the following chapters about the location of certain brain functions related to visual perception or cognition, our use of words should be understood in the light of the preceding remarks.

2 Early Concepts of Visual Perception and Cognition: Historical Observations

Introduction

Before we deal with the experimental and clinical observations of visual perception and cognition, we will begin with a short historical survey of this field. We will examine the development of Western thought leading up to the 'modern' scientific investigations of the visual system which took place in the nineteenth century. A discussion of the historical roots of modern vision and agnosia research during the nineteenth and early twentieth centuries will be treated subsequently in the relevant chapters.

Ancient Greek Thought on Visual Perception

Western thought stems essentially from two sources, ancient Greek philosophy and Judaeo–Christian religion. Both of these sources, in turn, had been influenced by the Babylonian, Sumerian and Egyptian cultures, which explains the dominance of the dualistic concept of body–soul interaction in Western thought. The ancient Greeks living at the time of Homer (second half of the eighth century BC) believed that the soul functioned as a breath-like, extremely rarefied substance (the pneuma), which, after the death of the body, wandered to Hades, the 'depth of the Ais' (Homer, *Iliad*, lines 853–855). One of the great philosophical schools of ancient Greece, that of Pythagoras of Samos (*c*. 580–496 BC), accepted this dualistic concept of a material body controlled by a transmaterial pneuma. The members of the Pythagorean sect believed in the transmigration of the soul and in reincarnation (metempsychosis). These ideas led to the question, addressed also by Plato, of precisely where the soul rested in the body during its lifetime on earth. The pre-Socratic

and post-Socratic philosophers of ancient Greece proposed two explanations:

1. Empedocles (*c*. 490–430 BC), and later Aristotle as well as several of the Stoics, thought that blood was the medium of the pneuma, and that the heart operated as the 'hegemonikon', the central organ of life and of all conscious functions.

2. Having observed that brain lesions led to impairment of perception and cognition, Alcmaeon of Croton (*c*. 530–470 BC) considered the brain to be the hegemonikon of the soul, a view also held and expanded upon by Plato and many of his followers (Theophrastus of Eresos, *De sensu*, Stratton, 1917).

Alcmaeon not only discovered the optic chiasm, but was also the first to describe deformation phosphenes, the 'fire' that is seen when the eye is pressed. In addition, Alcmaeon developed the first reported model of vision. He believed that the optic nerve connected the eyes with the brain, and that pneuma could move in efferent and afferent directions from the sense organ to the brain and then back again. Most members of the school of Hippocrates (Kos, *c*.460–377 BC) as well as the leading anatomists at the school of medicine in Alexandria (which flourished around 300 BC), such as Herophilos and his somewhat younger colleague Erasistratos, supported Alcmaeon's hypothesis. This was also true for the most influential philosopher in Greece, Plato (Athens, 427–347 BC). He divided the soul into three parts: the mortal, vegetative soul, located in the liver and diaphragm; the mortal, animalic soul, located in the spinal cord and the thorax region; and the human-specific, immortal, divine soul, located in the brain (Plato, *Timaios*, 73 B–C).

The pre-Socratic philosopher and physician Empedocles, who lived in the Greek colony of Agrigent in southern Sicily (the ancient Akragas), followed the lead of his colleague Alcmaeon and assumed that the sense organs were

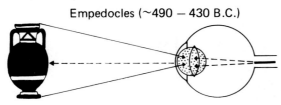

Empedocles (~490 – 430 B.C.)

Fig. 2.1 *According to Empedocles's extramission theory of vision, efferent light is generated in the eye, leaves it, touches the object, and is then reflected back to the eye (Grüsser, 1986).*

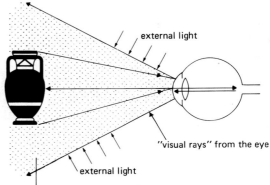

"body of vision" formed by external light and visual rays

Fig. 2.2 *Plato's interaction theory: efferent visual rays are emitted from the eye and interact with external light to form the 'body of vision', which touches the objects. The results of these interactions are then reflected back to the eye (Grüsser, 1986).*

connected with the hegemonikon by means of 'channels' inside the nerves. In order to explain vision, he hypothesized that pneuma, which he believed to be specific only to this sense, not only moved from the hegemonikon to the eye, but even left the eye for the purpose of vision. This efferent pneuma was radiated from the eye into the extrapersonal space, similar to the way in which the light of a lantern illuminates its surroundings on a dark night (Aristotle, *De sensu et sensato*, 437b). This 'extramission theory', or 'interaction theory', was most likely first conceived by Pythagoras: it is reported that he believed that a warm breath (pneuma) was emitted from the eye for the purpose of vision (Diogenes Laertius, VIII, 29).

Empedocles' interaction theory (Fig. 2.1) may be considered to be an early description of one important property of visual perception: namely, that it is not a passive but rather an active event depending on the activity of the organism, as is the case with perception in general. In contrast to the ideas advanced earlier by Parmenides (*c.* 540–480 BC), Empedocles recommended trusting the messages received from the sensory organs as a sound basis for thinking and cognition (Sextus Empiricus, *Adv. Math.*, VII, 125). To explain the specificity of the different sensory modalities, Empedocles hypothesized that channels of specialized size and shape exist in the sense organs:

> *Perception arises when something fits into the passages of any of the senses. Thus one sense cannot judge the objects of another, since the passages of some are too wide, of others too narrow for the objects perceived...* (Theophrastus, *De sensu*).

In his explanation of vision, Empedocles suggested the existence of four basic colours: white, black, red and yellow; all other colours corresponded to various mixtures of these four colours. According to this theory, 'black' and 'white' would, for example, fit different 'passages' in the sense organ, thereby evoking opposing visual processes (Theophrastus, *De sensu*, 7).

Diogenes of Apollonia (*c.* 460–390 BC) modified the interaction theory of vision. He proposed that the outer image mixes with inner air in the pupil of the eye at the point where one can see a small mirror image of the visual surroundings. This mixture would then be transmitted through the optic nerve to the brain (Theophrastus, *De*

sensu, 40). Although Aristotle rejected the extramission theory, Plato elaborated on the interaction between afferent light (the light of the sun or any other light source) and efferent light, the visual pneuma. Plato believed that the combination of both types of light formed a 'cone of vision' (Fig. 2.2). In his opinion, visual perception arose through a process in which the cone of vision 'touched' the objects. This interaction caused a modification of the cone of vision, which was then transferred back to the eye, and from there to the brain. This idea found wide acceptance among most ancient and medieval physicians and philosophers until the thirteenth century, when Albert the Great integrated several critiques of this interpretation, which had been published earlier by Alhazen, Avicenna and other Arabian scientists, into a new concept of visual perception (Albertus Magnus, cf. p. 29).

The pre-Socratic philosophers put forth two general physiological principles explaining perception. Several believed that the physiological process was similar to the signals received by the organism from the outer world; others, such as Anaxagoras of Klazomenai (500–428 BC), believed that perception was made possible only by a functional contrast between the signals from the objects and the physiological mechanisms transducing these signals. Anaxagoras was convinced that vision was caused by light reflection within the eye as well as by colour contrast produced by the dark pigments found in the eye (Theophrastus, *De sensu*, 27–29). Anaxagoras also discussed the problem of visual threshold, e.g. the subthreshold change in the colour of a white paint when small amounts of black paint are added and then evenly distributed. From such observations, Anaxagoras developed a rather sceptical viewpoint regarding the reliability of sensory perception: 'From the weakness of our senses we cannot judge the truth'. (Sextus Empiricus, *Adv. Math.*, VII, 90).

Democritus (~460 – 370 B.C.)

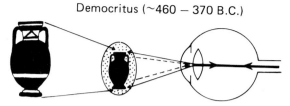

Fig. 2.3 *Democritus modified the extramission theory somewhat: after the efferent light (pneuma) is emitted from the eye, it interacts with the signals produced by the object in the near-distant extrapersonal space (located between the object and the eye), where small 'impressions' of the object are generated in the air (Grüsser, 1986).*

Like Empedocles, the first materialistic philosophers of Greece, Leucippus (fifth century BC) and his pupil Democritus (*c*. 460–370 BC), who both lived in Abdera (Thracia), also supported the extramission theory. They believed that in the process of vision 'small imprints' were generated in the air between the eye and the observed objects, and that the emitted visual pneuma interacted with these imprints (Fig. 2.3). As in the case of all extramission theories, Aristotle and his followers ridiculed this idea (Aristotle, *De sensu et sensato*, 440 a; Theophrastus, *De sensu*, 82). Democritus also argued that colour is not a property of objects, which were supposedly composed of atoms having no sensory qualities. In his opinion, the order and organization of the atoms from which the objects were composed produced the different colours after interacting with light or pneuma. Like Empedocles, he proposed four basic colours: white, black, red and yellow. He also thought that the different chromatic percepts would correspond to different properties of the colours, for example white being 'smooth' and black being 'rough' (Capelle, 1953).

Aristotle (384–322 BC) considered the soul to be the 'entelechy of a natural organic body', which guided and organized the living organism. It was characterized by four properties: nutrition, perception, movement and thinking (Aristotle, *De anima*, 412a, 27). As mentioned above, Aristotle rejected the idea that perception and cognition were somehow correlated with brain function. Nevertheless, through his careful analytical psychology, he significantly contributed to the basic concepts underlying the perception theories elaborated during the following two thousand years. He argued that signals from the five sensory systems were integrated by the common sense of the hegemonikon, which extracted the general properties of objects. Vision, in his opinion, was made possible only by means of a transparent medium such as air or water. He expanded Empedocles' four-colour theory into a seven-colour theory, according to which black and white were the first two basic colours, which were in turn complemented by five others: yellow, red,

green, blue and violet (Aristotle, *De sensu et sensato*, 438a, b). The appearance of a certain colour depended on the object's properties as well as on the process of perception. Pleasant colours were generated by a harmonic mixture of the basic colours, analogous to the harmony produced by a musical chord. Through this interpretation, Aristotle transposed Pythagoraean ideas about the aesthetics of music onto those of colour perception and painting (Aristotle, *De sensu et sensato*, 440a).

After the two Alexandrian anatomists Herophilos (*c*. 335–280 BC) and Erasistratos (*c*. 310–250 BC) had discovered the ventricles of the brain, the theory explaining the correlation between cognitive and brain functions became more complex. These two physicians at the school of medicine in Alexandria argued that the breath-like pneuma operated within the ventricular system of the brain. Because it was not yet known at the time that this system is filled with cerebrospinal fluid, Greek physicians generally accepted this hypothetical correlation between the ventricular system and pneuma activity.

The medical schools of Kos, Knidos and Alexandria made several important observations about visual perception. According to Galen, Hippocrates (*c*. 460–377 BC) had observed hemianopia and had reported the case of a patient 'who, whenever he wants to fixate something, is not able to do so and has the impression that he perceives only half of the person he wants to see' (Kühn, II, 221; Hirschberg, 1899). Galen also informs us that Hippocrates had described nystagmus and the *mouches volantes* that are visible during eye movements (Kühn, VII, 96). He also observed visual or multimodal hallucinations connected with delirium tremens:

> the patient reported that worms, animals of different species as well as fighting soldiers appear in front of him. The patient believed himself to be fighting with these soldiers and described this as if he observed it directly . . . . (Kühn, I, 151).

In addition to such complex hallucinations, simple phenomena, such as migraine phosphenes, were observed as well: "a patient, when strolling through the market places, had flickering sensations and could not see the sun" (Kühn, III, 667; Hirschberg, 1899, p. 109). The inducement of vertigo through intermittent flicker stimulation as well as the feeling of motion caused by vertigo were also well known to Greek physicians.

Claudius Galenos (Pergamon, Rome, 129–201 AD) provides us in his summary of the medical tradition of the preceding centuries with a clear account of earlier ideas about the correlation between brain function and the different properties of the soul (Falk, 1871; Siegel, 1970). Galen held the cerebrum to be the seat of the perceiving, thinking and moving *anima rationalis*, to which he attributed – as Aristotle had taught – three main functions: the 'phantasticon' (power of imagination), the 'dianoeticon' (judgement) and the 'mnemoneuticon' (memory and recognition). He believed that these different functions were correlated with various cognitive parts of the brain or ventricular system. The ventricular system was supposedly filled with the pneuma psychicon (spiritus animalis), formed in the ventricles of the brain through a process of distillation of the spiritus vitalis, which was, in turn, generated in the heart and pumped through the arteries into the brain. According to Galen's model, the 'phantasticon' performed a function essential to Aristotelian psychology: the integration of signals from the different sense organs. The *sensus communis* was thought to extract the general properties of the percept as categorized by Aristotle: size, shape, number, movement or non-movement, and unity (Aristotle, *De anima*, 424b). The 'dianoeticon', however, performed those functions in which the perceived information was evaluated, behavioural consequences drawn, and judgements made. This description reminds us of the more modern classification of perception, apperception and associative cognition used in nineteenth century psychology (Wundt, 1904).

Church Fathers, Arabian Scientists and Theologians Discuss Vision and Brain Function

In the following centuries, the three main psychological functions described in the preceding paragraph were attributed, with some modifications, to the ventricles of the brain. This is illustrated in the theory developed by the Christian bishop Nemesios of Emesa in the fourth century AD (Fig. 2.4). The 'first cell', i.e. the two lateral ventricles of the brain, was thought to contain the multimodal integrative power of the soul necessary for the perception of objects, the *sensus communis*. Aurelius Augustinus (354–430 AD) modified Nemesios' cell doctrine somewhat:

> *Thus three cells are found in the brain. The anterior one towards the face integrates all sensory signals; the posterior one towards the neck is the seat of memory, and from the third one in between the two, all movements are generated.*

(Augustinus, *De genesi ad litteram*, VII, 18.)

The cell doctrines put forth by Galen, Nemesios and Augustinus, which were incorporated into the anthropological chapters of many theological works, evidentally attributed the elementary visual functions to the eye. According to these doctrines, only multimodal integration and a higher-order analysis of the sensory signals of vision were thought to involve brain activity.

The medieval cell doctrines were modified by the leading Arabian physicians and philosophers, such as Costa ben Luca (864–923 AD), Al Kindi (803–873 AD), Alhazen (965–1040 AD), Avicenna (980–1037 AD) and Averroes (1126–1198 AD). Although each of these scientists

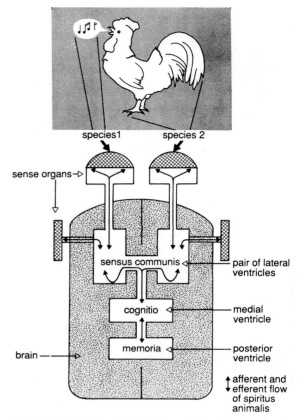

Fig. 2.4 *The 'cell-doctrine' of Galen and Nemesios of Emesa. The significant signals of the object (the 'species') interact with the spiritus animalis in the sense organs. The spiritus transfers the result of this interaction to the cellula prima (the lateral ventricles of modern anatomy). The sensus communis operates within the first cell, performing multimodal integration and extracting the general properties of the stimulus. The spiritus animalis transfers this information to the cellula secunda, where general judgements are derived through an interaction with information stored in the memory located in the cellula tertia. The result of the operations within the cellula secunda, which are transmitted to the cellula tertia (the fourth ventricle of modern neuroanatomy) for storage, can later be recalled (Grüsser, 1990a).*

assumed that modality-specific operations were executed selectively in the sense organs, the sensus communis was believed to be the first cerebral integrative mechanism which operated on a multimodal basis (Fig. 2.4). Cognitive operations followed this integration and allowed for judgement and control of the organism's movements. It was believed that these cognitive operations depended not only on the signals received from the sensus communis, but also on experience, which was supposedly stored in the memory and activated during the process of cognitive evaluation. Avicenna (Ibn Sina), like Aristotle, argued

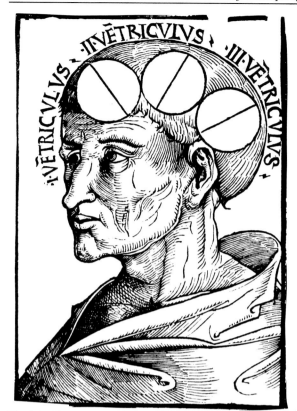

Fig. 2.5 *Illustration of the head of a learned monk, showing the three ventricles of the brain, each divided into two compartments. This figure, which was used as an illustration in a late printing of Albert the Great's 'Philosophia naturalis,' was presumably intended to be a portrait of the author (Basel, 1506). It was believed that the cerebral spiritus animalis, which supposedly controlled cognitive functions, operated within the ventricles. For this reason, large ventricles were thought to be a sign of high intelligence.*

against the old extramission theory of vision, refuting the idea of efferent visual rays as well as the pneuma theory (Wiedemann, 1913; Akdogan, 1984). In his book on optics, *Kitab al-Manazir*, Alhazen (Ibn al-Haytham) carefully described the structure of the eye. He also tried to explain the process of vision on the basis of the physical properties of light and of the morphology of the eye. By demonstrating the linear expansion of light as well as through his experiments with a simplified camera obscura, a dark chamber with a variable, slit-shaped aperture, he laid the foundations for the optics of the eye. However, when trying to integrate Galen's anatomy with optical theories dating back to the Greek opticians and mathematicians, Euclid (first half of the third century BC) and Ptolemy (second century AD), he had to struggle in order to find a functional explanation of the different parts of the optical system. He believed that the optical image was

transformed by the crystalline lens into a physiological process, which was then transmitted to the optic nerve and optic chiasm, where binocular fusion supposedly occurred (Bauer, 1911). Alhazen's twenty-two cognitive categories (described below, p. 35) were especially important for the understanding of higher visual functions. Alhazen's *Optics* was often translated during the Middle Ages; several manuscripts from the thirteenth and fourteenth centuries are still extant. Printed in book form in 1572 (*Opticae thesaurus ...*), it considerably influenced Western optical and visual theories up until the seventeenth century.

Albertus Magnus (*c.* 1198–1280 AD, Fig. 2.5), the major scientific figure and theologian of the thirteenth century, tried to bring some order to the psychological and biological knowledge of his time. In doing so, he elaborated extensively on the traditional brain localization theory, citing as his main sources the Arabian scientists discussed above. In addition to his commentary on Aristotle's scientific scripts, he included in his works his own observations on perception and the laws of nature (particularly in *Summa de creaturis* and *De anima*). Like Aristotle and the great Arabian philosophers, Albert was an empiricist, believing that sensory percepts have greater relevance to reality than does theory in the absence of experience. He realized, however, that theoretical concepts could of course transgress the limits of experience (*De anima*, Ed. Col., t. 7, pp. 2–3). Albert developed a rather sophisticated theory of perception and cognition, including the process of vision. He believed that the brain was the central organ of all sensory percepts, and divided its matter into three groups: the convoluted cortex (velum), the white matter (medulla) and the ventricles (*De animalibus*, I, t. 3, C1). Like Avicenna and Alhazen, he believed that a close correlation existed between brain function and the various psychological abilities: the signals generated by a given object corresponded to different sensory systems ('species'), and reached the respective sense organs by means of a medium located in the extrapersonal space. Each sense organ contained a specific spiritus sensibilis. The spiritus visibilis found in the eye was instrumental in transforming the signals produced by material objects (the 'species') into a physiological process (Fig. 2.6). The 'species' produced by the objects altered the spiritus visibilis, which was then transported from the crystalline lens through the hollow optic nerves into the cellula prima of the brain. According to this model, the cellula prima was the seat of the sensus communis ('common sense'), which integrated all sensory data perceived by the five external senses. The sensus communis, the first inner sense, extracted the above-mentioned Aristotelian perceptual categories from the external sensory data. Hence, the sensus communis supposedly formed the relay to the other four inner senses.

The second inner sense, the imaginatio or vis imaginativa, transposed the sensory data to a higher level of

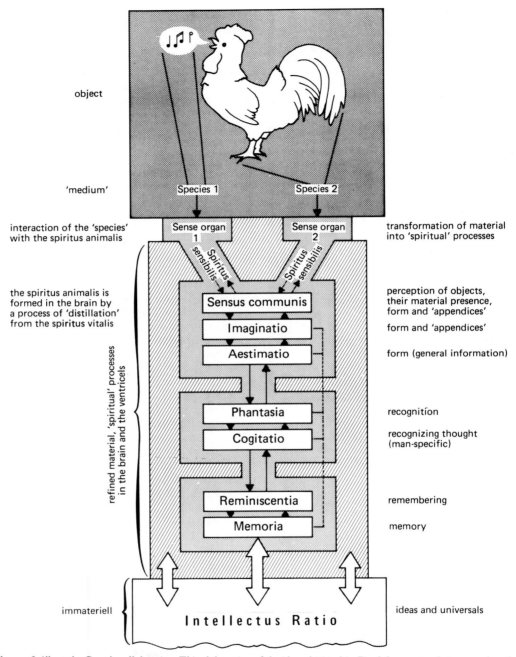

Fig. 2.6 *Scheme of Albert the Great's cell doctrine. This elaboration of the ideas depicted in Fig. 2.3 corresponds in general to the teaching of the Arabian scientist Alhazen. The three cells (cellula prima, secunda and tertia) are subdivided into functionally different regions, as indicated. For a further explanation see text (Grüsser, 1990a).*

abstraction. The same was true for the third inner sense, the estimatio or vis estimativa. Sensus communis, imaginatio and estimatio were all located either in the cellula prima or within its walls. After these three functions processed the sensory data, the general meaning of the percept was available. All processing was performed by the spiritus animalis, which also transmitted the data from the cellula prima to the cellula secunda, which corresponds to the third ventricle of modern anatomy (Fig. 2.6). Albert believed that the human-specific cognitive abilities, phantasia and cogitatio, were located in this part of the brain. Finally, a 'channel' (the aquaeductus Sylvii of modern anatomy) extending from the cellula secunda connected the second cell with the cellula tertia, in which reminiscence and memory (reminiscentia and memoria) operated.

Albertus Magnus attributed various precognitive and cognitive operations to the inner senses (illustrated in Fig. 2.6): the sensory organs transformed the external signals of the material world into a 'spiritual' process representing the different modalities of an object (for example, the visual shape, colour and movement of a rooster as well as the auditory signals of its crowing). The sensus communis combined sensory inputs and operated in the presence of the material stimuli. The imaginatio, however, did not require further material presence of the external signals; rather, it functioned with a short-term memory, elaborating on the perceived shapes and 'appendices' of the observed object (for example, elaborating on the rooster's different shapes and on the actual colour of its feathers). The vis aestimativa extracted only the general shape and meaning of the stimulus, not its 'appendices'. Signals from memoria, i.e. former experiences, were then integrated at this early level of precognitive operations, thereby enabling the organism to recognize the observed object. The presence of the visual object was no longer necessary during the next steps of phantasia and cogitatio; the duration of these 'elaborating' functions depended on the complexity of the cognitive task. Once again, information stored in the memory was activated by reminiscentia and integrated into the process of cognition. Through this process, man could extract the general properties of a stimulus and ultimately represent that stimulus with an appropriately chosen word.

Up to this level, all processes of perception and cognition were 'physiological' and therefore did not require a non-material soul. Albert, however, attributed the highest cognitive functions – the formation of ideas and universals – to a human-specific, immaterial process: ratio and intellectus. In his model of cognition, these belonged to the immortal part of the soul and were believed to interact with the physiological mechanisms described above. The specific nature of this interaction remains as enigmatic in Albert's works as in all earlier and later dualistic models.

Albert also elaborated on the theory of vision he learned about in the writings of the Arabian scientists. He discriminated between light coming from self-illuminating light sources (lux) and light reflected from illuminated objects (lumen). Albert suggested that colour was generated in three ways:

1. by the effect of colour pigments (surface colours),

2. by chromatic filters (coloured glass, mist or clouds), and

3. by the properties of the self-illuminating light sources.

The specific colour generated in the last category depended on the temperature of the light source (*Summa de creat.*, Quaest. XXI). Albert also rejected the extramission theory; like Alhazen, he believed that the interaction between the 'species' of vision and the spiritus visibilis took place in the crystalline lens of the eye, to which the spiritus visibilis flowed from the brain via the optic nerve and retina. On its way back, the spiritus visibilis transmitted the visual signals through the optic chiasm, and from there to the sensus communis located in the cellula prima, the first cell of the brain. Binocular integration of the signals from both eyes was performed in the optic chiasm.

Albert investigated the order of perceived colours by mixing chromatic pigments. Since he spoke about 'symmetrical colours' (*Summa de creat.*, Vol. II, Quaestio XXI), it is probable that he represented the 'natural order' of colours in a colour circle. Albert argued that because of the ordering of the colour space, one could move along different paths from white to black, for example via blue, red, green or yellow (*De anima*, II, tr. 3, cap. 29). Albert repeatedly distinguished between light–dark perception and colour perception, and evidently knew of people who were totally colour blind. These colour-blind persons, who showed the symptom of photophobia characteristic of monochromats (*De anima*, II, tr. 3), could see only by moonlight, not by daylight. As a result, Albert distinguished between two states of vision: "in the light [the visual process] accepts colours, in the dark only the splendour" (*De anima*, II, tr. 3, cap. 7).

The cell doctrine elaborated in the works of Albertus Magnus was accepted by the physicians of his time, and was also used as a diagnostic tool by following generations of physicians: it was believed that a patient suffering from blindness had lesions either in the eye or in the optic nerve or in the optic chiasm. Patients suffering from perceptual disturbances (including hallucinations) were thought to suffer from brain lesions around the cellula prima; someone who had normal perceptual abilities but exhibited thought disorders, such as a paranoia, was thought, however, to have brain defects in the region around the cellula secunda. Memory defects, observed more frequently in the elderly, were attributed finally to diseases of the spiritus animalis operating in the cellula tertia. The leading anatomist of the early fourteenth century, Mondino de Luzzi (Mundinus, *c.* 1275–1326 AD, Bologna) also accepted Albertus Magnus's model and elaborated on it by differentiating between the functions located within the first cell. Mondino believed that the spiritus flow was

LIBER DECIMVS TRACT.II.

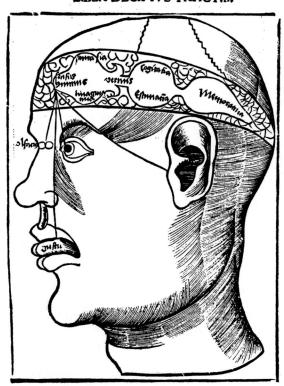

Fig. 2.7 *This illustration of the cell doctrine from the book of Gregor Reisch Margarita philosophica (1506) displays the ideas on brain function as expressed by Mondino de Luzzi (1316). The first cell contains the functions sensus communis, fantasia and imaginativa and is connected with the second cell by means of a valve-operating channel (vermis). In the second cell the two functions cogitativa and estimativa are located. The separate third ventricle, finally, is for the functions of memory (memorativa).*

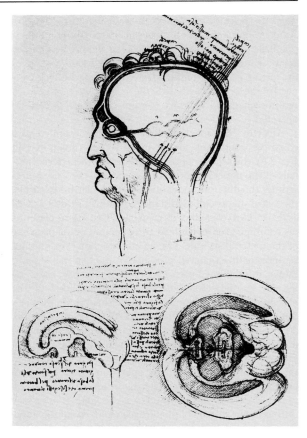

Fig. 2.8 *Upper part: Leonardo da Vinci's illustration showing a sagittal view of a section of the skull (about 1490). The ventricles of the brain are depicted as three oval cells. In this illustration, Leonardo followed the traditional cell doctrine. Lower part: Leonardo changed his opinion, however, after having reconstructed a realistic figure of the shape of the brain's ventricular system by injecting melted wax into the ventricle, a technique he knew from wax moulds applied in the creation of bronze sculptures. This is illustrated in the sagittal and horizontal sections running through the brain of an ox. Compared with (a), this is a fairly naturalistic depiction of the shape of the ventricles. (From Vangensten et al., 1911–1916.)*

mediated by 'channels' and controlled by 'valves' (Fig. 2.7; Mondino: *Anatomia*, 1316). Mondino published sketches in which the shape of the lateral ventricles, the compartment of the cellula prima, were more realistically depicted than in any medieval medical descriptions.

Representation of the Visual World by Brain Functions: A Renaissance Approach

The first realistic description in modern anatomy of ventricle shape is found in one of Leonardo da Vinci's manuscripts. Leonardo (1452–1519; Fig. 2.8), who grew up on a

farm in Tuscany, was the illegitimate son of a Florentine lawyer. His close contact with nature in his early years combined with his ingenious gifts later played a major role in his ability to make highly precise observations. After receiving his training in Andrea del Verrocchio's workshop in Florence, he soon became interested in engineering techniques and in the field of anatomy. In addition to his many animal dissections, he claimed to have obducted and examined approximately thirty human corpses. Although Leonardo had planned to publish an anatomy textbook with the anatomist Marcantonio della Torre

(1473–1506) from Verona, the book was never finished because of the young anatomist's premature death. In addition to realistic drawings of the ventricular system (Fig. 2.8), Leonardo's extant manuscripts contain a sophisticated model of vision. Presumably having read Alhazen's book *Optics* in Latin translation, Leonardo followed this scientist's lead in assuming that the dioptric apparatus of the eye generated a small upright image of the visual world on the papilla of the optic nerve, which clearly required a double inversion of the visual rays (Fig. 2.9). Leonardo believed that the optic nerve was located precisely at the spot where the optical axis of the eye cuts the retina. To prove his hypothesis, he built a glass model of the human eye in which he could indeed see a small upright image in the region of the papilla (Fig. 2.9).

Through his anatomical research, Leonardo learned that the eye was connected via the optic nerve to the optic chiasm, from which further connections reached the brain. He hypothesized that a spatial representation of the visual image was created by this projection along the walls of the ventricles, where visual impressions (impressiva) were supposedly formed. He assumed that the area of this physiological spatial representation of the visual image was some 10,000 times as large as the area of the pupil in the human brain:

> *The central organ of visual perception of man is like a big hall which receives light through a small hole while the corresponding organ of the owl is a much smaller room with a large opening.*
> (Codex D, 5r)

Leonardo's experimentation with the camera obscura (MS A, 21r) probably accounts for his metaphorical description of the visual image's central representation. If we assume a small pupil area of about 4 mm², the ventricular surface of the brain would require, according to Leonardo's figures, about 400 cm² projection space, i.e. in each lateral ventricle about 200 cm². This value is, however, too large for a human lateral ventricle. Leonardo presumably arrived at this value by extrapolating from his measurements of ox brain ventricles (Fig. 2.8) to find that of the human brain. He may also have based his deduction on findings from a human brain with a hydrocephalus internus. The ventricular system schematically drawn in a sketch of the human head was much too large (Weimar; Fig. 6 in Weale, 1988).

Leonardo's most important idea was his assumption that the representation of the visual image was achieved by the formation of a physiological, material 'image' (in which the geometrical order of the field of vision was maintained) on the walls of the lateral ventricles. Since the region of the fovea centralis actually projects onto a much larger part of the corpus geniculatum laterale and visual cortex than does the periphery of the retina, modern neurophysiology has confirmed Leonardo's idea with the

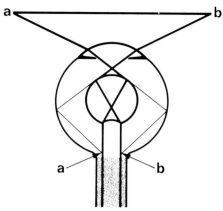

Fig. 2.9 *Redrawn scheme of one of Leonardo's drawings of a horizontal section through the eye and his construction of an optical image on the back of the eye. Leonardo assumed a twofold inversion of the image generated in the eye and constructed a small upright image falling onto the optic nerve (according to manuscript D 10r).*

modification that this representation follows a non-linear geometry (see Chapter 3). Although Leonardo da Vinci did not to our knowledge elaborate on visual cognitive functions, he was indeed the first to attribute modality-specific functions to a certain part of the brain, an idea which was not appreciated by his contemporary anatomists. The fact that Leonardo was not interested in publishing his own work offers one explanation for this social neglect of his ideas. For this reason, his contemporaries had not discussed most of his technical inventions, scientific theories, philosophical thoughts or anatomical discoveries.

With his idea of a geometrical representation of the visual image formed on the walls of the cerebral ventricles, Leonardo reshaped the more general ideas proposed by Nicolaus Cusanus (1401–1464) on perception and representation of the perceptual world in cognition. Cusanus, a cardinal of the Roman Catholic Church born at Kues on the Mosel, became one of the most influential philosophers of his time. After receiving a university education in Heidelberg and Padua, he worked in Cologne, the centre of the Dominicans, where the teachings of Albertus Magnus were highly regarded. He adopted the Sceptic tradition in his method of teaching, and taught that the cognitive abilities of man, like those of other animal species, correspond to species-specific behavioural needs (Cusanus, *De conjecturis*). He compared the human intellect to a cosmographer who constructs a simplified 'inner map' of the world by means of the sense organs, and conceived a four-level process of assimilation and abstraction. In this cognitive map all essential properties of the world were represented in a geometric order (Cusanus, *Compendium*, 1464).

Cusanus also developed a general theory of signs in

which he discerned 'natural' signs understood inherently by man by means of effective congenital mechanisms. 'Perception of colour and sound, of laughing and crying' were such natural signs. By contrast, 'artificial signs' had to be learned: their meaning was arbitrarily chosen and defined by learned convention (Cusanus, *Compendium*). Cusanus's ideas set the tone for modern semiology as well as for all brain theories which considered visual cognition to be a representation of the material world as transformed by brain functions. It is not known whether Leonardo was acquainted with Cusanus's published works.

Leonardo also made several new and interesting observations about the psychophysics of vision. He believed that each object possessed ten properties which could be perceived by the visual system: light, dark, colour, shape, size, position, distance and nearness, movement and rest (Codex Atlanticus, 90 r/b). He described the response of the iris to light: it constricts its pupil upon illumination. By rotating a burning coal in a large circle as stimulus, he demonstrated the 'inertia' of the visual perception process which is caused by retinal afterimages and cortical mechanisms (which correspond to the 'iconic memory' of modern psychophysics jargon). Leonardo demonstrated his knowledge of the generative power of visual imagination when he recommended to his pupils, who evidently showed a dearth of creative fantasy in painting, to sit in front of a rock cliff and watch the objects and scenes generated on its face by the pupil's visual fantasy.

Leonardo did not determine which physiological mechanisms lead to the geometrical representation of the visual world on the walls of the ventricles. Renaissance anatomists, however, slowly modified the Galenic tradition and developed their own thoughts on the perceptual and cognitive functions of the brain. Johann Fernelius (Fernel, 1497–1558), anatomist at the St Barbé college in Paris, discussed cognitive functions of the brain in *De naturali parte medicinae* (1542), a compendium of the medical knowledge of his time. For Fernel, the brain was the domicilium of all psychological functions. He believed that the spiritus animalis provided the material basis for these functions, and that it operated as a direct medium in the transfer between the immaterial soul and the material body. Thus, he still accepted the spiritus theory proposed by Galen as well as the cell doctrines described in the preceding sections. According to Fernel, the refinement of cognitive functions from perception of symbols to thoughts (Fig. 2.6) was accompanied by the repeated physical refinement of the spiritus animalis by means of mechanisms similar to the process of distillation. He no longer attributed the spiritus flow through the ventricular system of the brain to a temperature gradient, as Galen had thought, but rather to the somewhat mysterious vis innata cerebri, an inborn power of the brain. Fernel believed that the sensus communis and cognitive func-

tions operated in brain matter, and that the spiritus animalis served only as a mediator for the signal transfer.

Jacopo Berengario da Carpi (*c*. 1470–1538), a surgeon's son from the small Italian city of Carpi who later became physician to Pope Julius II and the Medici family in Florence, was also interested in developing a realistic picture of the brain and the ventricular system. He treated Lorenzo de Medici the Younger, who had received a gunshot wound in the skull. In his '*Tractatus de fractura calvae sive cranei*' (1518), Berengario discussed the various neurological symptoms associated with lesions in different parts of the brain. From his clinical observations, he came to the conclusion, which he published in his commentary about the anatomy developed by Mondino (Mundinus, 1513, pp. 425–428), that processes of perception and cognition were not located in the ventricles, which were supposedly filled with the spiritus animalis, but rather in the brain matter. Like Fernelius, he also attributed the function of signal transmission to the spiritus.

With the publication of *De humani corporis fabrica*, the classical work of Andreas Vesalius (1514–1564), a new era in brain anatomy dawned. In various diagrams, Vesal presented realistic portrayals of the ventricular system and its relation to the septum pellucidum, and of the brain's vascular system. After Archangelo Piccolomini (1526–1586) had distinguished between grey matter (cerebrum) and white matter (medulla), a distinction also recognized by Albertus Magnus, scientists eventually came to the opinion that while white matter performed signal transmissions (i.e. transmissions of the spiritus animalis), grey matter might be more important in the process of signal storage and complex signal processing.

Hieronymus Fabricius ab Aquapendente (*c*. 1533–1619), who belonged to the generation of anatomists following Vesal, carefully elaborated on the anatomy of the eye and on the physiology of vision. He was trained by the University of Padua's famous Falloppio, whom he succeeded to the chair in anatomy. Fabricius was well aware of the ideas of vision discussed above. Although he still used the concept of the 'visual pyramid', a modification of Plato's cone of vision, he believed that it only represented each eye's field of vision, i.e. a geometrical construct. He used pyramids of vision to explain binocular vision, and clearly separated the binocularly overlapping visual field seen by both eyes from the monocular components (Fig. 2.10). He recognized not only that the size of the visual fields was larger in binocular vision than in monocular, but also that binocular vision improved visual accuracy. For the mechanisms of binocular interaction, however, he assumed that the brain elaborated upon the monocular percepts alternatingly in short intervals. He originally thought the retina, which he knew to be sensitive to light, to be a possible organ of vision, but finally rejected this idea in favour of the traditional opinion,

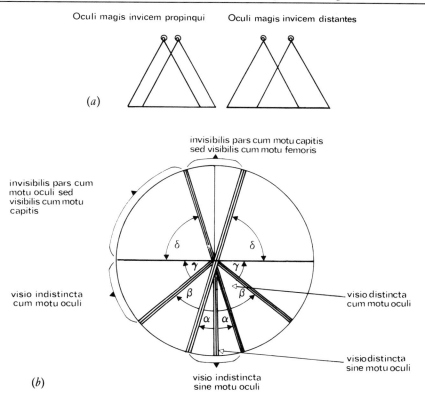

Fig. 2.10 *(a) Fabricius ab Aquapendente recognized that the binocular visual field consists of two monocular components and a medial overlapping section in which both eyes receive signals from the same objects. This binocular overlapping part of the visual field changes its size when fixation shifts from a near (left) to a distant object (right). (b) Schematic representation of the different sectors of the extrapersonal space perceived visually. In the centre of the visual field a small part exists within which the extrapersonal space is seen distinctively without eye movements (visio distinctiva sine motu oculi). The region (α) represents that part of the visual field seen indistinctly without eye movement (visio indistincta sine motu oculi). The region (β) depicts that part of the visual field distinctly seen when the eyes move and the head remains still (visio distincta cum motu oculi), while the sectors (γ) represent indistinct vision under these conditions. The regions (δ) represent those parts of the visual field which are seen when the eyes and head move together. A small part of the extrapersonal space, finally, can be seen only by body movements (visibilis cum motu femoris). (Redrawn from Fabricius ab Aquapendente, Opera omnia anatomica et physiologica: De actione oculorum pars secunda, 1687).*

which held that the crystalline lens was the actual instrument of vision. He thought that the retina served to conduct signals from the lens to the optic nerve.

Fabricius supported Alhazen's theory that twenty-two primary qualities ('intentiones') of visual perception existed: light, colour, distance, spatial localization, three-dimensionality, figure, size, continuity, interruption, number, movement, rest, roughness, smoothness, transparency, density, shadow, darkness, beauty, ugliness, similarity and difference. Besides these primary visual categories, Fabricius suggested several secondary visual percepts which he believed to be characterized by a certain order and shape, such as script, paintings and sculptures. For the recognition of a given figure's shape, he postulated four suborders which he considered to be qualities neces-

sary for perception: rectilinearity, curvature, concavity and convexity. He regarded rarity and abundance as subcategories of visual numbers, equality and augmentation as subcategories of similarity. Laughing, sadness, crying and cheerfulness were described as visual perception qualities of the 'shape of the face', which Fabricius considered to be a special operation specific to the sense of vision. This categorization of the process of vision, which reflected the Arabian tradition in Renaissance thought, sounds very 'modern' (cf. Chapter 1). Finally, Fabricius made another important contribution to the overall anatomy of the central visual system by indicating that behind the optic chiasm, the fibres of the optic nerves do not run towards the lateral ventricles but rather towards the 'posterior part of the brain'.

From Johannes Kepler to René Descartes: The Creation of Modern Physiological Optics

A change in theoretical visual concepts took place after the Swabian astronomer Johannes Kepler (1571–1630) had successfully applied the laws of refraction of optical surfaces to the dioptric apparatus of the eye, and proposed that an inverted image of the object was projected onto the inner surface of the retina (Fig. 2.11). Kepler based his optical investigations on the improved anatomical model of the eye published by the University of Basel's great clinician and anatomist Felix Platter (1536–1614). Platter assumed that the retina was the structure in which light was transformed into a physiological process. He also published anatomical figures of the structure of the eye, with which Kepler became familiar through his collaboration with the Prague anatomist Johannes Jessen (1566–1621). Kepler first published his ideas about image formation by the dioptric apparatus of the eye in *Ad Vitteloni paralipomena* ... (1604); he developed them further in a second book, *Dioptrice* (1611). As he did not consider retinal signal transduction to be a problem of physics, Kepler restricted his research to the optics of the eye, preferring to leave to the biological scientists all further investigations of the physiological process of transduction of light signals into retinal signals. Interestingly, Kepler still discussed the question of whether deformation of the eyeball would lead

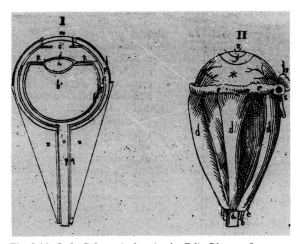

Fig. 2.11 *Left: Schematic drawing by Felix Platter of a horizontal section of the human eyeball (1583). Right: Outer view of the eye with some of the eye muscles (from Platter, 1583, plate 49). When Kepler developed his concept of retinal image formation, he used and reprinted these as well as other figures published by Platter.*

to the generation of 'real' light. He maintained that a mechanical irritation of the iris through deformation of the eyeball might induce 'sparks' which would stimulate the retina and lead to perception of phosphenes. The Jesuit father Christoph Scheiner (1579–1615), a contemporary of Kepler, also supported the idea that physical light was generated in the eye during the perception of deformation phosphenes; however, he believed that it was produced by mechanical irritation of the crystalline lens. When this stimulation released a large amount of internal light, it would become visible. Scheiner carefully observed the development and position of deformation phosphenes. He noted that phosphenes evoked in darkness not only differed from those seen in light, but that the initial phosphene was always perceived opposite the site of deformation, an observation that corroborated Kepler's idea about the functional reversion of the retina (Grüsser and Hagner, 1990; cf. Chapter 9). Scheiner also cleared up a misconception held by generations of anatomists before him, namely that the optic nerve head corresponded to the optical axis of the eye: he recognized the fact that the point where the optical axis of the eye meets the retina was considerably shifted towards the temporal side of the papilla nervi optici (Fig. 2.14; Scheiner, 1619).

In 1613, several years after the appearance of Kepler's two books on the optics of the eye, Franciscus Aguilonius (1567–1670), the rector of the Jesuit college of Antwerp, published one of the most important textbooks on vision written in the first half of the seventeenth century. Evidently, Aguilonius had not grasped Kepler's revolutionary concept of image formation in the eye, for he still regarded the tunica aranae, i.e. the lens capsule, as the site of image transduction into a physiological process. Nevertheless, Aguilonius's book shows some remarkable insight into the process of vision. It is still famous today because of the accompanying illustrations by Peter Paul Rubens (1577–1640), one of which is shown in Fig. 2.12 (Jaeger, 1976, 1990).

In discussing binocular vision, Aguilonius elaborated on the concept of the horopter and described the condition of crossed and uncrossed double images for objects placed inside or outside the horopter circle (Fig. 2.12). He erroneously maintained, however, that the optic nerves do not cross at the optic chiasm, but remain separated along the path leading to the ipsilateral brain (Aguilonius, 1613, p.15). Thus, it remained an enigma how signals perceived by both eyes were unified. Like Kepler, Aguilonius believed that the deformation phosphenes were generated by internal light evoked within the eye by mechanical irritation and the liberation of spiritus animalis. He did not, however, accept the idea that spiritus animalis left the eye for the purpose of vision.

Although Aguilonius's description of the order in colour perception did not transgress traditionally held

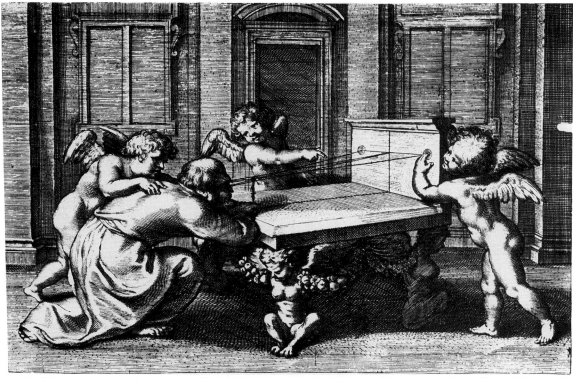

Fig. 2.12 *Illustration showing the generation of the double images appearing when one observes a near distant object while fixating upon a point further removed. Illustration by P. P. Rubens for F. Aguilonius's* Opticorum libri sex, *etched by Theodor Galle (Aguilonius, 1613).*

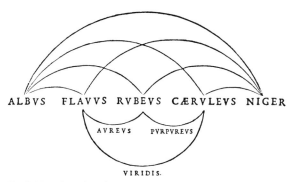

Fig. 2.13 *The order of perceived colours as depicted by Aguilonius (1613). A mixture of the three basic colours, yellow (flavus), red (rubeus) and blue (caeruleus), produces orange (golden, aureus), purple (purpureus) or green (viridis). Saturation of the chroma depends on the amount of white (albus) or black (niger) added to the mixture.*

ideas (Fig. 2.13), he introduced in his theory of order in the colour space the concept of more or less saturated colours generated by a mixture of white or black with one of the three elementary colours, yellow, red or blue. Mixtures of these three elementary colours produce purple, orange (aureus) and green. His representation of the colour space (Fig. 2.13) may be considered to be a first attempt at combining trichromatic colour vision with light–dark mechanisms (Aguilonius, 1613, pp. 38–41). It is evident that this structure contained more colours than Aguilonius had observed when separating the chromatic components of white light using triangular glass prisms.

Aguilonius correctly related visual acuity to a threshold determined by a minimal angle of size, and recognized that the intensity of illumination as well as the clarity of the medium existing between object and image both had a considerable impact on visual acuity (*l.c.*, p. 60). Finally, he discussed the cognitive components of visual perception and, referring to Aristotle, defined the following general 'objects' of vision: quantity, figure, site, position, distance, continuity, interruption, movement and rest. In his discussion of movement, he thought carefully about the formal condition of visual movement perception induced by a change in the position of the stimulus observed in the visual space (observer's eyes remaining still). For this condition he recognized a lower and an upper threshold for movement perception. Interestingly,

Aguilonius clearly discriminated between what today we know as 'afferent' and 'efferent' visual movement perception (Dichgans and Brandt, 1973; cf. Chapter 16), and also recognized the validity of the reafference principle, which was rediscovered in modern physiology by Steinbuch (1811) and Purkinje (1823), and which is discussed in Chapter 21. According to Aguilonius, the velocity of a moving stimulus could be estimated through a process in which the speed of the 'gaze' movements following the moving object were innerly measured; he assumed that the soul ('anima') had the faculty to perceive this eye movement and, from this value, to deduce the speed of the object. (*l.c.*, p. 21). In addition, he carefully elaborated on movement perception in the case of an object altering its distance from a stationary observer; he further believed that changes in distance were perceived not only by variations in object size, but also by internal signals correlated to the vergence angle of the eyes (*l.c.*, p. 188).

Although Aguilonius assumed that the brain was the organ of the sensus communis, he still accepted the idea that spiritus animalis was necessary for sensation, perception and movement. Without the sensus communis no visual cognition was possible; only the central cognitive abilities, the vis cognitiones of the brain, were able to recognize the presence and identity of objects (*l.c.*, p. 94). Expanding upon traditional conceptions of the hierarchy of cognitive processes (Fig. 2.6), Aguilonius discussed the problem of presence or absence of visual stimuli for the activation of visual imagination ('phantasia'). He emphasized the importance of previous experience in visual object recognition, but did not go beyond the traditional

ideas concerning the impact of 'memoria' on cognitive abilities.

When the eminent French philosopher René Descartes (1596–1650) began to develop a new concept of visual perception, he was aware of Kepler's ideas on image formation on the retinal surface. In his books *Dioptrique*

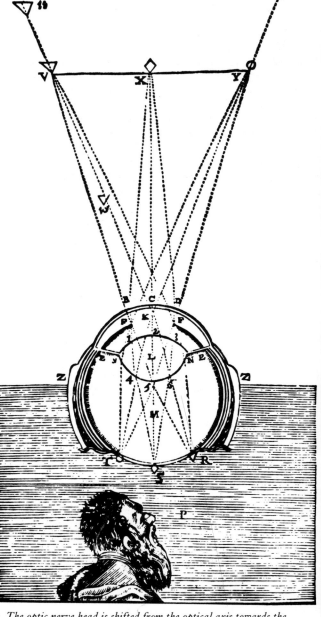

(a)

(b)

Fig. 2.14 *(a) Schematic drawing of a horizontal section of the eye. The optic nerve head is shifted from the optical axis towards the nasal side, and the position of the lens is shifted more anteriorly than in Platter's scheme (see Fig. 2.11). (Ch. Scheiner: Oculus, hoc est fundamentum opticum, 1619). (b) Kepler's construction of the inverted image of the retina as presented in Descartes's Dioptrique, 1637.*

(1637) and *Tractatus de homine* (*Traité de l'homme*, 1662/64), Descartes postulated that light acted on the retina by a direct mechanical effect leading to 'vibration' of the optic nerve fibres. According to the law of mechanics, this vibration was transmitted by means of small fibres inside the tubular nerve channels to the central projection region of the optic nerve, the walls of the ventricles. Like Leonardo da Vinci a century earlier, Descartes assumed that the representation of the optical image along the walls of the lateral ventricles followed simple geometric rules (Fig. 2.14). The small strings inside the optic nerve were supposed to open miniature valves on the ventricular walls, thereby controlling the outflow of spiritus animalis into efferent, tubular structures, i.e. motor nerve fibres, which in turn led to muscle contraction achieved by means of a valve-controlled pneumatic device. The respective muscle which 'contracted' was supposedly inflated by the spiritus animalis. A sophisticated valve system directed the flow of the spiritus from the 'relaxing' muscle to the corresponding contracting muscle. Descartes evidently introduced a new concept into the physiology of vision and other sensory functions. Instead of the old Galenic model of afferent and efferent spiritus flow driven by temperature gradients, Descartes gave preference to a mechano-pneumatic model, reminiscent of the sophisticated mechanics of an organ, an instrument made very popular at that time by great composers and organists such as Jan Pieters Sweelinck (1562–1621), Heinrich Schütz (1585–1672) and Samuel Scheidt (1587–1654). In Descartes's model the visual signals were not only 'mapped' onto the inner surface of the lateral ventricles where they interacted with many valves, but were then projected further into another brain structure, the pineal organ. Knowing of no other non-partite structure, Descartes considered this organ to be the central organ of the brain (cf. Zrenner, 1987). In this brain theory, the pineal organ played an important role in three different operations:

1. In vision, it coordinated binocular fusion (Fig. 2.15), thereby maintaining the geometrical organization of the visual world in the physiological processs.

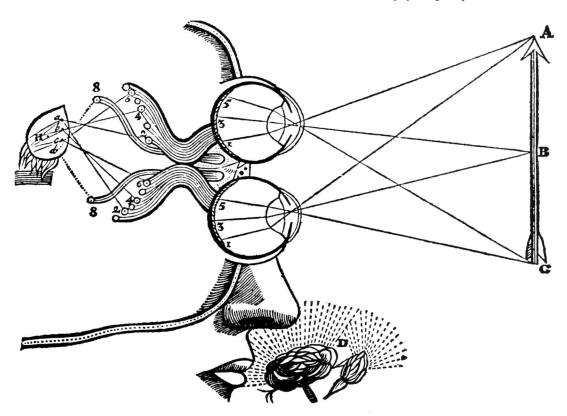

Fig. 2.15 *Illustration from Descartes's* L'homme *(1664) demonstrating the modality specific representation of the visual and olfactory signals located on the inner wall of the lateral ventricles of the brain. There are separate projections for each optic and olfactory nerve. Binocular fusion occurs at the surface of the pineal organ through mechanical interaction of the signals. The geometrical order of the binocular image is maintained during this process. Multimodal integration is also performed in this structure.*

2. It was responsible for the multimodal integration necessary for object perception.

3. Finally, this little structure was the relay station where the immortal and immaterial soul interacted with mechanisms of the brain; it was the 'liaison brain', where the immaterial res cogitans and the material res extensa communicated with each other. Thus in contrast to earlier models (e.g. that of Albertus Magnus), Descartes's focused the discussion of brain–mind interaction on a distinct anatomical structure.

Upon reading Descartes's concept of vision in his *Dioptrique*, one realizes how difficult it was to give a consistent mechanical explanation of vision:

> *The power of movement acts in those parts of the brain from where the small strings of the optic nerve originate and evokes in the soul the sensation of light. In this process the different types of movement lead to different chromatic sensations. In a similar manner, the movements of the auditory nerve cause the soul to hear tones, and the movements of the nerves of the tongue evoke gustatory sensations . . . . It is not necessary for any similarity to exist between the images the soul receives and the movement* [of the small nerve strings] *which produce these images' (Dioptrique).*

Progress in Neuroanatomy: New Models of Visual Perception and Cognition

The experts in neuroanatomy did not accept Descartes's concept because they could not find any direct connections between the lateral ventricles and the pineal organ. For example, the Danish anatomist Nicolaus Steno (1638–1686) argued in a lecture held in 1664 in the home of Melchisedec Thévenot (1620–1692), a highly educated Maecenas of sciences in Paris, that Descartes's theories were anatomically impossible. Steno supported Descartes's general mechanistic concept and discussed it in his *Discours sur l'anatomie du cerveau* (1669). He also supported the idea that a geometrical projection of the physiological representation of the retinal image was formed in the brain, and that this principle was not only maintained after binocular fusion, but that it continued to act at the cognitive level of multimodal interaction which was necessary for object and space perception.

Soon after the publication of Descartes's *Tractatus de homine*, several scientists in the seventeenth century, such as the Roman mathematician G. A. Borelli (1608–1679) in his book *De motu animalium* (1680), and the Dutch scientist Jan Swammerdam (1637–1680) in *Biblia naturae* (1737), disproved the existence of a spiritus animalis necessary for muscle contraction. Steno not only recognized that the white substance of the brain was composed

of fibres, but evidently also had the idea that this fibrous structure had something to do with sensation and movement as well as with the interaction between these two processes (*Discours . . .*, pp. 4, 8).

The English physician Thomas Willis (1621–1675), who in 1660 became Sedleian professor of natural philosophy at Oxford, published two important books in which he discussed several new ideas about brain mechanisms and their relation to perception and cognition: *Cerebri anatome* (1664) and *De anima brutorum* (1672). Like Borelli, Willis believed that the Spiritus animalis was indeed a fluid transported to and from the grey matter through the hollow nerve fibres of the white substance. He thought that signals from the sense organs reached the corpora striata, where the sensus communis was presumably located, through afferent nerve fibres (Fig. 2.16). The objects in the extrapersonal space were functionally mapped on both sides of the brain's corpus striatum in a manner similar to the way in which images of objects are projected by an optical lens onto a white wall. This was yet another model that used the idea of geometrical representation in order to explain visual cognition. Based on his observations of patients suffering from hemianopia who also had anatomical lesions on one side of the corpus striatum, Willis came to the conclusion that the corpus striatum must be the centre of visual functions. He interpreted the striatal lesions as the cause of visual field defects.

Nervous signals reach the corpus callosum from the corpus striatum. Since fibres from all parts of the brain were meshed together in this structure, Willis regarded the corpus callosum as that part of the brain in which perception was transformed into imagination. Furthermore, he believed that it sent signals to a large variety of different 'memory areas' located in the cortical grey matter, where information was then 'imprinted'. During the process of object recognition or 'remembering', these imprints were supposedly reactivated. Willis assumed that all voluntary motor actions originated in the grey matter of the hemispheres; he also argued, however, that a visual stimulus or any other sensory stimulus could evoke a subconscious motor 'impulse'. He presumed that such a motor response was automatically executed as a sort of sensory-motor reflex: '*Motus est reflexus qui a sensione praevia dependens illico retroquetur*' (in *Cerebri anatome*; 'movement is a reflex that, in its response, depends on the preceding sensation'). Willis did not attempt to include the higher-level cognitive abilities of man in his model of brain function. He left this problem to the 'authority of the theologians', whose task, he believed, was to think about the ways in which the immaterial soul and the material brain processes interacted with each other.

The function of the brain's grey matter remained a mystery for many seventeenth-century anatomists. Some scientists, such as the French anatomist Raymond Vieuss-

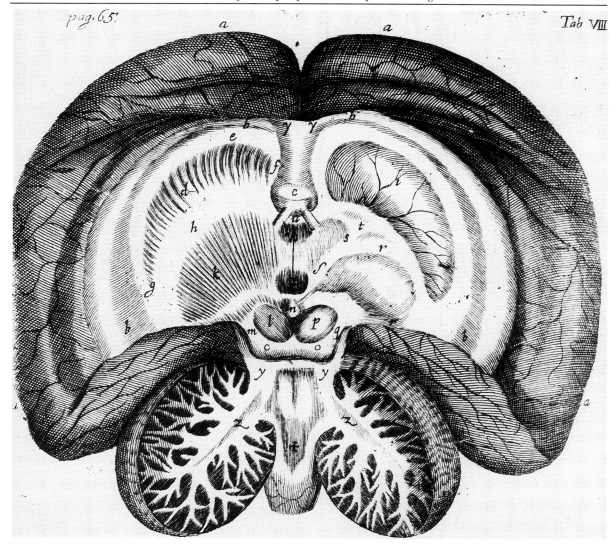

pag. 65.

Tab VIII

Fig. 2.16 *Thomas Willis's illustration of an oblique section of the human brain through the corpus striatum and the thalamus. The corpus callosum (c), the corpora striata (d, i), the thalamus (k), the pineal organ (n), and the corpora quadrigemina (l, p, c, o) are all designated. The cortical grey matter (a), the cerebellum (z) and the fourth ventricle (+) are also indicated, but only rather schematically. (From Willis: De anima brutorum, 1672.)*

ens (1641–1715) and the Italian anatomist Marcello Malpighi (1628–1694), believed that the grey matter consisted of many miniature glands. Using magnifying lenses, Vieussens discovered that the grey matter was composed of an innumerous quantity of small, intertwined oval-shaped structures (*Neurographia universalis*, 1664, p. 54). Malpighi, who boiled the brain in oil or in water before cutting it into slices, published similar findings. The little 'glands' described by Malpighi and Vieussens were probably not nerve cells but rather preparation artifacts. Towards the last quarter of the eighteenth century, Giovanni Maria della Torre published drawings of the cerebral grey matter, of the cerebellum, and of retinal flat mounts based on microscopic observations. In addition, he described regularly organized, small, ball-like structures found in the retina and the brain ('globetti', Fig. 2.17(a)–(c), *Nuove osservationi microscopicche*, 1776). We think that these globetti were, indeed, retinal ganglion cells and nerve cells found in the brain. No concepts for a cellular structure of the brain (nor for the visual centres) were put forth, however, until Purkinje's discovery in 1837 of nerve cells (as well as of the nucleus and nucleolus) in the cerebellum and in other structures of the brain (Fig. 2.17(d)).

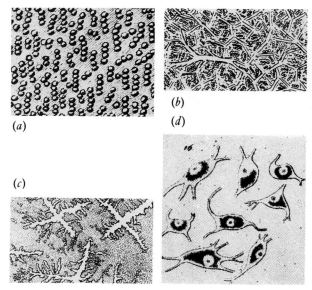

(a)

(b)

(d)

(c)

Fig. 2.17 *Several illustrations from G. M. della Torre's Nuove osservazioni microscopicche (1776). (a) Section of the grey matter of the brain. One recognizes the columnar organization of the 'globetti', which are presumably somewhat simplified drawings of nerve cells. (b) Flat mount of the retina showing vessels and small 'globetti' (here presumably retinal ganglion cells). (c) Section of part of the cerebellum. The small 'globetti' were probably Purkinje cells. (d) Purkinje's 1837 drawing of nucleus ruber nerve cells (including the nucleus and the nucleolus of the cell) located in the brain stem.*

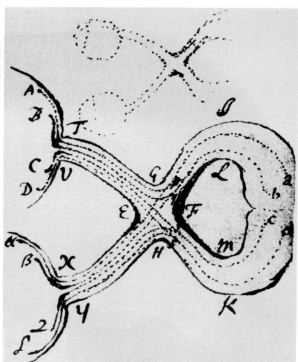

Fig. 2.18 *A page section from Isaac Newton's Opticks manuscript illustrating Newton's ideas on hemidecussation of the optic nerves found in the optic chiasm. While optic nerve fibres from the nasal half of the retina cross to the other side, those from the temporal retina remain on the same side. Note that Newton thought that binocular fusion occurred by axon fusion immediately after crossing. The geometric order of the two halves of the visual field is maintained on the left and right projection sites (Corpus geniculatum laterale) of the optic nerve fibres located in the brain (a, b, c, d). (From p. 10 of the manuscript Add.MS 3975; reproduced with permission of the Cambridge University Library.)*

A Physicist and a Mathematician Contribute to the Physiology of Vision: Newton and Mayer

Interestingly, it was two mathematically gifted scientists who developed new theories on visual function. In his book *Opticks*, Isaac Newton (1642–1727) described for the first time the hemidecussation of the optic nerve in the chiasm. Up until Newton's time, it had been thought that although the optic nerves touched each other in the optic chiasm, they remain separated along the central path, connecting to the side of the the the brain ipsilateral to the eye of origin. Since Newton's discovery of the hemidecussation of optic nerve fibres in the chiasm, we know that one half of the visual field of each eye is represented in the contralateral part of the brain, the other half in the ipsilateral (Fig. 2.18). This not only represented a new principle of neuronal organization, but also offered a novel representation of the visual world within the brain. Newton wrote:

Are not the Species of Objects seen with both Eyes united where the optick Nerves meet before they come into the Brain, the Fibres on the right side of both Nerves uniting there, and after union going thence into the Brain in the Nerve which is on the right side of the Head, and the Fibres on the left side of both Nerves uniting in the same place, and after union going into the Brain in the Nerve which is on the left side of the Head, and these two Nerves meeting in the Brain in such a manner that their Fibres make but one entire Species or Picture, half of which on the right side of the Sensorium comes from the right side of both Eyes through the right side of both optick Nerves to the place where the Nerves meet, and from thence on the right side of the Head into the Brain, and the other half of the left side of the Sensorium comes in the like manner from the left side of both Eyes (*Quaerie* 15, book 3, part I).

As one of Newton's drawings demonstrates (Fig. 2.18, manuscript add. MS 3975, p. 10, Cambridge University Library), he believed that binocular fusion occured in the optic chiasm, and that the projections travelling from there to the thalamus maintained the geometric organization of the image found on the retina. Newton did not hesitate, as Kepler had, to speculate about the physiological mechanisms that lead to visual sensation. He believed that 'the Rays of Light in falling upon the bottom of the Eye excite Vibrations in the Tunica Retina', which are then 'propagated along the solid Fibres of the optick Nerves into the Brain, [and] cause the Sense of seeing . . .' (*l.c.*, Quaerie 12). In this process, the size of the vibrations determined which colour was perceived, the 'shortest vibrations' producing a sensation of deep violet, the largest deep red. Newton evidently considered the frequency of nerve-fibre vibration to be the coding mechanism used in colour perception. For example, he argued that the afterimages seen after a flash of light were caused by the persistence of vibrations produced by the flash. Although Newton leaned toward a physical interpretation of colour vision, he realized that hues existed in subjective colour perception that were not present in the white light spectrum. Like Aguilonius, he knew for example that purple was a mixture of blue and red. He was the first to draw the obvious conclusions from this observation in proposing a closed geometrical figure, i.e. a circle, to represent human colour perception (Fig. 2.19).

In his physiological interpretation of signal transmission through optic nerve fibres, Newton also speculated

about the effects produced by changes in the amount of excitation ('vibrations'). The next step taken towards quantifying the processes of perception was the scaling of sensation relative to the strength of the stimulus, an approach which is still used today in visual psychophysics. Once again, it was a mathematician and astronomer who took the lead in this direction. Tobias Mayer (1723–1762) born into a family of craftsmen from southern Germany, was well known in his time as a cartographer, mathematician and astonomer. He was a professor of 'economics' (applied mathematics) and headed the astronomical observatory at the University of Göttingen (1751–1762). Mayer became famous for his precise astronomical measurements as well as for his high-quality maps of the moon (Forbes, 1980). In his everyday work with astronomical instruments, he was confronted with two major problems: visual acuity, and the dependence of visual resolution on illumination. In order to measure more precisely the angles on his astronomical instruments, which were equipped with special micrometres, he developed several technical innovations. He further tried to enhance their precision by repeating his readings and by computing algebraic means. This method, with which every scientist nowadays is familiar, was novel in Mayer's time. While trying to develop a theory of error measurement, he encountered the problem of visual acuity, which he decided to measure in human observers. He published his results in 1755 in his *Experimenta circa visus aciem*, using two interesting arguments to justify his measurements: the inadequate science of error evaluation, and the limited knowledge of the 'most important source of errors', namely 'the weakness of the human senses'. Mayer did not ask whether it was possible to measure psychophysical thresholds, or whether one could deduce quantitative rules from such measurements. He considered this problem a priori as the 'natural' way in which a scientist should solve such practical problems, an attitude prevalent among many scientists during the early Enlightenment period.

To measure visual acuity, Mayer used different-sized dots, black-and-white gratings, and chequerboards. He apparently did not know that the English astronomer and physicist, Robert Hooke (1635–1703), the 'Curator of Experiments' at the Royal Society in London, had demonstrated as early as 1674 at a Society meeting that visual acuity could be measured by means of black-and-white gratings. Hooke speculated that visual acuity was the result of the 'diameter of the optic nerve fibres forming the inner layer of the retina' (Hooke, 1705, p. 98). Other attentive observers had also noted that visual acuity depended on the strength of illumination. George Berkeley (1685–1753) mentioned this fact, for example, in his 1709 treatise, *An essay towards a new theory of vision* (section LIV). The German philosopher and mathematician Christian

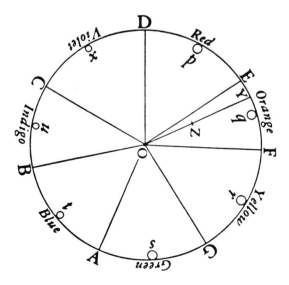

Fig. 2.19 *'Colour circle' designed by Newton (Parkhurst and Feller, 1982).*

Wolff (1679–1754) noted that visual acuity decreased moving from the centre of the visual field towards the periphery. Like Hooke, Wolff assumed that under optimal illumination conditions, the minimum visibile was related proportionally (1 : 1) to the density of the 'optic fibres' found in the retina (Wolff, 1725, pp. 381–382). Tobias Mayer was obviously acquainted with Wolff's work, having recommended Wolff's mathematics textbooks to his students. From his comparative studies using the above mentioned patterns, Mayer concluded that measurements of visual acuity that had been determined using gratings and chequerboard patterns were reliable; he then carried out a number of psychophysical experiments aimed at determining the dependence of the minimum visibile on the strength of illumination of the stimulus pattern. Using a candle as his source of light, he varied the distance (d) of the candle from the stimulus pattern, thereby changing the intensity of illumination. By also varying the distance between the observer and the stimulus pattern, he measured the minimum visibile α, i.e. the grating period, in visual angle seconds, and found a fairly constant relationship between α and the illumination intensity (I):

$$\alpha = k\, I^{-1/6} \tag{2.1}$$

Since the visual acuity (V_α), measured in (seconds of visual angle)$^{-1}$, can be defined as the minimum value of the minimum visibility,

$$V_\alpha = 1/\alpha = k * I^{1/6} \tag{2.2}$$

Mayer carefully tabulated his data and discovered a very close relationship between equation 2.2 and the empirical results. The data are replotted on a log–log coordinate system in Fig. 2.20, which clearly demonstrates that Mayer's power functions given by equation 2.2 closely matched his empirical data, and that the constant (k^*) depended on what type of gratings he used (Grüsser, 1989).

Mayer performed other metrical studies as well related to visual perception. As in his investigation of visual acuity, these studies were also attempts to solve practical problems. He struggled, for example, with the difficulties that craftsmen face in producing identical colours on multicolour maps. Frequently, the results did not meet the expectations of the scientist who had charted the map. In 1757 Mayer taught a course at the University of Göttingen on 'The drawing and colouring of geometrical diagrams, fortifications and architectonic schemes'. It is likely that he developed his quantitative description of a three-dimensional colour space in preparing for this course. At a meeting of the Royal Society of Sciences at Göttingen in 1758, Mayer reported on his efforts to construct a 'colour triangle' with the three 'main colours', red, yellow and blue: by adding white or black to the colour mixture, he

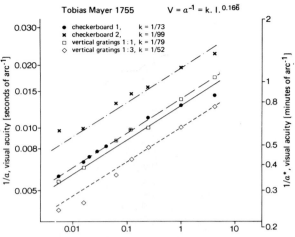

Fig. 2.20 *The relationship of visual acuity (ordinate axis), as measured in seconds of arc (left side) or minutes of arc (right side), is plotted as a function of the illumination of the stimulus pattern (abscissa). Mayer's data from 1755 are plotted in a logarithmic coordinate system. The straight lines correspond to the power functions described by Mayer. The slope for the function obtained with two types of checkerboards or vertical gratings remains constant (Grüsser, 1989.)*

was able to construct a three-dimensional hexahedric colour space (Mayer, 1758). Mayer summarized his studies on colour vision in a manuscript, *De affinitate colourum commentatio*, which was published in 1775 by Lichtenberg in the *Opera inedita Tobiae Mayeri*. In this treatise, Mayer addressed several questions, including: which and between how many hues man can discriminate, and whether a quantitative relationship could be found for this ability when the various hues (C_i) were produced by mixing different coloured pigments. In his experimental studies, he mixed the three elementary pigments (R = red, Y = yellow, B = blue) according to the following formula:

$$C_i = R^n\, Y^m\, B^{12-n-m} \tag{2.3}$$

whereby $n + m \leq 12$. The exponents used in this notation represented the quantitative mixture of the three colour pigments which Mayer used to obtain a subtractive colour mixture.

Mayer postulated with this equation that every mixed colour (C_i) was composed of twelve 'parts' that could be distributed in any proportion using the 'primitive' colours red (R), yellow (Y) and blue (B). In Mayer's notation, $R^4 Y^4 B^4$ represented the neutral colour grey, which was placed in the centre of his 'colour triangle'. Mayer deduced from this equation a two-dimensional geometrical representation of the 'pure' mixed colours, an early

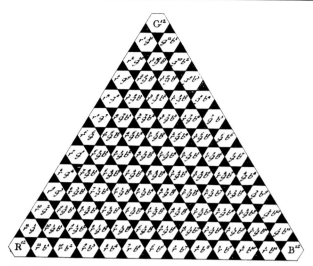

Fig. 2.21 *Mayer's colour triangle. For further explanation see the text. (From* Tobiae Mayeri Opera Inedita, *ed. G. F. Lichtenberg, 1775.)*

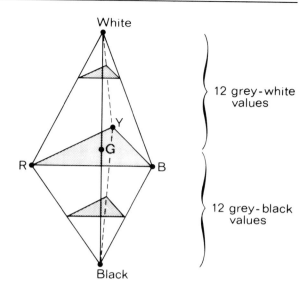

R = Red, B = Blue, Y = Yellow, G = medium Grey

Fig. 2.22 *Mayer's hexahedric colour space. The coloured triangle in Fig. 2.21 forms the triangle which separates the upper 'light' and lower 'shadow' part in Mayer's hexahedric colour space (Grüsser, 1989).*

version of the colour triangle (Fig. 2.21). Black and white were not considered primary colours, although Mayer knew, of course, that adding black or white pigments to a subtractive colour mixture would change the chroma. He considered the addition of black and white as a way in which to change a given colour's 'degree of light' or 'degree of shadow'. To represent the white or black components within a colour space, he added another dimension to his colour triangle, constructing a hexahedron with a black–white axis that was placed orthogonally to the plane and that passed through the centre of the colour triangle. The tips of the hexahedron were 'pure white' or 'pure black' (Fig. 2.22). Any colour (C_i) mixed with black (S) or white (W) could be assigned to one point in the colour hexahedron according to the following equations:

$$C_i = W^d \, R^a \, Y^b \, B^c \tag{2.4}$$

for the white half of the hexahedron, and

$$C_i = S^e R^a Y^b B^c \tag{2.5}$$

for the 'shadow part' whereby $(a+b+c+d)=(a+b+c+e)=12$. Illustrating his hexahedron colour space in tabular format, Mayer pointed out that the colour space was composed of 91 'perfect colours' corresponding to the colour triangle, 364 'pale colours' in the light part of the colour space, and 364 'dark colours' in the shadow part of the hexahedron. Thus, Mayer's colour space consisted of 819 different positions, each corresponding to a different hue. In Mayer's opinion, a human observer could easily distinguish between these different hues.

Mayer's efforts to construct a colour space using the results of a subtractive colour mixture was a first step towards developing an experimentally supported theory of colour vision. Using the limited techniques of his time, Mayer attempted to develop a metrically defined colour system with a specific position for each hue, something that was later done with more precision by Wilhelm Ostwald (1853–1927) and by Munsell (Krantz, 1972).

Mayer's two psychophysical publications were the 'by-products' of a creative scientist whose main field was astronomy. His research was strongly influenced, however, by an attitude prevalent at that time in most major European universities, namely the belief in applying the simple strategy of measuring everything that is measurable in order to render those operations and functions measurable, which, until this point, had been regarded in scientific circles according only to their qualitative aspects. Human performance was thus compared to that of a machine-like system. That such endeavours should have occurred at this time should not be surprising considering that, for example, J. O. La Mettrie (1709–51) had published his famous book *L'homme machine* in 1748. It was not until many generations later, however, that quantitative psychophysics and measurements of visual performance were introduced as systematic research tools in the study of human vision.

Paths and Wrong Tracks Leading Towards Localization of Higher Brain Functions

The problem of whether it was possible to attribute distinct cognitive functions to certain parts of the brain dominated eighteenth-century anatomical discussions. During this period, localization theories were opposed by several very influential scientists, such as Herman Boerhaave (1668–1738), professor of medicine at Leyden, and his pupil Albrecht von Haller (1708–77), professor of anatomy and physiology at Göttingen. Towards the end of the eighteenth century, Erasmus Darwin (1731–1802) argued in his famous book *Zoonomia* (Vol. 1, 1796) in favour of a general representational concept that would relate cognitive functions to brain mechanisms. He believed that objects in the extrapersonal space were mapped in both perception and recognition processes to brain functions, especially those operating in the brain stem. This was also assumed to be true for percepts related to one's own body. While experimenting on birds, Jan Evangelista Purkinje (1787–1869), together with his doctoral student H. C. G.

Krauss (1823), observed that unilateral lesions in the superior colliculi of pigeons led to circular flight paths in the direction ipsilateral to the lesion. Without elaborating in detail on these observations, they also wrote in their study, which was devoted mainly to the cerebellar structures controlling equilibrium, that 'instinctive responses' and 'intellectual functions' were affected in animals with 'control lesions' in the cortical grey matter.

Towards the end of the nineteenth century, Franz Joseph Gall (1758–1828) and his pupil Johann Caspar Spurzheim (1775–1832) proposed a rather speculative brain localization theory. Gall's *Phrenology* was based on comparative neuroanatomical studies, on observations of patients suffering from mental diseases, and on comparative measurements of the skulls of criminals or abnormal men. Gall believed that the human character was formed by the relative efficiency of several psychological entities, the 'faculties', which depended on the function of certain areas of the cortical grey matter ('organs'). Gall discriminated between those organs common to man and animals, and those serving higher-order social and cognitive functions found only in humans. He believed that the visual functions were located in three organs: the sense of colour

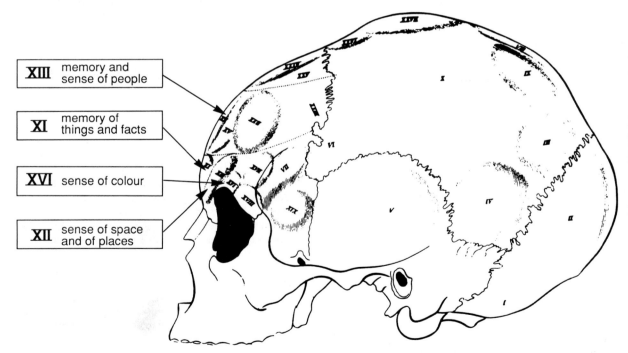

Fig. 2.23 *The first schematic projection of brain 'organs' onto the surface of the skull as performed by F. J. Gall. The development of these different regions can be judged by measurements or palpations ('cranioscopy'). Examples of correlation of the organs with the 'faculties:' I — reproduction, instinct; II — love of children; III — friendship; IV — self-defence; V — aggression; XV — language; XVII — musicality; XXIII — poetic talent; XXVI — religiosity. Gall localized the visual functions in the supraorbital region; they are indicated here separately. (From F. J. Gall,* Anatomie et physiologie du systeme nerveux en generale et du cerveau en particulière, *Paris, 1810–1819; Clark, Dewhurst, 1972.)*

in the frontal supraorbital brain (Fig. 2.23), the sense of places and of spatial orientation in the immediate vicinity of the sense of colour, and the memory and sense of people (recognition of persons) in the frontal brain. None of these speculations was later confirmed, however, by the symptoms produced by lesions in the respective parts of the brain. Gall's phrenology achieved importance nevertheless because of three essential assumptions that subsequently became significant in later studies of the cognitive functions of the brain as well as in the field of neuropsychology.

1. The brain, which acts as the organ of the soul, is the functionally and structurally subdivided centre of all perceptual and mental faculties of man.
2. Perceptual, intellectual and moral faculties of man are affected by brain lesions. Circumscribed brain lesions should lead to cognitive defects depending on the site of the lesion.
3. The left and the right hemisphere of the human brain do not necessarily serve the same functions.

While theorem 1 is a more general statement, theorem 2 could be verified through empirical observation. The French anatomist J. B. Bouillaud formulated theorem 3 more explicitly in 1825, writing that man possessed a 'double intelligence', one on the right side of the brain, the other on the left (cf. Harrison, 1985). In his book, *A New View on Insanity: Duality of the Mind* (1844), A. L. Wigan strongly emphasized this view.

Because of his speculative phrenology, which had even been ridiculed by several of his contemporaries, one often forgets nowadays that Gall was also an excellent neuroanatomist, having contributed to the multilocal representation of retinal signals in the brain. In the book *Recherches sur le système nerveux en général, et sur celui du cerveau en particulière* (1808), Gall and Spurzheim elaborated on the concept of retinal projections into the brain. Referring to Santorini, Hildebrand, Soemmerring and Boyer, who already were 'of the opinion that a large part of the anterior quadrigeminal bodies was the source' of optic nerve fibres, they reported their own observations of projections of the retina onto the superior colliculi:

> *On several occasions we have also observed that atrophy of one of the optic nerves, following a lengthier period of blindness, visible from one side in front of the meeting point of the two optic nerves, is found on the opposite side beyond this point. The optic thalamus corresponding to the atrophic nerve appears flatter ... we have only found a reduction in the latter attributable to the atrophy of the optic nerve ... however we have always observed a distinct deterioration in the anterior quadrigeminal body corresponding to the atrophic nerve* (pp. 102, 103).

On the basis of these observations, Gall and Spurzheim formulated an important new principle explaining multiple projections from a sensory organ into the brain. Nearly 80 years later in 1885, Edinger suggested the pulvinar as a third region containing optic nerve fibre terminals (cf. Edinger, 1904, p. 263); he emphasized that the pulvinar received afferent fibres not only from the retina, but also from the occipital part of the brain, the 'Sehzentrum' of Hermann Munk. The concept of a feedback loop in the brain's visual system was another new principle: corticofugal fibres found in the visual regions in the occipital part of the cortical grey matter were supposedly connected to the subcortical visual centres.

It is interesting that the physiological and clinical consequences of Newton's demonstration of hemidecussation of the optic nerves in the optic chiasm were not drawn. For example, F. Magendie, professor of physiology and medicine at the Collège de France in Paris, still reported in 1834 that unilateral hemispherectomy in mammals led to blindness of the contralateral eye. This did not take into consideration the position of the optical axis in animals with lateral eyes as opposed to those with frontal eyes: animals with lateral eyes possessed an overwhelming majority of crossed optic tract fibres; however, approximately 40% to 50% of optic tract fibres in animals with frontal eyes, such as cats, monkeys and men, originate in the ipsilateral eye and do not cross in the optic chiasma. Significantly, Magendie observed that while unilateral destruction of one of the superior colliculi did not lead to blindness in mammals, it destroyed vision of the contralateral eye in birds. He correctly described the colliculi superiores and the corpus geniculatum laterale as the two main projections sites of optic nerve fibres, and suggested the tuber cinereum as a third site where optic nerve fibres are found. He presumably discovered the hypothalamic root of the optic nerve. Magendie reported about an experiment with rabbits, in which he caused blindness in the contralateral eye by cutting the optic tract behind the optic chiasm. These experiments clearly proved that in animals with lateral eyes, the majority of optic nerve fibres cross to the other side. Although hemianopia caused by cerebral lesions was repeatedly reported in the early eighteenth century, human hemidecussation had evidently still not been correctly interpreted by the clinicians.

The Discovery of the Visual Cortex: Early Concepts of Optic Agnosia

Although the primary visual cortex (the area striata of the occipital lobe) was described as an anatomical entity in 1776 by Gennari, it took another hundred years until this peculiar part of the cortical surface was recognized as the primary cortical visual centre. Francisco Gennari (1752–1797) began his studies on the human brain while still a

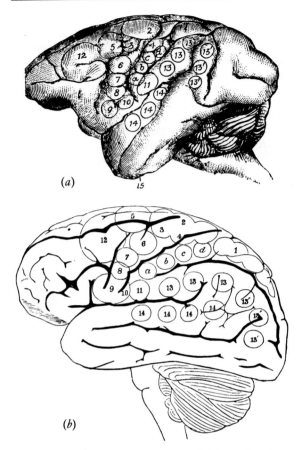

Fig. 2.24 *(a) Schematic representation of different functions at
the surface of a monkey brain according to electrical stimulation
and lesions. Circles with number 13 represent the visual
functions. (b) The scheme of the localization of cerebral
functions as found in experiments in monkeys and depicted in (a)
was projected by Ferrier onto the surface of a human brain (from
Ferrier, 1876).*

here the borders of what is nowadays called 'area striata', a
structure identical with the primary visual cortex.

Gennari's discovery of the morphological subdivisions
of the cortex, which were made visible by the thickness of
the stripe of Gennari, was first understood more than a
hundred years later, when researchers and clinicians
began to investigate the cortical areas more systematically.
This took place after Fritsch and Hitzig had demonstrated
in 1870 that electrical stimulation of certain parts of the
cortical grey matter led to motor responses, and furthermore that the site of stimulation determined where the
movement occurred and what type of movement was
evoked. David Ferrier was able to evoke eye movements in
dogs and monkeys by electrically stimulating a region
around the parietal end of the lateral fissure in the parietal
and temporal occipital bank (Fig. 2.24). He observed that
the animals became functionally blind after bilateral
removal of that cortical region, thus concluding that he
had discovered the visual centre of the cortex. He dared a
direct prediction of where the human visual cortex is
located, by assuming simple homologies for the brain of
man and monkeys (Fig. 2.24; Ferrier, 1876). Later, Ferrier
realized his error and reported that animals in which the
gyrus angularis region had been removed bilaterally
slowly regained reduced vision. What he had discovered
was evidently the impact of these parieto–occipital regions
on visual attention and on visually guided motor functions.

Hermann Munk (1839–1912), professor of veterinary
physiology at Berlin, was luckier than his colleague in
London. By systematically removing cortical grey matter
from dogs and monkeys, he came to the conclusion that
the most occipital part of the cortical grey matter was the
visual cortex. Examining various degrees of grey matter
removal, he demonstrated that bilateral removal of the
occipital cortex led to cortical blindness ('Rindenblindheit') while partial removal of the visual cortex
caused mind blindness ('Seelenblindheit') (Munk, 1878,
1880, Fig. 2.25). From his experiments in monkeys he
concluded that restricted lesions in the occipital grey
matter led to 'spot-like cortical blindness of both retinae'
(Fig. 2.25; Munk, 1880). Munk found in later experiments
performed in 1881 that electrical stimulations of the occipital visual cortex also evoked eye movements, an observation confirmed by the British physiologist Schäfer, who
also confirmed Munk's theory about the location of the
visual cortex (Schäfer, 1888). The academic feud between
Ferrier and Munk over the issue of cortical visual centres
seems today rather superfluous, for both were correct:
Munk on the one hand had discovered the primary visual
cortex, Ferrier on the other hand had found extrastriate
visual regions which served higher-order precognitive
visual functions (Glickstein, 1985)

At the same time that Munk performed his experiments

medical student at the University of Parma, where he
carefully inspected and drew sections of frozen human
brains. In 1782 he published his findings in *De peculiari
structura cerebri nonnullisque ejus morbis*, which also
included his ideas about brain pathology. Gennari found
that 'in addition to the cortical and medullary substance,
there is in the brain another substance, which I am accus-
tomed to call the third substance of this organ ...'
(Glickstein and Rizzolatti, 1984). This 'third substance'
was a thin white layer which divided the grey matter of the
cortex located parallel to the cortical surface. In sections
perpendicular to the cortical surface, this layer appeared as
a whitish stripe. Gennari observed that this stripe was
most pronounced on the mesial surface of the occipital
lobe of the human brain. The 'stripe of Gennari' marks

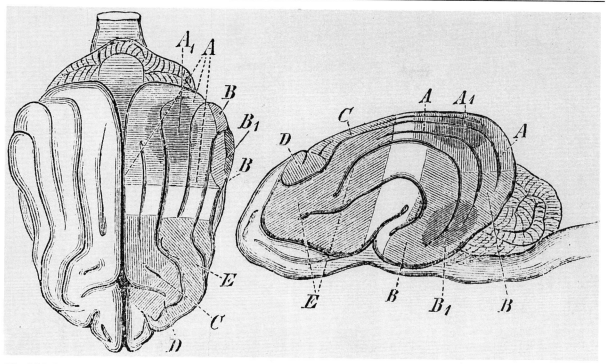

Fig. 2.25 *Brain of a dog. Extended bilateral removal of the occipital part of the cortical grey matter (A) led to cortical blindness. When only circumscribed parts of the cortical grey matter were removed (A_1), the lesion gave rise to destruction of visual responses in parts of the contralateral visual hemifield in both eyes. B and B_1 are auditory regions (from Munk, 1878).*

with animals, the Viennese physiologist Sigmund Exner (1846–1926) summarized all clinical descriptions of cortical lesions and functional defects in human motor and sensory systems published up to 1880 (Exner, 1881). By mapping out all cortical lesions found in postmortem examinations and by superposing the lesions onto schematic brain diagrams, he came to several conclusions about the cerebral localization of various sensory and motor functions. In Exner's sketch of human visual areas (Fig. 2.26), the shades of grey represent the frequency of a cortical lesion affecting visual functions; the grey areas represent the percentage of those patients suffering from visual defects who have lesions at these sites. Although the major visual symptom exhibited by most patients reported on in Exner's study was hemianopia, several clearly exhibited signs of visual agnosia and/or visual hallucinations caused by brain lesions. At the same time as Exner performed his work, the eminent French neurologist Jean-Martin Charcot (1825–93) emphasized the frequency of visual hallucinations occurring in the presence of lesions of the occipital lobes (Charcot, 1878–80). Exner concluded from his studies on the visual centres of the brain: 'The cortical area of the sense of sight is located in the occipital lobe and the most important part of it is at the upper end of the gyrus occipitalis primus.' Exner's work was the first

step toward quantitative statistical research on the functional localization of perceptual and cognitive visual operations in the cortical hemispheres; moreover, it represented a watershed in modern intellectual endeavours aimed at understanding the different brain functions involved in visual perception and cognition. His work was followed by another very systematic study conducted by the Swedish neurologist Salomon Henschen, who, like Exner, collected all reports on postmortem findings on patients who had suffered from hemianopia. He was an excellent anatomist and thought that the area striata, i.e. the region characterized by a thick stripe of Gennari in the medial part of the occipital lobe, was the visual area of the human brain. Using the location of the lesions, he also tried to map the projections of the retina onto the cortical region around the calcarine fissure, but erroneously assigned the visual field periphery to the occipital pole of the cortex (Henschen, 1892).

The Japanese ophthalmologists T. Inouye had more luck in similar efforts. He investigated 29 Japanese soldiers who had received occipital bullet wounds during the Russo–Japanese War in 1905. In order to determine precisely the location of the lesion, he invented a 'cranio-coordinator' with which he correlated the visual field defects and the position of the lesions in relation to the

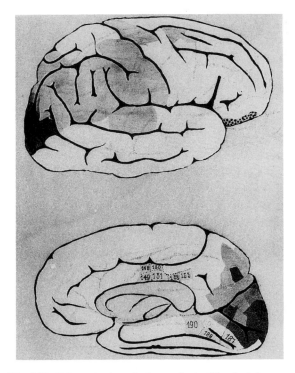

Fig. 2.26 *Schematic view of a human brain. The shaded areas indicate regions where lesions led to impairment of vision. Exner superposed findings in different patients onto the surface of the right hemisphere. The darker the area, the more frequently visual disturbances such as hemianopia, hallucinations, and visual agnosia occurred. Upper part: outer surface, lower part: mesial surface (from Exner, 1881).*

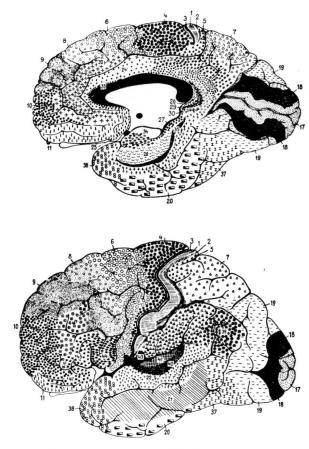

Fig. 2.27 *Cytoarchitectonic map of the human cortex as designed by Brodmann (Brodmann, 1909).*

fissures of the skull. He realized that the foveal region was represented at the occipital pole of the area striata; in addition, he also observed macular sparing with hemianopic field defects (cf. Chapter 9). Furthermore, he was the first to point out the non-linear mapping of the visual field onto the area striata, demonstrating that the fovea centralis occupied a much larger part of area striata than the parafoveal or peripheral visual field having the same angular size (Inouye, 1909; Glickstein and Whitteridge, 1987). Inouye's findings were later confirmed in studies of soldiers who had fought in the First World War who had also suffered from visual field defects caused by occipital brain lesions. (Holmes 1916, 1919; Wilbrand and Saenger, 1917). The systematic investigation of soldiers who had received brain wounds during the First World War contributed to the development of twentieth century concepts for the cerebral representation of visual functions, as well as to a bettter understanding of the causes of the different classes of visual agnosias (e.g. Poppelreuter, 1917; Gelb and Goldstein, 1920, 1923).

Parallel to the clinical studies a systematic investigation of the occipital brain took place applying rules of cytoarchitectonics and myeloarchitectonics, to subdivide the cortical surface into separate areas. Theodor Meynert (1833–1892) was the first to point out correlations between function and structure of different cortical areas. His view was supported by Paul Flechsig (1847–1929), who introduced developmental thoughts on myelinization of the cortical afferent and efferent fibre system into cortical architectonics (Flechsig, 1896, 1928). Cecile and Oskar Vogt, their co-worker Korbinian Brodmann and the Australian neuroanatomist Walter Campbell laid during the first quarter of this century the foundation for the 'classical' cytoarchitectonic maps, from which the one published by Brodmann (1909) is the most frequently reproduced (Fig. 2.27). This map illustrates the primary visual cortex (area 17) being located in the mesial part of the occipital lobe above and below the fissura calcarina. The area striata is surrounded by the visual areae 18 and 19 extending also to the outer surface of the occipital lobe, forming a relay to the parietal lobe area 7, the gyrus angularis region, the posterior limbic structures and the temporal lobe areae 20, 35 and 37. Only during recent years was this 'classical' cytoarchitectonic concept further elaborated; the extra-visual areae 18 and 19 are nowadays no longer believed to form functional homogeneous structures.

Note

This chapter is based on Grüsser (1990a). Further literature on the topic is found in Clarke and O'Malley (1968), Clarke and Dewhurst (1972) and Jung (1984).

3 The Functional Organization of the Human Eye and the Lateral Geniculate Nucleus

Introduction

As the early australopithecines 3–4 million years ago slowly developed upright gait and altered their living patterns from an arboreal to an earth-based mode, no essential phylogenetic adaptation of the eyes and the central visual system was necessary, except for the recalibration of vestibular–visual interaction. As compared with arboreal locomotion, walking upright through savannah increased some stimulus pattern asymmetries regarding the upper and lower visual fields, but otherwise few changes took place between the visual stimulus conditions of an arboreal hominid, such as *Ramapithecus* 10–12 million years ago, and those of the early earth-bound hominids, e.g. *Australopithecus afarensis* or *Homo habilis*. Thus the hominid and therefore also the human eye and its motor apparatus, including the brain stem oculomotor and gaze-motor neuronal mechanisms, represent typical primate structures adapted to the size of the head. Owing to the larger size of the eyeball in man compared with typical laboratory primates such as the Old World macaque or the New World squirrel monkey, man moves his eyes with somewhat slower saccades than the smaller primates. Moreover, the upper angular velocity of smooth pursuit eye movements and the slow phase of optokinetic nystagmus (OKN) is faster in the smaller primates. Otherwise the general principles of structure and function in the eyes and retinas of Old World monkeys are very similar to those in man and other primates: the anatomy of the eye and the eye muscles, the spatial frequency modulation transfer function (MTF) of the eye's optical apparatus, the trichromatic function of daylight vision (photopic vision) with its genetic variety of anomalous trichromacy, dichromacy and monochromatic vision in man, the duplicity of cone daylight and rod achromatic night vision (scotopic vision), the development of a fovea, the retinal blood supply, the primary projections of the optic nerve fibres into the visual centres of the brain stem and the cerebral gaze and eye motor control mechanisms.

Primate colour vision is a phylogenetically very old adaptation. 20–30 million years ago, when many primates which had developed from more elementary, predominantly nocturnal mammals occupied ecological niches of daylight activity in an arboreal habitat, and trees with leaves of different shades of green formed the visual background of this habitat. Primates collected coloured fruit in trees with green leaves and enriched their diet with frequently colourful insects, eggs and occasionally also the flesh of other mammals. Primate colour vision was primarily a phylogenetic adaptation for better form vision and object recognition, especially of red, orange and yellow fruits on a green background, and for fine colour discrimination of different shades of green leaves. Another characteristic of hominoid and hominid social life became important for phylogenetic adaptation of the central visual system: their life was characterized by organized social group activity which made visual recognition of the individual group members necessary and led to sophisticated cerebral mechanisms for the understanding of facial and gestural expressions, which became richer and richer during the development of hominids and *Homo*.

Toolmaking, which developed during the last 2 million years from *Homo habilis* to *Homo sapiens sapiens*, required adequate visual acuity, a precise eye–hand coordination, good 3-D vision in the grasping and near-distant action spaces and rapid matching of sensorimotor signals with visual signals. Before being able to make a stone tool, man had to be able to develop a mental visuo-spatial concept of what the tool should look like. Visual conceptualization was also necessary in organizing group activity within a hunting range. The hunting habits of *Homo habilis* and *Homo erectus* certainly utilized the preserved excellent spatial orientation from primate ancestors and were strongly dependent on the long-range planning abilities of

Homo, which required visual imagination and visual memory. The same was true for seasonal changes in the habitat. When *Homo presapiens* built the first huts about 300,000 years ago, visual-constructive imagination and visuo-praxic abilities were required. It is against this phylogenetic and ecological background that we will discuss in the rest of this chapter the basic principles of the human eye and visual system.

The Spatial Frequency Modulation Transfer Function of the Eye Optical Apparatus and its Importance for Form Vision

Visual perception of shapes depends on the correct formation of a retinal image as an 'input signal', which is received in the human eye by about 125 million photoreceptors and transformed into a complex pattern of neuronal activity in about 1 million optic nerve fibres at the output level of the human retina. This 'neuronal image' is generated anew after each shift in the fixation point, which occurs by means of saccadic eye movements about every 0.18 to 0.6 seconds. The short saccades last 0.03 to 0.08 s. Angular velocity of eye movements during saccades may exceed 600 deg s^{-1}. When a saccade is performed across a well-structured visual pattern, the flicker stimulation frequency of each retinal photoreceptor is then far above flicker fusion frequency. Consequently the retinal stimulus during a saccade corresponds to a short grey interval. Therefore visual signals relevant to object and space recognition are sampled during the fixation periods between the saccades. Eye movements during fixation periods are minimal ('eye tremor', cf. Ditchburn, 1973), and eyelid blinks are correlated in time predominantly to saccades. The sampling rate (1.5–5 per second) of the saccade intervals (fixation periods) characterizes the temporal frequency limits in which essential visual operations for space, object and colour perception are performed.

The spatial resolution of visual information about the objects and structure of the extra-personal space depends on the quality of the retinal image formed by the dioptric apparatus and the spatial raster of the retinal photoreceptor array. The dioptric apparatus consists of the cornea, the anterior chamber, the iris forming the pupil, the lens and the vitreous body. It is a composite optical system, which projects an inverted image of the visual world on the receptor surface of the retina. The inversion of this image was first postulated theoretically by the astronomer Johann Kepler (1571–1630), who relied in his considerations on the anatomical data provided by Felix Platter

(1536–1614) (Kepler, 1611; Platter, 1583; cf. Chapter 2). Kepler and a few years later the Jesuit priest Christoph Scheiner (1575–1650) confirmed the concept of the inverted image experimentally by cutting a window into the sclera near the optic nerve and covering it with an eggshell (cf. Chapter 2). With this method they could see the inverted image directly. When the visual image is 're-inverted' on the retina by means of prisms or mirrors, the world is perceived upside down only transiently, and within a few days of adaptation 'normal' vision is regained, provided the subject can move and interact with objects in his surroundings (Stratton, 1897; Erismann, 1948; Kohler, 1951). From such experiments one can conclude that the cerebral visuo-motor and perceptual mechanisms which signal the egocentric coordinates of the extra-personal space, namely up and down, left and right, forward and backward, relative to the head and/or body of the observer, are highly adaptable. The same is true for changes in retinal image magnification with eyeglasses. Even binocular fusion adapts to different retinal image sizes, provided the refraction differences between the optical systems of the two eyes do not exceed 2–3 dioptres. From these facts one can conclude that inversion and also a limited variation in retinal image size have little effect on visual form, object and space perception, provided the necessary time for cerebral adaptation was allotted. Greater magnifications such as are applied in surgical binocular microscopes (up to 40 times in microsurgery) require special training to adapt the new relation between hand movements and the perceived size of the objects under the microscope. This learning process becomes more and more difficult beyond 30 years of age.

The precision of the retinal image depends on correct accommodation of the lens, adequate pupil size and the quality of the optic components of the dioptric apparatus (cornea, aqueous humour of the anterior eye chamber, lens and vitreous body). The overall spatial modulation transfer function (MTF) of the dioptric apparatus characterizes some aspects of the image formation qualities. The MTF of the human eye is somewhat below the theoretical optimum which an optical system with a comparable aperture and focal length could achieve with optimum optics (Fig. 3.1). It is well adapted to the theoretical and empirical limits of visual acuity as determined by the receptor mosaic of the inner fovea (Fig. 3.2). Since the MTF depends on pupil size, the decrease in average pupil size with age compensates in part for the reduction in the quality of the optical media, which decreases with age owing to structural changes in the cornea, lens and vitreous body.

In judging symptoms of visual agnosia in elderly patients, one has to keep in mind the 'physiological' diminution in visual acuity due to changes in the dioptric apparatus (e.g. the beginning of a cataract) with ageing.

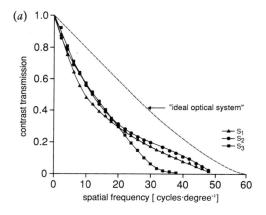

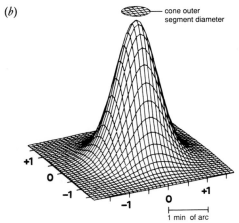

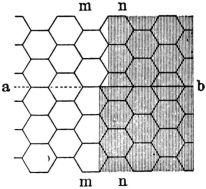

Fig. 3.2 *Schematic diagram of the hexagonal array of the receptor mosaic in the human fovea. Owing to this geometrical regularity, vernier acuity, measured as a break in a contour (shaded area), results in better values than two-point acuity (from Nagel, 1905).*

Fig. 3.1 *(a) Spatial modulation transfer function (MTF) of the human eye as measured by Campbell and Gubisch (1966). Data are from three different subjects (S₁–S₃). Pupil diameter was 2 mm. The dashed curve is the MTF of an ideal optical system. (b) Optical point-spread function of the human eye for a 2-mm pupil, calculated from the appropriate line spread function as published by Campbell and Gubisch (1966). The diameter of a foveal cone outer segment is schematically added to illustrate that the point-spread function is considerably wider than a single cone outer segment (Geisler, 1989, modified). The optical point-spread function is a transformation of the MTF from the frequency domain to the space domain. It summarizes the combined effects of an image formation of chromatic and spherical aberrations, pupil diffraction and light scatter in the optical media and the retina.*

One should also consider the rather frequent occurrence of reduction in visual acuity owing to retinal degenerative processes (e.g. macular degeneration), diabetic retinopathy or glaucoma. Furthermore, myopia or presbyopia in the elderly must be corrected precisely when tests on visual agnosia are to be performed. It is recommendable to test *Gestalt* perception of agnosic patients by means of visual patterns which do not push the limits of MTF or of

visual acuity. Pseudo-agnosic symptoms appear in patients suffering from foveal retinal degeneration accompanied by a considerable loss in visual acuity (Chapter 11) and are easily mistaken, by an inexperienced observer, for signs of impairment in cerebral visual signal processing. Elderly patients should also be alotted enough time in visual recognition tasks. The reader with normal visual acuity can imagine the problems patients have in visual form perception by comparing his ability to recognize faces or complex visual structures – such as the present text – with his vision in the visual field outside the range of foveal vision. In addition, glare, which occurs with unsuitable types of illumination, affects the performance of patients suffering from cataracts much more than that of normals. To evaluate visual agnosic symptoms adequately, it is therefore strongly recommended that the investigator should know the results of a thorough ophthalmological investigation beforehand. During testing of the patients' visual abilities, adequate illumination in the middle photopic range is advised.

Classes of Photoreceptors: Spectral, Spatial and Temporal Response Properties

In the modern neurophysiology of vision the concept of quality-specific 'channels' as proposed by Wilbrand (1887) has become popular and been applied to the experimental data in two respects:

1. The signal transfer of elementary qualities of the visual modality, like colour, contrast, luminance and

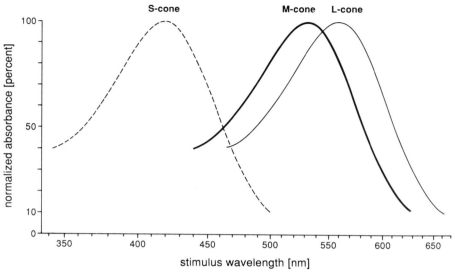

Fig. 3.3 *Spectral absorption curves of the three classes of cones in the human retina (L-, M- and S-cones). Schematically redrawn from data published by Dartnall* et al. *(1983).*

movement, is attributed to different classes of neurones, which form in part separate connections between the photoreceptors and the cerebral visual centres.

2. Within one of these elementary qualities, specific sub-properties are also attributed to different 'channels'. Interpreting data from contrast vision, for example, led to the assumption of 7 to 10 different spatial frequency channels existing within the afferent visual system, which are tuned to different regions in the spatial frequency domain. For colour vision the signals originating in the three classes of cones are transformed within the neuronal network of the retina and the lateral geniculate nucleus into red–green, yellow–blue and black–white messages, each represented in the activity of different classes of nerve cells.

The input layer of the human retina consists of two large classes of photoreceptors, rods and cones. These two receptor classes reach their operative optimum at considerably different luminance levels ('duplicity theory', Schultze, 1866). The cone system is adapted to conditions of daylight illumination (photopic vision). The 'colour-blind' rod system operates best at a luminance level of moonlight (scotopic vision, 0.01–0.0001 cd m^{-2}). In the human retina, rods outnumber cones by about 20:1. In a transitional luminance state, corresponding to the natural stimulus conditions about half an hour before sunrise or after sunset (mid-European geographical latitudes), i.e. at an average luminance level between 0.01 and 1 cd m^{-2}, both photoreceptor systems are active (mesopic vision). Since mutual retinal inhibitory mechanisms exist for cone vision and rod vision, mesopic vision, characterized by

reduced colour vision, is certainly not recommendable in testing visual agnosic patients.

Nearly all studies on visual agnosia were performed under photopic stimulus conditions, i.e. the patients were normally tested in the daylight or by a room illumination corresponding to moderate photopic illumination conditions. Little is known of how visual agnosic patients perform under scotopic stimulus conditions. We will therefore restrict our considerations of retinal receptor functions to photopic vision, i.e. to the operation of the cone system. In testing visual agnosic patients, glare and blinding conditions of the visual stimuli have to be prevented. As in most visual patterns generated by the natural habitat, luminance variations in the test patterns should not exceed 1:60.

In the normal human eye about 6 million cones can be divided into three functional classes, characterized by three different photopigments with different spectral absorption curves (Fig. 3.3). These photoreceptors are called for short red, green and blue cones or long- (L), middle- (M) or short- (S) wavelength receptors (cf. this series, Volume 2). The molecules of the photopigments are accumulated in the membranes of the multi-layered outer segments of the photoreceptors. The absorption of a photon by a photopigment molecule leads with a probability of 0.65–0.7 to change in the steric configuration of this molecule ('photoisomerization' and 'bleaching'), a mechanism which in its initial stages quickly and repeatedly activates G_1-proteins in the photoreceptor membrane. This activation leads to a reduction in cyclic 3′–5′-guanidine monophosphate (cGMP), which causes in turn

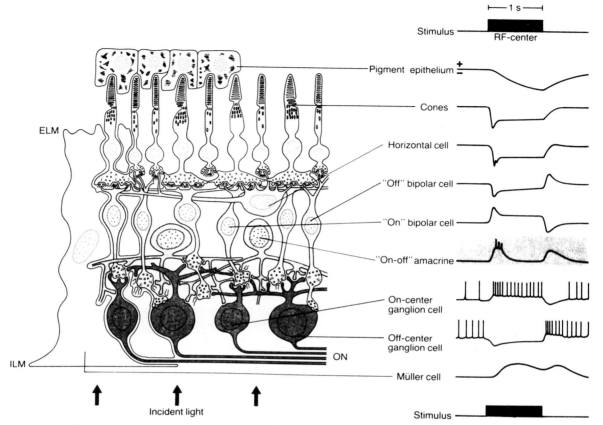

Fig. 3.4 *Schematic and highly simplified diagram of the neuronal connections of the mammalian retina and the corresponding responses of the different retinal cell classes, when a white spot of light is projected to the receptive field centre of the respective neurone. The morphological scheme is taken from Dowling and Boycott (1966). Colour-specific responses are not shown (from Grüsser, 1983, modified).*

a reduction in sodium conductivity of the photoreceptor cell membrane, since cGMP keeps the sodium channels of the cell membrane 'open'. By this mechanism photon absorption is amplified and finally evokes a hyperpolarizing receptor potential at the photoreceptor cell membrane (Fig. 3.4).

This change in photoreceptor membrane potential affects in turn the release of transmitters at the synaptic contacts of cone pedicles formed at two classes of retinal nerve cells: bipolar cells and horizontal cells (Fig. 3.5). Horizontal cells transmit their signals to bipolar cells, to other horizontal cells and back to the photoreceptor pedicles. By tight junctions of their membranes horizontal cells form a 'horizontal' neuronal network within which the membrane potential changes are transmitted far beyond the borders of an individual cell. There is good evidence to assume that horizontal cells form the first neuronal layer of 'lateral connections' within the afferent

visual pathway, which coordinates the light adaptation of the extended parts of the retina and also contributes to the 'centre–surround' antagonism of other neurones. In the case of the horizontal cells, the H-cell activity helps to shape the centre–surround organization of bipolar cells, as explained in Fig. 3.5.

Changes in the photoreceptor membrane potential are also transmitted through receptor–receptor contacts to other cones or rods. Depending on the wavelength composition (chromaticity) of the retinal image at each cone outer segment and the chromatic adaptation of the region of the retina from which an individual cone is a small part, the optic image creates a triplicate 'receptorial image', i.e. a spatial distribution of membrane potential changes in the set of S-, M- and L-cones of the receiving retinal surface. This triplicate representation of the visual image in the receptor layer constitutes the 'sensor space', the physiological input signal for all further neuronal data processing

(a)

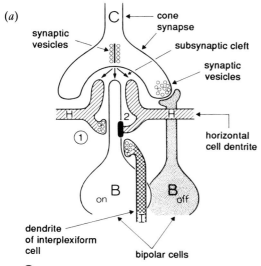

① chemical synapse
② electrical synapse

(b)

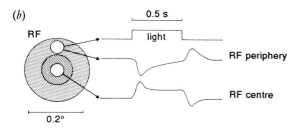

Fig. 3.5 *(a) Scheme of the connections between a cone synaptic pedicle (C), horizontal cells (H) and on-bipolar and off-bipolar cells (dark); the synaptic terminals of horizontal cells (1 = chemical, 2 = electrical) and of synapses originating presumably in interplexiform amacrines are illustrated (from Grüsser, 1979). (b) Diagram of the organization of an on-bipolar cell receptive field. Illumination of the RF centre leads to a depolarization, illumination of the RF periphery to a hyperpolarization of the cell membrane potential. The hyperpolarization is mediated by the horizontal cells (H in (a)), whereby light also leads to a hyperpolarization of the horizontal cells. 'Light off' in the RF centre evokes a transient hyperpolarization of the on-bipolar membrane potential, 'light off' in the RF periphery, however, a transient depolarization. Off-bipolar cells exhibit approximately a mirror-symmetric behaviour.*

in the visual system under photopic stimulus conditions. There exist no rods within the inner part of the human fovea, and rods in the parafoveal region do not transfer any essential visual signals under daylight adaptation since they are 'saturated'.

The upper limits of spatial resolution for the physiological process by which the retinal image is transformed into a threefold receptor image are determined by the diameter of the cone outer segments, the distance between the individual cones and the geometrical array of the cone mosaic at a given part of the retina. The outer segment diameter of cones and the distance between neighbouring cones increase in size from the centre of the fovea (foveola) to the periphery of the retina, while the spatial density of the cones decreases with the distance from the centre of the fovea centralis. Within a diameter of about 250 μm, corresponding to about 0.86 degrees of visual angle, the inner part of the fovea centralis contains only cones. It is this part of the retina which is used for visual recognition functions requiring optimum visual acuity, such as fine structure analysis or reading small print, and which represents for normal vision the centre of the visual field. Under photopic stimulus conditions, foveal vision normally also guides sampling gaze movements, and during fixation periods the 'attentive' fovea corresponds to the retinal fovea. It is possible, however, to separate spatially directed attention from the centre of the visual field and to suppress saccadic eye movements which normally occur when visual attention is shifted to a stimulus appearing in the periphery of the visual field.

L-, M- and S-cones are not equally distributed across the retina. The human retina seems to have about equal amounts of red and green cones, while blue cones are considerably less frequent (about 15 per cent of all cones). In addition, blue cones appear to be rare or even absent in the inner foveola. In a tangential section, the cone outer segments form within the fovea a regular hexagonal matrix (Fig. 3.2), similar to the section through a honeycomb. This matrix improves the upper limits of visual acuity, provided an integrated network of neurones exists, performing adequate computational operations on neighbouring cone signals. If we apply the Nyquist–Küpfmüller sampling theorem for the estimation of the limits of visual acuity, the minimum visual angle of resolution α_{min}, measured in degrees, would be

$$\alpha_{min} = 2d_p \qquad (3.1)$$

where d_p is the average distance between adjacent photoreceptors, i.e. the reciprocal value of the average spatial density of photoreceptors $1/d_p$ at a given retinal site. Thus the limiting spatial frequency $f_c = 1/\alpha_{min}$ (cycles $\deg^{-1}$) would be

$$f_c = \tfrac{1}{2}d_p \qquad (3.2)$$

Ewald Hering (1874) recognized that owing to the hexagonal matrix of foveal cone outer segments this theoretical limit is improved by a factor of about 3–4, provided regular contours are used to measure visual acuity (e.g. vernier acuity). Under optimum stimulus conditions this 'hyperacuity' (Westheimer and McKee 1977; Westheimer

1979) can indeed be demonstrated, where approximately α_{min}, measured in degrees, is given by the formula

$$\alpha_{min} = 0.5d_p \qquad (3.3)$$

This is the optimum reached under the best conditions of photopic illumination. Within photopic vision this minimum angle of resolution α_{min} depends on the luminance (I) and the contrast of the stimulus patterns used to determine visual acuity (Mayer, 1755; cf. Chapter 2).

Visual acuity values express receptor *and* visual nerve cell functions. When moderate photopic light sources are used while testing visual gnosic functions with objects of everyday life, the limiting factors of visual acuity are not of elementary importance, as a rule, but the investigator should always be aware that not only loss of foveal vision but also inadequate luminance conditions affect the results of his visual tests. In judging symptoms of visual agnosia, one has to know the visual acuity of the patient and also has to investigate whether the patient suffers from visual field defects affecting foveal vision, or from other diseases reducing visual acuity. A simple test with Snellen charts, Landolt rings or gratings of different spatial frequencies is generally sufficient to test visual acuity. Perimetric exploration of the visual fields is recommended in all patients suffering from visual agnosic symptoms (Chapter 11). Since patients showing signs of visual agnosia frequently have impaired elementary visual functions, some investigators (e.g. Bay, 1953; Critchley, 1964; Bender and Feldman, 1972) were led to conclude that impairment of elementary visual abilities might cause visual agnosia. On the other hand, many patients with cataracts or retinal malfunctions leading to reduced visual acuity, or visual problems due to lesions within the afferent visual system, show no sign of visual agnosia, provided the tests are adapted to their visual acuity. Therefore most research workers support the arguments of Ettlinger as against Bay's opinion (Ettlinger, 1956).

Different types of perceptive and associative agnosias affect colour vision (achromatopsia, colour agnosia, colour anomia). Before applying tests on 'cerebral' colour perception, one must explore whether the patient suffers in addition from congenital, 'retinal', colour vision defects, such as protanopia, deuteranopia, tritanopia or the corresponding colour vision anomalies. To rule out the most frequent, red–green, colour deficiency, the determination of the 'colour mixture' equation in a Nagel anomaloscope is adequate in many patients, with the exception of those suffering from cerebral achromatopsia. In the Nagel anomaloscope the Raleigh equation

$$a\lambda_1 = b\lambda_2 + c\lambda_3 \qquad (3.4)$$

is used, where a, b and c are the weighting factors for the three narrow bands of the visible spectrum (λ_1, yellow = 589 nm, λ_2, red = 671 nm, λ_3, green = 546 nm). Anam-

nestic exploration of performances in colour vision in professional or army health examination tests may be helpful in excluding colour anomalies or dichromacies existing before the brain lesions leading to visual agnosias and cerebral achromatopsia, in which the data obtained with Equation 3.4 can no longer be used as indicators of peripheral colour vision anomalies.

The temporal response properties of the visual system are determined by peripheral (photoreceptors and retinal neurones) and central factors. To measure the temporal response properties, flicker stimuli are traditionally applied. At the psychophysical level for a given background adaptation level, the critical flicker fusion frequency (CFF; measured in hertz) depends on luminance (I), depth of modulation (m) and area (A) of the flickering stimulus (for reviews see Landis, 1953; Kelly, 1972; van de Grind et al., 1973). For a single cone, CFF (measured in Hz) is at a constant depth of modulation and small light spots described by

$$CFF = aI/(1 + bI) \qquad (3.5a)$$

with the constants a and b.

At the niveau of retinal ganglion cells, LGN cells or 'simple' nerve cells of area 17, a more complex relationship is valid, which is also found in psychophysical studies:

$$CFF = c_1 \log I + c_2 \log A + c_3 \qquad (3.5b)$$

The constants c_1, c_2 and c_3 depend on whether rod vision (maximum CFF about 25–28 Hz) or cone vision is explored. The CFF and the constants of Equations 3.5a and b also depend on the location of the stimulus within the visual field. Furthermore, binocular CFF is somewhat higher than monocular CFF. Since maximum CFF of the rod system in man does not exceed 28 Hz, CFF above this value indicates that cones are efficiently stimulated and transmit their signals to a cognitive level. This is an important statement, especially in the case of cerebral achromatopsias in which all colour vision has disappeared and the investigator can ask the question whether any cone signals are still processed by the visual brain. Maximum cone flicker rate is at about 110 Hz. To reach this value in man, one has to apply very high stimulus intensities and large stimulus fields. Under 'normal' stimulus conditions maximum CFF is in a range below 80 Hz. Considering the average luminance modulation in a natural habitat under good daylight conditions, flicker fusion frequency is at maximum 40–45 Hz. As one can see on a television screen, 50 or 60 Hz are usually sufficient to suppress flicker sensations, and the intermittency of the image generated on the screen can be detected only with peripheral vision or when saccades are performed across the screen which 'divide' the temporal sequences of the generated images into a temporo-spatial event: one then perceives 2 or 3 images on the television screen in different parts of the visual field.

The signal transfer properties of the three cone types vary only slightly at low temporal frequencies (below 5 Hz), while the upper frequency response properties differ. At moderate stimulus intensities, the CFF of chromatic flicker stimuli correlates fairly well with the photopic sensitivity curve. As a consequence, monochromatic stimuli of equal subjective brightness and otherwise constant physical parameters reach the same CFF. The CFF measured under standard conditions with white light decreases somewhat when the patient suffers from cerebral lesions, even from those located outside the central visual system (for reviews see Landis, 1953; van de Grind *et al.*, 1973). This 'unspecific' factor in determining CFF is presumably caused by the fact that general and spatially directed attention are necessary requirements for precise decisions on the state 'flickering/non-flickering', which the subject has to make when his CFF is determined. It was demonstrated, for example, that the CFF of neurones located in the area 17 of cats was increased with electrical stimulation of intrathalamic nuclei (Creutzfeldt and Grüsser, 1957; cf. Chapter 4).

In testing agnosic patients' contour orientation, shape perception and recognition of visual objects or surrounding, the temporal frequency transfer properties of the three cone systems are usually not stressed. The *Gestalt* perception operates at a frequency limit below 8 Hz and reaches a maximum between 2 and 5 Hz. The '*Gestalt* fusion frequency' (cf. van de Grind *et al.*, 1973) is fairly independent of stimulus luminance and size and does not exceed 7 Hz. This low *Gestalt* fusion frequency is well adapted to the fact that we sample information on objects during the 0.18–0.6-second fixation periods in between the fast saccades.

Temporal response factors play a role when tachistoscopic tests are applied in agnosic patients. One has to keep in mind that correct responses in shape recognition may decrease in brain-lesioned patients when the duration of tachistoscopic presentation is too short. Temporal frequency properties of cones also become relevant when movement perception is tested at higher speeds and when, moreover, moving stimuli consist of different hues. Patients who have difficulty recognizing shapes or colours may exploit the temporal frequency properties of their photoreceptors by moving the stimulus slightly back and forth (an example is described in Chapter 20). Problems with temporal signal processing in the central visual system can interfere with movement perception, with the perceived stability of the visual space, and with the stability of object perception. It is therefore advisable in object agnosia to also explore the temporal integration properties of the central visual system, i.e. to measure CFF under standard conditions, *Gestalt* fusion frequency and the frequency properties in seeing real or apparent contours.

The Generation of Task-specific Neuronal Channels by Signal Processing within the Retina

In each eye the signals from about 120 million rods and 6 million cones are compressed into the impulse pattern of about 1 million retinal ganglion cells, which may temporarily modify their impulse rate between 0.5 and 650 impulses per second. Retinal ganglion cells send their axons through the optic nerve to different primary visual centres of the brain (Fig. 3.6). A large portion of retinal ganglion cells deal with signals from rods and cones; a minority, however, namely those processing the signals from the foveola, receive only cone signals. With photopic stimulus conditions, however, all nerve cells transmitting signals from the retinal image into the brain rely only on cone vision, since with daylight adaptation, rods are predominantly saturated and therefore not operating.

The numerical relationship between cones converging by direct excitatory contacts via bipolar cells on one retinal ganglion cell is relatively small for the fovea centre and amounts to about 2 to 5 cones per ganglion cell. In the parafoveal retina the spatial compression of the cone signals converging onto a single retinal ganglion cell could reach values of more than 200:1 for photopic vision. When one considers the fact that in addition to the 'direct' excitatory convergence (photoreceptors–bipolar cells–ganglion cells), lateral inhibitory and excitatory convergence exists via the connections of horizontal cells and amacrines (Fig. 3.4), effective signal convergence in the fovea is in a range of 20–30 cones per ganglion cell in the fovea to several hundred in the retinal periphery.

As elaborated in other volumes of this series (Volumes 4, 5 and 6), the operation of the retinal neuronal network, consisting of photoreceptors, several classes of bipolar cells, horizontal cells, amacrines and several morphologically distinct classes of ganglion cells (as recognized by cell soma size, dendritic arborization, synaptic connections and axon diameter or myelinization respectively), creates functionally different types of retinal ganglion cells characterized by distinct organizational properties of their receptive fields (RF). These different classes of retinal ganglion cells constitute the 'neuronal channels' at the output of the retina, where a multiple representation of the visual signals reaching the surface of the photoreceptor layer is found. Its main visual features for photopic conditions are brightness–darkness, local light–dark contours, general brightness, movement and chromatic properties (red–green, blue–yellow, black–white) (Fig. 3.7). The primary visual centres of the brain (Fig. 3.6), i.e. the projection sites of the retinal–ganglion-cell axon terminals, receive an unequal number of axon collaterals from the different classes of retinal ganglion cells and represent the

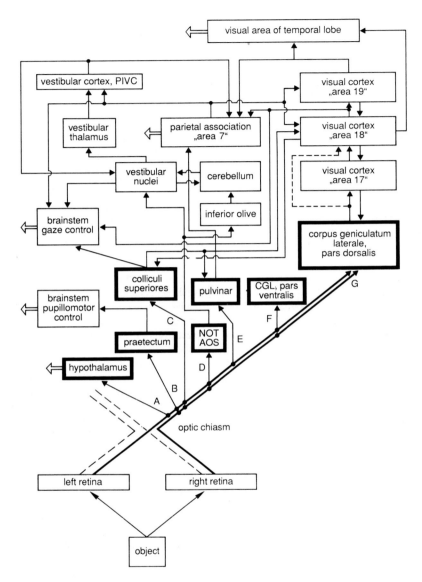

Fig. 3.6 *Scheme of the projection sites of the afferent optic tract axons. Seven main projection sites of the optic tract fibres are shown. (A) The 'hypothalamic root' of the optic tract consists of optic nerve fibres transmitting signals which induce the general vegetative effects of light. (B) Optic tract axons ending in the praetectum serve the pupillo-motor control and connect the retina with the Edinger–Westphal nucleus, the nerves cells of which send axons with the oculomotor nerve to the ganglion ciliare of the orbita. (C) Retino-tectal connections to the superior colliculi set the coordinates of goal-directed and reflectory saccades. (D) Connections of the retina with the nucleus of the optic tract (NOT) and the nuclei of the accessory optic system (AOS) project to a relay between the retina and the vestibular nuclei and the cerebellum respectively. Brain stem nuclei intercalated between the NOT and the vestibular nuclei are not drawn (nucleus reticularis tegmenti pontis and nucleus praepositus hypoglossi). (E) Connections between the retina and the pulvinar. (F) Some optic nerve axons project directly to the corpus geniculatum laterale, pars ventralis, and transmit like the connections with the pulvinar visual movement signals. These signals are finally integrated into the neuronal network of the parietal and parieto-temporal association cortices. (G) Connections between the retina and the corpus geniculatum laterale, pars dorsalis (lateral geniculate nucleus, LGN) constitute the main projection stream of the retina to the brain. In particular, the axons originating in foveal and parafoveal ganglion cells serve conscious object recognition, surface and texture perception, colour vision, movement recognition and stereoscopic vision. The sites onto which these primary visual centres project in the human brain are grossly simplified.*

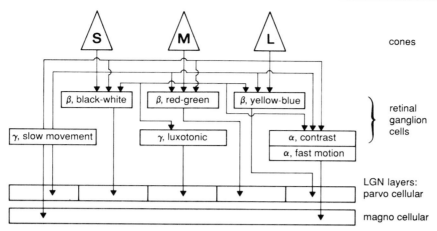

Fig. 3.7 *Scheme of the functional division of classes of retinal ganglion cells projecting to the parvocellular and magnocellular layers of the lateral geniculate nucleus. The connections of the slow-movement-sensitive neuronal system (gamma-neurones) are still under debate.*

information carried by the different visual 'channels' in different proportions. Some of the subcortical visual centres indeed process only signals from one or two classes of highly specialized retinal ganglion cells. For example, nerve cells of the nucleus of the optic tract (NOT), which transmit retinal signals via the dorsal cap of the inferior olive to the cerebellum and via the nucleus reticularis tegmenti pontis (NRTP) to the brain stem vestibular nuclei, receive only axon collaterals from small (γ-type) movement- and direction-sensitive retinal ganglion cells.

Projection Sites of Retinal Ganglion Cell Axons for Conscious Visual Processing

With respect to conscious visual cognitive functions in primates, the retino-geniculate-cortical pathway plays the key role, while the other visual pathways mainly serve unconscious and visuo-motor reflex functions, as indicated in Fig. 3.6. The six different layers of the lateral geniculate nucleus (LGN, corpus geniculatum laterale, pars dorsalis, Fig. 3.8) receive excitatory input signals from one half of the ipsilateral (3 layers) and the contralateral retina (3 layers). The relay cells of these 6 layers transmit the visual signals via axons running through the visual radiation to the primary visual cortex (area V1) of the occipital lobe and perhaps also send a few axons from the magnocellular layer to area V2 (Chapter 14). The LGN cells receive in turn a strong corticofugal input predominantly via interneurones located within the LGN or the perigeniculate regions. Furthermore the LGN neur-

ones receive non-visual signals from the brain stem reticular formation. Within the LGN, neuronal connections representing different functional channels are partly separated into different layers, as explained in Fig. 3.8.

Still a matter of controversy is whether other central visual pathways also contribute, at least marginally, to conscious visual sensation. This is especially disputed for the connections of the retina with the colliculi superiores (Fig. 3.6), a pathway which was discovered in the human brain as early as 1809 by Gall and Spurzheim (Chapter 2). In addition to the axons projecting from the colliculi superiores to the visual parts of the pulvinar and from there to the extrastriate visual cortices, direct retinal connections to the pulvinar may also contribute to subconscious visual sensations. Visual movement may be sensed indirectly by signals reaching the cortex via the pathway from the retina to the nucleus of the optic tract and from there to the vestibular nuclei. This visual-vestibular signal flow is integrated into the afferent vestibular pathway, reaching the vestibular cortex via vestibular neurones in the somatosensory thalamic relay nuclei and the magnocellular part of the corpus geniculatum mediale.

Signal Processing in the LGN

When analysing the signal properties of LGN relay cells, one can again find 'channels' corresponding to those discovered in retinal ganglion cells. The three chromatic channels present at the retinal ganglion cell level, forming the neuronal basis for a chromatic red-green, yellow-blue or black-white neuronal system, are represented by fairly small retinal ganglion cells (β-cells). These cells have

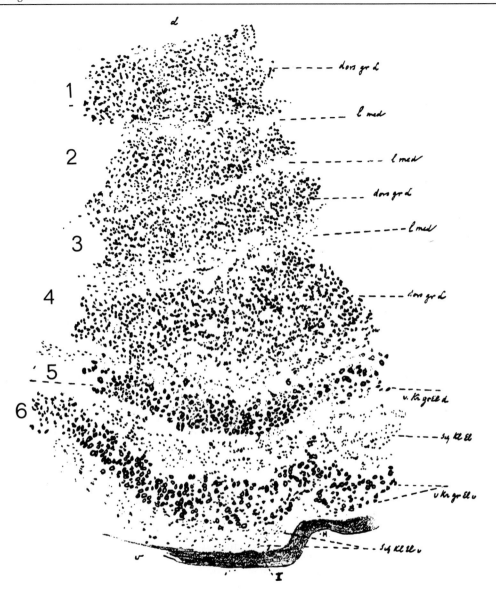

Fig. 3.8 *Section through the corpus geniculatum laterale of a human brain. Four parvocellular layers (1, 2, 3, 4) are separated by intermediate layers from each other and from two magnocellular layers (5, 6). The intermediate layers contain interneurones which connect layers 1/2, layers 3/4 and layers 5/6 with each other. The optic nerve axons of the contralateral eye project to layers 1, 4 and 6, those of the ipsilateral optic nerve to layers 2, 3 and 5. Parvocellular layers receive axons from the small retinal β-ganglion cells, magnocellular layers from the large retinal α-ganglion cells. The retinal γ-ganglion cells presumably project to both the parvocellular and the magnocellular layers (from von Monakow, 1905).*

axonal terminals predominantly in the parvocellular layers of the LGN (Fig. 3.8). An achromatic neuronal system represented by large α-ganglion cells of the retina integrates all three cone signals and transmits information about light–dark contours and fast movement to the central visual system through the magnocellular layers of the LGN. Another achromatic system monitors the average stimulus intensity ('luxotonic units') in a non-linear manner, enabling the primate brain to judge the level of average luminance in its habitat. Also a neuronal channel specialized for slow-movement perception (originating in the γ-ganglion cells of the retina) seems to be represented in the LGN. Axon collaterals of α- and γ-ganglion cells of the retina also project to the superior colliculi.

In the achromatic and chromatic neuronal systems, neuronal activity in the retina and the LGN depends on stimulus intensity relative to a background adaptation level. An equation first proposed by Ewald Hering (1874) for brightness and darkness perception can be adapted to describe the relationship between the average neuronal activity R measured in impulses per second, and the stimulus intensity I within the receptive field of a retinal ganglion cell or LGN neurones. Hereby R_0 represents the spontaneous dark activity:

$$R = R_0 + aI/(1 + kI) \qquad (3.6)$$

where a and k are constants. This equation, akin to the equation describing the Michaelis–Menten kinetics in biochemistry, has to be modified for some neurones according to an idea of Naka and Rushton (1973), who derived this modified Hering equation from their data on the intensity function of retinal horizontal cells:

$$R = R_0 + aI^\sigma/(1 + kI^\sigma) \qquad (3.7)$$

with the exponent $\sigma \leqslant 1$. Equations 3.6 and 3.7 hold for about 2.5 to 3 decadic logarithmic units of I relative to a general background adaptation level. For the light-activated on-centre ganglion cells or on-centre LGN neurones the constant a is positive; for the dark-activated off-centre neurones, a is negative, i.e. in these neurones a decrease in local retinal luminance leads to an increase in neuronal activity.

In addition to a neuronal system monitoring the average local stimulus intensity relative to the background adaptation level, a separate channel transmits information about light–dark contours ('fast' α-ganglion cells, some β-ganglion cells and corresponding relay cells in the magnocellular layer of the LGN). Another 'achromatic' neuronal channel monitors movement signals (α- and γ-retinal ganglion cells, predominantly cells of the magnocellular layer of the LGN). Fast movement signals are transmitted by nerve cells which operate in a temporal frequency domain at the upper limit of cone temporal frequency transfer properties. From the CFF of these nerve cells and the diameter of their receptive fields, one can estimate the upper limits in processing stimulus angular velocity.

For the movement- and velocity-sensitive neuronal systems of the afferent visual pathway, the relationship between neuronal activity R, in impulses per second, and stimulus angular velocity v (stimulus contrast and stimulus size constant) is best described by a power function:

$$R = R_0 + kv^b \qquad (3.8)$$

where k and b are constants and v is the angular velocity of the moving visual pattern (for details see Grüsser and Grüsser-Cornehls, 1973).

As mentioned above, the activity of nerve cells located in all layers of the LGN depends on efferent corticofugal signals (mainly from area V1, layer VI pyramid cells) as well as on non-visual inputs originating in the brain stem reticular formation. The latter input modulates the signal's transfer through the LGN according to different

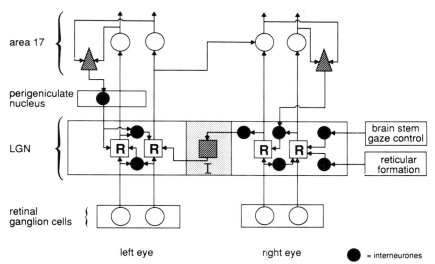

Fig. 3.9 *Schematic diagram of the main connections of the nerve cells located in the lateral geniculate nucleus. About half of the nerve cells are relay cells (R) sending their axons into the optic radiation, the other half of LGN cells are interneurones. Non-visual input signals reach the interneurones or the relay cells from brain stem nuclei belonging to the ascending reticular system or to the systems of gaze motor control. Other inputs to the LGN originate in the perigeniculate nucleus, in layer VI nerve cells of the primary visual cortex (area V1) and of the secondary visual cortex (area V2). These 'non-visual' inputs to the LGN modify the retino-cortical signal transfer by the LGN relay cells. I is a nerve cell of the intermediate layers (cf. Fig. 3.8).*

states of arousal and reduces neuronal responses during sleep. The corticofugal signals seem to modify the receptive field properties of the LGN neurones, and, perhaps, also have something to do with spatially directed attention. Details on these functions are still to be explored.

Furthermore some binocular interaction occurs between the 'monocular' layers of the LGN through interneurones located mainly in the intralaminar layers of the LGN. These interneurones most likely connect relay cells representing the same classes of operations in corresponding areas of the left and the right retina. Presumably these connections are inhibitory ones, serving the first stage of binocular interaction, i.e. 'binocular rivalry' (Fig. 3.9).

The responses of LGN neurones are thus not a simple repetition of retinal ganglion cell activity. The interneurones located in the six main layers of the LGN interact with the relay cells, shaping the receptive field properties of the latter. Interneurones also serve as targets for the non-visual input to the LGN. They are smaller than relay cells, as a rule, but their number seems to be equal to those of the main relay cells (Minkowski, 1920). Estimates of the number of LGN relay cells indicate that the signals transmitted by about 1 million optic tract fibres are sent by about 1 million visual radiation fibres to area V1. The factor of synaptic convergence and divergence varies within the LGN between 1:4 and 1:20.

The spatial projection scheme of the retina via the LGN and from there to area V1, the primary visual cortex, follows a simple geometrical rule: the geometrical properties of the retinal image are preserved in a non-linear fashion in the spatial representation of neurones in the LGN and area V1. This geometrical order is called a retinotopic map. The non-linearity of this retinotopic organization is especially characterized by a much larger representation of the fovea as compared with other areas of the retina. The non-linearity disappears to a great extent when, instead of the reference value of degrees^2 mm^{-2} neuronal area, the spatial density of retinal ganglion cells (ganglion cells mm^{-2} retina) is taken as a reference value. Then, an approximately linear representation of the retinal ganglion cell layer is found in the layers of the LGN and, with some limitations, also in the projection of the LGN to the surface of the visual cortex.

4

The Primary Visual Cortex, Signal Processing for Visual Perception of Shapes, Space, Colour and Visual Movement

The Representation of the Visual Field in Brain Structures: Retinotopic Projections and the Retino-cortical Magnification Factor

The image of the three-dimensional world is projected by the optical apparatus of the eye onto the almost spherical surface of the retinal receptor layers, where it is transformed into three different 'physiological images' related to the cone system and one such image related to the rod system. To understand visual acuity in photopic vision and the retinotopic organization of the central visual system, it is necessary to know that the cone density decreases with retinal eccentricity and its corollary, the spatial density of ganglion cells, also decreases with the distance from the fovea centre. Except for the ganglion cells related to the fovea centre, another simple rule applies for the further projection of the 'neuronal image' within the central nervous system: the retinal ganglion cell layer is linearly mapped to the lateral geniculate nucleus and the primary visual cortex. Every retinal ganglion cell projects to about the same numbers of LGN or cortical nerve cells. Thus the essential non-linearities of visual field representation in the brain are induced to a large extent by the ganglion cell density decreasing with eccentricity in the retina. As a consequence, the small fovea – small in terms of angular size – is projected onto a much larger part of area V1 than a corresponding area in the parafoveal or peripheral part of the retina.

Owing to the efforts of Richard Förster (1825–1902), Salomon E. Henschen (1847–1930), Hermann Wilbrand

(1851–1935), Gordon M. Holmes (1876–1965) and others, by the end of the 1920s a generally acknowledged concept of the 'projection' of the retinal image onto the primary visual cortex of man had evolved, as illustrated in Figs 4.1 and 4.2. That is, the right half of the right eye visual field is projected optically to the nasal hemiretina of the right eye and the right half of the left eye visual field is projected to the temporal hemiretina of the left eye. The anatomical projections of the two 'neuronal images' through the optic nerve, optic chiasm, lateral geniculate nucleus and visual radiation finally create a non-linear map of the right visual hemifield of both eyes within the primary visual cortex (area V1 = area striata) of the left occipital brain. The same projection rules are applicable for the left visual hemifields of the left and right eye, which are represented in the area striata of the right occipital cortex. The upper half of the retina, corresponding to the lower visual field, projects to the supracalcarine part of area 17, the lower part of the retina correspondingly to the infracalcarine part of area 17. The foveal region of the contralateral visual hemifield is represented at the area striata around the occipital end of the calcarine fissure and on a small part of the outer convexity of the occipital cortex. The anatomical projections of the retinal periphery are buried deeply around the anterior end of the calcarine fissure. Figure 4.2 illustrates that the principle of a regular but non-linear retinotopic projection is maintained throughout the afferent visual pathways, whereby owing to rotation of the fibre tracts in the optic chiasm, the optic tract and the visual radiation a somewhat complex geometry is generated. In addition, beyond the optic chiasm, fibres originating from geometrically corresponding areas of the left and right retinas are associated loosely with each other (for details see Polyak, 1957). At the level of the

left area striata   visual field, right eye

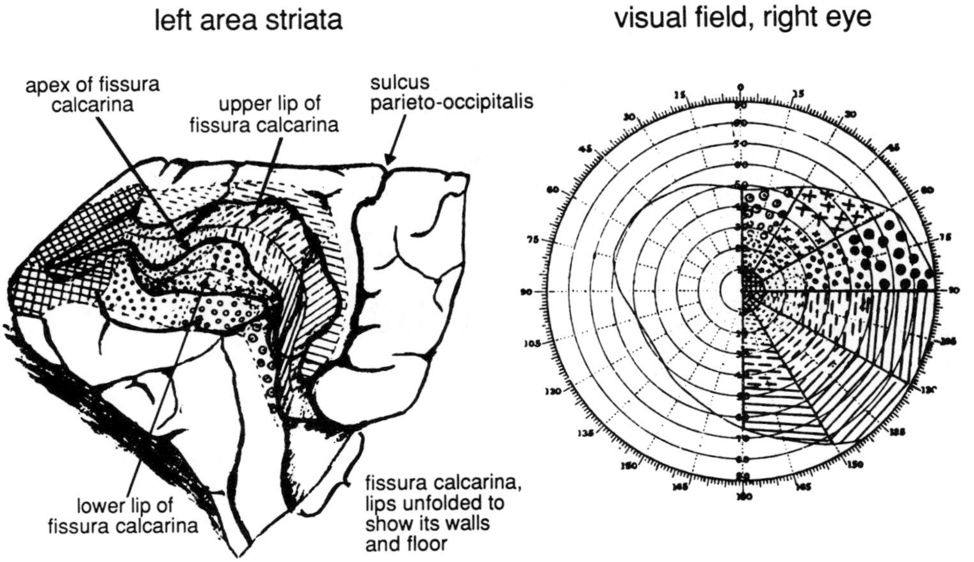

Fig. 4.1 *Schematic representation of the visual field of the right eye and the projection of the temporal part of this visual field onto the area striata located around the fissura calcarina on the mesial surface of the left occipital lobe. The upper and lower lips of the fissura calcarina are unfolded to show the walls and floor of the calcarine fissure. The relationship between visual fields and area striata surface is indicated by different symbols. The foveal halves of the visual field are projected to the occipital end, the peripheral parts to the anterior end of the area striata. This figure was derived from clinical observations on visual field defects caused by penetrating gunshot wounds (Holmes, 1918a).*

input to the LGN, the corresponding axons of retinal ganglion cells of the left and right eye separate from each other and project according to the retinal origin to layers 1, 4 and 6 for the contralateral retina and 2, 3 and 5 for the ipsilateral retina, as mentioned in Chapter 3. A somewhat loose retinotopic organization is preserved in the rather complex course of the optic radiation. Finally, the axons from nerve cells located in the ipsilateral and contralateral layers of the LGN contact nerve cells of the primary visual cortex, whereby projections related to geometrically corresponding retinal areas of both eyes 'meet' each other and form in part synapses at the same 'binocular' nerve cells of area V1.

The geometry of the fibre bundles of the optic tract and the optic radiation explains the clinical observation that circumscribed lesions within these retrochiasmatic structures of the afferent visual system lead only to approximately homonymous visual field defects in both eyes. In careful clinical investigations measuring the visual fields of the left and the right eye, one always finds small but distinct differences between the scotomata present in the left and right visual fields. A similar observation is made for lesions of the area V1, since with lesions of the cortical grey matter, parts of the afferent visual radiation fibres are also practically always destroyed. Thus lesions within the afferent visual system including area V1 lead only to

approximative and not geometrically precise homonymous visual field defects, which will be discussed in detail in Chapter 9.

As mentioned above, there exists a progressive diminution with retinal eccentricity of the size of a cortical area representing 1 square millimetre of retinal area. This change is described by the retino–cortical magnification factor (Daniel and Whitteridge, 1961). Rolls and Cowey (1970) demonstrated that in rhesus and squirrel monkeys the density of ganglion cells is approximately proportionate to the square of the retino–cortical magnification factor, whereby the foveal region deviates from this rule. The unidimensional cortical magnification factor M (mm diameter of cortical surface/degree of visual angle) is closely correlated to the visual acuity. Both decrease with retinal eccentricity according to a hyperbolic function, i.e. M^{-1} increases linearly with retinal eccentricity and is proportionate to the minimum visibile. When the retino–cortical magnification factor is taken into account, certain visual functions become uniform across the visual field. This M-scaling equates the spatial and temporal frequency contents of the visual stimulus patterns in terms of the calculated cortical image for different retinal eccentricities (Virsu and Rovamo, 1979). Thus visual patterns can be made equally visible if they are M-scaled. The same was found to be true for contrast sensitivity, which

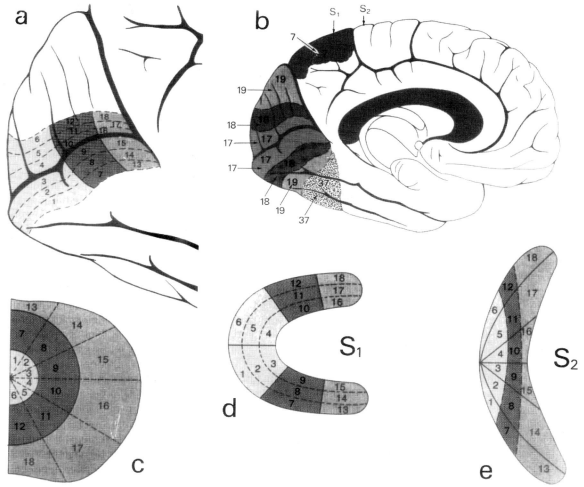

Fig. 4.2 *(a) Schematic view of the retino–cortical projection onto the surface of area striata of the left occipital cortex. The numbers refer to the sectors of the visual field as illustrated in (c). Brodmann's cytoarchitectonic areas 18 and 19 surrounding area 17 are functionally subdivided (b). (d) and (e) illustrate the projection of the axons related to the contralateral visual hemifield at different coronal sections through the left hemisphere (S_1 and S_2) as indicated in (b) (from Spalding, 1952a, b; redrawn and modified).*

follows the same power function at any eccentricity when the cortical area is stimulated by an *M*-scaled grating. Similarly, *M*-scaling of drifting random dot patterns unifies movement sensitivity across the visual field (Koenderink *et al.*, 1988; van de Grind, 1990; cf. Chapter 19). The data from which the retino–cortical magnification factor *M* of the human visual system was deduced were obtained by electrical stimulation of the visual cortex and a comparison between the location of the cortical stimulation electrodes and the corresponding location of phosphenes in the visual field. These experiments are discussed in detail in Chapter 10.

Elementary Rules of Signal Processing Within the Primary Visual Cortex

The major morphological subdivision of the afferent visual pathways from the retina to the primary visual cortex (area 17 = area V1) is expressed by the three classes (α, β and γ) of retinal ganglion cells and the magnocellular–parvocellular layer subdivision of the LGN. Functionally it is characterized by different colour channels, contrast channels, presumably two movement

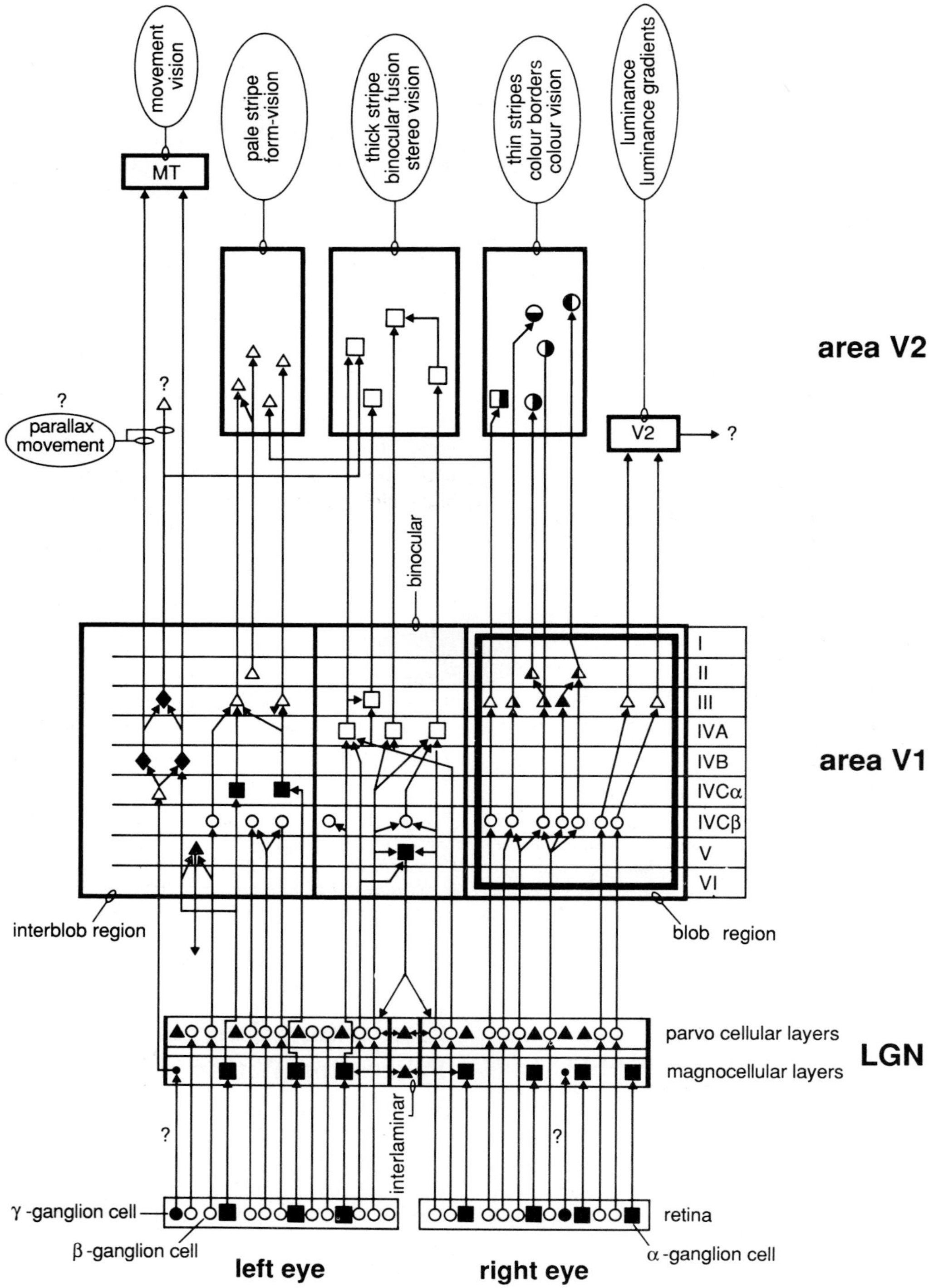

movement vision

pale stripe form-vision

thick stripe binocular fusion stereo vision

thin stripes colour borders colour vision

luminance luminance gradients

MT

area V2

?

parallax movement

?

V2 → ?

binocular

I	
II	
III	
IVA	
IVB	
IVCα	
IVCβ	
V	
VI	

area V1

interblob region

blob region

parvo cellular layers

magnocellular layers

LGN

interlaminar

?

?

γ -ganglion cell

retina

β -ganglion cell

α -ganglion cell

left eye

right eye

channels and 'luxotonic' neurones, i.e. nerve cells which convey signals about visual field luminance or luminance gradients. The axons of the geniculate relay cells extend through the visual radiation into area V1 of the occipital lobe. In primates some LGN neurones also send axon collaterals to the extrastriate visual cortex (area V2) (Benevento and Yoshida, 1981; Yukie and Iwai, 1981). The subdivision of the afferent 'channels' related to different qualities of vision is maintained and further elaborated in area V1 by a complex microparcellation of axonal projections. Small blocks of cerebral cortex, a few millimetres in diameter, form functional units in which the information content of the different types of LGN relay cells is preserved by the activity of small neuronal nets. Within some of these cortical 'modules', new combinations of the signals from different retino-geniculate 'channels' are created. Several morphological and physiological observations illustrate this functional parcellation (Hubel and Wiesel, 1968, 1972, 1974a, b, 1977; Hubel and Livingstone, 1981, 1987, 1990; Creutzfeldt *et al.*, 1987):

1. Most neocortical areas consist of 6 main tiers of nerve cells parallel to the cortical surface. The cell density and eventually additional subdivisions of these layers vary for different cytoarchitectonic cortical areas. In Brodmann's area 17 (area V1, Fig. 2.27) layer IV is particularly well developed and can be subdivided into the sublayers IVA, IVB, IVC α and IVCβ.

2. In addition to these layers, a columnar organization perpendicular to the 'horizontal' tiers and the cortical surface was found. Axons originating in the relay cells of the parvocellular LGN layers terminate predominantly in the cortical layer IVCβ, while neurones from the magnocellular layer of the LGN have axons which terminate mainly in layer IVCα. According to Livingstone and Hubel (1987, 1988, 1990), the main interlaminar connections of these two IVC sublayers within area V1 are also different, as is illustrated in Fig. 4.3.

3. Wong-Riley (1979) discovered another interesting principle shaping the columnar organization of area V1: when cytochrome oxidase staining is applied, densely stained 'blobs' oriented perpendicularly to the cortical surface appear, especially in the cytoarchitectonic layers I–III of area V1 (Horton and Hubel, 1981; Horton, 1984). Between these columnar 'blob' regions, less intensely stained 'interblob' structures appear. A high cytochrome oxidase activity correlates with high metabolic activity, since this mitochondrial enzyme serves the oxidative phosphorylization of glucose. The histochemical subdivision into 'blob' and 'interblob' regions also has some impact on the functional properties of nerve cells in layers IVCα and IVCβ.

4. Layer IVCβ neurones, which receive colour-coded signals from the cells of the parvocellular LGN layers (1–4), project within area V1 in turn predominantly to the blob regions of layers 2 and 3. These connections indicate that neurones located in the 'blob' regions of area V1 are involved, at least in part, in processing chromaticity signals. Direct microelectrode recordings from cells located in the blob region confirmed this assumption.

5. Some of the layer IVCβ neurones, however, also project to interblob regions, where many neurones have only weak chromatic selectivity, but exhibit responses characterized by their spatial orientation selectivity and narrow spatial frequency tuning (Figs 4.4, 4.5). Thus a new quality of visual signal processing is created in some of the area V1 neurones: orientation selectivity. This means that nerve cells are optimally activated when light–dark contours of a certain spatial orientation are projected to the receptive field (RF), while the neuronal activity decreases when the contour orientation changes. As careful exploration of the RF properties of these orientation-sensitive nerve cells has revealed, not only the orientation but also the width and length of a light or dark bar may be critical stimulus parameters, as illustrated schematically in Fig. 4.5.

Fig. 4.3 *Scheme of the projection of the axons originating in the parvocellular (1–4) and the magnocellular (5–6) layers of the lateral geniculate nucleus (LGN) into the different cell layers of area V1. Colour-coded neurones and luminance coded neurones of the parvocellular layers project into layer IVCβ of area V1. From there, connections exist predominantly to layers II and III of area V1. Cells of these layers elaborate on colour contrast (red–green and yellow–blue) mechanisms and send axons predominantly to the thin dense stripes of area V2. Some of the colour-coded cells of area V1 respond best to colour border contrasts. The system mediating luminance and luminance gradients most likely also projects from layer IVCβ and layer III to area V2 and beyond. Cells mediating binocular fusion and cells sensitive to stereo depth receive their input through the parvocellular and the magnocellular layers. Binocular fusion and a first step in stereo vision are achieved. The cortical nerve cells (layer IVA and III) which process binocular signals project to the 'thick dense stripes' of area V2. Within these structures a further elaboration on binocular fusion and stereovision is performed. In the 'interblob' regions of area V2 signals from parvocellular and magnocellular pathways converge on cortical nerve cells, which elaborate on light–dark contours and contour orientation. Projections exist from the interblob regions of area V1 mainly to the 'pale stripes' of area V2, where signals on form and contour vision are further processed. Cells from the magnocellular layers of the LGN project to the interblob regions of area V1, layer IVB. From there the signals are transmitted to area MT, where the information on visual movement is further elaborated upon. Presumably also a 'slow movement' signal mediated by the γ-ganglion cells and the small LGN cells is projected to layer IVB and beyond. 'Pale', 'thick' and 'thin' stripes of area V2 are discriminated by cytochrome oxidase staining, like the 'blob' and 'interblob' regions of area V1.*

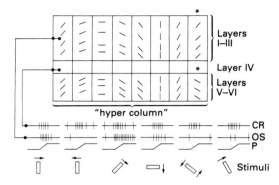

Fig. 4.4 *Scheme of orientation tuning of contrast cells in area V1 (layers I–III, V–VI). Most cells of layer IV do not show orientation tuning. The responses of an orientation-tuned (OS) nerve cell of layer II and of a nerve cell of layer IV non-selective for orientation tuning are shown. The stimulus, a 0.5 × 2-degree light bar, is oriented and moved in different directions (arrows). The movement is indicated by a change in position of the stimulus (P) and lasts about 0.2 seconds. The orientation tuning changes systematically from column to column. The nerve cells located in the column marked with an asterisk have a different optimum orientation sensitivity when they are located in layers I–III rather than in layers V–VI.*

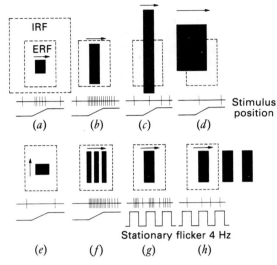

Fig. 4.5 *Scheme of responses of an area V1 nerve cell, which has an orientation-tuned excitatory receptive field (ERF) surrounded by an inhibitory receptive field (IRF). (a) Responses to a horizontally moving, vertically oriented, small dark bar. (b) The response increases considerably when the stimulus elongates in the vertical direction. Movement direction is indicated by arrows. (c) and (d) The stimulus extends from the ERF into the IRF. This leads to a reduction of neuronal activity. (e) When the dark rectangle is horizontally oriented and moved in the vertical direction, no response is obtained from the excitatory receptive field. (f) Several small black bars placed in optimal orientation and moved horizontally evoke a strong neuronal response. (g) The surroundings of a stationary, optimally oriented, black bar are illuminated intermittently at 4 Hz. This leads to strong responses. (h) In contrast, a pattern of three bars, one positioned in the ERF, the other two in the IRF, only evoke a weak response when illuminated intermittently or moved coherently.*

6. Many of the orientation-selective nerve cells in area V1 are activated best by a moving contour, whereby the optimum movement direction is usually perpendicular to optimum orientation (Fig. 4.4). Activation of orientation-selective nerve cells is also possible, however, when a stationary contrast contour is placed in the RF and the contrast pattern is illuminated intermittently. Flicker frequencies between 3 and 8 Hz were found to be especially effective in activating orientation-tuned area V1 nerve cells (Grüsser and Grüsser-Cornehls, 1969, in van de Grind *et al.*, 1973). The movement sensitivity of many of these 'contour-oriented' neurones is in our opinion an adaption to the fact that the retinal image is shifted every 0.18–0.6 seconds due to saccadic eye movements across the retinal surface, and the signal uptake relevant to the activation of cortical visual neurones occurs during the short fixation periods.

7. In addition to spatial frequency tuning, many of these orientation-selective cells have an 'end-stopped' response (Fig. 4.5) and some of them seem to measure curvature, as illustrated schematically in Fig. 4.6. In the responses of area V1 neurones the 'extraction' of information on contours (contrast borders), contour orientation, movement direction and stimulus angular size is not dependent on the chromatic properties of the stimulus nor on stimulus–background brightness contrast. This invariance in the activity of some area 17 neurones with respect to luminance contrast is illustrated in Fig. 4.7. Invariances

of this type do indeed suggest that the relevant information extracted by these neurones from the visual signals is spatial contour orientation.

8. Orientation-selective nerve cells are functionally organized into 'columns' perpendicular to the cortical surface. The orientation selectivity of neighbouring 'orientation columns' changes according to simple rules, as indicated in Fig. 4.4. Repeatedly the uniformity of the optimum orientation of the nerve cells located in a single orientation column of area V1 was questioned (e.g. Bauer, 1982). For the majority of the columns in monkeys, Bauer *et al.* (1983) found that the preferred orientation within one column shifts at the border of layers IV/V by 45 to 90 degrees (Krüger and Bach, 1982; von der Heydt and Peterhans, quoted in von der Heydt, 1987).

The regular geometry of orientation preference, as illustrated in Fig. 4.4, led to the concept of 'hypercolumns' composed of several 'orientation columns', which, taken together, cover all possible orientations of a contour on the retinal surface (Hubel and Wiesel, 1968, 1972, 1974). It should be emphasized, however, that only nerve cells of layers I–III and V–VI participate in this functional organization. In layer IV many neurones have RFs with a fairly symmetric and spatially non-oriented organization.

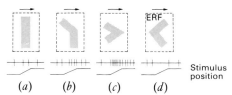

| (a) | (b) | (c) | (d) | Stimulus position |

Fig. 4.6 *Scheme of the responses of a cortical visual neurone (area V1) which has an excitatory receptive field (ERF) sensitive to the curvature of a contour. A black bar forming a contour with different angles is moved through the receptive field in the direction indicated by the arrows. The neuronal activation is dependent on the curvature, movement direction and orientation of the tip.*

9. It is now well established that not only the magnocellular input contributes to the excitation of cortical nerve cells with orientation selectivity, but also signals originating from the parvocellular layers of the LGN. Their projection to the interblob regions of layers 2 and 3 are presumably responsible for some 'shaping' of the RF properties of the orientation-selective cortical nerve cells. With this convergence of magnocellular and parvocellular input signals, chromatic specificity seems to be lost, which has led to the somewhat misleading statement that the signals of chromaticity present in our natural habitat do not contribute to visual *Gestalt* perception (cf. Chapter 3). On the other hand Michael (1978a, b, c) reported on colour-sensitive, orientation-tuned neurones in the monkey striate cortex which otherwise possessed typically 'complex' or 'hypercomplex' receptive field properties. Thus it seems fairly probable that in addition to achromatic contrast borders, chromatic contrast borders are also represented in an orientation-tuned fashion in the subclasses of visual cortex neurones (Michael, 1979, 1985).

10. As mentioned above, many neurones in layer IVC have more or less concentric, non-oriented, receptive

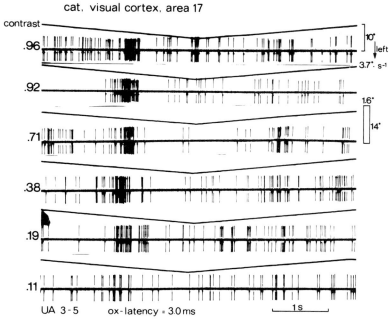

Fig. 4.7 *Recordings of the action potentials of a nerve cell located in the cat primary visual cortex (layer III according to depth measurements) which respond best to a vertically elongated slit of light or a vertical dark bar moving in a horizontal direction through the excitatory receptive field. The response to a 1.6 × 14-degree vertical light bar moving at a constant speed of 3.7 deg s⁻¹ left and right through the ERF (movement amplitude 5 degrees) leads to a strong neuronal activation with movement towards the left but to rare neuronal activity with movement to the right. The neuronal activation was not dependent on the contrast between the stimulus and the background for contrast values between 0.15 and 0.96. Only with a very low contrast (0.11) did the responses decrease considerably. This neurone was activated by optic tract electrical stimulation with a latency of 3.0 ms. The data illustrate neuronal response invariance regarding stimulus contrast (from an experiment of U. Grüsser-Cornehls and O.-J. Grüsser, unpublished, 1971).*

fields. Estimates of the frequency of primate area 17 neurones with non-oriented receptive fields vary between 20 and about 40 per cent, whereby non-oriented cortical nerve cells seem to be occuring more frequently within the cortical projection area of the fovea centralis (for further discussions see von der Heydt, 1987). Of course, the sampling properties of the recording microelectrode have a considerable effect on the percentage of different neuronal classes recorded during one penetration of the visual cortex. With micropipettes, for example, many more small cells having non-oriented receptive fields are found than with tungsten microelectrodes. Furthermore many orientation-selective nerve cells can be activated by diffuse flicker stimuli tuned to a certain range of temporal frequencies. This activation corresponds on the psychophysical level to the perception of flicker patterns seen in a large homogeneous but flickering field (e.g. van de Grind *et al.*, 1973). The application of different microelectrodes and different levels of anaesthesia (or no anaesthesia) led to contradictory reports on the presence of single neurones in the visual cortex (of cats) responding to diffuse light stimuli. Hubel and Wiesel (1962) claimed that the cat primary visual cortex does not contain neurones responding to large-field, diffuse light stimuli, while the Freiburg group (Jung *et al.*, 1952, 1957; Baumgartner, 1955, 1961; Grüsser and Grüsser-Cornehls, 1961, 1962) found about 50 per cent of cat area 17 neurones responding to diffuse light stimulation, especially flicker stimulation. The existence of cortical 'luxotonic' neurones, as Doty (1977) called them, processing information on large-field luminance and presumably also luminance gradients in the visual field, seems to be now well established. Neurones belonging to this class are found predominantly in layer IVC.

11. Another 'channel' present at the retinal and LGN output level is also maintained in the cortical microparcellation system. According to Livingstone and Hubel (1988, 1989), the majority of layer IVB neurones are highly movement-sensitive and most of them exhibit directional selectivity with respect to optimum movement direction. It seems that directional selectivity is one of the new properties attributed to the 'movement channel' of the retino-geniculate pathway at the level of area V1. For subcortical projections of the retinal γ-ganglion cell axons, directional selectivity seems to be present even at the retinal level (e.g. projections to the NOT and to the AOS, Fig. 3.6), but so far no directionally selective, movement-sensitive neurones have been found in the primate LGN. Movement-sensitive neurones of area V1 do not seem to have special chromatic selectivity, but one can expect the chromatic composition of a stimulus to affect movement responses, since the frequency transfer properties of the red–green and the blue–yellow system differ somewhat. Movement-selective neurones receive their main input

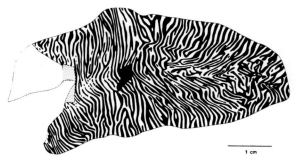

Fig. 4.8 *Ocular dominance stripes in area V1 of a macaque monkey were labelled by autoradiography after injection of [^{3}H]-proline into one eye. The stripes were reconstructed as projections onto the flattened cortical surface, whereby many autoradiographs were used for the reconstruction (from LeVay et al., 1985; by permission of the Society for Neuroscience).*

from the magnocellular layer of the LGN. Their activity increases with the angular velocity of the moving stimulus. As in other biological systems dealing with visual movement perception, a power function between angular velocity and neuronal activity is a good description within a certain range of angular velocities (Grüsser and Grüsser-Cornehls, 1973). A portion of the cortical movement-selective neurones exhibit clear signs of velocity selectivity and different velocity ranges are represented in several classes of 'velocity-tuned' cortical nerve cells (e.g. Orban, 1984; cf. Orban, Volume 4, Chapter 8 of this series).

12. The binocular interaction of retinal signals at the LGN level seems to be predominantly of the inhibitory type, mediated by cells located in the 'intralaminar' zones of the LGN. Binocular signal integration attains a new quality in some of the nerve cells of area V1. In addition to orientation tuning, area V1 columns are also functionally subdivided according to their 'ocularity'. In parts of a hypercolumn, which is composed of several orientation columns, either the ipsilateral or the contralateral retina dominates the neuronal activation. In between these 'monocular ocularity columns' one finds distinct zones in which the majority of nerve cells exhibit binocular activation for all layers except IVCα and IVCβ. Ocularity seems to 'interdigitate' with the other channel properties mentioned above. The binocular signal integration by area V1 neurones is a necessary condition for perceiving one visual world with two eyes. Physiological and anatomical techniques have led to converging results regarding the geometry of the monocular and binocular zones of area V1. The striate cortex of macaque monkeys, when viewed from its surface, is subdivided into many ocular dominance stripes, i.e. layers oriented perpendicular to the cortical surface. An ocular dominance column receives its main afferent visual input from the LGN layers connected with either the left or the right retina respectively. Left

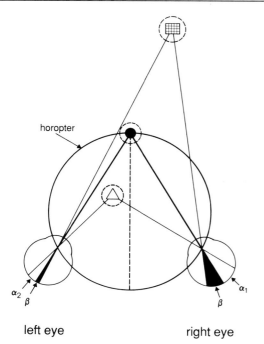

left eye   right eye

Fig. 4.9 *Response schemes of binocular nerve cells in the monkey areas V1 and V2, sensitive to stereoscopic depth. The RFs of three classes of neurones are illustrated: neurones activated optimally when geometrically corresponding retinal regions were stimulated synchronously, i.e. the stimulus was placed on the horopter circle (dot). The 'far neurones' responded best when the stimulus was placed outside the horopter (triangle), i.e. the receptive fields in both retinas were placed in uncrossed non-corresponding regions. The 'near neurones' (squares) responded best when the stimulus was between the horopter circle and the eyes. Their receptive fields were located in crossed non-corresponding regions of the two retinas (scheme drawn according to the data of Poggio, Fischer and their co-workers).*

(β) Neurones which were optimally activated when the stimuli were placed in a region between the eyes and the horopter circle ('near neurones'). Correspondingly, the location of their receptive fields in the two retinas was characterized by a certain crossed disparity.

(γ) Neurones which had an optimum response when the stimulus was outside the horopter ('far neurones') and showed a corresponding uncrossed disparity of the respective receptive fields in both retinas (Fig. 4.9).

When we move our head while fixating a stationary target in our visual surroundings, parallax movement of objects outside the actual horopter circle is evoked. This parallax movement varies slightly for the left and the right eye and, consequently, identical visual stimuli of the extra-personal space are projected to geometrically corresponding retinal areas with some temporal delay. It is therefore meaningful to also investigate the impact of temporal aspects of the binocular stimuli on cortical neurone activity. In such studies it was indeed found that the temporal delay between the visual stimuli projected to the left and the right retina has some effect on the activation of binocularly driven nerve cells of area 17 (Fig. 4.10; Grüsser and Grüsser-Cornehls, 1961, 1965; Cynader *et al.*, 1978). One can safely assume that binocular signal properties, especially parallax movement, are represented in the network of cortical nerve cells as a spatially and temporally structured field of excitation.

13. Up to a few years ago the temporo–spatial distribution of excitation and inhibition within extended networks of area V1 neurones could only be estimated indirectly by comparing the responses of different nerve cells recorded sequentially in the same cortical region while applying identical visual stimuli. With the development of multiple micro–electrode recording techniques (e.g. Reitboeck, 1983 a,b) simultaneous recordings of the activity of several neurones located in nearby cortical regions became feasible. Considering the 'horizontal' anatomical connections within area V1 or the 'higher-order' visual cortices, it is not surprising that with this recording technique a stimulus-related synchronization of neuronal activity was found. Two classes of neuronal synchronization were discriminated: synchronous activity induced directly by the visual stimulus and synchronous neuronal activity triggered, but caused only indirectly by, and therefore loosely related in time to, the visual stimulus. Synchronization of cortical neuronal activity in the latter case was interpreted as a consequence of short-range or long-range connections within the visual cortices (e.g. Mitzdorf, 1985). In addition to stimulus-forced synchronizations in cell assemblies of area V1, stimulus-induced late oscillations in a frequency range between 35–80 Hz were discovered. These stimulus-specific oscillations were evidently synchronized among distributed nerve cell assemblies located either in the immediate neighbourhood within area V1 or in distant

eye–right eye ocular dominance stripes alternate with a spatial period of 0.9–1.2 mm (Fig. 4.8). The transient zone between a left eye and a right eye ocular dominance stripe consists of a band containing binocularly activated nerve cells ('binocularity stripes').

In addition to simple binocular fusion, a new quality of vision is established for a portion of the neurones located in the binocularity stripes: stereoscopic depth. In alert monkeys, Poggio and Fischer (1977) and Poggio *et al.* (1985, 1988) found neurones in layer IVB responding to stereoscopic disparity. They could classify the responses of these neurones into three different groups:

(α) Nerve cells which had their optimum responses (binocular facilitation) when geometrically corresponding areas of both retina were stimulated, i.e. the binocular stimulus was a visual pattern positioned on the horopter (Fig. 4.9).

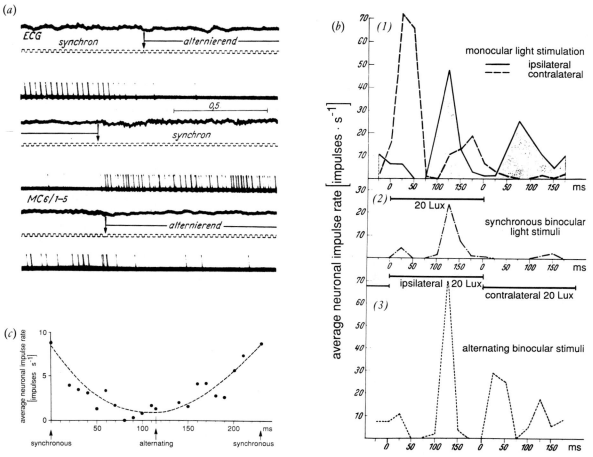

Fig. 4.10 *(a) Reponses of a nerve cell located in area 17 of the cat (encephale isolé preparation) to diffuse monocular flicker stimulation of each eye. This neurone exhibited a strong binocular facilitation when synchronous flicker stimuli were applied. When the flicker stimulation was 180 degrees out of phase ('alternierend'), the response decreased considerably. Flicker frequency in this example was 36 Hz. (b) Neuronal activity of a binocularly driven nerve cell of cat area 17. (1) Responses to monocular stimulation of the contralateral eye (dashed curve) or to monocular stimulation of the ipsilateral eye (solid curve). Diffuse large-field light stimuli. (2) Synchronous binocular stimulation diminished the neuronal response considerably. (3) When the binocular stimuli were 180 degrees out of phase, the response was again facilitated and binocular summation occurred. Stimulus frequency was 5 Hz. (c) The activity (ordinate) of a neurone which responded only to binocular stimulation and not to monocular stimulation of the ipsilateral or contralateral eye depended on the time delay between the light stimuli applied to the left and the right eye (abscissa). Recordings were as in (a) and (b) from the cat area 17. Duration of the light–dark period was 250 ms. Diffuse large-field light stimulation was 20 lux, white light (from Grüsser-Cornehls and Grüsser, 1961).*

neuronal assemblies in area V1 and V2, but referring to the same part of the visual field (Eckhorn *et al.*, 1988 a, b, c; Gray *et al.*, 1989; Eckhorn and Schanze, 1991; Engel *et al.*, 1991; Gray *et al.*, 1991). It is believed that these oscillatory responses not only reflect inter-columnar synchronization of neuronal activity but also represent certain generalizable properties of the stimulus. To date it is certainly premature to draw conclusions about shape perception

from this very interesting work done in the cat visual cortex. Data from the visual cortex neurones in awake, behaving monkeys have to be collected with the multiple-electrode, single-unit recording technique, before one can confirm whether or not the stimulus-locked and stimulus-induced synchronizations of neuronal activity spreading across the visual cortices encode invariant stimulus features.

stimuli

LGN

off-centre
neurone

on-centre
neurone

Area 17

simple RF

simple RF

complex RF

complex RF

hyper-
complex RF

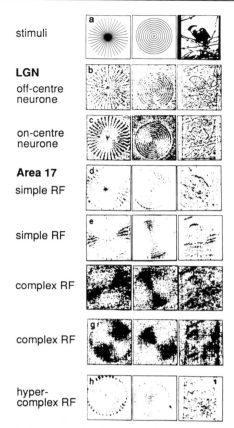

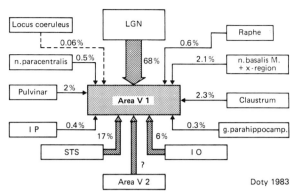

Fig. 4.12 *Scheme of the different inputs to the monkey primary visual cortex (area V1) as found in neuroanatomical tracer studies by Doty (1983). According to this work, about 68 per cent of the axons having terminals at nerve cells of the primary visual cortex originate from the afferent visual radiation fibres connecting the lateral geniculate nucleus (LGN) with the primary visual cortex. Non-visual inputs from other brain regions are also given in estimated percentages. No values are known for the 'efferent' connections from area V2 to area V1.*

Fig. 4.11 *Two-dimensional representation of neurone activity as recorded from the LGN and the area striata of cat. To activate the neurone the three different stimuli (a), a star, a set of concentric circles and a photograph of a bullfinch were slowly moved along a straight path line by line in random succession over the receptive field of the respective recorded neurone, i.e. the RF scanned systematically the whole picture. Whenever the neurone recorded was activated, a black dot appeared on the oscilloscope screen. By this method an image of the spatial representation of the stimulus pattern in a network of functionally identical nerve cells was represented. (b) Responses from an off-centre neurone of the lateral geniculate nucleus. (c) Same from an on-centre neurone. In (d)–(h) corresponding spatial response patterns are shown for nerve cells recorded from the area striata, having simple, complex and hypercomplex receptive field properties as indicated. It is evident that different cortical neuronal classes represent different features of the stimulus pattern moving slowly across the visual field (from Creutzfeldt and Nothdurft, 1978, modified). It is fairly probable that similar responses can be generated from the different nerve cells of area V1 of the primate brain.*

This modern aspect of visual cortex function is of extreme importance, since it leads away from the all-too-simple models in which a direct 1:1 correlation between the activation of a certain class of nerve cells and a certain percept was postulated (e.g. the 'grandmother cells' or 'red Volkswagen cells' mentioned in Chapter 1).

There are good reasons for assuming that within the primary visual cortex the neuronal representation of an individual object, which is perceived by us as a whole, corresponds to the spatio–temporal excitation pattern of many different classes of coherently activated nerve cells. The degree of coherence may depend on the state of alertness, the state of spatially directed attention and the features of the object seen. A summary of this distributed activity related to the visual stimulus or its retinal image respectively is given in Fig. 4.11.

Non-visual and 'Efferent' Visual Signals Reaching Area V1

So far we have discussed the principles of neuronal data processing in the primary visual cortex related to the stimulus patterns appearing in the visual field. In addition to the geniculo–cortical axons, however, the nerve cells of the primary visual cortex receive signals mediated by a considerable number of non-visual axons originating in other structures of the brain. Moreover, the 'higher-order' visual cortices, onto which area V1 projects, send 'efferent' axons back to area V1. Little is known about the functional importance of these connections, illustrated schematically in Fig. 4.12, but the anatomical data available suggest that

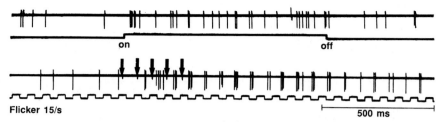

Fig. 4.13 *Responses of a nerve cell recorded from area 17 of the cat (encephale isolé preparation) evoked by diffuse binocular flicker stimuli. The critical flicker fusion frequency (CFF) was reached at 10 stimuli per second, i.e. above 10 light stimuli per second the neurone failed to respond to every light stimulus. At a flicker rate of 15 stimuli per second, the neurone responded only irregularly to the light stimuli. When five 16-per-second electrical stimuli (arrows) were delivered to non-specific intralaminar thalamic nuclei, an increase in neuronal activation was regularly evoked and for a period of 2–3 s the neuronal responses to the binocular flicker stimuli were facilitated (from Creutzfeldt and Grüsser, 1957).*

in a free-moving, active animal a considerable modification of the visual signal flow through area V1 should occur under the control of these feedback connections. In Fig. 4.12 the findings of Doty (1983) are summarized; he estimated the percentage of non-visual input to area V1 by means of anatomical methods (retrograde tracer studies). It is quite likely that the percentage of non-geniculate axons reaching area V1 nerve cells is even underestimated somewhat by the percentage values given in Fig. 4.12. The non-visual and the 'efferent' visual connections reaching area V1 from areas V2, V3 and V4, together with the inputs from non-visual parts of the brain, characterize the striate area located around the calcarine fissure of the occipital cortex as an 'association area', which selects the visual inputs and is more than a simple elementary visual relay structure.

Finally, it should be mentioned that non-visual input signals also reach area V1 from non-specific structures of the thalamus and the brain stem. Figure 4.13 illustrates the responses of a nerve cell located in area 17 of the cat to the binocular flicker stimuli and simultaneous electrical stimulation of non-specific intralaminar thalamic nuclei. As was regularly observed in these experiments, the non-visual activation facilitated the flicker responses of cortical nerve cells, indicating the modifying influence of non-visual, non-specific, thalamic signals on cortical structures. Most nerve cells in the primary visual cortex of cats responded to electrical stimulation of non-specific thalamic nuclei, whereby a slow temporal facilitation of neuronal activation was the rule (Akimoto and Creutzfeldt, 1957; Creutzfeldt and Akimoto, 1957).

5 Extrastriate Visual Areas: Examples of Higher-Order Visual Data Processing

Introduction

Clinical observations of patients suffering from lesions in the posterior part of the brain but having intact visual fields led to the conclusion that large cortical regions outside the area striata contribute to visual perception and cognition. Kleist (1934) summarized these observations by indicating that with respect to visual space orientation and object recognition, brain functions seem to be divided between extrastriate areas by two principles: space-related visual information is processed in the occipito–parietal cortex, object-related signals in the occipito–temporal cortex. In addition, Kleist attributed visually guided motor behaviour (oculomotor, gaze motor, grasping and locomotor activity) to distinct parts of the parieto–occipital and frontal lobes. During the last 15 years several hundred publications have appeared in which extensive and successful neurophysiological and neuroanatomical studies were reported, demonstrating the existence to date of more than 25 extrastriate visual and visuo-motor areas for the primate cortex. We owe this knowledge to the efforts of Allman, Andersen, Baumgartner, Creutzfeldt, Desimone, Dürsteler, Goldberg, Gross, Hubel, Hyvärinen, Livingstone, Lund, Mishkin, Mountcastle, Newsome, Optican, Peterhans, Poggio, Richmond, Rizzolatti, Robinson, Ungerleider, van Essen, von der Heydt, Wurtz, Zeki and their co-workers. For details, the reader is referred to Volumes 3–6 of this series.

Criteria for Cortical 'Visual Association Areas' or 'Visual Integration Areas'

In any discussion of visual association cortices, criteria have to be selected for defining an area as 'visual':

1. The majority of neurones in the area should respond well to 'adequate' visual stimulation. Adequate can sometimes mean the selection of rather specific visual stimulus patterns. To establish a predominance of visual input signals over all other non-visual signals is not a trivial task. Such a predominance is easily proven for the LGN or the primary visual cortex. More than 80 per cent of the synaptic contacts of the LGN relay cells are visual, i.e. are axon terminals of retinal ganglion cells, and the neurones respond easily to diffuse large-field stimuli. In the primary visual cortex, 'specific' visual synaptic contacts amount to about 65 per cent. In area V4 (Fig. 5.5), however, only about 35 per cent of the input signals are conveyed by 'visual' axons, originating predominantly in areas V1, V2 and V3. Evidently, for the signal processing within the 'higher-order' visual cortices, the dominance of the visual input from the 'lower-order' visual areas has disappeared or is at least weakened. Nevertheless, one finds brisk visual responses in neurophysiological recordings, provided adequate stimulus configurations are presented in the visual field.

2. Typical visual association areas contain several different classes of neurones, which all require rather elaborate visual stimuli with regards to chromatic composition, contour orientation, shape, movement or binocular stereoscopic disparity. Frequently nerve cells belonging to the same distinct class of visual data processing are organized together in 'columns' or 'patches'.

3. For many, but not all, of the recently discovered visual association cortices, the visual function was established through the existence of a systematic retinotopic organization, i.e. a fixed geometric relationship between the contralateral half of the visual field, or at least part of it, and the surface of the cortical area. The retino–cortical map valid for a given visual association cortex may extend beyond the vertical meridian separating the ipsilateral and contralateral visual fields. This extension is caused by projections originating in the homologous contralateral cor-

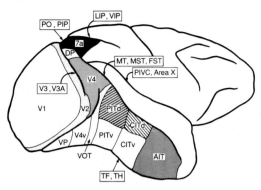

Fig. 5.1 *Aspect of the outer surface of the right hemisphere from a macaque brain. The location of the visual association areas visible at the outer surface are schematically drawn. Abbreviations: AIT, anterior infero-temporal area; CIT, central infero-temporal area, ventral (v) and dorsal (d) part; DP, dorsal prelunate area; FST, fundus of the superior temporal sulcus; LIP, lateral interparietal area; MST, medial superior temporal area; MT, middle temporal area; PIP, posterior intraparietal region; PIT, posterior infero-temporal region, ventral (v) and dorsal (d) part; PIVC, parieto-insular vestibular cortex; PO, parieto-occipital area; TF, temporal field F; TH, temporal field H; VIP, ventral intraparietal area; VOT, ventral occipito-temporal area (drawn according to figures published by Maunsell and Newsome, 1987, and van Essen, 1985).*

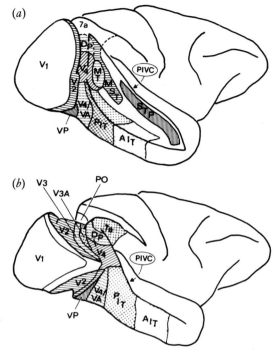

Fig. 5.2 *Schematic representation of the visual areas buried within the walls of the sulci of the occipital, temporal and parietal lobe. In (a) the superior temporal sulcus is unfolded. In (b) the lunate, intraparietal, parieto-occipital and inferior occipital sulci are unfolded. Abbreviations as in Fig. 5.1; STP, cortex around supratemporal sulcus (from Maunsell and Newsome, 1987, modified).*

tical areas and reaching the respective cortical areas through the corpus callosum. The 'grain' of the retinotopic map increases in coarseness the 'higher' is the level of visual data processing. In some visual association cortices only the foveal and parafoveal part of the visual half-field is represented.

4. In microscopic investigations, the spatial organization, size and distribution of the nerve cells located in the different cortical layers (I–VI) should enable the expert to discriminate distinct cytoarchitectonic or myeloarchitectonic borders, which clearly separate the visual cortical area in question from the neighbouring cytoarchitectonic fields. This task sometimes seems to be too difficult.

5. Tracer studies should provide evidence that the area in question receives axons from areas V1, V2 or V3. Evidently, the non-visual input increases with the 'order' of a visual association area in the hierarchy of visual data processing.

6. All visual association areas project 'downstream', i.e. back to visual areas V1, V2 and/or V3. Many of them have efferent connections to subcortical visual centres, such as the medial and the inferior pulvinar, the superior colliculi, the nucleus of the optic tract (NOT, Chapter 3) or the gaze motor complex of the brain stem (e.g. Fries, 1981, 1984, 1990; Glickstein et al., 1980, 1985; Lynch et al., 1985).

7. When visual responses are still evident in a cortical field, but no longer follow a retinotopic scheme, because the representation of the visual world on the cortical area is organized in a spatiotopic map (i.e. related to head or body coordinates), we will designate this cortical region as 'visual integration cortex'. The same term is applied when the visual area in question represents spatial relationships within the extra-personal space without any body-related map or when the visual response is not organized at all in spatial coordinates, but is related to categories of visual objects or events, independent of their place in the extrapersonal space.

Projections from Area V1 to 'Higher' Cerebral Visual Centres

Figure 5.1 illustrates the distribution of the visual areas of the occipital, temporal and posterior parietal lobe as seen from the outer surface of the right hemisphere of a macaque monkey brain. A considerable portion of these

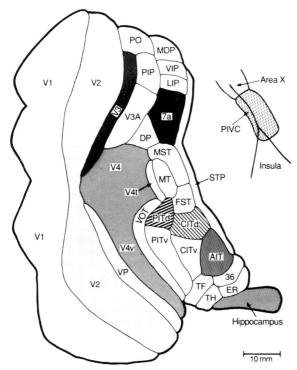

Fig. 5.3 *Flattened surface of the primary visual cortex (V1), the extrastriate visual cortices and the visual integration areas of the temporal and the parietal lobe. The different visual association cortices are schematically displayed. Abbreviations as in Fig. 5.1; ER, entorhinal area; MDP, medial dorso-parietal area. In the retroinsular region, the parieto–insular vestibular cortex is schematically drawn and the area X (corresponding approximately to the cytoarchitectonic area T3) is also depicted. In both regions, large-field visual stimuli lead to excitation or inhibition of the nerve cell activity (from Sereno and Allman, Volume 4, Chapter 7, slightly modified).*

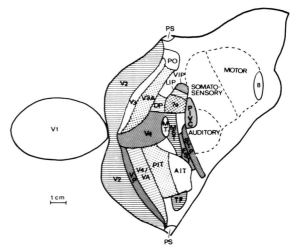

Fig. 5.4 *Schematic representation of the flattened surface of a macaque brain hemisphere illustrating area V1 and the visual association and integration areas. Note that more than half of the cortical surface is integrated in visual data processing. Abbreviations as in Fig. 5.1; PS, posterior sylvian area; VP, ventro-posterior area. (from Maunsell and Newsome, 1987, modified). (Note that in Figs. 5.1–5.4 the subdivision of the inferior temporal lobe deviates from the scheme used in Fig. 7.1.)*

cortical areas is hidden in the sulci of the occipital and temporal lobe, becoming visible when the cortical surface is unfolded as shown in Figs 5.2(a) and (b). Another way to demonstrate the large extension of the visual cortices across the posterior parts of the brain is a 'flat-mount' of the cortical surface, i.e. a graphical flattening-out of the cortex, which is normally folded into the walls around the sulci. When the whole neocortical structure of one hemisphere is unfolded in such a manner (Figs 5.3 and 5.4), at a first glance a somewhat surprising fact becomes evident: the primary visual cortex (area V1) together with the visual association cortices covers more than half the neocortical surface of one hemisphere. The functional significance of many of the distinct visual association areas shown in Figs 5.1–5.4 is only partially known. Microelectrode data are often available only from qualitative studies which were performed to delineate the borders of a suspected visual

association area. Nevertheless, some of the microelectrode data indicate a subspecialization for visual data processing in the different areas shown in Figs 5.1–5.4. It should be emphasized that the art of subparcellation of the posterior part of the brain into distinct visual association areas is still in progress. In a recently published review (Douglas and Martin, 1991) a diagram of van Essen *et al.* (1991) is included in which 32 visual association and integration cortices with their mutual connections are displayed. From this diagram we deduced that area V1 is connected with 9 other higher-order visual areas, area V2 with 13 visual areas, area V3 with 15 other visual areas, and area VP with area V1 and 14 'higher' visual association areas. Considering the complexity of such a 'wiring' diagram and the fact of 'backward' projections, a straightforward conclusion comes to mind regarding the physiological interaction within such a system: 'anything goes'. In quoting Feyerabend's (1975) 'anarchistic' epistemological view of science, however, we do not wish to express a certain pessimism regarding a future comprehension of the functions of the many visual association and integration areas of the brain. It becomes evident, however, that 'wiring diagrams' like those worked out by van Essen and his co-workers provide a basic anatomical framework which has to be filled in by physiological studies before its relevance can be established. Recordings of the physiological activity (preferably with multiple microelectrodes) in the awake monkey brain, under conditions in which the animal can interact with its surroundings or perform specific visual tasks, will be necessary in understanding the functions of many of the visual association cortices and their connections. Concerning the research efforts of numerous laboratories studying this task, one can expect that within the next generation the functional meaning of the complex connections between many visual cortical areas will be grasped.

To bring an elementary order into the many visual association cortices, Ungerleider and Mishkin (1982) proposed a simple 'construction rule' for the distribution of visual functions over the different visual association areas: those located in the temporo–occipital region mainly serve the identification and differentiation of various visual objects by analysing shape, colour and movement. In contrast, the parieto–occipital visual association areas serve the location of the object in the extrapersonal space and its movement through that space. A third operational task, namely the control of visuo–motor actions, related to the pursuit of objects by the gaze, to grasping objects visually guided by the hand or moving the whole body under visual control, can be clearly attributed to some parietal and prefrontal visual integration areas (e.g. Rizzolatti *et al.*, 1983). Ungerleider's and Mishkin's discrimination of an occipito–temporal 'what' system and an occipito–parietal 'where' system correlates well with the division made by Kleist (1934) for the human extrastriate visual cortices as mentioned above. From neurophysiological and anatomical data it seems rather probable that this dichotomy develops in steps. The visual areas V1 and V2 still contain information related to both object and space perception, while area V3, which receives input from areas V2 and V1, seems to connect predominantly to the occipito–parietal system, and area VP (Fig. 5.1) projects mainly to temporal visual association and integration cortices, particularly through areas V4 and VOT (Fig. 5.1). Area V3 and area V3a project via area PIP and area PO and DP respectively to the movement-sensitive regions MT and MST as well and through area VIP to the parietal region 7a, in which the extrapersonal space is represented. Area 7, however, according to van Essen's diagram mentioned above, also has direct connections with area V2.

All visual association cortices shown in Figs 5.1–5.4 receive strong non-visual inputs, which are related in part to the gaze motor system, in part to attentional mechanisms controlled from frontal lobe and limbic structures. Some of the signals reaching the visual association cortices of the parietal lobe from gaze motor regions are important for stabilizing the relationship between retinotopic and spatiotopic representations of the visual world within the visual association areas.

In addition to visually dominated association and integration areas, multimodal integration areas exist, in which the visual input is only one of several modalities activating

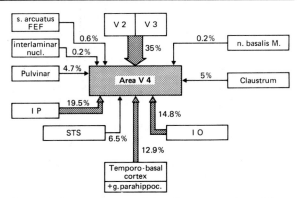

Fig. 5.5 *Schematic overview of the afferent connections of the visual area V4. IO, inferior occipital region; IP, inferior parietal lobule; STS, supratemporal sulcus region (drawn according to data published by Tanaka* et al., *1990).*

the neurones. Multimodal responses are, for example, typical for some of the superior temporal sulcus integration cortices, for area 7 neurones and for the visual vestibular integration areas located in the parieto–insular vestibular cortex (PIVC), located at the posterior end of the insula and the retroinsular region. 'Area X' (area T3) bordering on area PIVC at its posterior end also seems to be a visually dominated multimodal integration region (Fig. 5.4). Non-visual inputs to a visual association or integration area are detected either in neurophysiological recording studies or by the application of retrograde tracer techniques. Figure 5.5 illustrates the result of such a study, which was devoted to the connections of area V4 in the monkey brain, a region in which visual contours and especially chromatic signals are further elaborated. Tanaka *et al.* (1990) provided good evidence that the majority of input connections to area V4 are of non-visual origin and only about 35 per cent of the axons reaching area V4 originate in cells of the visual areas V2 and V3. According to the diagram of van Essen *et al.* (1991), area V4 also receives a direct input from the primary visual cortex.

From neurophysiological studies of the parietal areas of the awake and partially conditioned monkeys, it became evident that the activity of nerve cells depends heavily on the general arousal level of the animal, on its spatially directed or object-directed attention and perhaps also on its emotional state. So far the importance of these conditions has only been investigated marginally for most of the visual association cortices depicted in Figs 5.1–5.4. Very little detailed information is available about how the activity of neurones in the visual association areas depends on these factors.

In early studies of the physiology of visual association cortices, immobilized and anaesthetized animals were used, or at least highly sedated ones. These experimental procedures seem to reduce the non-visual input much more than the afferent visual signal flow, and one gains the impression that a 'skeleton' of visual data processing at best is preserved. In the following we will illustrate the function of the visual association cortices in a few examples selected according to their relevance to the general topic of this Volume.

Elaboration of Contour Perception in Area V2

As Mach emphasized (Chapter 1), the second derivative of the spatial light distribution on the retina determines the outer contours of the objects visible in a natural visual world. Neuronal mechanisms elaborating on contour detection are found in the secondary visual cortex (area V2) of the primate brain. Area V2 forms a part of the cytoarchitectonic area 18 of Brodman. In man and monkeys it is located in the immediate vicinity of area V1 (Figs 5.1, 5.3 and also Fig. 2.27). In most old-world primates, this visual area is partially hidden in the lunate sulcus region (Fig. 5.2(b)). Cytochrome oxidase staining revealed an interesting pattern characterizing this visual association cortex: instead of the 'blobs' and 'interblobs' found in area V1, parallel bands extending over the whole surface of area V2 appear in cytochrome–oxidase–stained brain slices. These bands are oriented perpendicularly to the cortical surface, whereby a more or less regular alternation of 'thick dense', 'thin dense' and 'pale' bands become visible in tangential sections. The spatial periodicity of these bands is coarser than in area V1 (4 to 4.5 mm; e.g. Tootell *et al.*, 1985). As Livingstone and Hubel (1987, 1988) emphasized, the main afferent visual input to area V2 originates in area V1. As in many cortico–cortical connections, the majority of afferent visual fibres projecting from area V1 to area V2 terminate in the upper half of layer IV and in the lower part of layer III with minor collaterals to layer V (Rockland and Virga, 1990).

A fairly regular projection of the different layers, 'blob' regions and 'interblob' regions, of area V1 onto the thick, thin and pale bands of area V2 was found (Fig. 4.3): the V1 neurones of layer IVB project to the thick dark stripes, where neurones were found to be particularly sensitive to stereoscopic stimulus conditions and responding in a manner akin to the three stereoscopic neuronal classes described for area V1 above (Fig. 4.9).

The majority of the thin dark stripes ('thin dense bands') contain nerve cells which respond to chromatic stimuli in a rather selective manner. These cells receive their main input signals from area V1 layer III neurones of the 'blob' regions. They seem to elaborate on chromatic signals, which will be discussed in detail in the following paragraph. The 'interblob' regions of layers II and III of area V1 project to the pale thin stripes of area V2. Within these stripes, nerve cells dominate which are characterized by strong orientation tuning and a rather limited size for optimally oriented light–dark bars, indicating a selective spatial frequency tuning, which can be interpreted as a first step to texture recognition and a further step to contour detection by neuronal networks. The cells found in the thin pale stripes seem to be insensitive to the chromatic properties of the stimuli. Within the pale thin stripes of area V2, as in area V1, orientation columns do exist, as recent studies applying the 2-deoxy-D-glucose method by Tootle and Hamilton (1989) have indicated.

Comparing the size of the excitatory receptive fields (ERF) of area V1 and V2 nerve cells, one gains the impression that the ERFs of area V2 neurones are at least two to three times larger than those of area V1 neurones and have their receptive field in the same part of the visual field. Correspondingly, the visual topography by which the contralateral visual hemifield is represented in area V2 is coarser than that of V1 (e.g. Rosa *et al.*, 1988), but the general rules for the retinotopic map remain similar to those of area V1. In this structure, as in area V2, the average ERF size increases with eccentricity and correspondingly the retino–cortical magnification factor decreases (van Essen and Zeki, 1978; van Essen *et al.*, 1986).

Subjective Contours

A further understanding of processing contour signals in area V2 stems from studies with so–called 'subjective contours', as illustrated in Fig. 5.6 (von der Heydt *et al.*, 1984; von der Heydt and Peterhans, 1989a, b; Baumgartner, 1990; Peterhans and von der Heydt, 1991). Orientation-tuned nerve cells located in area V1 do not respond to illusionary contours, while nerve cells from area V2, which clearly exhibit orientation tuning to 'real' contrast borders, also respond to patterns generating in man the perception of illusionary contours, as illustrated in Fig. 5.6. Not surprisingly, however, the neuronal response is weaker than that to real contours. This corresponds to the reduced precision of a subjective contour (Fig. 5.7). Illusionary contours are subject to certain rules in order to be optimally perceived, and the same is true for responses of area V2 orientation-tuned nerve cells when patterns evoking illusionary contours are used as stimuli. For example, the responses obtained in an area V2 nerve cell, the RF of which was stimulated by an illusionary contour as shown in Fig. 5.6(b) or (c), increased in activity with the number of line-ends meeting each other. A maximum neuronal response was obtained with about 10 line-ends (Fig. 5.8; von der Heydt and Peterhans, 1989a). This finding correlates very well with the maximum apparent border illusion

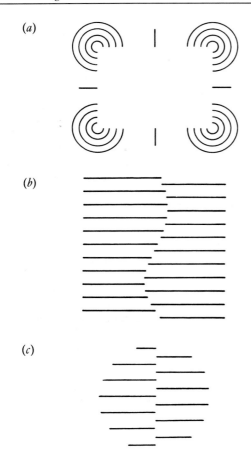

(a)

(b)

(c)

Fig. 5.6 *(a)-(c) Illustration of three different types of illusionary contour as published by Kanizsa (1979). ((a): from Varin, 1971).*

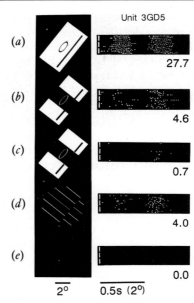

Fig. 5.7 *Responses of an orientation-tuned area V2 nerve cell to a black bar moving through the ERF (a) and a pattern creating an illusionary black bar across the gap (b). The neuronal response disappeared when the bar illusion had disappeared (c). (d) Response to a pattern generating an illusionary contour; movement direction was perpendicular to the illusionary contour. (e) Spontaneous activity was zero (from von der Heydt and Peterhans, 1989, by permission of Elsevier).*

which a human observer can attain with that type of pattern (Petry and Meyer, 1987).

Peterhans and von der Heydt (1991) provided logical schemes of how contour perception is elaborated upon by the neuronal networks of area V2. They postulated two mechanisms acting in the network of orientation-tuned neurones located in the thin pale stripe regions of area V2: a first process detecting 'real' contrast borders and a second one elaborating on pattern discontinuity. As with real contours, the patterns generating subjective contours also altered their efficiency in activating orientation-tuned neurones when the pattern was brought into such a position that the subjective contour deviated from the direction of optimal orientation sensitivity of the cortical neurone investigated.

Subjective contours are sometimes also called 'cognitive', suggesting a man-specific mechanism. Since cats also perceive subjective contours of the type shown in Fig.

5.6 and can be conditioned to recognize them (Bravo *et al.*, 1988), subjective contours are certainly not a man-specific phenomenon. Baumgartner (1990) summarized the conclusions drawn by the findings of the Zürich laboratory as follows:

Illusionary figures were often considered of cognitive origin and hence called cognitive figures. They were thought to be the result of a judgement of the visual input based on likelihood. Our findings show, however, that they are a consequence of the inherent organization of the system, which modifies the incoming information and generates perceptive values of its own. In evolution, this may have resulted for reasons of neuronal economy. An illusionary contour corresponds in nature mostly to an overlapping object and is so generated including its associated features as field contrast and depth, by a minimum of neuronal activity . . . .

The response of area V2 orientation-tuned neurones to patterns generating illusionary contours is a clear sign of a more elaborate visual data processing in area V2 as compared with area V1. The neurophysiological findings described in this section are in our opinion an indication that further studies of agnosic or non-agnosic occipital brain-lesioned patients should use patterns leading to illusionary contours as stimuli. It is expected that the outcome

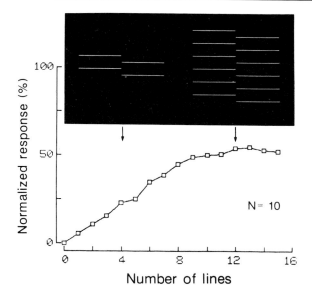

Fig. 5.8 *The subjective strength of an illusionary contour increases with the number of stripes generating the contour pattern (upper part). The same is true for the average activity of area V2, orientation-tuned nerve cells: the activity (normalized relative to real contour) increases with the number of lines in the pattern (from von der Heydt and Peterhans, 1989, by permission of the Society for Neuroscience).*

of these experiments will differentiate the mechanisms related to the occipito-temporal object recognition system and the occipito-parietal visual space recognition system.

Cerebral Neuronal Mechanisms of Colour Perception

As mentioned above, colour-specific signals reach area V1 by means of three main 'channels' related to the parvocellular pathway from the retina to the visual cortex. This is schematically illustrated in Fig. 5.9: The three different 'cone-images' are transformed by steps into a 'double-opponent' red–green, blue–yellow and black–white system. 'Double opponency' means that not only the receptive field centre but also the receptive field periphery exhibit opponent responses with regard to the chromatic composition of the stimulus. A typical cortical red–green neurone is for example activated by long-wavelength stimuli in the RF centre and inhibited by a medium- or short-wavelength stimulus. Chromatic stimulation of the RF periphery evokes just the opposite response: light stimuli in the medium-wavelength range lead to an excita-

tion and long-wavelength stimuli to an inhibition. Colour-specific neuronal data processing is attributed predominantly to layer II and III neurones in the blob regions of area V1. These neurones project to the 'thin dark stripes' of area V2 (Fig. 4.3). Nerve cells located in the thin stripes of area V2 are not sensitive to orientation of a contrast border and about 50 per cent are wavelength-selective, the other neurones presumably belong to a system sensitive to greys of different shades. Orientation-tuned cells in area V2 are found predominantly in the thick dense stripes and are for the most part not wavelength-selective (DeYoe and van Essen, 1985; Shipp and Zeki, 1985; Hubel and Livingstone, 1987, 1989).

According to Zeki (1973, 1977, 1983a) and Desimone and Schein (1987), a further, rather complex, colour-specific, data processing occurs in area V4 (Figs 5.1–5.4): this part of the occipital cortex receives projections from the thin stripes of area V2 as well as a direct input from the blob regions of area V1 (Fig. 5.9). Area V4 constitutes, besides areas V2 and VP, the main input structure to the visual integration areas of the inferior temporal lobe. For man we assume that on the basis of clinical observations, area V4 has in addition a direct or indirect input to the limbic system, in particular to the gyrus parahippocampalis, which is located in man in the vicinity of area V4. Owing to the shift of the striate cortex during phylogenesis of the hominid brain from the outer surface of the occipital lobe to the mesial surface, the extrastriate visual cortices have also been rotated in part around the occipital pole of the brain and therefore occupy a portion of the lower and inner surface of the mesial occipital lobe (cf. Fig. 2.27).

In addition to neurones sensitive to the chromatic properties of the stimulus, area V4 contains many cells selective for stimulus orientation, whereby the orientation selectivity was less pronounced than in corresponding cells of area V1 (Desimone and Schein, 1987). In this study, a considerable number of area V4 neurones were also found to be selective for direction of motion. The majority of neurones in area V4 were sensitive to the shape, i.e. the length and/or width, of simple visual stimuli like bars, and in addition, many of the cells were tuned to certain spatial frequencies when sinewave gratings were applied as stimuli. Since area V4 receives a strong input from the thick stripes of area V2, it seems fairly probable that in the cells not selective for colours, the chromatic properties of a stimulus are integrated in a system which elaborates on contour and shape. This would seem to be fairly meaningful, since the different surface colours of objects certainly help us to discriminate one from another and from their background (cf. Chapter 20). There is now converging evidence from several studies (for a discussion see Zeki, 1990) that some area V4 neurones exhibit an overlapping sensitivity to spatial and chromatic properties of the visual stimulus patterns. Systematic work related to oriented

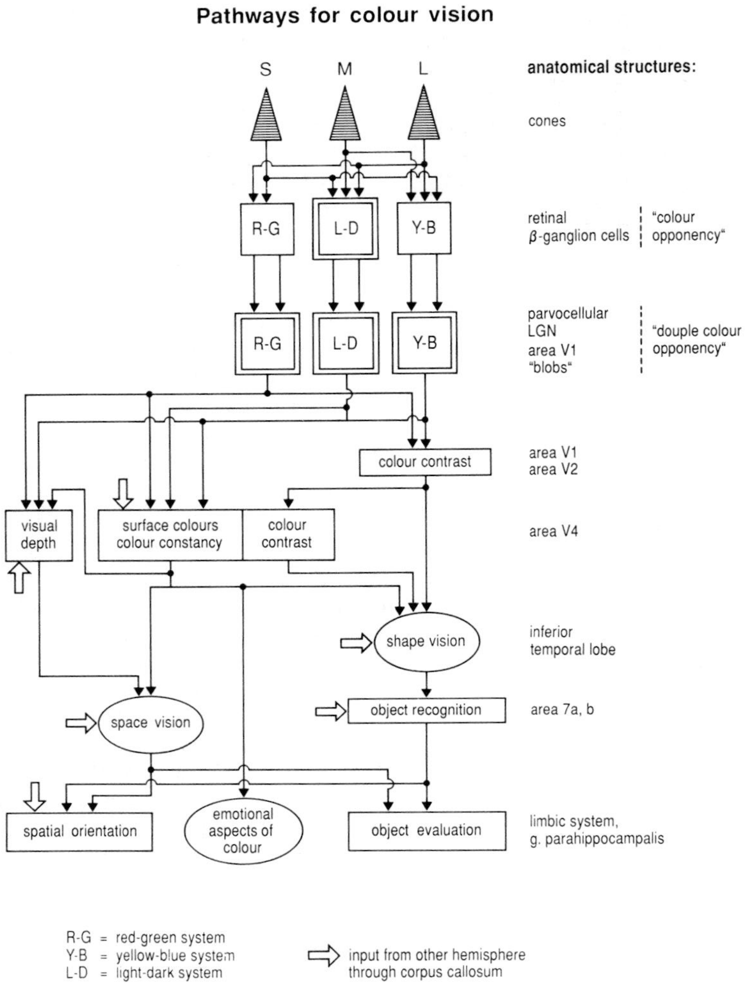

Pathways for colour vision

Fig. 5.9 *Schematic drawing of the different stages of colour processing in the peripheral and central visual system.*

chromatic borders, as has been done with black–white borders for area V1 and V2 neurones, is still lacking.

Most interesting and highly relevant for the interpretation of cerebral achromatopsia (cf. Chapter 20) are the findings regarding a further transformation of the cerebral colour signals performed by some of the area V4 neurones. First of all, we have to mention that a somewhat fuzzy retinotopic organization is still present in area V4, but in contrast to the retinotopic organization of its two main input regions, areas V1 and V2, several modifications were noted:

1. Only about 30 degrees of visual angle related to the contralateral visual hemifield seem to be represented in area V4. The retinotopic projection is precise enough, however, to predict a loss of colour vision in only part of

the visual field with small circumscribed lesions of area V4. Clinical observations confirm this view (Chapter 20).

2. In the foveal and parafoveal regions of area V4, a retino–cortical map extends about 5 degrees into the ipsilateral visual field. This extension is due to a strong transcallosal projection from area V4 of the contralateral hemisphere. Since these transcallosal connections seem to be the only input of area V4 related to the ipsilateral visual field, a complete unilateral lesion of area V4 should still lead to loss of all colour vision in one hemifield (hemi-achromatopsia, cf. Chapter 20).

3. When penetrating area V4 with the microelectrode perpendicular to the cortical surface, a columnar organization with respect to receptive field locations was found: one small region of area V4 'looks' to the same part of the

visual field. The size of the ERFs is considerably larger, however, compared with areas V1 and V2 at corresponding retinal eccentricities.

4. A systematic exploration of area V4 neuronal responses revealed that parcellation and segregation of visual functions also characterizes this visual association cortex: colour-sensitive neurones, frequently of the same type of colour selectivity, are organized in patches or columns. Other patches of this cortical region contain neurones which are sensitive to shape and contours.

5. Zeki reported on an interesting 'new' property found in some of the colour-selective nerve cells of area V4. Their activity was found to be related to the spectral reflectance of the object surfaces and not to the composition of the wavelength illuminating the respective receptive field. For example, when a human observer judges the colour of a certain particle of a complex multi-coloured pattern as being 'red', a 'red neurone' of this subclass of area V4 nerve cells is activated irrespective of the spectral composition of the light falling onto the receptive field. This spectral composition is the product of the spectral reflectance of the object surface and the wavelength composition of the illuminating light. Perception of surface colours, irrespective of the spectral composition of the illuminating light, is called 'colour constancy'. Colour constancy indicates that within the neuronal structures involved a 'long-range' integration process regarding the chromatic composition of a region is performed. At the level of a single V4 neurone, this means that a long-range neuronal integration in a visual area surrounding the respective ERF has occurred. Such an operation may be akin to what Land (1977) postulated from observations in psychophysics of colour perception. His subjects viewed a multi-coloured, two-dimensional stimulus pattern (a 'Mondrian pattern'), whereby the chromatic composition of the illuminating light was changed systematically. Land found colour constancy and explained it by assuming an integration of colour contrast processes occurring across the whole visual pattern. He attributed colour constancy to a long-range process effective within a large variability of chromaticity changes of the illuminating light. In Land's experiments at least for selected particles of the Mondrian pattern, the perceived chroma (corresponding to the surface of an object in the natural world) remained constant over a wide variety of chromatic illumination. As Zeki had found, selected neurones in area V4 responded similarly within a certain range, independent of the chromatic composition of the illuminating light, and coded the surface colour of the particle in the Mondrian pattern. It is therefore plausible that some area V4 neurones do indeed perform the necessary operation for attaining colour constancy by integrating the chromatic composition and chromatic contrast borders across a large part of the visual field. Since colour constancy as measured in a multi-

particle Mondrian pattern (Land, 1974) has considerable restrictions (O.-J. Grüsser and T. Caelli, unpublished 1985), one can expect that the same will be true for the 'selective' colour units of area V4.

6. As mentioned above, area V4 neurones have their receptive field near the fovea and frequently extend their excitatory receptive field into the ipsilateral visual hemifield. Chromatic stimuli contribute to depth perception and are also evaluated for binocular stereovision. Therefore it would be interesting to explore area V4 neurones with respect to binocular interaction, stereo vision and depth perception in further studies.

7. Finally it should be mentioned that Zeki (1990) in his recent review assumes that the 'visual area 4 complex' is functionally subdivided. Using visual field projection as a criterion, he found that an independent 'area V4a' exists as a region through which area V4 neurones project to the inferior temporal lobe visual integration cortices.

Neuronal Networks for Visual Motion Perception

Visual motion is an independent quality of the modality of vision. As discussed in detail in Chapter 19, visual motion is not only perceived when 'real' objects move across the extra-personal space or artificially created patterns are moving through the visual field; visual movement perception is also induced in a large variety of motion illusions ('apparent visual motion'). According to the basic rules that are believed to exist between brain activity and our perceptions (Chapter 1), one has to assume that visual movement neurones are also activated when illusionary motion is perceived. Visual movement signals are processed in a special afferent 'visual movement channel', by which at least two distinct classes of movement signals are mediated through the afferent visual system and the primary visual cortex: perception of 'local' movement and of 'global' movement. Local movement refers to a change in position of a distinct object or a local artificial pattern, while global movement under natural conditions is predominantly evoked when the gaze moves across a structured visual pattern. In our modern technical world, however, many types of global visual movement affect our visual system (cf. Chapter 19).

When one records movement-selective neurones within the visual or visuo-motor system, one should be aware that 'movement sensitivity' is not necessarily correlated with any visual movement perception. It is somewhat likely that the 'movement sensitivity' of many visual neurones is nothing other than an adaptation to the fact that the signals representing the stationary visual world in the brain are extracted from a retinal pattern, which because of eye saccades shifts across the retina every 0.18–0.6 second (cf. Chapter 1). Furthermore, many movement-selective neurones are involved in unconscious visuo-motor control, as in visual pursuit by eye and gaze movements in reflex saccades, in reflective visually guided stabilization of body position and in visually guided grasping (see Volume 8). In the following we will discuss, however, predominantly movement-selective neuronal responses, related presumably to the conscious perception of visual motion.

The segregation and parcellation within the afferent visual system, which was found for the visual qualities brightness, contrast and colour, is also valid for the quality movement. The retinas of many lower vertebrates contain a large number of ganglion cells particularly sensitive to small moving objects. The different neuronal classes of the frog retina became paradigmatic in this respect (for a review see Grüsser and Grüsser-Cornehls, 1976). The primate retina presumably contains two classes of ganglion cells sensitive to visual movement: (a) the 'achromatic' α-ganglion cells, which also respond to high-contrast, light–dark borders and flicker stimuli, and (b) a subclass of γ-ganglion cells, which respond selectively to slow movement. Whether these retinal ganglion cells, which are especially sensitive to movement of low angular velocities, are also directionally selective in the primate retina (as found in the rabbit and cat retina; for a review see Collewijn, 1981) is still an open question. It is plausible to assume, however, that ganglion cells which project from the retina to the nucleus of the optic tract (cf. Chapter 3) belong also in the primates to the γ-system and are, as in the rabbit retina, direction-selective. Primate NOT neurones exhibit a distinct horizontal directional selectivity corresponding to similar behaviour in lower mammals. The γ-ganglion cells of the primate retina also project to the LGN, but little is known about their functional role. So far, no movement-selective reponses were reported from the primate LGN, but the frequency transfer properties of the fast magnocellular on-centre and off-centre neurones make this class of nerve cells especially sensitive, of course, to stimuli moving at a higher speed across the receptive field. Hereby the optimum stimulus velocity activating a retinal ganglion cell or LGN nerve cell depends, as in the cat retina and LGN, on the RF diameter, stimulus contrast and stimulus size. Optimum angular velocities usually are in a range between 50 and 150 deg s^{-1} (for a review see: Grüsser and Grüsser-Cornehls, 1973).

Movement sensitivity and directional selectivity are frequently found in the responses of neurones of the primary visual cortex, whereby a considerable portion of orientation-selective neurones responded best when a contrast border was moved through the receptive field along a path oriented perpendicularly to the movement direction (cf. Fig. 4.5). The segregation of 'true' movement selectivity occurs within the primary visual cortex by a class of neurones located in layer IVB, which receives a predominantly magnocellular input from the lateral geniculate nucleus and has axonal projections to an area usually called MT ('middle temporal visual area', area V5 of Zeki, 1975). Lund et al. (1975), injecting horseradish peroxidase into small regions of area MT, found V1 nerve cells labelled in layer IVB and the upper part of layer VI. It is to date well established that the velocity-tuned nerve cells of area V1 constitute the main input to the movement-selective area MT, whereby the axons from area V1 form terminals predominantly in layer IV of area MT. A second input to MT originates in area V2. Due to the large number of movement-selective nerve cells in area MT, one has to assume that a movement-selective input from area V2 is also evaluated in area MT and integrated into visual motion information. In anaesthetized monkeys, 80–90 per cent of area MT nerve cells exhibit clear movement selectivity and most of them are also directionally selective (Zeki, 1974; Maunsell and van Essen, 1983,a, b, c; Albright, 1984; Komatsi and Wurtz, 1989).

The central role of area MT in visual movement perception is confirmed by experimental lesions of this area. Visual pursuit movements and optokinetic nystagmus are seriously impaired following chemical lesions of area MT (Dürsteler and Wurtz, 1988; Dürsteler et al., 1987). Discrimination of movement direction is also abolished by lesions of area MT (Newsome and Paré, 1988). Electrical stimulation of the MT foveal projection region led to a modification of trained eye pursuit movements in macaque monkeys. Stimulation during pursuit was accompanied by an increase in eye speed towards the side ipsilateral to the stimulated cortex and a decrease in pursuit velocity towards the contralateral side (Komatsu and Wurtz, 1989).

Area MT exhibits a retinotopic organization. Its cortical extension is not very large – 16 mm^2 or about 7 per cent of the area V1 in macaque monkeys (Weller and Kaas, 1983). The contralateral visual hemifield is represented in a somewhat loose retinotopic order, where the receptive fields are much larger in size than the corresponding ones in area V1. Myeloarchitectonic and cytoarchitectonic properties together allow a discrimination of area MT from the areas bordering it (Ungerleider and Mishkin, 1979; van Essen et al., 1981; Gattass and Gross, 1981).

The output of area MT is directed mainly towards the adjacent medial superior temporal area MST and to area FST (Figs 5.4 and 5.10). The parallel access of movement-selective visual signals to area MT, originating in the α-ganglion cells of the retina and using the neurones in the magnocellular layers of the LGN, the layer IVB neurones of area V1 with a sidepath via area V2, is also illustrated in the response latencies of movement-selective

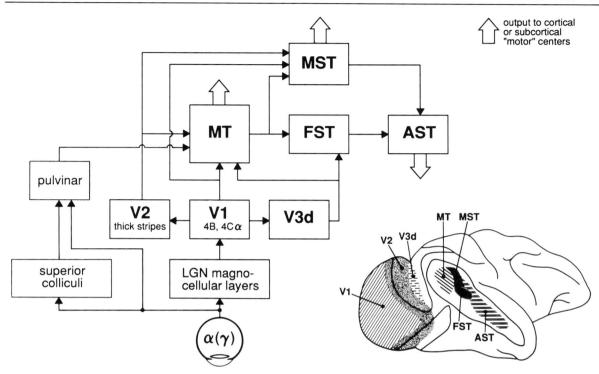

Fig. 5.10 *Schematic representation of the complex of movement-sensitive areas located around the superior temporal sulcus (MT, MST, FST and AST) and their inputs from the eye via the magnocellular layers of the lateral geniculate nucleus or via the pulvinar. For the preparation of this figure we used information concerning the areas FST and AST (anterior superior temporal region) from the laboratory of Dr L. Ungerleider, Bethesda.*

neurones located in the different structures of the visual cortex (Raigel *et al.*, 1989): in measuring the responses to light and dark slits moving at different angular velocities through the ERF, the response latencies were calculated to be 85 ms for area V1 movement-selective cells, 96 ms for area V2 movement-selective cells and 94 ms for area MT cells. If these data – obtained in anaesthetized and paralysed macaque monkeys – are applicable to the awake brain, the direct connection V1-MT plays a more important role in responses to moving stimuli than the indirect V1-V2-MT.

Area MT projects not only to higher-order cortical movement selective regions, but also to subcortical structures like the pontine gaze motor system, the NOT and the superior colliculi (Ungerleider *et al.*, 1984). In extensive studies it was demonstrated that area MT-neurones respond not only selectively to movement and movement direction, but cover a large range of velocities, being tuned neurone by neurone to different maximum angular velocities (Maunsell and van Essen, 1983; for further literature see Orban, Volume 4, Chapter 8). Rodman and Albright (1987) studied the interaction of the movement direction and the angular velocity of the moving stimulus. For a

given cell, the shape of the directional tuning curve was similar at different stimulus speeds, indicating a reasonable invariance of directional selectivity. When studying the invariance for the angular velocity tuning curves, Rodman and Albright discriminated two classes of movement-sensitive neurones according to the responses when the stimulus was moved in the non-preferred direction: 'S1 neurones' responded only in certain speed ranges with an inhibition of spontaneous activity when the stimulus was moved in the 'non-preferred' direction through the ERF (Fig. 5.11). This non-preferred direction (or 'anti-preferred' direction) was, as a rule, 180 degrees away from the optimum movement direction but some of the MT neurones evidently had two preferred directions about 180 degrees apart and a non-preferred direction shifted by 90 degrees (S1b neurone of Fig. 5.12). Rodman and Albright named those cells S2 neurones which responded in a wide velocity range with an inhibition, provided the stimulus was moving across the ERF in the non-preferred direction. The optimum velocities found for different MT ganglion cells were very variable. Figure 5.12 illustrates how direction and speed of the stimuli (photopic adaptation level, moving light slit oriented per-

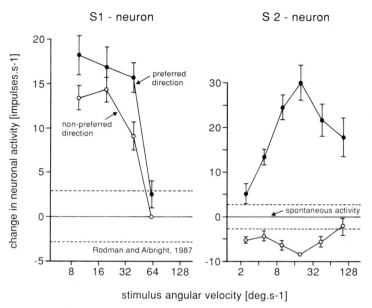

Fig. 5.11 *Two examples of velocity-tuning curves obtained in macaque area MT nerve cells. The type S1-neurone velocity tuning curves were parallel for the preferred and the non-preferred direction, but activation evoked by movement into the non-preferred direction was lower. For the type S2-neurone stimulus movement in the preferred direction led to a velocity tuning curve with a maximum activation at an anglular velocity of about 20 [deg s⁻¹]. The inhibition evoked by movement of the stimulus through the ERF in the non-preferred direction mirrored the velocity tuning curve found for movement in the preferred direction (from Rodman and Albright, 1987; modified).*

pendicularly to the movement direction) interacted with each other in three selected neurones.

In addition to the pathways from the retina via area V1 to area MT mentioned above, another visual input is present in area MT neurones: the retina projects directly or via the superior colliculi to the pulvinar and from there to MT (Cragg and Ainsworth, 1969; Ungerleider and Mishkin, 1979; Maunsell and van Essen, 1983; Standage and Benevento, 1983). The connections between MT and a crescent-shaped region of the pulvinar including the inferior and the lateral pulvinar presumably have reciprocal connections with area MT (Standage and Benevento, 1983). Further experimental work is needed to evaluate the impact of the retino–tecto–pulvinar pathway on the responses of area MT neurones.

To understand the function of area MT neurones, microelectrode data from MT nerve cells were compared with psychophysical data on movement perception in man (Newsome *et al.*, 1984). In addition to MT cells, area V1 nerve cells were selected for comparison, which exhibited movement sensitivity and directional selectivity. Their responses to phi movement were tested. Small rectangular slits of light, 2 or 3 degrees in length, were flashed while moving across the ERF. The rate of the stroboscopic

flashes and the speed of the stimulus movement across the ERF were varied. Thus the spatial intervals between the successively presented slits could be varied between 0.01 and 10.2 degrees. The responses to this apparent phi movement were compared with the responses to real movement. When the displacement speed of a stimulus was increased, directional selectivity was found to be lost beyond a certain value. This finding corresponded to similar observations made by Grüsser and Grüsser-Cornehls (1973) in movement and direction-selective nerve cells of the cat visual association areas (Fig. 5.13). Newsome *et al.* used the disappearance of directional selectivity to phi movement as a threshold criterion and plotted this 'critical spatial interval', as found in the responses of MT and V1 neurones, as a function of angular velocity. These data were compared with the psychophysical performance of five human observers and a fairly good overlap was established (Fig. 5.14). This study fulfilled one of the requirements for proving that a certain neurone is, with a high probability, part of a visual movement-coding system: The correspondence between phi data of area MT neurones and the perceptions of a human observer in a similar task supports the view that area MT activity is correlated with perceived local visual motion.

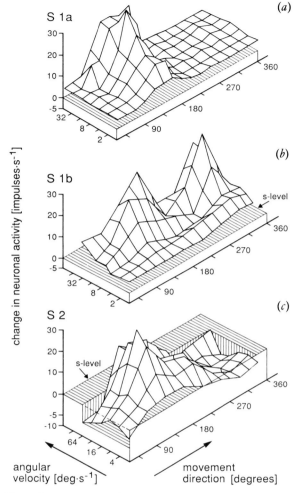

Fig. 5.12 *The activity of area MT nerve cells depended on the speed of the stimulus moving through the ERF and the direction of that movement. In the S1a nerve cell (a) preferred and non-preferred direction (null-direction) were 180 degrees apart. In the S1b nerve cell (b) the non-preferred direction was shifted 90 degrees from the preferred direction. This circumstance led to the two peaks shown in this diagram. In both S1a and S1b nerve cells, movement in the non-preferred direction did not lead to an inhibition of the neuronal activity below spontaneous level (grey plane). This was not the case for the S2 nerve cell (c): the movement in the preferred direction led to a movement in the non-preferred direction, which was 180 degrees from the preferred direction, causing an inhibition of the spontaneous activity (from Rodman and Albright, 1987; modified).*

In an extensive review on the relationship between the activity of single neurones in area MT and the perception of visual motion, Newsome *et al.* (1989) applied another experimental paradigm to correlate neuronal activity and psychophysical data. Their visual stimuli were dynamic random dot patterns in which a certain proportion of the dots were in coherent motion while spatially dispersed irregularly moving dots (random noise) were added. With this stimulus, two limiting conditions existed: complete coherent motion and complete random motion (Fig. 5.15). A forced-choice psychophysical procedure was used to measure the threshold values (coherent/incoherent motion) at which the monkeys could successfully detect the direction of the coherently moving dots. Simultaneously, single units in area MT were recorded and their preferred direction was determined. Thereafter the stimulus field with the random dot pattern (Fig. 5.15) was centred to the ERF centre and the size of the stimulus field aperture was adjusted approximately to the size of the ERF. The neuronal and psychophysical sensitivity in this task was compared (Fig. 5.16). As expected, at coherent motion of more than 10 per cent of the dots, area MT neurones indeed responded with a significant increase in neuronal activity when the coherent dots were moving in the preferred direction. A corresponding decrease in neuronal activity was observed when the coherent spots moved in the non-preferred direction. The bias between the responses to preferred and non-preferred direction increased considerably with coherence increase (Fig. 5.16). The performance of the monkey discovering correctly the coherent motion transgressed chance level at about 2 per cent movement coherence, and reached more than 90 per cent correct performance when about 10 per cent coherence of the moving dots was present. Newsome *et al.* (1989) concluded from their data that they had indeed identified the neurones providing the critical signals for the perceptual decision in the psychophysical task and that area MT is necessary in performing psychophysical tasks of the type applied.

In summary, one can conclude that area MT is indeed a crucial region in processing signals on local movement occurring in the visual field. Here the following properties of neuronal reponses are especially notable:

1. MT nerve cells respond to moving stimuli and are activated mainly by signals originating from the fast magnocellular input relayed through layer IVB of area V1. The indirect input via area V1–area V2 may exert a modifying effect, and the same is true for the retino-tecto-pulvinar signals reaching area MT.

2. The excitatory receptive fields of movement-sensitive neurones of area MT are larger than the corresponding receptive fields of area V1, but ERF size is still small enough (several degrees up to 15 degrees) to support the interpretation that MT neurones process local movement signals primarily.

3. All MT neurones are directionally selective, whereby the preferred direction and the non-preferred

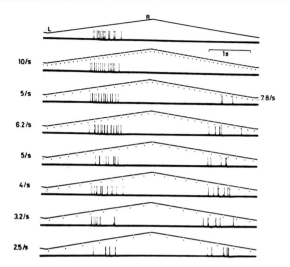

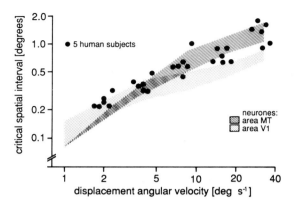

Fig. 5.13 *Activity of a movement-sensitive and directionally selective neurone recorded from the medial suprasylvian cortex of the cat (encephale isolé preparation). Responses to a round spot of light of 2.8 degrees diameter moving across the ERF in the preferred and in the null direction (amplitude of movement 22 degrees, angular velocity 9 deg s^{-1}). Action potentials appeared only when the spot moved in the preferred direction (upper row). The same was true for phi movement (next seven rows). The stimulus was intermittently flashed (15 ms flash duration). At a stimulus frequency below 8 flashes s^{-1} the directional selectivity of this neurone disappeared and it responded to movement in both directions. At a flash frequency below 4 flashes s^{-1} the responses elicited by the apparently moving phi stimuli were about the same for both movement directions (from Grüsser and Grüsser-Cornehls, 1973).*

Fig. 5.14 *Results from experiments with phi-movement stimuli in macaque monkeys: recordings from area MT and area V1. The apparent speed of the stroboscopically illuminated stimulus and the flash frequency were varied. The spatial interval between flashes (ordinate) could thus vary between 0.01 and 10.2 degrees. In every neurone, the spatial interval was determined at which the neurone failed to give directionally selective responses to the phi-movement stimuli at a given angular velocity (abscissa). The hatched area indicates the range of spatial intervals at which MT neurones, on the average, lost directional selectivity (above the envelope). The stippled region illustrates the same conditions for macaque area V1 neurones. The dots illustrate the maximum spatial interval for the perception of apparent phi motion as found in 5 human observers (from Newsome et al., 1986; redrawn).*

direction (null direction) are usually 180 degrees apart.

4. The neurones are velocity tuned, whereby optimum stimulus speed varies from neurone to neurone and depends evidently on the size of the receptive field and on retinal eccentricity of the ERF.

5. Area MT neurones also respond to apparent phi movement.

6. Randomly distributed moving stimuli masked the responses to coherent motion stimulation, but the sensitivity to coherent random dot movement was surprisingly high. A good correlation between simultaneously measured neuronal activity and psychophysical responses in the monkey supports area MT as being crucial for local movement detection.

7. Area MT neurones respond best to optimally oriented, small stimuli moving across the receptive field in the preferred direction at optimum velocity. When stimuli are applied extending the excitatory receptive field, a reduced neuronal response is observed, indicating a large spread of lateral inhibitory mechanisms.

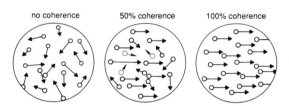

Fig. 5.15 *Illustration of the experimental paradigm applied by Newsome et al. (1989) in experiments leading to the results shown in Fig. 5.16. The stimulus was a dynamic random dot pattern in which a certain proportion of the dots moved coherently (here illustrated for horizontal coherent motion). Complete random motion is shown on the left side, complete coherent motion on the right and a partially coherent motion is illustrated in the middle of the figure. Coherent movement of the dots meant movement in the same direction with the same speed. For the random incoherent movement the dots were moved in different directions and at different speeds. The arrows illustrate speed vector.*

8. Area MT neurones project to other cortical movement-selective regions, especially areas MST, FST and VIP, and to the frontal eye field. These regions form reciprocal connections with area MT. Such connections

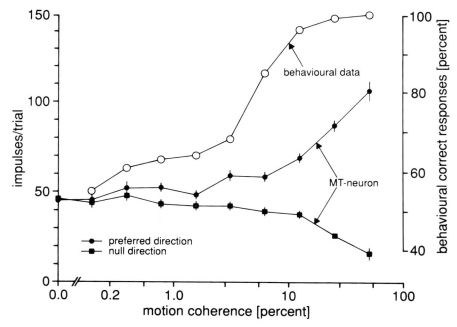

Fig. 5.16 *Example of responses obtained in a directionally selective nerve cell of macaque area MT with a stimulus pattern as illustrated in Fig. 5.15. With increasing coherency of the moving dots (abscissa) the MT neurone responded with an increase in activity when the coherent dots were moved in the preferred direction and with an inhibition when the coherent dots moved in the non-preferred direction (null direction). This directional selectivity increased with coherence. Measurements of neuronal activity were made during behavioural responses of the monkey, which had to decide in which direction the coherent spots moved. The monkey exceeded chance level (50 per cent) in deciding on coherent motion when the coherence was larger than 1–2 per cent and reached performance values above 90 per cent at a coherence of about 15 per cent. Ordinate for the behavioural data is on the right side of the graph for the neuronal data on the left (from Newsome* et al., *1989; redrawn).*

also exist between area MT and subcortical structures like the pulvinar, the superior colliculi, the pontine gaze motor centres and the nucleus of the optic tract.

From 'Local' to 'Global' Movement

Area MT projects to area MST, where the receptive field diameters of the nerve cells increase considerably. Projections to FST from MT and indirect projections via MST to FST and from there to area AST (Fig. 5.10) indicate that a complex neuronal structure exists along the upper bank of the superior temporal sulcus of the monkey brain in which further elaboration on visual movement signals seems to be the main task of the neuronal networks:

1. Local rotatory movement is discriminated from local translatory movement (MST).

2. Global but no longer local visual movement activates some of the neurones in FST, a neuronal response pattern observed for the 'vestibular' regions of the PIVC (Figs. 5.3 and 5.4).

3. Parallax movement is most likely evaluated.

4. Discrimination between visual movement in different directions is one of the neuronal tasks of these higher-order, visual, movement-selective brain regions.

5. Efference copy signals related to these motor signals are probably evaluated in areas MST and FST, leading to different responses evoked by retinal movement signals when the shift of the image across the retina was caused by active eye or gaze movements or by 'passive' large-field motion in the extrapersonal space.

6. Presumably an integration of 'afferent' visual motion signals (caused by a shift in the stimulus pattern across the retina) and 'efferent' visual motion, which is represented by efference copy signals of gaze-motor commands, may also be attributed to these higher-order visual movement areas.

Since a detailed description of these problems is beyond the scope of this Volume, the reader is referred elsewhere in this series (Volumes 4 and 8).

6 The Posterior Parietal Lobe and the Cerebral Representation of the Extra-personal Visual Space

Introduction

As will be elaborated in Chapters 21 and 22, the posterior parietal lobe plays a key role in visual spatial orientation. Some of the symptoms observable after posterior parietal lobe lesions are understandable in the light of modern neurophysiological data obtained by single unit recordings from the primate inferior parietal lobule. Other symptoms observed in patients suffering from parietal lobe lesions such as constructional apraxia, alexia, agraphia or acalculia, however, are man-specific deficits, correlated with the dysfunction of parietal lobe brain stuctures which developed during hominid brain evolution. In the following we will concentrate on the description of neuronal mechanisms related to the transformation of retinotopic into spatiotopic or 'egocentric' coordinates. This transformation, which is essential for our orientation in the visual world and which we share with other primates, is for the most part a task of the inferior parietal lobules. However, we will not deal with other aspects of primate parietal lobe functions in detail, as they have been competently reviewed by Lynch (1980), Hyvärinen (1982a, b), Andersen (1987) and Stein (1989).

The Anatomical Subdivision and the Connections of the Primate Area 7

The cytoarchitectonic analysis and the investigation of the connections of the posterior parietal lobe, especially the inferior parietal lobule, have led to a subdivision of the primate areas 7 into five main structures, the areas 7a, 7b, 7ip, 7op and 7m (Fig. 6.1). This subdivision follows the

Brodmann (1907, 1909) and Vogt and Vogt (1919) tradition. Other subdivisions and notations have been proposed (e.g. von Bonin and Bailey, 1947; Pandya and Seltzer, 1982). Figure 6.2 is a highly schematic summary of the main cortico-cortical connections of areas 7a, 7b and 7ip. The posterior part of the intraparietal sulcus (area 7ip corresponding to area POa of Seltzer and Pandya, 1978, 1980) is nowadays subdivided into the more lateral intra-

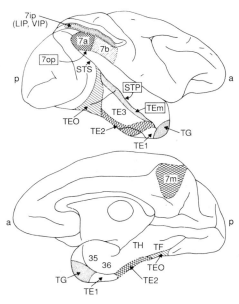

Fig. 6.1 *Schematic representation of the outer and inner surfaces of a macaque right hemisphere, illustrating the location of the different parts of area 7. The intraparietal sulcus is unfolded to display the areas 7ip. The areas LIP and VIP are contained in area 7ip. Area 7op (arrow) is hidden in the parietal operculum of the Sylvian fissure.*

92

Main ipsilateral connections of area 7a

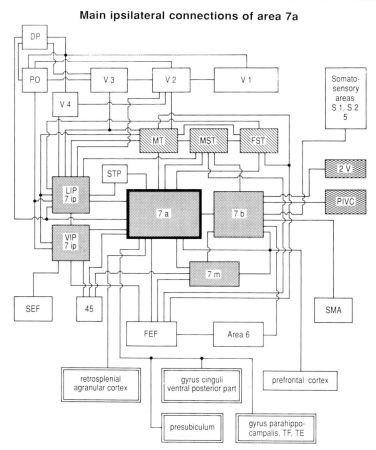

Fig. 6.2 *Schematic diagram of the connections between areas 7a, 7b, 7m and 7ip. Most of the connections drawn are bidirectional.*
Abbreviations: FEF: frontal eye field; FST: fundal superior temporal sulcus region; LIP: lateral intraparietal area; MT: medial temporal area; MST: medial superior temporal sulcus area; PIVC: parieto-insular vestibular cortex; SEF: supplementary motor eye field; SMA: supplementary motor area; STP: superior temporal polysensory area; VIP: ventral intraparietal area.

parietal area LIP and the ventral intraparietal area VIP. The connections illustrated in Fig. 6.2 are usually bidirectional and were identified by the application of antero- grade and retrograde tracer substances (Mesulam *et al.*, 1977; Seltzer and van Hoesen, 1979; Seltzer and Pandya, 1980, 1984; van Essen and Maunsell, 1983; Ungerleider and Desimone, 1986b; van Essen, 1985, 1990; Cavada and Goldman-Rakic, 1989a, b; Andersen *et al.*, 1990; Baizer *et al.*, 1991).

In addition to the ipsilateral intercortical connections of area 7 shown in Fig. 6.2, a major projection exists to the corresponding homotopic regions of the contralateral cor- tical hemisphere as well as to heterotopic areas. Bidirec- tional thalamo–cortical connections of area 7 were found, whereby various nuclei of the pulvinar complex including the lateral posterior thalamic nucleus were the main tar-

gets. The lateral and the inferior pulvinar relay retinoto- pically organized visual signals predominantly to area 7a. The medial pulvinar, however, is connected with the visuo–motor layers of the superior colliculi (Benevento and Standage, 1983) and has its main interconnections also with area 7a. The oral pulvinar, believed to be a soma- tosensory relay, ultimately projects to area 7b. The rather complex connections in the scheme of Fig. 6.2 are never- theless a simplification. Considering some of the physiolo- gical findings, one can postulate the following gross rules for a functional interpretation of these anatomical connec- tions, which are nearly always bidirectional:

1. Areas 7a and 7ip (LIP, VIP) of the monkey cortex have more visual and visuo–motor connections than soma- tosensory connections, while the reverse is true for area 7b,

which receives a strong somatosensory input from the somatosensory areas S1 and S2 and the parietal somatosensory association area 5.

2. The vestibular cortices (area 2v and the parieto-insular vestibular cortex PIVC) are connected with areas 7b and 7op and not directly with area 7a or 7ip.

3. In contrast, the visual cortical areas in which the contralateral visual hemifield is represented (V1, V2, V3, V4, PO) have a strong input to area 7ip but fewer direct connections to area 7a. The peripheral part of the visual field seems to have a stronger input to area 7ip than the foveal part.

4. The cortical regions processing visual motion information (MT, MST, FST, cf. Chapter 5) have bidirectional connections with areas 7ip and 7a. Functionally, these motion-processing cortical regions are parts of the posterior parietal lobe system, i.e. they are a part of the cortical structures representing the extra-personal space. The same principle to be discussed for area 7a neurones applies to neurones of MT, MST and FST: with the level of visual data processing, i.e. processing of visual movement in the extra-personal space, the retinotopic representation is lost and a spatiotopic one is established instead. Since the perceived depth of the extra-personal space depends on parallax movement, the close connections between the movement-sensitive regions along the superior temporal sulcus with area 7a are functionally understandable.

5. The frontal eye field is connected with areas 7a and 7ip and not with area 7b, which, however, has connections to the prefrontal area 6, a brain region involved in visually guided grasping.

6. Extended connections exist between area 7a and the other subfields of area 7. Thus area 7a plays an important role in integrating the incoming signals from other brain regions which enter different subfields of area 7, as illustrated in Fig. 6.2.

7. Extended connections exist between areas 7a and 7ip and some limbic structures like the agranular retrosplenial cortex, the ventral posterior part of the gyrus cinguli, the presubiculum and the gyrus parahippocampalis (e.g. Mesulam *et al.*, 1977; Cavada and Goldman-Rakic, 1989a). These limbic connections of area 7a and 7ip may be important for space-related functions guiding visual attention according to internal needs or drives. On the other hand, connections between area 7 and the limbic system may also provide input to limbic structures in which the spatiotopic representation of the actual percept of the visual world interacts with the stored spatial maps of early experience which are necessary for topographic memory.

8. The projections of areas 7a, 7b, 7m and 7ip to prefrontal regions are fairly widespread, but each of the area 7 subdivisions seems to have its own 'sectors' inside the prefrontal and premotor cortical regions to which it is connected. Within these prefrontal sectors only a small overlap exists of the projections related to the various area 7 subdivisions. The premotor regions of the frontal cortex connected with the subdivisions of area 7 are the supplementary motor area (SMA), the supplementary motor eye field (SEF) and the frontal eye field (Cavada and Goldman-Rakic, 1989b; Andersen *et al.*, 1990). Thus the inferior parietal lobule forms a relay between prefrontal and limbic structures which are only partly directly connected with each other (Fig. 6.2).

9. The functional homologies of the posterior parietal cortical regions in man and monkey are not easy to determine, since the posterior parietal cortex extended considerably during hominid phylogenesis. There are some arguments that in the human brain the areas 5 and 7 are homologous to the superior parietal lobule of the monkey, i.e. the primate areas 5a and 5b. Areas 7a and 7b, located in the inferior parietal lobule, are believed to have their homologues in areas 39 and 40 of the human parietal cortex (von Bonin and Bailey, 1947; for a discussion see Stein, 1989). We have some doubts about these homologies, because according to the comparative cytoarchitectonic studies of Brodmann (1907, 1909) the homology of primate and human area 7 seems to be well established. Thus areas 39 and 40 are most likely phylogenetically new cortical fields with man-specific functions.

Functional Deficits after Inferior Parietal Lobe Lesions in Primates

As will be discussed in Chapters 21 and 22, distinct symptoms related to human space perception are observed when the posterior parietal cortex is lesioned in one hemisphere: hemispatial neglect and inattention to the contralateral visual hemifield, constructional apraxia, difficulties in visual orientation, defects of visuo-spatial memory, disturbances in visually guided grasping and object-related eye movements in the visual exploration of the extrapersonal space or impairment of smooth pursuit eye movements when following moving single targets are typical parietal lobe symptoms. Considering the phylogenetic growth of the human parietal cortex in comparison with the monkey parietal cortex (compare Figs 2.27, 15.1 and 6.1), it is not surprising that parietal lobe lesions in man produce to a certain extent symptoms other than those occurring in monkeys. The clinically clear differences in defects following area 7 and gyrus angularis lesions in man support the opinion that Brodmann's areas 39 and 40 of the human brain (located in the gyrus circumflexus and the gyrus angularis of the lateral parietal and parietotemporal lobe) are man-specific regions which have developed during hominid evolution and are involved in predominantly man-specific visuo-constructive abilities. For these defects no animal model is available to date, whereas after area 7 lesions in monkey one can observe symptoms which are loosely related to those observed in man area 7 lesions. In the following we will briefly summarize the deficits found after posterior parietal lesions in monkeys.

Visual Hemineglect

Following acute lesions of area 7, monkeys show a transient visual neglect of the contralateral extrapersonal hemispace, but this hemineglect seems to be less pronounced than in man (Denny-Brown and Chambers, 1955; Ettlinger and Kalsbeck, 1962; Ettlinger, 1977; Heilman *et al.*, 1971). With simultaneous bilateral visual stimulation in the extrapersonal space, the phenomenon of 'extinction', i.e. attention only towards the stimulus in the extrapersonal space ipsilateral to the parietal lobe lesion, was also observed in monkeys (Schwartz and Eidelberg, 1968; Eidelberg and Schwartz, 1971; Heilman *et al.*, 1971; Lynch and McLaren, 1979b, 1982). It should be mentioned that lesions of the inferior area 6 in the frontal cortex also lead to hemineglect symptoms. Area 6, which receives a strong input from area 7b, plays an important role in guiding visually controlled hand movements, especially hand–mouth (Godschalk *et al.*, 1981; Rizzolatti *et al.*, 1981a, b). Correspondingly, destruction of premotor area 6 produces motor and attentional defects (Rizzolatti *et al.*, 1983): usage of the contralateral hand in visually guided movements within the grasping space is greatly reduced and the monkey is also no longer able to grasp food with its mouth when presented from the side contralateral to the lesion. Similarly, attentional deficits are especially strong in the peripersonal contralateral space around the mouth region. Responses to visual stimuli are not affected when they appear outside the grasping space (cf. Rizzolatti and Gallese, 1988).

Impairment of Visually Guided Grasping

Area 7 lesions in monkeys induce a pronounced inability to use the contralateral fingers, hand and arm adequately in visually guided reaching tasks, while non-visually guided, goal-directed hand and finger movements, especially when performed in coordinated locomotion or other automatic motor actions (e.g. climbing), were not seriously affected. The reaching inaccuracy with the hand contralateral to the parietal lobe lesion was not restricted to the contralateral hemifield but was also observed for manipulation in the ipsilateral hemifield (Wilson, 1957; Ettlinger and Kalsbeck, 1962; Moffett *et al.*, 1967; Hartje and Ettlinger, 1973; Faugier-Grimaud *et al.*, 1978; Lamotte and

Acuna, 1978; Glickstein and May, 1982). It seems rather probable that an impairment of area 7b in particular leads to these symptoms.

Gaze-control Defects

Gaze apraxia and considerably reduced eye movements to the contralateral part of the extra-personal space were observed in monkeys suffering from area 7 (especially 7a) lesions. Saccade latencies and precision as well as pursuit eye movements were impaired (Lynch and McLaren, 1979, 1982; Lynch, 1980).

Changes in spontaneous explorative eye movements were observed in monkeys by Munk (1881) after he destroyed their posterior parietal cortex. With bilateral frontal eye field lesions or posterior parietal cortex lesions Latto (1978) found a strong reduction in oculomotor search activity in Rhesus monkeys. Stein (1978, 1979) reported on a diminution and slowing of eye movements directed towards the contralateral side when area 7 was cooled in macaque monkeys. Simultaneously visually guided hand movements were impaired, a symptom presumably caused by dysfunction of area 7b. With bilateral posterior parieto-occipital lesions the oculomotor responses as measured in saccade latencies were slowed down, but visual fixation of a stationary target was in the range of normal behaviour (Lynch and McLaren, 1979; Lynch, 1980a, b). The optokinetic nystagmus of monkeys was affected by unilateral area 7 lesions, whereby the gain of the slow phase of OKN was reduced predominantly in the direction of the lesion. Bilateral parietal lobe lesions produced a reduction in OKN towards both sides (McLaren and Lynch, 1979; Lynch, 1980; Lynch and McLaren, 1982). Ventre and Faugier-Grimaud (1986) reported that area 7 lesions led to a change in the vestibular ocular reflex (VOR) in monkeys. VOR gain was reduced for horizontal rotation in the contralateral direction to the lesion and increased with horizontal rotation in the ipsilateral direction.

The involvement of area 7 in guiding eye movements was also demonstrated by electrical stimulation of this region. Ferrier (1886) was the first to observe eye movements when electrically stimulating the inferior parietal cortex of monkeys (cf. Chapter 2). C. and O. Vogt (1919, 1926) justified their subdivision of areas 7a and 7b (Fig. 6.1) not only on the basis of cytoarchitectonic criteria, but also on the outcome of electrical stimulation. Finger movements were evoked when area 7b was stimulated, eye movements when area 7a was stimulated. Convergent eye movements in connection with pupil constriction and accommodation were reported as a symptom of area 7 stimulation (Jampel, 1960). In their early study, C. and O. Vogt (1926) reported that eye movements can also be elicited by electrical stimulation of areas V1 and V2, the upper bank of the superior temporal sulcus, and areas 6 and 8 of the prefrontal cortex, i.e. brain areas connected with area 7 (Fig. 6.2). The Vogts obtained these data in *Cercopithecus* monkeys; similar results were later reported in *Rhesus* macaques by Wagman (1964).

Visuo-spatial and Visuo-motor Neuronal Data Processing in Area 7

Since the pioneer work of Hyvärinen, Lynch, Mountcastle and their co-workers in the 1970s (for reviews see Mountcastle, 1978, 1981; Lynch, 1980; Hyvärinen, 1982a, b) many reports have been published dealing with the problem of multisensory integration and visuo-spatial data processing in the inferior parietal lobule. The recordings were obtained either in monkeys sitting with the head restricted in a monkey chair but which could otherwise act spontaneously, or in monkeys systematically trained to perform certain fixation, pursuit, saccade or attention tasks related to stimuli projected to a tangent screen placed at some distance from the monkey chair. The latter experiments were usually designed to separate motor, visuo-motor, visual and attentional mechanisms which exert cooperative effects in many area 7 neurones. First of all it was demonstrated that the subdivisions of area 7 mentioned above were also functionally relevant at the single unit level. Corresponding to the anatomical connections with area 5 and the somatosensory cortices S1 and S2, area 7b receives a very strong input from the somatosensory system, while visuo-spatial signals reach this area predominantly through the connection with the neighbouring area 7a. It seems rather probable that area 7b in turn provides 7a with the input for sensorimotor signals necessary for visually guided actions in the grasping space. Since area 7b has connections with the supplementary motor area and with area 6 of the prefrontal cortex, a region which controls hand–mouth interaction by means of visual and somatosensory signals (Rizzolatti *et al.*, 1981a), area 7b is presumably involved predominantly in the visual and sensorimotor representation of the grasping space and the actions within that space. Area 7a, in contrast, like areas 7m and 7ip, seems to process the visual aspects of the distant extra-personal space. Area LIP most likely plays a key role in visuomotor activity, a function supported by the strong input from prestriate visual regions representing the peripheral visual field (e.g. Baizer *et al.*, 1991). Gnadt and Andersen (1988) reported that area LIP contains many more saccade-related neurones than area 7a. The important role of area LIP in oculomotor control is supported by the direct anatomical projections of this area to the oculomotor deep layers of the superior colliculi (Lynch *et al.*, 1985).

To date little is known about how the visuo-spatial activity of area 7 neurones is related to the different compartments of the extra-personal space: grasping space, near-distant action space and far-distant space (cf. Chapter 21). In a pilot study (U. Büttner and O.-J. Grüsser, unpublished, 1973) single cells were recorded in macaque monkeys areas 7a/b which responded to visual stimuli and visuo-motor tasks only when the stimuli were presented in the grasping space and not beyond. Other area 7 cells responded, however, to movement of interesting objects or persons in the near-distant action space. Interestingly, some area 7a cells were found which responded to visual stimuli restricted to a distinct direction within the extrapersonal space. The spatial response region of these neurones was independent of the position of the chair in which the animal was placed and the drum surrounding the chair onto which the stimuli were projected ('East–West neurones'). This finding suggested that area 7 neurones may also be involved in the transformation from spatiotopic to spatial coordinates. In one of these peculiar neurones the restriction of the responses to certain directions of the extra-personal space was abolished when the chair with the animal was rotated several times in the dark. Thereafter the visual response could be evoked from all directions of the extra-personal space.

The neurones of areas 7a and 7ip may be functionally subdivided into four large response classes:

1. Visual neurones, for which the responses are related predominantly to a certain part of the visual field.
2. Visuo-motor neurones, which are activated by visual stimulation in the extra-personal space and simultaneously by goal-directed eye movements related to a visual stimulus.
3. Gaze-motor neurones, which react predominantly in connection with eye or gaze movements directed towards a certain part of the extra-personal space.
4. 'Attentional' neurones, which indicate the animal's spatial shifts in attention which also occur without a shift in gaze position, which was kept constant in the experiment by a fixation task.

The different classes of neurones found in areas 7a and 7ip are not separated into distinct parts of these fields, but are intermingled throughout the two fields. There may be a local accumulation in cortical 'patches' or 'columns' of neurones belonging to the same response class.

In the following we will illustrate 'typical' responses of neurones located in area 7a or 7ip.

Gaze Movement Neurones

Figure 6.3(a) illustrates a neurone activated during pursuit eye movements. The monkey was following an interesting target, namely a raisin, which was moved either to the

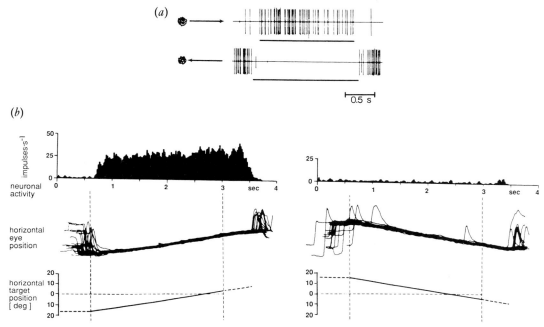

Fig. 6.3 *(a) Activity of a neurone recorded from area 7a which was sensitive to direction of movement and eye pursuit. An interesting object (a raisin) was moved to the right and left within the grasping space in front of the animal. The animal pursued the target with his eyes. Movement to the right led to an activation, movement to the left to an inhibition of neuronal activity (Hyvärinen and Poranen, 1974). (b) Tracking neurone activity recorded from area 7a of the macaque monkey. Trained eye pursuit movements were performed horizontally to the right or left. Movement to the right led to an activation of the neurone, to the left to an inhibition. In addition to the average neuronal activity and the stimulus position (lower trace), superimposed recordings of eye position illustrate the precise pursuit movements performed by the animal (from Motter and Mountcastle, 1975, modified).*

right (activation of the neurone) or to the left (inhibition of the neuronal activity; Hyvärinen and Poranen, 1974). The preferred direction of these 'visual tracking neurones' (Mountcastle *et al.*, 1975) may point in any direction in the extra-personal space. Systematic quantitative studies in these neurones, for which an example is illustrated in Fig. 6.3(b), revealed that not only the direction of the tracking movement but also its speed affected neuronal activity. Some of the tracking neurones responded when the visual stimulus approached the animal or moved away from it (Fig. 6.4, Hyvärinen, 1982a). Typically visual tracking neurones are activated during smooth pursuit eye (or gaze) movements, but not during saccades or a fixation task. When the monkey fixated a target and suppressed gaze movements, however, gaze neurones could be activated when a visual pattern moved across their visual receptive field, provided the correct movement direction was selected. Gaze neurones of area 7 responded in part similarly to neurones recorded in areas MT and MST (Wurtz and Newsome, 1985; for further discussion see Andersen, 1987). It seems rather likely that the activity of area 7a gaze neurones is controlled by the input from areas MT and MST (Chapter 5).

Vestibular Responses

About 2–5 per cent of area 7a neurones responded to vestibular stimulation (sine wave movements of the monkey in a yaw, pitch or roll direction; Java monkeys: O.-J. Grüsser, M. Pause and U. Schreiter, unpublished, 1980; squirrel monkeys: S. Akbarian, O.-J. Grüsser and W. Guldin, unpublished, 1989–1991). Kawano *et al.* (1984) studied the effect of vestibular stimulation (horizontal rotation only) in area 7a visual tracking neurones (vestibulo-ocular reflex, VOR, and VOR suppression). Visual tracking neurones responding with a preferred horizontal direction were selected. Three different response types were found, as illustrated in Fig. 6.5, they were as follows.

Type A Tracking Neurones

These responded only to visual tracking of a small target moving horizontally back and forth in total darkness and not to vestibular stimulation in the dark (horizontal sinusoidal rotation of the monkey chair). When target and chair were moved together, however, and the monkey cancelled the VOR by fixating the target, type A visual track-

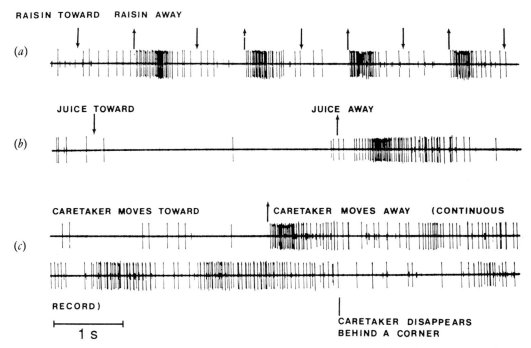

Fig. 6.4 *Visual responses of a cell in area 7 (perhaps 7b) to object movement towards and away from the animal. (a): The neurone was activated whenever an interesting object, a raisin, was moved away from the monkey, while neuronal activity was reduced when the raisin was moved towards the monkey. Change in movement direction illustrated by arrows. (b): The same experiment, performed with a spoon filled with orange juice. (c): When the attendant moved towards the monkey, the neurone was inhibited, when he moved slowly away, a maintained activity was recorded. As soon as the attendant disappeared from the monkey's visual field, neuronal activity returned to the spontaneous level (Hyvärinen, 1982a, by permission of Springer Verlag).*

ing neurones were directionally activated. For example: while the monkey suppressed the VOR, some of the neurones became activated during movement towards the right and inhibited when the chair moved towards the left. The same neurones were normally activated when the eye pursued a target moving horizontally towards the right. Sinusoidal rotation and fixation of an earth-fixed target led only to a weak activation of type A neurones. Thus it appears as if type A neurones contribute to visual movement perception related to the extra-personal space.

Type B Tracking Neurones

These were activated by visual tracking and by chair-rotation in the dark. They also responded when the animal suppressed VOR by fixating a target which was rotating with the chair. When, however, an earth-fixed target was fixated during chair rotation, the neuronal response was weak. Thus the activity of type B responses was related to visual movement relative to head or body coordinates.

Type C Tracking Neurones

These responded to sinusoidal rotation in darkness in the opposite direction to that eliciting activation by visual

target movement. When VOR was suppressed by fixating a target rotating together with the monkey chair the neuronal response was reduced, whereas a facilitation of the neuronal response was observed when an earth-fixed target was fixated during sinusoidal chair rotation (Fig. 6.5). The activity of type C tracking neurones seems to be related predominantly to eye movements.

Tracking Neurones and Extra-personal Space Perception

It is evident that by means of the information contained in the responses of these three classes of neurones a neuronal network should be able to judge whether a visual stimulus remains stationary in space during head rotation, is moving with the animal, or travels independently across the extra-personal space. From these findings it also became evident that vestibular signals originating in the semicircular canal receptors reach area 7a and interact in a meaningful manner with gaze controlling neurones. Access is gained presumably through the parieto-insular vestibular cortex (PIVC), which has anatomical connections with area 7op and 7b (Pause and Schreiter, 1980; Akbarian, *et al.*, in preparation, 1991). In our opinion the

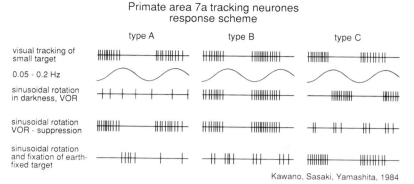

Primate area 7a tracking neurones
response scheme

Fig. 6.5 *Response scheme of area 7a tracking neurones. Four different stimulus conditions: the eyes pursued a small, sinusoidally moving target, the animal was in horizontal sine wave rotation in darkness (VOR), horizontal rotation with VOR suppression, or fixation of an earth-fixed target. Scheme drawn according to the data published by Kawano et al., 1984.*

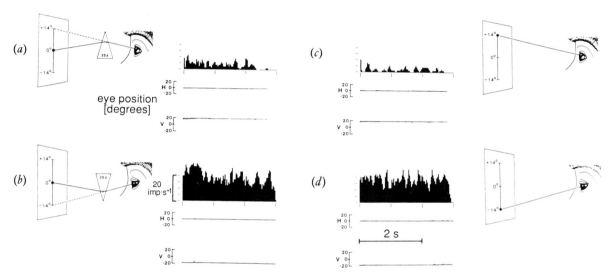

Fig. 6.6 *The activity of this area 7a neurone depended on eye position in the orbit and not on eye position relative to the extra-personal space. In (a) and (b) the animal, with his head fixed, fixated a light target placed in the centre of the screen through a 25-dioptre prism, either with base down (a) or base up (b). To fixate the target the monkey had to shift his optical axis 14 degrees up or down as illustrated. In (c) and (d) the prisms were removed and the animal looked 14 degrees up or 14 degrees down at the target on the tangent screen. In all conditions the neuronal activity depended on the position of the eyes in the orbit and not on the position of the target relative to the surroundings. The horizontal (H) and vertical (V) eye position traces indicate precisely how the monkey performed the fixation task (from Andersen et al., 1987; by permission of Springer Publishing Company).*

vestibular input to areas 7a and 7b is utilized predominantly to provide the signals which 'stabilize' the coordinates of the perceived extra-personal space.

Fixation Neurones and the Control of Gaze Position

Gaze-related neuronal activity was observed in another class of area 7a neurones, called fixation neurones. It was first reported that the activity of these nerve cells depended very little on eye position, but was maintained when the animal gazed at a stationary target. Mountcastle *et al.* (1975) characterized the operational meaning of fixation neurone activity as a 'command function' related to the extra-personal space. Whenever the monkey fixated a stationary target, these neurones were activated. Sakata *et al.* (1980), Lynch *et al.* (1985) and Andersen *et al.* (1987) found that the activity of typical 'fixation cells' depended

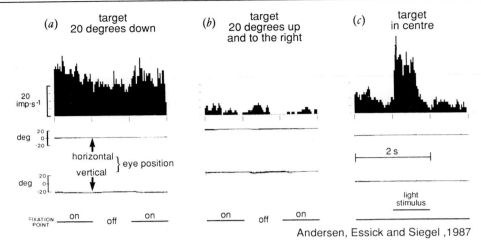

Andersen, Essick and Siegel ,1987

Fig. 6.7 *Experiment to separate the visual and eye position responses of an area 7a neurone. (a) The animal fixated a target located 20 degrees down from the centre of the screen in otherwise total darkness. The animal was trained to also maintain his eye position when the fixation point was turned off ('off', lower trace). The neuronal activity depended essentially on eye position and not on the presence of the fixation target. (b) The animal was fixating the target shifted on the screen 20 degrees upwards and 20 degrees to the right. Note the low neuronal activity corresponding approximately to the spontaneous neuronal discharge rate. (c) The animal fixated the fixation target placed in the centre of the screen. In addition to the fixation target a light spot was flashed into the visual excitatory receptive field of the cell (marked as 'light stimulus' in the lower trace). This neurone clearly increased its activity during light stimulation. This example illustrates the experimental separation of 'visual fields' and 'gaze fields' (Andersen et al., 1987; by permission of Springer Publishing Company).*

on the position of the target looked at in the extra-personal space. These fixation cells were thus gaze-position cells and activated whenever gaze was directed to a certain region in the extra-personal space ('gaze field'). Andersen *et al.* (1987) designed a clever experiment which indicated that eye or gaze position and not the stimulus position in the extra-personal space is the relevant parameter in the neuronal activity of fixation neurones (Fig. 6.6). In exploring whether the relative position of the visual surroundings or the eye position determines the activity of fixation neurones, the monkey was trained to fixate a small target either directly or through a 25-dioptre prism. With the prism base downwards the monkey had to look 14 degrees above the straight-ahead position, and with the prism base upwards 14 degrees down, to fixate the target. When the prism was removed and the fixation target was displaced 14 degrees up or down, the neuronal activity was still clearly dependent on the eye position, as with the prism, and not on the general background seen outside of the prism (Fig. 6.6).

In fixation neurones the eye position and the visual stimulus in the fovea or near-foveal region evidently interact with each other (Robinson *et al.*, 1978). Some fixation neurones were also activated when the animal fixated a recalled target in total darkness, i.e. targets for which the position was stored in a short-term visuo-spatial memory (Andersen *et al.*, 1987; Fig. 6.7). Fixation neurones not only had an optimal region in the extra-personal space (or

eye in orbit position), the fixation of which led to maximum activation, but also a visual field (relative to the fixation target) from which stationary flashed-light stimuli evoked a distinct neuronal activation (Fig. 6.7).

Saccade-related Neurones

Some of area 7a and 7ip cells were activated when the monkey performed goal-directed saccades to a target in the extra-personal space. Neuronal activation could begin shortly before or during a saccade and was maintained after the eye had reached the new position. The amplitude and the direction of the saccade in the field of gaze as well as the end position of the eye in the extra-personal space seemed to modify the neuronal activity. The majority of these saccade-related area 7a cells had in addition a visual receptive field. Thus, their activity was determined by both the gaze direction and the visual stimulus (Fig. 6.8; Robinson *et al.*, 1978; Andersen *et al.*, 1987).

Visual Neurones

A considerable portion of area 7a and 7ip neurones were dominated by the visual stimulus, i.e. they exhibited a 'visual excitatory receptive field' (VERF), related to a distinct part of the visual field. As a rule, this visual activation was possible through either eye and no selective ocular dominance was found. In these experiments the VERF

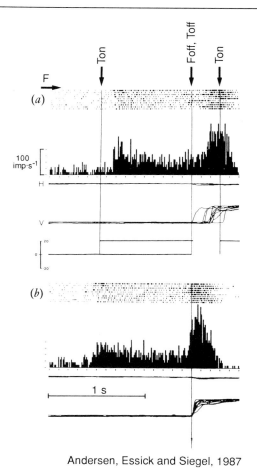

Andersen, Essick and Siegel, 1987

Fig. 6.8 *Area 7a neurones are also activated when saccades are performed to a remembered location in total darkness, provided this location corresponds to the gaze field. (a) The animal fixated a central target (F). The target to which a delayed saccade had to be performed (20 degrees upwards) was turned on at the arrow 'T on'. At the arrow 'F off, T off' the fixation target and, 60 ms later, the saccade target were turned off. This was a sign for the animal to execute a saccade. After the saccade was performed the target to which the saccade was directed was turned on again (arrow 'T on'). (b): The same neuronal activity as in (a) is temporally aligned to the beginning of the saccade towards the saccade target. Note that the neuronal activity is increased as compared with the 'fixation level', while the saccade target is visible, but the saccade is not performed. Performance of the saccade led to a further saccadic and postsaccadic increase in neuronal activity (Andersen* et al., *1987; by permission of Springer Publishing Company).*

was explored after the animal was trained to fixate a stationary target. During this fixation task another visual stimulus either was flashed as a stationary target into different parts of the visual field or was moved through the

visual field. Whenever the stimulus appeared in the VERF, a distinct neuronal activation was observed. In all of these studies, the VERF size was found to be large, whereby the VERF could be located either in the ipsilateral or the contralateral visual hemifield. Frequently, however, the VERF covered regions in both hemifields. A considerable number of these neurones exhibited 'foveal sparing' (Motter and Mountcastle, 1981). Foveal sparing suggests that the neurones monitor visual stimuli located within the respective extrafoveal part of the visual space. This property of the visual neurones perhaps indicates their role in preparing goal-directed eye movements.

In some of these 'visual' neurones directional selectivity could be demonstrated when an object was moved through the VERF, but no clear dependencies on other elementary visual qualities like size, contrast, intensity or composition of the stimulus were established. Many of these neurones seemed to alter their visual sensitivity with the angle of gaze (Andersen *et al.*, 1985), a fact which indicates that even in these 'visual' neurones of area 7 gaze motor conditions modify the response.

Movement and Direction-sensitive Area 7a Neurones

As illustrated in Fig. 6.2, areas 7a and 7ip receive a strong input from the parieto-temporal visual areas selectively responding to smaller or larger visual patterns that are moving in a certain direction across the visual field. It is therefore not surprising that movement-selective neuronal responses were found in area 7a (Robinson *et al.*, 1978; Motter and Mountcastle, 1981). Directional selectivity was best illustrated when the monkey fixated a small stationary target. In our opinion, two different classes of visual movement-selective cells should be discriminated (as for the area MT and MST neurones): cells responding selectively to 'local' movement and cells selective for global movement, i.e. stimuli which induce optokinetic responses under normal conditions. Area 7a cells responding to local movement are frequently activated optimally when the movement deviates from a simple linear translocation. Figure 6.9 illustrates a cell responding to object rotation. Other cells have a maximum activation when a visual stimulus located within the VERF is expanding or contracting, corresponding to the change in stimulus size when the objects move towards or away from the animal. Tanaka *et al.* (1986) discriminated between local and global (wide-field) visual movement responses of area 7 cells and could indeed demonstrate that relative movement between object and background ('induced' movement) modified the neuronal activity as if the object had moved across the ERF.

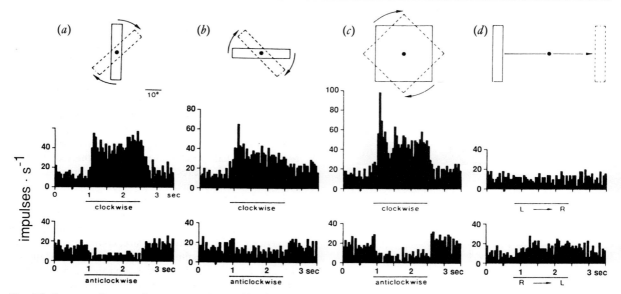

Fig. 6.9 *Response of an area 7a neurone sensitive to 'local' movement of the target. This neurone was sensitive to a clockwise rotation of a stimulus, while counterclockwise rotation led to an inhibition (a, b, c), and horizontal displacement (d) did not change neuronal activity significantly. The stimuli, light bars (a, b, d) or a light square (c), rotated around the fixation target (a, b, c) or moved across the visual receptive field (d) while the animal kept his eyes stationary by fixating the target (black dot) (from Sakata et al., 1986, modified; by permission of Springer Publishing Company).*

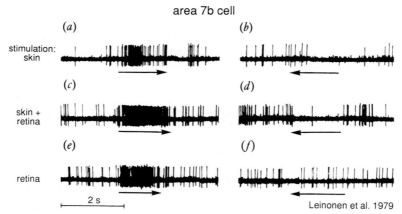

Fig. 6.10 *Multimodal cell recorded from area 7b in the macaque monkey. (a) The monkey's eyes were covered and his chest was stroked with a finger from right to left. This led to a strong activation of the neurone. (b) The stroking was performed along the same path but in the reverse direction: inhibition of neuronal activity. (c) and (d) The same tasks as in (a) and (b) were performed but the monkey could see the moving tactile stimulus. This led to a facilitation of neuronal activation when the stimulus was moved in the preferred direction. (e) and (f) The same movement stimulus was applied but without touching the skin. The investigator's hand moved from left to right (e), arrow, or from right to left (f), at about 15 cm from the chest (Leinonen et al., 1979a, by permission of Springer Publishing Company).*

Bimodal Responses

In addition to visual and visuo-motor signals, somatosensory signals modify the responses of area 7 neurones. 'Bimodal cells' are located predominantly in area 7b, but some have also been found in area 7a. Responses of two such cells are illustrated in Figures 6.10 and 6.11. Cells in area 7b were found to be sensitive to visual and cutaneous stimuli, whereby the responses illustrated in Fig. 6.10 were prototypical. This neurone was activated when the

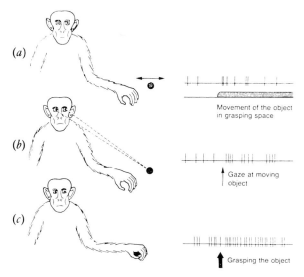

Movement of the object
in grasping space

↑ Gaze at moving
object

⬆ Grasping the object

Fig. 6.11 *Response scheme of a neurone recorded from area 7 of the awake Rhesus monkey. (a) An object is moved in the grasping space near the hand. (b) Back-and-forth movement of the object is continued, but now the monkey gazes at the moving object (arrow). This leads to an increase in the neuronal activity. (c) The monkey grasps the object. During grasping the neuronal activity increases and is maximal at the moment the monkey touches the object with its hand (arrow). (Unpublished observations of U. Büttner, O.-J. Grüsser and V. Henn, 1975; from Grüsser, 1978.)*

investigator moved his finger across the monkey's chest from left to right, while movement in the reverse direction inhibited the response. The spontaneous neuronal activity was greatly enhanced, moreover, when the monkey could also see the moving finger. A strong activation was further obtained when an object or the observer's hand moved at a distance of about 15 cm from the chest and the stimulus was thus monomodal visual movement near the region of somatosensory sensitivity. Neurones of this type indicate that area 7b activity seems to represent, at least in part, structures of the grasping space.

Figure 6.11 illustrates that neuronal activity may be modified by the object position in the grasping space, by eye position related to the object, by intended hand movement and by somatosensory stimulation while grasping the object. To explore the responses of the neurone illustrated in Fig. 6.11, an 'interesting' stimulus (a raisin fixed on a thin plastic rod) was moved laterally in the extra-personal space contralateral to the recording site about 20 cm away from the hand. When the stimulus appeared in the lateral lower grasping range, the spontaneous neuronal activity increased. It increased further when the monkey gazed at the object and reached maximum activity when the monkey moved its hand and grasped the object. Thus

goal-directed hand movement increased neuronal activity, which was further augmented when the object was successfully grasped. Neuronal activity also increased when the monkey tried to grasp the interesting target without directly looking at it, a custom acquired by the monkey very early in this explorative study. Multimodal area 7b neurones of this type are thus activated by visual movement stimulation, goal-directed gaze-motor activity, goal-directed hand and finger movement and somatosensory stimulation when touching the object in a certain part of the visual space. When the interesting visual target was shown in another part of the extra-personal space, e.g. ipsilateral to the recording site, the spontaneous neuronal activity was not changed. In our pilot study (Büttner *et al.*, 1975) we found that more multimodal neurones were activated from the extra-personal space contralateral to the recording site than from the ipsilateral. To understand the neuronal representation of the grasping space in more detail, one has to design machine-controlled stimulation in which object position, gaze motor and hand motor responses are monitored and the type of object is also variable. Considering the connections between area 7 and the limbic structures (Fig. 6.2), it is not unlikely that the relevance of the stimulus moving in the grasping space also has some impact on the neuronal activity.

Quantitative Evaluations of Area 7 Neuronal Responses: Gaze Fields, Visual Receptive Fields and First Steps Towards a Model of Cerebral Space Representation

The different response types of area 7a and 7b neurones described in the preceding paragraph are based mainly on qualitative studies related to the different stimulus parameters possible in such experiments. Some quantitative functions were investigated such as, for example, the dependency of the neuronal activation on visual stimulus position, on speed, or on gaze position. Data on the distribution of the different neuronal responses in a larger cell population, however, were not available. Statistical data on areas 7a, 7b, LIP and DP neurones were recently published by Andersen *et al.* (1990). In this study emphasis was put on the problem of location and size of the 'gaze fields' of area 7 neurones and in addition on the visual responses of 'gaze cells'. Andersen *et al.* (1990) analysed altogether 405 cells recorded from the cortical regions mentioned. Fifty-one per cent of the cells tested showed a clear dependency of their excitability level on eye position. The monkey fixated a small light target in an otherwise

(*a*) gaze field (eye position)

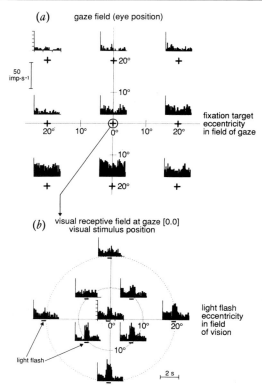

(*b*) visual receptive field at gaze [0.0]
visual stimulus position

Fig. 6.12 *Responses of a macaque area 7a neurone. (a) The neuronal activity depended on the position of the fixation target, i.e. on the eye in orbit position. Maximum activity was obtained when gaze position (head fixed) was downwards. Recordings of this type resulted in 'gaze fields' of area 7a neurones, as illustrated schematically in Fig. 6.13. (b) At gaze position (0, 0), i.e. in the centre of the field of gaze and considerably removed from the maximum sensitivity of the 'gaze field' of this neurone, the visual receptive field was tested. The sensitivity of the visual excitatory receptive field (VERF) was maximum in the right lower part of the visual field. The visual receptive field was not concentrically organized (Andersen* et al., *1990, modifed).*

gaze field and visual receptive field
of area 7a neurone

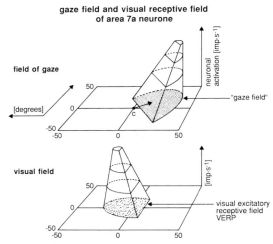

Fig. 6.13 *Scheme of a gaze field and a visual excitatory receptive field of an area 7a neurone. In the upper half of the figure part of the field of gaze is drawn . When the monkey shifts his centre of gaze (arrow) to the gaze field of a neurone, the activity of the neurone increases, whereby the distribution of neuronal excitability across the gaze field may be less regular than in this example. Whenever the gaze fixates a stationary target, visual responses are also elicitable in many neurones (lower part of the figure). The average activity evoked by visual stimuli depends on the position of the optical axis within the gaze field and of the light stimulus on the retina. The visual excitatory receptive field of some area 7a neurones may be less regular than the one illustrated in this scheme.*

dark room. This target was systematically shifted on a vertical tangent screen placed in front of the monkey. By this method, illustrated in Fig. 6.12, the 'gaze field' of individual neurones was explored. A 'gaze field' consists of all gaze positions in the overall field of gaze at which the neuronal activity was increased above the spontaneous level. Since the monkey's head was fixed, the gaze position was identical in these experiments with the eye-in-orbit position. The position of most gaze fields was considerably off the centre of the overall field of gaze. The neuronal activity declined from the 'gaze field maximum' towards the centre of the field of gaze and also towards the further periphery. This is schematically illustrated in Fig. 6.13.

In the study of Andersen *et al.* (1990) the visual receptive field, or better the 'visual excitatory receptive field'

(VERF), was determined for selected gaze positions in the following manner. The monkey fixated a target and a flash of light covering about 1 degree of visual angle was projected to different parts of the visual field. All those light spot positions from which the neuronal activity was increased by the flash stimulus above the spontaneous rate were defined as part of the VERF. This is illustrated in Fig. 6.12. As one can see from these recordings, the visual receptive field was typically not concentrically organized (Fig. 6.13). Sixty-four per cent of area 7a or LIP neurones with a clearly defined gaze field responded to light stimuli and had a circumscribed visual excitatory receptive field. Just as the gaze field was large, so the size of the VERFs was itself 20 to 40 degrees, and as a rule was not concentrically organized. Nothing is known of the effect of stimulus intensity, contrast and area on the visual responses of these neurones. For the overall response of the gaze neurones, the activity of which clearly depended on the visual stimulus pattern present within the VERF, one can only guess that the following condition may be applicable for the neuronal impulse rate R, measured in impulses per second:

$$R = k a_g \, i [f(a_r) * f(i_r)] \qquad (6.1)$$

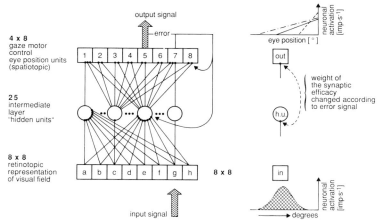

Fig. 6.14 *Scheme of the Zipser–Andersen model (1988) simulating the responses of area 7a neurones. The retinotopic input layer (e.g. area V2) is simulated by an 8 × 8 matrix of input units (here reduced to a row of units, a to h), which have a visual receptive field within which excitability is distributed approximately according to a 3-D Gaussian function. All input units are connected with all 25 intermediate layer units ('hidden units', h.u.), which in turn are connected with all output units. The output units represent eye-in-orbit position by linear functions of different slopes in a matrix of 4 × 8 units (here also reduced to a row of 8 units, 1 to 8). The model computation begins with an equal weight for all 'synaptic' contacts. Depending on the average error of model performance (shifting the output layer to the input stimulus position), the weight of the synaptic contacts at intermediate layer and output layer units is increased or decreased. After several thousand runs with this 'back-propagated programming' the hidden units were reported to acquire properties similar to those of area 7a cells regarding gaze field and visual excitatory receptive field.*

where a_g is the sensitivity level at a given gaze position, $f(a_r)$ the sensitivity distribution within the VERF and $f(i_r)$ a function of the spatial light distribution i_r within the visual field. The sign * stands for a convolution between the two functions. To our knowledge no information is available about spatial summation within the VERF; therefore the proposed convolution is indeed hypothetical, but seems plausible from the data provided by Andersen *et al.* (1987, 1990).

Andersen *et al.* (1990) explored systematically the spatial distribution of the gaze fields and of the VERFs in the cells recorded and found no correlation between the two functions. Furthermore, no systematic dependency of retinal eccentricity of the VERF on the location of the neurones within area 7a seems to exist. The gaze fields indeed constitute a kind of 'spatial gain field' for the visual ERF, but its function within the network of gaze neurones in area 7a also seems to still be enigmatic.

Zipser and Andersen (1987) tried to model the neuronal responses obtained in the macaque area 7a gaze neurones by a computer simulation using a 'back-propagating' programmed network consisting of three layers (Fig. 6.14). They assumed correctly that the visual signals are first processed by the visual brain regions in retinotopic coordinates, while the motor output controlling the gaze motor performance, i.e. goal-directed movements, is available in spatiotopic (egocentric) coordinates. The eye or gaze position layer consisted of a matrix of 4 × 8 units coding hori-

zontal or vertical gaze position. The neuronal activation was assumed to be a linear function of eccentricity of eye position, whereby the slope of the linear function between neuronal activation and eccentricity varied from unit to unit. The question raised in this investigation was whether a back-propagated programmed network with a layer of units intercalated between the retinotopic input and the spatiotopic output might learn to adapt its output to the required task, namely, to transfer a stimulus from retinotopic to spatiotopic – or, more precisely, 'craniotopic' – coordinates, since the data simulated stem from experiments in which the heads of the animals were fixed during the recording sessions. By back propagation the sensitivity of the individual synaptic contact at the intermediate layer of 'hidden units' and at their connections with the output layer was varied according to the performance of the network at the output level, as represented by an average error signal. In the initial state, every input unit had equally sensitive connections with all units of the intermediate layer and every hidden unit of the intermediate layer projected to all output neurones with the same synaptic gain (Fig. 6.14). When such a model was implemented on a digital computer and sufficient training was applied, the hidden units acquired very similar properties to those found in area 7a cells. This was true for the VERF properties and the gaze fields of hidden units.

From the similarity between the properties of post-training hidden units of the intermediate layers and the area 7 neurone reponse characteristics, the authors concluded that neuronal responses like those shown in Fig. 6.13 indeed form an essential step in the transformation of the signal pattern present in retinotopic coordinates at the visual input level of area 7 into spatiotopic coordinates present at the motor output level of the cerebral centres controlling gaze.

We think that other models still have to be explored before conclusions on area 7 network functions can be drawn from which new experimentally testable hypotheses may be deduced. The efforts of Zipser and Andersen, however, are an important step in understanding one of the main functions of area 7a, namely, the transformation of the visual percepts from the visual field coordinates to those of the perceived extra-personal space. This operation is still performed in area 7 predominantly for the contralateral half of the extrapersonal space, but some overlapping of operations related to the left and right area 7a certainly exists.

Acknowledgement

This chapter was written in collaboration with Dr S. Akbarian, Berlin.

7 Visual Object Recognition and Temporal Lobe Functions: the Evidence From Experiments in Primates

Introduction

When Karl Kleist (1879–1960) summarized his observations in brain-lesioned patients (Kleist 1923, 1934), principally those suffering from gunshot or shrapnel wounds from the First World War, he emphasized the difference between visual defects following temporal and parietal lobe lesions. Parietal lobe lesions led to visuo-spatial defects, temporal lobe lesions to disturbances in visual object recognition. Considering the interaction of the subject with the visual objects of his extra-personal space by means of visuo-motor, handmotor and locomotor goal-directed movements, however, a meaningful synthesis of object recognition and object location is nearly always necessary. This synthesis seems to involve premotor structures of the frontal lobe.

Kleist's concept of two visual systems, one devoted to space representation, the other to object recognition, was confirmed by animal experiments and led to the idea widely applied at present that the parallel signal processing present in the retina and the afferent visual system ('parvocellular' and 'magnocellular' pathways, cf. Chapters 3 and 4) separates into two cerebral visual systems as soon as the signals leave the peristriate, retinotopically organized, visual areas and enter parietal or temporal lobe structures (Ungerleider and Mishkin, 1982; Ungerleider, 1985).

From animal experiments performed during the last 30 years it became evident that the cortical visual pathways from area V1 through the peristriate and parastriate belt to the inferior temporal lobe play a key role in primate object recognition. In general, one can discriminate four different behavioural fields where visual object and dynamic signal recognition is highly relevant in primates:

1. Interaction with objects which may serve as food or prey.
2. Recognition of objects which are potentially threatening, like predators, poisonous plants or fruits.
3. Communication with partners in the social field, i.e. other primates of the same or different species, and recognizing visual signals relevant to group coordination.
4. Perception of 'neutral' objects, which become behaviourally important, however, as 'landmarks' in spatial orientation, or as 'shelters' or 'watchtowers' in everyday behaviour.

It is still debatable whether the differentiation of the inferior temporal lobe (IT) function with regards to signal processing related to different object classes is expressed by a difference in location extending beyond small patches or columns of neurones and by neurones highly selective in their responses to one stimulus class only (detectors of 'universals' or 'grandmother cells'), or whether different objects are represented by different spatio-temporal states of excitation in neuronal networks widely distributed across the IT. We assume the latter to be the case.

Historical Review

In monkeys, following bilateral temporal lobe lesions, Brown and Schäfer (1888) observed 'psychic blindness', i.e. despite normal visual acuity their animals were no longer able to recognize objects or to understand their functional meaning. This defect corresponded to the 'Seelenblindheit' concluded by Munk (1881) to be present in his brain-lesioned animals, which did not recognize objects but avoided obstacles when moving about (cf. Chapter 2). 'Seelenblindheit' soon became important in the interpretation of visual agnosic symptoms observed in patients suffering from temporo-occipital brain lesions (cf. Chapter 11). When Klüver and Bucy (1937, 1938, 1939; cf. Klüver, 1951) performed bilateral temporal lobectomies in monkeys, visual object agnosia was evident; these animals also lost their visual learning and visual object memory ability. In addition, they lost all social fear, became 'tame' and exhibited signs of hyperphagia and hypersexuality. Klüver and Bucy (1937) summarized their finding as follows:

> *The animal does not exhibit the reactions generally associated with anger and fear. It approaches humans and animals, animate as well as inanimate objects without hesitation and although there are no motor defects, things are examined by mouth rather than by use of the hands. There is a general slowing down of movements; the quick, jerky movements characteristic of the normal rhesus monkey have almost entirely disappeared. Various tests do not show any impairment in visual acuity or in the ability to localize visually the position of objects in space. However, the monkey seems to be unable to recognize objects by the sense of sight. The hungry animal if confronted with a variety of objects, will, for example, indiscriminately pick up a comb, a bakelite knob, a sunflower seed, a screw, a stick, a piece of apple, a live snake, a piece of banana, and a live rat. Each object is transferred to the mouth and then discarded if not edible .... These symptoms of what appears to be 'psychic blindness' are not present in four other monkeys which are being studied at present and in which only one temporal lobe has been removed. However, these cases seem to respond less easily and less strongly to a variety of stimuli which in monkeys with one or both frontal, parietal or occipital lobes extirpated, or in normal monkeys, call forth extreme excitement as evidenced by motor or vocal behavior.*

Klüver and Bucy (1939) tried to differentiate the contribution of different temporal lobe areas to the 'Klüver–Bucy syndrome' as mentioned above, which is indeed now considered to be a combination of impaired functions attributed to limbic structures, to inferotemporal (IT) or to supratemporal sulcus (STS) regions. By destroying the outer surface of the temporal cortex subtotally, Klüver and Bucy could not evoke gross changes in the animal's behaviour (Klüver, 1951). Studies by Ades and Raab (1949), Blum et al. (1950), Chow (1951) and Pribram and Bagshaw (1953) provided further evidence that bilateral ablation of the inferior temporal lobe led to a 'selective impairment of the animal's ability to solve simultaneously presented problems of visual discrimination' (Pribram and

Bagshaw, 1953). This observation was confirmed and extended by Mishkin (1954) and Mishkin and Pribram (1954). Lesions of the superior temporal gyrus and of the limbic parts of the ventral and mesial inferior temporal lobe (mainly gyrus fusiformis and gyrus parahippocampalis) did not impair the ability to solve visual discrimination tasks (Pribram, 1967; Gross, 1973). The involvement of the outer surface cortical areas of the inferior temporal lobe in visual discrimination learning was confirmed by later studies, in which elementary visual functions, visual acuity, contrast and colour vision were demonstrated on a quantitative basis to be intact (Ettlinger, 1959; Cowey and Weiskrantz, 1967; Cowey and Gross, 1970; for review see Gross, 1973; Mishkin, 1982; Mishkin et al., 1983).

The first microelectrode recordings from the inferotemporal cortex (Gross et al. 1967, 1969) did not contradict the concept that the primate inferior temporal lobe contains neuronal networks elaborating on 'higher-order' visual signal processing: however, only the recordings performed later in awake, behaving and interacting animals led to a deeper understanding of the IT function. These pioneering microelectrode recordings were preceded by electroencephalographic studies which also indicated that the inferior temporal lobe is involved in visual discrimination learning. For example, Bailey et al. (1943) demonstrated that the EEG recorded from the inferior temporal lobe did not change with auditory stimuli, as the EEG did which was recorded from the superior temporal lobe of macaques and chimpanzees. Furthermore, local strychninization led to a rather narrow projection of strychnine spikes in the EEG within areas 20 and 21 of Brodmann, corresponding roughly to the areas TEO and TE of the scheme used in the present volume (Fig. 6.1). This finding indicated the existence of rather effective local intracortical connections in the inferior temporal lobe. Chow (1961) found a decrease in EEG wave amplitudes and an increase in EEG frequency while recording from IT in monkeys learning a visual discrimination task. When epileptogenic lesions were applied to IT, visual learning and retention of visual discrimination tasks were reduced (Stamm and Pribram, 1961). The EEG changes in the IT recordings observed during learning tasks may have been signs of general arousal. However, the question of how well EEG recordings may assist in the experimental analysis of IT function was addressed by Gerstein et al. (1968), who recorded EEG visual evoked responses in monkeys during visual discrimination tasks. With implanted EEG electrodes these authors could find no correlation between the evoked potentials and the class of visual stimuli, their structural complexity or the monkey's response (right/wrong). Thus EEG recordings did not seem to be appropriate for exploring IT function. Indeed, progress in understanding inferior lobe function came from systematic microelectrode studies which will be discussed below.

The Inferior Temporal Cortex: Structure and Neuronal Connections

Brodmann (1905, 1919), von Bonin and Bailey (1947) and Seltzer and Pandya (1978; cf. Fig. 6.1) distinguished different areas of the monkey inferior temporal cortex on cytoarchitectonic and myeloarchitectonic grounds. In the following we will use the scheme of Baylis *et al.* (1987), who relied on the cytoarchitectonic concept of Seltzer and Pandya (1978) and subdivided the temporal lobe region around the superior temporal sulcus (STS) and in the IT region as illustrated in Figs 7.1(a) and (b). This subdivision of the lower bank of the STS and of IT into different areas was justified not only by the cytoarchitectonic and myeloarchitectonic arguments but also by functional differences found in single unit recordings. What Baylis *et al.* deduced from the responses of more than 2600 neurones recorded from these regions is added schematically to the maps of Figs 7.1(a) and (b). These maps suggest that, similar to the peristriate visual association cortices, IT is parcellated into many functionally diverse subregions, within which the neuronal responses differ in their statistical distribution regarding the most effective stimuli. While auditory responses dominate in the upper part of the superior temporal lobe, an extended region in the upper bank of the supratemporal sulcus contains polymodal neuronal networks (STP, 'supratemporal polymodal area', upper STS region). Neurones located in the inferior bank of the supratemporal sulcus and in the extended substructures of area TE, however, are dominant visual, whereby the different visual qualities (shape, movement, movement direction, colour) and a higher-order complexity of the visual stimuli determine the neuronal responses. This is only roughly summarized in Figs 7.1(a) and (b) and is discussed in detail in the following paragraph.

The pathways from V1 to the different IT areas have been studied repeatedly (e.g. Desimone *et al.*, 1980). The schematic diagram of these pathways shown in Fig. 7.2 follows the arguments presented in a recent publication by Baizer *et al.* (1991): cells from the primary visual cortex (V1), primarily those related to the regions representing the central part of the visual hemifield and belonging to the parvocellular system, project to areas V2, V3, V4 and DP and from there to area TEO and the different regions of area TE of the inferotemporal lobe. Areas V4, V4t and the dorsal prelunate area (DP; Figs 5.1–5.3) seem to form the main afferent visual relay structures to areas TE and TEO. In addition, the parts of area V2 and V3 which represent foveal vision also project to area TE. From the regions around the upper STS which were found to be particularly involved in visual movement detection (cf. Chapter 5), only area FST (Figs 5.1–5.3) is directly con-

nected with TE. Besides area V2, area V4 seems to play a key role in 'distributing' the pathway to the inferior temporal lobe and to the parietal and STS regions. Gattas *et al.* (1988) provided evidence that the V4 cells which project to the parietal cortex are predominantly those representing the peripheral parts of the visual field, while cells projecting to the temporal cortex correspond to the representation of the foveal and parafoveal parts of the visual hemifield in area V4. Thus the distribution of the two visual pathways not only follows the division of the magnocellular/parvocellular system but also that of foveal/peripheral vision, at least to a certain degree. In the 'hierarchy' connecting V1 with IT regions area TEO seems to be intercalated, at least in part, between V2, V4 and TE (see below).

In addition to the 'visual' inputs just mentioned, some connections from the frontal eye field (FEF) to area TE were found. In an earlier study Pandya and Kuypers (1969) demonstrated, by means of the Nauta silver-impregnation technique of degenerating fibres, a pathway from the prefrontal region inferior to the principal frontal sulcus (IPFS) to area TEm. Several non-visual inputs to TE originate in area TG of the temporal pole (Fig. 6.1) and in structures belonging to the limbic system like areas TF and TH of the gyrus parahippocampalis and the presubiculum. Area TEO (Figs 6.1, 7.2) is connected with the lateral nucleus of the amygdala, area TE with the lateral and basal nuclei of the amygdala (Webster *et al.*, 1991). Both TEO and TE are connected with the perirhinal areas 35 and 36. Interestingly, some of the limbic connections are greatly changed during postnatal development. 'Both elimination and refinement of projection thus appear to characterize the maturation of axonal pathways between the inferior temporal cortex and medial temporal lobe structure in monkeys.' (Webster *et al.*, 1991).

The limbic connections, like the other connections of area TE, are presumably reciprocal. They may convey the 'internal' needs or drives from the hypothalamic–limbic structures to area TE, since the search for appropriate objects is dependent on the internal state of the animal. Furthermore, efferent connections from the different subfields of TE to limbic structures may serve visual object-related memory. Finally the different substructures of area TE, as illustrated in Figs 7.1(a) and (b), are interconnected with each other, whereby details still have to be explored by very small, circumscribed tracer applications.

Inferior Temporal Cortex

The distribution of the neuronal response characteristics in the different regions of STP and IT is described sche-

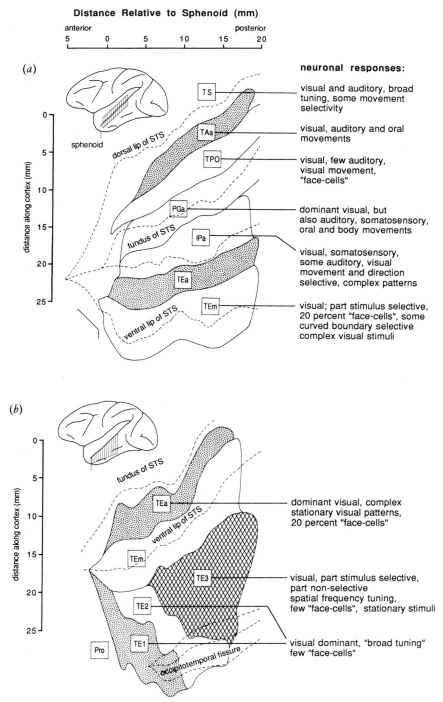

Fig. 7.1 *Scheme of the extension of the different cortical areas around the supratemporal sulcus (a) and at the outer surface of the inferior temporal lobe (b). In (a) the cortex around the supratemporal sulcus is unfolded and stretched in a direction perpendicular to the fundus of the sulcus. In (b) the lower bank of the supratemporal sulcus and the surface of the inferior temporal lobe are stretched out. On the right hand of the figures the main neuronal response properties deduced from recordings in the different cytoarchitectonic areas are summarized (from Baylis* et al., *1987, modified).*

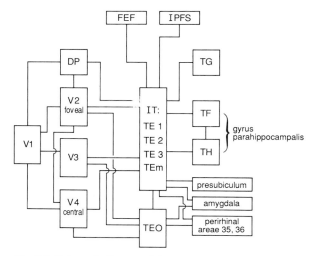

Fig. 7.2 *Schematic diagram of the connections of the areas TE of the macaque inferior temporal lobe. Only the connections with cortical areas on the ipsilateral hemisphere are drawn.*

matically in Figs 7.1(a) and (b). In the following we summarize some of the most important properties of neuronal responses recorded from the inferotemporal cortex and mention more details of stimulus features required to obtain a strong response from IT neurones. We also try to deduce from the neurophysiological data more general conclusions related to visual object recognition. The contributions of multimodal areas to object recognition, especially those located in the frontal lobe, are not discussed, because this task is beyond the scope of this volume. One of the multimodal integration areas, however, seems to be dominated by visual signals and therefore deserves a short description (Bruce *et al.*, 1981). Along the upper bank of the supratemporal sulcus the 'superior temporal polysensory area' (STP) extends over a large part of cortex. More than half of the neurones of this area responded to more than one sensory modality: 21 per cent to visual and auditory stimuli, 17 per cent to visual and somatosensory stimuli, 17 per cent had trimodal responses and 41 per cent were exclusively visual. The ERFs frequently covered both visual hemifields. Moving stimuli were often more effective than stationary patterns, but movement direction was crucial only in a few neurones. Some of the movement-sensitive neurones had preferable responses for stimuli moving either towards or away from the animal. About 30 per cent of STP neurones were stimulus-shape selective, in the other 70 per cent of visually responding cells no particular effect of stimulus size, site, orientation, contrast or colour was found. A small percentage of STP nerve cells responded rather selectively to face stimuli. This will be discussed in detail

in the next paragraph. In pattern-selective STP cells stimulus orientation was generally more important than stimulus shape. We presume that area STP may contribute to object recognition and social interaction, but further recording and lesion studies seem to be necessary to understand the significance of this multimodal cortical field.

In the following we will restrict our review to neurones of the inferior temporal lobe which are nearly selectively responding to stimuli of the visual domain (Fig. 7.1(b)).

Properties of Visual Input Signals to Inferior Temporal Cortex

Before we discuss the receptive field properties of TE neurones, it seems appropriate to summarize the properties of the neuronal receptive fields of the peristriate input areas (cf. Chapter 5). Continuing the work of Zeki (cf. Chapter 5), Tanaka *et al.* (1986) and Desimone and Schein (1987) demonstrated that the most important peristriate visual input area to TE, namely area V4, contains a considerable number of neurones selectively responsive to certain shapes and colours, but restricted in their responses to rather small ERFs. Movement and directional selectivity (about 10 per cent of the recorded neurones), sensitivity to the length and width of the stimulating light bar, variable size of the most effective stimuli (about 0.05 to 6 degrees), as well as spatial frequency tuning (between 0.12 and 8 cycles per degree), were found in V4 neurones. In spatial-frequency-tuned neurones the optimum grating period corresponded frequently to the ERF size. Since most V4 cells responded rather selectively to certain wavelengths, some showed sensitivity to spatial colour contrast and some exhibited even colour constancy effects (i.e. these neurones responded to surface colours rather than to wavelength mixtures; see Chapter 5 and Zeki, 1990). Evidently spatial and chromatic stimulus properties are combined within the retinotopically organized area V4 before retinotopic organization is lost in further visual signal processing within the inferior temporal lobe (Schein and Desimone, 1990). A combination of spatial and chromatic response properties seems to be one of the important measures performed by the neuronal network, providing a major input to essential brain areas in object recognition. We suppose that a similar integration is true for contours and spatial luminance changes in area V2, which provides another important visual input to areas TE and TEO. For both areas V2 and V4 mainly signals from the foveal representation are transmitted to areas TE, while the visual field periphery seems to play an inferior role.

Very recently Boussaoud *et al.* (1991) studied receptive field properties and connections of nerve cells located in area TEO. This area is a 10–15-mm-wide band of cortex extending from the lower lip of the STS towards the occipito-temporal sulcus at the basal temporal surface of the brain (Fig. 6.1). It is now considered to be a visual area which still possesses a loose retinotopic organization and is characterized by neuronal receptive fields intermediate in size between those of area V4 and area TE. The foveal and parafoveal parts of the visual field project to the lateral convexity of TE.

Receptive-field Properties of TE Neurones

IT cell data, as measured by single unit recordings, were predominantly from area TE, where areas TE1, TE2 and TE3 responses were lumped together in most studies. The responses of these inferior temporal lobe structures are dominated by the visual input, but in awake animals object-related or space-related attention, the type of behavioural task and the animal's experience seem to play a role in determining the strength of the neuronal response. It is therefore not easy to obtain reliable quantitative data on the receptive field properties of TE neurones.

In anaesthetized and paralysed monkeys Gross *et al.* (1967) found responses to diffuse visual stimuli in about 25 per cent of TE neurones, provided slow, repetitive light flashes were applied (e.g. 2 flashes per second). Moving small stimulus patterns were effective only in a few TE cells. Even in this preparation complex visual patterns were found to be selectively effective in some neurones, but later studies in conscious and behaving animals led first to the recognition of a highly complex response pattern to objects of different shapes. Receptive fields of TE neurones were large in comparison to those found in peristriate neurones.

All peristriate regions connected with area TE are retinotopically organized and transmit visual signals predominantly from the contralateral visual hemifield (cf. Chapters 3, 4 and 5). Only a small percentage of peristriate neurones also include a narrow part of the ipsilateral visual field within their ERF, provided their ERF centre is located along the vertical meridian. Under these conditions callosal fibres connecting homologous areas of the two hemispheres contribute to the neuronal responsiveness of peristriate neurones. The ERF size and the contribution of the ipsilateral visual field to the neuronal responses are changed dramatically in TE neurones: the retinotopic organization has disappeared in the areas of IT, while the ERFs of individual neurones are large, usually more than 10 degrees in diameter, some even extending across the greater part of the visual field and many far into the ipsilateral visual field. Clearly, the ERFs of TE neurones extend much more into the ipsilateral visual hemifield than the ERFs of V2, V3, or V4 and TEO neurones. As a rule, the fovea is part of the ERF of TE neurones. Ocular dominance has also disappeared in most TE neurones. Whenever an 'adequate' stimulus pattern is selected, the neuronal response depends very little upon whether the right or left eye is stimulated, or both.

Gross *et al.* (1977) determined the pathway through which visual signals from the ipsilateral visual hemifield reach TE neurones: a transection of the splenium corporis callosi and the anterior commissure abolished all neuronal responses to stimuli projected to the ipsilateral visual hemifield, while transection of the extrasplenial corpus callosum fibres had no effect on TE neurone reponses. Transection of the splenium alone led to a reduction of about 50 per cent in ipsilateral visual responses. In contrast, sectioning the anterior commissure alone led to no measurable changes in TE neurone response properties. These findings indicate the importance of the callosal fibres running through the splenium in integrating the two visual fields for the purpose of object recognition. This observation is helpful in understanding some of the symptoms occurring in patients suffering from unilateral brain lesions, including an impairment of the connections through the splenium. Such lesions affect the patient's ability in colour perception, object recognition or reading in both hemifields (cf. Chapters 11, 14, 18 and 19; see also Doty and Negrão, 1973).

Non-visual Experimental Conditions Modify Responses of TE Neurones

The response properties of TE neurones depend essentially on the experimental conditions. In anaesthetized (pentobarbital or nitrous dioxide) animals only about 25 per cent of the TE neurones respond to slowly repeated diffuse flashes and very few neurones to small moving or complex visual stimuli (Gross *et al.*, 1967). The characteristic selectivity of TE cells regarding stimulus shape, colour, movement direction etc. found in awake animals is lost not only under anaesthesia but also by immobilization. Gross *et al.* (1979) reported that uniocular eyeball immobilization (by sectioning all oculomotor nerves) led to an alteration in neuronal responses similar to that observed with general anaesthesia and total immobilization. This result is somewhat surprising and depended presumably on the visual stimulus conditions. In man, unilateral immobilization of the eyeball led to a disappearance of all visual pattern perception, sparing only a central foveal region, for which the small movements of the eyeball synchronous with the heartbeat were sufficient presumably to prevent the visual percept from fading. With the disappearance of pattern vision the appearance of a homogeneous medium grey filling the visual field from the periphery towards the centre was noted, provided the head was immobilized tightly by a head holder. Under this stimulus condition disappearance of visual objects is understandable. Intermittent retinal stimulation, however, restored

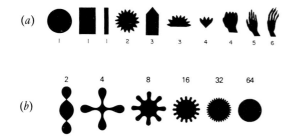

(a)

(b)

Fig. 7.3 *(a) Silhouette stimuli used to test the responses of a 'hand cell' of the inferior temporal lobe (Gross, 1973). (b) Silhouettes of 'Fourier descriptors' used as stimuli to activate TE cells (Desimone* et al., *1984).*

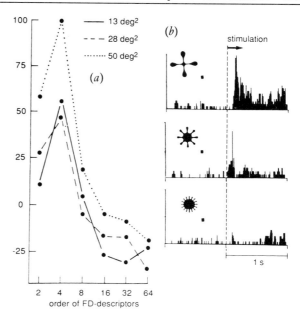

Fig. 7.4 *(a) The activity of TE neurones tested with silhouettes of 'Fourier descriptors' (Fig. 7.3(b)) depends on the number of the lobes as well as on the average size of the stimulus pattern as indicated in one example (13, 28 and 50 deg²) (Desimone* et al., *1984). (b) Example of the responses of a TE neurone, displayed in peristimulus time histograms, to 'Fourier descriptors' projected to the ERF (From Gochin* et al., *1991).*

visual form and object perception immediately (observations of O.-J. G., cf. Grüsser *et al.*, 1981). Intermittent opening and closing of the eyelids at 2–3 short blinks per second was easily sufficient to maintain pattern vision. Pattern vision was also preserved when the stimulus pattern was moved slowly across the visual field.

The general attention level was found to have considerable effects on TE neurone activity. Gross *et al.* (1972) reported that the visual response properties of TE neurones depended on the general cerebral activity as expressed by the frequency and amplitude distribution of the EEG waves. The best responses of TE neurones were found with a desynchronized EEG.

Search for Optimum Visual Stimulus Patterns and an Adequate Quantitative Description of TE Neurone Visual Responses

In the awake animal the activation of TE neurones depends on the shape, colour and visual context of the stimulus pattern, but very little on size, contrast and stimulus position within the ERF. Whenever a unit is 'specialized' to respond to a certain shape or movement direction, these stimulus conditions are invariant with respect to stimulus position within the ERF. In searching for the optimum stimulus activating a TE cell, experimental fantasy and some luck seem to be necessary. A minority of TE neurones responded only to very restricted stimulus patterns such as faces, parts of faces or hands. The responses of such 'face cells' will be discussed separately in the next paragraph. Many of the TE cells responded less selectively. When a TE cell exhibited narrow shape selectivity, however, it was not only valid for the whole ERF, but also remained invariant with respect to those stimulus parameters which still have some effect on the neurones of the peristriate belt, like contrast, stimulus size, chromatic composition, etc. (Schwartz *et al.*, 1983; Gross, 1991).

To elaborate on shape selectivity of inferior temporal lobe neurones in a more quantitative manner, a special set of stimulus patterns was selected: 'Fourier descriptors' (FD stimuli) as illustrated in Fig. 7.3(b). About 70 per cent of the TE cells were reported to be systematically tuned to these FD stimuli, i.e. response maxima were obtained with 2, 4, 8 or 16 'lobes', whereby the neuronal response varied minimally with stimulus size (Fig. 7.4; Desimone *et al.*, 1984).

Pollen *et al.* (1984) recorded from IT neurones in the owl monkey and applied as stimuli a special set of Gabor functions, namely one-dimensional spatial sinewave gratings, the amplitude of which decreased perpendicularly to the gratings according to a Gaussian function of variable width. The authors reported that IT neurones responded fairly selectively to the different stimulus classes generated by changing the grating spatial frequency and the spatial width of the Gaussian envelope. Pollen *et al.* concluded that under their stimulus conditions 'only one orientation band and one spatial frequency band provide an input onto each inferotemporal neuron.' This result suggests a highly selective filter function appearing between area V2, V4 and TEO neurones and the TE neurone output. Interesting and somewhat difficult to understand is the

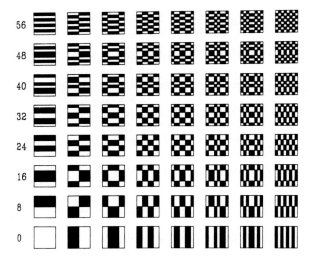

Fig. 7.5 *Set of Walsh functions as used to stimulate TE neurones in the experiments of Richmond* et al. *(1987).*

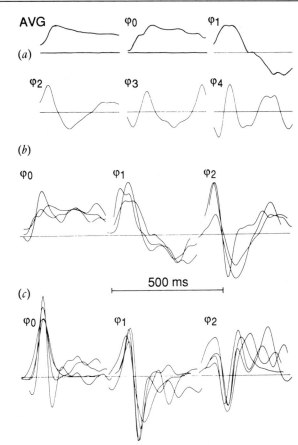

Fig. 7.6 *(a) Computation of the average response (AVG) and of 'principal' components in the responses of a TE neurone to a set of Walsh patterns as illustrated in Fig. 7.5. The first 5 principal components (phi 0, phi 1, phi 2, phi 3 and phi 4) computed from the data are displayed. (b) and (c) The first 3 principal components (phi 0, phi 1, phi 2) of 7 TE neurones are illustrated. The data of 3 neurones are superimposed in (b), that of 4 other neurones in (c). The common characteristic of the 3 neurones in (b) was a sustained first principal component (ϕ_o); that of the 4 neurones in (c) was a phasic first-principal component (from Richmond and Optican, 1987, modified).*

finding that the preferred spatial frequencies were very low (0.2–0.6 cycles per degree), leaving little opportunity for object specification by narrow contours or fine texture.

A rather ambitious and highly interesting approach to a quantitative analysis of TE neurone responses was made by Richmond *et al.* (1987), who explored the responses of TE neurones to a set of 64 Walsh functions. These are two-dimensional patterns as illustrated in Fig. 7.5. Walsh functions have the property that with a resolution visible in the highest spatial frequency chequerboard of the set, every black-and-white visual pattern can be represented by an adequate combination of Walsh patterns. Richmond and his co-workers analysed the temporal structure of the impulse sequences of TE neurones evoked by the different Walsh patterns, which were projected to the respective receptive fields. They found that the temporal sequence of action potentials conveyed a considerable amount of information related to the pattern used as a stimulus. To describe these findings quantitatively the temporal structures of the action potential sequences in the responses were analysed quantitatively by computing an orthogonal set of temporal waveforms, the so-called 'principal components', which were determined for every neurone from the responses to all Walsh patterns (Richmond and Optican, 1987). The first principal component (0th order) was related to the average neuronal impulse rate, a measure usually applied to evaluate neuronal responses. Higher-order principal components existed, however, which were not related to the average neuronal impulse rate at all and which were nevertheless essential properties of the neuronal responses. On average, 3 to 4 principal components could be determined with sufficient reliability. Their tem-

poral shape was found to be fairly similar across different classes of IT neurones (Fig. 7.6). Finally, an information theoretical analysis of the information transmitted by the first three principal components as compared with the information about the stimulus transmitted by the neuronal impulse rate was performed (Optican and Richmond, 1987). The most important result of this analysis was the finding that the highest number of impulses (i.e. the strongest increase in neuronal impulse rate) did not necessarily correspond to the highest transinformation flow values.

These important analyses put a strong caveat on the traditional (and technically easy) evaluation of neuronal responses by using averaged peristimulus time histograms or average impulse rates, as illustrated in many figures of this book. The work of Richmond and Optican, which to our knowledge was not pursued by other groups, opened the possibility that perhaps some of our difficulties in understanding the contribution of IT neurones to object recognition may not be due to a lack of experimental data but rather to an insufficient method of data analysis, which discards, as a rule, the temporal structure of the action potential sequences evoked by the visual stimulus patterns.

Network Responses

A further complication in the understanding of TE neurone responses may be caused by the fact that in most animal experiments for technical reasons the action potentials of only one or two neurones were recorded at one time. On the basis of the close interconnections found in tracer studies for the neuronal network of area TE, one could expect the neuronal responses to depend not only on the input stimulus patterns but also on gross interactions within area TE. Using the multiple-microelectrode recording technique and applying a cross-correlation and autocorrelation analysis of the neuronal impulse trains, Gochin *et al.* (1991) found that two classes of neuronal cojoint activation appeared: (a) a 'shared-input' activation with discharge coupling restricted to a rather small cortical area a few hundred μm in diameter and (b) a distributed correlated activity across longer intracortical distances, which led to input-independent correlations of neuronal activity. These findings support the hypothesis expressed above, of course, that object recognition is an achievement of the spatio-temporal activation of extended neuronal networks and not elaborated by an object-selective class of neurones. Thus in addition to the 'temporal structure complication', as illustrated by the work of Richmond and Optican, future generations of neuroscientists who wish to better understand our brain mechanisms underlying object recognition will most likely also have to analyse the spatial and temporal network properties of the inferotemporal lobe before they can honestly claim to have comprehended the function of this structure. A serious test of whether this goal has been achieved is the sufficiently precise mathematical or computer simulation of the neuronal network activity. We hope that these critical remarks will not prevent the reader from studying further what is known about TE-neurone response properties.

The Dependency of the TE Neurone Responses on Mechanisms of Attention

Richmond *et al.* (1983) studied the responses of area TE neurones in awake macaques which had been trained to detect the dimming of a fixation target. As long as the monkey was involved in the detection task, TE neurone responses to other visual stimuli projected to the respective ERF were reduced. When the fixation target was turned off and the trained monkey maintained its gaze position, the responses to the test stimuli increased. Evidently the functional diameter of the TE neurone–ERF shrank during the fixation and dimming detection task and re-expanded when the fixation target was turned off. In the same animals the typically large ERFs were found for TE neurones when the animals were anaesthetized; under these conditions the neuronal responses corresponded to those described in the early studies of Gross *et al.* (1969, 1972). From the findings of Richmond *et al.* it became evident that the 'visual context' and presumably object-related attention play an important role in TE neurone activation.

Sato (1988) elaborated on these properties of TE cells. He trained his monkeys to release a lever in a matching or in a dimming detection task. During these tasks a 'neutral' light bar, i.e. a stimulus to which the monkey was not required to respond, was projected to the respective ERF. When the pattern to be discriminated was located at or near the fovea, about 50 per cent of the TE neurones responded less to the 'neutral' stimulus when the latter was presented during the discrimination tasks than when it was presented in between the tasks (Fig. 7.7). This suppressive effect also depended, however, on the location of the neutral stimulus relative to the attended stimulus and the visual field. When the neutral stimulus was located in the ipsilateral visual field and the attended pattern was located in the contralateral, the response to the neutral stimulus was suppressed. The closer the attended stimulus pattern to the fovea, the greater was this 'extinction effect', but it was not present for reversed stimulus conditions (attended stimulus ipsilateral, neutral stimulus contralateral).

Moran and Desimone (1985) demonstrated that not only cell responses in the TE region but also the responses of area V4 neurones depended greatly on the animal's attention to a certain stimulus projected to the ERF. The unattended stimulus had a considerably lower efficacy in activating V4 neurones than the attended one. This was true for stimuli of various colours, orientations and sizes. The attentional effect may have been transmitted by a 'backward' connection from area TE to area V4.

More recently Spitzer *et al.* (1988) investigated the area V4 response properties in a monkey trained in a visual discrimination and delayed matching task of two difficulty

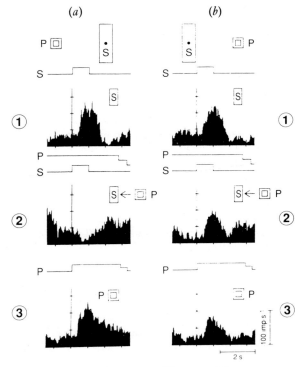

Fig. 7.7 *Responses of a macaque TE neurone. The responses to a light bar P projected to the foveal region are illustrated. (a) The pattern S attended was projected to the contralateral visual field. 1, Response to S stimulus. 2, Response to S stimulus is suppressed when task-relevant stimulus P was turned on. 3, Response to task-relevant stimulus alone. In (b) the same paradigm was applied for 1 to 3, but the task-relevant stimulus P was shifted to the visual hemifield ipsilateral to the hemisphere from which the recording was made (Sato, 1988, modified).*

levels. Stimuli were small bars of differing orientation and colour optimized in size for the response properties of the respective neuronal ERF. The task difficulty in colour discrimination or stimulus spatial orientation was set at two levels, with large or small orientation or hue differences. The neuronal responses became more selective with the more difficult discrimination conditions. This experiment demonstrated that a task-specific adaptation in the neuronal network necessary for object recognition, which one can expect in TE neurones, is present at earlier stages of cerebral visual signal flow.

Visual Memory Effects on TE Neurone Responses

Not only simultaneous presentation but also short-term and long-term visual memory affects the responses of TE

neurones. Fuster and Jervey (1982) tested the responses of TE cells during a visually delayed matching to sample task in 7 macaque monkeys. The animals sat in a primate chair facing a panel with a translucent stimulus and response buttons. First a central button lit up in one of four colours. The animal had to press the sample button and after a delay one of the four colours appeared as a stimulus to which the animal had to respond in the case of sample match identity in order to receive a juice reward. Thus in this task a coloured stimulus appeared twice in the foveal region of the visual field. Most TE cells were activated when the sample stimulus appeared, whereby the activation of many cells was dependent on the colour of the sample stimulus, in some cells restricted to one of the four colours (Fig. 7.8). Many TE cells showed a maintained discharge for a specific colour during the retention period between sample and match stimuli (Fig. 7.9(a)); other cells increased their activity only after the sample stimulus had disappeared. These cells increased their firing rate further when the animal performed the matching task (Fig. 7.9(b)). The findings of Fuster and Jervey indicate that all information necessary for performing the behavioural task was present in the TE neurone responses: colour-specific initial responses during sample presentation, retention of that colour by maintained activation, 'expectation activity' related to the matching colour and 'confirmation activity' when the sample and matching colour were the same. Of course, nothing can be said as to whether the response was indeed colour-specific or only class-specific (i.e. 'the 3rd of 4 possible classes') in the matching to sample task.

A very interesting experiment was designed by Miyashita (1988). He used computer-generated coloured fractal patterns (Fig. 7.10). The fractal patterns had a low similarity to each other. In a preceding study by Miyashita and Chang (1988) these patterns were found to evoke highly selective responses in some TE neurones, a fact expected from the data of Richmond *et al.* (1987). Since such fractal patterns had never been seen by the monkey before, TE neuronal selectivity indicated a basic general pattern sensitivity, independent of selective experience in the TE neuronal network. With the same type of patterns, however, Miyashita (1988) tested the effect of pattern learning on TE neurone responses. He presented a set of 97 coloured fractal patterns in a delayed matching task, always in the same sequence till this order was 'overlearned' by the animal. During the recording session these 97 learned patterns were applied in addition to 97 'new' coloured fractal patterns. Only a few of both the overlearned and the new fractal patterns led to an activation of a particular TE neurone during the delayed matching to sample task. A very interesting difference appeared, however, when the responses to the overlearned or the new fractal patterns were compared. The probability that a

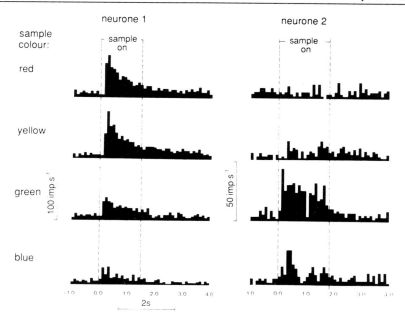

Fig. 7.8 *Responses of two TE neurones during a matching-to-sample task. Responses to onset of the sample stimulus which could have 4 different colours (red, yellow, green or blue, as indicated). The 2 neurones exhibited different chromatic sensitivities (Fuster and Jervey, 1982, modified).*

new fractal pattern activated a TE neurone was independent of the order of that pattern in the set, while for the fractals in the overlearned pattern it depended on the order, i.e. on the 'distance' from a pattern which led to a strong neuronal activation. This amazing result is illustrated in Fig. 7.11. In other words, the activity of a TE cell evoked by an abstract and meaningless stimulus pattern depends not only on its structural properties or the attention of the animal, but also on the learned context sequence in which this pattern appears. The consequences are obvious: TE neurone responsiveness is dependent – at least in part – on the visual experience acquired by the animal sometime before the experiment. One is tempted to correlate this statement with the morphological observations of Webster *et al.* (1991) mentioned above, and also with the problems in visual object recognition experienced by patients which had acquired pattern vision late in life after a longstanding pattern deprivation in childhood and adolescence (cf. Chapter 1).

Face-responsive Neuronal Activity in the Temporal Cortex of Primates

Non-human primates live like man in social groups, which may comprise a few family members, as with the orang-

utan, or several hundred loosely coordinated group members, as with some macaques or squirrel monkeys. Recognizing the face of a group member may be one way to detect its individuality. Understanding facial expression (and other averbal signs like gestures), recognizing the position of a certain group member in the social hierarchy and judging by recognizing the individual to which subgroup it belongs are abilities important for group coordination and may be deduced, at least in part, from static and dynamic face signals. Other face signals such as the direction of gaze may guide the attention of other animals to certain objects or events in the common extra-personal space, a behavioural pattern which is amplified by body posture and in man also by pointing. Monkeys are known to be able to discriminate other monkey faces well (Rosenfeld and van Hoesen, 1979) and evidently respond to facial expressions displayed by other group members. Hereby facial expression is only one component of socially relevant averbal signals of body language. The expression of a monkey face may attain a wide variety of finely tuned combinations, as illustrated in the 'Lorenz matrix' of Fig. 7.12. One can assume that monkeys are able to perceive these expressional changes and guide their own behaviour and expressions accordingly.

As is discussed in Chapter 14, circumscribed brain lesions may lead to the symptom of prosopagnosia. Patients suffering from prosopagnosia are no longer able to recognize the individuality of other people by face signals,

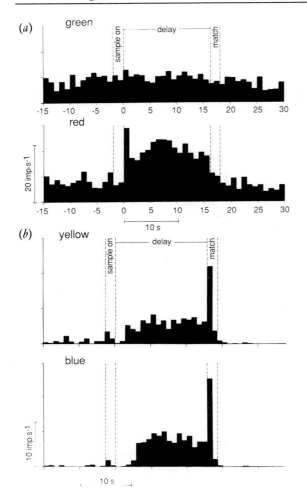

(a) green

(b)

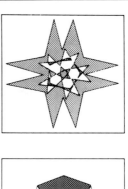

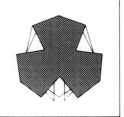

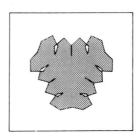

Fig. 7.10 *Schematic black-and-white drawings of 3 out of 97 multicoloured, computer-generated fractal patterns used in the experiments by Miyashita (1988).*

Fig. 7.9 *Responses of macaque TE neurones during a matching-to-sample task. (a) The neurone was activated during the delay period when the stimulus was red, but not when the stimulus appeared in other colours (e.g. green). The neuronal activation ceased when the monkey matched the sample to the delayed stimulus. (b) This TE neurone was activated independently of the colour of the sample stimulus during the entire delay period and produced a short burst of activity during the match (from Fuster and Jervey, 1982, modified).*

despite being able to recognize a face as a face, and may use other visual signals (e.g. typical body movements) or auditory cues. Some, but not all prosopagnosic patients are at a loss to recognize and judge facial expressions, and in some, but certainly not in all, social gaze interaction may be visibly disturbed.

In the following we will summarize the main findings on 'face-responsive' neuronal activity patterns recorded in single neurones of the superior temporal sulcus region

(STS) and of area TE of the inferior temporal lobe. As illustrated in Figs 7.1(a) and (b) 'face-cells' were found by means of microelectrode studies throughout a large part of the cortex around STS and in extended regions of areas TEm, TE1, TE2 and TE3. Face cells are neurones responding especially strongly to faces from a certain angle, parts of faces such as eyes or hair, or to facial expression. Rolls (1991) summarized what the experts defined as 'face-responsive' neurones. These cells, found among many others in a wide area of the temporal lobe, 'respond 2–20 times more (and statistically significantly more) to faces than to a wide range of gratings, simple geometrical stimuli, or complex 3-D objects.'

The first observation on IT neurones possibly sensitive to a face pattern was mentioned by Gross *et al.* (1969), who recorded from 226 TE neurones of macaque monkeys anaesthetized by nitrious oxide, and found that 'for at least three TE units, complex coloured patterns (e.g. photographs of faces, trees) were more effective than the stan-

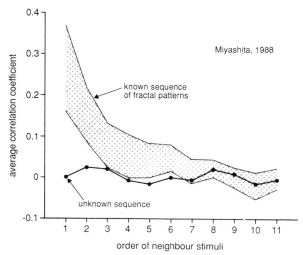

Fig. 7.11 *The neuronal activity evoked by a set of 97 learned multicolour fractal patterns (Fig. 7.10) of TE neurones depended on the stimulus configuration. It depended, however, also on the order of successive stimuli, i.e. on the temporal context of a stimulus pattern. This dependency was expressed by computing the average correlation coefficient between the neuronal activations evoked by the different patterns. The average correlation coefficient is plotted as a function of the order of neighbouring stimuli (abscissa). For an unknown sequence of 97 multicolour fractal patterns the average correlation coefficient of the responses to successive stimuli was around 0. The hatched area represents the variation of the correlation coefficients found in different TE neurones (from Miyashita, 1988, modified).*

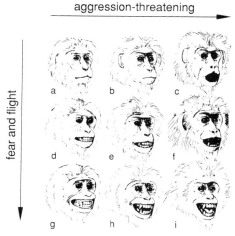

Fig. 7.12 *'Lorenz matrix' of facial expression in a macaque monkey. In the matrix, the degree of aggression increased from left to right, while fear and flight tendency increased from above to below. (a) Neutral expression, (b) mild threatening, (c) open threatening, (d) low tendency to flight, (e) mild aggression and fear mixed, (f) aggressive expression with some hesitation, (g) preparation for flight, (h) preparation for flight with some tendency to aggression and (i) balanced high tendency for aggression and flight (Chevalier-Skolnikoff, 1973; from Ploog, 1979, modified, with permission of the Springer Publishing Company).*

dard stimuli, but the crucial features were never determined.' In one unit the silhouette of a hand (Fig. 7.3(a)) was the most effective stimulus and the activation of this neurone by other silhouettes was clearly correlated to their similarity to a hand. Few 'face cells' were found in a later study exploring the responses of the 'superior temporal polysensory area' (STP) located in the upper bank and the fundus of the STS (Bruce *et al.*, 1981). Figure 7.13 illustrates the responses of such a face cell, which is still considered a 'typical' example: removing the eyes from the face stimuli led to a reduction of neuronal activity, and the same was true when instead of a 'realistic' face stimulus a highly schematic face was presented to the monkey.

A systematic search for face cells and the exploration of the stimulus features required to activate them has been continued by the work of Rolls, Perret and their co-workers up to the present. Studies by Kendrick and Baldwin (1987, 1989) demonstrated that nerve cells specialized in the processing of signals related to faces or people are also found in the inferior temporal lobe of sheep, i.e. IT face-responsive neuronal networks have also developed in

non-primate mammals. In the following we will summarize some of the main properties of primate temporal lobe neurones active in the processing of face signals.

Where Are 'Face Cells' Found?

Figure 7.14 (see below) summarizes the location of face-responsive neurones as recorded in the macaque brain by several research groups (Perret *et al.*, 1992). Three main cortical regions can be distinguished: the anterior part of the upper bank and a small fundal region of STS, the anterior third of the lower STS bank and the anterior half of the inferotemporal cortex (Perret *et al.*, 1982, 1985a, b, 1987; Desimone *et al.*, 1984; Baylis *et al.*, 1985; Hasselmo *et al.*, 1989; Rolls and Baylis, 1989). Owing to the massive projection of areas TE to limbic structures, one can also expect face-related responses in these structures (Fig. 7.2). So far, face cells have been recorded only from the amygdala (Rolls, 1984; Leonard *et al.*, 1985). In reading through the different studies on STS and TE face cells, one finds two properties in general: in none of the regions depicted in Fig. 7.14 does the average density of face cells presumably exceed 10 per cent and in all regions face cells are accumulated in small patches 0.5–3 mm across. As for

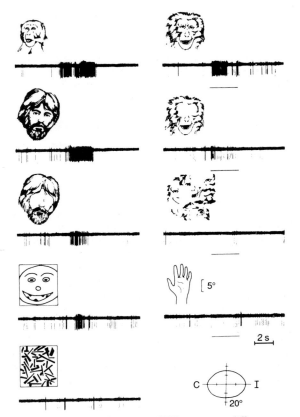

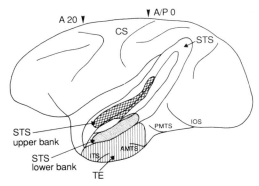

Fig. 7.14 *Schematic view of the three areas in the monkey temporal lobe from which 'face cells' were recorded in different laboratories by means of microelectrodes (Figure drawn by using a figure of Perret et al., 1992; supratemporal sulcus unfolded).*

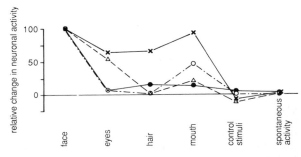

Fig. 7.13 *Responses of a primate STP neurone to different stimulus patterns as illustrated. Note that faces without eyes led to a reduced neuronal activation, while scrambled faces, random patterns and a hand did not evoke a significant change in spontaneous neuronal activity (from Bruce et al., 1981, by permission of the American Physiological Society).*

Fig. 7.15 *Response profile of four different 'face cells' recorded from macaque STS region. The relative change in neuronal activity (ordinate) to five different stimulus patterns (face, eyes, hair, mouth and non-face control stimulus) are shown. This figure illustrates that different STS cells respond differently to face components (from Perret et al., 1989, modified).*

neuronal networks responding rather selectively to other complex visual patterns, very narrow neuronal pools seem to be specialized for face-responsive tasks.

Receptive Field Properties

The size and location of the STS and TE face-responsive neurones are typically within the wide range of IT cell ERFs, as described above. Response properties are uniform across the respective ERF, which always includes the foveal part of the visual field. Some face-responsive neurones respond better to movement of the relevant stimuli and some prefer 3-D stimuli. All face cells respond to monocular stimulation of each eye and little binocular facilitation was observed.

Optimum Stimulus Features

Either the whole face or parts of it evoke a strong neuronal activation (Fig. 7.15). The 'response profiles' obtained when a full face is seen in front view, or eyes, hair or mouth are presented alone, may vary from neurone to neurone (Fig. 7.15; Perret *et al.*, 1982). Yamane *et al.* (1988, 1990) concluded from responses of TE neurones recorded in monkeys trained to discriminate three specific human faces out of a large set that face-responsive neurones detect the relationship (or the combination) of certain face-specific distances like hair–eyes, eye–eye, eyes–mouth, and that the overall neuronal activation is a function of these distances, which are weighted differently from cell to cell. This interesting work is a formal structure-analytical approach to understanding the peculiar selective response properties of face cells. It should be the goal of future work

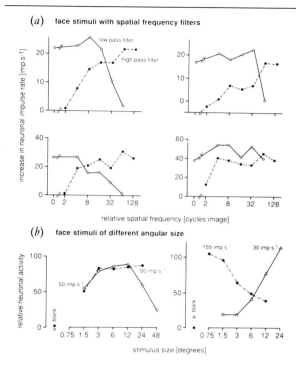

(*a*) face stimuli with spatial frequency filters

(*b*) face stimuli of different angular size

relative spatial frequency [cycles/image]

stimulus size [degrees]

Fig. 7.16 *Responses of macaque STS neurones. (a) The neuronal response (ordinate) depended on spatial frequency filtering of face stimuli. The effect of low-pass filtering or high-pass filtering is illustrated in four neurones. On the abscissa the limits of the respective low-pass or high-pass filtering of the face limits are given in cycles/image. Note that the responses of the four different neurones depended in a variable manner on spatial frequency filtering (from Rolls* et al., *1985, modified). (b) The response of macaque STS neurones to face stimuli also depends on the angular size of these stimuli as illustrated. On the ordinate is plotted the relative neuronal activity evoked by the face stimuli, on the abscissa the overall stimulus size in degrees of visual angle. The responses of the four STS neurones selected depended rather variably on stimulus size. A certain size invariant response was found only for stimulus sizes between 3 and 24 degrees in the neuronal responses plotted in the left-hand diagram (Rolls* et al., *1985, modified).*

to evaluate this model with respect to changes in neuronal responses due to stimulus view, size and relative spatial frequency, stimulus properties which will be discussed next.

During the last few years Perret and his co-workers (Perret *et al.*, 1986–1991) have provided good experimental evidence that STS face-responsive neurones may be divided into at least 4 different classes according to the preferred view of the face stimuli: frontal full face, right profile, left profile and back view. Furthermore, some of

the face cells seem to be sensitive to facial expression (Fig. 10.12), others not (Hasselmo *et al.*, 1989). Turning the head (of the stimulus) forwards or backwards or about 60 degrees to the left or right respectively still leads to an activation of face-position-sensitive face cells, but the activity level decreases with increasing angle of deviation from optimum view.

Performance in human face recognition depends very little on size and absolute spatial frequency content as long as the stimulus is not beyond the elementary visual acuity range. Perret *et al.* (1984) and Rolls *et al.* (1987) addressed this question for face cells and reported some dependency of STS neurone responses on the size and the spatial frequency of the photographs used as face stimuli (Fig. 7.16(a), (b)). It is evident from Figs 7.16(a) and (b) that the individual neuronal response remains invariant only within a rather limited stimulus range. Since the size and spatial frequency dependence of the neuronal responses exhibit a considerable variability between different 'face cells', the overall network response may be more stable with respect to spatial frequency and stimulus size variation than the individual cell responses.

A similar statement is true when the stimulus pattern is rotated in the projection plane around the optical axis of the animal. As everyone knows, a face seen upside down is more difficult to recognize than a face in the upright position. Sensitivity of face cells to rotation varies. Under certain conditions the response hardly depends on stimulus orientation (Fig. 7.17). Other cells, however, are highly sensitive to any positional change of the head in space (see below). As expected, the stimulus–background contrast also had some effect on the face cell reponses, especially when the contrast values were below 0.3 (Rolls and Baylis, 1986).

Cells Responding to Individual Faces

Occasionally face-responsive STS neurones were recorded which 'preferred' one out of many faces, i.e. one face evoked a much stronger response than all others in the stimulus set. According to the model of Yamana and his co-workers, mentioned above, this can be expected whenever an individual face fits best in the structural template of the neurone defined by the characteristic inner-face distances. Despite such apparently selective responses, this observation also does not support the idea of 'grandmother cells'. Although one particular class of face cells may respond rather selectively to an individual face, many other cells respond in a rather variable manner to the same face. Furthermore, no one so far has claimed the existence of 'face-only' cell reponses, since most face cells also respond at least mildly to non-face stimuli. Figure 7.17 illustrates the different responses of a highly selective face cell to two faces known to the animal. Typically the

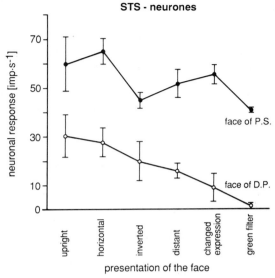

Fig. 7.17 *Response profile of a macaque STS neurone which responded differently to the faces of two subjects known to the animal (P. S. and D. P.). The neuronal activation above spontaneous activity (ordinate), however, was also dependent on the position of the respective face (upright, horizontal, inverted) or its angular size reduced by greater distance, on facial expression and whether it was seen through a green filter, as indicated (from Perret et al., 1989, modified).*

response of this cell also depended on the rotational position of the faces.

Modification of Neuronal Responses by Experience

In the daily recording of face cell activity, the experimenter naturally uses his own face as a readily available stimulus. He or she is well known to the experimental animal, however. Are face-responsive neuronal networks sensitive to experience? Rolls *et al.* (1989) studied whether STS neurones changed their responses to a set of faces when the latter were presented to the animal repeatedly. Six out of 20 neurones studied altered the strength of their reponses during the progress of familiarity with the set of faces. Figure 7.18(a) illustrates two examples. In a second set of recordings 26 neurones were tested as to whether their response properties changed when a novel face was added to a learned set of familiar faces. Five neurones altered their response strength to the familiar faces according to the scheme illustrated in Fig. 7.18(b): When a novel face was added to the set, most familiar faces led to an increased neuronal activity, a few to reduced activity. The novel face evidently changed the 'context' within which the familiar faces were perceived.

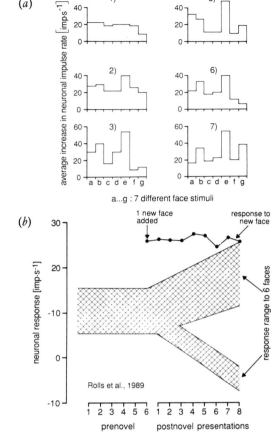

Fig. 7.18 *(a) Responses of a monkey STS neurone. The average neuronal response (ordinate) to seven different face stimuli depended not only on the faces used as stimuli but also on the degree to which the monkey became acquainted with the stimuli. The response profile related to the 7 different face stimuli (a–g) changed significantly with the number of presentations. The average activity evoked by the first, second, third, fifth, sixth and seventh presentation of the face stimuli sequence is illustrated and shows the effect of repetition on the neuronal responses. (b) Schematic diagram of the response range of a macaque STS neurone to a set of familiar faces before ('prenovel') and after ('postnovel') a new face was added to the set of known face stimuli. By the addition of the new face, which evoked by itself a fairly strong neuronal response, the responses to the other faces were changed. The neuronal activity evoked by 2 faces of the set declined, while that evoked by 4 other faces in the set increased. The hatched area indicates the range within which the neuronal activations were found in this experiment (from Rolls et al., 1989, modified).*

Gaze Direction as a Stimulus Parameter

Recent studies by Perret and his co-workers (1989, 1990, 1991, 1992) on STS face cells provide important new insight into the response properties of these neurones,

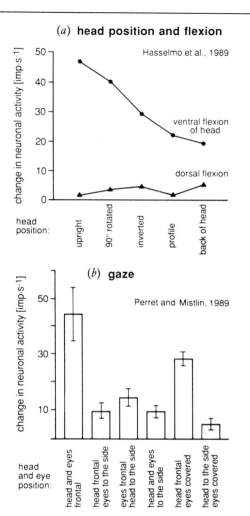

(a) head position and flexion

Hasselmo et al., 1989

ventral flexion of head

dorsal flexion

change in neuronal activity [imp·s⁻¹]

head position:

upright | 90° rotated | inverted | profile | back of head

(b) gaze

change in neuronal activity [imp·s⁻¹]

Perret and Mistlin, 1989

head and eye position:

head and eyes frontal | head frontal eyes to the side | eyes frontal head to the side | head and eyes to the side | head frontal eyes covered | head to the side eyes covered

Fig. 7.19 *Responses of primate STS neurones. (a) This neurone was most sensitive to ventral flexion of the head seen by the monkey, while dorsal flexion of the head led to very few changes in neuronal activity. This ventral–dorsal flexion bias in neuronal response was modified by the position of the head seen by the animal (upright, 90 degrees rotated sideways, upside down, profile or seen from the rear) (from Hasselmo et al., 1989, modified). (b) Responses from a macaque STS neurone sensitive to gaze of the stimulus relative to the experimental animal. The neurone was activated best when the stimulus was a face in frontal view with gaze towards the animal. Head and eye position of the stimulus modified the neuronal activity. When the head was maintained in the frontal position but the eyes looked to the side, the neuronal activity decreased. The same was true when the eyes looked straight ahead but the head was turned to the side, or when both were turned to the side. When the head was placed in the frontal position but the eyes were covered, the neuronal activity was also reduced in comparison with the initial condition. The weakest response was recorded when the head was turned to the side and the eyes were covered. (From Perret and Mistlin, 1989, modified.)*

with the possibility that the face-related neuronal responses discussed so far may constitute only the 'background' of another function, namely social gaze contact or perception of another social meaning of gaze direction. Gaze of the social partner has a striking effect on the responses of STS neurones, which are sensitive to the position of the seen head in space and/or the eye in head. More than 60 per cent of the STS cells responsive to the sight of a head were found to be also sensitive to the gaze direction of the head (Perret *et al.*, 1985b, 1987c; Hasselmo *et al.*, 1989; Perret and Mistlin, 1989; Perret, 1992). Presumably the direction of deviation of gaze from the frontal straight-ahead view is evaluated by many STS cells. The activity of these face cells depends on which direction and how strongly gaze deviates upwards, downwards, to the right or to the left. Figure 7.19 illustrates some of the findings relevant to this task.

Cells which monitor the gaze position of a social partner have reached a higher level of stimulus abstraction than face-reponsive neurones. They inform the observer's brain about properties of visual objects independent of the view of the observer. Some STS neurones evidently fulfil this condition. The hypothesis that the cortex around the STS contains a field involved in social gaze evaluation and not in face recognition is supported by a recent study by Cowey and Heywood (1991, 1992). These authors found that the monkey's ability to discriminate between pictures of faces and non-faces, to select the odd face from a group of known faces, to perform a matching to sample task with faces, to identify faces and to discriminate between known and unknown faces, was not impaired by bilateral destruction of the STS region.

All these findings lead to the interesting question of whether the 'face-responsive' network of the STS region is recognizing faces at all, or rather the gaze movements and gaze position of the partners in the social field instead. If this hypothesis is true, it will be of some relief to those trying to understand human brain function in the context of hominid evolution. No morphological or functional homologies between a region around the gyrus fusiformis, highly relevant for face recognition in man (cf. Chapter 14), and the face-responsive neurones in monkey STS have to be sought. Furthermore, the phylogenetically highly improbable hypothesis that the STS area moved during hominid evolution around the outer surface to the inner surface of the temporal lobe and hereby of necessity 'jumped' across several well-established cytoarchitectonic areas to reach the region around the gyrus fusiformis can be abolished. In our opinion, when one attempts to find areas homologous to the human face-detecting neuronal system, one has to search in the inferior medial part of IT for primate face cells which were shifted during hominoid and hominid phylogenesis towards the mesial temporo-occipital region near the fusiform gyrus.

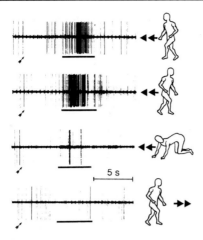

Fig. 7.20 *Some neurones in the inferior temporal lobe region TE respond to the body posture of the stimulus and the direction a person is moving relative to the animal. This recording was made from the temporal lobe of a sheep, but similar responses were also obtained in STS neurones of macaque monkeys. Note that the approach of the person led to an activation of the neurone, but only when the approaching person moved in a bipedal and not in a quadrupedal position (from Kendrick and Baldwin, 1989, by permission of Elsevier Publishing Company).*

In addition, these thoughts lead to a testable hypothesis, namely the prediction of a 'new' symptom appearing in patients suffering from lower medial temporal lobe lesions: social gaze agnosia, which should dissociate from prosopagnia, but may be associated with difficulties in recognizing facial expression.

Facial Expression

Rolls (1986a, b, 1990) repeatedly emphasized that within STS different neurones respond to faces as structural stimuli and to facial expression. The neuronal reponses were measured with face stimuli of 3 monkeys and with 3 different facial expressions for each face (Hasselmo *et al.*, 1986b, 1989). 15 TE neurones out of 45 showed response differences to different face identities but not to facial expression, and 9 neurones recorded from the STS region responded with the reversed dissociation. Hasselmo and his co-workers also discussed the possibility that these cells responded predominantly to social facial signals like changes in gaze position (Rolls, 1991).

The dissociation between neuronal mechanisms of recognizing face identity and those relevant to the perception of facial expressions seems to be meaningful in the light of clinical observations (chapter 14). It is still too early, however, to attribute these two functions to different distributed networks, one in the STS region, the other in the inferotemporal lobe area TE.

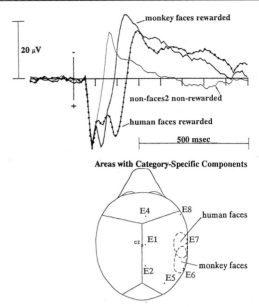

Fig. 7.21 *Averaged evoked potentials from the electroencephalogram of a Java monkey who was trained to discriminate monkey faces, human faces and non-faces of different classes. With chronically implanted electrodes above the temporal lobe (E7, E6) the EP related to non-faces had only one early peak at about 95 ms. This peak also appeared with faces as stimuli, but with monkey faces a second peak appeared at about 120 ms and with human faces a third peak appeared at about 190 ms. These two face-related peaks were independent of which stimulus was rewarded. The late peak, appearing typically when human faces were stimuli, was maximum above the inferior temporal lobe in more anterior regions as compared with the second peak appearing when both monkey and human faces were used as stimuli. The stimulus consisted of a sudden change (< 6 ms) in the stimulus patterns without a change in the overall pattern luminance (Fuhry and Grüsser, 1990).*

Beyond Faces

Averbal social communicative signals comprise more than just faces and facial expression. It is therefore not surprising that in addition to the 'hand cells' encountered in area STP (see above), expressive gestures and movements of an entire person have some impact on the responses of some STS cells. Body posture, a socially important sign in a monkey colony, was found to be a parameter having an effect on STS cells as well as movement on the part of the investigator towards or away from the animal. Thus head position was only one of the signals evaluated, since the neuronal activity evoked by seeing a human subject in quadrupedal as opposed to bipedal position was only modified but not determined predominantly by head position. The neuronal activity changed significantly when the body position of the stimulus changed from the quadrupedal to bipedal position even when the head was not seen by the monkeys (Perret *et al.*, 1991). Such signals also determine cell responses in the sheep temporal lobe, as illustrated in Fig. 7.20 (Kendrick and Baldwin, 1989) and are therefore not primate-specific responses.

It seems fairly probable that STS cells located in the region where face cells are found process a large variety of signals related to socially relevant body gestures used and understood by the monkeys in their social field.

Face-related Components in the Visual Evoked Potentials (VEPs)

Monkeys trained to discriminate monkey faces from non-faces and/or human faces served as experimental subjects for recording evoked potentials in the electroencephalogram through electrodes chronically implanted above one cortical hemisphere. As Figs 7.21 and 7.22 illustrate, face-responsive components appeared in the evoked potentials recorded through the electrodes above the inferior temporal lobe. These face-responsive components were generated independently of which class of visual stimuli was rewarded (non-faces, faces, monkey faces only or human faces only). When human faces were used as stimuli, a VEP component appeared which was not observed in the responses evoked by monkey face stimuli. The spatial distribution of this component was somewhat different from the face-responsive component in the VEP common to the

responses evoked by monkey and human faces (Fuhry and Grüsser, 1989a, b; Grüsser and Fuhry, 1990).

Visual Signal Recognition and the Temporal Lobe

The data described in the preceding paragraphs led to the following conclusions regarding the function of temporal lobe structures in visual signal processing:

1. The excitatory receptive fields increase in diameter by approximately a factor of 3 for every cortical relay area. For the pathway V1–V4–TEO–TE an increase in the ERF by about 25–30 would be the result. For the pathway V1–V2–V4–TEO–TE a more than 80-fold increase follows. ERFs 20 to 80 times larger than in V1 were indeed found in TE neurones.

2. With the increase in the ERFs the retinotopic organization of an area in the occipito-temporal (O-T) pathway becomes coarser and coarser till it disappears with the transition from TEO to TE. Correspondingly, specialization of the neuronal responses generalizes across the ERF.

3. Signals from contrast, colour and movement 'channels' are successively integrated along the O-T pathway. It is to date not clear how surface colour and texture are integrated into object perception, but evidently this inte-

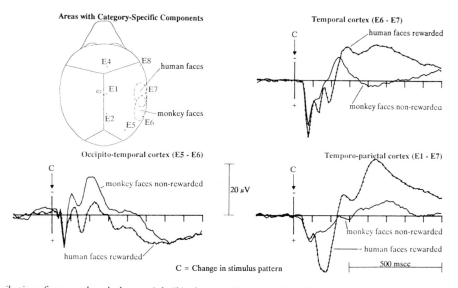

Fig. 7.22 *Distribution of averaged evoked potentials (bipolar recordings as indicated) in a monkey trained to discriminate between monkey faces, human faces and non-face stimuli. A prominent 'third' peak characteristic of human face stimuli appeared in bipolar recordings between temporal electrodes E6 and E7. Differences between responses to monkey faces and human faces were also evident in recordings E1–E7, but minimally in E5–E6. The peak appearing after about 160–170 ms was independent of which class of stimulus was rewarded (from L. Fuhry and O.-J. Grüsser, 1990, unpublished).*

gration has occurred along the O–T pathway before the signals reach the inferior temporal cortex.

4. There is no experimental evidence whatsoever that the items we perceive in the world of visual objects and signals as distinct classes ('universals') are represented by the activity of a single or very few classes of IT neurones (cf. Barlow, 1972). All experimental evidence supports the hypothesis that objects and other complex visual signals are represented by a widespread activity of IT neurone ensembles, whereby the contribution of different functional classes varies. We still do not understand the significance to be attributed to the activity of different neuronal classes in the generation of a percept in which the objects are perceived highly independent of the elementary stimulus parameters. It seems fairly probable that, as in the frog visual system where the occurrence of neuronal 'worm or bug detectors' has been claimed without the necessary experimental evidence, in primate IT neuronal networks also the spatio-temporal co-operation of manifold different nerve cell classes represents the objects. The model proposed for the frog may also be applicable to IT function: each neuronal class represents an elementary informational 'letter', whereby many 'words' can be constructed out of the finite set of elementary letters. The spatio-temporal combination of different neuronal 'words' into a distinct 'sentence' finally represents the unique object recognized at the perceptual level (cf. Grüsser and Grüsser-Cornehls, 1978 and Chapter 1).

5. IT neurone activity evoked by a distinct object or complex visual signal depends on the context within which the object appears, i.e. the neuronal activity varies with the set of other visual stimuli presented simultaneously or shortly before. IT neurone activity also seems to depend on the 'expectation' set by previous object learning, either in a sequential context or by individual familiarity with a particular object. Finally, IT neurone responses depend on past experience and on longstanding learning processes, but little is known about the 'sensitive' periods of visual object learning.

6. The complexity of the correlation between object representation and IT neurone activity is not surprising for those who have had experience with patients suffering from visual agnosias or other disorders of higher visual brain functions. Despite extended brain lesions leading to considerable defects in the construction of a meaningful visual world, the patients impress the neurologist again and again by their 'detour' strategies in overcoming their cerebral deficits in daily life. Furthermore one gains the impression that such a strategy is all the more successful the 'higher' the lesion is located in the hierarchy of cerebral visual data processing. Regarding the widely distributed neuronal networks interacting with each other within the inferior temporal lobe, such 'detour' abilities seem to be readily available in all those patients who have not lost the whole inferior temporal lobe or its afferent and efferent connections.

8 Brain Lesions: Grey or White Matter – It Matters

In this chapter we summarize briefly the principal events with which one must be familiar in order to understand the differences present when a brain lesion affects predominantly the white matter, the grey matter or both.

The Telephone Network – An Early but Misleading Brain Function Model: Neuronal Connections and Associations

In science, facts that are quite evident sometimes remain obscure or neglected for generations before they reach the cognitive level of scientists. This happened with the visible compartments of the brain. When one cuts a piece of fresh calf brain into slices to prepare 'cervelles de veau', a delicacy in South German, Swiss and French cuisine, the 'grey' matter and 'white' matter are evident, except that a 'naive' observer would use other names: the grey matter appears reddish, the white matter has a slightly yellowish tint. The gourmet discriminates between both and also between cerebrum and cerebellum. In the thirteenth century Albert the Great – of south German background – differentiated between the grey and white matter of the brain ('velum' and 'medulla'), but for generations neuroanatomists did not integrate this observation into their teaching until the Roman professor Archangelo Piccolomini emphasized the distinction between grey and white matter in an anatomy book published in 1586 (cf. Chapter 2). Thereafter, the neuroscientists also began to look into the functional meaning of these two compartments of the brain.

The anatomists of the Renaissance attributed two functions to the white matter.

1. Transport of the 'spiritus animalis' or the 'succus nervosus' through 'small tubuli' believed to run through the white matter;

2. Functional association of signals by means of branching and confluence of many white-matter tubuli (Chapter 2).

Only after the neurone doctrine was established towards the end of the nineteenth century were the associative mechanisms of the brain sought in the grey matter. Between the generation of Purkinje, Schwann and Schleiden in the first half of the nineteenth century and that of His, Waldeyer, Flechsig and Cajal in the second half, the basic principles now accepted by neuroscientists regarding the functional differentiation between grey matter and white matter were established. Nowadays, for the first examination in neuroanatomy every medical student has to know that a functional dichotomy exists between the two compartments of the brain: the grey matter is the highly organized cellular structure where nerve cells are ordered into layers and columns, receive synaptic contacts at the surface of their somata and dendrites, and send off an axon that branches either within a rather narrow cortical region or enters the white matter to reach other parts of the brain. The white matter consists of glial cells and efferent and afferent axons of different diameters and different degrees of myelinization. Cortical nerve cell axons connect one cortical area to the next (U-fibres), to the mirror area or other parts of the other hemisphere through the corpus callosum, and to other areas of the ipsilateral hemisphere by means of long fibre bundles, which frequently join together forming distinct tracts. Cortical axons also project through the internal and external capsule to subcortical and spinal centres or to the cerebellum. Afferent axons running through the subcortical white matter originate in the brain stem, the thalamic nuclei or the basal ganglia.

Axons send signals from their nerve cell to their many synaptic terminals by means of action potentials. These action potentials are transmitted along the axon membrane with a speed of about $0.5–150 \, \mathrm{m \, s^{-1}}$. The velocity of axonal conduction depends on the diameter of the axon and its myelin sheath. The nerve cell transmits its messages by means of the change in the temporal sequence of successive action potentials leading to different 'impulse rates', measured in impulses per second [imp s^{-1}]. In addition to this fast electrical signal transmission by action potentials, chemical messages and particle transport use a slower, intra-axonal transport system. For example, by the 'fast' anterograde transport (about 400 mm/day) vesicles are exported from the nerve cell soma to the synaptic terminals. The vesicles are produced by the endoplasmic reticulum and the Golgi apparatus of the cell body and contain precursors of the synaptic transmitter. In addition to the fast anterograde transport a slow axoplasmic flow exists, transporting soluble proteins, peptides and so forth from the cell soma to the axonal terminals. Besides the anterograde transport, fast retrograde transport is present by which vesicular structures (lysosomes) are moved from axonal terminals towards the cell body. This transport has in part a 'scavenger' function; it also moves polypeptides with messenger functions as nerve growth factors from the axonal periphery to the cell soma. These polypeptides interact with the DNA or the mRNA system of the cell. Retrograde and anterograde transport is used in numerous neuroanatomical studies to trace connections from one part of the brain to the next by means of tracer substances (Schwartz, 1979; Grafstein and Forman, 1980; Ochs, 1982).

After the difference between the two classes of brain compartments for signal processing and signal conduction had been generally accepted towards the end of the nineteenth century, the telephone network was taken as an obvious model of brain function. The white matter was considered as a structure of 'wire' bundles, the grey matter as the switchboard and dialogue 'centre' as served by the assistants of the telephone network. The telephone was invented in about 1860 by Philip Reis of Gelnhausen and Alexander Bell of Edinburgh and was widely used by industry, state admininistration, military organizations and private households of European bourgeois society during the last decades of the nineteenth century. The telephone network fitted very well as a model in the interpretations of brain function as summarized by Wilhelm Wundt (1874/1893) in five general statements:

1. Each nervous element is connected with other nervous elements. Physiological functions are meaningful only in the context of these connections (the principle of the connections of elements).

2. No single element of the nervous system has any specific function. The specificity of the function of a nerve cell is dependent on its connections to and relations with other nerve cells (the principle of functional indifference).

3. For every element (nerve cell) that loses its function or is inhibited in its function, other elements can act as substitutes, provided sufficient connections are present (the principle of substitution).

4. Every distinct function is correlated with a certain region of the central organ (the brain), provided that connections are present. Whenever a certain function is sufficiently complex, it is related to activity of a certain complex of brain regions, the nerve cells of which are connected with each other (the principle of localized functions).

5. Every element improves its aptitude for a certain function the more frequently it has to serve this function (the principle of training).

In the light of today's knowledge, of course, the telephone network model looks like a somewhat insufficient model of brain function. Nevertheless, the development of diagrams with 'centres' representing certain functions and their afferent and efferent connections was an important step in understanding the higher brain functions of man. Carl Wernicke (1848–1905) was, along with Ludwig Lichtheim, the most prominent 'connectionist' in early clinical neuropsychology, then called 'clinical brain pathology'. Wernicke tried to bring some order to the manifold symptoms of aphasia by separating subcortical from cortical aphasias, caused by lesions of the motor or sensory speech centre located in the grey matter of the foot of the third frontal gyrus (the Broca centre) or the planum temporale region of the upper temporal gyrus (the Wernicke centre). Subcortical aphasias were believed to be caused by a disconnection of the projection fibres reaching the cortical speech areas from non-speech regions of the brain. The third type of aphasia, the transcortical aphasia, was thought by Wernicke to develop after an interruption of association fibres between the cortical speech centres (conduction aphasia). Lichtheim published 'wiring diagrams' corresponding to these ideas, and since then more than three generations of neuroscientists have tried to elucidate their findings by brain function models represented by 'telephone network' diagrams: grey matter centres connected by signal–conducting white matter. As the reader will realize, we also prefer such diagrammatic schemes as graphic metaphors to summarize essential properties of central nervous functions.

In our generation, Norman Geschwind and his coworkers took up this nineteenth–century concept and generalized it by differentiating neuropsychological defects caused by focal lesions of the cortical grey matter from those caused by local interruption of the white matter. The latter were called disconnection syndromes (Geschwind, 1965). This clinically meaningful schematic subdivision of higher brain function disturbances was also applied to lesion-induced defects of visual perception and cognition. When one reads papers dealing with disconnection syndromes, one frequently gains the impression that the old telephone network model is still believed to be literally true. This was certainly not suggested by Geschwind, since he was aware that axotomy leads to a rather

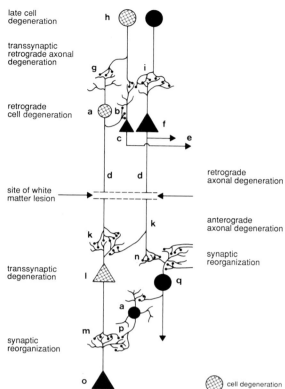

late cell
degeneration

transsynaptic
retrograde axonal
degeneration

retrograde
cell degeneration

site of white
matter lesion

transsynaptic
degeneration

synaptic
reorganization

retrograde
axonal degeneration

anterograde
axonal degeneration

synaptic
reorganization

cell degeneration

Fig. 8.1 *Schematic pictorial summary of the events happening when axons running through the white matter of the brain are disconnected by an acute white-matter brain lesion. Two large classes of degenerative processes are observed operating in either an anterograde or a retrograde direction relative to the signal flow from the nerve cells through the axons to the synaptic terminals. In the retrograde direction the degenerative process commences with an axonal degeneration affecting the axon (d), and the myelin sheath. It finally reaches the nerve cell (a), which may degenerate completely. The axonal collaterals (b) of the degenerating axon experience a complete synaptic degeneration, which leads to a reorganization of the synaptic surface of the contacted nerve cell (c) not directly affected by the lesion. When the axon interrupted by the white matter lesion is only a side branch (d) of another uninjured main axon (e) of a nerve cell (f), the process of retrograde degeneration does not seriously affect the nerve cell and the main axon, but only the interrupted axonal branch (d). Retrograde cell death of a nerve cell (a) leads to transsynaptic retrograde changes in the synapses (g) that contact the nerve cell (a). Whenever the majority of synapses of a nerve cell (h) activating the degenerate nerve cell (a) undergo retrograde transsynaptic degeneration, eventually the nerve cell (h) is also affected. If this nerve cell degenerates then synaptic reorganization in the nerve cell layer of nerve cells (c) and (f) may occur (i). Anterograde degeneration occurs in the axons of the white matter cut (k) and ultimately leads to a dissolution of all synapses belonging to the axonal branches of the axons cut (k, n). When a postsynaptic nerve cell (l) has been predominantly under the synaptic control of the axons cut,*

transsynaptic anterograde degeneration of this nerve cell, its axon and synaptic terminals (m) probably occurs. If only part of the synaptic input to a postsynaptic nerve cell is removed, synaptic reorganization occurs (n). Owing to the synaptic degeneration in (m), higher-order postsynaptic nerve cell synaptic surfaces may change as well and synaptic reorganization will be the consequence (p). Synaptic degeneration (k, n) most likely activates local growth of axonal branches of nerve cells not directly involved in the degenerative process (q).

complex mechanism of anterograde and reterograde degeneration, followed by adaptive mechanisms involving cortical and subcortical grey matter. In the following we provide a rather schematic overview of the mechanisms one has to consider when investigating patients suffering from 'focalized' lesions in the white or grey matter of the brain, as seen by the modern imaging techniques such as X-ray computerized tomography (CT) or magnetic resonance imaging (MRI).

Anterograde and Retrograde Degeneration after Axotomy

The axons of retinal ganglion cells form the optic nerve and connect the retina with several subcortical visual centres (Chapter 3). The optic nerve is not a peripheral nerve but a central tract, since the retina is embryogenetically and morphologically a part of the brain. Interruption of optic nerve fibres can thus serve as a handy experimental paradigm to investigate the events occurring after white-matter disconnection. Optic nerve axotomy is is achieved by xenon or laser light coagulation of the retina or the optic disc, by direct cutting of the optic nerve, or by electrical coagulation by means of electrodes inserted stereotactically into the optic chiasm or the optic tract. When an axon is interrupted, nerve cell function and structure change proximal and distal to the axotomy site. Such anterograde and retrograde degeneration effects will be illustrated in the following and are summarized schematically in Fig. 8.1.

Anterograde Degeneration

After optic nerve axotomy all recordable activity from the axons ceases, but the electrical excitability remains intact for about 4 or 5 days. Therefore electrical stimulation of the optic tract leads to synaptic activation of cells in the lateral geniculate nucleus (LGN) as long as the synaptic terminals are functioning. The morphological and functional changes that were observed during the first week after optic nerve axotomy can be divided into the following stages:

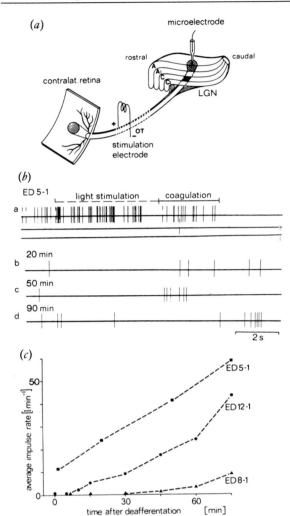

Fig. 8.2 *(a) Schematic drawing of the experimental situation after acute deafferentation by local retinal photocoagulation of the cat retina. The coagulated area of the retina (hatched region) causes a cylindrical population of cells in the layers A and C of the contralateral LGN to be deafferented. The response of the deafferented cells can be tested by electrical stimulation of the optic tract (OT). (b) Spontaneous activity and light activation of a latency class I on-centre LGN cell recorded before, during and at selected times after acute deafferentation. Note the slow recovery of activity with time after deafferentation (20, 50 and 90 min). (c) Changes in the spontaneous impulse rate (ordinate) of three neurones recorded after acute deafferentation by photocoagulation of a small retinal area including the receptive field. The average impulse rate (imp min^{-1}) is plotted as a function of time after deafferentation. The respective impulse rates before deafferentation were for ED 5–1 latency class I, on-centre neurone): 13 imp s^{-1}, ED12–1 (latency class II, off-centre neurone): 15.5 imp s^{-1}, ED 8–1 (latency class I, on-centre neurone): 8.5 imp s^{-1}. (From Eysel and Grüsser, 1978.)*

1. The nerve cell soma activity in discharging action potentials was not immediatedly affected when the axon a few millimetres away was cut. For example, neuronal activity of retinal ganglion cells is not seriously impaired when the optic nerve is cut behind the eye. When the retina is removed from an excised eye and placed into an appropriate bathing solution, nerve cell activity goes on, despite retinal ganglion cells having lost the main part of their axons.

2. When the optic nerve axons were interrupted, the spontaneous activity of LGN cells dropped immediately from an average of 17 impulses per second to < 0.1 impulses per second.

3. Within the first hours after axotomy the spontaneous activity of LGN cells recovered to a level of about 5–10% of the pre-axotomy values without any signals reaching the LGN cells from optic nerve fibres (Fig. 8.2; Eysel and Grüsser, 1974, 1975, 1978).

4. Stimulating the optic tract or optic chiasm electrically led after axotomy to an increased excitatory postsynaptic potential and increased postsynaptic action potential activity. This effect was presumably due to the accumulation of synaptic transmitters in the otherwise not activated optic nerve fibre terminals (Fig. 8.3).

5. In electronmicroscopic studies of the optic nerve axon synapses at the LGN relay cells during the day 1 after axotomy, no changes were observed in the synaptic terminals. During the following 3 days, however, the synaptic structures formed by the optic tract fibres on the LGN cells underwent a characteristic morphological and functional change: about 24 hours after interruption of the axoplasmic flow, the volume of the degenerating synaptic endings increased slightly (terminal swelling) and the number of synaptic vesicles began to decrease. With further degeneration, the number of synaptic vesicles and mitochondria found within the synaptic endings decreased (Fig. 8.3), and the average diameter of the synaptic vesicles and the variability in vesicle size increased. Neurofilaments appeared within the degenerating synaptic terminals (Eysel et al., 1974a, b, c).

6. Parallel to these morphological changes in axons and axon terminals, the signal transmission by the degenerating synapses underwent a fairly rapid change. Whereas during the first hours after axotomy a single electrical shock applied to the optic tract evoked 2 or 3 action potentials of single LGN nerve cells instead of 1 action potential, synaptic signal transmission decreased from day 2 after axotomy onwards. Between days 2 and 4 of degeneration, the statistical fluctuation of the synaptic signal transmission increased, and the same was true for the amplitude of the excitatory postsynaptic potentials (EPSP) recorded intracellularly from LGN cells activated by degenerating synapses. On day 4 of degeneration the amplitude of the EPSPs was greatly reduced. Simultan-

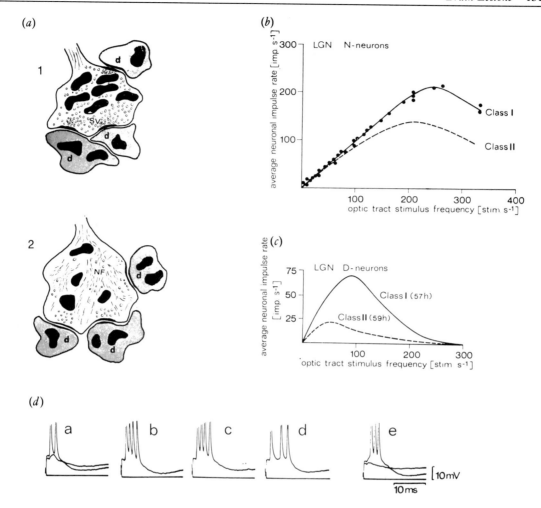

Fig. 8.3 *Morphological and physiological effects of acute deafferentation and degeneration on cat LGN relay cells. (a) Schematic drawing of a normal optic axon terminal (1) in the LGN and 60 to 80 hours after interruption of the axoplasmic flow (2). M = mitochondria, NF = neural filaments, SV = synaptic vesicles, d = dendrites from relay cells. (b) Frequency diagrams of a latency class I and class II relay cell in the normal LGN. The neuronal activity imp s^{-1} is plotted as a function of optic tract electrical stimulus frequency (abscissa). (c) Frequency diagrams of a latency class I and a latency class II LGN relay cell activated by degenerating optic tract terminals and recorded about 60 hours after interruption of the optic nerve. Note the difference from (b). (d): Intracellular recordings from an LGN relay cell about 15 minutes after acute destruction of the retinal receptive field area. Note the normal subthreshold excitatory postsynaptic potentials, EPSPs (a, e), and multiple discharges (a–e) evoked by suprathreshold EPSPs. In normal LGN relay cells a single electrical optic nerve stimulus elicits only one postsynaptic action potential under comparable stimulus conditions (From Grüsser, 1978; (a–c) from Eysel et al., 1974; (d) from Eysel and Grüsser, 1978).*

eously with these changes in the synaptic terminals, the upper frequency limit for the signal transmission between the optic nerve terminals and single LGN cells was lower, the longer the interruption of the presynaptic axoplasmic flow (Fig. 8.3). On day 4, the last day of effective signal transmission through the degenerating synaptic terminals,

the synaptic efficacy was greatly reduced and on repetitive stimulation of the optic tract a pronounced exhaustibility of EPSPs was found.

7. Recordings from optic nerve axons indicated that during days 1–4 of degeneration all electrical stimuli led to a conducted action potential, i.e. the degeneration of signal

transmission through synaptic terminals occurred several days before the final degeneration of the axons began (days 5–8) and their ability to conduct action potentials ceased.

8. Five days after axotomy a significant shrinkage of the optic axon terminals occurred and 'black degeneration' of synaptic terminals was observed in electronmicroscopic slides (Eysel *et al.*, 1974a, b, c). Finally the degenerating synapses disappeared.

9. It became evident that the degenerative events described occurred somewhat faster in terminals of the smaller, latency class II optic nerve axons originating from the β-ganglion cells than in the larger, latency class I axons of the optic nerve (α-ganglion cell axons). Thus the size of the axon and its myelinization had an effect on the speed of degenerative processes in the axonal terminals occurring after axotomy.

10. The final optic nerve axonal degeneration in the LGN and the dissolution of the optic tract fibres combined with growth of glial elements lasted several weeks.

11. During the following weeks these presynaptic degenerative events led to the next response step of the nervous system: for many weeks, signs of postsynaptic adaptation of LGN nerve cells and synaptic reorganization became observable. Finally, however, in the overwhelming majority of LGN relay cells a postsynaptic degeneration occurred, indicated by a cell shrinkage and finally cell death. From day 1 to about day 30 after axotomy, the spontaneous activity of LGN nerve cells increased. This finding may be interpreted by the assumption that during this period the efficiency of non-visual synapses formed at the surface of LGN cells by corticofugal fibres, LGN interneurones and axon terminals running from the nerve cells of the brain stem to the LGN increased. About 6 to 8 weeks after axotomy, the spontaneous activity of deafferented LGN cells reached values of about 50% of the pre-lesion activity (Eysel, 1977). During this period of postsynaptic adaptation, the size of the cell soma of deafferented LGN cells decreased slightly. It seems fairly probable that the relative size of synaptic surface occupied by non-visual synapses and some local sprouting of axonal terminals led to the much higher efficacy of non-visual synaptic input to deafferented LGN cells as compared with normal conditions.

12. Finally, about 3 to 4 months after optic nerve axotomy the third step of postsynaptic adaptation to presynaptic degeneration became visible: the majority of deafferented LGN relay cells degenerated, including their axons, which extended through the visual radiation to the primary visual cortex. As a consequence of these late transsynaptic degenerative events, the synaptic terminals formed by LGN relay cell axons at cortical nerve cells also degenerated. Thus the 'disconnection' of the retina from the LGN had finally led to transsynaptic effects influencing the synaptic pattern of the next step of signal pro-

cessing at the surface of cortical nerve cells (Fig. 8.1). We may assume that a reorganization of the synaptic structures at many cortical nerve cells has finally taken place.

Retrograde Degeneration

Interruption of the optic nerve axons also exerted retrograde effects. The cut axons degenerated and within 2 weeks most of the retinal ganglion cells shrank and disappeared (Maffei and Holländer, 1978). This disappearance of most of the ganglion cells led to a reorganization of the synaptic contacts formed by bipolar cells and amacrines. Thus transsynaptic retrograde degeneration also affects the neuronal network beyond the neurone directly involved (Fig. 8.1).

Transsynaptic retrograde degeneration was also observed when the optic radiation fibres were interrupted or the primary visual cortex was removed. After such procedures, about 50% of all LGN cells underwent retrograde degeneration. Presumably most LGN relay cells were affected by this retrograde degeneration. Finally, the process of retrograde degeneration continues transsynaptically and also affects retinal ganglion cells. Size and myelinization of optic nerve axons change and the number and size of retinal ganglion cells is eventually also affected months after the visual cortex has been removed (Cowey, 1974). This transsynaptic retrograde process is the reason why ophthalmologists, since the application of retinoscopy, have made the observation that years after extended lesions of the visual radiation or visual cortex, part of the optic nerve disc becomes pale, a sign that the transsynaptic retrograde degeneration has reached the retina.

Brain Lesions of the Cortical Grey Matter and Plasticity of Cortical Neuronal Circuits

A cerebral infarct, i.e. a complete interruption of the blood flow to a circumscribed part of the cortex or a restricted mechanical lesion, leads to the death of nerve cells and glial cells, which results finally in a dissolution of the totally ischaemic cortical region. Along the borders of the lesion a glial scar develops, and within the transitional zones, where only some of the nerve cells were chronically affected by the local ischaemia, an increase in glial cells is observed and a reorganization of cortical nerve cell activity occurs. Such a region can develop pathologically increased nerve cell activity and later affect cortical function by generating a focus of epileptogenic activity, which disturbs cortical function in regions far outside the locus of a direct lesion.

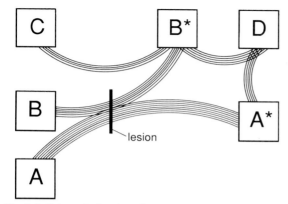

Fig. 8.4 *Schematic drawing of a circumscribed lesion within the white matter of the brain. Such a lesion may destroy all mutual connections between a few cortical regions (A–A*, B–B*), but may leave other connections totally unimpaired (C–B*, D–B*, D–A*).*

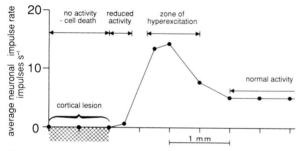

Fig. 8.5 *Activity profile through a cortical region adjacent to a small cortical lesion about 1 mm in diameter produced by laser light coagulation in the cat primary visual cortex. The activity within the lesioned region is, of course, zero. Immediately adjacent to the lesioned area one finds a ring of reduced cortical activity, followed by a zone of hyperexcitability and increased spontaneous activity. At a distance of more than 2.5 mm from the small cortical lesion, cortical activity is again normal (Modified after Eysel and Schmidt-Kastner, 1991).*

Experimental studies on microlesion of the cat visual cortex indicated that adjacent to the 1-mm-diameter cortical lesion there exists a ring of reduced neuronal activity, which is surrounded by a zone of hyperexcitability in which spontaneous nerve cell activity is not only increased but also characterized by high-frequency discharge groups of nerve cell activity. Further away from the locus of the cortical lesion, normal activity is recorded (Fig. 8.5; Eysel and Schmidt-Kastner, 1991).

All efferent axons belonging to nerve cells destroyed by the local cortical lesion degenerate, of course, and the same is true for afferent axons forming synapses at the nerve cells of the infarcted area, if their main axon projected to the destroyed cortical area. Retrograde degeneration as illustrated in Fig. 8.1 occurs and, as in white matter, lesions can produce long-lasting retrograde transneuronal degenerative effects. As mentioned above, extended lesions of the primary visual cortex lead finally to degenerative effects of retinal ganglion cells. Secondary changes can be expected in all those cortical areas to which the nerve cells of the destroyed cortical area projected. Anterograde axonal degeneration and synaptic degeneration as illustrated in Fig. 8.1 lead to a change in the synaptic surface of the receiver neurones in the respective cortical areas. In these areas only those nerve cells degenerate that were predominantly activated by the axons from the destroyed region. In general, owing to the very large variety of synaptic convergence in visual cortical association areas, one can expect very little anterograde trans-synaptic death of nerve cells, but mostly a reorganization of the synaptic input at the cells of the higher-order visual cortices. The dendritic surface occupied by the degenerated synapses either shrinks or synaptic reorganization occurs, owing to local sprouting of axonal terminals from other inputs. Since cortical areas are connected, as a rule, with many others, destruction of the cortical grey matter in the primary visual cortex or higher visual association cortices leads to a much more widespread cerebral reorganization than a corresponding small white-matter lesion, which might affect only one or two intracerebral tracts, as illustrated in Fig. 8.4.

Acute destruction of a cortical region leads quite frequently to a hyperexcitability of some of the receiver areas. This effect may lead within the central visual system to the spontaneous sensations of phosphenes or photisms, as discussed in Chapter 9. The adaptive responses of the receiver areas are presumably also dependent on the age of the subjects suffering from the local lesion of the cortical grey matter. It is well known that in the brain of humans older than about 22 to 25 years neuronal plasticity decreases and spontaneous nerve cell degeneration is greater than in the earlier years of life. Spontaneous nerve cell death presumably depends on unknown genetic factors, but is facilitated by chronic drug abuse, extensive alcohol consumption and heavy smoking. Such 'physiological' losses of nerve cells distributed over the neocortical regions and man-specific cortical association areas do not induce dramatic effects, since a local reorganization of neuronal connections seems to occur, which is of course much more discrete than those observed with local cortical microlesions as mentioned above. The 'biological ageing' of a certain brain region, however, certainly influences the neuronal adaptation processes occurring after a grey-matter or white-matter lesion.

During the ontogenetic development of the central visual system (discussed in Chapter 1) cortical plasticity decreases with age. This circumstance leads to the well-

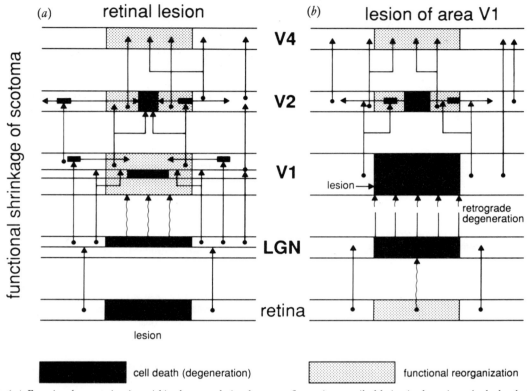

Fig. 8.6 *(a) Functional reorganization within the central visual system after a circumscribed lesion in the retina. At the level of the retina the nerve cells degenerate (black area). Synaptic connections from nerve cells outside the destroyed area lead at the LGN level, owing to axonal branching or interneuronal activity, to a slightly smaller functional impairment and transsynaptic degeneration than would be expected from the retinal lesion. This mechanism of lateral compensation continues at the level of the primary visual cortex, area V1. Finally, at the secondary and tertiary visual cortices no gross morphological changes are observable and nerve cell activity seems to be normal. Illumination of the destroyed retina does not lead to neuronal activation, of course, but the respective cortical neurones (stippled area) are activated by retinal stimulation outside the destroyed retinal region ('filling-in' mechanism). With unilateral retinal lesions only the nerve cells in the layers correlated with the lesioned retina are affected at the level of the LGN and in layer IV of the visual cortex. This is schematically illustrated. (b) Scheme of the effects of a circumscribed lesion in the primary visual cortex (area V1). Retrograde degeneration occurs in the relay cells of the LGN and – with a long temporal delay – also in the retinal ganglion cell layer. Anterograde postsynaptic changes in neuronal activity occur initially in a region of area V2, which is somewhat smaller than the lesion in area V1. Owing to synaptic reorganization and the 'horizontal' network of cortical interneurones, the region impaired in V2 shrinks with time, while in higher-order visual cortices such as areas V4 or MT even smaller functional changes may appear. One does not observe, however, a scotoma-type abolition of neuronal activity. The spread of signals through lateral conduction by interneurones leads, as in (a), to a functional 'filling in' of the cortical scotoma.*

known clinical observation that a brain lesion occurring during childhood or early adolescence can be functionally 'compensated', while the same lesion incurred beyond the age of 16 to 20 years leads to a non-compensated chronic defect.

Plasticity of neuronal networks in the central visual system is also the reason why visual field defects change with time. Figures 8.6(a) and (b) illustrate schematically the adaptive processes leading to such changes: when a

scotoma is caused by a lesion in the retina or the optic nerve fibres (Fig. 8.6(a)), the extension of that lesion determines the size and extension of the scotoma for simple light–dark stimuli. Interestingly, with time (months or years), a functional shrinkage of the scotoma was observed, which is characterized by 'filling-in effects' caused predominantly by the increasing receptive field sizes in areas V1, V2 and the higher cortical visual association areas. Furthermore, when a certain portion of LGN nerve cells degenerates owing to retinal lesion, the neurones in V1 that received direct excitatory contacts from these LGN cells can reorganize their synaptic input since they still receive signals from non-visual afferents and a widespread cortical lateral network.

Figure 8.6(b) illustrates schematically the effects following a circumscribed lesion of area V1, which leads to a distinct contralateral homonymous scotoma in the visual fields of both eyes (cf. Chapter 9). A retrograde degeneration of LGN relay cells corresponding to the destroyed cortical area occurs throughout the LGN in all 6 layers, and finally even a transsynaptic retrograde retinal degeneration of ganglion cells. As with cortical scotoma due to the large receptive fields of the nerve cells located in area V2 and higher-order visual cortices, a functional 'filling in' occurs. When large-field stimuli of a similar structure are applied as mentioned in Chapter 9, the scotoma disappears functionally, owing presumably to a reorganization of the connections between areas V1 and V2.

9 The Visual World Shrinks: Visual Field Defects, Hemianopias and Cortical Blindness

Introduction

The concept of homonymous and heteronymous visual field defects and their precise measurement by means of perimetry are fairly recent medical developments which took place during the nineteenth century. Perimetry is an important tool used to diagnose lesions located between the photoreceptors of the retina and the visual cortex; it relies on the relatively small interindividual variability in the topography of the afferent visual pathway and on the interindividual similarity of retino–cortical mapping of the visual field on the surface of the mesial part and the pole of the occipital lobe where the primary visual cortex is located (Chapters 3 and 4).

Historical Background

The notion of an ocular visual field can be traced back to the idea of the 'visual cone' or 'visual pyramid', a concept that first appeared in early Greek writings dealing with physiological optics in the time of Plato and Euclid. A distinction between field of vision and field of gaze and between monocular and binocular visual fields was clearly made during the fifteenth and the sixteenth centuries and was specifically elaborated upon by Fabricius ab Aquapendente. Greek physicians were familiar with hemianopia caused by cerebral brain lesions. The great seventeenth century anatomist and physician Thomas Willis attributed hemianopia to lesions of the corpus striatum (Chapter 2). In his *Adversaria anatomica omnia*, Morgagni (1719) described a case of homonymous hemianopia caused by a unilateral brain lesion. Vater and Heinicke (1723) provided the first correct explanation of hemianopia, pointing to the partial decussation of optic nerve fibres found in the optic chiasm, which had first been recognized by Newton in 1704 (Chapter 2). The British ophthalmologist John Taylor popularized Newton's ideas in his book *An Account of the Mechanism of the Eye* (1727, 1750). Since then, the existence of an ipsilateral (uncrossed) and a contralateral (crossed) projection of about half of the optic nerve fibres leading to a contralateral representation of the left and the right visual hemifield of each eye in the brain has been generally acknowledged; the detailed optic nerve projection sites were first elaborated upon towards the end of the eighteenth and the first half of the nineteenth centuries. Visual field defects have been under discussion and considered to be useful signs indicating the location of cerebral brain lesions only since the second half of the nineteenth century, however. Early visual field studies were reported by Alexander (1867), Förster (1867), Jackson (1875), Charcot (1875), Baumgarten (1878), Wilbrand (1881) and Harris (1897). More recently, functional differences between the upper and lower halves of the visual field, between the nasal and temporal halves, and between the left and the right visual field have been explored in greater depth.

To our knowledge, the first perimeter was designed by Purkinje in 1825 (Fig. 9.1). He determined the outer boundaries of the monocular visual field using this small portable device, and recognized that a kinetic stimulus was much more effective for this purpose than a stationary one. He correctly explained the superiority of kinetic – as opposed to stationary – testing by referring to the rapid local adaptation in the visual field periphery (Troxler effect, 1804). Purkinje, who was interested in the properties of 'indirect vision' ('*indirectes Sehen*') outside the foveal region of the visual field, noted that colour recognition was restricted to a much smaller, inner part of the visual field than was light–dark perception. He also

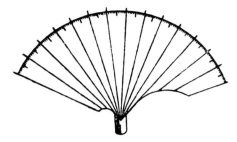

Fig. 9.1 *Small portable perimeter as designed by Purkinje (1825). It consisted of a segment of a 140-degree-periphery circle, 7 inches in diameter, made from white cardboard and graded to read off the stimulus position at the periphery of the circle. This perimeter was constructed to measure the visual field of the right eye, whereby the small piece cut out left of the handle corresponded to the nose and the larger cut out right of the handle to the right cheek. The handle was fixed perpendicularly to the plane of the cardboard. In a sufficiently darkened room, the limits of the visual field were measured by means of a small flame, while the eye fixed a target in the middle of the sector. Purkinje also measured the chromatic visual field borders. For perception of light stimuli, he found the horizontal borders of the right-eye visual field to be 100 degrees to the right, 60 degrees to the left (nasal) side, 60 degrees upwards and 80 degrees downwards. Similar data were reported by Young (1802).*

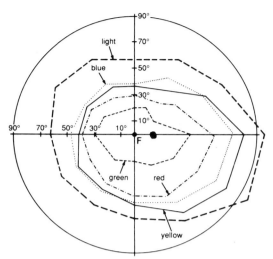

Visual field of right eye

Fig. 9.2 *Examples of correct recognition of achromatic and chromatic stimuli within the monocular visual field. The size of the visual field for correct blue, yellow, red and green recognition differed. Most observers recognized green better than red, i.e. the inner-most border for chromatic recognition represents the red recognition and not the green recognition as in this example (from Höber, 1934).*

found that one could recognize the 'true' colour of a chromatic target, i.e. the colour seen with foveal vision ('*directes Sehen*'), only up to a certain eccentricity – the visual field for blue and yellow being the largest, that for red the smallest, and that for green somewhere in between (Fig. 9.2). Purkinje, an extremely meticulous observer, realized furthermore that the transition between the achromatic peripheral parts of the visual field, on the one hand, and the regions with full colour vision on the other, was a gradual one. Therefore, the hue and distinctness of the perceived colour of a slow moving target change along its path from the colour-blind visual field periphery through a transitory region to the inner part of the visual field with full colour vision.

Using his perimeter, Purkinje also plotted the position of the blind spot, i.e. the projection of the papilla nervi optici within the visual field. Described for the first time by Mariotte in 1668, the blind spot was a discovery of such great public interest that Mariotte was asked to demonstrate his findings to the King of England (Helmholtz, 1896), which illustrated that leading politicians also have blind spots! The discovery of the blind spot spawned a discussion about whether visual perception in the region of the blind spot corresponded to the perception of 'dark'

or 'black', or whether a 'filling-in' of the percepts from the area surrounding the blind spot occurred (see Fig. 9.3; Purkinje, 1825).

A generation later, Albrecht von Graefe (1856) introduced to the field of ophthalmology the systematic exploration of the visual fields through his use of a tangent screen; two other researchers, Aubert and Förster (1857), recommended using a graded, semicircular, rotatable perimeter based on the principles applied by Purkinje. In the next 25 years, several perimeters were designed as tools allowing for more or less precise measurement of visual fields and visual defects. Engineering technology worked toward two different goals: to either a handy, portable perimeter like Purkinje's, or an 'autometric, self-recording perimeter' (e.g. Albertotti, 1884). These efforts ultimately led to the construction of the Goldmann perimeter, or the Tübingen perimeter, and more recently to computer-controlled 'automatic' perimeters (Fig. 9.4). A better evaluation of the results of perimetry first became possible after a more precise neuroanatomy of the afferent visual pathways and of the topographic organization of the primary visual cortex had been worked out (Wilbrand, 1881; Henschen, 1923; Walsh and Hoyt, 1969a, b).

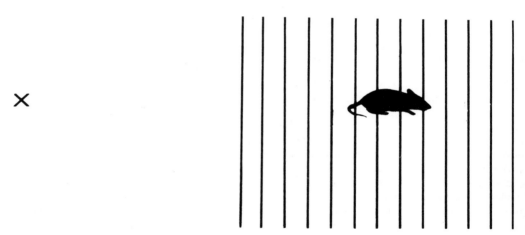

Fig. 9.3 *Two demonstrations of the blind spot. In the upper pattern, monocular fixation with the right eye on the cross at an adequate distance (about 35 cm) leads to a disappearance of the white spot and a 'filling in' of the blind spot, which is seen in the same black chroma as the surroundings (Helmholtz, 1896). In the lower part, fixation of the cross leads to a disappearance of the mouse within the blind spot but completion of the vertical stripes. No empty space is seen at the place of the blind spot (Grüsser and Grüsser-Cornehls, 1977).*

Principles of Perimetry

The goal of modern perimetry is to evaluate quantitatively simple visual sensations within the visual field, which should lead to a 'quantitative determination of the functional capacity of the visual system in the perceptual field' (Aulhorn and Harms, 1972). Perimetry depends on the co-operation of the patient, on his general attentiveness and on his ability to restrict eye movements by concentrat-

ing on a small 'fixation' target. Although this procedure has remained basically the same over the years, modern semi-automatic perimetry is able to adjust the variability of the data by recording the patient's eye movements.

By continuing Purkinje's study of the difference between light and colour perception in different parts of the visual field, Aubert and Förster (1857) laid the basis for colour perimetry (Aubert, 1857; Förster, 1867). Between 1856 and 1940, as Aulhorn and Harms emphasized in their

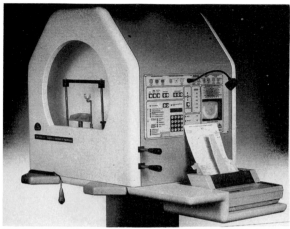

Fig. 9.4 *Photograph of an automatic Tübingen perimeter, kindly provided by the manufacturer (Oculus, Wetzlar, Germany). Chin- and head-rest and the holder for a correcting lens are visible. The patient's eye is centred in the geometrical centre of the perimeter half-globe. Stimuli are selected on the panel on the right side.*

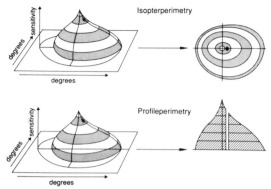

Fig. 9.5 *Three-dimensional representation of luminance sensitivity within the monocular visual field as revealed by quantitative perimetry. Upper row: representation of isoluminant threshold lines (isopter perimetry). Lower row: same, but representation in profiles along a selected diameter (profile perimetry) (modified from Aulhorn and Harms, 1972).*

1972 study, clinical perimetry was predominantly based on the so-called 'kinetic examination technique', in which, as Purkinje had recommended, the target was moved from outside the visual field towards its centre. Because evaluation of visual perception within the inner 20 degrees of the visual field as well as a rapid appraisal of visual field defects are, in many cases, necessary and of special importance, an examination using a tangent screen ('Bjerrum screen') on which black-and-white or small coloured discs on thin sticks are moved against a white, grey or black background, provides useful data (e.g. Glaser, 1978). Five classes of instrumental perimetry are currently defined as follows.

Static Light Perimetry

At well-defined background adaptation light, the subject has to discern a small spot of light having a certain intensity and angular size which is flashed for about 0.2 to 0.5 second onto the visual field. The position of this stimulus is varied systematically. The investigator has to make sure that during the examination the patient concentrates on a 'fixation' target placed in the centre of the perimeter. In many clinical centres, this 'static perimetry' has replaced the older 'kinetic perimetry,' in which the small spot of light was slowly moved across various diameters of the visual field. The term 'static' is somewhat misleading, since the method relies on the transient appearance of a small flashed target, i.e. on the dynamic response properties of the visual system.

Measuring threshold values along different diameters allows for more precise perimetry. The results are combined and plotted together in two ways: 'isopter perimetry' or 'profile perimetry' (see Fig. 9.5). One can of course combine both evaluations, but this type of quantitative perimetry is somewhat time-consuming. Therefore, a shorter examination is used for routine clinical diagnostics: standards of background adaptation, stimulus size and stimulus intensity are selected for basic isopter perimetry, and interesting meridians are selected for profile perimetry (Fig. 9.6; Aulhorn and Harms, 1972). By this method, changes in visual field defects taking place over a certain period of time can be carefully evaluated. A comparison of perimetry performed under photopic as well as under scotopic adaptation levels is helpful for certain clinical diagnostic decisions.

Colour Perimetry

Aubert and Förster introduced the detection of colour – as opposed to light and dark – into perimetry in 1857; nowadays this is done mainly using 'static' perimetry (colour isopter perimetry). To obtain reliable results, the following variables have to be defined: adaptation level, size, intensity and spectral composition of the small chromatic spot of light. The results are displayed in the 'chromatic visual fields' (Fig. 9.2). The visual field for detection of the colour blue is normally larger than that for green and red. The interindividual differences in detecting red or green targets are rather large. Colour perimetry is especially useful in the diagnosis of optic neuritis or suprasellar tumours exerting pressure on the optic chiasm. The thinner latency class II axons (X-system), which transmit

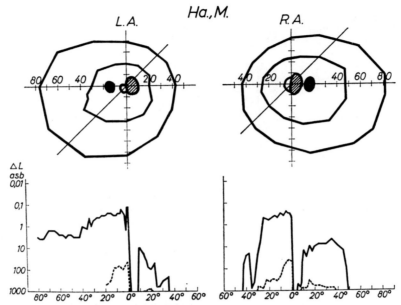

Fig. 9.6 *Combined isopter and profile perimetry adapted to the needs of a fast examination. Data from a patient suffering from a small paracentral homonymous scotoma. Upper row: isopter perimetry for the left (L.A.) and the right (R.A.) eye leads to the discovery of the scotoma (hatched area). Lower row: profile perimetry along a selected meridian. Continuous curve: light difference thresholds (ordinate). Dotted curves: thresholds of pupillomotor responses (Aulhorn and Harms, 1972).*

colour signals (Chapter 3), are more sensitive to demyelinization and local pressure than the axons of the achromatic, latency class I neurones (Y-system). Colour perimetry also aids in the detection of cortical achromatopsy (Treitel, 1879; review: Ziehl and Mayer, 1981; cf. Chapter 20).

Dynamic Perimetry

This type of visual field evaluation is performed with small flickering light targets projected onto different parts of the visual field. The subject has to decide whether or not the stimulus (steady light or intermittent stimuli, 10–30 Hz) is flickering. Flicker perimetry can also be used to measure the local flicker frequency (critical flicker frequency, CFF). Background adaptation and definition of the flicker stimulus (average luminance, size and depth of modulation) are especially necessary for this type of measurement because all of these parameters have an effect on the local CFF (review: van de Grind *et al.*, 1973; Kelly, 1973). For photopic adaptation conditions and small flickering targets (having a diameter of 0.5–1 degrees), the CFF decreases from the centre of the visual field to the periphery. With large flickering fields the peripheral CFF is higher than the foveal CFF (Fig. 9.7). The reader can easily observe

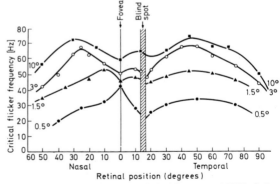

Fig. 9.7 *Dependency of critical flicker frequency (CFF, fusion-frequency ordinate) on stimulus location along one selected diameter (horizontal) through the visual field (abscissa). (Redrawn from Hylkema, 1941.)*

this effect on a 50 or 60 Hz TV screen: flicker is not perceived by foveal vision, but when the TV screen is shifted at some distance into the periphery of the visual field, a flicker sensation is observed. In regions with impaired visual function, the CFF decreases below normal values.

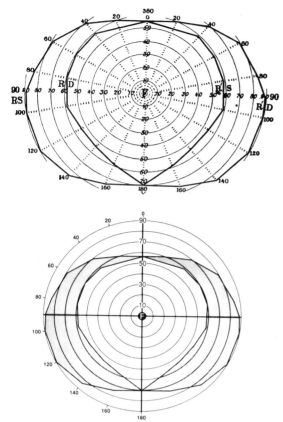

Fig. 9.8 *Binocular visual field composed of the monocular visual fields of the right (RD) and the left (RS) eye. Hering called the overlapping part of the two monocular visual fields 'binoculares Deckfeld'. Upper part: Förster's (1861) description (from Wilbrand and Saenger, 1917). In the lower part, a simplified version of the upper figure is presented. The outer, monocular, quartermoon-shaped parts of the binocular visual field are represented in grey, the binocular 'Deckfeld' in white.*

Shape and Visual Acuity Perimetry

The perimetric investigation of visual acuity at different areas in the visual field, another more specialized type of perimetry, uses gratings of varying orientation and spatial frequency, Snellen charts, Landolt rings (C) or simple shapes such as round or square spots of light having equal area and luminance (Aulhorn and Harms, 1972; Anstis, 1974). This type of 'structural' perimetry is restricted, as a rule, to scientific investigations of visual perception at different parts of the visual field. In the course of studies investigating possible functional differences between various compartments of the visual field (upper/lower, nasal/temporal, left/right), even more sophisticated stimuli were applied (see below). The goal of using such stimuli is, as a

rule, to explore higher order visual data processing performed by visual areas beyond the primary visual cortex.

Although perimetry is normally performed separately for each eye, it is useful to apply binocular perimetry in certain cases. In order to interpret the data obtained in such studies, including perimetry with stereoscopic targets, one must note the structure of the binocular visual field (Fig. 9.8). It is composed of two temporal monocular quarter moon-shaped parts and a binocular overlapping inner part (Hering's '*binoculares Deckfeld*').

Noise-field Campimetry

Co-operation between Professor Elfriede Aulhorn, an ophthalmologist at the University of Tübingen, and one of her patients led to the discovery of a new method of perimetry. The patient, who was suffering from a Bjerrum scotoma, was examined at the Tübingen eye clinic with a Tübingen perimeter. When he saw the results of the examination, he immediately told the ophthalmologist that he thought the results were correct. Questioned about his judgements, he reported that the outlines of the scotoma plotted by the perimeter were exactly like the ones he could see on a TV screen filled with 'visual noise' (Aulhorn, personal communication, 1987). Under this condition, the patient perceived his scotoma as a homogeneous grey field. Aulhorn and Köst (1989) did indeed find that pathological scotomata were clearly perceived by their patients when a field of small, irregularly distributed, black-and-white dots flickering at random at a high temporal frequency ('white noise') was used. They generated the noise field onto the screen of a black-and-white computer monitor by means of a program that allowed for variations in the temporal frequency, luminance and size of the pixels. The best description of the scotoma was obtained at a flicker rate of 50 Hz, a luminance variance between 0.8 and 60 cd. m^{-2} for the pixels, and a pixel diameter having a visual angle of 0.25 degrees. Sitting at a distance of 30 cm from the monitor with his head placed on a chin rest, the patient could outline his scotoma when concentrating on a target on the screen; the results fitted very well with traditional perimetry. With this method, the ophthalmologist can use a computer mouse to draw on the screen the scotoma reported by the patient; the visual field defect on the TV screen can be easily transformed into traditional polar coordinates in the visual field. The advantage of this method is that patients can also plot their scotoma at home on a TV screen. After having investigated 250 patients, Aulhorn and Köst (1989) came to the conclusion that visual field defects caused by pregeniculate lesions (of the retina, optic nerve, chiasm or optic tract) could be detected by this method, independent of the time that had passed since the defect had developed. Lesions of the visual radiation and the visual cortex led to noise-field campimetry field defects corresponding to those found using traditional perimetry only when the lesion occurred during the last few months prior to testing. Scotomata older than two years exhibited the phenomenon of 'filling-in' when tested with noise-field campimetry. Similarly, blind spots cannot be discovered using this method (monocular stimulation). In Fig. 10.21 an acute migraine scotoma is depicted as seen on a random-dot noise field.

Functional Differences in the Different Parts of the Visual Field

The Upper and the Lower Visual Fields

When standing or sitting outdoors on a sunny summer day in a natural habitat – for example, in a meadow with many flowers, some trees, mountains in the background and some clouds in a blue sky – one notices under such conditions that there are some asymmetries in the structure of the visual signals within the visual field. When gazing towards the horizon, objects that are closer are located primarily in the lower half of the visual field (LoVF). More distant objects, on the other hand, are usually found in the upper half of the visual field (UVF). Furthermore, the variability in object chromaticity is greater in the LoVF than in the UVF. In addition, the variability of structure and the mixture of low, middle and high spatial frequency stimuli are considerably richer in the LoVF than in the UVF. The retinal image of small distant objects more frequently seen in the UVF contains fewer low spatial frequency components. Furthermore, the parts of one's own body visible within the visual field are mainly in the LoVF. When one tries to grasp an object, the hand, as a rule, approaches the object more frequently through the LoVF than the UVF. When we walk, the distribution of the visual flow field angular velocity in the LoVF differs from that in the UVF, with higher velocities, on the average, in the former. When one walks along an unfamiliar path and fixes on a target on the ground several metres ahead, a vertical optokinetic nystagmus is caused while moving forward, guided during its downward slow phase predominantly by the proximate visual flow and structures of the LoVF. Fixation on a new target by an upward saccade, however, is controlled by the stimulus constellation in the UVF.

These considerations prompt one to ask whether or not a functional difference can be detected between the UVF and LoVF. Histological analysis of the retina tells us that in the primate, eye receptor density is larger on the average in the upper than in the lower hemiretina (e.g. van Buren, 1963; Perry *et al.*, 1984; Skrandies, 1987). Correspond-

ingly, the density of the retinal ganglion cells is higher for the upper hemiretina, but only outside a parafoveal region of about 8 degrees; the retinotopic organization of the macaque striate cortex indicates a somewhat larger representation of the LoVF than of the UVF (van Essen *et al.*, 1984; Tootell *et al.*, 1988). When one looks at the overall area of the LoVF and UVF, one finds that the upper half of the visual field is about 7–8 degrees smaller than the lower half (not taking into consideration the functional reduction of the nasal LoVF caused by the Caucasian nose).

Some functional differences exist as well between the upper and lower visual hemifields. For example, reaction times are shorter in the LoVF by about 8–10 ms for light stimuli placed along the vertical meridian, and by more than 20 ms for stimuli in the nasal hemifield (Payne, 1967; Rizzolatti *et al.*, 1987; Gawryszewski *et al.*, 1987). In general, chromatic sensitivity is somewhat better in the LoVF than in the UVF (Skrandies, 1987). Tysen and Lisberger (1986) found that initiation of smooth-pursuit eye movements is somewhat better developed in man in the lower than in the upper half of the visual field. Murasugi and Howard (1986) reported that horizontal optokinetic nystagmus in man is evoked with a higher gain from the lower than from the upper part of the visual field. This finding was corroborated by Collewijn *et al.*'s observations (1982) that sigma-OKN is evoked with a higher gain when attention is shifted towards the stimulus in the LoVF than when it is shifted toward the stimulus in UVF (Fig. 9.9).

For low and medium spatial frequencies, contrast sensitivity is higher in the lower part of the visual field (Rijsdijk *et al.*, 1980; Lundh *et al.*, 1983; Skrandies, 1985). Temporal resolution (as measured by the critical flicker fusion frequency) seems to be higher at corresponding points in the LoVF than in the UVF (Hylkema, 1942; Skrandies, 1987). A LoVF superiority was also reported for perception of in-depth motion (Regan *et al.*, 1986).

Prevec (1990) has recently suggested that the bias for far and near vision determines the functional differentiation between the upper and lower visual fields. We think, however, that this is a rather exaggerated view: when one observes an object from some distance, half of the object is seen, on the average, with the upper, the other half with the lower visual vield. Similarly, the upper and lower parts of the parafoveal and foveal visual fields participate fairly equally when one works with or without tools on an object within the grasping space. Although a stronger functional difference is expected, of course, for the peripheral parts of the upper and lower visual fields, these differences, in our opinion, do not justify Prevec's conclusions relating perception in the grasping space to LoVF information, and perception in the near-distant and far-distant action space to the UVF. Furthermore, one must keep in mind that

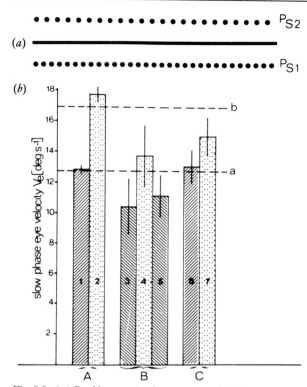

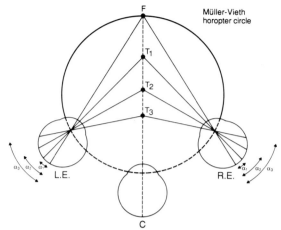

Fig. 9.10 *Schematic construction of the Müller-Vieth horopter circle determined by the fixation point F and the two nodal points of the left- and right-eye optical system. All targets T_1, T_2, ... T_n, which are placed along a sagittal plane perpendicular to the horopter circle and aligned to the hypothetical axis of the cyclopean eye (C), have their respective retinal images on points equidistant from the fovea but on opposite sides. The cortical representation of these visual points located mirror symmetric to a vertical line in the binocular visual field are functionally interconnected with each other. For further explanation, see text.*

Fig. 9.9 *(a) Double-row stimulus pattern used in the experiments with sigma-optokinetic nystagmus (sigma-OKN). Some of the results are shown in (b). The spatial period of the upper row P_{S2} was 1.1 degrees, that of the lower row P_{S1}, was 0.84 degrees. (b) Angular velocity V_e of sigma-OKN slow phase was averaged from 15–20 single measurements (algebraic means ± s.e.). Different stimulus conditions as follows. A: foveal schaunystagmus, when the centre of gaze attentively pursued the sigma movement of the P_{S1} dot row (A1) or P_{S2} dot row (A2). Flash frequency, 15 flashes s^{-1}. The values $P_{S1}.f_S$ and $P_{S2}.f_S$ are indicated by the horizontal dashed lines 'b' and 'a' (corresponding to gain 1 of the OKN slow phase). B: foveal stiernystagmus. The centre of gaze pursued the P_{S1} dot row (B_3), the P_{S2} dot row (B_4) or the midline (parafoveal stiernystagmus, B_5). C: parafoveal attentive nystagmus. The centre of gaze moved along the horizontal midline between the dot rows. The subject payed attention to either the P_{S1} dot row (C_6) or the P_{S2} dot row (C_7). Note that the OKN evoked by the stimuli in the lower visual field reached gain 1, while this was not the case for the OKN evoked by the stimuli in the upper visual field (from Collewijn et al., 1982).*

visually guided action is primarily related to extra-personal space, not to visual fields (cf. Chapter 22).

Nasal and Temporal Visual Fields

A second possible division of the visual field is a vertical separation forming nasal and temporal visual fields. As is

evident from the visual field charts in Fig. 9.2, the nasal part of the visual field is hardly greater than 50% of the temporal visual field's areal size when measured in degrees squared. There is also some functional difference between the nasal and the temporal visual fields when both eyes cooperate, which is illustrated in the horopter construction (Fig. 9.10): all objects in the extra-personal space which are located within the 'triangle' between the fixation points and the two nodal points of the eye are perceived with the temporal retinas of each eye. Those objects which are in the extra-personal space positioned more or less along a straight line between the fixated target and the subject's 'cyclopean eye' are especially important for space perception. Their retinal images fall on those non-corresponding areas of the temporal retinas, which are symmetrical with respect to the vertical meridian of the binocular visual field. The cortical representations of field areas horizontally equidistant from the vertical meridian are functionally connected with each other through the corpus callosum (cf. Chapters 4 and 5). All objects located outside the plane of the horopter are projected onto non-corresponding and non-symmetrical areas of the retina except those positioned on the line between fixation target and cyclopean eye and in a plane perpendicular to the horopter circle through this line. Depth perception of the visual space is dependent not only on retinal disparity but essentially also on parallax movement. The evaluation of parallax movement of objects seen with the two nasal visual hemifields seems to be especially important for the perceptual structure of the grasping space and the near-distant action space (Fig. 21.1).

Left and Right Visual Fields

A third subdivision of the visual field relates to head coordinates: left and right visual fields (LVF, RVF) have some functional differences that are predominantly caused by the hemispheric asymmetry of higher order visual signal processing. Since a detailed analysis of differences in signal processing in the LVF and RVF is beyond the scope of this book, we shall just summarize some of the essential findings. For further information, the reader is referred to recent reviews by Davidoff (1982) and Beaumont (1982). A general left-visual-field advantage (LVFA) was observed for right-handed subjects asked to perform 'simple' visual tasks. A 'visual hemifield advantage' was defined when reaction times were faster, when the probability of correct responses was higher or when the response thresholds were smaller. In relation to 'natural' visual stimuli, visual field advantages are marginal. They were found to be consistent effects when investigated in the laboratory in 'divided visual field experiments'. LVFA was found for the simple task of detecting a flash of light (Poffenberger, 1912; Jeeves and Dixon, 1970), provided that the stimuli were placed near the vertical midline of the visual field (Berlucchi *et al.*, 1977). Similarly brightness perception indicated a LVFA: from two physically equal spots of light projected onto areas symmetrical to the vertical midline, the one in the LVF appeared to be brighter (Dallenbach, 1923; Davidoff, 1975). Perception of light bar orientation revealed LVFA if the bar appeared in the not verbally labelled vertical and horizontal orientation (Umilta *et al.*, 1974).

An LVFA was found for the discrimination of spatial phase (Fiorentini and Berardi, 1984) however only for stimulus pairs differing also in contrast magnitude; no visual field advantage was observed for the detection of mirror-symmetric grating pairs (Rentschler *et al.*, 1986). Colour discrimination revealed LVFA, provided that a 'difficult' task was performed (Davidoff, 1976; Hannay, 1979). In regard to motion perception, LVFA was observed for velocity discrimination (Bertolini *et al.*, 1978), while a right-visual-field advantage (RVFA) was found for the perception of apparent phi-movement (Jasper, 1932). For the localization of small dots, LVFA also seemed to be present (Kimura, 1969; Levy and Reid, 1976). LVFA was prominent for face recognition provided that no verbalization of the faces (such as in the case of 'famous' faces) was necessary (e.g. Rizzolatti *et al.*, 1971; Marzi and Berlucchi, 1977). Further findings on visual

hemifield differences regarding face recognition are discussed in Chapter 16.

In contrast to LVFA for simple visual tasks, RVFA was found for complex recognition tasks, especially in tachistoscopic studies in which words, nonsense strings of letters, single letters or numbers were used as stimuli (e.g. Beaumont, 1982). These findings are discussed in detail in Chapter 17. The advantage of visual signal processing in the left or right visual hemifield for complex stimulus material is certainly caused by a difference in the left and right hemisphere neuronal data processing beyond area V1. The same is true for the correlation of RVFA or LVFA with the 'handedness' of the subject (Annett, 1982), and for the still controversial interpretation of positive or negative findings regarding different degrees of cerebral lateralization caused by gender (reviews: Fairweather, 1982; Springer and Deutsch, 1989).

On Visual Field Defects and Their Topical Diagnostic Values

Figure 9.11 illustrates rather schematically the direct afferent visual pathways running from the retinae to the striate cortex (area V1) via the optic nerves, the optic chiasm, the optic tracts, the lateral geniculate nucleus (LGN) and the visual radiation. Area V1 is located at the mesial surface of occipital cortex and at the posterior end of the outer surface of the occipital lobe (Chapter 4). Figure 9.11 depicts the gross retinotopic relationship along the afferent visual pathway and on the surface of the primary visual cortex. Lesions are located at different sites in the afferent visual pathway from the retina to area V1, the pathway important for conscious perception of form, colour, depth and movement, and can be discovered using light perimetry. The lesions lead to characteristic heteronymous or homonymous visual field defects, as illustrated in Fig. 9.11. Monocular scotomata or binocular heteronymous scotomata are observed both in retinal lesions and in lesions of the optic nerves. Lesions of those optic nerve axons crossing within the optic chiasm cause heteronymous bitemporal hemianopia. This is most frequently seen in tumours found in the pituitary gland region (e.g. craniopharyngeomas, meningiomas or adenomas of the pituitary gland; Walsh and Hoyt, 1969). A pituitary adenoma occasionally breaks through to the left and/or right side and grows around the lateral parts of the chiasm, leading also to nasal visual field defects of one or both sides. Homonymous field defects occur in 'retrochiasmatic' lesions of the optic tract, the LGN, the visual radiation or the primary visual cortex. Because of the spatial arrangement of the axons found in the optic tract or in the

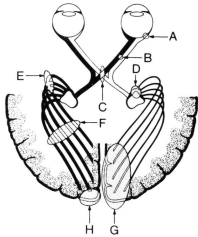

Fig. 9.11 *Schematic illustration of the afferent visual pathway from the retina to area V1. Different sites of lesions (a) and the corresponding visual field defects (b) are depicted. A: retinal lesion. B: lesion of the right-eye macular optic nerve fibres as found in optic neuritis. C: bi-temporal hemianopia as found in a pituitary adenoma pressing against the optic chiasm. D: lesion of a part of the right lateral geniculate nucleus (LGN). E: lesion of parts of the visual radiation near the LGN. F: complete lesion of the visual radiation white matter below the left visual cortex. G: destruction of the right primary visual cortex (area 17). H: lesion of the most occipital, supracalcarine part of the area 17.*

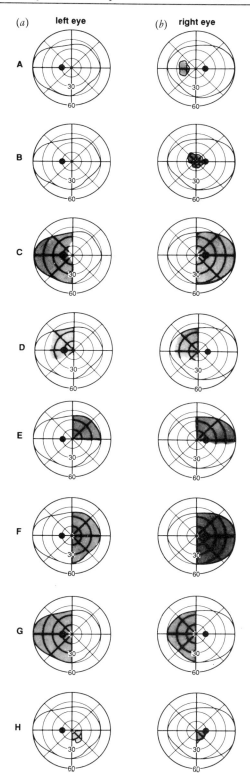

visual radiation, however, the visual field defects do not exhibit a perfect congruency in the left and right eyes (Behr, 1909, 1916, 1931; Brouwer, 1936; Dubois-Poulsen, 1952; Polyak, 1957; van Buren and Baldwin, 1958).

Variability of Homonymous Field Defects in Cortical Lesions

Extensive summaries of visual field defects occurring in the presence of cortical lesions have been published by Inouye (1909), Axenfeld (1915), Holmes and Lister (1916), Wilbrand and Saenger (1917, 1918), Holmes (1918, 1919, 1934, 1945), Fleischer and Ensinger (1920), Bender and Teuber (1947, 1949) and Teuber *et al.* (1960). These studies were based on examinations of soldiers suffering from brain injuries incurred during the Russo-Japanese War (1905/06) or the First and Second World Wars (cf. Glickstein, 1988). Cortical lesions did not always produce precisely overlapping field defects in both eyes, as Henschen had claimed (1910, 1911, 1923, 1926a, b). Teuber *et al.* (1960) emphasized the fact that they could not confirm Henschen's finding of an 'almost mathematical congruence' of homonymous field defects caused by area V1 lesions. Rather, incongruent field defects seemed to be correlated with the tendency of defects to be larger in the nasal part of the visual field than in the corresponding part of the other eye's temporal visual field. Interestingly, the patients did not actually notice serious defects in the temporal half as smaller, but, on the contrary, considered the temporal defects to be more serious (Teuber *et al.*, 1960). In general, the outlines of homonymous field defects lack precise congruence, regardless of where the cortical lesions develop. Teuber *et al.* thought that 'the most probable interpretation of this incongruence would be that, contrary to current anatomic conceptions, corresponding elements in the visual system are not perfectly aligned, even at the level of the striate cortex'. In light of modern neurophysiology, the following explanation is more plausible: incongruence is probably caused by different degrees of impairment of the afferent fibres spreading laterally through the stripe of Genarri and of the 'monocular' sublayers 4a, b of area V1 (Chapter 4). Furthermore, a 'mixed' lesion of the cortical grey matter and of the geniculo-cortical axons below the grey matter might also lead to some incongruencies in the monocular visual field defects, especially when brain tumours are the cause of the defects (Cushing, 1922).

Except for some 'claw-shaped parafoveal defects', pathological scotomata produced by cortical lesions are, like the 'physiological scotoma' of the blind spot, not perceived as dark areas or as empty parts of the visual field (Teuber *et al.*, 1960). 'Completion effects' across smaller scotomata are rather common, as moving stimuli or Gestalt completion demonstrate. Several patients suffering from perifoveal defects who had been investigated by Teuber and his associates reported under certain conditions positive sensations from their visual field defects: on a red background, for example, their visual field defect had a greenish hue. This complementary 'filling-in' effect was even observed in afterimages forming around the scotoma: when an afterimage evoked by a red stimulus was projected by the patient onto a neutral grey background, it was perceived as green and the scotoma as red. Large cortical visual field defects or hemianopias have been described by intelligent patients as akin to the perception of the extrapersonal space without direct visual sensation, similarly as normal subjects perceive the region outside of the binocular visual field, i.e. the region 'behind the head'. The integration of visual field defects into a 'full' extrapersonal space, corresponding to that perceived by a normal subject with unimpaired vision, contrasts with the change in extrapersonal space perception occurring in the presence of parietal lobe lesions, which produces the symptom of spatial hemineglect (Chapter 22).

Figure 9.12(a)–(g) illustrates various visual field defects caused by lesions of the occipital lobe. They are all taken from the extensive collection published in 1917 in Wilbrand and Saenger's pioneering work. Figure 9.12(a) illustrates a right homonymous hemianopia with macular sparing caused by a vascular incident in the left posterior artery of a 57-year-old patient. 'Macular sparing' is the most frequently observed deviation from precise hemianopia. Teuber *et al.* (1960) attributed macular sparing to

> *a combination of four factors*; (a) *slight irregularities of fixation during perimetry*; (b) *persistent pseudo-foveae*; (c) *lack of congruence between the monocular fields; or* (d) *lower vulnerability of central as against peripheral fields, owing to the widespread macular representation in optic radiation and cortex, and, possibly to better vascular supply of the cortical macula* (p. 65).

Figure 9.12(b) (published by Inouye) shows the homonymous visual field defects of a Japanese soldier caused by a shell wound in the occipital pole of both hemispheres that had evidently affected the supracalcarine parts of areae V1 more than the infracalcarine parts. Figure 9.12(c) depicts a complex homonymous visual field defect affecting both halves of the fovea that consequently led to a considerable reduction in visual acuity. This comes from a soldier who received a bullet wound during the First World War that affected both occipital lobes. E is the entrance site, A the exit site of the bullet. Figure 9.12(d) illustrates a left upper quadrantanopia, caused by a vascular disease in the territory of the right posterior cerebral artery. The field defect spared foveal vision. Wedge-shaped homonymous field defects caused by only minor occipital brain trauma were also observed, as in the case of a 47-year-old hunter suffering from a small buckshot wound in the left occipital lobe (Fig. 9.12(e)). Bullet wounds in the occipital lobe could cause rather bizarre visual field defects (Hegner, 1915), such as those illustrated in Fig. 9.12(f): this 25-year-old soldier was shot through the occipital part of his brain from the right upper to the left lower part of the occiput. His visual field defects also exhibited marked incongruities. Bullet wounds affecting the occipital pole regions only cause bilateral homonymous central scotoma (e.g. Abelsdoff, 1916; Putnam and Liebman, 1942; Bender and Furlow, 1945). Finally, cases were repeatedly reported in which foveal vision was not affected although bilateral hemianopias were observed. This is illustrated in the visual fields of a 60-year-old lady suffering from arteriosclerosis, which first caused a vascular event leading to a right homonymous hemianopia together with transient right-sided hemiplegia. A small foveal visual field was all that remained after a second vascular lesion had occurred (Fig. 9.12(g)). Patients with such tunnel vision have some difficulties with rapid visual orientation, walking and standing, as well as with reading and motion perception. Finally, the very rare ring-shaped visual field defect deserves mention. Figure 9.12(h) illustrates Gelb and Goldstein's obser-

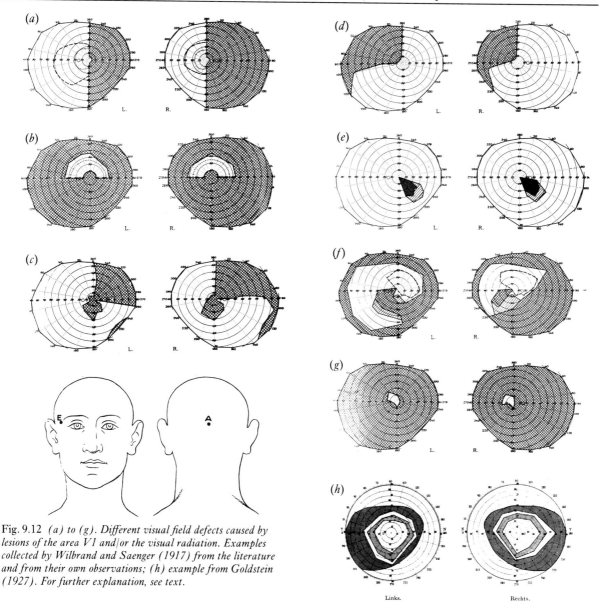

Fig. 9.12 *(a) to (g). Different visual field defects caused by lesions of the area V1 and/or the visual radiation. Examples collected by Wilbrand and Saenger (1917) from the literature and from their own observations; (h) example from Goldstein (1927). For further explanation, see text.*

vation of a patient suffering from a bilateral occipital brain lesion. Goldstein (1927) emphasized that the functional aspect of these ring-shaped visual field defects are not related to distinct 'ring-shaped' brain lesions, but rather to a more diffuse occipital lesion which leads to a high variability and reduction in sensitivity to light stimuli (cerebral asthenopia) and to attention difficulties during the perimeter examination. In such patients, the field defects evidently also depend on the duration of the examination.

Cortical Blindness

On the basis of the results of animal experiments, Munk (1881) differentiated between two different types of 'blindness' caused by cerebral lesions: cortical blindness ('*Rindenblindheit*') and psychic blindness ('*Seelenblindheit*'). Cortical or cerebral blindness (Berger, 1885; Förster, 1890; Marie and Chatelain, 1915) is a loss of all conscious vision due to lesions of the visual radiation or the primary visual cortex. It can appear suddenly as a transient or a chronic symptom, but can also develop from bilateral hemianopia, whereby the blindness in the two hemifields occurs at different times. Cerebro-vascular disease (basilary artery occlusions, bilateral posterior cerebral artery infarcts) is the most common aetiology in cortical blindness (e.g. Gloning *et al.*, 1962). Approximately 20% of patients who became hemianopic because of a unilateral infarction in the territory of the left or right posterior cerebral artery became blind (not always completely, however) because of an infarction of the posterior artery located on the other side (Bogousslavsky *et al.*, 1983). Other causes of cortical blindness are subarachnoid haemorrhage, extended occipital glioblastomas, transient cardiac arrest, or carbon monoxide (Adler, 1944) or mercury (Evans *et al.*, 1975; Landis *et al.*, 1982) poisoning. In rare cases, cortical blindness might appear as an ictal manifestation (Sadeh *et al.*, 1983; Aldrich *et al.*, 1985). In modern medicine, there is a further risk that cortical blindness will occur in the course of cardiac surgery or cerebral angiography (Prendes, 1978; Aldrich *et al.*, 1987). From the observations of Silverstein and Krieger (1960), Aguilar *et al.*, (1971) and Smith and Cross (1983), one realizes that occipital lobe infarctions occurring as a complication of open heart surgery indicate a poor prognosis.

Subsequent to transient cortical blindness, a small visual field frequently recovers, especially in the region of the foveae (tunnel vision). The occipital alpha rhythm of the electroencephalogram disappears or is greatly reduced as a result of complete cortical blindness. It reappears when small islands of the visual field recover (Bergmann, 1957; Aldrich *et al.*, 1987). Although visual evoked potentials (pattern reversal potentials) are not always a reliable sign of recovery from cortical blindness (Bodis-Wollner, 1977; Spehlmann *et al.*, 1977; Hess *et al.*, 1962), the initial absence of visual evoked potentials in cortically blind patients is not always a sign of a poor prognosis, as has been suggested by Abraham *et al.* (1975) Bodis-Wollner *et al.* (1977) found pattern-reversal visual evoked potentials in a blind boy and attributed these potentials to extrastriate cortex activation which does not go through area V1. In 'islands of vision' during recovery from a completely blind visual field, one often finds achromatopsia, but cases have also been reported in which very small islands of vision ('*inselförmiger Gesichtsfeldrest*') have absolutely normal colour vision.

Negation or unawareness of cortical blindness was first described by Anton (1898, 1899); it was not found in all cortically blind patients, however, by Redlich and Bonvicini (1907, 1909). Babinski (1914) referred to this unawareness or denial as anosognosia. Anosognosia of cortical blindness or of extended visual field defects is most likely a sign that the bilateral lesion extends beyond the visual radiation or the primary visual cortex. Analysis of CT-scans in forty-one patients indicated that those who are partially or fully aware of their hemianopia had lesions restricted to the occipital cortex in the region of area V1 (Koehler *et al.*, 1986). Cerebral lesions interrupting the pathways from area V1 to the visual association cortices led to unawareness of the hemianopic defect. On the basis of the neuropathology of patients suffering from cortical blindness reviewed by Wilbrand and Saenger (1917), anosognosia does indeed appear to be a symptom associated with cortical blindness only when the cerebral defect extends beyond area V1. Frequently accompanying the denial of cortical blindness are vivid complex visual hallucinations, whereby the patient is unaware of the mismatch between possible tactile percepts and the visual hallucinations. The latter can be explained as a disinhibition phenomenon (Cogan, 1973; see below). Patients recovering from cortical blindness caused by poisoning or cardiac arrest frequently experience a transient state of cerebral asthenopia and visual agnosia. Pötzl (1928) described the following stages of recovery from cortical blindness (cf. Gloning and Tschabitscher, 1969):

1. low-level light sensations without perception of shape, contour orientation, visual space or colour
2. diffuse perception of visual movement
3. hazy object perception, i.e. the objects are seen as in a fog ('psychic Tyndall phenomenon')
4. spontaneous flicker sensations; moving, unsteady contours of the objects, fading away (pseudo-agnosic disturbances of Faust, 1947)
5. slow return of colour perception: red first, followed by yellow and green, and finally by blue and violet
6. normal light producing dazzling effects
7. cerebral asthenopia with blurred vision and visual fatigue, fading out of colours and difficulties in visually controlled eye and gaze movements.

Blindsight

As is discussed in Chapter 10, electrical stimulation of the 'second' afferent visual pathway leading from the retina via the superior colliculi to the pulvinar, and from there to the extrastriate cortical regions, either caused patients to see flashes of light or inhibited visual percepts and evoked eye movements. In light of these observations, it was meaningful to investigate possible visual percepts or responses to visual stimuli projected to a hemianopic field. In addition, since Munk's (1881) observations, animal experiments have repeatedly indicated that recovery of visual function after ablation of the striate cortex was possible, varying however from species to species. There was, therefore, no *a priori* reason why 'extrastriate' or 'extrageniculate' vision should not exist in patients who had lost their primary visual cortex.

Animal Experiments

Typical laboratory animals such as rats, rabbits or cats clearly exhibit visually guided and goal-directed behaviour after bilateral removal of area 17. Three factors explain this phenomenon:

1. The subcortical visual system controls the observed visuo-motor responses.

2. The extrastriate visual cortices receive direct afferent visual inputs from LGN relay cells, of which the axons project to prestriate cortical areas, a projection also found in primates (Fries, 1981).

3. One or more extrageniculate afferent visual pathways exist which connect the retina with the cortex. The connection of the retina to the pulvinar either by direct optic nerve axons or by a disynaptic pathway via the superior colliculi is the most likely candidate for this function. The pulvinar also projects into extrastriate visual areas in primates. Munk (1881), who initially believed that ablation of monkey striate cortex would lead to complete blindness (Chapter 2), later became convinced that elementary visual functions could 'regenerate'. The recovery of residual visual functions could take several months, during which visual functions remained at a level beyond precise object recognition and object–space correlation at a fairly low level. The residual visual functions certainly approach the level of elementary sensation, as Luciani (1884) had deduced from his observations of monkeys after performing an ablation of the visual cortex:

> *When some time had elapsed after the removal, their visual sensation became perfect again; they were able to see minute objects, but they lacked the ability to discern objects and to correctly judge their properties and nature; they lacked, in a word, visual perception. For example, if small pieces of fig, mixed with pieces of sugar, are offered to them, they are incapable of choosing by sight alone, but first take the sugar in their hand and then put it in their mouth in order to reassure themselves.... The animal is not able to distinguish meat from sugar using only its visual impression.* (p. 153)

The fact that a part of residual vision is entirely subcortical was even acknowledged in physiology textbooks by the end of the nineteenth century. For example, Wundt (1893) described the behaviour of animals who had undergone bilateral hemispherectomy: 'Birds, rabbits and even dogs without a cortex respond to tactile and visual stimuli not only goal-directed, but, like normal animals, they adapt their locomotion to impressions from external stimuli. They avoid obstacles...' (p. 214). The problem of residual vision was taken up again by Klüver (1942), who performed bilateral occipital ablations in monkeys. His animals, who could only respond to changes in the overall luminance of the habitat, did not show any signs of pattern-recognition recovery. Weiskrantz (1986) explained these findings by suggesting that visual areas

beyond area V1 had been destroyed in these monkeys. Denney-Brown and Chambers (1955) observed that monkeys with bilateral area V1 damage responded to or even followed moving objects with their eyes. This was an important observation since it indicated that space-related behaviour activity could occur in the absence of area V1.

Pasik and Pasik (1971) demonstrated that monkeys without area 17 could learn to discriminate simple shapes presented in stimulus sets with equated stimulus luminance. Miller *et al.*, (1980) tested the ability of such animals to discriminate between black and white gratings having different spatial frequencies. Although they noticed reduced spatial contrast sensitivity, which had also been found in cats after ablation of area 17 by Orban *et al.* (1988), the Pasiks still observed remarkable performances in their monkeys. The same was true in a study of grating orientation recognition, in which a threshold orientation value of about 8 degrees was found (Pasik and Pasik, 1980). Even residual colour discrimination was observed in monkeys having no primary visual cortex (Schilder *et al.*, 1972).

Humphrey (1974) and Humphrey and Weiskrantz (1967) also reported a remarkable recovery of residual visual abilities in sufficiently trained animals after the removal of area V1. Humphrey (1974) carefully trained a macaque monkey after an almost perfect bilateral removal of the primary visual cortex. This animal could avoid obstacles, grasp goal-directed small objects and move with visual guidance through a fairly large outdoor environment. These observations were confirmed by Weiskrantz *et al.*, (1977), who also pointed out that after striate cortex ablation, monkeys could locate small stimuli in the extrapersonal space even when the presentation had been so short that the stimulus disappeared before eye or head movements could have been possible.

In summary, all these findings suggest a remarkable recovery of residual visual function in monkeys lacking area 17, provided that the animals are given enough time to adapt to 'cortical blindness' and to relearn visuo-motor coordinations.

A Controversial Issue: Blindsight in Hemianopic Patients

After the introduction of systematic perimetry into ophthalmology and neurology, observant clinicians noticed that some of their patients exhibited residual visual functions in the blind hemifield. For example, Poppelreuter (1917) ultimately came to the conclusion that a blind hemifield did not necessarily mean the loss of all visual functions. Riddoch (1917) observed residual movement perception in the blind visual field in patients suffering from hemianopia. Furthermore, it was repeatedly observed that scotomata caused by occipital lesions did indeed shrink even years after the acute brain lesion had occurred. After the examination of many soldiers with occipital brain injuries received during the First World War, it was generally acknowledged that an absolute scotoma, at least in the acute phase, was accompanied by surrounding regions of reduced visual perception (amblyopia). In the acute state, collateral oedema that had developed near the cortical lesion could explain these regions of reduced vision. Fields of amblyopia surrounding absolute scotomata were, however, described as a chronic result of cerebral lesions, which indicated that a partial recovery of the function required for visual field representation was possible. As mentioned above, a state of 'blurred' vision, reduction of visual acuity and temporary loss of colour vision could also accompany recovery from cortical blindness caused by intoxication or ischaemia.

It has been demonstrated only recently that some unconscious visual functions may still be present within absolute scotomata in man: this has been called blindsight (Weiskrantz *et al.*, 1974). Blindsight is still a controversial issue, and even those who strongly accept the idea of blindsight within an 'absolute' hemianopic visual field admit that it can only be demonstrated in some patients, and that it depends on training and time after the cortical lesion occurs.

Poppelreuter's and Riddoch's observations were not further pursued until the first modern research on blindsight conducted by Pöppel *et al.*, (1973). These authors questioned the general belief 'that total destruction of visual cortex and optic radiations in men should lead to blindness, and that regional (subtotal) destruction should correspondingly produce circumscribed areas of blindness (scotomata) in the visual field'. Suspecting that the responses leading to absolute scotomata might depend on the requirements of the task, Pöppel and his co-workers looked for other types of visual stimulation that would evoke responses in the blind hemifield. On the basis of their data, they claimed that they had 'found evidence for the processing of information about the locus of light stimuli presented in areas of the visual field which are 'blind' by the traditional definition. They selected oculomotor responses as a test case, knowing that ter Braak *et al.*, (1971) had found reduced optokinetic nystagmus in a patient suffering from total cortical blindness. After determining the visual field defects using the Tübingen perimeter (Fig. 9.4), Pöppel *et al.* asked the patients to perform a saccade from the small, central fixation point to a spot of light having a diameter of 19 degrees (10 millilambert) flashed for 100 ms to different eccentricities from the fixation point. A click stimulus used simultaneously with the light stimulus indicated to the patient that he now had to guess the position of the unseen light stimulus and to perform a saccade as quickly as possible toward that

stimulus. A somewhat surprising response was obtained after the patient had overcome the difficulty of looking at something not readily visible: a small but significant increase in average eye-movement amplitude with increasing eccentricity of up to 30 degrees was found. Of course, the question of stray light or other possible cues that might have influenced the results was not experimentally addressed in this seminal paper. Since then, however, the data have been repeatedly confirmed, at least in selected patients; nevertheless, other patients have evidently never shown any signs of blindsight or residual vision.

Weiskrantz *et al.* (1974) performed further research on blindsight visuo–motor response. They asked a hemianopic patient, D. B., to reach for rather than gaze at an unseen target that appeared for two seconds or less within the hemianopic field. The patient, whose ability remained consistent or even improved over several years, performed this task remarkably well (Fig. 9.13). The patient, whose data are shown in Fig. 9.13, suffered from a vascular malformation at the pole of the right occipital lobe. This led to repeated migraine headaches, scintillating light sensations and scotoma of variable extent and duration in the left hemifield from age 14 (which suggests an abnormal adaptation of the central visual system early in life) until age 26,

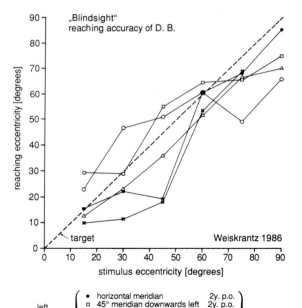

Fig. 9.13 *Examples of reaching accuracy of the patient D. B. illustrating 'blindsight'. The patient was investigated 2, 6 and 10 years postoperatively (p.o.). The stimulus eccentricity of a flashed target (abscissa) was varied within the blind visual field along a horizontal meridian or a 45-degree meridian left downwards. (Selected data from Weiskrantz, 1986.)*

when he underwent surgery that removed 'a major portion of the calcarine cortex . . . on the medial surface of the right hemisphere' (Weiskrantz, 1986, p. 21). This surgical intervention resulted in a nearly complete left hemianopia without macular sparing, but with small amblyopic islands in the upper quadrant. Visual field defects improved considerably over many months following the operation, leaving a left lower quadrantanopia that extended into the parafoveal region of the upper quadrant. Repeating the experiments performed by Pöppel *et al.* (1973), Weiskrantz *et al.* (1974) found 'a weak but significant effect of target position on eye position out to an eccentricity of 25 degrees.' Eye movements were less accurate than reaching with the left or right hand.

While investigating two patients with bilateral field defects, Pöppel and Richards (1974) found that residual visual function could be demonstrated in that part of the hemianopic visual field corresponding approximately to the vertical axial mirror region of a small scotoma in the opposite visual hemifield. Their patient was able to detect moving targets in his blind hemifield. This observation indicated that a hemispheric interaction might occur on the level of the superior colliculi, which would, under these conditions, lead to facilitatory responses. This view was supported by one of Sprague's earlier observations, demonstrating that hemianopia caused by unilateral ablation of area 17 in cats could be considerably improved by performing a secondary ablation of the superior colliculus contralateral to the cortical lesion (Sprague, 1966). Sprague speculated that the functional hemianopia was caused by intertectal inhibition. Since superior colliculi neurones respond preferentially to moving targets, Pöppel and Richards' discovery (1974) of a disinhibited zone of movement perception becomes more meaningful if one assumes that such a cortico-tectal and tecto-tectal interaction is also present in man.

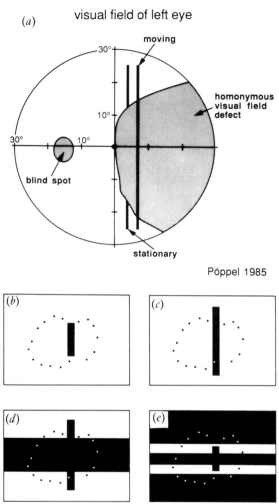

Pöppel 1985

Fig. 9.15 *Perception of a contour within the blind visual field generated by moving stimuli. (a) A stationary vertical light bar of 0.15 degrees width and 50 degrees height is not seen within the homonymous visual field defect (left occipital lobe lesion). When the bar is moved horizontally backwards and forwards, the patient perceives the whole bar (completion effect); (redrawn from Pöppel, 1985). (b–d) Such a completion effect is also seen with illusionary contours, provided that the inducing visual patterns are in part visible within the 'good' visual field (from Landis et al., unpublished, 1990). Illusionary contours (e) as real contours (c), which are restricted to the scotoma, are not seen. The borders of the scotomas are indicated by dots.*

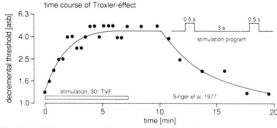

Fig. 9.14 *Time course of increase in threshold to a stationary target flashed periodically, as indicated by the inset (Troxler effect). Target diameter 1.93 degrees. Target eccentricity 30 degrees in the temporal visual field of the right eye. Abscissa: time from onset of adaptation procedure in minutes. Ordinate: decremental threshold luminance of target. The adapting stimuli were presented for 7 minutes. Three minutes after the repetitive stimulation was turned off, the threshold decreased slowly (data from Singer et al., 1977, redrawn).*

The work of Singer *et al.* (1977) also suggested a tecto-tectal interaction in humans having some impact on visual perception. They tested this concept by using the Troxler effect: when a retinal area at constant eccentricity was continuously activated by intermittent or moving light stimuli, the threshold (as measured in target luminance) increased with time and recovered with a slow time constant of about 5 minutes (Fig. 9.15). The size of the adapted retinal area (the flashed target had a diameter of 1.9 degrees) increased with the horizontal eccentricity of the target. Resetting the increased threshold to normal values was possible when an area of the visual field located mirror-symmetrically along the vertical midline axis was stimulated. This effect could have been transmitted either between cortical visual areas through the corpus callosum or through subcortical, e.g. tecto-tectal, commissures. The resetting effect was also observed in hemianopic patients when an area was adapted in the good hemifield and a mirror-symmetric resetting stimulus was applied to the blind hemifield. Resetting also occurred when normal subjects or a hemianopic patient performed saccadic eye movements directed towards the target used for adaptation. Thus, two mechanisms seem to have played a role: a feedback signal from the oculomotor system and a visual signal transmitted by the intertectal or other subcortical commissures, which in the case of the hemianopic patient also remained effective even when the resetting mirror stimulus was not consciously perceived. This observation suggests the existence of a rather interesting subcortical residual visual capacity.

Two further examples of blindsight effects are illustrated in Fig. 9.15. The completion effects observed in homonymous scotomata caused by lesions of area 17 may be one of the mechanisms also important for blindsight. For example, these completion effects induce colour contrast in the scotoma due to the function of cortical visual areas beyond area 17. Pöppel (1985) illustrated a completion effect across the scotoma by comparing the patient's report of seeing a stationary vertical light bar with that when the bar was moved. Completion of the bar across the visual field defect was attained when the bar was moved back and forth, as illustrated in Fig. 9.15(a). This completion effect was presumably due to the activation of neurones located in area V2, which respond especially well to moving contours. This explanation is supported by the observation that even illusionary contours lead to completion effects across a homonymous scotoma when the inducing stimuli are moved. These inducing stimuli only have to be partly outside the blind visual field, as illustrated in Fig. 9.15(b)–(e) (Landis *et al.*, 1990).

After having repeatedly investigated the above-mentioned patient D. B., Weiskrantz published an extensive report of his findings (1986):

1. Whether or not D. B. could or could not detect an object was tested 3 years after the brain surgery. Correct recognition decreased with retinal eccentricity through the scotoma, reaching chance level at about 45 degrees eccentricity. Six years after the neurosurgical intervention, however, 100% correct detection of a 1.75 degrees target

of 1.18 foot lambert was present along the same meridian through the scotoma. All detection was performed without conscious perception (meridian 45 degrees downwards).

2. Weiskrantz tried to estimate residual visual acuity by measuring responses to contrast gratings: the patient had to guess whether the stimulus was a grating or a homogeneous field of equal luminance and size. Visual acuity was estimated to be less than 1.0 cycle/degree at 6.25 degrees eccentricity; surprisingly, it improved to 2.5 and 2.9 cycles/degree at 16.5 and 25.8 degrees of eccentricity. Thus, while visual acuity in the parafoveal region was less than 10% of the values obtained in the corresponding regions of the normal right visual hemifield, blindsight responses at 6.5 and 25.8 degrees eccentricity were about 1/4 and 1/3 of normal visual acuity respectively. Under these stimulus conditions, the patient did not consciously perceive the stripe patterns; under certain conditions, however, he was fairly sure that his guess was correct.

3. Movement thresholds (as measured by the threshold amplitude of a circular spot moving on an oscilloscope screen) were considerably elevated for the perifoveal and medium eccentric regions in the blind hemifield, but decreased and approached normal values (i.e. those measured in the good hemifield) at eccentricities between 17 and 90 degrees. One can attribute these findings to an increasing efficiency of the tecto–cortical input with increasing eccentricity within the visual field.

4. Discrimination of single bar orientation was also tested, and revealed some residual capabilities: the threshold difference for orientation was about 10 degrees at an eccentricity of 45 degrees. Discrimination of shape and form was first tested using the letters 'X' and 'O' under two different contrast conditions, i.e. white letters on a black background or black letters on a white background. Correct estimation of the fairly large stimuli (7×9 degrees to 11×16 degrees) was greater than chance at medium eccentricities, despite the patient's report that 'it was 100% guesswork. I was not aware of anything.' The patient failed, however, to discriminate between 'X' and a closed triangle of the same size. His ability to differentiate between squares and equal-sized rectangles of different lengths and widths also indicated the presence of rudimentary shape perception in the blind hemifield.

The findings on residual vision in a blind hemifield provoked hefty opposition, such as that voiced in a 'target article' written by Campion *et al.*, (1983), 'Is blind sight an effect of scattered light, spared cortex and near-threshold vision?', in which the authors tried to reduce blindsight to stray light artifacts, criticized the methods of several groups involved in this task and added their own observations of hemianopic patients. Although the pros and cons in the 'open peer commentary' were balanced, new experimental evidence would meanwhile indicate that blindsight might be more than just an experimental artifact (cf. also Meienberg *et al.*, 1981). Furthermore evidence was accumulated indicating that some plasticity exists in the visual cortex of patients suffering from long-lasting central visual field defects (Pöppel *et al.*, 1987) which even exhibit diurnal variation (Zihl *et al.*, 1977). Such findings led to some optimism regarding the probability of therapeutic success in the rehabilitation of patients suffering from visual field defects caused by cerebral lesions (Zihl *et al.*, 1978; Zihl, 1988).

Stoerig and Pöppel (1986) applied fairly strict methodological criteria deduced from signal detection theory in their investigation of eccentricity-dependent residual target detection by patients suffering from visual field defects of cortical origin. The subjects had to detect a 0.7-degree spot of light projected for 200 ms onto three spots in the perimeter hemisphere: one within the blind field at 10 or 20 degrees eccentricity, another onto the blind spot within the blind hemifield, and the third at 35 or 40 degrees eccentricity in the blind hemifield. The eye with the temporal visual field defect was chosen and the other covered; fixation was carefully controlled by a built-in telescope. Half of the presentations, intercalated randomly, were blank. The patient was asked to indicate each time he heard an acoustic signal sounding at the same time that a light stimulus or blank stimulus was flashed. Four of the 5 patients detected the eccentric spot of light at a high significance level, but not the one projected onto the blind spot or onto the parafoveal region of the scotoma. Although this finding refuted the argument that residual visual function is supposedly a stray-light artifact, it still does not settle the question of why all patients with cortical lesions do not perform equally well in these tasks.

Stoerig and Cowey (1989), who continued this work, tested whether and how target diameter and intensity affect correct response probability (same patients and method tested as in Stoerig *et al.*, 1985; Stoerig and Pöppel, 1986). Curves relating the 'hit' rate to the 'false alarm' rate were obtained at different eccentricities (10 degrees to 20 degrees) and angles varying from 0.17 to 1.9 degrees diameter for the subjects. Interestingly, the residual detectability was above the chance rate for the 0.17 degrees and 0.45 degrees spot and again for the 1.15 degrees and 1.9 degrees spot, but did not exceed chance performance for the 0.7 degrees spot of light. This study expanded upon work carried out earlier by Barbur *et al.*, (1980), in which spatial summation for stimulus detection in a blind hemifield was tested for stimulus diameters between 2 degrees and 13.9 degrees. Under these conditions, target detectability increased with stimulus area. Perhaps the decrease in stimulus detectability at about 0.7 degree stimulus diameter indicates that two different classes of neurones are involved in the task, one presum-

ably operating on an on-activation, the other on an off-activation basis; both inhibit each other and have different receptive field sizes.

Finally, the residual vision ability to detect stimulus targets with different wavelength compositions was also tested (Stoerig, 1987; Stoerig and Cowey, 1989). Evidence for residual vision with respect to chromatic stimuli had been reported previously by Bender and Krieger (1951), but questioned by Perenin *et al.*, (1980) in a case of cortical blindness. In Stoerig and Cowey's experiments, the tests were performed monocularly, so that the visual field defect was on the temporal side; the relationship between false alarm rate and hit rate was then plotted. In 5 of the 10 patients studied, either the red or the green target was detected; the achromatic target presented at the same retinal position could not be detected, however. In 6 of the 8 patients explored for the texture of red and green targets, discrimination between red and green was found for stimuli projected onto the blind field. This work was expanded upon by Stoerig and Cowey (1989), who tested chromatic sensitivity within the scotoma at an eccentricity of 10 degrees in three patients, and found that chromatic opponency remained at least partially active in blindsight. This finding posed a new problem for blindsight: chromatic opponent neurones have not been detected so far in the retino-tecto-pulvinar-cortical pathway. Evidently colour-sensitive parvocellular neurones of the lateral geniculate nucleus (Chapter 4) send axons to cerebral regions beyond area V1 of the occipital lobe.

Recently Rafal *et al.* (1990) elaborated upon oculomotor effects on blindsight stimulation, exploiting the phylogenetically old asymmetry of the retino-tectal pathway,

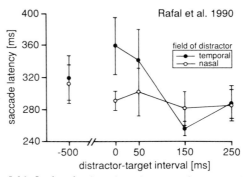

Fig. 9.16 *In three hemianopic patients saccades were evoked by a target projected into the intact visual field (monocular stimulation). The latency of these saccades (ordinate) was modified by a distractor target projected into the blind visual hemifield. A significant increase in saccade latency was only found when the distractor was projected into the blind temporal hemifield of the one eye and not into the blind nasal hemifield of the other. Beyond a distractor target interval (abscissa) of 150 ms, no inhibiting or facilitating distractor effect was observed (redrawn from Rafal et al., 1990).*

which contains many more crossed fibres from the contra-lateral than uncrossed fibres from the ipsilateral retina. In normal subjects, saccades briefly inhibit responses to visual signals at a recently noted location (Rafal *et al.*, 1989). This effect was also tested in hemianopic patients, whereby a consciously not perceived visual signal presen-ted to the temporal or the nasal blind hemifield was used. CT-scans of all three patients showed extended lesions of area V1 caused by an interruption of the calcarine branch of the posterior cerebral artery. No sign of any uncon-scious perception (blindsight) in the blind hemifield was noted for different stimulus conditions; when forced to guess whether or not a stimulus was applied, correct responses for these patients were at chance. In the main experimental paradigm, the subjects fixated monocularly on a central target and were asked to perform a saccade as fast as possible towards a light stimulus appearing at 10 degrees horizontal eccentricity in the normal visual field. A distractor stimulus of the same size (1.8 degrees squared) was presented at different temporal delays rela-tive to the target stimulus, either to the blind temporal or to the good nasal hemifield. As Fig. 9.16 illustrates, the consciously not seen stimulus led to an increase in saccade latency when projected to the blind temporal visual hemi-field and synchronously presented with the target stim-ulus. This latency increase pointed to the effect of the distractor stimulus projected into the blind visual field on the voluntarily performed saccades. It disappeared when the distractor–target interval was 150 ms or more. When the blind nasal hemifield in the other eye was tested, this distractor-induced increase in saccade latency was absent (Fig. 9.16). These findings indicate a left–right inter-action, which could have occurred, of course, entirely at the brain stem level, since sufficient connections exist from the colliculi superiores to the gaze motor system of the brain stem.

Open Questions

We think that the accumulated experimental evidence supports the idea that visual information is available at a subconscious level from a scotoma or hemianopic visual field caused by lesions of the visual radiation and/or of the primary visual cortex. Assuming that in those cases in which blindsight could be statistically proved, prestriate areas are functionally intact and the lesion is more or less restricted to area V1, besides a direct projection of LGN cells to pre-striate areas, the following pathways are most likely to bring information to the extrastriate visual regions:

1. The retino–tecto–pulvinar–prestriate connection (as discussed above).
2. The retino–pulvinar–prestriate pathway.

3. The retino–vestibular pathway, i.e. the connections from the retina to the nucleus of the optic tract. From there, there are connections to the dorsal cap of the inferior olive and to the nucleus prepositus hypoglossi or the nuc-leus reticularis tegmenti pontis, and from there to the ves-tibular nuclei. From the vestibular nuclei, afferent pathways exist via vestibular thalamic neurones to the parieto-insular vestibular cortex (Grüsser *et al.*, 1982, 1990a, b; Akbarian *et al.*, 1989). The neurones of this pathway respond to large-field, horizontally moving sti-muli. When the projections of the retina to the medial terminal nucleus of the accessory optic system of the brain stem are included, neuronal responses in vertically moving visual fields join the retino–vestibulo–cortical connec-tions, since from this brain stem, nucleus connections to the vestibular nuclei exist as well.

4. Little is known about possible connections of the retina via the pars ventralis of the lateral geniculate nuc-leus to the prestriate cortical regions of the human brain. A small projection from the lateral geniculate nucleus (pars dorsalis) relay cells to extrastriate visual areas seems to exist in monkeys (Fries, 1981) and might also be present in man.

Although rarely discussed, the most striking problem arises, however, when one assumes that the 'blindsight' signals reach the cortical level although they are not con-sciously available. Why, for example, are illusionary con-tours generated at the level of area V2 consciously perceived by primates and man (von der Heydt and Peter-hans, 1989), while a presumed activation of the same cor-tical region via the extrastriate pathways does not lead to conscious perception? Perhaps the answer to this problem lies in the connections between the colliculi superiores, the thalamus and the frontal regions of the cortex, which nor-mally function for eye movements and visually guided hand movements. While solving a task, the patients activate such mechanisms by specifically directing their attention towards the blind hemifield. If this hypothesis is valid, blindsight would improve when targets move within the blind hemifield towards the subject's face, and target recognition would also increase if the patient moved towards the target himself.

Another explanation would be that conscious visual perception requires the simultaneous activation of area V1 and of the extrastriate visual cortices. One argument in support of this hypothesis could be the strong backward projections of the striate cortex's extrastriate visual areas (Chapter 5). This hypothesis is weakened, however, by the fact that hemianopic patients might spontaneously per-ceive phosphenes and visual pseudo–hallucinations within the blind hemifield, as discussed in the next section. Finally, in interpreting blindsight, one has to take into consideration that lesions of the primary visual cortex or the visual radiation not only lead to retrograde degeneration of the relay cells of the lateral geniculate nucleus, but also to transsynaptic retrograde degeneration of optic nerve fibres in the long run and finally to atrophy of retinal ganglion cells (Hoyt and Kommerell, 1973; Cowey, 1974).

Spontaneous Visual Sensations in Cortical Blindness or in the Hemianopic Visual Field

Patients suffering from cortical blindness due to a bilateral loss of area V1 or from cortical hemianopia may report four different classes of spontaneous visual sensations not related to any external visual stimulus:

1. Phosphenes, like those described for migraine attacks (Chapter 10).
2. Structured photopsias, i.e. simple but more or less regular achromatic or chromatic visual patterns, which are perceived in some cases as 'scintillating'.
3. Visual pseudo-hallucinations of figures (often repetitive ones), or schematic scenes which are recognized as images ('bildhaft') not really existing in the external world.
4. Visual hallucinations of achromatic or coloured scenes, which are perceived, at least temporarily, as being 'real' ('leibhaft') and are not experienced as contradictory to the tactile percept of objects in the extrapersonal space.

All these abnormal visual sensations can be interpreted as being caused by a pathological activation of visual cortical structures beyond area V1, which remains at least partially intact. The phosphenes and photisms are presumably caused by an activation of neuronal networks in areas V2, V3 and V4, while more complex, visual pseudo-hallucinations and hallucinations are evoked by abnormal stimulation of occipito-temporal and temporal visual regions. They are generated by the activation of visual memory functions, whereby the abnormal neuronal activity seems to be able to combine old visual material with new, not previously experienced visual scenes, as in dreams. Henschen (1911, 1925) emphasized the different localization of the pathological processes leading to phosphenes and photisms (striate and peristriate areas) and to complex visual hallucinations, the latter indicating the involvement of occipito-temporal regions. It is interesting that scenic hallucinations are more frequently observed by patients suffering from cortical blindness than from hemianopia. On the other hand, one has to keep in mind that visual hallucinations are also observed after several days of bilateral eye occlusion. Thus a gradual transition seems to exist between the *phantastische Gesichtserscheinungen* of Johannes Müller (1826) seen by normal subjects, visual images perceived after days of visual deprivation and vivid hallucinatory experiences after the formation of bilateral area V1 lesions. Any chronic disconnection or reduction in activation of the visual cortex evidently facilitates scenic pseudo-hallucinations or hallucinations. Consequently, Weinberger and Grant (1940) rejected any locational value of visual pseudo-hallucinations. In our opinion, one should differentiate between two classes of aetiologies leading to visual sensations in patients suffering from brain lesions:

1. Abnormal visual sensations which are caused by local pathological processes leading to epileptic discharges of nerve cells still active in the region near the brain lesion (including regions occupied by collateral oedema).
2. Abnormal visual sensations caused by disinhibition, i.e. by the interruption of the afferent visual signal flow from area V1 to 'higher' visual centres beyond area V1. In the following section, we shall discuss some of these spontaneous visual sensations occurring in the blind visual field (Gloning *et al.*, 1968).

Phosphenes Caused by Abnormal Excitation of Area V1

These phosphenes appear typically during migraine attacks and are therefore discussed in Chapter 10. They may also be evoked by an excitation of area V1 neurones in cases of hemianopia caused by lesions of the optic tract, the lateral geniculate nucleus or the visual radiation. In some patients extended scintillating phosphenes accompany the sudden occurrence of cortical blindness, as described by Schirmer (1895, mentioned by Wilbrand and Saenger, 1917). Postmortem examination revealed a bilateral infarct of the occipital lobes. Similarly, Gloning *et al.* (1968) reported the occurrence of simple phosphenes and photisms in 23% of their patients suffering from occipital lesions. 67% of the visual sensations were achromatic, 23% revealed some chromatic structures. Wilbrand and Saenger (1917) mentioned one of Westphal's patients who suffered from hemianopia and focal epilepsia of the Jacksonian type; during the early stages of his disease, he perceived undulating lines of red, green and blue colours as epileptic equivalents moving across the later blind hemifield.

Photopsias in Cortical Hemianopia

Photopsias are simply structured, coloured or achromatic visual sensations which exhibit different levels of spatial organization: regular geometric shapes often organized into repetitive geometrical patterns of rhomboids, squares, circles, etc., which frequently appear in bright colours. While about two-thirds of the phosphenes and photopsias

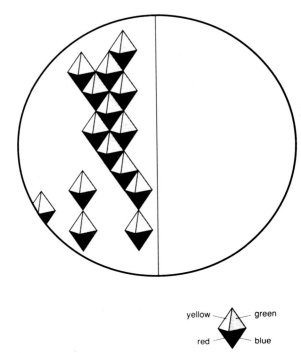

yellow — green
red — blue

Fig. 9.17 *Kaleidoscope-type of coloured geometrical photisms as seen by a patient suffering from a left homonymous hemianopia. The patient described the geometrical figures as regular and saw them in saturated colours (yellow, green, red and blue), as indicated (redrawn from Kölmel, 1984).*

movement were reported, indicating a continuous transition from migraine-type phosphenes to photisms (Vorster, 1893; Uhthoff, 1899, 1915; Wilbrand and Saenger, 1917; Henschen, 1925; Gloning *et al.*, 1968). These achromatic photisms are presumably caused by a pathological activation of area V2 (cf. Chapter 10).

Visual Pseudo-hallucinations

Visual pseudo-hallucinations of complex structures seen in the hemianopic field are, as a rule, visual sensations which do not appear before or immediately after the acute onset of hemianopia. It frequently takes several days before these spontaneous visual sensations appear. Naturally structured, stationary or moving objects, persons or faces appearing for seconds in the foveal or parafoveal part of the hemianopic field are characteristically reported. They can be chromatic or achromatic and are frequently repetitive, building, for example, rows of identical figures. Lamy (1895) emphasized that in regard to these visual sensations, most patients realize that their hallucinations are not real, i.e. that they belong to the class of pseudo-hallucinations. In many patients, these pseudo-hallucinations recur as identical or very similar patterns which are sometimes rather bizarre. Lamy reported on a 35-year-old luetic woman who suffered from a right homonymous hemianopia; she repeatedly saw an upside-down child. While the simple geometrical photisms are suppressed, as a rule, by saccadic eye movements, eye movements do not usually have such an effect in complex visual pseudo-hallucinations occurring in the hemianopic field.

About 10 years ago, by courtesy of Dr Kölmel, one of the authors (O.-J. G.) saw a 34-year-old ophthalmic nurse who, early one morning, suddenly suffered a painful headache on the left side; upon looking into the mirror she realized that she was suffering from a right hemianopia. Two days later an ophthalmologist confirmed a right homonymous hemianopia with macular sparing. During the first day of hemianopia, she was evidently emotionally disturbed as well and reported having seen stars, light nebula, patches and some geometrical patterns in the hemianopic field, which sometimes flashed in pure, bright, scintillating colours. After several days, as the hemianopia gradually decreased, she suddenly noted a visual pseudo-hallucination like a movie scene in the hemianopic field: a man with a hat, coat and briefcase was seen from behind crossing a street at a traffic light. She could not remember having seen such a scenario in real life; she repeatedly observed precisely the same scene for 4 days. Thereafter, the visual pseudo-hallucinations did not return. During the first days after the acute hemianopia, the patient occasionally heard an unknown voice speaking to her. This auditory hallucination was much more upsetting than the visual pseudo-hallucination of the man with

in the study of Gloning *et al.* (1967) were reported by the patients as achromatic, Kölmel (1984) described very colourful photisms in the blind hemifield in the majority of 60 hemianopic patients whom he investigated. 25 of his patients saw only repeated coloured geometrical structures, 17 reported only achromatic photisms and 10 observed both coloured and achromatic visual sensations. Figure 9.17 illustrates such a brightly coloured, geometrically repetitive structure, as described by one of Kölmel's patients. It is interesting that such patients usually report fairly pure colours (Wilbrand and Saenger, 1917), the two antagonistic colour pairs red–green and yellow–blue seem to be preferred. Characteristically, repetitive chromatic pattern photisms appear as brief events seen for seconds or minutes and occur generally during the first days following the acute hemianopia. Some patients reported having seen these geometrical photisms hours before they became aware of their hemianopia.

Achromatic geometrical photopsias are, as a rule, less geometrically organized than the coloured ones: bright stars, zigzag structures, moving flashes, spirals, light nebula and spots of light which usually move with eye the briefcase. She was frightened and did not report this experience to her physician. The auditory hallucination indicated an involvement of the left temporal lobe; it disappeared a few days after the vascular incident.

Landis *et al.* (1986) reported on a patient suffering from a left hemianopia, prosopagnosia and mild topographic disorientation. About 4 weeks after the acute incident, the patient experienced photisms and scenic pseudo-hallucinations: she repeatedly observed the same man walking from left to right across her left, visually not perceived, extrapersonal space. Scenic visual pseudo-hallucinations in the hemianopic field can be interpreted as epileptic equivalents affecting occipito–temporal visual association areas. Paillas *et al.* (1965) reported that 17 out of 36 patients suffering from occipital lesions experienced complex visual hallucinations or pseudo-hallucinations. Allen (1930) observed this symptom in 25% of 40 patients suffering from occipital tumours. Visual pseudo-hallucinations restricted to faces will be described in Chapter 17, which deals with prosopagnosia. Gloning *et al.* (1968) pointed out that patients with occipital lesions may also see doubles ('heautoscopy') in the blind hemifield (Chapter 16).

Complex Visual Hallucinations

Literature describing complex visual hallucinations lasting for hours or days in the hemianopic visual field is rare (cf. Hoff and Pötzl, 1937b). It is interesting that visualization of people and animals is most common, as is the case in acute Korsakoff psychosis. Laehr (1896) cited the report of one of his hemianopic patients who saw moving figures such as men and women donning fashionable hats, as well as animals, in particular elephants and rhinoceroses; the animals were a grey colour, the humans a muddy yellow. Zihl and von Cramon (1986) reported on a patient suffering from a left homonymous hemianopia, who while reading a newspaper, noticed a black-and-white striped cat sitting on the lower left end of the breakfast table. He interrupted his reading, headed towards the kitchen to get a piece of sausage for the animal, then suddenly became aware that this percept must have been an illusionary one.

Wilbrand (1890) observed a patient suffering from a left homonymous hemianopia who reported vivid, scenic visual hallucinations in the blind hemifield over a period of days. The scenes changed frequently (landscapes, heads, cats, furniture, corridors, etc.) and were observed with open or closed eyes. Postmortem neuropathology revealed an infarct in the right occipital lobe without any impairment of the left side. In general, visual scenic hallucinations in the hemianopic field seem to be reported more frequently with a right occipital lobe lesion than with a left one (cf. the review of Wilbrand and Saenger, 1917).

Visual hallucinations appear only in a minority of cortically blind patients (Aldrich *et al.*, 1987) and are a sign of involvement of the cortical areas beyond the striate cortex (Horrax, 1923; Horrax and Putnam, 1932). Patients experience vivid visual scenes, begin to interact with people or objects seen at least partially and are usually not aware that they are blind.

10 Light Not Illuminating the World: Phosphenes and Related Phenomena

Introduction

Phosphenes are non-figural achromatic or coloured light sensations which are caused by inadequate stimulation of the retina, the optic nerve or the central visual system (area V1 and V2). They are stable within the visual field, as a rule, and therefore are perceived as moving with saccades or smooth pursuit eye movements, similar to long-lasting retinal afterimages. In the following we will classify phosphenes according to their site of origin and the type of inadequate stimulus. If not otherwise mentioned, the phosphenes described are light sensations in the dark. Under these conditions, phosphenes are not seen against a black background, since when one perceives 'nothing' in the dark one in actual fact spontaneously sees dark-grey clouds, light nebula, and sometimes very fine-grained amorphic structures. This 'Eigengrau' or 'Eigenlicht' is caused by the spontaneous activity of the nerve cells in the retina and the central visual system. Several days or weeks after acute loss of both retinae, the 'Eigengrau' appears brighter than under normal conditions. One of us (O.-J. G.) observed a patient who about three weeks after losing her sight due to prolonged retinal ischaemia reported 'dazzling' light sensations filling the whole visual field, without any distinct structures except for some 'clouds' which differed in brightness from the background. 'Eigengrau' and 'Eigenlicht' form the perceptual background on which the phosphenes described in the following appear in the dark when no visual input is present.

Retinal Phosphenes

Light sensations caused by non-photic stimulation of the retina are easily experienced by normals, provided the inadequate stimulus is effectively applied (Benedict, 1830). The retinal phosphene most frequently observed is evoked by mechanical irritation of the eyeball and is also seen when one holds the eyelids tightly shut.

Deformation Phosphenes

When the eyeball is pressed or indented in total darkness, within less than 200 ms, an oval or quartermoon-shaped spot of light is perceived in the visual field part corresponding to the indented region of the retina, i.e. in the visual field opposite the site of indentation (Fig. 10.1(a)). In the seconds following, this phosphene extends across the whole visual field and changes its appearance during further eyeball indentation: irregular, large bright spots of light, finely structured moving light grains ('light nebula') and stationary bright stars are seen. In some amblyopic subjects (squint amblyopia), regular geometrical patterns appear when one eyeball is deformed. Purkinje was such a case and he described phosphene patterns which are normally seen only when both eyes are indented simultaneously (Purkinje, 1825; Tyler, 1976; Grüsser et al., 1984; Grüsser et al., 1989). When the eyeball deformation with monocular stimulation is released, part of the retina again lights up for 1 to 2 seconds and curved light lines are seen following the course of the larger retinal vessels (Fig. 10.1(d)). The deformation or 'pressure' phosphene was first described in the Fifth century BC by Alcmaeon of Croton and led to the development of the theory of 'efferent' light involved in the mechanisms of vision (Chapter 2). The name 'phosphene' was coined in 1838 by the French physician Savigny (cf. Serre d'Uzèz, 1853). Grüsser and Hagner (1990) have provided an extensive review of the history of deformation phosphenes and their role in the development of theoretical concepts of vision over two millenia.

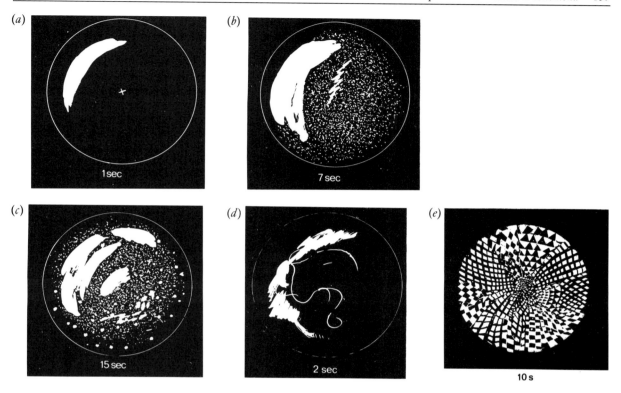

Fig. 10.1 *(a–d) Development of deformation phosphenes after indentation of the temporal side of the right eyeball at different intervals following indentation (a–c) and after release of eyeball indentation (d), as seen by one of the authors (O.-J. G.). (e) With simultaneous bilateral indentation of both eyeballs on the temporal side of the eye a patterned deformation phosphene is observed, flickering at about 10 Hz. (e) represents the impression after about 10 s of indentation. The grain of the triangular, rhomboid and rectangular flickering patterns increases with the distance from the centre of the binocular visual field. (From Grüsser et al., 1984.)*

When the eyeball is indented, the surface of the eye is increased and the retina is stretched locally. In accordance with the elastic–plastic properties of the retina, this stretch extends slowly and inhomogeneously across the retinal surface. The mechanical properties of the retina are different along the larger vessels, i.e. the branches of the arteria centralis retinae and the larger retinal veins, than in the other parts of the retina. These inhomogeneities explain the appearance of phosphenes along the retinal vessels when the indentation is released. Part of the perivascular retinal tissue is then stretched again. Within several seconds, the eye regains its 'normal' shape.

Single unit recordings from optic tract axons revealed that during eyeball deformation the great majority of on-centre ganglion cells, normally activated when the retina is illuminated by light and inhibited when the light is turned off, increase their neuronal activity after a latency of 0.2 to 3 s during constant eyeball deformation in total darkness. This activity is maintained for 10 to 20 s and decreases thereafter due to retinal ischaemia. The off-centre gang-

lion cells, which are normally inhibited transiently by illumination of the retina, are inhibited by eyeball deformation with a delay of 0.2 to 4 s. When the deformation is discontinued, off–centre ganglion cells slowly return, as a rule, to the pre-deformation activity level. Some of them exhibit a transient excitation. This response scheme together with the presumed responses of other retinal neurones evoked by eyeball deformation are shown in Fig. 10.2.

The deformation of the eyeball stretches and increases the retinal surface, whereby the horizontal cell structures, in particular the dendrites of horizontal cells and of certain amacrines, are affected. This leads to an increase in the cell surface of these structures, accompanied by an increase in sodium conductivity, and consequently to a depolarization of the resting membrane potential. In the model of Fig. 10.2, it is assumed that horizontal cells (H-cells) are especially affected by this mechanism. A depolarization of H-cells causes in turn a depolarization of on-bipolars (BP_{on}) by activating sodium and chloride channels and a

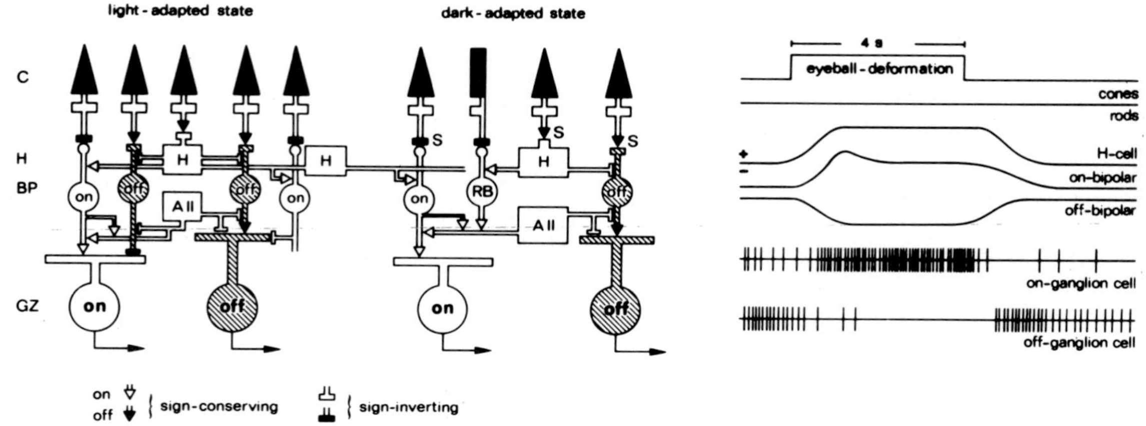

Fig. 10.2 *Scheme of the effect of eyeball deformation on the activity of retinal neurones. The deformation stretches and increases the retinal surface, whereby the horizontal elements in particular (horizontal cells and amacrines) are affected. This leads to an increase in cell surface of these structures and to a depolarization of the horizontal cells (H), which in turn causes a depolarization of on-bipolars (BP_{on}) and a hyperpolarization of off-bipolars (BP_{off}). A similar depolarization of the amacrine cells (AII) could also lead to a modification of the ganglion cell responses, an activation of the on-ganglion cells and an inhibition of the off-ganglion cells of both latency classes I and II (corresponding to Y-cells and X-cells). In the dark adapted retina, the horizontal cell depolarization is presumably mediated through the rod bipolar cell (RB), which activates AII-amacrines, activating in turn on-ganglion cells and inhibiting off-ganglion cells. Excitatory ('sign-conserving') synapses are drawn as arrows, inhibitory ('sign-reversing') synapses as bars. Since the synaptic endings of the rod amacrine cell AII leads to an activation of on-ganglion cells and an inhibition of off-ganglion cells depolarization in the dark-adapted state is qualitatively and quantitatively not significantly different from depolarization responses in the light-adapted state. (From Grüsser and Hagner, 1990.)*

hyperpolarization of off-bipolars (BP_{off}) by activation of potassium channels. These changes are transmitted to the corresponding ganglion cells (G), which are activated (on-centre ganglion cells) or inhibited (off-centre ganglion cells). It is not yet clear whether a similar depolarization of the amacrine cells, especially those of class AII (Fig. 10.2), also leads to a modification of the ganglion cell responses. Owing to their antagonistic innervation of on- and off-ganglion cells, the amacrines of type II are, as horizontal cells, candidates for the mediation of direct stretch responses. It seems fairly likely, however, that in the light-adapted retina the responses of retinal ganglion cells during and after eyeball deformation are dominated by the horizontal cell depolarization. In the dark-adapted retina, the horizontal cell depolarization is perhaps mediated through the rod bipolar cells (RB in Fig. 10.2), which activate AII-amacrines, exciting in turn on-ganglion cells and inhibiting off-ganglion cells.

Figure 10.3 indicates that, provided the experiment was performed in darkness, the deformation activation of on-ganglion cells was not dependent upon the state of dark adaptation. The same was true for the inhibition of the off-ganglion cells evoked by eyeball indentation. The deformation activation of on-centre ganglion cells and the corresponding inhibition of off-ganglion cells was about the same in a 'closed' system in which the intraocular pressure increased during eyeball deformation and in an 'open' system in which the intraocular pressure was maintained at a constant level during deformation (Grüsser *et al.*, 1981; 1984; 1989a,b).

When light stimuli and eyeball deformation were combined, the deformation responses of on-ganglion cells depended on the light intensity (diffuse illumination). At low-level retinal illumination (< 0.01 cd m^{-2}), the eyeball deformation still led to an activation of on-ganglion cells. At photopic illumination conditions, however, the on-ganglion cell activity was inhibited by eyeball deformation. The results obtained by 'titration' of light and eyeball deformation led us to conclude that the activation of the chloride channels of the on-bipolar cell membrane by horizontal cell depolarization explains this light-dependent change in deformation effects. Off-centre ganglion cell inhibition by eyeball deformation, however, was scarcely dependent on the intensity of the light stimulating simultaneously the retina, a fact foreseeable through the assumption that H-cell depolarization leads to an increase in potassium conductivity of off-bipolar cells (Przybyszewski *et al.*, 1990; Chung, *et al.*, 1991). The corresponding psychophysical observation fits well with the neurophysiological data: when one deforms the eyeball and looks simultaneously at a homogeneously illuminated white screen, within a few seconds eyeball deformation

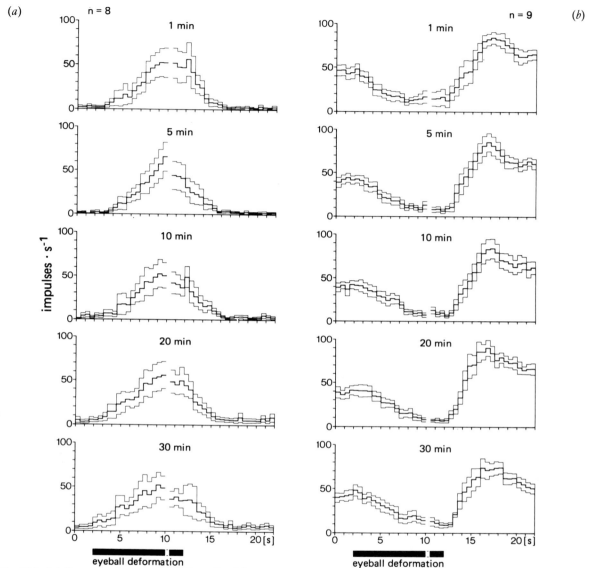

Fig. 10.3 *(a) Responses of on-centre ganglion cells of the cat retina (latency class I) to eyeball deformation at different levels of dark adaptation. (b) Same, but for off-centre ganglion cells (latency class II). (From Grüsser et al., 1989.)*

diminishes the brightness of the light perceived and within another three to four seconds it is replaced by a dark-grey field with finely grained light spots. When the same deformation is applied in darkness, however, phosphenes as described above are perceived (Fig. 10.1).

Binocular eyeball deformation leads to a characteristically patterned phosphene with finely grained squares, rhomboids or triangles in the visual field centre. The angular size of these structures increases towards the periphery of the visual field (Fig. 10.1(e)). The binocular phosphene pattern shows a somewhat irregular and not completely synchronous flickering at about 10 Hz (cf. Tyler, 1978). The binocular deformation phosphene pattern is explainable by the columnar organization of the visual cortex (Chapter 4) and the afferent neuronal signals reaching it: with binocular eyeball deformation, all off-centre ganglion cells in both retinae and the afferent visual system cease to discharge, while latency class I and II on-ganglion cells respond with a sustained activation. This creates an afferent input pattern to the cortical nerve cells of area V1 which is normally not present. Evidently, the cortical network responds with an oscillatory resonance, whereby neurones belonging to individual hypercolumns are coordinated in activation and inhibition. In a pilot experiment Grüsser (unpubl. 1982) found periodic burst activation of area 17 cortical nerve cells in anaesthetized cats when both eyes were deformed simultaneously in total darkness.

Jordan and Baumgartner (1960) reported that after a sudden increase in intraocular pressure above arterial systolic blood pressure, cortical on-neurones of cat area 17 increased and decreased their activity periodically, while the activity of off-type cortical nerve cells ceased after 15–20 s of retinal ischaemia.

Accommodation Phosphenes

When one shifts the fixation point in darkness from infinity to an imagined object very close by, e.g. the tip of the nose, eyeball convergence and strong accommodation of the lens is the consequence; in addition one perceives an illumination of the visual field periphery (Purkinje, 1825; Czermak, 1858; Berlin, 1874; Helmholtz, 1896; Hellner and Gauri, 1986). Due to the mechanical connections between lens zonule of Zinn, ciliary body and retina, the retina is stretched during maximum near accommodation. This leads, as in the case of deformation phosphenes, to an activation of the neuronal on-system, whereby the maximum retinal stretch is exerted, of course, in the periphery of the retina. Correspondingly one perceives a diffuse ring of light illuminating the periphery of the visual field. The mechanisms generating the accommodation phosphenes are the same, in principle, as those described for the deformation phosphenes.

Saccadic Phosphenes

Saccadic phosphenes were first described by Aristotle, who also discussed the mechanisms leading to deformation phosphenes (*De sensu et sensato*, 437a, b). Owing to the somewhat unequal forces exerted by the extraocular eye muscles on the eyeball during a saccade, particularly when the eyelids are closed, the eyeball is slightly deformed and the region where the optic nerve enters, moreover, is stretched. This stretch is transmitted to the peripapillary retina. As in the case of deformation phosphenes, retinal stretch leads to activation of the neuronal on-system and, as a consequence, an incomplete ring-shaped phosphene is seen around the blind spot. When large voluntary saccades are executed and the eye position is maintained at the far right or far left of the orbit, the saccadic phosphene is seen for about half a second shifted approximately 10 degrees laterally from the centre of the field of vision.

For those interested in clinical pathophysiology it should be pointed out that saccadic phosphenes are noted by intelligent patients in all those diseases which lead to an increased mechanical sensitivity of the retina to stretch in the peripapillar region. This is the case, for example, in oedema of the optic nerve head caused by optic neuritis, in some retrobulbar tumours as well as in tumours affecting the optic chiasm (cf. Swerdloff *et al.*, 1981). Furthermore, stretch-induced phosphenes are evoked when the venous pressure in these patients is increased transiently, as in the case of heavy coughing or sneezing. Under these conditions, mild phosphenes are also observed by normals. In patients suffering from optic neuritis or other diseases affecting the optic nerve, saccadic phosphenes and 'coughing phosphenes' can be so strong that they are noted not only in total darkness but also in dimly lit rooms. A patient seen by one of the authors (O.-J. G.), for example, reported peculiar strong phosphenes when coughing in the dark. These phosphenes were the first symptom of a pituitary adenoma and preceded all other neurological symptoms by more than a year. It is therefore advisable for a clinician to ask his patients about such light sensations.

Electrical Phosphenes

Electrical stimulation of the eyeball also leads to light sensations. Electrically induced phosphenes were first described in 1755 by Le Roy (Helmholtz, 1896). As soon as galvanic piles became available, several physiologists experimented extensively with constant voltage stimulation of their own eyes, whereby either the positive or the negative pole was closer to the corneal surface. It was soon discovered that chromaticity of the electrical phosphenes depended on the direction of the current flowing through the eyeball. In most experiments one stimulation electrode was fixed to the eyelid, the other to the skin of the neck or in the mouth. Early systematic studies on electrical phosphenes were performed by Pfaff (1795), Ritter (1800, 1802, 1805) and Purkinje (1819, 1825), who reported the following properties:

1. When the eyeball was near the negative pole and the direct current turned on, the phosphene was perceived as white-violet and the blind spot was seen initially as a dark disc in the illuminated visual field.

2. When the direct current was turned off, darkening of the visual field was seen with a transient yellow-red colouring of the blind spot.

3. Reversed polarization led to a decrease in the *Eigengrau*, which in addition took on a yellow-red chroma. The blind spot region was seen as a light-blue disc on a dark background.

4. When direct current was turned off, a transient illumination of the visual field with some bluish chroma appeared and the blind spot was seen as a dark disc.

These descriptions of direct current phosphenes, as summarized by von Helmholtz (1896), indicate that antagonistic retinal light–dark mechanisms as well as chromatic

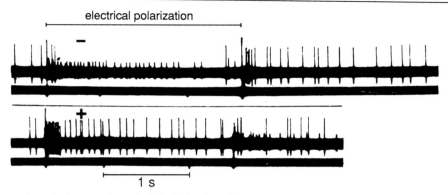

Fig. 10.4 *Responses of a retinal on-ganglion cell of the dark-adapted cat retina to electrical polarization of reversing directions as indicated. (Modified from Granit, 1948.)*

antagonistic processes are involved, determining the appearance of the electrical phosphenes.

This general idea was pursued in later studies on electrical phosphenes (e.g. Schliephake, 1874; Schwartz, 1889; Finkelstein, 1894) and confirmed by recording the responses of single retinal ganglion cells evoked by electrical polarization of the retina. Gernandt and Granit (1947) found that *anodal polarization* of the cat retina led to an activation of the on-ganglion cells and inhibition of the off-ganglion cells. When the direct current was turned off, the reverse responses were observed. *Cathodal polarization*, however, led to the opposite responses: inhibition of on-ganglion cells and activation of off-ganglion cells (Granit, 1947, 1948, 1950; Fig. 10.4). Owing to the antagonistic responses of on-centre and off-centre neurones, the conclusion is plausible that the interference of near threshold direct current with the physiological retinal signal flow occurs not at the level of the ganglion cells but at the site of the outer plexiform layer, i.e. in the synaptic region between the pedicles of the photoreceptors and the dendrites of bipolar and horizontal cells (Chapter 3).

After a.c. sources became available, extensive studies were also conducted on electrical phosphenes evoked by a.c. stimulation of the eyeball with different stimulus frequencies and amplitudes. When intermittent sinewave or squarewave rectangular electrical stimuli were used, the threshold strength of the phosphene seen by normal subjects was found to be a function of stimulus frequency (F. Schwarz, 1940; Lohmann, 1940; Barnett, 1941; Motokawa and Iwama, 1950; Abe, 1951; Bouman *et al.*, 1951; Baumgardt and Bujas, 1952; Clausen, 1955). Minimum threshold values were reached in the light-adapted eye at frequencies around 20 Hz (Fig. 10.5(a)). An approximate linear relationship between the logarithm of phosphene threshold Θ above and below 20 Hz and the logarithm of stimulus frequency f was found:

$$\log \Theta = a \log f + c \qquad (10.1)$$

from this the power function, for the threshold Θ, measured in milliamps, is obtained:

$$\Theta = k f^a \qquad (10.2)$$

The constants of these power functions depended on the background illumination (Fig. 10.5(a), F. Schwarz, 1944; Meyer-Schwickerath and Nagun, 1951). The constant a was negative below 20 Hz and positive above. Motokawa and Ebe (1953), measuring the threshold-frequency relationship in much smaller steps than Schwarz had done, found several subminima for the threshold curves at about 7.5, 27.5, 35, 42.5 and 47 Hz (Fig. 10.5(b); cf. Motokawa and Iwama, 1950; Abe, 1951; Motokawa, 1970). Enhancement of electrical excitability at selected a.c. frequencies (corresponding to some of the minima shown in Fig. 10.5(b)) was found for illumination of the retina with monochromatic light. Hereby the electrical flicker threshold for 36-Hz a.c. was reduced maximally at about 460 nm wavelength, for 42 Hz at 550 nm and for 77 Hz at 650 nm (Takahashi *et al.*, 1956, as quoted by Motokawa, 1970). Motokawa and Ebe (1953) reported even two or three peaks for the facilitation of electrical flicker threshold when the wavelength of monochromatic illumination was changed between 400 and 700 nm. At a.c. frequencies between 20 and 42 Hz these peaks were found in the short wavelength range below 550 nm, while with a.c. frequencies between 53 and 92 Hz these peaks appeared at about 550, 600 and 650 nm. These findings indicate that chromatic mechanisms of the retina are sensitive to temporal factors of excitation concerning the neuronal mechanisms proximal to the photochemical process (for further discussion see Motokawa, 1970).

The maximum stimulus frequency at which distinct flicker phosphenes were elicitable reached values between 100 and 150 Hz, significantly above the critical flicker fusion frequency (CFF) of intermittent light. Measurements at higher frequencies require stimulus intensities above the pain threshold. From animal experiments, per-

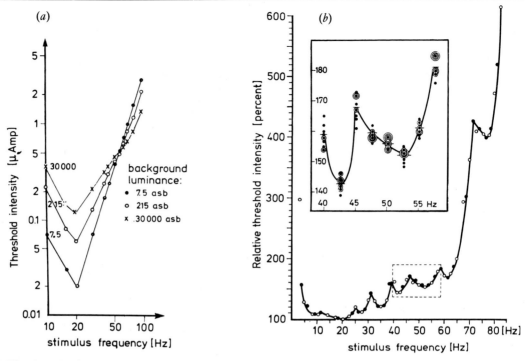

Fig. 10.5 *(a) Phosphene threshold intensity (ordinate), obtained with a.c. stimulation of the eye of a human observer adapted to three different levels of background illumination (Schwarz, 1944. (b) Relative phosphene threshold intensity (ordinate) obtained with a.c. stimulation of the human eye at different stimulus frequencies (abscissa). Data represented by different marks were obtained from the same subject on different days. Inset: part of the threshold curve obtained between 40 and 60 Hz a.c. enlarged (Motokawa and Ebe, 1953).*

formed in deep anaesthesia, it became evident that single retinal ganglion cells can follow sinewave electrical stimulation of the retina up to 180 Hz (Grüsser *et al.*, 1984).

In the light-adapted eye, electrical flicker phosphenes could be elicited at higher stimulus frequencies than in the dark-adapted eye. The minimum threshold frequency was shifted by dark adaptation from about 20 Hz to 3–10 Hz (Lohmann, 1940; Bouman and ten Doeschate, 1969). At stimulus frequencies above 110 Hz, spatially structured phosphene patterns were evoked by the alternating current (Lohmann, 1940). These non-flickering patterns disappeared only at stimulus frequencies above 320 Hz: regularly or irregularly oriented grids, star-shaped figures, etc. were reported which frequently appeared to be coloured. The higher the temporal stimulus frequency, the smaller the spatial difference between the particles of the phosphene.

The hypothesis mentioned above, that the site of interaction between the electrical stimuli and the physiological signal processing is the outer plexiform layer, was corroborated by results obtained in experiments with simultaneous stimulation of the eye by sinewave electrical stimuli and intermittent light stimuli (Brindley, 1955, 1960;

Clausen and Vanderbilt, 1957). When electrical and light flicker stimuli at diverse frequencies were applied, visual beats corresponding to the frequency difference appeared. By this method, Brindley (1962) could demonstrate that above the psychophysically determined photopic critical flicker fusion frequency the overall output signals of the photoreceptors of the human retina evidently still follow the light stimuli up to about 110 to 120 Hz. Corresponding to Brindley's beats, Veringa (1964) reported that sinewave-modulated a.c. enhanced or suppressed the flicker perception of a sinusoidally modulated test field when the phase angle between current and light was appropriately adjusted. The suitable phase angle depended on flicker frequency. It increased with the frequency of flicker and electrical stimuli and depended as well on the adaptation state of the retina (Veringa and Roelofs, 1966; review: van de Grind *et al.*, 1973).

Correlates of the properties just described for the subjective appearance of electrical phosphenes evoked by a.c. stimulation were also found when the activity of single retinal on-centre or off-centre ganglion cells was measured by recording action potentials of single optic tract axons in anaesthetized cats. In these experiments electrical stim-

(a)

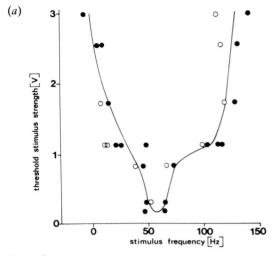

(b)

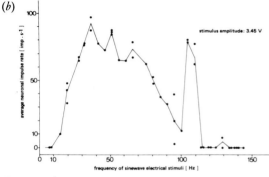

(c)

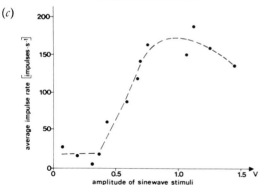

ulation was applied to the eyeball by means of a ball-shaped electrode fixed in a corneal contact lens. Figures 10.6 and 10.7 illustrate some of the findings (Grüsser *et al.*, 1985, 1986, 1987). As expected from the direct current data of Gernandt and Granit mentioned above, low-frequency, sinewave, electrical stimulation led to an antagonistic activation and inhibition in on-centre and off-centre ganglion cells. With increasing frequencies, intermittent responses of the ganglion cells were evoked up to 150 to 180 Hz. This response was not caused by direct electrical stimulation of ganglion cells or optic nerve axons, since by a simultaneous increase in intraocular pressure above arterial blood pressure the light responses and the responses to the a.c. were abolished simultaneously owing to retinal ischaemia (cf. Grehn *et al.*, 1981, 1984). Increasing electrical stimulus strength 15 to 20 times led to a neuronal activation caused by the direct electrical stimulation of retropapillar optic nerve fibres. At this stimulus strength, on-centre and off-centre neurones responded similarly. This response was not suppressed by retinal ischaemia and was therefore generated outside the retina.

When intermittent light stimuli and sinewave electrical stimuli were applied simultaneously at slightly varying frequencies, the 'beats' observed in psychophysical experiments were also found in single ganglion cell responses (Fig. 10.7). Hereby the beat frequency of ganglion cell activity corresponded to the difference between the two stimulation frequencies applied. These findings

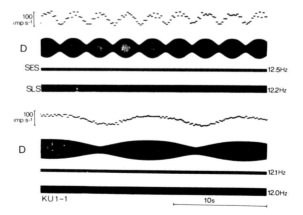

Fig. 10.6*(a)* *Threshold curves of a retinal on-centre ganglion cell (latency class II) to sinewave electrical stimulation at different stimulus frequencies (abscissa). Cat retina, pentobarbital anaesthesia. Active corneal contact lense electrode; indifferent electrode was placed at the frontal skull (Grüsser et al., unpubl., 1984). (b) Responses (average neuronal activation) of the same ganglion cell as in (a) to electrical sinewave stimuli at different frequencies (abscissa). (c) Cat retina, on-centre ganglion cell, latency class I. Stimulus strength–response curve obtained at 120 Hz sinewave electrical stimuli. Electrodes as in (a). (From experiments performed in collaboration with R. Kusel and A. W. Przybyszewski.)*

Fig. 10.7 *Beats in the activation of an off-centre retinal ganglion cell (latency class I) to sinewave light flicker stimuli (SLS, 12.2 and 12.0 Hz) and simultaneous sinewave electrical stimulation (SES, 12.5 and 12.1 Hz). According to the phase change of the slightly different stimulation frequencies for electrical a.c. and light stimuli, the neuronal response consisted of an increase and decrease of the neuronal activity at beat frequency. The relative difference signal D of light and electrical stimuli is shown in the second recording line (Grüsser et al., 1984).*

confirmed Brindley's assumption that interaction of light and electrical current occurs at a level distal to the ganglion cell layer.

Electromagnetic Phosphenes

Strong electromagnetic alternating fields also induce flicker sensations (Loevsund *et al.*, 1980). These magnetophosphenes were studied at frequencies between 10 and 50 Hz in particular. The threshold values reached minima at frequencies between 20 and 30 Hz, provided that a broad-spectrum white light was used for background stimulation. Then the minimum threshold flux density was between 10 and 12 mT. This threshold intensity increased during dark adaptation. It also depended upon the spectral composition of the background luminance. It is interesting that the stimulation frequency for electrical phosphenes and magnetic phosphenes leading to maximum sensitivity is in the same range. Raybourn (1983) reported on the effects of strong d.c. magnetic fields on the light-induced signals in the turtle retina. Magnetophosphenes are without clinical relevance. The strength and frequencies of the magnetic fields applied in clinical studies, for example in the measurement of eye position by means of the electromagnetic search coil technique (Robinson, 1964; Collewijn, 1984) and in the diagnostic techniques of MRI for imaging of body parts, are far below the range within which retinal magnetic phosphenes are induced.

Single Flashes Seen in Space

Astronauts and high-altitude pilots have repeatedly reported seeing short light flashes in darkness or when the eyes are closed. Two explanations are possible. These 'flashes' are saccadic phosphenes evoked at lower thresholds owing to the stronger filling of venous vessels in the retro-orbital tissue in the state of weightlessness. Or, the short punctiform flashes reported could be caused by high-energy particles absorbed in photoreceptor outer segments. Their energy dissipates and might lead to bleaching of packages of photopigment molecules, a mechanism which in turn evokes a short change in the membrane potential of photoreceptors and a corresponding activation of retinal neurones, ultimately noted as a short flash sensation.

X-ray-induced Retinal Responses

The interpretation in the preceding section is supported by neurophysiological findings on the effects of X-rays on the retina and rhodopsin bleaching (Doly *et al.*, 1979, 1980a,b). Strong X-rays induce electrophysiological responses comparable to those induced by light, as for example those measurable by the electroretinogram (ERG). In order to obtain the same X-ray retinogram amplitude as for a light-induced ERG, the incident energy

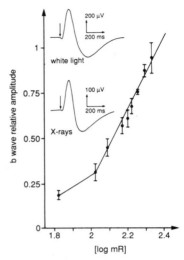

Fig. 10.8 *Relationship between b-wave amplitude of X-ray-induced electroretinograms (see inset) and log stimulus intensity (abscissa, mR). X-ray stimulus duration 80 ms. The inset demonstrates the similarity of the electroretinogram evoked by light flashes (1 ms duration) and X-ray flashes (80 ms, 230 mR). (Modified from Doly* et al., *1980a.)*

on the retina for X-rays had to be about 50 million times that for visible light (Fig. 10.8). It is assumed that X-rays act directly on the rhodopsin molecule, but not primarily as photons at the chromophore *Retinal* but at the protein component *Opsin*. After energy absorption by the protein component, the energy is shifted to the chromophore group, the 11-*cis*-retinal, and leads to a *cis-trans*-stereoisomerization, which induces the physiological chain leading to visual sensation.

Presumably also related to high-energy particle phosphenes are light sensations induced by therapeutic high-energy radiation. We obtained a report from a physicist treated for a pituitary adenoma with 20 MeV high-energy radiation. He perceived transient light sensations in the direction of the radiation source. This observation points to the retinal effects of short-range secondary electrons (about 1 MeV) generated by the calcium atoms of the orbital bone absorbing energy from stray radiation.

Phosphenes and Inhibitory Effects Evoked by Electrical Stimulation of the Afferent Visual System during Neurosurgery

Electrical stimulation of the optic nerve leads to a short coloured flash percept. Similar responses are obtained by

(a)

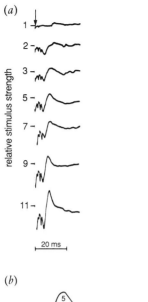

(b)

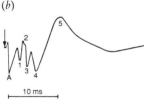

Fig. 10.9 *(a) Electrocorticogram of the primary visual cortex (cat, encéphale isolé) evoked by electrical stimulation of the ipsilateral optic nerve. The amplitude of the evoked potential increases with increase of the stimulus strength (indicated in threshold units). The time constant of the electrical stimulus was about 0.2 ms. (b) Electrocorticogram potential evoked at five times threshold strength by a single electrical stimulus applied to the optic nerve as in (a). Waves 1 and 2 represent presynaptic, waves 3, 4 and 5 postsynaptic potentials. (Modified from Grützner et al., 1958.)*

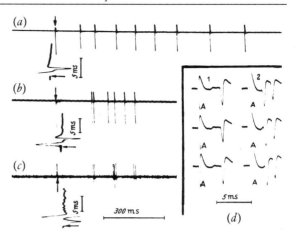

Fig. 10.10 *Responses of four different neurones of the primary visual cortex to electrical stimulation of the contralateral optic nerve (single electrical stimuli of about 0.2 ms time constant). Note the inhibition period after the first neuronal discharge evoked by the electrical stimulus. Stimulus intensities in (a) and (b) were seven times the threshold, in (c) four times the threshold and in (d) 1.5 times the threshold (1) and 3.5 times the threshold (2). 'A' in (d) indicates the stimulus artefact. The stronger stimulus evokes two action potentials. (From Grützner et al., 1958.)*

electrical stimulation of the optic tract or the visual radiation. Tasker *et al.* (1980) studied visual phenomena evoked by electrical stimulation of the human brain stem. They were able to identify two afferent visual pathways sensitive to electrical stimulation which led to phosphenes, i.e. short light sensations perceived only during the electrical stimulus trains. Stimuli applied to the pathway from the optic tract to the lateral geniculate body or to the successive pathway through the visual radiation to area 17 evoked predominantly coloured flash phosphenes in the contralateral visual hemifield. Electrical stimulation of the pathway from the colliculi superiores via the pulvinar to area 18 or 19 evoked contralateral or bilateral achromatic phosphenes, but could alternatively also cause an inhibition of the visual percept in limited parts of the visual field (cf. also Nashold, 1970). Occasionally visual movement

sensations were evoked by electrical stimulation of this pathway. Fedio and van Buren (1975) investigated the effect of electrical stimulation of the pulvinar region in 40 patients. No visual effects were reported when the left pulvinar was stimulated, while electrical stimulation (60 Hz, biphasic squarewave pulses of 2.5 ms duration) of the right pulvinar frequently led to inhibition of the discrimination and recognition of complex visual patterns, like drawings of horses, keys, cups, hands, etc.

Electrophysiological investigations of the responses of area 17 nerve cells in cats provided an explanation for these phosphene sensations: a single shock applied to the optic nerve or the optic tract led to a complex response of the epicortical electroencephalogram, as illustrated in Fig. 10.9 (Chang and Kaada, 1950; Malis and Kruger, 1956). Single cortical nerve cells of area 17 responded with 1 to 3 discharges, a succeeding inhibition period of about 50 to 200 ms duration, followed by a rebound activation when the optic nerve of the dominant eye was stimulated. However, if the activity of a 'monocular' cortical neurone was recorded and the non-dominant optic nerve was stimulated, a primary inhibition period of 80 to 300 ms duration followed by a post-inhibitory rebound was observed (Grützner *et al.*, 1958; Fig. 10.10). Short series of high-frequency optic nerve stimuli led to repetitive discharges of area 17 nerve cells, as illustrated in Fig. 10.11(a) (Grüsser and Grützner, 1958). At the subjective level short trains of electrical stimuli were most effective in leading to phosphenes. Responses of area 17 neurones to trains of electrical stimuli applied to the optic nerve or the optic tract depended on stimulus frequency as indicated in Fig. 10.11(b).

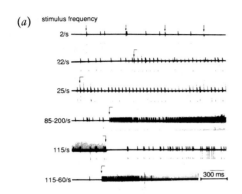

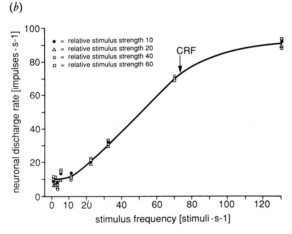

Fig. 10.11 *(a) Action potentials recorded from a single neurone of the primary visual cortex (cat, encéphale isolé preparation). Electrical stimulation was at different stimulus frequencies as indicated. The electrical stimuli applied to the ipsilateral optic nerve were at about five times threshold values for the evoked potential (Fig. 10.9). Stimulus time was constant at about 0.2 ms. Stimulation frequency was as indicated. The beginning and end of a stimulus series is marked by arrows. Note the decrease in response probability with a duration of the stimulus train. (b) Relationship of the neuronal impulse rate (ordinate) of a primary visual cortex nerve cell as a function of optic nerve stimulus frequency (abscissa). CRF is the 'fusion frequency' obtained between 75 and 80 stimuli/s. Above this frequency not every electrical optic nerve stimulus was followed by a neuronal response. Relative stimulus intensities were as indicated. Stimulus strength '1' was about twice threshold for the evoked response in the electrocorticogram (Fig. 10.9). Time constant of the electrical stimulus was about 0.2 ms. (From Grüsser and Grützner, 1958.)*

Light Sensations Evoked by Electrical Stimulation of the Primary Visual Cortex

Direct Cortical Stimulation

After Fritsch and Hitzig (1870) had successfully introduced electrical stimulation of cortical regions to explore the functions of different cortical areas in animals, and Munk (1880) had reported eye movements evoked by electrical stimulation of the visual cortex in monkeys, this method was also applied by neurosurgeons to humans. It brought new insight into the function of the human brain and was applied in open brain surgery by the first generation of modern neurosurgeons more frequently than today, since many brain operations at that time were performed under local anaesthesia and the surgeon could ask his patient about stimulus-induced sensations. Löwenstein and Borchardt (1918) stimulated the left occipital lobe of a patient electrically, while repairing a bullet wound and removing bone fragments above the occipital lobe. The patient reported flicker sensations in the right half of his visual field. More systematically, the neurosurgeons Fedor Krause (1924) and Otfried Foerster (1929) applied focal electrical stimulation to cortical areas around the calcarine fissure in conscious patients undergoing neurosurgery (cf. also Krause and Schumm, 1931). The patients reported on small visual phosphenes, the location of which varied with the cortical site stimulated. When the extreme occipital pole was stimulated, a small phosphene appeared motionless directly in front of the patient, i.e. in the foveal part of the visual field. When the electrodes were placed at the medial surface of the occipital lobe near the calcarine fissure, a parafoveal phosphene appeared during stimulation. The patient reported on movement of this phosphene, but his eye movements were not controlled. Involuntary eye movements could have been the cause of the perceived movement of the phosphene. Later Foerster (1936) described similar observations in other patients.

Penfield and Rasmussen (1952) stimulated predominantly the outer surface of the occipital cortex and also placed electrodes above area 17 (area V1) and extracalcarine regions anterior to area V1 (area 18 and 19 of Brodmann). Stimulation of area 17 led to the perception of circumscribed small phosphenes, many of them coloured. Stimulating the extracalcarine visual cortex also evoked phosphenes located in the contralateral visual field, many of them colourless. Movement of the phosphenes was more frequently reported when area 18 was stimulated; 'a star moving' and 'dancing lights' were characteristic notations in some of the protocols. However, it was again not ascertained whether these movements were correlated with eye movements. When the cortex at the occipital end of the calcarine fissure was stimulated, no distinct lateralization was reported by the patients, a finding which corresponds well with the projection of foveal vision into that part of the cortex. Penfield and Rasmussen came to the following conclusion:

> *Excision of the primary visual cortex produces complete homonymous hemianopic blindness. Excision limited to the secondary visual cortex does not produce such a blindness. And yet electrical or epileptic stimulation in the primary and the secondary fields produces visual phenomena, which are identical in character. It might therefore be suggested that the essential function of the secondary visual cortex cannot be demonstrated by stimulation.... It seems probable that the secondary visual cortex is a field for visual elaboration, elaboration of visual impulses coming in from both fields of vision.*
> (Penfield and Rasmussen, 1957, p. 146, 147)

Krause and Schumm (1931) described a patient who was hemianopic for more than eight years owing to a bullet wound of the left visual radiation. Nevertheless phosphenes were elicitable in the hemianopic field by electrical stimulation of the visual cortex. This finding demonstrated that deafferentation of the visual cortex did not lead to functional inexcitability. Also, Button and Putnam (1962) pointed out that electrical stimulation of the visual cortex in blind patients led to phosphene perception. So arose the idea of constructing a prosthesis for the blind (cf. Brindley, 1970; Sterling, 1971). Marg and Dierssen (1965) reported on visual percepts from stimulation of the occipital brain in conscious patients by means of microelectrodes inserted during neurosurgery. From their work it became feasible to think about chronic implants as a visual prosthesis. Owing to glial cell responses to chronically implanted fine wires in the cortical grey matter, only epicortical electrode implants for the purpose of visual prosthesis are recommendable. Recently Bak *et al.* (1990) reported on visual sensations evoked by intracortical microstimulation in patients who were undergoing occipital craniotomies under local anaesthesia for excision of epileptic foci. All stimulation locations were within 2 cm of the occipital pole, i.e. within the project region of the parafoveal visual field. Two- or three-electrode arrays were used with tip spacing between 250 and 1000 μm. The small phosphenes evoked by short electrical pulse trains (100 pulses s^{-1}) were precisely mapped into the contralateral visual field. In contrast to surface stimulation, no phosphene flicker was reported. Thresholds were minimal at a depth corresponding to the lower cortical layers 4 to 6. Most phosphenes were circular and about 1–2 degrees of visual angle, almost all coloured deep blue or yellow, and occasionally red. Raising stimulus strength increased the phosphene brightness but reduced the size. Simultaneous stimulation of electrodes 0.7–1 mm apart led to fusion of two phosphenes. These data were not

surprising in the light of earlier studies with microstimulation of the visual cortex in awake macaques (Bartlett and Doty, 1980). The animals could be conditioned to respond to the percepts evoked by cortical microstimulation. Minimum thresholds were between 1–5 μA, as compared with 10–20 μA in the experiments of Bak *et al.* in humans. The higher thresholds in man might have been caused by the sedation during surgery.

Brindley and Lewin (1968) applied the first working visual prosthetic implant, to our knowledge, in a 52-year-old woman, who was almost blind from glaucoma and retinal detachment. The implant consisted of 81 regularly arranged platinum electrodes on the pial surface above the occipital pole and the posterior part of the medial surface of the patient's right hemisphere. Electrical stimulation was achieved by radio receivers implanted between the skull and the scalp and connected with the individual stimulation electrodes. In Fig. 10.12 the positions of 39 electrodes through which phosphenes were evoked are shown,

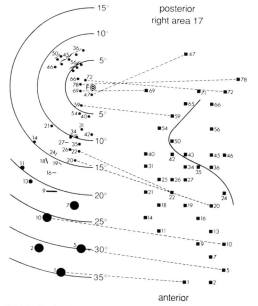

Fig. 10.12 *Right: Position of effective electrodes in the electrode array implanted in the first patient of Brindley and Lewin (1968). Those electrodes by which no phosphene could be evoked are deleted. Left: Phosphene position and approximative size evoked by short electric pulse trains delivered through the electrodes depicted on the right side. Perimetric projections to the left visual hemifield are presented by the position of the dots or bars. To clarify the relationship between phosphenes and stimulating electrode, dashed lines are drawn for some of the corresponding pairs. On the right, the curved line represents the presumed position of the calcarine fissure. The smallest distance between the electrodes was about 3 mm. On the left, the circles represent the distance in degrees from the fovea centre (F). (Redrawn from Brindley and Lewin, 1968.)*

including the presumed location of the calcarine fissure, and the corresponding positions of the phosphenes perceived in the left visual hemifield. From these findings Cowey and Rolls (1974) tried to calculate the retino-cortical magnification factor M, defined as the 'linear extent of visual striate cortex to which each degree of the retina projects' (cf. Talbot and Marshall, 1941). From the interelectrode distance applied in Brindley's experiments and the perceived position of the phosphenes within the left visual hemifield, M was computed by connecting pairs of neighbouring electrodes as illustrated in Fig. 10.13(a). Cowey and Rolls found that M decreases continuously from about 4 mm/degree at 2 degrees eccentricity to 0.5 mm/degree at 25 degrees eccentricity. Since the nearest phosphene to the fovea was observed at about 1.6 degrees eccentricity, the foveal magnification factor could not be directly determined. By inference from extrapolation a value of about 10 mm/degree would result from Cowey and Rolls's measurements (Fig. 10.13(b)). When the value $1/M$ is plotted as a function of eccentricity in the visual field a linear relationship results. Cowey and Rolls therefore concluded that the reciprocal of M is directly proportionate to retinal eccentricity. In addition, a linear relationship between $1/M$ and the minimum visible α valid for photopic vision at different retinal eccentricities, resulted from this study (cf. Wertheim, 1894; Weymouth *et al.*, 1928; Weymouth, 1950).

In a second patient, blind for 30 years, Brindley *et al.* (1972) implanted arrays of electrodes over the left and right calcarine cortex and plotted the phosphene position in a manner similar to that described for their first patient. In their report they emphasized the rather strong irregularities in phosphene location and discussed the discontinuities in the correlation between visual field and surface of area V1 (cf. also Brindley, 1973, 1982; Rushton and Brindley, 1977). One has to keep in mind, however, that such irregularities may not only be caused by the sulci of third order, but also by changes in local electrical impedance due to tissue responses to the metal electrodes. To our knowledge, no systematic study corresponding to that of Cowey and Rolls was performed on the data of this second patient.

The group of Dobelle at the University of Utah and later at Columbia University, New York, continued Brindley's work in a more extended approach to obtain data also useful in the development of a visual prosthesis for the blind. They performed the study in blind and in newly hemianopic volunteers and placed the epipial electrode array over the mesial surface of the occipital lobe above or below the calcarine fissure (Dobelle and Mladejovsky, 1974; Dobelle *et al.*, 1974, 1976, 1979a, b). The brightness of the phosphenes evoked through different electrodes depended on the electric current and between 1.8 and 5 mA was approximately a logarithmic function of stimulus current (Evans *et al.*, 1979). Phosphene brightness also increased with the frequency and number of stimuli in a short pulse train (Henderson *et al.*, 1980). In general, Dobelle *et al.* (1976, 1979) confirmed the findings of Brindley and Lewin: electrical stimulation of one point of cortical surface at just suprathreshold stimulus intensities produced one phosphene ranging in size from a tiny punctuate sensation like 'a star in the sky' seen in the centre of the visual field up to a fuzzy light spot of about 3 degrees diameter in the visual field periphery. Local electrical stimulation substantially above threshold led to a second conjugate phosphene seen at a mirror site above or below the horizontal meridian. Occasionally, multiple phosphenes were perceived. The amount of colour appearing in a phosphene and the occurrence of short flicker sensations varied from stimulation point to stimulation point. With continuous trains of electrical stimuli, phosphene sensations were maintained for no longer than 10 to 15 seconds, indicating a central adaptation phenomenon. As Dobelle and Mladejowsky (1974) reported, 'the position of phosphenes in the visual field corresponded only roughly with expectations based on classical maps ....' (Chapter 4). In general, however, the visual field position of the phosphene and the electrode position in the occipital lobe in the data of Dobelle *et al.* (1979a) agreed with those reported by Brindley and Lewin (1968).

An analysis of the data obtained in the experiments of Dobelle and associates, which were similar to those performed by Cowey and Rolls (1974), was published by Dobelle *et al.* (1979a,b): phosphene eccentricity was reported to be a linear function of the estimated distance

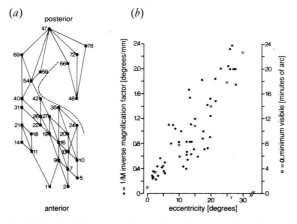

Fig. 10.13   *(a) Examples of the pairs of electrodes from the experiments of Brindley and Lewin (1968) used by Cowey and Rolls for computing the relationship between electrode distance and phosphene distance (Fig. 10.12). (b) From this relationship, the inverse magnification factor 1/M was computed and was plotted as a function of eccentricity in the visual hemifield. (Redrawn from Cowey and Rolls, 1974.)*

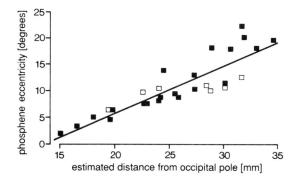

Fig. 10.14 *According to Dobelle* et al. *(1979a), the electrode distance from the tip of the occipital lobe of a human subject correlates well with the phosphene eccentricity, i.e. the distance of the phosphene from the centre of fovea (ordinate). This is a finding which is hard to interpret in the light of other experimental data.*

from the occipital pole (Fig. 10.14), a statement valid at least for the region between the fovea and 15 degrees eccentricity. As in the data of Cowey and Rolls, the retino-cortical magnification factor *M* exhibited a rather large scatter and decreased with retinal eccentricity, from a maximum of about 6.3 at 4 degrees eccentricity to values considerably below 0.5 at eccentricities above 12 degrees. The statement on a linear relationship between the distance of the stimulus electrodes from the occipital pole and retinal or visual field eccentricity respectively, which was deduced from the results of these stimulation experiments, is at variance with the corresponding findings based on single unit recordings and the localization of receptive field centres in the visual field of monkeys as discussed in Chapter 4. It is difficult, however, to transpose the monkey data directly to area V1 of man. Microelectrode recordings from the visual cortex of man have as yet not provided sufficient data regarding electrode position and the corresponding visual field location (Marg *et al.*, 1968, 1970; Marg and Adams, 1970; Marg, 1973).

Electrical or Magnetic Stimulation Through the Skull

Strong electrical stimuli (0.1 F) charged to about 2000 V and applied to the skin over the occipital region led in human volunteers to electrical stimulation of the visual cortex and corresponding phosphenes about 5 degrees wide near the fixation point. Phosphene position changed with electrode position. A few sharp, bright, sinewave lines were observed within the phosphene. Single electrical shocks evoked phosphenes only in some of the subjects;

in others a short inhibition of the visual percept was reported (Merton and Morton, 1980a, b). With such strong stimuli, in addition to the activation of pain receptors, stimulation of the retina has to be excluded. Indeed, pressure blinding of both retinae was reported not to abolish the phosphene.

Strong focal percutaneous magnetic field stimuli were also applied to the occipital region of the skull (Barker *et al.*, 1985; Barker *et al.*, 1988). When adequate coil combinations for magnetic stimulation were applied, the induced stimulation of the cortical surface is believed to have been restricted to a few square centimetres. Stimulation of the visual cortex at the occipital pole of the skull led to phosphene perception in some of the subjects, but in others none at all. This was presumably due to the fact that only *single* strong magnetic field stimuli were applied so far and no repetitive stimulation was possible. When magnetic coil stimulation is combined with light stimulation, the former can interrupt light sensation (Day *et al.*, 1987). Amassian *et al.* (1989) reported that such a suppression occurs when the interval between the visual stimulus and the succeeding magnet coil stimulus is between 60 and 120 ms. Letters were used as visual stimuli. They were perceived as either blurred or not at all when adequate intervals for the two different stimuli were chosen. This observation indicates the dominance of inhibitory effects evoked by strong focal magnetic field stimuli in the human visual cortex.

Responses of Single Visual Cortex Neurones to Epicortical Electrical Stimulation

Baumgartner and Creutzfeldt (1955), Baumgartner and Jung (1955) and Pollen (1977) reported on the responses of single nerve cells of cat area 17 to epicortical electrical stimulation. A single electrical shock evoked a short activation of the nerve cells consisting of 1 to 3 action potentials, followed by a short inhibitory period of 50 to 100 ms and an 'after-discharge' during which neuronal activity level was increased above spontaneous activity. When repetitive cortical stimulation was applied, depending on the duration and frequency of the stimulus train, a high-frequency burst of cortical nerve cell activity was evoked. The activity of single nerve cells depended on stimulus strength, frequency and numbers of stimuli in a stimulus train. Prolonged electrical stimulation led to high frequency 'epileptic' afterdischarges or even to focal epileptic high-frequency neuronal activity. Below threshold for focal seizure activity, these neurophysiological data correspond well, we think, to the phosphenes observed by human subjects mentioned above. The long inhibition period following the short initial excitation after an electrical pulse, however, also indicates that electrical stimulation of the visual cortex leads not only to excitation but also to an activation of longer inhibitory effects.

Migraine Phosphenes

Phenomenology of Migraine Phosphenes

So many people are afflicted with migraine headaches and phosphenes prior to attacks that the phenomena are subjects for discussion even in magazines for the general public (Zimmer, 1989). Competent reviews on migraine are available (e.g. Ad hoc committee, 1962; Friedman, 1968; Pearce, 1975; Dalessio, 1980; Raskin, 1980, 1988; Sacks, 1985; Olesen, 1986; Jerusalem, 1988). The scintillating migraine phosphenes and accompanying scotoma as symptoms of 'classical' migraine attacks were well known to Greek physicians (Chapter 2) and have a long history in clinical neurology (Friedman, 1972; Pearce, 1986). According to Bäumler (1925), the English physician J. Fothergill (1778) was the first to describe the typical 'fortification' patterns of the scintillating migraine phosphenes, also mentioned by Parry (1825). The first pictures of the typical 'fortification' patterns of migraine phosphenes were published in 1870 by Airy (Fig. 10.15). The migraine phosphenes, evidently encountered fairly frequently by neurologists, have provided manifold interesting investigations in modern clinical and pathophysiological research. Figure 10.16 illustrates the shape

and temporal course of migraine phosphenes, also described by Jolly (1902), Lashley (1941), Hare (1966), Pöppel (1973), Bücking and Baumgartner (1974), Baumgartner (1977, 1982) and Jung (1979). From such protocols, one can deduce the following main properties of migraine phosphenes, appearing in darkness or on a homogeneous grey background illuminated at a low light intensity:

1. Most of the migraine phosphenes begin at or near the fovea centralis and extend slowly into the visual field periphery of one hemifield. Less than 5 per cent begin in the outer parafoveal region of the visual field and move towards the fovea.

2. Migraine phosphenes can travel into the upper or lower quadrant only or into the whole hemifield. Migraine attacks in the same patient on different days can affect different hemifields and/or quadrants.

3. Fairly constant typical 'fortification patterns' are reported which flicker at a rate corresponding to about 10 Hz as compared with the flicker sensation evoked by an intermittent light stimulus placed in the intact part of the visual field. Richards (1971) judged the flicker frequency of migraine phosphenes to be 5 Hz, but did not report how he had reached this estimation. Pöppel (1973) gauged a scintillation frequency 'above 5 Hz'. Our own observations in comparing migraine scintillations with flicker stimuli on an oscilloscope screen led to an estimate of 10–12 Hz. The low values reported by Richards are most likely due to the fact that a regular frequency of flicker stimuli is underestimated above 3 Hz (Forsyth and Cha-

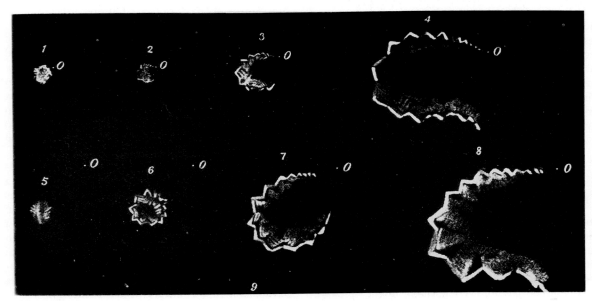

Fig. 10.15 *First illustration of the fortification scintillations seen in migraine phosphenes. The small dot marked 0 is the fixation target, i.e. the centre of the fovea. (From Airy, 1870.)*

(*a*)

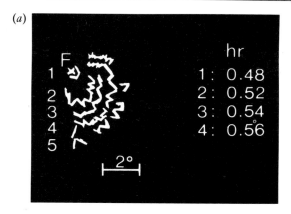

(*b*)

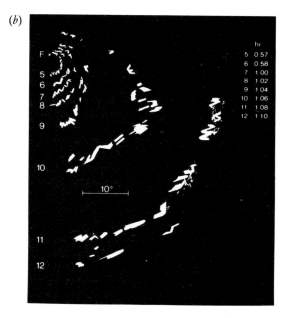

Fig. 10.16 *Drawing of the development of a migraine phosphene observed by one of the authors (O.-J. G.) in 1984. From protocols of this type, the data illustrated in Fig. 10.18 were derived. Note the two different size scales in (a) and (b).*

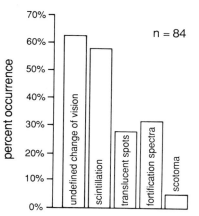

Fig. 10.17 *Frequency of different visual disturbances observed by 84 patients suffering from migraine with visual sensations (modified from Baumgartner, 1977).*

panis, 1958; van de Grind *et al.*, 1973).

4. Other visual sensations during migraine attacks are 'defective vision' at the beginning of the aura, which might be associated with foveal blurring, monocular double or triple vision for the inner fovea and cracking of contour vision (Fig. 10.17; Baumgartner, 1977).

5. The speed at which the migraine phosphenes slowly move across the visual field increases from fovea to periphery when measured in degrees s^{-1} (Fig. 10.18(a) and (b)). Simultaneously, the size β of the flickering 'particles' forming the fortification patterns increases. A linear increase in the size of the fortification lines ('bars') with

retinal eccentricity was found in two independent studies (Fig. 10.19(a),(b)).

6. A quartermoon-shaped scotoma moves with the flickering fortification pattern at its 'rear' end. It becomes visible when one tests visual perception by means of a small light spot or the tip of a pencil (Fig. 10.20(a), (b)).

7. Lashley (1941) reported a structural difference between the fortification patterns seen in the upper and lower quadrants, with finer line structures in the upper quadrant of the visual field: 'The coarser and more complicated figures are generally in the lower part of the field' (Fig. 10.20(b), Lashley, 1941, p. 335). In our experience this difference disappears with normalization of the distance of the fortification patterns from the fovea centre.

8. Some of the fortification patterns are seen in colours; often achromatic stripes alternate with chromatic ones. Small sectors are then seen in colours which appear very 'pure'; red and blue are more frequently reported than the other colours of the spectrum.

9. When the migraine phosphene is seen on a background of dynamic visual noise (e.g. a TV screen), characteristic changes in the fortification patterns appear: parts of the bar-shaped substructures are seen as flickering, bright, white or very brilliant black bars; others appear as striated chromatic structures with narrow coloured and non-coloured stripes. With such a dynamic noise background, chromaticity is increased but non-chromatic fortifications are still dominant (Fig. 10.21). On the rear side of the fortification pattern the absolute scotoma becomes visible on the dynamic background noise, corresponding to the technique of noise-field campimetry (Chapter 9), and is seen as a very smooth, homogeneous, medium-grey quartermoon. This grey area corresponds to the negative scotoma found with perimetry during a migraine attack (cf. Lashley, 1941).

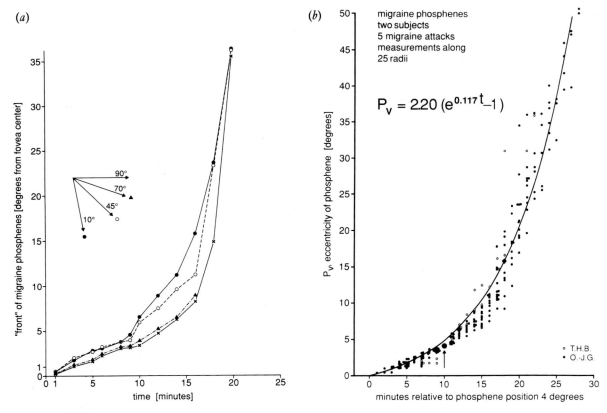

Fig. 10.18 *(a) Measurements from migraine phosphenes observed in 1984 along different radii as indicated. (b) Relationship between duration of the migraine phosphene attack (abscissa) and the position of the scintillating fortification pattern (ordinate). Protocols were evaluated from the moment the migraine phosphene reached 4 degrees eccentricity. Protocols obtained during 6 years by one of the authors (O.-J. G.) with a time interval of at least 10 months. The circles are measurements from a protocol of a migraine phosphene kindly provided in 1990 by Prof. T. H. Bullock of San Diego.*

10. By active saccades or smooth pursuit eye movements, the migraine phosphene is moved across the field of gaze, i.e. the fortification pattern remains stable within the field of vision. Jung (1979) also observed translocations of the phosphenes during horizontal vestibular stimulation (acceleration or deceleration when sitting in a rotating chair) and during perrotatory or postrotatory nystagmus. According to Jung, this type of stimulation also causes deformation of the whole fortification pattern and shifts the phosphene in the direction of the vestibular nystagmus slow phase. In contrast to voluntary eye movements, however, the vestibular translocation of the phosphenes during postrotatory nystagmus, according to Jung's own observation, did not transgress the midline. The migraine phosphene also follows tilting of the head or the whole body and is shifted back and forth when the subject sits or lies on a horizontal swing (authors' own observations).

11. When a migraine phosphene is seen in the perifoveal region and a lasting afterimage is imprinted simultan-

eously onto the fovea, during saccadic or pursuit eye movements the perceived shift in both is always in parallel and no relative movement between the two is seen (Grüsser *et al.*, 1987).

12. Rapid, acoustically triggered, horizontal, back-and-forth saccades lead to a reduction in the apparent horizontal shift of a parafoveal migraine phosphene, similar to that observed in foveal afterimages. At a saccade rate of above 1.5 saccades per second doubling of the foveal or near parafoveal migraine phosphene was observed. With increasing saccade frequency, the distance between the two parafoveal migraine phosphenes decreased and at a saccade rate above 3.5 saccades s^{-1}, despite undiminished saccade amplitudes of 30–40 degrees, the migraine phosphene became stationary. Thus the saccade-induced translocation and disappearance with back-and-forth saccades at a high rate was the same for cortical migraine phosphenes as for an enduring retinal afterimage (Grüsser *et al.*, 1987).

13. As in the case of retinal afterimages, the apparent

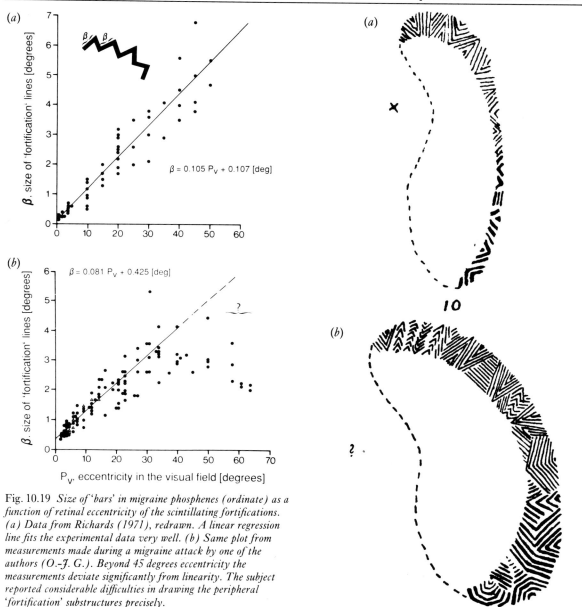

Fig. 10.19 *Size of 'bars' in migraine phosphenes (ordinate) as a function of retinal eccentricity of the scintillating fortifications. (a) Data from Richards (1971), redrawn. A linear regression line fits the experimental data very well. (b) Same plot from measurements made during a migraine attack by one of the authors (O.-J. G.). Beyond 45 degrees eccentricity the measurements deviate significantly from linearity. The subject reported considerable difficulties in drawing the peripheral 'fortification' substructures precisely.*

Fig. 10.20 *Two drawings from Lashley (1941) of his migraine phosphenes. In (a) the fixation target is indicated by a cross. In (b) no fixation target is given. (b) was illustrated by Lashley to indicate the grosser structure of the fortification patterns in the lower half of the visual field. We assume that as in (a) the fixation target was not symmetrically positioned relative to this figure. A question mark is placed at the presumed site of the fixation target. (From Lashley, 1941.)*

size of the migraine phosphene changes with the fixation distance (Richards, 1971). This phenomenon is explained in part by the findings of Marg and Adams (1970) that 'zoom' effects, modifying the receptive field size of visual cortex neurones, are indeed induced by changes in the fixation distance.

14. Migraine phosphenes disappear when the cortical process responsible has reached the area 17/18 border. Otherwise, 'jumps' and backward movements towards the centre of the visual field would be expected. Such

phenomena have not, to our knowledge, been reported in the literature. The migraine process can extend, however, beyond the visual cortex: paraesthesia, sometimes spread-

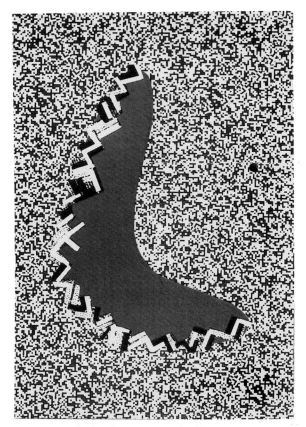

Fig. 10.21 *Drawing of a migraine phosphene observed by one of the authors (O.-J. G.) on the background of a blank TV screen (dynamic random noise). Some of the bars (stippled) were coloured in a pure chroma. The scintillation frequency of the migraine phosphenes did not change when seen on the dynamic random noise background, in contrast to a homogeneous white or a dark background. One difference, however, was the appearance of 'brilliant' deep black fortification structures, which were not seen on a light/dark background. Simultaneously, the negative scotoma (not seen on a grey or black background) became visible and had the appearance of an absolutely homogeneous neutral grey (Grüsser, unpublished, 1987).*

ing across half of the body surface like the fortification patterns spread across the visual field, motor dysfunction and even aphasic symptoms might appear (Baumgartner, 1977; Jensen *et al.*, 1986). This extension beyond the primary visual cortex is presumably due to vascular events and cannot be explained by a further extension of spreading depression.

15. With active, horizontal, sinewave head movements in darkness and the eyes closed, a parafoveal migraine phosphene moves in the opposite direction. This is especially observable at about 0.3 Hz pendular horizontal head movements and corresponds to the eye movements caused by the vestibulo–ocular reflex. When goal–directed fast gaze 'saccades', i.e. combined active eye and head movements, are performed, the fortification pattern moves in the direction of the voluntary gaze movements, similar to that of a foveal afterimage (protocol of O.-J. G., 1981).

16. When the migraine phosphene is combined with a binocular deformation phosphene by means of simultaneous indentation of the left and right eyeballs (Fig. 10.1(e)), the flickering migraine fortification pattern suppresses the binocular deformation phosphene locally and is not inhibited by it in its lateral spread. The oscillation frequency of the patterned binocular phosphenes and the migraine phosphenes seems to be at about the same frequency. On the rear side of the fortification pattern, the binocular pattern deformation phosphene is not visible within a quartermoon-shaped region corresponding to the scotoma. This region appears dark grey (observations in total darkness, protocol O.-J. G., 1983).

17. During migraine attacks patients have reported other light sensations in addition to the typical fortification patterns: diffuse coloured flashes, diffuse dazzling white light with reduced visual acuity, bright stars and light spots distributed across the visual field. Occasionally distortion of the visual world has been reported, such as polyopia (Bender, 1945), macropsias or micropsias, and heautoscopy with or without vestibular sensations could also appear (Klee, 1975; Chapter 16). Atkinson and Appenzeller (1978) described the migraine attacks of an artist, who saw a fairly distinct pseudohallucination, i.e. the figure of a woman in great detail. Even déja vu, the experience that the present scene, complete in every particular, has already taken place some time ago, has been correlated with an acute migraine attack. These complex visual sensations indicate the involvement of temporal lobe dysfunctions in these certainly rare cases of migraine.

18. As demonstrated for the blind spot in Fig. 9.3, completion of figures across migraine scotoma has also been observed. Lashley (1941) gave a vivid report of this fact:

> Talking with a friend, I glanced just to the right of his face, whereon his head disappeared. His shoulders and necktie were still visible, but the vertical stripes in the wallpaper behind him seemed to extend right down to the necktie. Quick mapping revealed an area of total blindness covering about 30 degrees, just off the macula .... (pp. 338–339).

Pathophysiology of Migraine Phosphenes

The phenomena described above indicate that the fortification scintillations characteristic of migraine phosphenes are caused by a hyperexcitability of cortical neurones, while the transient scotoma at the rear of fortification pattern corresponds to a cortical region of neuronal inactivation. The fortification pattern and its scintillation are explained by a local hyperactivation of neurones belonging to certain cortical orientation columns and an inhibitory interaction between columns of the same optimum orientation. The temporal oscillation is most likely induced by the fact that only the layers I–IV are in a state of hyperexcitability and the interneurones connecting layers V and VI to the upper layers provide an inhibitory feedback signal.

Presumably local ischaemia and some functional impairment of the sodium-potassium exchange pump of glial cell membranes lead to a local increase in the extracellular potassium and a decrease in the calcium concentration, which in turn – according to the Nernst or Goldman equation – causes a depolarization of cortical nerve cells, triggering a high-frequency action potential sequence. This high-frequency activation leads to a further loss of intracellular potassium. As in the case of focal epileptic activity (Frederking *et al.*, 1968), a further increase in extracellular potassium concentration finally leads to a depolarization inactivation of cortical nerve cells. When the membrane potential is depolarized more than 40 mV above the resting value, the fast sodium channels necessary for discharging action potentials at the axon hillocks or the nerve cell membrane are inactivated. Then the nerve cell discharge ceases. The locally increased extracellular potassium is not transported quickly enough, however, into the glial cells and from there to the vascular system, but diffuses into the surroundings, triggering there a new increase in nerve cell activity. This mechanism corresponds to that described by Leao (1944, 1947) as *spreading depression* (Ochs, 1962). Grafstein (1956a, b) and Morlock *et al.* (1964) observed an electrical hyperactivity zone of single neurones along a front of spreading cortical depression, whereby hyperactivity was followed by a period of neuronal inactivation. As signs of repeated local ischaemia, multiple small foci were found by means of magnetic resonance imaging in the brains of patients suffering at an early age (9 to 39 years) from migraine attacks (Kuhn and Shakar, 1990).

The similarity between the time course of spreading depression and the movement of the migraine phosphene across the visual field is rather striking (Milner, 1958). Lashley (1941) estimated that the speed of the pathophysiological process leading to a fortification scintillation in migraine spreads at about 3 mm per minute across the primary visual cortex, a value similar to that found in spreading depression, while Richards (1971) preferred a value of about 3.3 mm per minute. According to the observations reported in Figs. 10.16 and 10.18 and Filimonoff's (1932) data on the overall extent of the area striata in the human brain (average anterior-posterior length 67 mm), the estimated speed of cortical pathophysiological mechanisms leading to the fortification phosphenes is 2.4 to 2.6 mm per minute.

More recent observations support the hypothesis that migraine phosphenes and spreading depression are related to each other. Spreading depression evokes a characteristic negative potential at the cortical surface, which is accompanied by a large increase in extracellular potassium and a decrease in calcium concentration (e.g. Kraig and Nicholson, 1978; Nicholson *et al.*, 1981). The potassium profiles measured during spreading depression only changed, however, in the superficial cell layers of the grey matter. Correspondingly, the slow negative potential recorded from the cortical surface during spreading depression decreased on penetration of the electrode. It reversed at about 250 μm from the cortical surface (measurements in the cerebellum, Nicholson *et al.*, 1981). From these findings one can deduce that in migraine as well, hyperexcitability is restricted to the upper layers of the cortical grey matter of area 17. Assuming this to be the case, one might also find the reason why the migraine phosphenes disappear, as a rule, when the pathological process reaches the area 17/18 border. At this border, the thick stripe of Gennari, separating the upper and lower cortical cell layers of area 17, decreases considerably in thickness. Presumably lateral diffusion of the increased extracellular potassium is facilitated by the horizontal structures of the stripe of Gennari and is thus stopped when it disappears at the area 17–18 border.

The reason why spreading depression starts preferably within the foveal or parafoveal projection region of area 17 is still debatable. The same is true for the relation of migraine and focal epileptiform discharges (cf. Basser, 1969). Changes in local blood supply and an increase in serotonin release are discussed as local factors starting the migraine phosphene. Electroencephalographic studies in migraine subjects revealed left–right differences in the occipital alpha- and theta-activity of the EEG during the migraine attack with a reduction in both frequency bands on the side contralateral to the visual or somaesthetic aura (Schoenen *et al.*, 1987). In some of the patients at least, visual pattern-reversal evoked potentials had an increased latency of the P100-wave when the recordings were performed during the migraine intervals (Raudino, 1988; Mariani *et al.*, 1990). Furthermore, an increased interhemispheric difference in pattern-reversal evoked potentials was noted (Nyrke *et al.*, 1990). These electrophysiological findings point to some elementary functional deviations of visual cortex metabolism in patients suffering from migraine.

Tepley *et al.* (1989) were able to study four patients during 'spontaneous' migraine attacks, three of them triggered by perfume inhalation, cheese consumption or strenuous exercise. In two patients, the magnetencephalogram was measured during typical fortification patterns (gradiometer technique). The signals recorded consisted of two components, 'short' biphasic waves of up to 10 seconds duration with amplitudes between 0.8 and 13 pT and a profound reduction in signal level lasting up to 10 minutes, which was explained by the authors as a sign of suppression of spontaneous neuronal activity during the spreading depression induced by the migraine. These findings indeed support the pathophysiological mechanisms discussed above.

Migraine Phosphenes and the Geometrical Organization of the Area Striata

Careful protocols, obtained by drawing the fortification patterns with a constant distance between eye and projection plane, led to findings like those presented in Fig. 10.16. One of the authors (O.-J. G.) used his protocols of five migraine attacks collected over a 7-year period to calculate the angular position of the fortification scintillations along different radii (mainly in the left or right lower quadrant at 10, 45, 70, 90 and 110 degrees to the left or right from the vertical meridian) and to plot the angular position of the fortification phosphenes as a function of onset time of the migraine aura. Some of the data obtained are shown in Figs. 10.18 and 10.19. It is interesting that despite the very long time span of 7 years, minimal data fluctuation was present and when the spread along the different radii was compared, the average change in position of the migraine scintillations did not vary significantly. It can be described by a simple hyperbolic function, as illustrated in Fig. 10.18. Interestingly, the data of a second observer (kindly provided by Professor T.H. Bullock, San Diego) fit the protocols very well.

Measurement of the size of fortification particles as illustrated in Fig. 10.19 showed that β, measured in degrees, increased linearly with eccentricity P_v in the visual field (Richards, 1971):

$$\beta = a + bP_v \qquad (10.1)$$

The local retino–cortical magnification factor M,

measured in mm deg^{-1} (cf. Rovamo and Virsu, 1979), is defined by

$$M = dP_c/dP_v \qquad (10.2)$$

In the case of a spreading migraine phosphene,

$$M = V_c/V_v \qquad (10.3)$$

where P_c is the distance of a given cortical point from the foveal centre projection in the area striata, V_c the cortical speed of the pathological process (spreading depression), P_v the eccentricity of the corresponding point in the visual field from the centre and V_v the speed of the migraine phosphene in the visual field. Since according to Cowey and Rolls (1974)

$$M^{-1} = a + bP_v \qquad (10.4)$$

one finds from equations (10.2) and (10.4)

$$dP_v/dP_c = a + bP_v = dP_v/V_c \, dt \qquad (10.5)$$

$$dP_v/dt = V_c a + V_c bP_v \qquad (10.6)$$

assuming V_c to be constant. The solution of this first-order linear differential equation is (cf. Sirk, 1956):

$$P_v = k_1(e^{k_2 t} - 1) \qquad (10.7)$$

for $k_1 = aV_c/b$ and $k_2 = bV_c$

As Fig. 10.18(b) indicates, the empirical data fit reasonably well to equation (10.7). The 'diffusion speed' V_c, assumed to be constant, can be estimated, provided the overall extension of the visual cortex is known and the time taken by the migraine phosphene to spread through the visual field considered. Using an estimate of 65 to 70 mm from the most occipital to the most anterior part of area 17 (Filiminoff, 1936), a lateral extension of the visual hemifield of 90 degrees and about 30 minutes maximum travelling time of the migraine phosphene from the foveal centre to the visual field periphery, the estimates for V_c would be about 2.2 to 2.3 mm min^{-1}. For further discussions see Grüsser (1991).

11 Agnosias of Visual Form, Object and Scene Recognition

Historical Introduction

Early Studies of Visual Agnosias

Bodamer (1947), in his brief historical review on research in agnosia, mentioned early anecdotal descriptions of visual agnosia in antiquity. Thucydides, for example, described agnosia developing in patients of a plague ravaging Athens in 430–429 BC, and Hippocrates alluded to agnosic symptoms in his book *On Sacred Disease*. According to Bodamer, the first modern description of a visual agnosia which meets today's clinical standards was made by Quaglino (1867). While there have been other early reports on disturbances of visual gnosis (e.g. the first case reported by Finkelnburg, 1870; Gogol, 1874 cited by Thiele, 1928), they did not trigger much interest in clinical neurology.

Unlike the study of aphasia, interest and research in visual agnosia started in the field of experimental physiology, and began with clinico-pathological observations in brain-lesioned dogs. In 1877 Munk (see Chapter 2) found that dogs behaved rather peculiarly after the ablation of parts of occipital cortical areas. While they behaved apparently normally during locomotion through the environment, avoiding or jumping over obstacles, they behaved in an abnormally indifferent manner in emotional situations, such as in the presence of their master, food or other dogs, or in normally frightening situations, such as in the presence of a whip or fire. These dogs could see but did not recognize objects. Since the ablation of adjacent visual cortical areas led to cortical blindness, Munk felt that the ablations leading to 'agnosic' behaviour caused a loss of previously acquired visual memories, a condition he termed '*Seelenblindheit*' (psychic blindness). '*Seelenblindheit*' has largely been replaced by the term 'visual agnosia' introduced by Freud (1891) and referring to the distinction between perception and recognition, a concept already used by Wernicke (1874).

The isolated loss of mental images, i.e. visual memories, as postulated by Munk (1877) later became the major theme in agnosia research, as exemplified by the cases described by Charcot (1883) and Wilbrand (1887) (discussed in more detail in the chapter on prosopagnosia (Chapter 14). In these years there also appeared the first descriptions of other isolated visual deficiencies, such as 'amnesic colour blindness' (Wilbrand, 1884), 'pure alexia' (Broadbent, 1872; Westphal, 1874; Dejerine, 1892) and the distinction between the 'optic agnosias' and 'optic aphasia' (Freund, 1889).

In their 1917 handbook, Wilbrand and Saenger summarized their view on visual agnosias and reviewed published cases of 'psychic blindness' with respect to the neuroanatomical site of the lesion, the presence or absence of hemianopias and the side of the hemianopias. (Wilbrand and Saenger, 1917, pp. 393–446). They reconfirmed Wilbrand's (1887) concept of a distinction between a visual centre for perception and an isolated field of visual memory, psychic blindness being the result of loss of visual memories. In their description of the clinical picture they emphasized the following groups of symptoms:

1. An unfamiliarity and strangeness which old and well-known visual stimuli evoke in the patient (loss of memory for persons, places, and images of word forms).
2. A loss or diminution of visual imagery and an alteration of mood dependent on such imagery, as well as reduced ability for visual expression (impairment of the ability to draw and to do craftwork, etc.)
3. A disturbance of associations in the usual sequence of visual images – 'inverted thinking'.
4. Impairment of the sense of time.
5. Disorientation as a consequence of the sudden and massive estrangement of visual percepts.
6. Dissociation between psychic blindness and deficits of the primary visual perceptive centres.

These six clinical criteria of visual agnosia are, with the exception of the last, somewhat surprising, because they do not correspond to many of the clinical case descriptions of 'psychic blindness' discussed below. Moreover, they corroborate many of the clinical signs and symptoms we have outlined in the chapters on prosopagnosia and top-ographical agnosia (Chapters 14 and 21), which are usually associated with right-hemispheric posterior lesions, and to which Wilbrand had been more exposed than to purely left-hemispheric posterior lesions. This discrepancy may explain some of the controversies over subsequent years.

In line with a modern view of vision, Wilbrand (1887) and Wilbrand and Saenger (1917) proposed that spatially distinct areas within the occipital lobe are concerned with the perception of light, space and colours. Wilbrand (1887) thought that for these different qualities of vision separate channels exist for the transfer of signals from the retina to the visual centres of the brain. Wilbrand and Saenger (1917) reviewed extensively most of the cases with psychic blindness known at that time, including a number of their own cases. Their special emphasis was on the location of the lesion at autopsy, the presence or absence of visual field defects, and the role of right versus left hom-onymous hemianopias. They found psychic blindness to be associated with bilateral hemianopias in 8 cases (6 with autopsy findings), with right hemianopia in 12 cases (9 with autopsy), with left hemianopia in 16 cases (12 with autopsy) and without any visual field defect in 11 cases (7 with autopsy).

Since virtually all authors at this time agreed that lesions must be in either or both occipital lobes in order to produce visual agnosia (Wilbrand and Saenger, 1917), they were struck by the fact that there were a number of patients who had lesions in the occipital lobes but did not suffer from psychic blindness. They reviewed 7 such cases and referred to Poppelreuter, who had seen only 5 patients with psychic blindness among 67 penetrating wounds of the occipital lobes.

Although Wilbrand and Saenger (1917) reviewed a large number of patients thought to have suffered from visual agnosia with respect to lesion site and associated symptoms, in particular visual field defects their final con-clusions were relatively meagre. Psychic blindness was accepted as a well-characterized symptom complex which may be transient or persistent and occurs only after organic lesion within the occipital lobes. Moreover, they stated that visual agnosia is not dependent upon bilateral lesions but can occur subsequent to unilateral lesions of either occipital lobe. They rejected the idea that psychic blindness is primarily a symptom of left posterior lesions, but emphasized that it may well occur subsequent to lesions of the right posterior lobe. However, they were not able to localize the lesions responsible for psychic blindness more precisely within the occipital lobes on the basis of their extensive pathological material.

Finally, they underlined the fact that the many reports of persistent psychic blindness appear to contradict von Monakow's (1905) statement that agnosia is a conse-quence of 'diaschisis', i.e. far-reaching but transient effects of brain lesions.

Among those interested in visual agnosia was Pick (1908), who described a 75-year-old patient who, subse-quent to atrophy of the occipital lobe, was no longer cap-able of recognizing large objects, though his visual acuity and colour recognition were normal. Pick thought that the main defect in his patient was an impaired faculty to fuse single impressions into a whole picture. This is probably one of the first descriptions of what nowadays is called 'simultanagnosia', and moreover is an early description of focal cortical atrophy leading to specific agnosic deficits similar to those recently published in reviews on the neuropsychology of focal cortical degenerations (e.g. Benson *et al.*, 1988; De Renzi, 1986; Cogan, 1985).

Liepmann (1908) has preferred a compromise interpre-tation of agnosias as diseases of single modalities. He dis-tinguished between *dissolutional* and *disjunctive* or *ideational* agnosia. In the development of the dissolutional agnosias he discriminated three steps:

> *1. a disturbance of the synthesis or 'fusion' of signals of a single modality;*
> *2. a disturbance of the memory functions related to a single sensory modality; and*
> *3. a disturbance of the association of object-related 'images' of one sensory modality to the 'images' of other sen-sory modalities.*

The first step of this dissolutional agnosia is of particular interest in the light of modern neuroanatomical and neuropsychological findings (see Chapter 4). It points to failure in recognition at the level of the signal integration ('fusion') of correctly perceived qualities, i.e. in the visual domain, colour, form, movement, and depth.

Lissauer's Patient

The most important step towards the present view of visual agnosias came from a case report by Lissauer, pub-lished with theoretical considerations in 1890.

Lissauer reported on a patient who suffered from what he called associative visual agnosia. The patient, attending Wernicke's outpatient clinic in Breslau, was an 80-year-old merchant. He had an uneventful medical history for his age, but reported on repeated attacks of vertigo for about 3 years, attacks which occasionally were so severe that he fell. He recovered quickly from these episodes, which were never associated with paralysis, speech or vision disturbances. About a year prior to his admittance to the clinic he began to suffer from memory problems, occasionally forgetting dates and names and sometimes mistaking his daughter for his daughter-in-law. However, it remained unclear whether these findings really ante-dated the event which brought him to the attention of Wernicke and Lissauer, since he was able to manage his business normally, travelled alone and wrote and read letters even without glasses. Three days prior to the event he felt unwell, weak and without appetite and interrupted a business trip. He stayed in bed for 3 days, but when he rose and started to move about, a number of symptoms were noted immediately by others. He bumped into doors and obstacles, could not orient himself outside his own room and had to be accompanied by someone. In the street he frequently stopped and looked around as if everything was completely new to him. Even in his home he could not find the most common things, mistook pictures which had hung on the wall for many years for cupboards, even attempting to search for things in them, and mistook different parts of clothing. When eating, he inverted the knife and fork, handled the spoon the wrong way around and once even put his hand into a hot cup of coffee. The patient could no longer read and gave all his mail to his daughter, complaining about his weak eyesight. During a short acute phase the patient did not recognize his daughter, called her 'Oscar' and told her incoherent stories. After a few days the episodes during which he did not recognize real familiar objects or persons became rare and he recovered his ability to orient himself in his room.

Only after a few weeks and solely because he complained about his worsened eyesight, he consulted the ophthalmologist Förster. The patient was first seen by the neurologist Lissauer about 6 weeks after the initial event. He reported the history of his illness correctly and adequately, but insisted that his only difficulty was his bad vision.

In fact the initial examination revealed that he was unable to recognize common objects visually, although he recognized and described everything correctly by touch or sound. Moreover, it was clear from the way he fixated that he could see and during the course of the examination it was possible to have him draw simple objects which he could not subsequently recognize. Lissauer was convinced that the patient was of normal intelligence.

Detailed examination showed the patient to be fully aware of his illness. Although he appeared to be of normal intelligence, interested in everyday events and as having adequate concern and insight into his personal and business affairs, he showed some memory problems, concerning mostly old and overlearned information, while his recall of recent events appeared intact. In particular there was no aphasic disturbance; his spontaneous speech was normal, as was auditory comprehension. Except for visual symptoms his neurological examination was completely normal.

The visual examination revealed a complete right-sided homonymous hemianopia with macular sparing. His visual acuity was about 0.6, estimated initially by having him count dots of different size and later by reading single letters of different size. The subjective disturbances of vision which the patient complained about were quite variable from day to day and consisted mostly of 'dimness of vision' and rapid visual fatigue when tested over longer periods. Concerning colours, he was at chance when naming coloured wools, but above chance when selecting colours according to a verbally given colour name. When asked to select finer nuances of colours, such as the yellow of a canary or the red of blood, he invariably failed and also described the colours he was looking for wrongly. However, he was correct in matching colours even of the finest hue differences. He was also able to categorize all the different hues of a certain colour, provided the colour name was not asked for.

Appreciation of space was tested by line bisection and by marking the centre of a closed figure, as well as by judging the size and distances of objects where he had to demonstrate the length or width by indicating size or distances manually. All these functions were unimpaired, but if the patient was asked to report verbally about distances or sizes in metres or centimetres he frequently made gross errors. Like his dealing with colours, his appreciation of size and distance was impaired only in relation to verbal descriptions or upon verbal request.

The patient appeared to use stereoscopic and/or parallax cues in his attempts to identify objects and during formal testing could distinguish depth differences of about 3 cm within the grasping range.

His visual memory was classified by Lissauer into newly learned visual information and old memory content. The patient was able to store new visual engrams, since he had learned to find his way in new surroundings and had learned to recognize previously unfamiliar persons. Moreover, whenever he had seen an object repeatedly he always remembered that he had seen it before, independently of whether he could recognize the object or not. For example, he was shown 50 pictures, to 2 of which his attention was specifically drawn. Six days later, when asked to indicate these 2 particular items, he pointed to them without hesitation.

His memory for visual events learned before his illness was poor. He usually failed to describe previously well-known topographies or the clothing, stature and hairstyle or hair-colour of well-known persons. He was, however, able to describe the form and size of fruits and animals but usually failed to draw from memory more than just a rudimentary sketch of objects, persons, fruits or geometrical figures. He could write normally, a fact which Lissauer interpreted as indicating intact older visual memories.

The patient copied simple objects correctly, even though he did not recognize them while drawing them. Copying of real objects with complicated forms and shadows, however, as well as the copying of drawings was poor and took an enormous amount of time; ultimately the patient stated that he did not like his drawings. While drawing from memory he got stuck with parts of the object

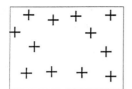 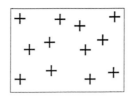

Fig. 11.1 *The pair of stimuli produced from Lissauer's (1890) description. The two textured items are rectangles both filled with an equal number of crosses, but different in that the texture on the right side has an empty space roughly in the middle. The patient was asked to judge whether these two textures are identical or different. While normal subjects detect the difference at a first glance ('pop-out-phenomenon'), Lissauer's patient took considerable time in serially comparing the crosses.*

and was unable to complete the whole. For example, when asked to draw a boot he correctly drew the leg, but completely failed to place the heel. Realizing his failure, he behaved as if the parts already drawn were meaningless to him and would not help him to complete the object.

Unlike his spontaneous drawings, this seemed not to be the case for spontaneous writing. He wrote flawlessly to dictation or spontaneously, and what he wrote seemed not to interfere with what he planned to write. He was, however, completely unable to read what he just had written. His reading was initially extremely poor for both printed and handwritten material and he was not able to discriminate between words or numbers. As in some cases of pure alexia (Chapter 18), he could occasionally read single words such as 'liberty', and was helped in the recognition of single letters by tracing them with his hand. During the time after the stroke when he was unable to understand a single written word, he usually did not acknowledge this inability but rather confabulated any text which passed through his mind. With the passage of time the patient improved his reading capacities; he learned to read single letters and occasionally could read single words correctly although he spelled them wrongly. Apparently it made no difference for him if letters were in lower or upper case, Latin or German print, or if they were letters or numbers.

Lissauer's most important contribution was his analysis of the patient's ability to perceive and recognize forms. He attempted to measure apperception by using the patient's faculty to discriminate differences between similar sensory stimuli. He wrote:

> *The magnitude of alteration which the content of a perception has to undergo to be realized consciously as a difference would constitute the measure for just this capacity.*

In practice, what he measured was the patient's ability to distinguish similar-but-not-identical visual forms. While the patient could easily recognize simple letter- or number-like figures, with details added or omitted, it took great effort and a long time for him to distinguish between

textured-item patterns, such as two rectangles both filled with an equal number of crosses, but different only in the spatial arrangement, leaving an empty space in the middle of one of the two textures (Figure 11.1), a task which is easily performed by normal subjects.

The capability of almost immediate texture discrimination, also called the 'pop-out phenomenon', as opposed to the serial screening strategy this patient was forced to use, has recently been extensively investigated in normal subjects (Julesz, 1975; Treisman,1982), and has also been reintroduced in the study of agnosic patients (Humphreys and Riddoch, 1987; Scheidler *et al.*, in press). It is noteworthy that Lissauer tested his patient in a similar way over a century ago.

To increase the degree of complexity in discriminating similar textures, Lissauer showed his patient two book covers with similarly complex though not identical ornaments and asked him to detect the details of one in the other. The patient succeeded only sometimes at this task and only after lengthy, effortful and tedious search, but usually abandoned his attempts. Since 'normal' hemianopic patients had much less difficulty with this task, Lissauer concluded that hemianopia alone could not account for this specific trouble of his patient.

To uncover the kind of difficulties this patient had in recognizing objects, Lissauer asked him to compare drawings of objects with a wide variety of real objects and to indicate whenever he felt that they corresponded. He was very slow and indecisive in performing this task and frequently envisaged similarities between very different shapes, such as a bottle and a pair of scissors or a brush, but he finally correctly indicated the correspondence between real object and drawing.

Although the patient could recognize neither the drawing nor the real object he needed much more time to reject the wrong combination of drawing and real object, than to accept the correct combination. When asked if he could recognize different objects or pictures he usually behaved in a very uncertain manner, advancing his ideas about the nature of the things as questions rather than as affirmations. Lissauer provided an extensive protocol concerning the performance of this patient in object recognition, documenting not only the severe and persisting impairments, but also the inconsistencies in different sessions. He also mentioned a striking improvement of recognition of objects when their use was demonstrated visually, i.e. when the objects were moved (see also Levin, 1978; Scheidler *et al.*, in press).

Since the patient totally lacked any symbolic understanding, object recognition was impossible, but a drawing and the corresponding real object were apparently more similar than the drawing and other objects, thus facilitating the comparison in a step-by-step analysis. To exemplify the importance which symbolic understanding has or

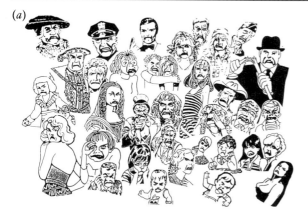

(a)

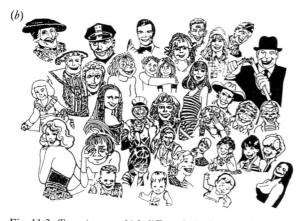

(b)

Fig. 11.2 *Two pictures which differ only in the sad (a) and happy (b) mood of the faces. These two pictures have been generated according to the example Lissauer (1890) provided to exemplify the difficulties a patient with a lack of symbolic understanding would have (see text).*

may have even at the level of the seemingly 'apperceptive' task of discriminating two patterns as being identical or different, Lissauer (Fig. 11.2) provides us with a fictitious example:

> *Imagine two identical pictures with human figures in the most complex situations, the only difference being that the physiognomies of the persons in one picture have happy expressions and those in the other picture are sad. Irrespective of any degree of complexity of the visual pattern no normal subject would have any difficulty in immediately discriminating the two pictures as not being identical. But imagine the enormous task for anyone who would see only meaningless forms and who would have to compare these two pictures in a step-by-step fashion.*

Unlike the patient described by Wilbrand (1887; 1892) Lissauer's patient had no topographical disorientation. Moreover, when based solely on visual information, his

performance in recognizing a wide variety of objects and pictures was strongly impaired and in a curious way variable across testing sessions.

Each time he recognized a number of single items immediately, but usually the same items were not recognized during the next session. Among the few objects which he recognized in almost all circumstances were objects belonging to himself such as his hat, his clothing and, curiously enough, a coloured picture of the Emperor, Wilhelm I. The faculty to recognize one's own belongings has recently been predicted to be selectively impaired in patients suffering from prosopagnosia (Damasio *et al.*, 1982; cf. Chapter 14) and appears to have been spared to some extent in Lissauer's patient. Another dissociated performance of this patient, as distinct from those suffering from prosopagnosia or topographical agnosia, was his relatively spared ability to recognize the identity of famous faces (e.g. the Emperor Wilhelm I and Bismarck), in spite of his inability to recognize single facial features of the same persons, such as their eyes and ears, and his inability to place them correctly. This appears to indicate a double dissociation of function as compared with prosopagnosic patients who, on the contrary, are able to recognize single facial features but cannot recognize the person's identity (cf. Chapter 14). It is tempting of course to attribute these functional double dissociations to distinct anatomical structures, such as the left hemisphere's visual system (damaged in Lissauer's case) as opposed to the right hemisphere's visual system, damaged in cases of prosopagnosia (cf. Chapter 14).

Five years after Lissauer's (1890) seminal publication, Hahn (1895) published the anatomo-pathological findings of the same patient. He found a large infarction covering almost the entire territory of the left posterior cerebral artery, including the cuneus, the calcarine fissura and the fusiform and lingual gyri, as well as the lower two-thirds of the splenium of the corpus callosum. The infarction involved not only the cortex but also extended deep into adjacent white matter. In the right hemisphere he found no infarction but, of course, secondary transcallosal degeneration along the forceps. The infarction in the left hemisphere thus covered completely the primary and associative visual cortex and interrupted the splenial connections of the right occipital cortex with the sensory speech areas.

It was not so much the symptoms and their interpretation by Lissauer as the theoretical distinction between *associative* and *apperceptive* agnosias which has provoked discussions and controversy up until today.

Lissauer (1890, 1898) summarized his concept as follows:

> *I will divide the process of recognition into two stages and will attempt, as far as possible, to differentiate these two stages from each other. They are:*

1. The stage of conscious awareness of a sensory impression. This I shall call apperception.

2. The stage of associating other notions with a content of a perception. This I shall call the stage of association.

Lissauer himself considered his patient to have suffered from a not absolutely pure but almost pure form of associative visual agnosia. While the latter has never posed a real problem, the concept of apperceptive agnosia has been interpreted in somewhat different ways and has even led Lissauer to express some caution:

There remains the question whether a selective impairment of the perceptive process can also result in the clinical picture of visual agnosia.

The controversy as to whether apperceptive agnosia exists as a clinical entity has continued for almost a century and seems to have originated in part in differences in the interpretation of Wundt's concept of apperception itself and also in differences in the tolerance of the concomitant presence of relative impairment of some elementary visual functions such as acuity, brightness contrast, colour, movement, depth or size, etc.

Von Stauffenberg (1914) admitted that a severe disturbance of form synthesis in isolation could theoretically lead to an apperceptive agnosia, but stated that no adequately documented case had yet been found. As a disciple of Von Monakow (1905) he did not accept agnosia as a clinical entity and dismissed it as an effect of diaschisis within the visual system. Poppelreuter (1914–1917) was one of the leading neurologists who analysed patients with traumatic brain lesions from the First World War. In his extremely careful investigations of the visual system he found only a few patients with occipital injury who failed to recognize objects, mostly during the acute or subacute stages or shortly prior to and after surgery. He believed that in no instance had he found a case meeting the criteria for either pure apperceptive or pure associative visual agnosia and thought that the acts of perception and recognition were interwoven with each other in a complex way. Brain damage would therefore lead to decomposition of these faculties into multiple individual defects.

The Patient Schn. of Goldstein and Gelb

During the second decade of this century, when the concept of visual agnosia as a true clinical entity was thoroughly questioned, the concept of apperceptive agnosia might have died but for the publication of a seminal and extensive, though extremely controversial, case report by Goldstein and Gelb in 1918 (for an abbreviated English translation see Ellis, 1938).

The patient Schn., a 24-year-old man with an average education and an unremarkable medical history, sustained a severe head injury due to shrapnel from a mine entering the occiput, which left him unconscious for 4 days. Despite purulence, the wounds closed within 6 weeks. One year after the injury the sequelae were reported to be primarily visual: he could not identify simple drawings and could read words only by tracing each letter. Attempts to visualize were distressing, causing fatigue, vertigo and headache. An 'acquired red-green colour blindness', mainly for subtle hue discrimination, was demonstrated and the patient himself stated that for many months after the injury he had not recognized any colour at all. He underwent extensive experimental investigation (for a recent summary see Landis *et al.*, 1982).

Mr Schn.'s visual fields were restricted bilaterally, leaving a roughly circular intact central field somewhat over 40 degrees of visual angle in diameter (Fig. 11.3), with sufficient visual acuity (L, 5/10; R, 5/15). Depth perception was intact, as weres colour naming, colour discrimination, colour matching and the naming of the colours of objects. Perception of movements was reported to be impaired. He failed to see movement in tests using the phi phenomenon and he described moving things in everyday experience as a series of different positions in space, very much in the same words as patient L. M. described by Zihl *et al.* (1983; also discussed in Chapter 19). Despite relatively preserved elementary visual functions Schn. was found to have severe visual recognition problems. Although he could write and draw spontaneously, he completely failed to read, to copy or to draw real objects. He had, however, developed some compensatory strategies using head and hand movement to decipher script in a letter-by-letter way or to discriminate between simple drawings, such as a circle and a triangle. He failed totally to recognize any letter or word when they were obscured by cross-hatches (Figure 11.4) or when tachistoscopic presentation at short exposure duration was used. His method of using motor feedback for visual recognition led him frequently to mistake background features as the meaningful figure. Perspective appeared meaningless to him and invariably a circle tilted away was described as an ellipse. Surprisingly he was not 'fooled' by illusory figures such as the Mueller–Lyer illusion and others. He also complained of having lost 'mental images'; he could not evoke the faces of close friends or relatives, or the mental picture of a well-known room, even though he could recite its contents.

Goldstein and Gelb (1918) concluded that Schn.'s deficits represented not only a visual agnosia of the apperceptive type but also a striking example of defective Gestalt vision in that he failed to 'see' objects at all. They believed that he 'saw' only coloured patches, recognizing their approximate size and location in space but being unable to integrate them into unitary 'whole' objects. Gelb and Goldstein concluded that Schn. automatically identified objects, letters, etc., through a system of kinaesthetic

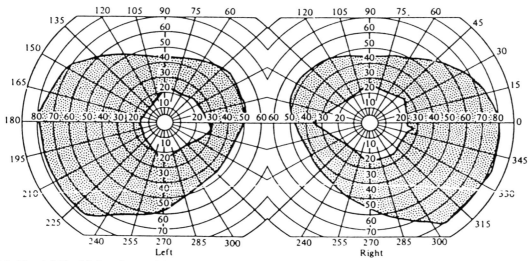

Fig. 11.3 *Visual fields of Schn., showing bilateral restriction (redrawn from Goldstein and Gelb, 1918).*

feedback that he was unaware of, but which consistently improved.

This famous case remained of importance for agnosia research for several reasons:

1. It was probably the first thorough clinico-experimental single case study in which clinical testing was guided by ideas derived from psychological experiments and a trenchant analysis was provided. Goldstein and Gelb's description has thereby set 'standards' for all subsequent reports on agnosic disturbances.

2. It revived the discussion on agnosia as a two-stage mechanism, namely visual form perception followed by a 'meaningful' process of association and recognition, as originally proposed by Lissauer (1890).

3. It opened a new road in agnosia research, namely that of putting it into the framework of Gestalt theory.

It is also noteworthy, however, that this case not only renewed interest in agnosia but has also created a great deal of controversy. In 1922 Benary examined Schn., noted a marked deficiency in calculating ability, and surmised that this represented a general deterioration in Schn.'s intellectual capacity. He stated that both number concept and number handling were limited, although the patient had developed a system for using numbers in everyday commerce. Benary applied the Gestalt explanation of Goldstein and Gelb and noted that Schn. relied heavily on kinaesthetic aids and dramatic gestures to aid communication.

In 1923 Poppelreuter discussed the psychology and pathology of visual recognition, using Schn. as a prime example. Poppelreuter had never examined Schn. personally and had to rely on details from the published reports of Goldstein and Gelb. In his lengthy (130 pages) and detailed discussion, Poppelreuter described experiments on normal subjects looking through tubular devices, demonstrating the loss of simultaneous recognition and problems in the recognition of amorphous forms. His subjects learned to improve their visual identification by tracing the outlines of figures with a finger. With this technique Poppelreuter could replicate in normals many of the findings described in Schn. and concluded that Schn. did not have a visual agnosia but, rather, a pseudo-agnosia based on elementary perceptual deficits and restrictions. He suggested that Schn.'s visual field deficit was the crucial finding.

In 1926, Gelb pointed out that, for several reasons, Poppelreuter's explanation was wrong:

1. Schn.'s visual field defect never touched the perifoveal regions so important for Poppelreuter's model.

2. Despite enlargement of the visual field over time, no improvement of visual recognition occurred.

3. Replication of Poppelreuter's tests in normals with tubular devices did not give the same results.

Some years later, Kleist (1935) compared Schn. with one of his own cases of visual form agnosia. He argued that Schn. must have perceived the outline of a form in order to trace the outline with his fingers, and therefore his problem was exclusively a disturbance of form recognition, a disturbance of higher processing, a visual agnosia or 'thing agnosia' ('*Dingagnosie*').

Goldstein (1943), in a reply to Brain's 1941 paper, refuted Kleist's interpretation by stressing the point that Schn. never recognized by hand movement alone, but only in combination with movement of his head. In addi-

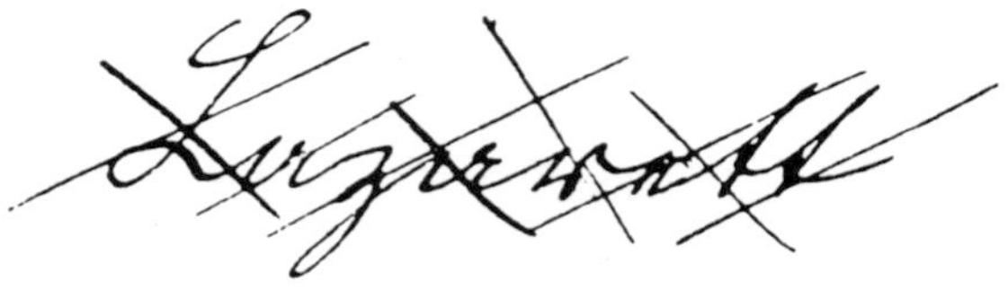

Fig. 11.4 *Schn. completely failed to read the German word 'Lazarett' when it was obscured by crosshatches (from Goldstein and Gelb, 1918, p. 23).*

tion, the tracing movements were shown to be without a special strategy and did not demonstrate 'form-perception'.

In 1928 Pötzl, in his monograph on visual agnosia, discussed the case of Schn. in detail, again without having personally evaluated the patient. In general, Pötzl accepted both the findings of Goldstein and Gelb and their conclusions. He emphasized that the Gestalt explanation was entirely psychological and that a more physiological explanation would be necessary before the case could be understood.

Maeki (1928) carefully studied Schn.'s visuo-motor activities and noted a strong ipsilateral predominance. Thus, a line drawing outlining a facial profile facing left was identified by head and left-hand movements but not by right-hand movements. A profile facing to the right was identified only by head and right-hand movements. Maeki asserted that the head movements were necessary for identification while the hand movements were used to ascertain fine details. There appeared to be no interhemispheric transfer of kinaesthetic information.

In 1931 Quensel reviewed the case of Schn. (without seeing the patient) and agreed with the findings and the general conclusions of the original authors, but expressed reservations about the Gestalt explanation. The following year Hochheimer (1932), in an extensive analysis of language impairment, reviewed the case of Schn. in great detail. He investigated the patient personally and added a number of original observations. He concluded that Schn.'s linguistic skills were normal in most respects, but that he often had problems in the organization of language-based verbal material, probably a residuum of the original brain injury, but compensated for through the use of a series of verbal stratagems (descriptive words, openings of poems, etc.).

In 1941 Brain published a case report of a patient with a visual object agnosia. He presented both the case of Schn. and a lucid outline of the discussion in the literature as a model for discussion of his own case. Brain also included material on visual perceptual and associative problems presented earlier by Riddoch (1917) and Holmes (1918a). Brain accepted the Gestalt explanation of Goldstein and Gelb and considered it a useful concept for understanding the problems in his own case. In response, Goldstein

(1943) noted that Schn. could not recognize real objects more accurately than drawings but, rather, was more successful in guessing because of the larger number of non-visual cues.

In 1936 Lange, in an article concerning visual agnosia prepared for the German *Handbook of Neurology* (eds Bumke and Foerster), discussed Schn. in some detail. Again, the author had not actually examined the patient, but he suggested that a number of the responses were unreal, 'unnatural' for an individual with visual disturbances, and possibly had been exaggerated by Schn. for the benefit of the examiners. He considered the Gestalt explanation of the patient's movements to be inadequate. For the first time in 20 years of examination and discussion, the reality of Schn.'s symptomatology was questioned.

Later investigators also questioned the reality of the findings. In particular, Bay (1953) believed that many of the findings described by Goldstein and Gelb and later discussed by others were either hysterical or grossly exaggerated. Bay examined Schn. personally, some 30 years after onset, and his opinion was partly based on the fact that he could not demonstrate many of the findings described in earlier examinations. Moreover, skull X-rays demonstrated that all of the iron splinters were outside the brain itself. Bay believed that Schn. had suffered increased intracranial pressure producing a 'chiasm syndrome' but had not sustained focal damage in the occipital region. He believed that some of Schn.'s symptoms were remnants of the chiasm syndrome but that others were an artificial product of repeated and suggestive examinations. Discussion of Schn. became a cornerstone of Bay's attack on the concept of visual agnosia; he eventually stated that every case of visual agnosia in the literature could be defined merely as a disturbance of visual perception aggravated by reduced intellectual capacity (Bay, 1953), a concept that receives strong support from eminent neuroscientists, such as Critchley (1964), Milner and Teuber (1968) and Bender (1962, 1972).

Jung (1949) also examined Schn. in the 1940s and noted that the typical head movements during object recognition were still present, although they disappeared with increased interest in the material and were enhanced during replication of the old Goldstein and Gelb experiments. Jung also doubted that Schn. had sustained focal brain damage and questioned explanations based on widespread brain abnormality. Thus, while demonstrating some ongoing problems, Jung refused to accept earlier theoretical explanations and suggested that some of the abnormal responses were overlearned. He concluded that a single case, particularly one with findings never seen before or since (despite extensive search), was too narrow a base for a neurological theory.

Critchley, in his book on the parietal lobes (1953),

reviewed the original case and discussed the literature without seeing the patient or taking a definite position, although he emphasized the views of Bay and co-workers. Finally, in a discussion of visual agnosia in 1954, Ajuriaguerra described a variety of visual problems and used Schn. as one example, again without examining the patient. Ajuriaguerra discussed both the pros and cons of the visual problems demonstrated by Schn., but did not give a definite opinion of his own view.

Thus, over a span of 36 years, the unique findings of Schn. were published in over a dozen reports and played a significant role in most discussions of visual agnosia and in the formulation of a major neuro-psychological theory of agnosia, but eventually came to be suspected of being unreal or exaggerated. Since post mortem study of the brain was not made, the case evaluation rests entirely on the clinical findings. On reading the original case report, one does gain the impression that Schn. exhibited some hysteriform exaggerations. However, Weigl (1978), who had repeatedly investigated Schn. in the 1920s, reported to one of the authors (O.-J. G.) that the original symptoms reported by Goldstein and Gelb had been very consistently observed. Furthermore, according to Weigl, Schn. did not exhibit any personality traits which would support the later interpretation of hysteriform symptom exaggeration. This was the retrospective judgement of one of the leading authorities in German neuropsychology.

Development of Concepts on Visual Agnosia

During the first 50 years of modern agnosia research, a sizeable number of patients thought to have suffered from psychic blindness were described and several attempts to review the clinical presentation as well as the underlying pathology were undertaken (e.g. Wilbrand, 1887; Von Stauffenberg, 1914; Von Monakow, 1914; Wilbrand and Saenger, 1917; Poppelreuter, 1917). Although these authors and many others used the same or similar clinical and experimental procedures and described very similar cases, they interpreted their results along two fundamentally different lines, as follows.

Hierarchical models

A popular attempt was to segregate functions according to 'hierarchical' models, which led to the postulation of different types of agnosia corresponding to the level of impaired function between sensory and motor areas. Deriving his concept from Finkelnburg's (1870) view of higher cognitive disorders as an impairment of symbolic representations (the so-called 'asymbolias'), Meynert (cited in Liepmann, 1900) introduced the idea of a separate sensory and motor representation of symbols in the brain. Wernicke (1894) considered impairments in visual recognition to be due to a loss of visual memory, a function which he considered to be necessary for the creation of the concepts of objects and visual events. Such patients could therefore not recognize objects because intact sensory information appeared foreign and meaningless to them. Wernicke made a distinction between two hierarchically linked processes of identification. The first step, primary identification, consisted of evoking sensory images from a real sensory experience; the second step, secondary identification, was the evoking of sensory images acquired by prior experience but not necessarily related to the current activation of a sensory channel.

In Wernicke's opinion, secondary identification, e.g. the activation of memories from different modalities associated with a sensory input, provided the concept of an object (cf. the discussion on Albertus Magnus in Chapter 2). Consequently, lesions at different sites and levels of sensory processing were thought to give rise to different clinical syndromes. Similar views have been expressed by Wilbrand (1887, 1892) and Freund (1889). Lissauer (1890) and Liepmann (1908) also advanced basically two-stage mechanisms, though these were somewhat different from those proposed by Wernicke or Wilbrand. Both Lissauer and Liepmann emphasized the importance of an early integration within one sensory modality, e.g. vision, rather than attributing an outstanding rôle to the evocation of multi-sensory memories. Lissauer concentrated upon the impairment of recognizing differences that distinguish two similar things, which he called 'apperception', while Liepmann (1908, p. 615) wrote:

> I will not say that the process necessary for recognition happens exclusively within one sensory modality (intrasensory), but demonstrate what a one-sided view it is to consider only the intersensory moment in the process of recognition.

Common to the way of thinking of all the authors cited above is that they have had a definable cerebral substrate in mind, which may be impaired at one or another stage in the processing of sensory information up to the level of object recognition. Such models can and have been tested by correlating clinical deficits to brain pathology. It has been found that the difficulties in 'apperception' or in the integration of intrasensory qualities (submodalities) are correlated with lesions of the occipital cortex itself, while difficulties in associating complete percepts ('*Gestalten*') within intra- or intersensory signals are associated with lesions of pathways connecting cortical visual areas beyond area V1.

Anti-localizationist arguments

The other line of argument was adopted by authors who, confronted with the complexity and variety of agnosic symptoms, rejected the notion of discrete lesions at strategically important places within the sensory processing lines. As Hécaen (1972, pp. 180–186) pointed out in his impressive synthesis of the history of visual agnosias and the relationships among theoretical positions, this anti-localizationist, or anti-associationist, tendency is quite old, but has been adopted by different authors for quite different reasons.

Goltz (1892), relying on extirpation experiments in dogs and arguing against the views of Munk, considered psychic blindness to be the combination of primary sensory visual disturbances together with a defect in general 'intelligence', a view shared some 60 years later by Bay (1950, 1952, 1953). Von Monakow (1914), in his authoritative treatise *Die Localisation im Grosshirn*, reviewed the different theoretical positions as well as the clinico-anatomical evidence of his time in a 50-page chapter on the localization of the agnosias, but rejected the notion of simple anatomical lesions disrupting different levels of processing on both theoretical and clinical grounds. He accepted that the clinical picture of 'psychic blindness' itself existed and was sufficiently homogeneous subsequent to bilateral occipital and occipito-parietal lesions to be described as a separate syndrome. On the other hand, since visual agnosias frequently did not last for long, and even extensive lesions of the occipital lobes did not always lead to the occurrence of visual agnosias, he argued that an additional factor beyond anatomically restricted lesions was necessary to create the syndrome. He therefore attributed the associative agnosias to far reaching but transient effects, the so-called diaschisis (cf. p.180). Moreover, he advanced a major theoretical counter-argument against the localizationists' view of agnosias, namely:

> ... *What appears basically doubtful in the Wernicke–Liepmann way of thinking is their silent supposition that purely anatomical disruption of fibre tracts (association fibres) could produce an adequate disruption of psychological processes. According to my view only physiological processes can be disturbed by anatomical lesions, but never psychological processes.*

Poppelreuter (1917) also rejected the associationist notion because he felt the interactions between different levels of perception were too complex to be explained on the basis of relatively simple theoretical models of the telephone network type (Chapter 8). He refrained from offering a new theory of agnosia, but rather emphasized the necessity to investigate and define experimentally perceptual levels in normals and in patients with lesions of the visual system. He distinguished several stages of visual form processing:

1. formless presence within the visual fields;
2. detection of its position in space;
3. differentiation of the surfaces of objects;
4. contour orientation;
5. estimation of overall shape and classification into small, large, elongated, or wide objects;
6. distinction of separate forms; and
7. form perception by distinction and integration of lines and defined shapes.

Poppelreuter not only took into consideration visual qualities such as light, colour, movement, depth and orientation, but also their relative position with respect to the visual fields. He emphasized that defects from central visual lesions are relative and rarely absolute, leading to 'amblyopia' and not to blindness. As such, lesions should lead to a wide variety of impairments of the process of visual integration. Thus, Poppelreuter was not concerned with inconsistencies and fluctuations of performance in visual agnosic patients, such as the observation that such patients fail to name a specific item but recognize its class, make within-class errors or arrive only at a global class concept. Of particular importance is Poppelreuter's rejection of a chain-like, one-way, successive activation which leads finally to visual 'reproduction' (imagination, *Vorstellung*). Although he considered sensation *('Empfindung')* to be not only in psychological terms different from imagination *('Vorstellung')*, but also in terms of *physiologically* underlying processes, he wrote:

> *The differentiation of these processes need not necessarily be a differentiation of the anatomical substrate, e.g. a different topological cerebral localization, but could well mean a different chemical behaviour of one and the same neural substrate.*

A large group of opponents of localizationist theories were adherents of the Gestalt theory (e.g. Goldstein and Gelb, 1918, 1920, 1924; Goldstein, 1939; Conrad, 1948). Their viewpoint, that cortical lesions which were not restricted to primary sensory areas caused disturbances across all higher cortical functions in different sensory domains (though in various degrees), was equally incompatible with the idea of strict cerebral localization of function. These authors considered the defect brought about by any prior cortical lesion – almost irrespective of its site – to cause a fundamental flaw in the differentiation of figure from ground, and to lead to a loss of the ability for abstraction, irrespective of the sensory modality.

By the mid-1920s, theories on the localization of higher cortical functions and their potential understanding by assuming a locally restricted breakdown of processing in the brain were seriously questioned by different concepts, which appeared to be mutually incompatible. Furthermore, an anatomical approach was neither possible within the framework of Gestalt theory nor compatible with the idea that agnosia could appear subsequent to any lesion at any level within a sensory system. W. Köhler

(1947) must have felt the shortcomings of Gestalt theory and tried to save Gestalt-theoretical ideas by postulating homomorphic spatially distributed electrical processes ('fields') in the brain, which accompany every successful act of Gestalt perception.

All four interpretations of the visual agnosias discussed in this historical review have been entertained over the last 50 years, and have in fact been defended by even more extreme proponents, but the basic theoretical positions are as outlined above. An almost cyclical change of general acceptance of these four viewpoints can be traced, and summarized in the following five stages.

1. The segregating, anatomo–clinical localizationist approach came to its extreme with the works of Henschen (1920–1922), Kleist (1934) and, for the Anglo–Saxon world, Nielsen (1937, 1946).

2. The approach of those who viewed visual agnosia to be no more than a combination of some elementary visual and general intellectual disturbances was pursued in the work of Bay (1953), but also by Bender and Feldman (1965, 1972), and has influenced and modified the viewpoint of others. For example, after reviewing the state of the art of agnosia research Critchley (1953, 1964), wrote:

It is tempting to state none the less that the traditional conception of 'agnosia' is one which is being drastically modified, if, indeed, it is not already in the process of being rejected altogether. In all probability, the term 'agnosia' will eventually be as discarded from the vocabulary of perception as 'aphemia' has been in the domain of language.

3. The third approach, originated by Poppelreuter, is a rather descriptive attitude which places emphasis on extremely careful analysis of the visual fields, the primary visual submodalities and their interference with visual 'recognition'. This approach has been pursued more recently by Gloning *et al.* (1968) and in particular by Zihl and von Cramon (1986). In line with their view of the visual system as being interwoven in too complex a way to allow higher visual disturbances to appear in isolation, neither group found a single case of 'pure' visual agnosia in their respective analyses of over 200 cases with posterior brain lesions.

4. The fourth approach, that of the Gestalt school, was taken to its extreme by a number of authors until the mid-1940s (e.g. Stein, 1928; Von Weizsäcker, 1928; Conrad, 1948; Kohler and Wallach, 1944). This approach has not yet had a revival in clinical agnosia research, but the imminent revival of this line of thought is suggested by the fact that visual stimuli generated by neo-Gestaltists (Kanizsa, 1979) in the search to discover the organization of vision are increasingly used by visual neurophysiologists studying vision on a single cell level in the monkey (e.g. Von der Heydt *et al.*, 1984; Peterhans *et al.*, 1990) or

to evoke visual potentials in humans (Landis *et al.*, 1984; Brandeis and Lehmann 1986, 1989).

5. Several somewhat different approaches to the problem of agnosia will be discussed briefly here but will later be considered in separate sections of this chapter.

Other Approaches to Visual Agnosias

Following the clinical observations of Poppelreuter (1917) and von Stauffenberg (1914), Wolpert (1924) presented a patient whose main difficulties in visual recognition were:

> *1. an inability, while viewing pictures which display an action scene, to grasp the whole, but an ability to recognize correctly the details;*
> *2. an inability to grasp the whole word while reading, but to be forced to fixate each letter and to form a word out of single letters (thus spelling) and to produce countless reading errors when abandoning the spelling strategy; and*
> *3. a disturbance of spatial orientation.*

Wolpert called this disturbance 'simultanagnosia' and explained it as 'a disturbance of grasping the whole'. It was not so much the case description by Wolpert but the term 'simultanagnosia' which attracted attention, together with the implication of a basic deficit in attention rather than in vision. Many authors until today have considered defective recognition in terms of an impairment of grasping the whole (for reviews see Luria, 1966/1980, 1973; Levine and Calvanio, 1978; De Renzi, 1982; Benson and Stuss, 1986; Farah, 1990).

Another major step in the history of the visual agnosias came from Pötzl (1928) in his monograph on 'Optic-agnosic Disturbances'. He attempted to classify visual agnosias by grouping partial agnosic defects according to common sites of lesions and introduced the concept of cerebral dominance – especially of the left hemisphere – for a number of visual agnosic deficits (cf. Chapter 18). In a later paper (Hoff and Pötzl, 1937) he emphasized the role of the left versus the right posterior part of the cerebral hemispheres with respect to pure alexia versus the memory for physiognomies, and introduced the concept of a dynamic interaction in the recovery of function between the higher visual systems of the two hemispheres. This approach has subsequently been pursued and extended with studies of large groups of patients and the introduction of statistical analysis by Hécaen and his group (Hécaen and Angelergues, 1957, 1961, 1962, 1963, 1965), De Renzi *et al.* (1966, 1967, 1968, 1969, 1970, 1972, 1987, 1991) and also by Warrington *et al.* (1967, 1973, 1985, 1988). By virtue of these studies a number of 'partial agnosic' syndromes became firmly associated with lesions of one or the other hemisphere. Thus deficits in the recognition of objects, colours and letters were associated with left-hemisphere lesions and deficits in the recognition of unusual views of objects, places and faces with right-hemisphere lesions (see Chapters 14, 18, 21). With the separation of these partial agnosias the term visual agnosia became more and more restricted to visual form agnosia and to some extent to visual object agnosia. We will subsequently concentrate in this chapter upon this narrowed definition of disturbances of recognition.

Pötzl (1928) has also re-emphasized the importance of cerebral metamorphopsias and visual perseverations in the consideration of disturbances of visual recognition (cf. Chapter 23). This work has been pursued by his pupils (for a review see Gloning *et al.*, 1968), but also by Hécaen and Angelergues (1963) and Critchley (1953) (for review see also Hécaen, 1972).

Finally, although the concept of visual agnosia has repeatedly been considered to have died or become obsolete, research on 'how we perceive and recognize visually' has gained momentum during the last 10 to 15 years. As a consequence, the number of visual agnosia publications in major neurological and neuropsychological journals has increased dramatically, and a number of recent books have been devoted solely to this issue (e.g. De Renzi, 1982; Zihl and von Cramon, 1986; Humphreys and Riddoch, 1987a, b; Brown, 1988; Brown, 1989; Humphreys and Bruce, 1989; Farah, 1990).

This interest is due, on the one hand, to new discoveries of the physiological and anatomical organization of the visual system (see Chapters 4–7), to the increasing interest of cognitive neuropsychologists in testing models in brain-lesioned patients (e.g. Riddoch and Humphreys, 1987; Davidoff and Wilson, 1985; Milner *et al.*, 1991), and to the interest of psychophysicists concerned with pattern recognition in real human deficits (e.g. Efron, 1968; Rentschler *et al.*, 1988; Scheidler *et al.*, in press; Treisman, 1982), together with, on the other hand, the increasing need of researchers in the field of artificial intelligence to realize visuo-spatial simulation (e.g. Watt, 1988).

Despite the enormous research effort on visual agnosia mentioned in this section, it appears that two statements by Teuber (1965) are still valid:

We are thus left, as we said initially, with a sharpened sense of ignorance regarding the nature of classical, modality-specific agnosias.

And:

Yet it remains true that the problem of agnosia lies close to the centre of any physiologic theory of perception, and that the continued lack of such a theory, in turn, may well account for our failures in coming to terms with the major classes of perceptual disorders.

Visual Form and Object Agnosia: Clinical Examination Strategies

An Early Methodological Approach

The standards for examination of visual form and visual object agnosias have been set by the extensive single case analysis of Goldstein and Gelb (1918) of the famous patient Schn., and by the sophisticated examination technique used and described by Poppelreuter (1917) on patients with occipital trauma sustained in the First World War. But even prior to those seminal publications, the psychologist Külpe (mentioned in Wilbrand and Saenger, 1917) had emphasized the need for a complete and methodological investigation of patients with 'mind blindness' and had outlined a test programme as follows:

1. This first section concerns the exact assessment of primary vision (visual acuity, visual field, movement, depth, colours, forms and size differences, etc.)

2. Assessment of perception:
(a) detection, observation, concentration, faculty of abstract reasoning, interest, attention, etc.;
(b) assessment of the relation of visual stimuli to other stimuli in space; localization, judgement of distances, judgement of an overall impression, judgement of real and apparent sizes and Gestalt, etc.;
(c) pure sensory judgements and analysis of complex visual scenes;
(d) differentiating familiar stimuli from unfamiliar stimuli (objects);
(e) differences between pure and mixed visual stimuli;
(f) observation of cueing by words and gestures;
(g) reaction to the perceived;
(h) operations of comparison, differentiation and value attribution;
(i) emotional impact and response.

3. Assessment of the faculty of imagination, in particular location of visual memories and imagination of new scenes
(a) description of such imaginations;
(b) drawing from memory;
(c) operations and reactions which are dependent upon visual imagination;
(d) assessment of rules of occurrence and of the time course of such imagery. In particular the following criteria must be considered:
(i) evocation of visual imagery responses to sensations (Empfindungen);
(ii) free imagery;
(iii) associative imagery;
(iv) attention during visual imagery;
(v) assessment of their clarity, completeness, and their degree of verisimilitude;
(vi) relation of these imagery contents to prior perceptions (objects);
(vii) differentiation between visual memories and associative creations;

(viii) assessment of the differences between a real object and its visual memory;

    (ix) differences between old and new visual memories (before and after recognition);

    (x) the influence of emotions;

    (xi) copying;

    (xii) the influence of will and imagery upon actions.

4. Assessment of the faculty of thought according to the following four criteria

    (a) description of thoughts (differentiation between 'non-visualizable' concepts and real objects to which they relate);

    (b) reference to objects to which thoughts have been directed (in particular abstract conceptions of their use);

    (c) performance in operations and reactions subsequent to thoughts;

    (d) observance of rules for the occurrence, the course and the coherence of thoughts.

A differentiation should be made between thoughts as conscious contents (Bewusstheiten) and thinking as a function.

5. Investigation of the faculty of recognition

    (a) recognition of primary conscious thought contents (sensation and imagination);

    (b) recognition of objects represented through such contents;

    (c) recognition of the meaning of such contents and objects;

    (d) distinguishing between levels of recognition;

    (e) analysis of misrecognitions;

    (f) analysis of the difference between recognized and non-recognized impressions;

    (g) do disturbances in recognition extend to imagery in the same way as to sensations?

    (h) investigation of the role of general intellectual functions (similarities, differences, etc.);

    (i) impairments of attention;

    (j) differentiating between cognition and recognition;

    (k) analysis of the impact of 'mind blindness' upon emotion (affect, mood, preferences and instinctive behaviour);

    (l) its influence upon will and action.

Külpe's protocol is probably the first attempt to formulate a standardized methodological programme to investigate 'mind blindness' and clearly illustrates the influence which ideas concerning visual imagery and memory had on early research in this field. Although parts of his list appear rather vague and perhaps outdated, others appear extremely modern in the light of recent experimental approaches to visual imagery (e.g. Farah, 1988; Goldenberg, 1989).

General Clinical Approach

Confronted with a patient suspected of having difficulties in visual recognition, two approaches must be taken. The first is a clinical bedside examination, which can be per-

formed within a reasonable time and serves as a screening method for uncovering specific disturbances in visual recognition, defining its specificity and distinguishing it from disturbances of other sensory modalities, of language, of abstraction and conceptual thinking, and from disturbances of primary visual sensation. Most of such a screening exam can be performed at the bedside with little technical equipment.

The second approach, which if the technical possibilities are available should follow subsequent to establishing diagnosis, consists of a time-consuming, partly experimental visual evaluation; this needs some technical equipment and, as a rule, an adaptation of some tests to the specific deficiencies of the patient.

Since later chapters will discuss the clinical examination of partial agnosias, such as pure alexia, prosopagnosia and agnosias for places or space (Chapters 14, 18 and 21), we will concentrate here on the clinical examination of a presumed deficit in the recognition of forms or objects.

Bedside Clinical Examinations

It is mandatory to perform a complete neurological examination in order to exclude primary sensory deficits in modalities other than vision. This examination includes fundoscopy, pupillary reactions, the ability to fixate, examination of ocular and gaze movements, accommodation and convergence, and methods to provoke a pathological nystagmus.

Bedside visual tests include those for visual acuity, for visual fields on confrontation with black and coloured targets, and for movement perception in the periphery and for the evaluation of extinction phenomena (Chapter 22). Depth perception may be tested with Julesz stereograms (binocular stereodepth), but also by judging the distances of objects within the room, their relative position in front of or behind each other and by similar tests in the far distance by looking out of the window (parallax depth). Movement perception can be assessed by judging the speed and direction of moving objects such as cars or people seen from the window. In the same way, size discrimination can be tested by comparing objects or surfaces of similar sizes in distant space, as well as by judging their relative sizes. The following can all easily be performed with paper and pencil: discrimination between straight and curved lines; ability to judge the shapes of forms made up by dotted lines; susceptibility to visual illusions such as the Mueller–Lyer illusion; ability to perceive illusory contours such as in the Kanizsa triangle (Kanizsa, 1979) (Fig. 11.5); presence or absence of a pop-out effect versus a serial search-strategy (Fig. 11.6); estimation of surfaces by pointing to the middle of a regular or irregular closed loop; presence or absence of neglect (see Chapter 22), using tests of line bisection or the copying of a complex figure; and judging line orientation (Benton, 1975). Equally, reading

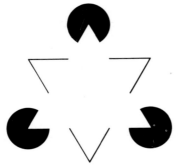

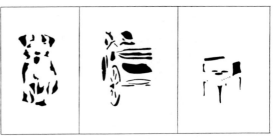

Fig. 11.8 *Examples of pictures from the Street Gestalt completion test, graded for degree of difficulty of identification (from Street, 1931).*

Fig. 11.5 *The 'Kanizsa triangle', an example of the perception of illusory contours. One does not see three black sectors and three angles, but rather a white triangle in front of the three black discs and an outlined triangle (from Kanizsa, 1979).*

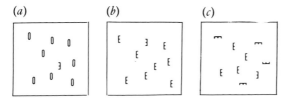

Fig. 11.6 *Examples of displays of nine items in visual search tests with the target 'a mirror-imaged E' present. The patient must decide whether a mirror-imaged 'E' is present or not: (a) among Os the 'pop-out-effect'; (b) among homogeneous distracters; (c) among heterogeneous distracters.*

of words crosshatched by lines (Goldstein and Gelb, 1918) (Fig. 11.4), reading of words rendered ambiguous by non-continuous lines (Landis *et al.*, 1982) (Fig. 18.4) or reading of words written in a discontinuous way by shadowing (Fig. 18.4), can be performed *ad hoc* using a sheet of paper. Simple tests for form constancy can easily be done at the bedside. For example, one can use the famous circle–ellipse test used by Goldstein and Gelb (1918), where a circle drawn on a sheet of paper or cardboard is still perceived as a circle when the sheet is tilted away from the

patient and therefore its retinal image corresponds to an ellipse. As with words, line drawings of objects may be crosshatched; or overlapping figures such as the Ghent (1956) or Poppelreuter (1917) figures may be used. The level of recognition in relation to segregation or perceptual degradation may be tested by using the Gollin figures (Fig. 11.7; Gollin, 1960) or the Street figures (Fig. 11.8; Street, 1931). Figure–background formation can be tested by using ambiguous figures such as the Rubin vase (Fig. 11.9: Rubin, 1921), unstable figures such as the Necker cube (Fig. 11.10; Necker, 1832) or hidden figures (Fig. 11.11; Porter, 1954; Landis *et al.*, 1982). The importance of context in recognition can be tested by presenting, for example, parts of a face in or out of context (Fig. 11.12; Palmer, 1975). A simple global versus local feature test consists of presenting a number made up by much smaller but different numbers or a letter by much smaller but different letters (Fig. 11.13). In a similar way, patients may be asked to solve puzzles of pictures of objects or faces (Fig. 11.14). A longer list of such perceptual, ambiguous and illusory figure tests could be given, but the interested reader is referred to the reviews in the books by Kanizsa (1979) and by Schober and Rentschler (1986). The patient should be shown line drawings of simple objects, stylized objects and objects drawn from unusual views (Warrington and Taylor, 1973; Warrington and James, 1986),

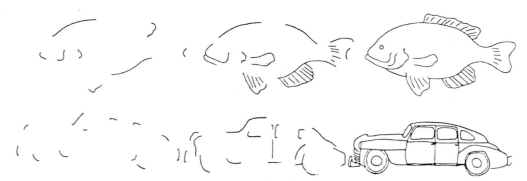

Fig. 11.7 *Examples of incomplete drawings of objects, graded for difficulty of identification from the Gollin's pictures test (1960).*

Fig. 11.9 *What is seen? A vase or two faces? An example of an ambiguous figure.*

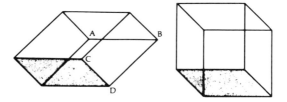

Fig. 11.10 *Two examples of perceptually unstable figures, known as Necker's rhomboid (left) and Necker's cube (right). The perceptual fluctuations of the rhomboid were first noticed by Necker in 1832 when he was examining crystals. The darkened surface in these two figures appears at one time to be an inner surface and at another an outer surface, or in other words sometimes the A is nearest and the C furthest and sometimes vice versa.*

also drawn action pictures and drawn scenes, as well as geometrical figures and 'meaningless' shapes. The same should be done with photographs of real objects, objects presented from unusual views (Fig. 11.5) and degraded objects. The patient should be asked to copy such drawings and photographs, and of course to draw real objects. Moreover he should be asked to draw objects from memory.

The patient should view real objects and be asked to name them and/or to describe their use. Care should be taken not to allow these objects to produce characteristic noises, since visually agnosic patients are extremely good at sensing non-visual cues. If the patient fails to identify the object, he should be asked to describe the material from which it is made. The use of the object may be gestured, and frequently serves as a good cue for recognition. Simple real objects should also be presented under a more prototypical and unusual view (e.g. Fig. 11.15(a)). Of course, real objects must be presented through other sensory modalities such as touch or hearing, because the patient should not be impaired in recognizing the same object via a non-visual modality. He should also be presented with silhouettes of objects and with a sheet of paper on which the silhouettes are missing ('negative shapes'). Finally, the patient should be asked to pick out of an array of similar items the one which belongs to him, such as his own glasses from an array of glasses, his own wallet from an array of wallets, and to distinguish between an array of similarly looking car-fronts or to make other within-class decisions.

Discrimination of simple or complex geometric shapes is easily done in bedside examination, and the same applies to the discrimination of very similar items differing by just one or more small details, as beautifully outlined by Lissauer (1890) (p. 182). Usually one finds a gradient of increasing difficulty of impairment in recognizing real objects, photographs of objects or line drawings of objects (for review see De Renzi *et al.*, 1987). If a patient fails to name an item, he should be asked to describe its use, to

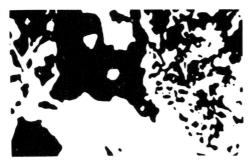

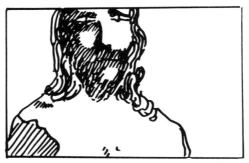

Fig. 11.11 *Example of the hidden figure of a bearded man (left). The picture on the right side provides the solution (modified from Landis et al., 1982).*

(a)

(b)

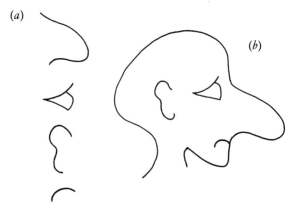

Fig. 11.12 *Example of parts of a face without (a) and within (b) context (modified from Palmer, 1975).*

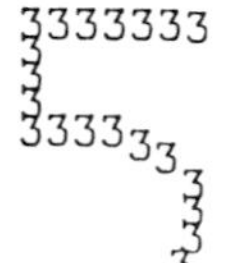

```
3333333
3
3333 3
3     3
      3
333333
```

Fig. 11.13 *An example of a 'global' number (5) made up from smaller 'local' numbers (3s).*

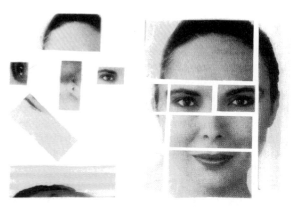

Fig. 11.14 *An example of a face puzzle. Right: correct solution; left: the unsuccessful attempt of a patient with prosopagnosia and agnosia for non-canonical views (cf. Chapter 14), despite her correct recognition of the individual facial parts (from Landis et al., 1988).*

pantomime its use, to pick out the item among an array of different items when the name is given or written, to match the item with its photograph or drawn picture from an array of different photographs and drawings and finally to match it with its identical twin. This, of course,

can be performed with real objects as well as with photographs and line drawings. These stimuli should include classes such as fruits, vegetables, tools, living or non-living things, etc., which may reveal the recently discovered class-specific naming disorders (e.g. Warrington and McCarthy, 1987; Goodglas *et al.*, 1986). Many of the items we have referred to here, including those used in testing for colours and famous faces, can be found in newspapers or journals which are present in almost every hospital room. For some of these tests the examiner must be prepared, possibly by making up a few sheets with some of the items of tests outlined above. Some tests will need to be manufactured *ad hoc* in relation to the defects suspected in a patient and are beyond the scope of this chapter.

Further Instrumental and Experimental Examinations

Once the provisional bedside diagnosis of a visual agnosic disorder is made, more extensive and partly experimental investigation is necessary, if time and equipment are available. Without claiming completeness, we will here attempt to outline some of the procedures to further evaluate such patients.

A clinical confrontation testing of visual fields, though quite reliable in the hands of the experienced, is not always sufficient to uncover small or partial visual field defects. The examiner is therefore recommended to perform formal quantitative dynamic perimetry (e.g. with a Tübingen perimeter, Chapter 9) using light, colours, different shapes and flicker stimuli. Most of the widely used perimeters are not equipped to test all these functions. In particular, the facility for perimetrical investigation of form and flicker fusion is often lacking, but may be of considerable importance in the assessment of visual agnosia (for a review see Zihl and Von Cramon, 1986). Besides the dynamic perimetry, static perimetry, for which automatized apparatus is present in most institutions today, should be used. It should however be kept in mind that automatized static light perimetry alone is not sufficient to exclude more elementary visual field defects in agnosic patients. For precise perimetric methodology, the reader is referred to the extensive specialized literature (e.g. Harms, 1969; Aulhorn and Harms, 1972; Fankhauser, 1969; Ellenberger, 1974; Harrington, 1976; Zihl and Von Cramon, 1986) and to Chapter 9. In addition to formal testing of visual acuity in near and far space and for vernier acuity, careful assessment of contrast sensitivity should also be made in such patients (Rentschler *et al.*, 1982). Moreover, experimental analysis of the discrimination of phase-altered textures (Caelli *et al.*, 1985) and the assessment of visual evoked potentials may be of use.

Threshold measurements for a whole variety of simple and more complex stimuli should be performed using

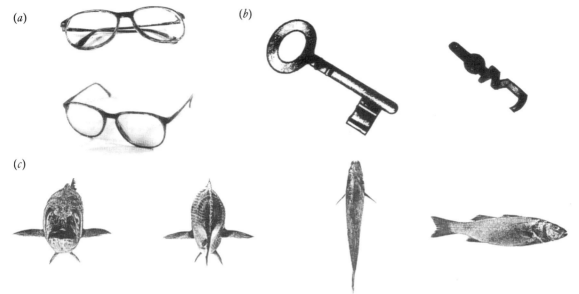

Fig. 11.15 *Examples of items represented at a different views (a) Real object: upper, non-canonical presentation of glasses; lower, canonical presentation of the same glasses. (b) Drawn object: left, prototypical view of a key; right, non-canonical view of the same key. (c) Fish photographed from different angles; the view at the right is the most canonical.*

increasing and decreasing exposure durations in tachistoscopic experiments. The stimuli which can be used are similar to those used in a clinical paper-and-pencil bedside testing, e.g. ranging from the relatively simple discrimination of straight versus curved lines to the estimation of different surfaces and to the analysis of complex patterns or the recognition of objects. By the use of a tachistoscope or by generation of the stimuli on a computer screen apparent movement (the phi phenomenon) or apparent depth may be assessed. The sensitivity of the patient in detecting moving dots among stationary ones or to recognize meaningful stimuli when motion is only transmitted by a few moving points (Johansson, 1973) should also be assessed. Tachistoscopic experiments may help to elucidate the question as to whether a patient chooses a matching by form or a matching by function strategy (Levy, 1974; Warrington and Taylor, 1978) (Fig. 11.16). Moreover, with the tachistoscope face- or object-superiority effects can be investigated (Davidoff and Landis, 1990) (Fig. 11.17).

Another class of experiments deriving from a psychophysical approach to perception concerns visual search tasks in which the search rate for a target among distractors may vary depending upon which stimulus is the target and which is the distractor (e.g. Treisman and Souther, 1985; Treisman, 1982) (Fig. 11.6). In such tasks the exposure duration is a critical variable in normal subjects in separating different kinds of search strategies and may well uncover similar search biases in agnosic patients.

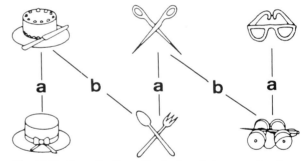

Fig. 11.16 *Example of matching by form (a), or matching by function (b) strategies (modified from Levy, 1974).*

Yet another experimental paradigm stemming from psychophysics and artificial intelligence research is 'supervised visual learning'. With this procedure a patient's ability to learn to classify stimulus material of different degrees of complexity can be evaluated (Caelli *et al.*, 1987; Watanabe, 1985; Ahmed and Rao, 1975). By this procedure the patient is trained to construct prototypes or class representatives by averaging over the samples of each of the classes. The recognition of learned or novel signals is then possible by selecting the prototype which is most similar, e.g. closest in feature space. Class prototypes of pattern recognition are not given a priori, but are acquired by means of interaction with the stimuli (Scheidler *et al.*, in press). The advantage of this procedure is that the

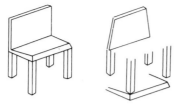

Fig. 11.17 *Example of a chair and a scrambled chair. Such stimuli can be used to test for object superiority effects (from Davidoff and Landis, 1990).*

breakdown of class concept formation can be observed in relation to physically defined stimulus properties, and that it can be assessed whether or not the learned concepts can be generalized.

In cases where visual form or object recognition must be assessed in a patient with highly concentrically restricted visual fields, i.e., with 'tunnel vision', the question sometimes emerges of a 'psychogenic' origin of these restricted fields. It is then helpful to test visual fields at different distances from the patient (Fig. 11.18) (Landis *et al.*, 1982). For a subject with 'psychogenic' visual field restriction, it is impossible to maintain a linear visual field extension over a distance of up to 10 metres.

The role of disturbance in ocular motion and fixation for the recognition of forms, particularly in simultaneous

form perception, has been emphasized by many authors (e.g. Luria *et al.*, 1963; Lhermitte *et al.*, 1969, 1973; Karpov *et al.*, 1979; Rizzo and Hurtig, 1987). Thus it is of considerable importance that patients suspected of suffering from visual agnosia undergo eye-movement recordings while attempting to recognize a wide variety of stimuli. Several methods of eye-movement recording are available. Virtually all techniques have their own disadvantages, be they technical or discomforting to the patient. However, the comparison of the ocular search strategies of such patients with those of normal subjects looking at the same pictures, in relation to their verbal report of what they recognize, is of considerable importance in distinguishing recognition deficits in 'spatial agnosias' or visuo-perceptuo-motor disturbances from those of 'true' visual agnosias in which the search strategy is very similar to that of normal subjects, but recognition fails (Lhermitte *et al.*, 1969).

Patient Interview

Common to both bedside clinical examination and extended clinical–experimental investigations is the need for a careful interview aimed at uncovering the patient's subjective experience of seeing and recognizing. The interview should in particular evaluate the degree of awareness the patient has about his own incapacitation. Disturbance of self-awareness of a visual deficit may range from active denial of a disturbance to mild misinter-

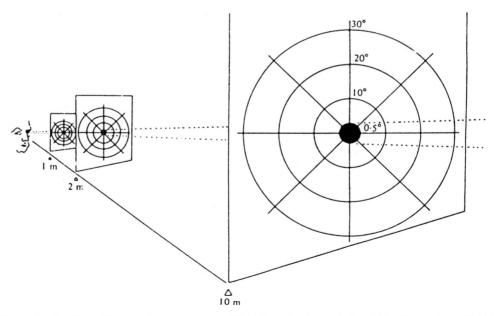

Fig. 11.18 *Perspective drawing to illustrate three separate visual field determinations at 1, 2 and 10 m in a patient with highly concentrically restricted fields, in whom a 'psychogenic' origin of 'tunnel vision' was suspected. In this case an intact visual field of about 0.5 degrees was demonstrated at all three distances (see the text) (from Landis et al., 1982).*

pretations, such as the commonly found reference by patients to their difficulty being a consequence of 'bad eyesight'. The degree of reduced awareness is related to the site of the lesion within the visual system: peripheral visual field defects, as a rule, are fully realized, while central visual field defects frequently are not or not completely realized. When peripheral and central field defects were present in the same patient, as described by Bender (1984), the peripherally impaired vision in one eye was spontaneously complained about and fully realized, while the concomitantly present left homonymous hemianopia subsequent to a right posterior cerebral artery stroke went unrecognized and was denied by the patient even after the quite explicit perimetric demonstration. But even with central lesions, the degree of awareness varies considerably. Impaired awareness appears clinically to be present much more frequently following posterior lesions in the right hemisphere than in the left. Lesions restricted to area V1 are more likely to come to awareness than lesions beyond V1. One of our patients clearly demonstrated this dissociated awareness with respect to left and right posterior lesions. He had suffered within the space of several days first from a left posterior cerebral artery stroke and then from a right. While the initial right homonymous hemianopia was fully realized and described adequately, the subsequent left homonymous hemianopia was not. His right hemianopia recovered within a few days but his left hemianopia remained dense. The only subjective complaint of this patient was that of a somewhat dimmer and imprecise visual ability in the partly recovered right visual field.

Denial of blindness, or 'Anton's syndrome' (Anton, 1898; Redlich and Bonvicini, 1909), sometimes referred to as anosognosia (Babinski, 1914), is a typical symptom subsequent to lesions in both occipital lobes (see also Gloning *et al.*, 1962). Denial or unawareness of visual defects in parts of the visual field should be carefully evaluated and their eventual presence kept in mind by the examiner, since such patients, as a rule, confabulate about the presence or absence of a stimulus in such areas, and may even confabulate about stimulus details. Unawareness on the part of the examiner about the possibility of denial has occasionally led to grotesque visual acuity values in cortically blind patients.

The 'incomplete Anton's syndrome' refers to a reduced self-awareness or denial of the defects in the visual fields, e.g. hemianopias (Gloning *et al.*, 1962; Gassel and Williams, 1963) associated frequently with a curious behaviour of the patients: they claim that objects into which they repeatedly bump have been placed in a wrong position, or blame people with whom they collide for having used the wrong side of the path. They cannot easily be convinced that they should attribute these events to their blind hemifield. Critchley (1953) has used the term

'anosodiaphoria' for the tendency to minimize the importance of visual field defects for everyday behaviour by patients who acknowledge the presence of the defect. He attempted to relate the different levels of impaired awareness in patients to visual field defects subsequent to different cerebral lesions (Critchley, 1949b) and distinguished six different levels of impaired awareness:

1. the complete absence of awareness even after the repeated demonstration of the visual field defect;
2. the absence of awareness of the defect itself, but the presence of awareness of its consequences (e.g. bumping into objects);
3. projection and rationalization of the disturbance (e.g. the perceived dimness is taken as a consequence of reduced illumination and not considered to be a consequence of the cerebral lesion);
4. a relative awareness but an inability to explain or adequately describe the visual disturbance;
5. the awareness of the defect, which can be described adequately but is given erroneous interpretation (e.g. disturbance of vision in one eye rather than one homonymous hemifield);
6. the awareness of the visual field defect, the adequate description of the defect and also an adequate awareness that this defect is due to a lesion in the brain.

Although an interview concerning the awareness of visual deficits and an attempt to have the patient describe his subjective experience of impaired vision is mandatory, it often remains frustating for the examiner. Patients are often incapable of describing how they reach 'wrong' conclusions, what exactly disturbs them, how they experience their visual world, and especially, in what way this experience is different from the experience prior to the occurrence of the visual disturbances. These difficulties in describing the disturbance are not as great when simple visual defects are concerned, but are more notable when a failure to recognize things or forms is concerned. Their description remains curiously vague, and terms like 'blurred', 'strange' and 'unfamiliar', 'moving' or 'fuzzy' etc. are often used. The examiner frequently has the impression of somebody describing a completely different sensory channel unknown to 'normals', thus rendering the possibility of sharing the experience impossible. Since many of the descriptions of patients with central visual lesions suggest the presence of metamorphopsias, palinopsias or other more elementary visual perseverations, the clinical interview must include questions concerning such phenomena.

One way of rendering evident such visual phenomena (cf. Chapter 23) is to present a white sheet of paper to the patient and ask him to describe the pattern he sees.

In experimental or clinical tasks in which the patient shows great difficulties in recognizing, e.g. line drawings of objects, one may intersperse blank white sheets and ask the patient to describe the 'line drawing'. If the patient fails to detect spontaneously the absence of a stimulus on the white sheet, the first step should be to have him learn to discriminate between the presence and absence of a target, before continuing the recognition task. This procedure has definitely helped one of our patients to learn to substract his own 'visual noise' and has thus improved his ability to recognize.

Five Dimensions Applied in Agnosia Classification

As the historical introduction to this Chapter has indicated, the classification of the different types of visual agnosia related to the perception of shapes, objects and visual scenes was not and still is not a simple task on which all investigators agree. For the purpose of classifying the different types of apperceptive and associative agnosias, different classification criteria have been applied. We will discuss five of those 'dimensions' along which a classification of the different clinical syndromes is possible:

Phenomenological Classification

Such a classification relies on the clinical observation of the symptoms found in visual agnosic patients, and uses five levels of sensory integration to bring the clinical observations into order: *sensation, perception, apperception, association* and *cognition*. This scheme was developed during the last decades of the nineteenth century and became very popular in psychology. It was proposed by Wilhelm Wundt (1896/1905), but much earlier Leibniz proposed a distinction between perception and apperception. As discussed in Chapter 2, a systematic phenomenological description of different levels of sensory integration leading to cognition was considered by Albertus Magnus and the Arabian scientists of the eleventh and twelfth centuries AD. This discussion shaped Western thinking on this matter by making use of Aristotelian thoughts.

Defects of visual sensation are due to diseases of the optical media of the eye and the optic nerve, which will not be discussed in detail in this volume. Defects in visual perception (elementary perceptual 'agnosias') are those disturbances in which the basic qualitites of vision, such as perception of lightness and darkness, contours, movement, colour and depth, are affected. Disturbances of visual apperception prevent elementary recognition of the shapes of objects, as in visual form agnosia, or impair the mental construction of a 'full' visual world, as in one type of simultanagnosia. Disorders of visual association affect the recognition of the meaning of an object, which, for example, can be outlined with the hand by the patient or

slavishly copied, but categorization and meaningful interpretation of what is seen is either abolished or at least incorrect. Visual object agnosia, prosopagnosia, topographagnosia and alexia may be combined into a class of associative visual agnosias. The cognitive agnosias extend beyond the boundaries of the visual modality. These are multimodal impairments of cognitive functions relevant for behaviour and for understanding the context of the signals from the external world.

The Cerebral Localization of Pathological Processes

This is another dimension of visual agnosia classification, by which focal lesions and global lesions are discriminated. 'Focal' lesions are, for example, circumscribed lesions in the visual radiation, a gunshot wound in the occipital pole of the primary visual cortex or a vascular lesion in the region of the left angular gyrus. Owing to retrograde or anterograde degeneration processes, all focal lesions also affect neuronal structures outside the destroyed brain area (cf. Chapter 8). Global lesions are those which have effects in widespread cortical areas, predominantly certain cell layers, without destroying the whole cortical field. Functionally, global lesions which are characterized by many 'patchy' circumscribed microlesions distributed over a larger cortical area should also be included in this group. Of course, owing to retrograde and anterograde degeneration which also occurs in global brain lesions, the functional impairment affects more of the brain than one can see in macroanatomical studies.

Visual Field

Visual agnosia classification related to the visual field is a classification dimension that is of course closely related to the site of the lesion. A defect in visual perception or cognition can occur in structures characterized by an almost retinotopic projection, i.e. it is restricted to certain parts of the binocular visual fields. The defect, however, can be related to spatiotopic (egocentric) coordinates as in hemispatial neglect. Further, an agnosic defect may be related to the external space independently of the patient's position. Topographagnosia is such a spatial defect. Finally, several classes of visual agnosias are non-spatial, since the perception of objects (object categories) or object meaning is affected.

The Aetiology of Disorders of Higher Visual Perception

This is a fourth classification, especially relevant for clinical diagnosis and the treatment of the patient: vascular diseases such as transient ischaemias or strokes, brain tumours or metastases within the brain, general ischaemia as in cardiac arrest, intoxication affecting brain cell metabolism as in mercury poisoning, demyelinization processes as in multiple sclerosis or in intoxication with organic solvents, diffuse brain encephalitis due to bacterial or viral infections, slow viral diseases and hereditary degenerative diseases of brain functions may all lead to visual agnosic symptoms.

The Neurological Classification of Different Visual Agnosias

This is based on the concept illustrated under 'Phenomenological classification', but includes the other aspects of the neurological status such as the impairment of motor functions, other sensory modalities, the state of consciousness or sensorimotor integration.

Support for the Classification

Formally, these five aspects of visual agnosia classification constitute a five-dimensional space, within which the symptoms of every well-examined patient with visual disturbances occupy a distinct subspace. In classifying many patients suffering from elementary visual perceptual deficits or from higher-order visual agnosias, one finds that certain ranges of this five-dimensional space are more densely 'filled', while others remain 'empty'. This classificatory grouping of data justifies the selection of special names for syndromes which are believed to constitute clinical entities, i.e. syndromes which occupy a defined space in the five-dimensional classificatory scheme.

As always with such efforts in classifying complex facts, much discussion and emotion have been invested in the pros and cons of such a scheme. For pragmatic reasons, however, it seems meaningful to select names and to avoid the use of the same name in describing different facts. In the history of agnosia research, however, it has been repeatedly questioned whether visual agnosic symptoms are more than a severe impairment of primary visual processes, and those who have attacked the concepts of selective impairment of higher visual cognitive functions have also argued with clinical observations.

Von Stauffenberg (1914), for example, reported 21 patients suffering from visual agnosia. Visual acuity was normal in only 4 patients while it was impaired in all the other 17. Could this reduction in elementary sensory functions explain part of the agnosic symptoms? Nature provides conditions which give a clear answer that this is not the case. When visual acuity is decreased in the elderly owing to the beginning of cataract formation or retinal degeneration, no symptoms similar to visual agnosia of objects or space perception are observed, even with a visual acuity below 0.1, provided that the general intellectual capacity is preserved. As one can easily recognize when studying patients over 80 years of age with reduced visual acuity due to cataract or retinal degeneration, but with no signs of cerebral disease, a rather reduced visual sensory input is sufficient for object recognition and when an object or a spatial relation between objects is not perfectly seen it is sufficiently well guessed and no typically agnosic errors are made. The same is true for the perception of colours, letters, words, faces, spatial relations, visual depth, figure–background relations, object separations and object meaning. These observations indicate that primary sensory defects, even when accompanying agnosic symptoms, do not explain those symptoms. Back in 1890 Siemerling had pointed out that even a reduction of visual acuity to 1/30 cannot explain the occurrence of visual agnosia. Behavioural interaction with the objects of the visual world is different in a patient suffering from low visual acuity as compared with visually agnosic patients. Amblyopic patients (e.g. those with large visual field defects due to retinal detachment, optic nerve diseases or visual radiation impairment), on the other hand, are able to use marginal cues to construct a rough but correct image of the visual world, and to compare this image with the mental images stored in memory. These patients are also able to correctly recognize object rotations, size changes and spatial relations between objects, whereas an agnosic patient may typically be disturbed in one or more of these tasks. Thiele (1928), referring also to the publications of Poppelreuter (1917, 1923), reported on 34 patients suffering from visual agnosia, of which 23 were in addition hemianopic. Homonymous hemianopia was observed 13 times for the right and 10 times for the left half of the visual field. Thiele pointed out that one has to take into consideration these visual field defects when evaluating the performance of the patients in visual object and space recognition, but also noted that these visual field defects do not explain agnosic symptoms. He observed patients with severe visual field defects due to lesions in the visual radiation or the striate cortex, who were able to use the visual information perceived through the good parts of the visual fields and to combine this information intelligently to attain correct object recognition. Characteristic adaptations in gaze movements during the exploration of the visual world were observed which compensated in part for the visual field defect.

The behaviour of patients suffering from elementary perceptive defects owing to lesions in the afferent visual system and in area V1 resembles that of elderly patients suffering from cataract or macular retinal degeneration. They recognize objects more slowly, but without the typical visual agnosic errors, and all such patients apply successfully compensatory mechanisms and use their visual memory effectively to make the best out of the rudimentary and temporally disjunct information received through the still functioning parts of their visual fields. Patients with peripheral sensory and central perceptive defects develop new exploration patterns to compensate their input difficulties, and as a rule are rarely helpless in making use of these input data. Quite in contrast, in observing responses of visual agnosic patients one realizes that they are at a loss with regard to the use of part of the sensory signals; their ability to construct a meaningful visual world, even a rudimentary one, is seriously affected.

In the light of these considerations, it is somewhat surprising that still after the Second World War, when again many brain-lesioned soldiers were investigated by neurologists and ophthalmologists, arguments were provided to suggest that a combination of elementary sensory and perceptive defects with general impairment of intelligence can lead to symptoms of visual agnosia. In Germany, Bay (1953) and his co-workers emphasized this point of view and explained visual agnosia as being caused by a combination of perceptual and memory defects. This view was contradicted by other researchers (Ettlinger, 1956; Best, 1952; Faust, 1955; MaCrae and Trolle, 1956; Hoff, Gloning *et al.*, 1962; Hécaen and Angelergues, 1963), but it gained a certain momentum, since Bay could indeed demonstrate that general cortical amblyopia was frequently observed in visual agnosic patients (cf. also Bender and Feldman, 1972; Critchley, 1964; Teuber *et al.*, 1958).

We think that many clinical observations of patients with reduced sensory and perceptual visual functions or with severe loss of memory (including visual memory) contradict Bay's view. Patients suffering from severe impairment of memory are still able to interact with the visual objects in a meaningful relation and to move adequately within the visual space with respect to the different objects; they separate objects from their backgrounds and even when they can no longer name the objects they still realize that they are different perceptual entities.

In summary, after careful evaluation of all accompanying sensory and perceptive defects as well as impairments in visual memory or sensory functions in agnosic patients, we concur with the majority of neurologists and neuropsychologists in the view that visual agnosias can be classified into clinical entities which appear when the structures responsible for visual signals processing beyond area V1 are lesioned. The following paragraphs are devoted to the admittedly somewhat difficult classificatory discrimination of apperceptive and associative visual agnosias, while later chapters will elaborate in detail on specialized types of cerebral disturbances of vision.

Apperceptive Visual Agnosia (Form Agnosia)

Concepts of Apperceptive Agnosias

The concept of apperceptive agnosia came to life as a theoretical prediction when Lissauer (1890) used Wundt's definition of apperception: 'a first stage of conscious awareness of a sensory impression', and speculated that a brain lesion might impair this level of visual signal processing. The very existence of an apperceptive agnosia was immediately questioned by Lissauer himself, who felt uncertain whether a selective impairment of the apperceptive process could result in the clinical picture of visual agnosia. Benson (1989) operationalized the concept of apperceptive agnosia as follows:

> *Individuals with apperceptive visual agnosia cannot name, copy, or recognize visually presented objects, but immediately identify the item following tactile or auditory cues. They fail at all constructional tasks, cannot copy drawings or writing and cannot identify faces. In sharp contrast, they correctly identify colour, light intensity, direction and dimension of visual stimuli; they only fail to recognize visual form.*

Farah (1990) rephrased Lissauer's thought in the following way:

> *Apperceptive agnosias are those in which recognition fails because of an impairment in visual perception, which is none the less above the level of an elementary sensory deficit such as a visual field defect. Patients do not see objects normally, and hence cannot recognize them.*

Liepmann (1908), in his somewhat different definition of the same concept of apperception, wrote:

> *. . . a disturbance of the synthesis or fusion of impressions in a single modality.*

This definition gave a new dimension to apperception, namely that of a defect in 'fusion', i.e. in the perceptual integration of correctly perceived visual *qualities*.

Baumgartner (1990) advanced the concept of apperception one step further when he stated:

> *The neuroanatomical and neurophysiological data make it likely that the different attributes of vision are processed in parallel and are perceived in spatially separate areas. This could explain the occurrence of isolated defects of colour, movement and depth perception or object recognition after focal cortical lesions in the prestriate regions. But the continuity and wholeness of our visual experiences are difficult to imagine under this assumption. It favours the postulation that different visual submodalities must converge somewhere. However, the clinical experience may indicate that this is not necessary, since in the case of convergence an isolated loss of one submodality should result in disturbances also in others. Partial unawareness could, however, be understood if submodalities are not only processed but remain perceptively independent. The integration of different submodalities to*

global perception could be the contribution of time. Time could serve as the unifying parameter by coincident activation (Phillips et al., 1984) of neuronal population with different spatial coordinates. The rich interconnections between and along the different processing lines could be thought to act as a time control device for correlating local features within the visual field to different submodalities.

Be it by 'fusion' or 'convergence' or by the facilitating factor of quasi-simultaneous activation of independent submodalities, it is clear that a disruption of this basic process cannot be due to a single circumscribed unilateral cerebral lesion and we do not even see the possibility that two circumscribed structural lesions, of vascular traumatic or tumour origin – one placed in each hemisphere – could reasonably be made responsible for such an interference. Only extended, diffuse damage preferentially interrupting intracortical signal transfer could lead to a failure to integrate adequate neuronal activity from spatially disparate visual centres, representing the visual qualities with different weights.

A few patients have been reported who fulfill all these criteria and may, in our view, be called apperceptive agnosics. The term apperceptive agnosia has, however, been used also for other conditions, such as simultanagnosia or defective perceptual categorization. These two conditions will be dealt with later in this chapter and we will restrict the term *apperceptive agnosia* to a small but relatively homogeneous group of patients. This group includes the case Schn. (Goldstein and Gelb, 1918; described in more detail above), and the patients A. C. (Adler, 1944, 1950), who after 40 years was shown (Sparr *et al.*, 1991) to suffer still in a virtually identical way from apperceptive agnosia; Mr S. (Efron, 1968; Benson and Greenberg, 1969), Mr X (Landis, *et al.*, 1982), E. S. (Alexander and Albert, 1983), R. C. (Abadi *et al.*, 1981; Campion and Latto, 1985), and D. F. (Milner *et al.*, 1991). A few more cases of carbon monoxide poisoning with visual impairments, which either improved rapidly or were less extensively studied, will not be considered here in detail (Schilder and Isakower, 1928; Solomon, 1932; von Hagen, 1941; Cobb and Lindemann, 1943). Despite individual differences these seven cases have many points in common. Considering the aetiology and anatomy of the lesions involved, 6 of the 7 patients suffered from acute or subacute onset of allegedly diffuse and widespread diseases, known to lead to extensive cortical disturbances, namely carbon monoxide intoxications in 5 cases (Adler, 1944; Benson and Greenberg, 1969; Abadi *et al.*, 1981; Alexander and Albert, 1983; Milner *et al.*, 1991) and an intoxication with inorganic mercury vapours in 1 other case (Landis *et al.*, 1982). Only one patient, the one reported by Goldstein and Gelb (1918) did not fit this pattern, having suffered from a penetrating 'mine splinter' wound, which left him comatose for 4 days. In the medical charts

severe bradycardia and intermittent myocloni of the legs were reported. Subsequent investigators (e.g. Bay, 1953) raised the question of whether this patient had suffered primarily from increased intercranial pressure and cerebral oedema, rather than from focal damage due to the penetrating wound.

Since no postmortem studies of carbon-monoxide-induced visual agnosia have yet been reported, the exact anatomical locus of damage remains unknown. However, carbon monoxide poisoning is known to damage the hippocampus and the basal ganglia, to produce subcortical white matter degeneration characteristically involving occipital and splenial fibres, and to lead to diffuse cortical damage – in particular laminar necrosis – as well as multifocal disseminated lesions (Hsü and Cheng, 1938; Schwedenberg, 1959; Richardson *et al.*, 1959; Plum *et al.*, 1962; Lapresle and Fardeau, 1967; Ginsberg, 1980; Lacey, 1981; Briereley and Graham, 1984). Moreover, in acute stages of anoxic injury, irrespective of the aetiology, severe cerebral oedema can occur, leading to herniation with impaired posterior cerebral artery circulation, which in turn would accentuate the anoxic effects of carbon monoxide in this vascular distribution bilaterally. Apperceptive visual agnosia in these patients is probably due to one or more of the following: cortical laminar necrosis interfering with intracortical signal interaction; patchy cortical lesions (salt and pepper infarcts); the cumulative carbon monoxide effect in a compromised posterior circulation; disseminated subcortical white matter lesions; however, the exact cause or causes must remain unknown until postmortem studies are available.

Less is known about the cerebral pathology subsequent to chronic mercury intoxication. On the basis of a few autopsy studies (Sabelaish and Hilmi, 1976; Hay *et al.*, 1963) it appears that mercury has a predilection for white matter, particularly the corpus callosum and the optic nerves, and that its cerbral effects are most prominent in the posterior brain region with a nerve cell loss in all layers, but particularly in layer IV and V. Part of these losses may be due to retrograde or anterograde degeneration after mercury degeneration of the axons (cf. Chapter 8).

The initial clinical picture in the cases with carbon monoxide poisoning was fairly uniform, mostly with an initial phase of coma followed by a wide variety of neurological and neuropsychological disturbances, including extrapyramidal signs, gate disturbances, agraphia, acalculia, amnesia and frontal lobe signs which usually disappeared or greatly improved. Adler (1944) gave some examples of this condition in her patient:

She talked almost incessantly during the first two weeks. Her talk was incoherent, but with clear pronunciation of words. There was marked reiteration. She was disoriented for a time and was unable to give the date of her marriage. She was unable to do simple calculation and could not read. She could write, however, although at first with perseveration and errors.

By far the most striking finding in these patients, however, is that they are considered blind. Adler (1944) wrote:

Several times she complained that she could not see. She had to be fed since she could not find her food, but she identified it by its taste. After two days she recognized nurses as such 'by their white uniforms', as she explained at that time. She was unable to name objects shown to her, and her gaze did not fix on them during the first week. However, she quickly identified people by their voices, and objects like keys by their sound.

Three months after the injury the patient herself gave a report of how she experienced the first days:

At first everything seemed dark to me. Then I could see white – nurses and doctors. I recognized them by their uniforms, and I could distinguish the doctors because of the odour of tobacco. Soon I could distinguish doctors from nurses by the way their hair was done. Doctors do not have curls. The voices helped a lot.

Adler (1944) saw the patient for the first time 5 days after the injury, when she was blind. Two days later she could tell white from dark but could not recognize colours. In the beginning she could not recognize letters or words but she could write. She had a complete acalculia and could not recognize objects, pictures or persons. Hearing, smell, taste, touch, articulation and understanding of words and motor abilities were not impaired.

After varying amounts of time, from a few days to several months, as in the case of Goldstein and Gelb (1918), elementary visual qualities such as colour, visual acuity, brightness discrimination and depth and movement perception returned to normal or improved and could be tested for the first time with some accuracy. One of the hallmarks of this syndrome is that, despite normal or relatively unimpaired elementary visual percepts, recognition of shape or form information may be grossly impaired, as exemplified by the patient of Benson and Greenberg (1969):

He identified a photograph of a white typewritten letter on a blue background as 'a beach scene', pointing to the blue background as the 'ocean', the stationery as 'the beach' and the small typewriter print as 'people seen on the beach from an airplane'.

and further:

He was unable to select his doctor or family members from a group until they spoke and was unable to identify family members from photographs. At one time he identified his own image in a mirror as his doctor's face. He did identify his own photograph, but only by the colour of the military uniform. After closely inspecting a scantily attired magazine 'cover girl', he surmised that she was a woman because 'there is no

hair on her arm'. That this surmise was based on flesh colour identification was evident when he failed to identify any body parts. For example, when asked to locate her eyes he pointed to her breasts.

On perimetry testing, this patient (Benson and Greenberg, 1969; Efron, 1968) had normal visual fields even for small white targets and only a minimal inferior constriction to small red and green targets. He was able to distinguish small differences in luminance (0.1 log unit) and wavelength (7–10 nm) of a test aperture subtending a visual angle of approximately 2 degrees and could detect even small movements easily, but failed to distinguish between two objects of the same luminance, wavelength and area when the only difference between them was in shape.

The inability to distinguish two structures similar in all aspects except for shape is one of the most prominent common denominators of all these cases with apperceptive agnosia and has given rise to the alternative term 'visual form agnosia'. Efron (1968) developed a test to evaluate this ability, which has subsequently been given to most of the patients considered to be apperceptively agnosic (Fig. 11.19). The pair of shapes A are identical, while pairs B–G are not, since the ratio of the lengths of the sides of one of the component figures is progressively increased. As one can see, the test is trivially simple for an individual with normal foveal vision and a 100 per cent correct recognition of the pairs B–G as being different is expected. The patient Mr S., however, was severely impaired at this task. On the one hand he considered the identical pair A to be different in 60 per cent of the trials while on the other the pairs with unequal shapes B–G were recognized as being different; in about 70 per cent of the trials for pairs B–E, and less than 90 per cent of the trials for the markedly different pairs F and G. Since in the very same patient foveal visual acuity, colour vision, discrimination of luminance, size and wavelength as well as movement perception were shown to be normal, Efron (1968) stated that:

The various tasks which Mr S. cannot perform are the identification of objects, geometrical figures, letters, numbers and people. Is there one attribute of these various existents which must be perceived for their identification? The answer is inescapable: they are all identified by their attribute of shape. The perceptual capacity to make discriminations between shapes is therefore a precondition for their recognition and identification.

While this is true for each of the patients in this small group, it is also true that in each of them not all elementary visual submodalities were found to have been processed normally, or to have been tested experimentally or sufficiently well. While foveal visual acuity was found to be normal or near normal in all, the visual field was restricted in the case reported by Goldstein and Gelb (1918) (Fig. 11.3), in our own patient (Landis *et al.*, 1982), the patient

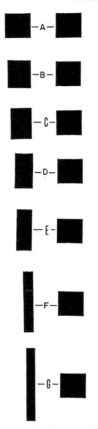

Fig. 11.19 *Efron shapes matched for total light flux and area. The patient is asked to decide whether the two members of a pair have the same shape or not. Pair A is identical; pairs B–G are not. The ratio of the lengths of the sides of one of the component figures is progressively increased (see text) (modified from Efron, 1968).*

reported by Abadi *et al.* (1981) and Campion and Latto (1985), as well as in the patient of Milner *et al.* (1991). With the exception of our own patient, who showed an extremely restricted concentric field defect, leaving a roughly circular field of 1 degree in foveal vision, all other cases showed an intact central vision of 20 degrees or more as measured in conventional dynamic perimetry. However, the functional validity of this measure was questioned by Campion and Latto (1985) on the basis of their patient, who showed only a right inferior field defect on dynamic perimetry, but a number of small patchy scotomatas and areas of reduced brightness sensitivity, when the central 20 degrees were looked at with static perimetry using an 800-dot matrix. Contrast sensitivity functions, when evaluated (Campion and Latto, 1985; Milner *et al.*, 1991), were abnormal in the low-frequency domain.

Colour discrimination, when clinically tested, was minimally abnormal in the patient of Goldstein and Gelb (1918), in whom a slight 'red–green' anomaly for the discrimination of subtle hues was noted; and was minimally abnormal with refined discrimination tests in the cases described by Campion and Latto (1985) and Milner *et al.* (1991). It should however be kept in mind that these patients were successful in identifying most of the colours of the dots of the Ishihara pseudo-isochromatic plates without perceiving the hidden digit, that they had no problem in naming colours or pointing to colours, and that all 7 patients relied heavily on the cueing value of colours in their attempts to recognize form. This point is exemplified by Efron (1968):

> *... his ability to learn the name of an object may suggest to some readers that Mr S. perceives objects normally but has either lost the memory of its name, or lost the visual memory of its appearance. Such a conclusion is not supported by the following experiments which show that Mr S. actually identifies these objects by a process of deduction. In the first place, after he had learned to apply the name 'playing card' to the red and white playing card, he was shown a playing card identical in every way except that it was blue and white. He was unable to identify it. Secondly, when he was shown a red and white postage stamp, he called this object a 'piece of a playing card'...*
>
> *Mr S. could learn to 'identify' correctly an object from a limited repertoire by its attributes of colour, reflectance and/or size, and not by any other attribute. Knowing the entire repertoire, he could deduce which object was before him from the attributes he could identify.*

Similarly, our own patient (Landis *et al.*, 1982) could not distinguish four-legged animals unless a salient feature was prominent. He recognized a line drawing of a female lion in his typical tracing strategy as an animal but guessed that it was a horse or a dog; when a yellow colour was added he identified it as a lion.

Brightness discrimination has been reported to be impaired in the patients of Milner *et al.* (1991) and of Campion and Latto (1985). The patient of Milner *et al.* (1991) was shown to be far better at discriminating colour hues than at discriminating equivalent Munsell achromatic (grey) series (Milner and Heywood, 1989). But even when impaired, such patients do rely on cues about reflectance.

Depth perception, as tested with Julesz (1971) stereograms, was normal when tested (Landis *et al.*, 1982; Milner *et al.*, 1991). Goldstein and Gelb's patient also showed an apparently normal depth perception in the near-distant space. In most of these cases there is no reference about distance estimation in the far-distant space, where appreciation of relative size, partial covering of objects by others and one's own body and head movements become important.

Movement perception was impaired in the patient reported by Goldstein and Gelb (1918) (see also Chapter

19). Clinically, roughly normal movement perception was reported in three cases (Alexander and Albert, 1983; Benson and Greenberg, 1969; Landis *et al.*, 1982). Particularly noteworthy is the fact that Mr S. was reported to rely heavily on movement cues and also to improve detection and to some extent size appreciation by movement (Efron, 1968). This patient could point efficiently to an object only if it was moved; only when two items (e.g. squares) were moved was he able to tell which of the two was larger, except when the differences in size were very small. Apparent movement (the phi phenomenon) was tested in three cases (Goldstein and Gelb, 1918; Landis *et al.*, 1982; Milner *et al.*, 1991) and was shown to be defective in all three. A careful analysis of movement perception with today's standards has only been undertaken by Milner *et al.* (1991). Their patient, D. F., reported great difficulty in estimating the speed of vehicles, which made it impossible for her to cross the road on foot. When initially tested she could accurately report the direction of movement of a random dot shape against a static random dot background, without being able to identify the shape that moved. Since this patient showed abnormal perception of apparent movement in an informal test using three LEDs spaced 1 degree apart and illuminated successively in various combinations, they tested movement systematically with a procedure in which the coherence of a moving dot pattern could be varied. Of 100 displayed dots either 10, 25, 50 or 100 per cent would move in a coherent manner. For normal subjects this task is trivial and only for the most difficult level with only 10 per cent of the dots moving was there less than 100 per cent correct performance (75 per cent). D. F., however, identified the movement direction perfectly when all 100 dots were moving coherently, but fell to chance when only half or less of them were moving. Moreover, when tested for 'biological motion' (Johansson, 1973) she could only detect the direction of the net translation of such 'walking figures', but was at chance on judgements of internal body-forms.

Finally, ocular fixation and pursuit was reported to be abnormal in one patient (Alexander and Albert, 1983) and to have been impaired in the initial phase of disease in two others (Adler, 1944; Milner *et al.*, 1991).

Although intact or only minimally impaired elementary perception of visual qualities stands in striking contrast to the severe impairment of the recognition, discrimination, matching or copying of simple visual forms in these apperceptive agnosics, the old idea has recently been revived that the concept of apperceptive agnosia is nothing more than some form of primary sensory impairment (Warrington, 1985; Warrington and James, 1988; Campion and Latto, 1985). Some observations, however, speak against this view:

1. An impairment or even a loss of a single elementary

visual quality does not lead to a profound effect on form recognition; it may even pass unnoticed by the patient, a fact which has been taken as an argument against a physical signal convergence of the different elementary visual processing lines (Baumgartner, 1990).

2. Alterations of different elementary visual functions in these patients make it unlikely that a relatively homogeneous syndrome would be produced, as is evidenced by the strikingly similar observations made in such patients over a time span of some 80 years by different observers.

The clinical similarities in these patients may be divided into two groups of observations, namely those which indicate an inability to use 'Gestalt grouping principles', and those which indicate the relative preservation of visuo-motor skills.

The Gestalt Aspect of Apperceptive Visual Agnosia

A number of basic figural properties are, according to Gestalt psychology, easier or harder to perceive. Correspondingly, these figural properties were found to be more or less impaired in patients. We will mention a few examples. Four patients (Goldstein and Gelb, 1918; Adler, 1944; Benson and Greenberg, 1969; Landis *et al.*, 1982) perceived straight lines much better than curved lines. Adler (1944) wrote:

Whereas the patient was not able to recognize any letter during the first two weeks, she occasionally succeeded in recognizing mathematical figures. While she did not recognize the figures 2, 3, 5, 6, 8 and 9, naming them interchangeably 6 or 5, she recognized the 1, 4 and 7 during the second week of her illness. The recognition first of figures with straight lines and later of those with curves is of special interest: the patient perceived only parts and guessed the rest. Since it is possible to guess where a straight line is going but not the direction of a curve, she was able to recognize the figures 1, 4 and 7 first. The first number with a curve that she recognized was 5. This she recognized by the combination of the two straight upper lines. At present, 7 months after the injury, she correctly recognizes any single number. She was conscious of the fact that she distinguished the individual numbers by their special characteristics. A few months ago she explained: 'In a 6 there is only a lower loop. If I find an upper loop, too, I know it is a 3. If there is only an upper loop it is a 9. There are two circles in the 8'.

When tested tachistoscopically for number recognition, this patient needed longer exposure times for an 8 than for a 1 when using this strategy. The following protocol reveals how she finally recognized the 8:

1/150 s. '. . . a 6?' She then corrected herself, saying 'a 3. I first thought the loops were in different directions. Or is it a 5?' When asked to draw what she had seen, she wrote a 5 without the vertical line. 1/100 s. '. . . a 6'. 1/50 s: '. . . 0; it is an 8. All the time I have seen only the lower loop, and therefore I thought it was a 6.'

This performance closely resembles the performance of our own patient (Landis *et al.*, 1982), who perceived simple shapes by tracing them with his left hand. He had much more difficulties with tracing curved than straight lines and had also devised a relatively complicated personal verbal code for individual letters such as:

M – *'two poles like an "H" but has a small "x" inside'.*
W – *'two poles and a half "x" at the bottom instead of the top, the reverse of an M'.*
S – *'two cups, one foward, one backward'.*
D – *'half of a ball'.*
P – *'a pole and a basketball hoop'.*

His own description of his failure to draw a bicycle (Fig. 11.20) offers a good example of the writing problem, and the coda provides an explanation for some of the mirror errors; note that the coda contains no direction to orient the elements and he was unaware of his mirror reversal errors.

The same kind of mirror and upside-down reversal errors in writing have also been described by Adler (1944) when 5 months after the injury her patient successfully formed from cardboard letters the word 'Tracy', where the letter sequence was correct but most of the letters were either upside down or mirror-reversed.

The temporal summing-up procedure observed in Adler's patient with tachistoscopic exposures is not unique. Both Goldstein and Gelb (1918) and the present authors (Landir *et al.*, 1982) have found almost identical effects:

This process can be illustrated by his (X's) identification of the block letter 'R'. At 200 ms exposure he gave no response. With a 1-s. exposure his left index finger began to move a vertical excursion and he said 'I'. With further exposure of 1.5 s. his left index finger made a partial circle and he said 'P'. With additional exposure his left index finger made a straight slanted motion and eventually he said 'R'.

Dissociations in the perception of straight versus curved lines were also reported by Benson and Greenberg (1969).

The recognition of figures composed of dots was especially hard for the patients of Goldstein and Gelb (1918), for our own patient (Landis *et al.*, 1982) and for those patients who used a visuo–motor feedback strategy. Crosshatching of meaningful figures or words (Fig. 11.4), a test originally introduced by Goldstein and Gelb (1918), made recognition impossible, since a slavish tracing would not distinguish between meaningful shapes and crosshatches. Similarly, discontinuation of lines should markedly alter or prohibit recognition with this method. Thus, words written with shadowing (Fig. 18.4) remained an utterly meaningless assembly of lines and edges, whereas the

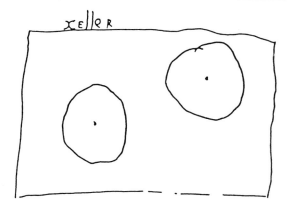

Fig. 11.20 *Attempt of the patient X to draw a bicycle on command, with his written explanation of his problem (see text) (from Landis* et al., *1982).*

word 'THIS', containing broken lines (Fig. 18.4) was never recognized as anything other than 7415 by the patient X (Landis *et al.*, 1982). This example, like many others, suggests that 'top-down mechanisms of perception', so powerful in normal visual recognition, do not act at the level of the disturbance present in these patients. Almost any English-speaking reader would immediately recognize the meaningful and highly overlearned word 'THIS', rather than the relatively meaningless letter combination 7415.

In concordance with Gestalt theoretical concepts, some of the patients suffering from apperceptive agnosia recognized contours of homogeneous surfaces better than line contours, real objects better than photographs of objects and photographs better than line drawings of objects. Furthermore, difficulties in figure–background discrimination are common in those patients. These effects ultimately led Goldstein and Gelb (1918) to conclude that their patient suffered from a basic disturbance of Gestalt formation. A similar conclusion, though worded differently, was reached by Milner *et al.* (1991) when interpreting the findings observed in their patient D. F.:

In order to identify a particular shape, the brain must deter-

mine the orientation of the component boundaries. To do this it can use many different visual submodalities, including intensity, colour, saturation, stereopsis and motion (through shear, occlusion or coherence). It is therefore necessary to conceive of edge orientation, not just as a primary quality extracted by luminance-based 'edge-detectors' but rather as a higher-level attribute. D. F. failed to perceive boundary shape or orientation accurately whether it was conveyed by colour, intensity, stereopsis, motion, proximity, good continuity or similarity: thus edge perception may be disrupted at a high level. She was unable to segment perceptually part of pattern on the basis of common textural properties of size, orientation, intensity or shape (e.g. + vs. T) of its component elements. Such texture discrimination does not require judgements of boundary orientation or shape per se. Perceptual grouping based on similarity in size and intensity would thus seem to be deficient independent of deficits in orientation processing. There therefore seems to be a generalized inability to perceive shape and 'shape primitives', that is, basic figural qualities that would serve in the recognition of many different objects. These would include the Gestalt grouping principles (proximity, closure, similarity, good continuity and common fate) and also other descriptors such as parallelism (Biederman, 1987; Lowe, 1987b). We would argue that D. F.'s form-recognition deficit derives not from a loss of particular input channels (edge detectors) but rather from a deficit arising at a higher level, at or beyond a general purpose mechanism for extracting shape primitives.

Preserved Visuo-motor Abilities in Apperceptive Agnosia

A striking phenomenon observed in four of these patients is the spontaneous use of tracing strategies to help, or to render possible, the recognition of visual form (Goldstein and Gelb, 1918; Adler, 1944; Efron, 1968; Landis et al., 1982). Goldstein and Gelb's patient traced contours both by employing head and hand movements and by using this feedback together with a highly verbalized coding system of figural elements, and succeeded in recognizing some forms. Using this strategy he could recognize a number of relatively simple items, including letters and, by summation, even words, provided they were written in print or in his own handwriting. Cross-hatching made this procedure meaningless and recognition was therefore abolished. Our own patient used a similar strategy and could recognize simple geometric figures, provided that the point of departure for tracing was unimportant (e.g. a circle or triangle). With more complex figures he was usually misled by unimportant details. He failed to recognize shapes if his hand was prevented from moving, if lines were interrupted or if cross-hatches covered the item to be recognized. Adler (1944) mentioned that her patient started to use the index finger to trace the contours of objects in order to facilitate perception about two weeks after the injury. Efron (1968) summarized similar findings:

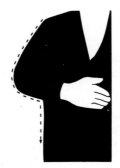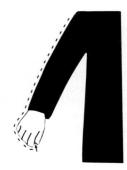

Fig. 11.21 *Attempt of the patient Mr S. to locate the hand (see text). The dotted line indicates the path traced by the patient when he was able to locate the hand (right), and when he failed to do so (left) (modified from Efron 1968).*

After he (Mr S.) has located an object, he can trace its contour with his finger ... he will often go around a simple figure many times, not knowing that he has completed the task ... in those cases in which he is asked to trace a complex object, he will almost always follow the contour of a single colour area ... when asked to find the examiner's hand, or the hand in a colour photograph of a person, Mr S. traced the outer (silhouette) contour of the body until he came to the region of the hand. On some occasions he stopped and indicated that he had achieved the goal; at other times he continued to follow the silhouette contour, apparently failing to recognize that he had passed the hand. On those occasions in which the arm and hand were not outstretched and thus did not appear in a silhouette projection, he never managed to locate them. (Fig. 11.21).

A somewhat similar aspect of preserved visuo-motor function was found by Milner et al. (1991) in their patient D. F. She was able to modify the posture of her hand to match the orientation of a slot towards which she was reaching, yet she was unable to perceive the orientation of the slot by visual cues alone. Moreover, in a recent study of D. F. by Goodale et al. (in press: cited in Milner et al., 1991) the patient was found to obtain implicit knowledge of the size and orientation of solid rectangular objects when asked to reach and grasp them. Goodale et al. compared their findings with those in patients with optic ataxia (Perenin and Vighetto, 1988), who showed the inverse dissociation. That is, they were able to judge the orientation of a visual slot, but failed to use such orientation information to guide their hand movements towards and into the slot. In both phenomena, the correct tracing, reaching or shaping of the hand indicates that there must be direct routes from early visual contour analysis to the cerebral areas of the posterior parietal lobes involved in visuo-motor coordination, bypassing visual areas involved in conscious pattern recognition. Milner et al. (1991) conjectured that there exists a direct route from visual boundary analysis in area V1 to the parietal areas important for visuo-motor coordination, which is responsible for this phenomenon and which, in some of these cases, appears to be the only way to 'see'.

Anatomical Findings in Cases with Apperceptive Agnosia

There is as yet no single patient with apperceptive agnosia who has come to autopsy. However, in several of these patients computer tomography (CT) and single photon emission computer tomography (SPECT) have been performed. One must keep in mind, however, that diffuse lesions, in particular cortical laminar necrosis, as observed in carbon monoxide or mercury intoxication, are usually not visualized using neuroimaging techniques. While in our case (Landis *et al.*, 1982) the CT scan was normal, a CT scan of R. C. (Abadi *et al.*, 1981; Campion and Latto, 1985) recorded three years after the injury showed a large low-density area in the left occipital lobe, involving predominantly lateral aspects of the striate and peristriate area, as well as a somewhat smaller low-density lesion in the lateral peristriate area of the right occipital lobe. Neuroimaging was most extensive in the case of Milner *et al.* (1991). Early CT scan (11 days after onset) was reported to show small, low-density areas on the right side at the level of the internal capsule and around the body of the left lateral ventricle, while a CT scan 9 weeks later was considered normal. Early SPECT (after 4 weeks) showed a reduced flow in the left posterior parietal and temporo-occipital region most marked at the temporo-occipital junction, together with widespread hypoperfusion in the frontal areas on both sides, while SPECT after 8 months was reported to have shown a symmetrical hypoperfusion bilaterally in the parieto-occipital regions without abnormality in the striate cortex, the frontal or the temporal lobes. The early MRI (after 17 days) was reported to have shown damage at the level of the lentiform nucleus bilaterally and, less clearly, in the temporo-occipital cortex on the left side. The most striking finding, however, became visible in MRI scans taken 13 months after injury: distinct and extensive alteration of both lateral occipital cortices was visible. It included the polar convexity and extended into the parasagittal occipito-parietal region. This lesion certainly would fit with the hypothesis advanced by Milner and Heywood (1989) and Milner *et al.* (1991) of a disturbance predominantly of the magnocellular projection system, damage to which they suggest is primarily responsible for the occurrence of apperceptive agnosia. However, it is difficult to imagine a completely intact parvocellular 'projection system' which does not provide enough information for pattern recognition to be possible. Moreover, depending on the weight one gives to the early SPECT findings, medial occipito-temporal areas have been involved as well.

Visual Associative Agnosia (Visual Object Agnosia)

Variability of Symptoms in Visual Asociative Agnosias

The term visual associative agnosia derives from Lissauer's distinction of a two-stage recognition process from apperception to association, association being: 'The stage of associating other notions with a content of apperception.' (see p. 184). Associative visual agnosia was rigidly defined by Teuber (1968) who would not accept either a distortion of visual percept or a disorder of naming to be present in this condition. Visual object agnosia thus is 'in its purest form a normal percept that has somehow been stripped of its meaning'. The controversies surrounding this concept are mentioned in another section of this chapter, but it was evident with such restrictions that a 'pure' visual object agnosia, if it exists at all, must be a very rare event. However, a small number of reported cases do fulfil the definition of Teuber (e.g. Rubens and Benson, 1971; Taylor and Warrington, 1971; Lhermitte *et al.*, 1972; McCarthy and Warrington, 1986).

Benson (1989) operationalized the condition in the following way:

Patients with associative visual agnosia cannot name on visual stimulation but easily copy figures or written material. Tactile or auditory stimuli are named normally. Routine language testing shows no significant abnormality and the IQ is normal except for those test modalities demanding visual identification. Of significance, individuals with associative visual agnosia do well on many visual tests such as hidden figures, block designs, etc.

There are three major requirements in order to make this diagnosis:

1. Elementary visual perception should be intact, or at least intact enough for the patient to be able to copy objects or drawings they cannot recognize, or to match pairs of them as being the same or different. The ability to produce an adequate copy of a visual stimulus is considered to be sufficient proof of an intact perception which then has the potential to allow for recognition.
2. The presented visual stimuli should be normally recognized through modalities other than vision, i.e., by touch or hearing characteristic sounds. This point is of considerable importance because extravisual recognition is frequently tested relatively loosely, but when it is tested formally (De Renzi *et al.*, 1987; Feinberg *et al.*, 1986; Ratcliff and Newcombe, 1982; Taylor and Warrington, 1971; Beauvois, 1982) impairment in tactile naming is not infrequently found. As with other clinical behavioural neurological syndromes, however, we feel that the relative impairment in one faculty in proportion to impairments in

other faculties should guide classification into syndromes, rather than a search for pure and 'absolute' defects.

3. The difficulty in recognizing meaningful visual stimuli should not be restricted to naming but should extend to classification into semantic and behavioural categories and also to recognition of meaning by function, e.g. gesturing. It is important to test semantic categorization and non-verbal indication of comprehension of meaning, since these functions may be preserved in patients suffering from 'optic aphasia', a condition similar to but distinctly different from visual associative agnosia (e.g. Freund, 1889; Lhermitte and Beauvois, 1973; for a recent review see Farah, 1990). Optic aphasia is a condition in which many more semantic than visual errors occur and which can be interpreted as the consequence of a disconnection between the higher visual association areas and the speech centres of the left hemisphere.

When the diagnosis of a 'pure' visual disturbance is made, failure of recognition of meaningful stimuli is ensured and optic aphasia is ruled out; the crucial test to distinguish apperceptive and associative agnosia is the ability of the patient to make a recognizable copy of a presented meaningful visual stimulus, thus verifying the patient's apperceptive appreciation of the shape of the stimulus. At first this test seems straightfoward, but as in the clinical examination of prosopagnosia and topographagnosia (Chapters 14 and 21), the question arises as to whether such a copy is performed in a 'normal' way, or whether compensatory or circumventing strategies are used by the patient. By means of such compensatory strategies an existing apperceptive agnosia can be disguised. A finding pointing in this direction has been reported by many observers. That is, agnosic patients use an enormous amount of time for copying in a slavish manner line by line, often losing track while drawing (e.g. Brown, 1972; Levine, 1978; Wapner *et al.*, 1978; Ratcliff and Newcombe, 1982; Humphreys and Riddoch, 1987). During such a prolonged time, the patients can correctly perform the copy test using a sequential strategy of copying bits and pieces one after the other – a result which would not be proof of 'normal' perception. Levine (1978) therefore proposed that normal visual perception can be assured only when accurate drawings of briefly exposed visual stimuli are performed. In fact, in some patients considered to be associative visual agnosics, the quality of performance drops sharply with decreased presentation time of stimuli on the tachistoscope (e.g. MaCrae and Trolle, 1956; Cole and Perez-Cruet, 1964; Levine, 1978). The increasing difficulty in recognition between real objects, photographed objects and line drawings (e.g. Boudouresque *et al.*, 1972; Mack and Boller, 1977; Cambier *et al.*, 1980; Ratcliff and Newcombe, 1982; Riddoch and Humphreys 1987a; Levine and Calvanio, 1989), and also the difficulty produced by covering parts of an object

(Rubens and Benson, 1971), indicates that in fact many 'associative' visual agnosics have difficulties in recognizing perceptual qualities or even shape-primitives p.206), a defect which is usually taken rather as a sign of apperceptive agnosia. It thus appears, that within the group of patients considered by the above criteria to suffer from associative visual agnosia there exists a considerable variation along a continuum of defects, rather than a sharp border between apperception and association. It should be kept in mind that in Lissauer's (1890) case, discussed earlier, Lissauer himself did not consider this patient to have suffered from a pure form of visual associative agnosia, but rather from a mixture of impairments of apperceptive and associative functions, in which the associative defect predominated.

The question of visual associative agnosia as a discrete entity is further rendered difficult by the fact that the lesions reported to create this syndrome are very heterogeneous with respect to localization as well as to aetiology, ranging from unilateral right posterior lesions to unilateral left posterior lesions and with a large number of bilateral posterior lesions with various degrees of asymmetry.

If one loosens the definition of visual associative agnosia to the point of accepting any relatively correct copy, irrespective of the way it was done, then it could be said that a large and increasing number of such cases have appeared in the literature (e.g. Lissauer, 1890; Mueller, 1892; Souques, 1907; Niessl von Mayendorf, 1935; Duensing, 1952; Hécaen and Ajuriaguerra, 1956; MaCrae and Trolle, 1956; Hécaen and Angelergues, 1963; Cole and Perez-Cruet, 1964; De Renzi and Spinnler, 1966; Scheller, 1966; Körner *et al.*, 1967; Lhermitte *et al.*, 1969; Rubens and Benson, 1971; Boudouresques *et al.*, 1972; Lhermitte *et al.*, 1973; Hécaen *et al.*, 1974; Albert *et al.*, 1975; Mack and Boller, 1977; Levine, 1978; Wapner *et al.*, 1978; Kertesz, 1979; Cambier *et al.*, 1980; Pillon *et al.*, 1981; Bauer, 1982; Ratcliff and Newcombe, 1982; Ferro and Santos, 1984; Gomori and Hawryluk, 1984; Morin *et al.*, 1984; Davidoff and Wilson, 1985; Larrabee *et al.*, 1985; Feinberg *et al.*, 1986; McCarthy and Warrington, 1986; Riddoch and Humphreys, 1987; Mendez, 1988; Levine and Calvanio, 1989). This list is incomplete, and does not refer to many of the cases in the older German and French literature which have been partly reviewed earlier. Nor does it include many of the patients with prosopagnosia or pure alexia which have been dealt with in separate chapters. For a more extensive list of such patients the reader is referred to Farah (1990).

Some Problems in Defining Clinically Visual Object Agnosia

Two points in visual associative agnosia need some further discussion: (a) the heterogeneity of clinical symptoms in patients who can still be considered to suffer from visual associative agnosia, and (b) the relation of the localization of lesions in cases of 'visual associative agnosias' to their symptom presentation and especially to their associated symptoms.

There exist some remarkably pure cases of visual associative agnosia. In none, however, was the disorder of recognition entirely restricted to objects; rather the object recognition difficulties are usually associated with either pure alexia or with prosopagnosia or with both. In some of the patients suffering from alexia or prosopagnosia, however, no or only minimal disturbances of the kind found in apperceptive agnosia could be demonstrated, as evidenced by their good performance in hidden figure recognition, detection of overlapping figures, discrimination between very similar shapes or the detection of gradually degraded stimuli (e.g. McCarthy and Warrington, 1986; Rubens and Benson, 1971).

Here we would like to illustrate the other end of the spectrum, namely, a patient who should still be considered as an associative agnosic, because he had *no* difficulties in tactile, auditory, gustatory and olfactory recognition, and maintained sufficient visual perception in order to adequately copy even quite complex drawings, though requiring considerable time. He failed to understand the meaning of visual stimuli and could neither name nor categorize by gesturing the objects shown to him. According to the definitions mentioned above, this patient suffered from associative agnosia. Extensive testing using supervised learning procedures, however, revealed disturbances which are difficult to understand in terms of a dichotomy of perception and cognition (Scheidler *et al.*, in press).

The patient, M., a 70-year-old man, had a severe reduction in eyesight following a brief loss of consciousness. Prior to this event he had suffered two transient episodes of blindness. Initially he was unable to detect more than bright light sources within a uniform dimness. Within 4 weeks this dimness disappeared and visual acuity improved. By the time of testing, 13 months after the incident, the patient showed a persistent bilateral upper hemianopia and a complete achromatopsia in the remaining lower fields, about which he made no spontaneous complaint. He was prosopagnosic, topographically disoriented, and his initially global alexia without agraphia had improved to single letter reading. He could read short, high-frequency nouns fairly well when they were written in upper-case block letters, but completely failed to read cursive writing and was quite unable to read the same words when they were written in a shadowing fashion or when these words were crosshatched. His ability to copy drawings of objects or geometric shapes as well as letters had been fairly good, though slow and slavish, early after onset, but had even improved later. Initially he did not

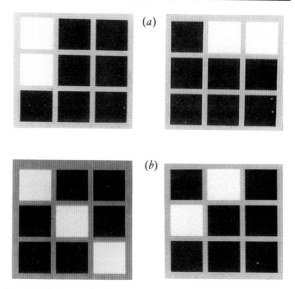

Fig. 11.22 *Examples of stimuli from different classes used in supervised learning (see the text). (a) Vertically and horizontally aligned white squares. (b) Two classes of diagonal alignment of white squares (from Scheidler et al., in press).*

recognize common objects, except by modalities other than vision. Later his visual recognition of common objects became fairly good, although he still had difficulties when these objects were presented to him from unusual perspectives. His ability to recognize photographed or drawn objects, especially from unusual views remained severely impaired. Computer tomography and MRI scans revealed extensive occipito-temporal infarctions bilaterally in the territory of both posterior cerebral arteries.

Supervised visual learning took place over a period of several months, during which the clinical condition of the patient remained stable. In all experiments, the supervised learning procedure consisted of a training phase during which all stimuli were shown to the patient three times, one at a time in a random sequence, and the patient was informed as to what class the stimulus belonged. This training period was followed by a test run where the patient had to identify the class membership of each pattern.

In a first experiment, modified chequerboard patterns were grouped into 2 classes consisting of vertically or horizontally aligned squares (Fig. 11.22(a)). The patient did learn to classify these patterns as quickly and accurately as normal age-matched controls. A modified version with obliquely aligned white squares, where the two classes were aligned on one or the other diagonal, took him only slightly longer to learn than normals (Fig. 11.22(b)).

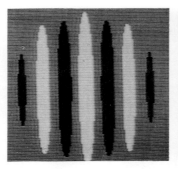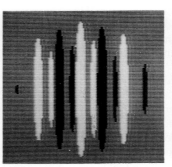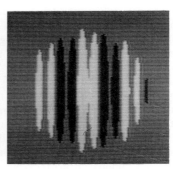

Fig. 11.23 *Examples of a stimulus of each of the three classes of compound Gabor signals used for supervised learning (see the text) (from Scheidler* et al., in press).

The success of the patient in classifying these chequer-board patterns shows (a) that elementary visual functions such as coarse spatial resolution and discrimination of simple geometric figures were relatively unimpaired, (b) that he was able to make decisions as to which category a given simple visual stimulus belonged, and (c) that he was able to synthesize a simple Gestalt out of individual elements.

In the next experiment the patient was given stimuli from three different classes of compound Gabor signals (Caelli *et al.*, 1987; Rentschler *et al.*, 1988) (Fig. 11.23). None of the age-matched controls took more than 3 training runs, while the patient needed 129 training and 43 test runs to successfully classify these patterns. However, he succeeded quite well in classifying stimuli of 1 but not of the other 2 classes. He thus succeeded in constructing an internal representation of this class of pattern by means of which he identified the corresponding test pattern. Such an internal representation is called a prototype in the pattern recognition literature (Ahmed and Rao, 1975; Watanabe, 1985). The behaviour of the patient towards the two remaining classes indicated that he related these patterns to very similar internal representations or prototypes and, moreover, that he had a bias toward the prototype of one of the two remaining classes.

Repeated testing after successful classification revealed that the learned classification performance did not remain stable, except for the class for which a successful prototype had been formed. When, however, he was given one member of each class to compare with as a 'classification aid' he was able to classify all stimuli correctly. From this performance it was deduced that the patient was unable to *construct* the prototypes for 2 of these 3 classes.

The issue of generalization of learned performance was addressed by training the patient to classify the initial pattern and by subsequently testing him with truncated versions of the same stimuli. Normal subjects have no difficulty whatsoever in classifying immediately the trun-

cated versions, once they have learned the original classes. The patient, however, performed very poorly in this task, a result which implies a difficulty in generalizing what he had learned before. Nevertheless, he could be trained with supervised learning to classify these truncated stimuli in much less time than he needed to classify the original pattern, but performance on these new classes was as unstable as with the original ones. This implies that the patient was, to a certain extent, capable of visual learning, but failed to capture similarity relationships between learned stimulus material and unknown test stimuli.

The patient, who was an enthusiastic card player, was now asked to classify cards, which are of course highly complex visual patterns. The patient's performance was tested on his ability to classify an individual card into one of four suits (using black- and white photographs). When this procedure was used for Swiss playing cards (Fig. 11.24(a)) well known to the patient, he not only had no difficulties classifying them according to the suits, but found it very easy to distinguish between individual cards. The performance was identical when a set of French cards, also known to the patient, was used. However, when German cards (Fig. 11.24(b)), very similar in appearance but unknown to the patient, were used, he could not be trained to classify them according to the suits. The experiment was repeated, with him now being provided with a classification aid, i.e. a member of each class (suit) for comparison. He then became capable of correctly stating whether the card which had been displayed was among the classification aids. For instance, if as an example of the spades suit he received the ten he was able to identify it on tachistoscopic presentation, but he could not recognize the spades on the jack of spades or the seven. In other words, the patient's internal representation of the Swiss card game was not as 'prototypical' as it would be in the case of a normal individual. Indeed, it was not generalizable and remained strictly linked to the concrete objects, namely, the Swiss playing cards. It can therefore be said that in this

(a)

(b)

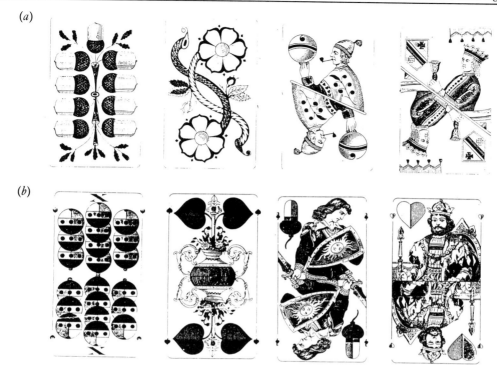

Fig. 11.24 *Examples of playing cards, each card from one of four suits, used as classes for supervised learning (see the text). (a) Swiss cards; (b) German cards.*

patient's visual perception the range of similarity was so narrow that no cards of the German and Swiss suits were perceived as being similar.

While this patient conform to the clinical definition of 'associative visual agnosia', it is nevertheless apparent that he had a number of problems at the ill-defined interface between apperception and association. The pattern recognition approach used in this patient was designed (a) to test his ability to create class representatives or prototypes, (b) to test his ability to relate sensory events to these prototypes in order to recognize, and (c) to test his capacity of generalizing prototypes. This procedure may represent an alternative approach to visual agnosic deficits.

Lesion Location, Contribution of Hemispheres and Varieties of Visual Associative Agnosias

Ever since the recognition of visual associative agnosia, attempts have been made to relate different agnosic symptoms to lesions in either the left or the right hemisphere (e.g. Wilbrand and Saenger, 1917; Hoff and Pötzl, 1937a; Hécaen and Angelergues, 1963; Gloning *et al.*, 1968; Newcombe, 1979; Farah, 1990). This contrasts with the

view of others (e.g. Alexander and Albert, 1983) who consider cerebral damage to be typically bilateral. However, while many cases with associative visual agnosias do in fact have bilateral occipito–temporal damage, there are some cases in which there has been only posterior unilateral left-sided damage (e.g. Hécaen and Ajuriaguerra, 1956; Boudouresque *et al.*, 1972; Pillon *et al.*, 1981; Feinberg *et al.*, 1986; McCarthy and Warrington, 1986) or unilateral right-sided damage (e.g. Levine, 1978; Boudouresque *et al.*, 1979). Moreover, as especially stressed by Hécaen, object agnosia subsequent to lesions in the left hemisphere's visual system is strongly associated with pure alexia, while agnosia associated with lesions in the right hemisphere's system is strongly associated with prosopagnosia. However, since associative visual object agnosia virtually never occurs without being associated with pure alexia or prosopagnosia and these syndromes, when present in isolation, are strongly associated with visual recognition of the visual system of the left or the right hemispheres, respectively (see Chapters 14 and 18), it is tempting to assume parallel but different ways of processing visual object information, one primarily subserved by the left and the other by the right hemisphere's visual processing lines. Obvious candidates for such dichotomies are 'semantic versus perceptual categorization' or 'name-able versus unnameable' object attributes. In the normally functioning individual, these parallel, hemisphere-dependent processes would have only relative dominance and would stand in a continuous dynamic interaction. It should be kept in mind that dynamic interaction with respect to recovery from pure alexia or prosopagnosia in relation to the hemispheric locus of lesion was suggested by Hoff and Pötzl as early as 1937. A discussion of the different cognitive models proposed for the processing of object information is beyond the scope of this book and the reader is referred to a recent review by Farah (1990).

The idea of distinct differences in the processing of object information between the two hemispheres is further supported by a few reports of cases in which subsequent to right or left posterior cerebral lesions parts of the contra-lateral visual field, mostly the inferior quadrant, remained intact and experimental tachistoscopic testing revealed the presence of agnosia only in one hemifield, the so-called hemiagnosias (e.g. Charnallet *et al.*, 1988; Mazzucchi *et al.*, 1985).

Visual Agnosia in Slowly Progressive Dementia

As mentioned earlier, a possible model for studying visual agnosia, i.e. a disorder of higher visual processing in the absence of disturbances of elementary visual qualities, would be a disease which affects associative cortex but leaves primary sensory cortex relatively intact, such as the cortical dementias (e.g. Alzheimer's disease). Although visual agnosias in the framework of degenerative dement-ing disease were recognized early in the history of agnosia research (Pick, 1908), they have received little attention until very recently. Magnani *et al.* (1982; cited in De Renzi, 1986) reported one patient with a slowly progres-sive visual agnosia developing over a 2-year period without major cognitive dysfunction in other areas. Thereafter in rapid succession 10 patients showing a very similar course were reported (Cogan, 1985, 3 cases; De Renzi, 1986, 2 cases; Benson *et al.*, 1988, 5 cases). Until late in the course of the disease all these patients showed intact elementary visual perception, as evidenced by full visual fields, normal visual acuity and good colour recognition. They all had disturbances in copying visual material and could not read though they could mostly still write early in the disease, and were unable to recognize objects, places or persons. Most of these patients also developed signs of unilateral or bilateral parietal disease, including in some cases a com-plete Balint's syndrome. Although their conditions were blurred by a number of additional features, especially those of visuo-motor disturbances, some of these patients

could be considered as having suffered from apperceptive visual agnosia. The clinical presentation, including the sometimes very slow course, is quite consistent in this group and suggests that this condition represents a subva-riety, or even a new entity of slowly progressive dementing disease. As yet these cases have not improved our under-standing of the anatomy or physiology underlying visual agnosias, but early detection of such patients, together with serial experimental study of the visual system, may provide a new approach to disturbances of higher visual processing.

Defective Perceptual Categorization: A Focal Disturbance of Apperception?

While apperceptive visual agnosia as discussed in the pre-vious sections is a syndrome which is devastating for the patient – leaving him in a condition close to 'blindness', with all the social consequences such a severe debility has – the syndrome of 'defective perceptual categorization' usually is not clinically apparent, and can be made evident only by clinico-experimental procedures, usually with photographed or drawn material in which the degree of perceptual difficulty is systematically varied. Again, unlike the apperceptive agnosia sufferers discussed above, such patients are afflicted by focal right-hemispheric posterior lesions and their symptoms, are, if at all, accompanied by various degrees of 'right posterior symptomatology' such as prosopagnosia, topographical disorientation, neglect or disorders of space explorations (discussed in the relevant chapters). Only rarely have difficulties in perceptual categorization *not* been uncovered by experimental investigation, instead becoming clinically apparent when patients could not recognize real objects in real situations if they saw them from unusual perspectives or under natural but perceptually degrading conditions (Levine, 1978; Landis *et al.*, 1988). We would like to emphasize that we consider it inappropriate, even for the sake of purism, to use the quite established term 'apperceptive visual agnosia' for the condition of impaired perceptual catego-rization as a consequence of right posterior focal cerebral lesions. It is of no service to behavioural neurology and neuropsychology where the nomenclature is already con-fusing to further enhance the confusion. Moreover, it makes little sense to call a person an apperceptive visually agnosic patient when they have no problems in reading, can recognize almost all real objects and can name cor-rectly almost all photographs or drawn objects (provided they are not presented under conditions of increased per-ceptual difficulty).

Early evidence for the existence of and concerning the cerebral lesions involved in the syndrome of defective perceptual categorization stems from a series of group studies that have compared patients with left and right unilateral cerebral lesions (e.g. Milner, 1958; De Renzi *et al.*, 1969; De Renzi and Spinnler, 1966b; Warrington and James, 1967a; Benton and van Allen, 1968; Newcombe and Russel, 1969; Kerschensteiner *et al.*, 1972; Warrington and Taylor, 1973a). These authors found difficulties in visual object recognition, usually in an experimental setting, to occur in patients without visual sensory deficits subsequent to postrolandic lesions in the right hemisphere. These difficulties extended over a wide variety of visual stimuli, such as anomalous pictures, faces viewed from different angles or under different shading conditions, overlapping drawings of familiar objects, photographs of objects viewed from unconventional angles, etc. In particular, the experiments performed by De Renzi *et al.* (1969) and Warrington and Taylor (1973) are of tremendous interest to the study of how objects are perceived and recognized. The former authors tested a large series of left- and right-hemisphere-damaged patients with tasks designed to uncover difficulties in either apperception or in association. They found that patients with right-hemisphere lesions do more poorly on apperceptive tests (overlapping figures, matching of faces photographed from different angles), but that patients with left-hemisphere lesions perform more poorly on associative tests (matching real objects to photographs of different items of the same class). The latter authors (Warrington and Taylor, 1973) showed that patients with right posterior damage perform poorly at identifying objects photographed from unusual perspectives (Fig. 11.15), while they performed identically to patients with left posterior damage in identifying objects photographed under 'normal', more 'prototypical' views. From these early experiments were born the dichotomies between left and right hemispheres in visual processing in terms both of apperception versus association and of perceptual categorization versus semantic categorization.

Subsequently, it has been the Warrington group in particular who in an impressive series of experiments using an array of simple and more complex visual stimuli, rendered perceptually difficult by various means (Fig. 11.25; see also Figs. 11.7, 11.8 and 11.15), has experimentally demonstrated the crucial role of the right hemisphere's visual system for perceptual categorization on the basis of data obtained from normal subjects and groups of brain-damaged patients, as well as from the analysis of single cases (Warrington and James, 1967, 1986, 1988; Warrington and Taylor, 1973, 1978; Warrington, 1982, 1985). This group and others (Humphreys and Riddoch, 1984, 1985; Shallice, 1988) have discussed these findings in the framework of Marr's (1982) theoretical approach to object

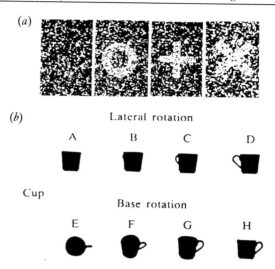

Fig. 11.25 *Two examples of how to render visual stimuli perceptually difficult. In (a) the contrast is altered by superimposing a fragmented character upon a fragmented background (the item on the left is a no-shape control) (modified from Warrington and Taylor 1973). In (b) there is lateral or base rotation of the stimulus (modified from Warrington and James, 1986).*

recognition (cf. Chapter 1). On the basis of their experimental and clinical evidence, Warrington and Taylor (1978) (Fig. 11.26) have proposed a model of visual object recognition with respect to the left and the right hemispheres's visual systems. The important and still controversial issue lies in the fact that, after an analysis of elementary visual submodalities, they introduced a step where all visual information must pass through the right hemisphere's visual system for perceptual categorization, which is then followed by a semantic categorization in the left hemisphere.

In light of the fact that patients with lesions within the right hemisphere's visual processing system can easily read and name real objects without any difficulty, and also can usually identify photographs and line drawings of objects with ease (provided they are not artificially degraded), it seems unlikely that the right hemisphere has an exclusive role in perceptual categorization. These functions are apparently also performed by the left hemisphere's visual system and imply at least some degree of perceptual categorization. It appears to us that the dominance of the right hemisphere for perceptual categorization is *relative* rather than absolute, and that perceptual analysis is done by both hemispheres in parallel, though perhaps not in the same way or with the same degree of success. This point is illustrated by two of our

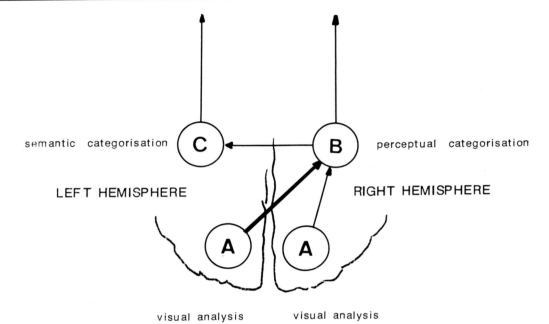

semantic categorisation

perceptual categorisation

LEFT HEMISPHERE

RIGHT HEMISPHERE

visual analysis   visual analysis

Fig. 11.26 *A model of the stages of object recognition proposed by Warrington and Taylor (1978). The important point in this model is that visual information at A from both hemispheres converges upon B in the right hemisphere (emphasized here by a thicker arrow from A to B) and that the semantic categorization unit (C) is not directly connected with A (modified from Warrington and Taylor, 1978).*

own patients (Campbell *et al.*, 1986, Landis and Regard, 1988b), one with a *right*, the other with a *left* posterior lesion. Given handwritten material, the one with a left posterior stroke could only analyse the text as to 'who' had written it but not what it meant while the situation was reversed for the patient with the *right* posterior stroke. Similarly, when analysing facial photographs the one with the *left* posterior stroke could only classify similar grimaces (facial expressions corresponding to different emotional states) across different persons, but could not classify according to the lip-read sound (facial expressions corresponding to the enunciation of vowel sounds), while the opposite applied for the patient with the *right* posterior stroke. These examples of double dissociation of performances irrespective of stimulus material (text, faces) imply different visual analysers at work, both with the ability to make perceptual categorizations.

To conclude this section we shall briefly present the case of a patient who showed clinically relevant difficulties in the recognition of non-canonical views and in whom autopsy findings demonstrated a unilateral lesion in the territory of the right posterior cerebral artery. In discussing this syndrome, we have not considered the numerous cases in which bilateral posterior damage was present, since the possibility of a hemispheric dichotomy of apperception versus association or of perceptual categorization versus semantic categorization cannot be evaluated in such

patients. Nevertheless, patients with bilateral posterior damage may, of course, show clinically relevant difficulties in perceptual categorization.

Our patient (for details, see Landis *et al.*, 1988) suffered from an acute onset of a left homonymous hemianopia subsequent to a large stroke in the territory of the right posterior cerebral artery. She was tested almost daily during the 10 days she was in hospital until she died of a pulmonary embolus. She was shown to be severely prosopagnosic and topographically agnosic but also showed some problems in recognizing objects.

When shown objects or pictures she always took considerable time for visual inspection and, as an initial response, usually denied knowing what they represented. However, she correctly named most of the objects presented in canonical views, that is, in prototypical representations (Fig. 11.15). When shown real objects and small-scale models she was unable to identify the non-canonically presented items (Palmer et al., 1981) but identified them correctly when the same objects were presented in a more canonical view. When shown, for example, a folded pair of glasses (Fig. 11.15(a)) she said 'something made of glass'; shown the same glasses in a more canonical perspective she recognized them. When presented with a toy trumpet from the front or from the top she said 'something made of metal'; when it was shown in a more canonical view from the side she identified it as a trumpet. Although she could not identify an object presented noncanonically, she almost always identified the material out of which it was made and sometimes misidentified it as an object of the same material, such as a key lying flat in the examiner's hand as tweezers.

We have referred here only to the clinically relevant difficulty of recognizing real objects in the situation of bedside examination, where alterations of context, background, viewing angle and position are necessarily achieved rather as they occur in real life situations. More formal testing with a variety of degraded 'artificial' stimuli, as mentioned above, confirmed the results. It must be mentioned though that colour perception, colour matching and colour naming were intact, as were matching of letters and words written in various typefaces, as well as reading and all language functions.

Postmortem findings showed a huge fresh infarct covering the entire territory of the posterior cerebral artery on the right side. The entire left hemisphere was free of lesions except for a barely visible *old* microinfarct in the occipital-parietal region which apparently passed clinically unnoticed (Fig. 14.2).

The present case shows that a unilateral large acute lesion in the right hemisphere's visual system may lead to even clinically relevant deficits in perceptual categorization, but also that this patient's intact left hemisphere's visual system was able to deal with a wide variety of visual stimulus materials quite adequately, a faculty which seems to imply at least some ability of perceptual categorization in the left hemisphere.

Optic Aphasia

Since the time when Freund (1889) distinguished a new entity of 'optic aphasia' from 'mindblindness', controversy has continued not so much about the existence of this special variety, but about where to place it in a functional or anatomical framework. Freund (1889) described a patient in whom naming was impaired only for stimuli in the visual modality. 'Optic aphasia' is, as the name says, a modality-specific anomia. The most representative case analysis of optic aphasia is probably that of Lhermitte and Beauvois (1973). Their patient could not name stimuli presented visually, but naming was intact in response to oral descriptions. The patient suffered not only from optic aphasia but also from agnosic alexia and colour anomia. Analysis of errors to visually presented items showed that there were predominantly semantic misnamings, i. e. the wrong name was situated in the same semantic field as the target item. This is one aspect distinguishing optic aphasia from visual associative agnosia, where predominantly visually similar errors occur. Lhermitte and Beauvois (1973) viewed optic aphasia as a visual–speech disconnection syndrome, in which visual information which has

already been processed in the visual system is prevented from reaching the language areas. Unlike visually agnosic patients, patients with optic aphasia may be able to semantically categorize a visually presented item or even gesture its meaning, while being utterly unable to produce its name. Such patients also frequently show a successful homing-in strategy (e.g. a grasshopper: 'a cricket, not a cricket, a grasshopper') (Lhermitte and Beauvois, 1973). Optic aphasia may be overlooked and erroneously be taken as visual associative agnosia if the above-mentioned points are not considered. Thus, semantic categorization should be tested and the frequency of semantic versus visual errors analysed; gesturing or a homing-in approach is suggestive of the presence of optic aphasia. Optic aphasia is relatively rare, but a number of recent cases can be found in the literature (e.g. Gil *et al.*, 1985; Larrabee *et al.*, 1985; Poeck, 1984; Riddoch and Humphreys, 1987b; Assal and Regli, 1980; Pena-Casanova *et al.*, 1985; Coslett and Saffran, 1989).

The relation between visual associative agnosia and optic aphasia has been viewed differently by different authors, ranging from visual associative agnosia being essentially an optic aphasia (Geschwind, 1965) to optic aphasia being a mild associative agnosia (e.g. Bauer and Rubens, 1985; Kertesz, 1987) or optic aphasia being an associative agnosia with entirely normal perception (Riddoch and Humphreys, 1987b). In the framework of cognitive neuropsychological modelling, optic aphasia is difficult to explain because one would have to postulate a direct route from vision to naming, without passing a step of semantically mediated object naming (Ratcliff and Newcombe, 1982).

Simultanagnosia

Variability of Associated Symptoms

The term simultanagnosia was coined by Wolpert (1924). He described a patient who, subsequent to probably several generalized seizures, complained of peculiar visual disturbances and an inability to read. While visual acuity was fair, Wolpert had difficulties assessing the visual fields of this patient because of his rather fluctuating attention. Although he could exclude a hemianopia, he thought that the patient suffered from a mild concentric bilateral restriction of the visual fields. There was no disturbance in colour perception, but an unusual disability which Wolpert termed 'simultanagnosia – a disturbance of overview'. While looking at pictures, the patient was unable to grasp the whole, although he usually recognized details correctly. Moreover, the patient was unable to read whole words; he fixated each letter individually in order to grasp the meaning of the word by summing up the letters. The patient also had a topographical disorientation. Wolpert interpreted the various symptoms of his patient as being due to a single unitary defect, that of an 'inability to perceive a whole as the sum of its parts'. Not only has the idea of such a unitary defect been criticized (see Weigl, 1964), but the term 'simultanagnosia' has also been used for different clinical syndromes.

Simultanagnosia is a clinical diagnosis made both on the basis of the patient's behaviour (i.e. the inability to grasp more than one visual stimulus at a time, irrespective of its size, and the failure to see the whole, but to recognize parts) and on the basis of the patient's subjective experience. Such patients may describe their difficulties in 'simultaneous perception' quite strikingly:

When observing a complex scene, the patient always stated that he saw but a single object. Thus looking out of the window of a car, he was able to see only one car, then a second, then a third, but always one at a time. ('I know there are many but I only see one'.)(Luria *et al.*, 1963)

While viewing the picture of the 'telegraph boy' (Fig. 11.27), another patient is reported to have said:

A bicycle with the wheel off, crank, pedals, back wheel, a young chap sitting on the bike, something he is carrying on the bike, that's the fork, brake. I can't see it all at once. It comes to me by casting my eye around.'(from Kinsbourne and Warrington, 1962)

The ability to grasp the *whole*, or to attend to more than one visual stimulus at the time may, however, be interfered with by disturbances of different mechanisms, caused by lesions in different structures.

While the two patients above gave almost identical descriptions of their disability and failed to recognize the *whole* scene, they nevertheless had quite different lesions and associated neurological symptoms. In the patient reported by Luria *et al.* (1963), the disease was slowly progressive, accompanied by bilateral pyramidal signs, cortical sensory impairment in the right hand, and a severe oculomotor disturbance (ocular apraxia), which rendered visual field testing impossible, indicating bilateral occipital, or occipito-parietal disease. In the case reported by Kinsbourne and Warrington (1962) there was an acute onset of a right sensorimotor hemisyndrome, a right homonymous hemianopia, alexia without agraphia, and some impairment of colour discrimination, indicating a stroke, most likely in the territory of the left posterior cerebral artery.

It is thus not astonishing to find that the patients reported in the literature to suffer from simultanagnosia form clinically and anatomically a quite heterogeneous group (e.g. Hécaen and Ajuriaguerra, 1954; Luria, 1959; Kinsbourne and Warrington, 1962; Luria *et al.*, 1963; Godwin-Austen, 1965; Tyler, 1968; Kase *et al.*, 1977; Levine and

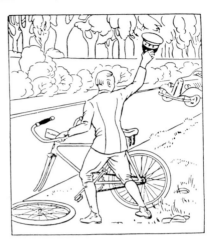

Fig. 11.27 *The picture of the 'telegraph boy' from the Binet scale (see the text).*

Calvanio, 1978; Girotti *et al.*, 1982; Goldenberg *et al.*, 1985; Rizzo and Hurtig, 1987).

Different Types of Simultanagnosia

Given the clinical and anatomical picture, one can discriminate three different classes of simultanagnosia, as follows.

Type (a): Integrative Simultanagnosia
Patients can discriminate single components of an object but are unable to integrate the components into a meaningful whole. For example, they can recognize the wheels, the pedals, the chainwheel and the handlebars of a bicycle, but are unable to recognize the whole bicycle. Patients suffering from this type of simultanagnosia are also not able to recognize an object when only a part is presented, i.e. they suffer from impairment of a visual *pars-pro-toto* function, as discussed in Chapter 15. One can interpret verbal alexia (spelling dyslexia, letter-by-letter reading) as a special case of this type of simultanagnosia, since letters are recognized, but words are not recognized, or only with great difficulty. Wolpert's (1924) patient, who had difficulty in picture interpretation and was alexic, probably had this variety of simultanagnosia. A few patients with this disorder have been described and experimentally investigated (Kinsbourne and Warrington, 1962; Levine and Calvanio, 1978). The threshold for single-letter recognition presented tachistoscopically is found to be the same in such patients as in normal subjects, but to be tremendously increased when more than one letter must be recognized.

The lesions in 'integrative simultanagnosia' are either

bilateral or unilateral *left*-sided infero-medial occipito-temporal. The disorder is not accompanied by optic ataxia (disturbances of visual reaching), nor by ocular apraxia (a disturbance of visual scanning). Such patients do *see* multiple things outside the focus of their attention, but they have difficulties recognizing more than one item at a time. They can walk around without bumping into obstacles and manipulate objects normally.

Type (b): Competitive Simultanagnosia

Patients accurately perceive a single object presented on a homogeneous background, and have no difficulties in object classification and object naming, but report severe difficulties maintaining the perception of one single object when many objects are presented simultaneously in the same part of the extra-personal space. This competitive mutual inhibition of object recognition is increased when part or all of an object moves.

There have been a few patients reported with this type of simultanagnosia. The three patients reported by Rizzo and Hurtig (1987) and the patient of Zihl *et al.* (1983) (cf. Chapter 19) correspond to this subtype of simultanagnosia. The patients of Rizzo and Hurtig (1987) complained that stationary objects in the visual environment would 'disappear' from direct view and this symptom was more pronounced for objects in relative motion. There was no optic ataxia, and analysis of ocular scanning of pictures revealed normal performance. They suffered from an isolated form of what Holmes (1918) called visual disorientation and Balint (1909) called 'spatial disturbance of attention'.

The location of the lesions in all patients suffering from 'competitive simultanagnosia' were bilateral latero-superior occipital. This lesion location, as distinct from the biparieto-occipital location in the full Balint–Holmes syn-drome (cf. Chapter 22), led Damasio (1985) to postulate different 'centres' for the structuring of the visual field as a whole as opposed to '[centres] capable of directing gaze toward interesting new stimuli that appear in panoramic vision and of guiding hand movements toward visual targets' in the superior-occipital and parietal association areas, respectively.

Type (c): Pseudosimultanagnosia

Simultanagnosia may appear in the context of a Balint–Holmes syndrome (cf. Chapter 22). The patients are neither able to shift their attention nor gaze across extra-personal space (ocular apraxia). They fixate their gaze at one object for many seconds. Meanwhile the other objects 'fade out' from the percept. This state has a retinal analogue: when a retinal image is stabilized on the retina it disappears within a few seconds. One of the authors (O.-J. G.) was once the subject in a study in which the effects of eyeball immobilization by retrobulbar injection of a local anaesthetic were tested. When complete external ocular palsy was achieved and the head was also immobilized, the visual world disappeared within a few seconds into a homogeneous neutral grey except for a small foveal field, where visual perception was maintained because of small movements of the eyeball in the orbit caused by heart-rate-synchronous and respiration-induced pulsations of the retro-orbital veins.

Most of the patients reported to suffer from 'pseudosimultanagnosia' have other features of the Balint–Holmes syndrome in addition to visual disorientations, in particular 'ocular apraxia' (Hécaen and Ajuriaguerra, 1952; Luria, 1959; Luria *et al.*, 1963; Godwin-Austen, 1965; Tylor, 1968; Girotti *et al.*, 1982; Karpov *et al.*, 1979). The location of the lesions in these cases is usually bilateral occipito-parietal.

12 Man as a Social Partner in the Visual World: Perception and Recognition of Faces and Facial Expression

Introduction

Since the appearance of Aristotle's book on physiognomy, scientific interest in faces and facial expression has been constant in Western thought and has periodically become a fashionable topic. In the days of Renaissance science, Giambattista della Porta's (1538–1615) book *De humana physiognomia* (1586) was the most famous one on this topic. Porta tried to evaluate different human physiognomies by searching for similarities with animal faces, and evidently produced a primitive characterological evaluation of the human face (Fig. 12.1). During the time of the Enlightenment studies of human physiognomy became especially popular. Since then, many people have believed that simple morphological features of the face are useful signs for making characterological evaluations. Johann Kaspar Lavater's (1741–1801) *Physiognomische Fragmente zur Beförderung der Menschenkenntnis und Menschenliebe* (Physiognomic fragments for furthering the knowledge and love of man; 1775–1778) and Johann Jacob Engels' (1794–1802) *Ideen zu einer Mimik* represent this tendency, which interpreted the body and its expressive movements as a visualization of the soul.

Of the nineteenth century anatomists, Charles Bell was one of the first to investigate the role played by the different facial muscles in facial expression (*Anatomy and Physiology of Expression*, 1806/1844). Charles Darwin's book *The Expression of the Emotions in Man and Animals* (1872) set the standard for further research on the physiology of expression. Darwin relied on data obtained by Duchenne, who described in his *Mécanisme de la Physiognomie humaine* (1862) the contraction of single face muscles evoked by electrical stimulation and its impact on facial expression. Darwin systematically classified different types of facial expression and tried to integrate them into a more general biological context. The same goal was pursued by Piderit (1858, 1867) in his books on physiognomics and facial expression and by Gratiolet (1865).

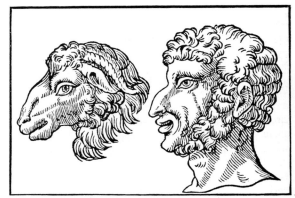

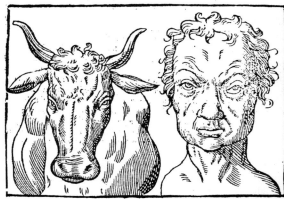

Fig. 12.1 *Two examples of della Porta's comparisons of human and animal faces (from 'De humana physiognomia', 1586).*

218

Modern research on human social interaction continues in the tradition of Bell and Darwin, interpreting the face and facial expression as visual signals important for spontaneous, averbal human interaction. Averbal human communication is based on the recognition of 'key stimuli' by elementary inborn releasing mechanisms. Although these mechanisms are heavily modified by learning during childhood and adolescence, they nevertheless seem to constitute a set of signals that can be generated and understood by all men (cf. Eibl-Eibesfeldt, 1972, 1988). There is a universally understood set of facial expressions and gestures signalling love, social aggression, the need for social help, farewell, social superiority or social submission, joy and sadness.

In this chapter we review some of the many neuropsychological studies dealing with perception and recognition of faces and facial expression. Since a huge amount of experimental data has been obtained in this field during the last 20 years, only a representative selection of data and interpretations is presented. For more extensive modern reviews, the reader is referred to the books edited by Bruyer (1986) and Ellis *et al.* (1986).

Is Face Recognition Distinct from that of Other Complex Visual Patterns?

Before we discuss impairments of perception and recognition of faces, facial expression and gestures caused by circumscribed or diffuse brain lesions, we shall present some facts and thoughts on 'normal' face recognition which are only in part deducible from neurobiological studies (cf. Grüsser, 1984). Visual identification of faces and facial expression is an important component of nonverbal, human social behaviour. As we shall discuss later on, man possesses several basic visual brain mechanisms allowing for perception of faces, facial expression and gestures, as do other primates which interact socially with one another (whereby the individuality of the group member plays an important role). Primates and many 'lower' mammals communicate their mood and social intentions partly by means of face signals and visual 'body language'; in many species, however, olfactory signals also play an important or even dominant role. In man, however, visual and auditory signals dominate group interaction.

In many primate species, and certainly in man, the individual structure of the face is the most important set of visual signals characterizing each group member. Face signals convey two types of information: static, structural signals, which indicate individuality, age, gender and race; and dynamic signals, which convey facial expression and indicate mood, intentions and and social eye contact. Dynamic face signals are frequently complemented by gestures. The elementary face signals can be modified by make-up or other paraphernalia such as glasses, earrings, a beard or a type of haircut. Face signals are always perceived in the context of who is interacting with whom, i.e. behavioural consequences depend not only on the signal, but also on whether or not the 'sender' and 'receiver' know each other and their respective social ranks. Nevertheless, some of the basic responses to face stimuli are 'rank-independent' and rely on presumably inborn mechanisms. A special class of visual face signals are those emitted by the mouth region during speaking. These signals are visually perceived by lip reading and modify the auditory perception of language in normal verbal communication (McGurk and McDonald, 1978; Campbell *et al.*, 1986).

Man can discriminate and recognize several thousand different faces, undoubtedly more than most people were able to see in their entire lifetime up to a few hundred years ago. Photography, movies and television have increased tremendously the number of individual faces seen by each member of our society. Although the capacity for face memory has not been investigated very thoroughly, one can assume that the number of faces appearing in the media is certainly beyond the average memory capacity of most people – even of those politicians who require a well-developed face recognition ability for their professional career.

Man's enormous capacity to discriminate and remember so many faces and shades of facial expression successfully raises the question of whether or not particular 'face-specific' perceptual and memory functions have developed in the human brain in addition to the cerebral perceptual mechanisms used for general object recognition. Several observations described in the following sections as well as prosopagnosia, which is discussed in Chapter 14, support the idea that the recognition of face structures and that of facial expression are related to two distinct classes of brain mechanisms that developed during primate and/or hominid phylogenesis. These two types of visual mechanisms also operate, however, for patterns other than 'real' faces. It seems plausible that animals and man-made structures which have 'physiognomic' properties, such as houses, cars, furniture, dishes, aeroplanes, etc., also belong to the class of visual signals which are processed by some of the 'face-specific' cerebral mechanisms, probably because they partly fit the neuronal face-template (cf. Chapter 7). This idea is supported by several recent studies (Bradshaw and Sherlock, 1982; Anderson and Parkin, 1985). Furthermore, some 'face-specific' cerebral functions may be 'specific' not only for faces alone, but also for other parts of the living body or for the shape of a whole person. The same cerebral mechanisms are also involved in the recognition of animal faces.

Similar considerations may also be true for the neuronal mechanisms contributing to the recognition of facial expression, i.e. the dynamic face signals, in that they extract information about the actual emotional state of the 'sender'. Certain 'expressions' supposedly seen in animal faces, which are produced by certain structural configurations, lead to erroneous judgements by non-expert human observers about the animal's character and mood. The well-known examples of the 'arrogant and supercilious' camel or the 'stupid' bulldog are a result of the fact that the structural patterns of animal faces fit into certain neuronal templates used in the recognition of human facial expressions. We think that these 'errors' indicate the flexibility as well as the limits of the two specialized neuronal mechanisms, which select from an infinite set of complex visual structures those fitting roughly into the template 'human face' and/or into one of several templates that recognize different emotional states. In addition, dynamic face signals may be used to transmit meaningful, non-emotional signals between human subjects. These signals must be learned, of course, in order to be correctly understood.

Under certain conditions, our ability to recognize faces and facial expression can be misled. Persons interacting with patients suffering from Parkinson's disease, for example, often misjudge the patient's mask-like facial appearance, which can easily be perceived to be depressive or unemotional. Similarly, people suffering from involuntary motor facial movements (tics) are often believed to be stupid, which constitutes another incorrect judgement of facial expression. One should also be very cautious when interpreting hypo- or paramimic face patterns such as those appearing in patients suffering from large right hemispheric lesions (Landis *et al.*, 1990). In everyday life, nevertheless, we rely on elementary and rather 'primitive' judgements of physiognomy and facial expression. The physician should at least be aware that under certain conditions, his simple, naive interpretation of the patient's face, facial expression or gestures can be misleading. Finally, disfiguration of the face caused by injuries, especially burn scars, evokes fear-like responses in the observer, which, even when consciously compensated for, still have an impact on social interaction. Reactive depressive states and social withdrawal may result on the part of the injured person.

Hominid Phylogenesis and Face Recognition

A part of our ability to recognize faces and facial expressions is shared with other primates, specifically with monkeys and the great apes (Rosenfeld and van Hoesen, 1979; Bruce, 1982; Vermeire *et al.*, 1983; Dietrich, 1984; Fuhry

and Grüsser, 1989a). Charles Darwin (1872) emphasized the homology of facial emotional expression in man and other primates (cf. also van Hoof, 1967, 1976; Redican, 1975). Some differences in facial expression between non-human primates and man are not caused by different innervation patterns, but rather by structural differences in the skull and facial muscles. Moreover, differentiation of face muscles is much more refined in man than in other primates, allowing for a greater variety of possible facial expressions. The basic emotion-related innervation patterns of homologous muscles are very similar, however, in man and other primates. Thus, with some training, behavioural biologists can learn to interpret the different facial expressions and gestures used by monkeys and apes (e.g. van Lawick-Goodall, 1971; Goodall, 1986, in chimpanzees).

Early hominids such as *Australopithecus afarensis*, which lived more than 3 million years ago, formed social groups of probably no more than 120 to 150 members. A similar estimate also holds true for early man (*Homo habilis*), who lived approximately 2 million years ago; even smaller numbers may be true for a 'tribe' of *Homo habilis* contemporaries, the australopithecines *A. africanus* and *A. robustus*, who lived up to 0.5 million years ago. Groups of early man certainly met other hominid groups, but one can assume that the overall number of other men seen by *Homo habilis* in a lifetime did not exceed several hundred. Similar numbers probably hold true for *Homo erectus* and *Homo praesapiens*. It was not until after the Neolithic period of *Homo sapiens sapiens* that the number of fellow men seen during a lifetime increased as a result of the expansion of settlements from villages into cities, and the development of trade across considerable distances. The structural variability of the skulls of *Homo erectus* and *Homo praesapiens* indicates that individual facial differences were indeed present and could be used to discriminate between other men and women.

Looking at endocasts of hominid skulls, one realizes that pre-frontal (supraorbital) and parieto-temporal cortical integration areas were less well developed in *Homo habilis* and *Homo erectus* than in modern man (e.g. Tobias, 1971, 1979, 1985; Delson, 1985; Fig. 15.1). One can therefore argue that *Homo habilis*, and presumably *Homo erectus* as well, were only in command of a rather restricted verbal language, and that non-verbal signals may have played a more important role in social communication than is the case today. The bilateral neocortical brain structures believed to be essential for face recognition and facial expression in modern man were well developed in these early men. These considerations suggest a phylogenetic priority of non-verbal over verbal hominid social communication. This idea is supported by the observation that a certain set of facial expressions and gestures is applied and understood universally, regardless of cultural background (e.g. Eibl-Eibesfeldt, 1967, 1972). The fact that rudimentary recognition and understanding of faces, facial expression and gestures is present during the first month of life also supports this interpretation (see below). A basic neuronal structure responsible for face recognition, facial expression and body language seems to be present in all men; its phylogenetic development preceded the development of the sophisticated neuronal mechanisms used for verbal communication. Of course, the operation of the structures controlling averbal social communication is heavily modified by cultural habits and social learning during the first two decades of life; presumably the learning process begins right at birth (see below).

Faces, Masks and Portraits

Palaeoanthropological artifacts demonstrate that artistic interest in human faces and the figure of the human body has been in existence since the oldest known documents recording the artistic activity of men (this does not include the sophisticated stone tools that functioned as pieces of art rather than as utensils). Man-made sculptures of human bodies have existed since the times of early *Homo sapiens sapiens*. The first sculptures that appeared in the Upper Palaeolithic Age (about 30,000 years ago) most likely depict mother goddesses. Most of the early Palaeolithic and Neolithic statuettes that have been found have highly schematic faces. Only a few exhibit – at least with some imagination – individual features: the impressive head of the small statuette discovered in La Grotte du Pape in Brassempouy, France, which dates from about 25–22,000 BC (Sandras, 1968; Fig. 12.2(a)), for example, or the caricatural engraving of a male face on the wall of a cave near Marsalon in France (Leroy-Gourhan, 1971; Fig. 12.2(b)) from about 15,000 BC (Müller-Karpe, 1968). As seen in the drawings of 4- to 6-year-old children, prominent facial features, i.e. eyes, nose and mouth, are frequently over-emphasized; this is also true not only for Neolithic cave drawings, but also for drawings on pottery or on the walls of Mediterranean houses or tombs dating back to the Bronze and Iron Ages (e.g. early Greek, Minoan or Etruscan art, Fig. 12.2(c)). Such schematic faces should not be interpreted as a lack of artistic skill. Rather, one should assume that only a minor artistic interest in the individual face existed at that time. Schematic faces and mask-like artistic objects are still considered attractive today; many of the face paintings produced by twentieth-century Western artists were evidently influenced by the structure and expressions of tribal masks (Rubin, 1984). A schematic or schematically deformed face as well as a 'realistic' face both fit into the same neuronal templates and therefore constitute an effective pattern attracting the attention of the observer

(leading to foveal fixation). This is even true when parts of the face, such as pairs of eyes or mouths, appear isolated, as is the case in many of Joan Miró's paintings, for example.

A selective enhancement of certain components of the human face (e.g. eyes, eyebrows, teeth, etc.) is also evident in the sculptures and masks that have been collected by anthropologists in nearly all parts of the world. These objects played an important role in the religious rituals of many Neolithic societies. Masks symbolizing demons, deceased ancestors, forest gods, etc. are still found in today's Neolithic cultures and are used during ritual dances and ceremonies (e.g. Kussmaul 1982; Fig. 1.5). Masks with an exaggerated eye–mouth region, for example, denote 'defensive' or 'aggressive' states. Dionysian dancers as well as the chorus members appearing in pre-classical and classical Mediterranean theatre wore schematic human face masks exhibiting stereotypical facial expressions; this was particularly true for the Greek tragedies written from the sixth to fourth centuries BC. Masks or mask-like face paintings are still worn today during Western carnivals and Hallowe'en festivities; they are also important, for example, in Japanese Kabuki and Noh theatre (Pound *et al.*, 1963). As in older religious dances, the individual actor disappears behind the mask. The make-up worn by actors in Western theatrical productions is a vestige of this tradition.

In Western culture, it was not until the fifth century BC that Greek artists began to sculpture individual faces. A similar development had begun 2200 years earlier in Egypt, where the representation of individual faces was usually restricted to members of the ruling families and high-ranking officials (Buschor, 1960; Rachewiltz, 1966). Their busts, which also served religious purposes, appear to be a combination of prominent individual and common idealized features (Fig. 12.2(d)). During the development of the first democratic or republican systems in Athens and Rome, stone portraits began to place emphasis on individuality. In the busts of Greek philosophers and politicians from the fourth and third centuries BC, individual features frequently outweigh idealized ones. One of the most important artists of this period, Lysippos, appears to have used plaster moulds of living faces as models for his portraits (Giuliani, 1980). Similarly, the sculptures of politicians living in Rome between the second century BC and the second century AD strongly express individuality: they were used not only as demonstrations of the power held by influential families but also as political propaganda aimed at procuring prestigious state positions.

Some individual features are also recognizable in the wall paintings found in Pompeii and Herculaneum (first century BC to first century AD). The sculptures of the late Roman emperors, dating from the first century BC to the fourth century AD, combine some individual features with

(a)

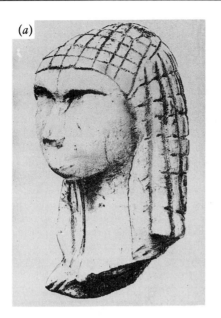

(b)

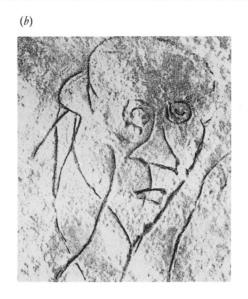

(c)

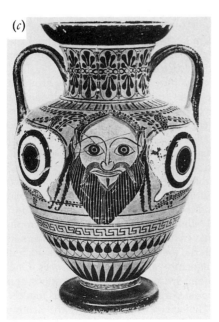

(d)

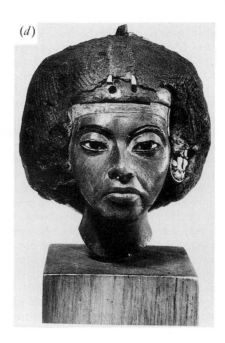

Fig. 12.2 *(a) Woman's head from Grotte du Pape, Brassempouy, France, about 25,000–22,000 BC. Retouched Xerox copy from a photograph published by Sandras (1968). (b) Cave drawing of a face in Marsoulas, Haute-Garonne, France, about 15,000 BC. Xerox copy from a photograph published by Leroi-Gourhan (1971). The engraved lines are amplified. (c) Vase from Attica, 6th century BC, Munich, Staatliche Antikensammlung. In addition to the head of a Silen, two large eyes enhance the threatening expression of the face. (d) Queen Teje. Egyptian, 18th dynasty, about 1370 BC, Berlin, Ägyptisches Museum, No. 21834, Müller and Settgast 1976 (from Grüsser, 1984). (e) The French caricaturist Charles Philipon was fined 6000 Francs for depicting the French King Louis Philippe (1753–1850) as a pear. In response to this sentence, he asked for which stage of transformation of the face portrait to the pear he was fined the 6000 Francs (from Charles Philipon: 'Les Poires' in the Journal 'Charivari', 1834). Note how the malicious facial expression increases with the degree of caricaturizing abstraction.*

(e)

LES POIRES,

Faites à la cour d'assises de Paris par le directeur de la CARICATURE.

Vendues pour payer les 6,000 fr. d'amende du journal le *Charivari.*

(CHEZ AUBERT, GALERIE VERO-DODAT)

Si, pour reconnaître le monarque dans une caricature, vous n'attendez pas qu'il soit désigné autrement que par la ressemblance, vous tomberez dans l'absurde. Voyez ces croquis informes, auxquels j'aurais peut-être dû borner ma défense :

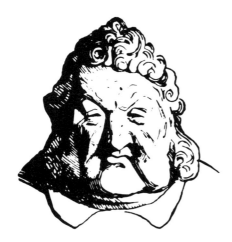 

Ce croquis ressemble à Louis-Philippe, vous condamnerez donc ?   Alors il faudra condamner celui-ci, qui ressemble au premier.

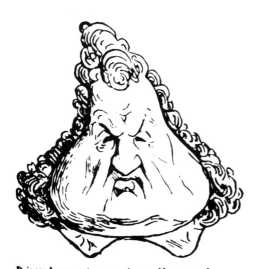 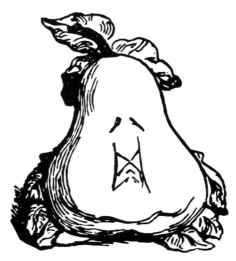

Puis condamner cet autre, qui ressemble au second   Et enfin, si vous êtes conséquens, vous ne sauriez absoudre cette poire, qui ressemble aux croquis précédens.

Ainsi, pour une poire, pour une brioche, et pour toutes les têtes grotesques dans lesquelles le hasard ou la malice aura placé cette triste ressemblance, vous pourrez infliger à l'auteur cinq ans de prison et cinq mille francs d'amende !!

Avouez, Messieurs, que c'est là une singulière liberté de la presse !!

a considerable degree of idealization. The latter was more pronounced the more power the particular emperor wielded and the more frequently these busts were used in religious state cults (e.g. compare the highly idealized busts of Augustus). Although individual features rarely dominated medieval and Romanesque paintings and sculptures, late Gothic and Renaissance portrait art soon reached an admirable degree of perfection in its depiction of individual characteristics (Bloch 1980; Bock and Grosshaus 1980; Severin 1980). Portrait painting and sculpture had very personal objectives: to preserve the memory of the subject for later generations, or to serve as a surrogate for an absent family member or friend living elsewhere.

A special art of portrait drawing is the caricature. It exaggerates typical features of facial structure and emotional expressions. An effective caricature still needs features fitting into templates for distinct facial expressions and some person typical properties of facial structure. This is nicely illustrated in Fig. 12.2(e).

With the development of artistic skill and a greater interest in painting or sculpting 'naturalistic' representations of individuals, the double social role of human face signals became more evident: 'public' faces (with a limited number of 'official masks'), and individual faces, with their many shades of emotional expression. These two aspects have become more accentuated with the development of photography and modern visual media (movies and television). Today, 'mask' manipulation using 'official' portraits of leading politicians plays an important role not only in totalitarian states but also in democratic societies. The 'leaders' are usually idealized and made more youthful in appearance. When these faces appear 'live' on television, heavy make-up is sometimes used for the same purpose. On the other hand, because of educational efforts aimed at producing well-developed individuals, modern democratic societies also favour the evolution of highly sophisticated portrait painting and portrait photography skills. When one examines the paintings or photographs produced by earlier generations, one easily recognizes that individual adult faces also represent the '*Zeitstil*' – if not the '*Zeitgeist*'. In the very young and very old, however, family characteristics, i.e. genetic factors, seem to dominate.

In light of these very recent cultural developments, it would seem meaningful for neuropsychological investigations to discriminate between the recognition of faces of relatives, friends and colleagues, individual faces of unknown persons seen daily in public places, and faces of politicians, actors or other people involved in show business, with whom most subjects are acquainted only indirectly through the media ('public' or 'famous' faces). In addition to neuropsychological studies of faces, facial expression and gestures, systematic tests of man's ability to recognize animal faces and man-made objects exhibiting physiognomic visual properties should contribute considerably to our knowledge of the operation of face-specific neuronal mechanisms in the human brain.

Faces as Visual Stimuli

The highly schematic woodcut of Fig. 12.3(b) and the highly sophisticated drawing of Fig. 12.3(a) are both perceived as faces. They fit into the same neuronal scheme of visual data processing in our brain. What makes the face a 'face' stimulus: eyes alone, eyes and eyebrows, eyes and nose or eyes, nose and mouth (Fig. 12.4)? The face scheme seems to be fairly stable, as Fig. 12.5 illustrates. This figure also represents the rank order of more or less deformed, schematic faces, chosen most often by adult subjects in a sorting test. This order is independent of the viewing distance, as long as the individual parts of the schematic faces can be seen clearly, i.e. it remains stable across a magnification factor of more than 1:20. Evidently, configurational factors are more relevant for 'face' recognition than are absolute spatial frequency components. Laughery *et al.*, (1971) found by analysing the introspective reports of their subjects that the following face components are, in rank order, the most important for recognition of 'faceness': eyes, nose, lips/chin, hair, ears.

Using computer quantization of face photographs, Harmon (1973) demonstrated that low spatial frequency components can transmit essential face signals (Fig. 12.6). Ginsburg (1978) reached the same conclusion using bandpass filter techniques. A finely drawn pencil sketch of a face contradicts, however, the general idea that only low-spatial-frequency signals convey the essential face signals. Figure 12.7 illustrates examples of faces depicted by different artists using different graphic techniques which led to face pictures with rather different spatial frequency contents (Fig. 12.8). Nevertheless, the observer can see faces in all of these pictures, and can do this from different viewing distances varying between 10 cm and more than 3 metres, i.e. when the frequency components of the pictures are shifted by about 1.4 decadic logarithmic units, the characteristic features of the faces or facial expression are not lost. This simple example illustrates that spatial frequency analysis does not offer much help in understanding face recognition, as some research groups have suggested (cf. the discussion by Sergent, 1986; Millward and O'Toole, 1986). The relative spatial frequency distribution scaled to the outlines of the schematic face may be relevant, however, in determining 'faceness'. Using sufficiently powerful high-spatial frequency band-pass filtered signals, Fiorentini *et al.* (1983) have demonstrated that face identification was better than was the case using low-pass filter signals. However, recognition of a face as a face

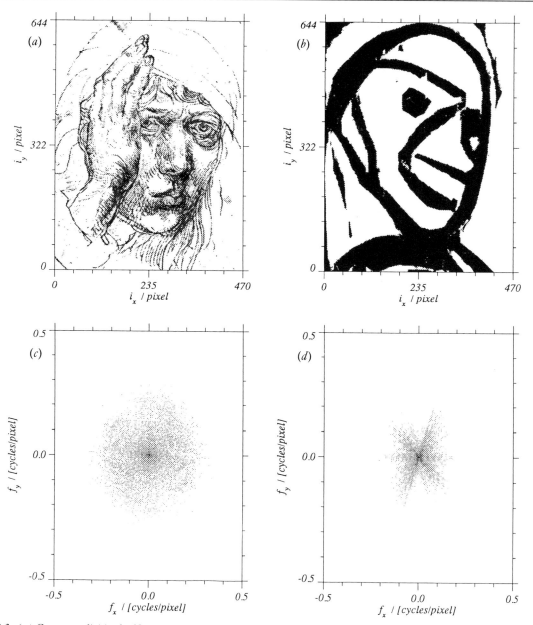

Fig. 12.3 *(a) Computer-digitized self-portrait of Albrecht Dürer (drawing, about 1492). (b) Face from a woodcut ('Männchen', 'little man') by Christian Rohlfs (1922). (c) Two-dimensional spatial frequency spectrum of (a). (d) Two-dimensional spectrum of (b). Despite the considerable difference in the spatial frequency composition of the two pictures, both are immediately recognized as faces. This recognition is fairly independent of a viewing distance between 10 cm and about 3 m. Thus the decision that both pictures represent faces certainly does not depend on their spatial frequency content.*

(as opposed to a non-face) and the ability to identify the face of a certain subject are two different tasks, which might explain the experimental discrepancies between the contribution of low- and high-spatial frequency compo-

nents of face recognition (for discussion see Sergent, 1983, 1986). Sergent and Switkes (1984) projected low-pass (0–2 cycles per degree) and broad-band (0–32 cycles per degree) filtered face stimuli onto the centre or lateral part

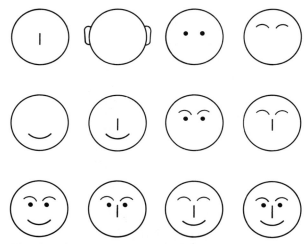

Fig. 12.4 *Set of highly schematic faces, by which the reader can judge which structural components contribute to the perceptual generation of a face scheme.*

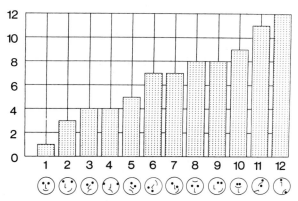

Fig. 12.5 *In a highly schematic face (1), the four internal components (eyes, nose, mouth) are shifted within the circle. 31 adult female and male subjects were asked to put the 12 stimuli in a rank order between the 'good face' (1) and the 'non-face' (12). On the abscissa the rank order is plotted, on the ordinate the median of the rank order from the decisions made by the group of 31 subjects (from an unpublished study of O.-J. Grüsser and B. Kaskas, 1985).*

of the visual field. They found reaction times to be significantly longer using low-pass filtered faces; recognition accuracy did not differ significantly between the two types of stimuli.

The suggestion that the inability to recognize familiar faces subsequent to the formation of cerebral lesions (e.g. prosopagnosia, Chapter 14) may be caused by an acquired impairment in the ability to perceive low-frequency channels, is not supported by the observational data: some

prosopagnosic patients have indeed been reported to have normal contrast sensitivity functions (Rizzo *et al.*, 1986). In one of our own prosopagnosic patients (Rentschler, Encke, Landis and Treutwein, unpublished data) we also observed normal contrast sensitivity functions; moreover, we found no difference in the impaired ability to recognize familiar faces – whether these faces were high- or low-pass-filtered. A corollary to this observation is the fact that, for the prosopagnosic patient, the ability to recognize face photographs is not facilitated by increasing size to a range beyond the limits of visual acuity.

The proportions and the detailed structure of human faces exhibit remarkable genetic and gender variability. Within genetically homogenous groups, however, sophisticated photographic superposition techniques have revealed that less than twenty face photographs superposed on each other produce very similar results, provided that the subjects were selected according to gender, age and intelligence (Katz, 1953; Fig. 12.9). It is interesting that such 'averaged faces' approximate rather closely the 'ideal' face of the social group in terms of social acceptance and beauty.

Like the structure of the face, facial expression also seems to fit into elementary schemes. One such scheme can be placed along a happy/sad scale. The idea that recognition of facial expression depends in part on the operation of neuronal schemes led to the creation of perceptual categories for facial expression which are used to evaluate the 'emotional content' of facial expression (Ekman, 1973, 1980; Ekman and Friesen, 1975). In a more recent study using computer-generated schematic faces, Musterle and Rössler (1986) confirmed this idea and published a set of 'Lorenz matrices' illustrating the different expressive states of the human face by simulating the effects of individual face muscle contractions (see Fig. 12.10).

Symmetry and Left–Right Laterality in Human Face Recognition

The structure of most faces deviates considerably from axial symmetry. In fact, a totally symmetric face looks boring in comparison with a slightly non-symmetric one. Asymmetry of the human face increases with age. When the asymmetry is too excessive, however, the face starts to look strange. Perceptive evaluation of faces is side-biased. When one compares photographs of faces with those having double-left or double-right halves (Fig. 12.11(a)-(c)), one finds that to a right-handed subject and to about half of all left-handers, 'double-right faces' have a

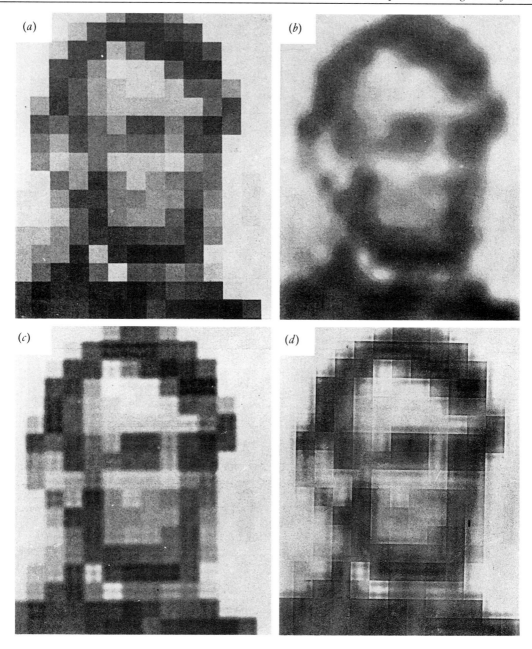

Fig. 12.6 *(a) A portrait painting of Abraham Lincoln was transformed into a 'block painting' of 14 × 18 squares of different shades of grey. Due to the size of the squares, the highest spatial frequency of the photographic signal is 9 (height) and 7 (width) cycles per picture. (b) The higher spatial frequencies extending above 10 cycles per picture (due to the squarewave block construction) are filtered out from (a). This procedure greatly enhances recognition of the portrait painting. By selective removal of the part of the spatial frequency spectrum above 10 cycles per second, one can determine the spatial frequencies which most effectively mask the image. (c) All frequencies above 40 cycles per picture have been removed. There is only a minor increase in face perception compared to (a). (d) Spatial frequencies between 10 and 40 cycles per picture have been removed. The face is recognized better than in (a) and (c), but not as well as in (b). This figure illustrates that certain spatial frequencies mask face perception effectively whenever phase information is also affected (from Harmon, 1973; by permission of Scientific American Inc., New York.).*

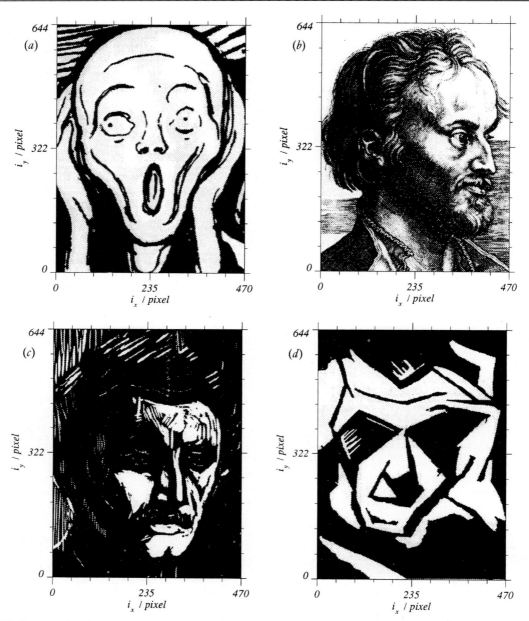

Fig. 12.7 *Four computer-digitized portraits. (a) Part of a lithograph by Edvard Munch 'The shriek', 1895. (b) Albrecht Dürer's etching of a portrait of* Philipp Melanchthon *(1526). (c) Self-portrait of Edvard Munch, a woodcut from 1911. (d) Self-portrait of Stanislav Kubicki, a woodcut from 1922. Without quantitative analysis it is evident by inspection that the spatial frequency content of these four faces is rather different. Furthermore all pictures are recognized as faces from a distance between 10 and 300 cm, i.e. when the spatial frequency content is shifted by 1.4 log units.*

greater similarity with the original photograph than double-left ones (Wolff, 1933; Gilbert and Bakan, 1973; Lawson, 1978; Milner, 1979; Overman and Doty, 1982; Fig. 12.11(d)). When measuring the centre-of-gaze pos-

ition of right-handed subjects inspecting human faces or face photographs (slide projection technique), one observes that the right side of the face is preferred about 60–70 per cent of the time – at least in face recognition

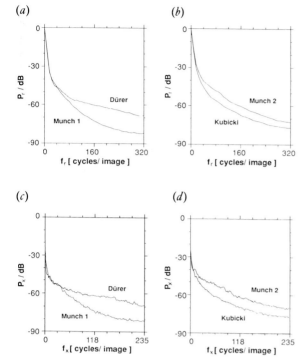

Fig. 12.8 *Quantitative analysis of the spatial frequency content of the four pictures shown in fig. 12.7. In (a) and (b) the spatial frequency distribution was averaged circularly. In (c) and (d) the spatial frequency distribution was averaged over the pixels of the X-axis. Note that large spatial frequency differences indeed exist for the four pictures of fig. 12.7. Munch 1 is (a) and Munch 2 is (c) of fig. 12.7. (Computations by K. H. Dittberner and W. Seidler.)*

tests, memorizing tasks, or tasks involving emotional decisions about the observed face (Grüsser, 1980, 1984; Fig. 12.12; Mertens *et al.*, 1991). This side preference is only in part face-specific, since under certain conditions a tendency also exists to scan objects placed in front of the subject with eye movements which shift more frequently towards the left field of gaze, i.e. to the right side of the object (M. Jeannerod, personal communication, 1980). The tendency for asymmetric scanning of a face has its correlate in the asymmetry of emotional expression: it is believed that the left half of the human face expresses the slightest emotional changes more readily than the right half, which is considered to be our more 'official' face half, somewhat akin to a 'public mask' (Campbell, 1978; Sackheim *et al.*, 1982; Moscovitch and Olds, 1982; Borod and Koff, 1983; Borod *et al.*, 1983; Dobson *et al.*, 1984). The tendency to explore the right side of a face more frequently has its corollary in the right cortical hemisphere's greater contribution to face recognition (Chapter 14). This scanning asymmetry is not found when photographs of decorative vases are used instead of face photographs in a learning paradigm (for explanation, see the caption of Fig. 12.12).

Interestingly, movements of the mouth region clearly exhibit 'dynamic' asymmetry during speech (right side more active) and non-speech action, e.g. singing without words or laughing (left side preference; Graves, *et al.*, 1982; Landis, 1982a, b; Graves and Landis, 1985; Wolf and Goodale, 1987; Wyler *et al.*, 1987; Cadalbert, 1990). It is claimed that winking with one eye is usually performed by the left eyelid (Moscovitch and Olds, 1982); in addition, the left side of the face is a target for hand–face interaction more often than the right side.

(a)

(b)

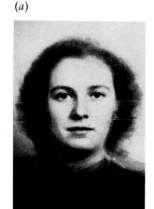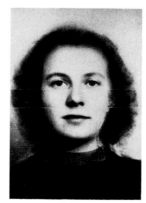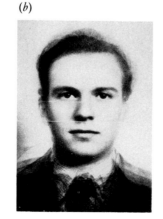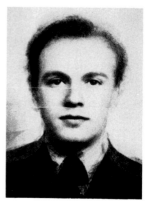

Fig. 12.9 *(a) Photographic averaging of portrait photos of 2 × 14 different Swedish female students of about 23 years of age. (b) Same for 2 × 14 different male Swedish students of about 24 years of age. Note the high similarity in the averaged faces, which was in part due to the genetically rather homogeneous population selected (from Katz, 1953; by permission of Schwabe Publishing Company, Basel).*

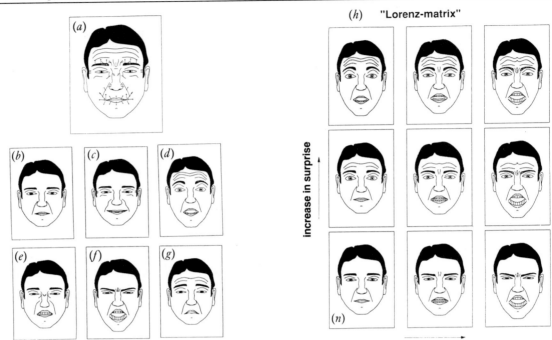

Fig. 12.10 *Computer-generated set of facial expressions which change along expressive 'dimensions' (from Musterle and Rössler, 1986; modified). (a) Neutral face with lines and 'muscle vectors' along which facial expression is generated. (b-g) Different pure and full facial expressions: (b) neutral, (c) friendly, (d) surprise, (e) disgust, (f) anger, (g) grief, (h) examples of 'mixtures' of facial expressions in a 'Lorenz' matrix (anger) × (surprise). Horizontal axis: increase in anger; vertical axis: increase in surprise.*

It is interesting that left–right asymmetry with respect to face perception has even had some impact on man's cultural productivity, as one notices, for example, in the portrait paintings of Western art. Paintings of the Gothic and early Renaissance periods exhibit a strong preference for depicting subjects with the head turned towards the right shoulder, thus displaying more of the left, 'emotional' half of the face than the right side. Although this tendency was significantly more pronounced in female portraits, it declined between the eighteenth and twentieth centuries in both male and female portrait paintings (Fig. 12.13; for details, see Grüsser *et al.*, 1983, 1988).

Hemispheric Specialization in Human Face Perception as Revealed by Tachistoscopic Tests

Traditionally, hemispheric superiority for visual pattern processing is tested by short monocular or binocular stimulus presentations in the left or right visual hemifields. As a rule, those who use this technique believe that 'better' results (as indicated by shorter reaction times or higher recognition scores) obtained with right-visual-hemifield stimuli indicate a left-hemisphere superiority, and vice versa. These findings do not exclude, of course, a strong contribution from the other cerebral hemisphere in performing the task, since a transfer through the corpus callosum takes no more than 5 milliseconds. In general, there is a slight tendency to perform better when verbal stimuli are projected into the right visual hemifield (RVH, Chapter 17). A similar preference was found for the recognition of averbal visual stimuli projected into the left visual hemifield (LVH). The idea that the right hemisphere is superior to the left in terms of averbal visual stimulus processing, especially for complex visual patterns, is accepted by the majority of neuropsychologists, whereby the degree of left–right difference depends on the complexity of the pattern as well as on the relative contribution of the memory processes to pattern recognition (for recent discussions see Moscovich, 1979; Springer and Deutsch, 1990).

A left–right difference is frequently but not always present when faces are used as stimuli. In tachistoscopic projection experiments, unknown face stimuli projected into

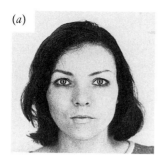

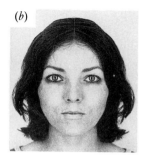

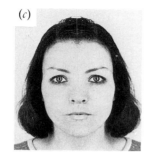

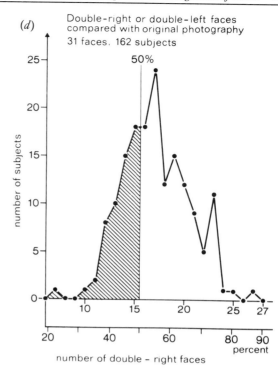

Fig. 12.11 *Photograph of a test slide with a normal face (a) and two artificial faces composed of double right halves (b) and double left halves (c). The observers had to judge which of the two lower faces best resembles the upper face. For this particular combination more than 90 percent of 162 medical students who were shown this slide in a set of 31 slides decided that the double-right face (b) looks more similar to the normal face than the double-left face (c). (d) Statistical results obtained in 162 male and female medical students with 31 slides of the type (a – c). The slides were projected for 6 seconds each with a pause of 6 seconds in between. The subjects had to decide whether the double-right or double-left face looked more similar to the normal face. They were not informed of how the different faces were constructed. Positions of double-right and double-left faces were varied at random. The figure shows the frequency distribution of the preference for the double-right face. The two data points on the left end of the distribution were from left-handed subjects. The data of 6 further left-handed subjects are intermingled at random with those of the other right-handed subjects (Grüsser, 1978, from Grüsser, 1984).*

the LVH of right-handers are recognized with greater accuracy and shorter latency (reaction time experiments) than those projected into the RVH, provided that names are not involved in the task (Rizzolatti *et al.*, 1970, 1971; Geffen, *et al.*, 1971; Gilbert and Bakan, 1973; Hilliard, 1973; Marzi *et al.*, 1974; Klein, 1976; Rizzolatti and Buchtel, 1977; Berent, 1977; Milner and Dunne, 1977; Marzi and Berlucchi, 1977; Leehey and Cahn, 1979; Landis *et al.*, 1979; Ley and Bryden, 1979; Bertelson *et al.*, 1979; Schwartz and Smith, 1980; St John, 1981; Natale *et al.*, 1983). Some of the variables influencing visual field asymmetries in face processing and some still yet unexplained inconsistencies are presented briefly in the next section.

With respect to accuracy in the recognition of famous faces, a right visual field superiority was found when verbal recognition was required (Marzi and Berlucchi, 1977). For example, Jones (1979, 1980) reported an RVH

advantage when either female or male subjects had to classify tachistoscopically presented faces as male or female. Rizzolatti and Buchtel (1977) have pointed to gender differences with regard to hemispheric specialization in face recognition: when stimuli were projected into the LVH, the reaction time for faces was faster for male subjects than when they were projected into the RVH. This finding depended on stimulus duration and did not appear in female subjects. The stronger lateralization of a certain brain function in male subjects corresponds to the general assumption that the two cerebral hemispheres of the human brain are more lateralized in men than in women for both spatial and verbal cognitive processes (e.g. Lansdell, 1962; Kimura, 1969; McGlone and Davidson, 1973; Hannay and Malone, 1976; Lake and Bryden, 1976). The presumed stronger hemispheric lateralization in the male brain with respect to face signal processing is not accompanied, however, by an overall better performance

(a)

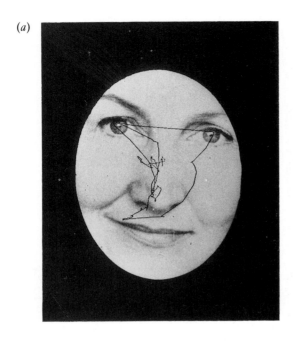

(b)

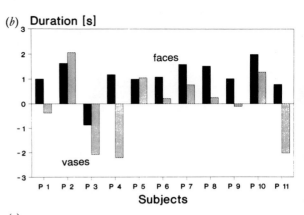

(c)

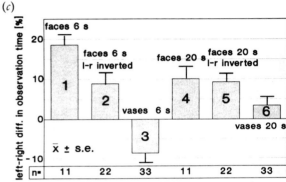

Fig. 12.12 *Slides of black-and-white photographs of ornamental vases or the inner part of faces were used as stimuli. The subjects, male and female medical students, inspected the items for 6 seconds and were instructed to remember the item for a later memory-test. By means of an infrared-reflection technique, the eye position was measured and later evaluated by different computer programmes (example in a). On the average, faces were inspected longer and with more saccades on their right halves (left field of gaze) than on their left halves, while for vases no significant deviation from approximate symmetrical inspection strategies was found (Mertens* et al., *1991). (b) Individual data from 11 subjects. Left-right difference in inspection duration in the left and right field of gaze. (c) Averaged data from different groups of subjects inspecting faces, left-right inverted faces and vases for 6 and 20 s.*

in face recognition tasks. In fact, the contrary is true: female superiority in face recognition was found in the majority of neuropsychological studies (cf. pp. 235–237).

Studies investigating the influence of the menstrual cycle upon cognitive tasks, particularly with respect to verbal and non-verbal performances, may provide some physiological insight into the differences between male and female performances for hemispheric lateralization tasks. Hampson and Kimura (1988) detected changes in performance related to the menstrual cycle of their subjects in investigations of the speed required to perform manual and non-verbal spatial tasks under conditions of normal vision. High levels of female sex hormones facilitated tasks which women generally perform better and hampered their performance for tasks in which men were usually superior. In a test battery of cognitive tasks, Gordon and Lee (1986) also found similar, though less clear, results in their investigations of the relation between

hormonal status and performance results. Follicle-stimulating hormone concentrations were negatively correlated with visual spatial tests and positively correlated with word fluency.

In a use of this approach to study functional cerebral asymmetry experimentally, performance in lexical and facial decisions was tested in a lateralized tachistoscopic double-simultaneous 'go/no-go' paradigm during the menstrual cycle of women who did not use hormonal contraceptives (Heister *et al.*, 1989). Although alterations in overall performance during the four phases of the cycle were found, no shift in functional cerebral asymmetry for the verbal lexical decision task was discovered. Hemispheric asymmetry in face perception did decrease during the menstruation cycle, however, from a large right-hemisphere superiority to a small left-hemisphere superiority during the premenstrual phase (Fig. 12.14). This result is considered to be relevant not only for the discus-

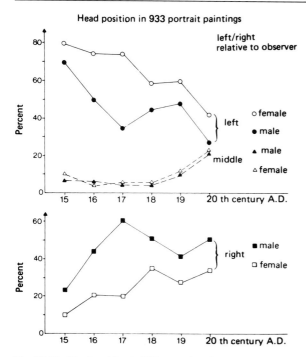

Fig. 12.13 *Head position in 933 portrait paintings originating between the 15th and 20th centuries (abscissa). Separate data for male and female portraits. Note that the historical trend over 6 centuries from an initial left-sided preference to right-sided preference is evident, but the left facial half is displayed more often in female portraits than in male through all centuries. Left means that the portrayed subject's head is turned to the right and displays more of the left half of the face to the observer (from Grüsser* et al., *1988).*

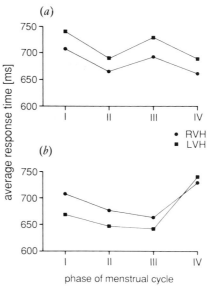

Fig. 12.14 *Average reaction time (ordinate) in a lexical decision (a) and a face-recognition decision (b) task for stimuli projected into the left (LVH) or the right (RVH) visual hemifield of female subjects at the four different phases of the menstrual cycle. Note the RVH-advantage (shorter reaction times) for lexical decisions (a) and the LVH-advantage for face recognition (b). This LVH-advantage, however, disappeared during the last week of the menstrual cycle (from Heister* et al., *1989).*

sion of gender differences in cerebral asymmetry but also for the concept of cerebral organization in general.

In a tachistoscopic test, Moscovitch *et al.* (1976) investigated the ability of subjects to match black-and-white photographs of famous singers with corresponding caricatures. An LVH advantage with respect to reaction time was observed for a same/different task. No hemifield differences were found, however, when two stimuli from the same graphic category (photographs, caricatures) were used.

We have applied a similar paradigm using conceptual matching, i.e. the capacity to associate two pictures which cannot be matched on the basis of physical features but rather only on the basis of their common meaning (Landis *et al.*, 1979). The performance of normal subjects matching photographs and stylized drawings of objects was compared with their performance matching profile photographs of facial expressions with stylized, front-view drawings of facial expressions exhibiting the same or different emotions. This study was performed in order to test the hypothesis that the left hemisphere is dominant for conceptual matching, and the right hemisphere for physical or apperceptive matching, i.e. matching by similarity of shape (De Renzi *et al.*, 1969; Levy, 1974). In this study, a RVH advantage, i.e. a left-hemisphere advantage, was found for the conceptual matching of objects; an equally strong LVH (right-hemisphere) advantage for the conceptual matching of emotional facial expressions was also observed. The results demonstrated that both hemispheres are able to make conceptual judgements, though probably by different means. Since the three emotional concepts 'angry', 'happy' and 'astonished' are easy to identify and name because of frequent daily experience, we conjectured that the LVH advantage was caused by a more efficient and faster process associating different facial features with a common emotional meaning (without using verbal concepts). Figures 12.15(a) and (b) illustrate some of the stimuli used, and Fig. 12.15(c) presents the mean differences between decision times for the two classes of stimuli projected into the left or right visual half-fields.

Although the ability to discriminate between faces and non-faces reveals, at least in male subjects, some hemi-

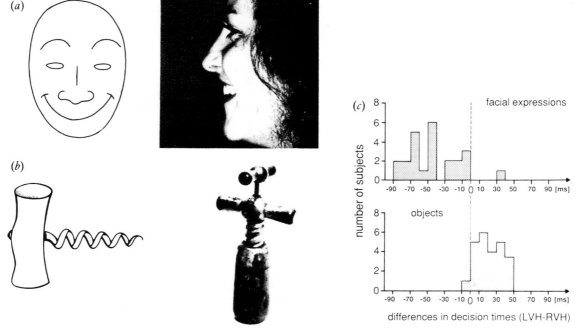

Fig. 12.15 *(a) and (b) Examples of the stimulus combinations used in the experiment of Landis* et al. *(1979). (a) The emotional expression 'happy' is common in the frontal schematic face and the side view of the face photograph. The stylized drawing was always presented in foveal vision and subtended a maximum visual angle of 3.4 degrees. The photograph of the same size was presented either to the left or the right side of the drawing and was placed within 2.2–5.6 degrees of visual angle as measured from the fixation point. (b) Example of the second stimulus category. In this example the drawing and the photograph belonged to the same category ('corkscrew'). The drawing was projected to the fovea, the photograph either to the left or right side of the drawing. The subjects had to judge in (a) whether the expressions were the same or different and in (b) whether the objects did or did not belong to the same category. For further explanation see text. (c) Distribution of the reaction time differences for the photographs presented to the left (LVH) and the right (RVH) visual field. For judging facial expressions, the majority of subjects exhibited an LVH advantage, i.e. their reaction times were shorter when the photograph which was compared with the drawing was placed into the LVH. The opposite was true for comparison of drawings and photographs of objects (from Landis* et al., *1979, modified).*

spheric laterality effects, recognition of certain facial properties is, in part, not lateralized. Marzi *et al.* (1985) performed three 'laterality experiments' at different cognitive levels in male and female right-handed students. In the first experiment, the subjects had to decide whether the face was that of a male or female person. Half of the faces used in this experiment were those of 'famous' persons. No statistically significant laterality effects were found for the vocal reaction time when the stimuli were projected for 150 ms into the LVH or RVH (eccentricity about 2.2 degrees). Female subjects were faster, however, than male subjects in responding to left or right visual hemifield stimuli (LVH 590 f/695 m, RVH 594 f/595 m [ms]). In a second experiment using the same stimuli, the subjects were required to decide whether or not the faces were those of famous or unknown people. Marzi *et al.* found a significant LVH advantage for both genders (LVH 951 f/908 m; RVH 963 f/956 m [ms]). In addition,

the verbal response time for famous faces (869 ms) was shorter than that for unknown faces (1020 ms). Finally, in the third experiment, the subjects were asked to say the correct name of each of the famous faces they recognized. Ninety-one per cent were correctly named. The unknown faces were named '*sconosciuto*' (unknown). Contrary to the authors' expectations, these face-naming experiments revealed neither a visual hemifield difference nor a reaction time difference for naming and designating known and unknown faces. In this task, female subjects again performed faster, on the average, than male subjects.

Anderson and Parkin (1985) noted an LVH advantage, not only for the processing of face stimuli, but also for pictures of hands and aeroplanes. Their subjects had to compare stimuli projected for 0.5 seconds onto the fovea with those projected for 0.2 seconds (after a delay of 1.1 seconds) 4 degrees laterally either within the LVH or the RVH. The subjects had to decide in a test of reaction time whether or not the second stimulus was physically the same item as the first, or whether it was another item belonging to the same category. The reaction times were shorter for faces than for hands and planes, and shorter for faces and hands seen in the LVH than for those seen in the RVH.

A Special Memory for Faces?

The existence of specialized neuronal mechanisms for face recognition is supported by the results of experiments in which memory and retrieval of previously presented faces and visual control stimuli were tested. In the majority of studies, short-term memory was tested either by immediate recall or several minutes after presentation. Most of these experiments, which were performed using brain-damaged patients, are discussed in Chapter 14. The high-precision performance for face recognition (e.g. Freedman and Harbor, 1974; Klabky and Forest, 1984) was explained by Goldstein and Chance (1980) as a consequence of man's more frequent exposure to many different faces compared to any other visual stimulus pattern. Goldstein and Chance (1971) demonstrated that faces were better recognized than any other symmetrical (snowflakes) or non-symmetrical (ink blots) visual patterns, while Scapinello and Yarmey (1970) reached the same conclusion using photographs of buildings and dogs as control stimuli.

We do not think, however, that these findings prove that it is only repeated exposure which leads to the fact that faces are better memorized than other comparably complex structures. Learning and the daily need to differentiate faces certainly improve the recognition mechanism, but there is good evidence that the neuronal schemata which operate in face recognition also rely on inborn recognition mechanisms, which are already present at birth (see below).

In the experiments performed by Zynda (1984) and Grüsser *et al.* (1985), subjects saw a set of black-and-white slides (6 seconds for each photograph) in an upright or upside-down position and had to indicate whether the faces appeared to them to be 'positive', 'neutral' or 'negative' (*'sympathisch'*, *'neutral'*, *'unsympathisch'*). During this test, the subjects did not know that other tests of recognition would be performed later. In the first experiment, 116 medical students (44 female, average age 24.3 years; 72 male, 23.9 years) and male police recruits (matched for age) served as unpaid volunteers. One hour after the inspection series, some of the slides were projected together with an unfamiliar partner; some of the stimuli were presented again upside down (test 1). A second test was performed 1 week later. Faces seen in this inspection series and in test 1 were presented with a new partner; 'partner faces' from test 1 were presented with a different partner; faces seen in the inspection series only were now presented with a partner (each for 6 seconds). The subjects had to decide which of the two items had been seen before. It was possible to conduct a third test 1 year after the inspection series with twelve of the subjects. Figure 12.16 presents some of the data collected. In a second experiment involving 126 subjects (female and male medical students), slides of faces as well as of vases and pairs of worn shoes were used as stimuli. The main results of these two studies were as follows:

1. Female subjects performed significantly better and made approximately half as many errors as male subjects when asked to recognize faces 1 hour or 1 week later. This female superiority was even greater for the subjects tested 1 year later.

2. Presenting or testing faces in an upside-down position affected recognition considerably (Fig. 12.16). This inversion effect was not observed for recognition tasks involving decorative vases or pairs of shoes, which indicates that the 'inversion sensibility' of face stimuli is different from that of non-face stimuli. Impairment of short-term face recognition by inversion had been consistently reported in several preceding studies (Hochberg and Galper, 1967; Yin, 1969; Scapinello *et al.*, 1970; Bradshaw and Wallace, 1971; Leehey *et al.*, 1978; Phillips and Rawles, 1979).

3. Female superiority was no longer true when faces were presented in an upside-down position (inversion) in both the inspection and test series.

4. Presumably school education had some impact on face recognition: male medical students performed better than male police apprentices of comparable age.

5. Female faces were better recognized than male faces by both female and male subjects. This effect might have been primarily a result of the stimulus material used.

6. Repeated presentation (inspection series and first test) decreased errors in face recognition after 1 week. Lengthening the time interval between inspection series and test increased slightly the number of erroneous responses. Minor effects related to the time interval between face presentation and test (2 or 7 days, respectively) were also described by Goldstein and Chance (1970) and Laugherty *et al.* (1971).

7. Emotional decisions made during the inspection series had no significant effects later on recognition of faces, vases or pairs of shoes.

8. Partner faces in test 1 were significantly less well recognized in test 2, as compared with faces seen in the inspection series but not seen in test 1. Selective attention during decision-making in test 1 seems to have had some effect on face recognition later.

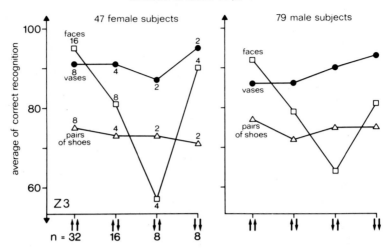

Fig. 12.16 *Effect of stimulus orientation (slides of black-and-white photographs) on recognition after one week. During the inspection session, every item (face, vase or pair of worn shoes) was shown for 6 seconds. Within the next 6 seconds, the subject had to note their emotional or aesthetic decision (+, 0, -). Recognition test performed after 8 days. The items were either in the normal position (↑) or upside down (↓). First arrow indicates the position during the inspection series, the second arrow during the test series. Note the strong effect of orientation on face recognition (O.-J. Grüsser and B. Zynda, unpublished observations, 1978).*

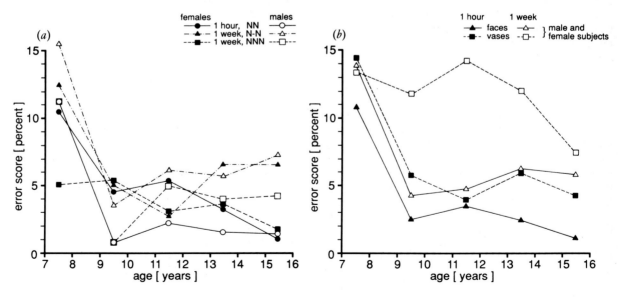

Fig. 12.17 *(a) Change in the error score (ordinate, percent) with the age and gender of the subject in recognizing faces (upright position) after one hour or one week (O.-J. Grüsser, Th. Selke and B. Zynda, 1982, unpublished). (b) The recognition scores obtained after one hour or after one week were similarly related to age of the subject, but faces were much better recognized than ornamental vases (O.-J. Grüsser, Th. Selke and B. Zynda, 1982, unpublished; see Grüsser et al., 1985).*

Long-interval face recognition was studied by Bahrick *et al.* (1975), who used faces from high-school yearbooks as stimuli; they tested subjects who had left high school sometime between 2 weeks and 50 years prior to testing. The initial recognition score (2-week delay) reached 89 per cent; it decreased only slightly to 73 per cent for subjects tested 50 years after high school leaving. From these results, it seems that the ability to recognize the faces of social partners who had once played an important role in one's daily activities is remarkably well developed in man. Female superiority in face recognition was also found by McKelvie (1981) for Canadian college students. In a similar test, the subjects tested by Witreyol and Kaess (1957) performed better only in recognizing faces of members of their own gender.

In comparison with other items, repeated inspection of faces leads to a greater improvement in recognition scores. Scapinello and Yarmey (1970) tested the recognition of faces presented seven times, compared with those presented only once. Similar results related to repeated presentation were found for face stimuli presented in the normal and upside-down positions.

Development of Face Recognition

The First Year of Life

Observational and experimental data indicate that some human face recognition abilities are determined by innate neuronal mechanisms, which use the configuration of a face as a 'key stimulus', as suggested by Mach (1906). His thoughts on key stimuli and the inborn releasing mechanisms which they triggered were later elaborated upon and experimentally supported by Konrad Lorenz and Nikolas Tinbergen. There are several reports in the literature claiming that neonates born at term respond differently to faces than to non-faces, even during the first days or weeks of life – although their visual acuity is certainly well below that of older children or adults (Braddick and Atkinson, 1979; Pirckio *et al.*, 1979). In neonates, the ability to track moving visual patterns of different configurations has been repeatedly used to study whether or not faces represent special stimuli in the set of patterns normally seen by a baby. Goren *et al.* (1975) explored neonates with an average age of 9 minutes (!), presenting them with a schematic face, two scrambled faces and a blank face. Each stimulus was moved to and fro about 180 degrees in front of the baby. Head and eye movements were observed, but not measured. A significant preference for looking at 'normal' face stimuli was noted. The results of this work were later confirmed by Dziurawiec and Ellis (1986), who used television tape recordings instead of direct observations. Field *et al.* (1982) presented 2-day-old

infants with a real face expressing joy, sadness or surprise (different durations). The infants' observation time decreased when the expression remained constant over a period of time, but interest increased again when a new facial expression was displayed. Carpenter *et al.* (1970) explored the ability of 2-week-old infants to discriminate the mother's face from a schematic face model and an abstract model. Their data suggest that the mother's face is 'imprinted' during the first two weeks of life. The surprising ability of young infants to imitate some facial expressions (opening of mouth, protrusion of lips or tongue) also indicates at least a rudimentary ability to perceive different facial expressions (Meltzoff and Moore, 1977, 1983). Fantz (1961, 1966) also reported that 13-week-old infants preferred fixating on a face pattern rather than on scrambled patterns with the same outlines.

Some studies tried to determine at what age infants can distinguish certain individual faces from other faces. Maurer and Salapatek (1976) investigated 4-week-old infants, who looked significantly more frequently at faces of unknown males or females than at their mother's face, provided that the faces were not moved. Different emotional responses to face stimuli, as indicated by pupil dilation, were found in 17-week-old infants when the face of the mother and that of a stranger were presented (Fitzgerald, 1968). These observations indicated an early learning ability for some structures of individual faces. Most studies agree that 4- to 5-month-old babies are also able to learn face structures under experimental conditions (Fagan, 1972; Cornell, 1974; Miranda and Fantz, 1974; Fagan, 1976; Dirks and Gibson, 1977; further discussion in Carey, 1981).

These conclusions about innate face recognition abilities in young babies are somewhat weakened by the reports presented by Maurer (1985) and Fagan and Shepherd (1981), who deduced from their experiments that the responses of babies younger than four months to schematic faces are not significantly different from those to other comparable test stimuli. Carey (1981) thought that the infant's attention to faces depends mainly on the complexity of the stimulus and not on innate face recognition mechanisms. Bower (1974) argued similarly, having observed that babies below 6 weeks of age smile with the same probability when shown two dots or a real face.

In early systematic studies of the face recognition abilities of babies, Kaila (1932), Bühler (1934), Spitz and Wolff (1946), Ahrens (1954a, b) and Spitz (1967) considered the infant's smiling response to be an indicator of face or facial expression recognition. Movement of the face stimuli increased the probability of reaction. With masks and schematic faces exhibiting different facial expressions, the eyes and mouth regions were the most likely to induce smiling. Ahrens (1954a, b) interpreted these findings to be an indication of an innate face recognition mechanism which matures during the first months of life. We think that this interpretation is the one best supported by experimental evidence.

Early mother–child interaction presumably introduces some left–right asymmetries into the infant's face recognition system. Because most mothers prefer to hold their babies in the left arm, the very first important face seen by most babies, i.e. that of the mother, is frequently shifted somewhat to the left of the baby's field of gaze (when it lies turned slightly to its right side and close to its mother's left breast). This left–right asymmetry is enhanced when the mother makes cheek-to-cheek contact with her baby – a behavioural pattern enjoyed by both mother and baby: she usually touches the left cheek of the baby held in her left arm with her left cheek. Thus with respect to possible face pattern learning in emotional face-to-face contacts early in life, some tactile and visual asymmetry is present in the infant's stimulus field. When a mother sits in the sun with her baby cradled in her arm, she turns herself so that the rays of sun do not fall directly on the baby's face. This means that the left side of the mother's face is more illuminated than the right, creating an asymmetric input stimulus for the infant's neuronal face templates (for details see Grüsser *et al.*, 1988).

Childhood and Adolescence

Normal children of early school age have no difficulty recognizing classmates, other children about their age, or those adults with whom they frequently interact. When children in this age range (6 to 8 years) report on similarities they have observed between different adults, one is surprised by the fact that these similarities are not discernible by the adult observer. Evidently, children under age 8 operate with less precise or with other structural categories than those used by adults to classify individual faces. This divergent observational faculty may be a result of daily experience, for most children interact more frequently with children of their own age group than with adults.

The development of the ability of kindergarten or school-age children to recognize faces was also tested using tachistoscopically presented stimuli. The results of these investigations clearly indicate an increase in correct face recognition (naming of known faces) correlated to an increase in age (Young and Bion, 1980, 1981). Correspondingly, reaction times to tachistostopically projected faces decrease with age in school children (Reynolds and Jeeves, 1978; Broman, 1978). A left visual-field advantage for tachistoscopic face recognition is not present in the 7- and 8-year-old groups, but does exist in the 13- and 14-year-old groups as well as in adults (where reaction time was used as a criterion) (Reynolds and Jeeves, 1978). A left visual-field advantage for recognizing tachistoscopically projected upright faces was also reported in younger boys

and girls (5 years and older) only when a small set of four stimulus faces was used (Young and Ellis, 1976), or when immediate recall was required (7 to 9 years; Marcel and Rajan, 1975). When the number of faces used was increased to 40, the left-visual-field advantage was observed only in boys of age 7 and older, but not in girls (Young and Bion, 1980). This observation corresponds to the age-dependent different degree of lateralization in male and female subjects, as discussed above. Most studies agree that in general, a considerable improvement in face recognition ability occurs during childhood development between ages 5 and 10 (Goldstein and Chance, 1964; Cross *et al.*, 1971; Ellis *et al.*, 1973; Ellis, 1975; Diamond and Carey, 1977; Blaney and Winograd, 1978; Carey *et al.*, 1980; Flin, 1980; Carey, 1981). In most tests of face recognition abilities, recognition was tested immediately after the first inspection of the items. Children of 8 years and younger encoded unfamiliar faces rather poorly, whereas the performance of children 10 years of age and somewhat older was almost on a par with that of adults. Carey (1981) argued that, in children up to age 10, the development of face encoding and recognition skills is restricted predominantly to increasing processing accuracy for upright faces, since no significant age dependence was found for recognizing inverted faces in the age range of six to ten years (Carey *et al.*, 1981; Young *et al.*, 1980). In contrast to Carey *et al.* (1981), however, Young *et al.* (1980) claimed an inversion effect in 6-year-old children, provided that a small set of target faces was used.

Grüsser *et al.* (1985) studied the ontogenetic development of memory for faces and of long-term face recognition abilities in school children and adolescents. The stimulus set consisted of 42 black-and-white photographs: 14 male and 14 female faces, and 14 decorative vases, each presented for 6 seconds. Each presentation was followed by a 6-second interval during which the children were asked to note their 'emotional' evaluation ('positive'/ 'negative'). Faces and vases were presented in random order. Boys and girls between ages 7 and 16 were tested, and the data were compared with the results obtained for medical students. One hour after the inspection series, a two–choice recognition test was performed; 1 week later, the second recognition test was performed (6-second presentations of each item). In all age groups, recognition was better for faces than for vases. For both items, the 7- and 8-year-old children had significantly higher error scores than did the other age groups. Boys reached adult performance levels at age 9 to 10. Only above ages 15 to 16 did female subjects demonstrate a significantly better face recognition ability than that of male subjects. The gender of the faces and the emotional responses during the inspection series had a slight influence on face recognition scores. Correct item recognition decreased after 1 week for both faces and vases seen in the inspection series only (and not in the first test 1 hour later). For items seen in the inspection series and in the test performed 1 hour later, no decrease in correct recall was observed 1 week later. Thus the second presentation on the day of inspection compensated for the memory decay found after 1 week for both faces and vases. As Fig. 12.17(a) and (b) indicate, a developmental factor exists for 'long-term' face recognition abilities, whereby faces are better recognized than decorative vases by all age groups. Female superiority in face recognition first develops after puberty.

Recognizing One's Own Face

The use of mirrors is a rather recent cultural innovation that first appeared during the Bronze Age. Before polished metal surfaces became available, women or men who wanted to see themselves had to look at water surfaces in pots or ponds. Interacting with one's own face is thus not a behavioural pattern for which any special neurobiological mechanisms might have developed. In human society, which frequently uses mirrors daily, one's own face is presumably one of those most frequently seen as compared with the faces of other people. A 6-month-old baby does not recognize himself in a mirror, and, when forced to look into the mirror, often cries. It is not really clear how early in life children really recognize the reflection in the mirror as being their own face. This presumably occurs sometime during the second year of life. Three-year-old

children like to 'play' with their own faces in the mirror and enjoy 'making faces' (own observations). Doing this in groups seems to enhance the fun. From this age on, it seems that children are able to recognize themselves in the mirror.

Animals are not able to recognize their image in a mirror, although they can use a mirror within a familiar environment for spatial orientation and to help them plan their movements (dogs, own observation). Macaque monkeys perceive their mirror image as the image of another monkey and repeatedly try to look behind the mirror for the 'other' animal (Trendelenburg, 1928; Hall, 1962; Gallup, 1968, 1970, 1977; Gallup *et al.*, 1971; Zazzo, 1979; Anderson, 1983, 1984a). Squirrel monkeys reveal typical display patterns towards their own mirror image because they do not recognize themselves (MacLean, 1964). Chimpanzees seem to be aware of who the mirror image belongs to. This indicates not only a rudimentary development of self-recognition but perhaps as well the existence of the concept of the 'self' (Gallup, 1970, 1977; Anderson, 1984b).

The average human observer becomes acquainted with the left–right asymmetry of his or her own face in the mirror. As a rule, this adaptation to one's own face is responsible for the alienation one experiences when seeing oneself for the first time in a movie or on television. Although the mirror effect is the same when one compares one's mirror image with sufficiently large photographs, the alienating effect is stronger when moving pictures are observed (e.g. Michel, 1978).

13 The Search for Face-responsive Components in the Visual Evoked Potentials (EPs) of the Human Electroencephalogram

Introduction

The symptom of prosopagnosia (Chapter 14) suggests the existence of a neocortical region located in the medio-basal, occipito-temporal cortex of the human brain in which face-specific neuronal operations are performed. These enable us to recognize other people by their faces, and to perceive their facial expressions, which indicate intentions and emotions. The existence of neocortical regions specialized for face recognition is also suggested by face-specific activations found in the neurones of the temporal lobe and amygdala of the monkey (Chapter 7). In the light of these findings, it seemed meaningful to investigate whether one could discover 'face-specific' or 'face-responsive' components in the evoked potentials of the human electroencephalogram by using suitable paradigms. One has to keep the following in mind when performing such an investigation: (a) the core regions that perform the task of face recognition and that evaluate facial expressions are located in cortical structures that do not belong to the outer cortical convexity areas; (b) the main projection sites of the neocortical face-responsive neurones seem mainly to involve structures of the limbic system that are also not located on the cortical surface.

Other restrictions with regard to the recording of face-responsive components in the evoked potentials or the 'event-related potentials' of the electroencephalogram limit the degree of freedom involved in the search for face-responsive components in the evoked potential:

1. The stimulus pattern should change instantaneously from one category to the next without a change in the average stimulus luminance.

2. About 40 visual evoked potentials (EPs) related to the same stimulus category have to be averaged in order to obtain sufficiently reliable data characterizing the responses of an individual subject. Therefore, only a maximum of 4 to 5 stimulus categories can be used during one recording session.

3. During the recording session, the stimulus-directed attention of the subject must be kept as much as possible at a constant high level. To this end, one has to invent certain tasks for the subject which do not interfere with the evoked potentials related to the stimulus categories investigated; one still has to make sure that the subject's attention remains directed on the stimulus pattern at a constant high level.

4. The set of non-face stimulus patterns used as controls have to be carefully selected in order to obtain meaningful EP data.

In the light of extensive research on the visual evoked potentials (EPs) recorded from the skull of man, we know that the EPs depend not only on the elementary properties of the stimulus, such as intensity, size, colour and retinal location, but also on the subject's 'internal' states, i.e. general and spatially directed attention, vigilance, expectation, etc. (for reviews see Regan, 1972, and Volume 10, Chapter 6, of this series). The spatial frequency content of the visual stimuli, their geometrical configuration, the contextual meaning, and the tasks that the subjects have to perform during stimulus presentation may also affect the EPs (for reviews see John et al., 1967; Johnston and Chesney, 1974; MacKay and Jeffreys, 1973; Neville et al., 1982). All of these factors that influence the EPs seem to interact in a more or less complex way with one another.

Methodological Approaches to Stimulation, EEG Recordings and Computerized Data Evaluation

With the difficulties just mentioned in mind, we decided about 10 years ago to build special stimulus equipment that would guarantee a very fast change in stimulus patterns without changing average stimulus luminance. Furthermore, we restricted the number of recording electrodes to 6 channels, and carefully selected the 4 stimulus categories that would be applied during 1 recording session. Visual, category-related evoked potentials have been recorded in more than 180 adult subjects over the last 9 years. Only right-handers, whose right-handedness had been confirmed by the Edinburgh Inventory (Oldfield, 1971), were chosen as subjects. Less than half of the subjects were paid; the others were mainly volunteer medical students who participated in the recording sessions because they wanted to learn more about the technique of EEG recording and about visual evoked potentials. None of the subjects was informed about the scientific goal of the experiments. All subjects had normal binocular vision and showed no signs of neurological, visual or oculomotor impairment. Myopic subjects were allowed to wear corrective eyeglasses, however. Apart from the experiments in which known or famous faces were used, the subjects were not informed until after completion of the series that faces were the crucial stimuli in which we were interested.

Each subject sat in a rather comfortable chair and rested their head against its back. The room they sat in was separated by a wall from the room containing the recording and stimulation equipment (Fig. 13.1). The subject was instructed to relax and to fixate either on a small, red spot of light located in the centre of a continuously visible projection field (3.9×5.9 degrees visual angle) or else just on the centre of that field. The stimuli consisted of a sequence of slides projected onto this field for 2.5–4.3 s each slide. The average luminance of the stimulus pattern was between 3 and 15 cd m^{-2} for the set of 'positive' stimuli (black line drawings on a white background, black-and-white photographs), and 0.5 cd m^{-2} for the 'negative stimuli' (white line drawings on a black background). The background luminance in the room was about 0.01 cd m^{-2}. The 1×2 m vertical projection screen placed at a distance of 2 m from the subject was considerably larger than the 3.9×5.9 degrees stimulus pattern.

The slides were alternately projected from one of two carousel slide projectors, and were precisely directed at the same spot on the screen. A shutter controlled by a pneumatic system and by computer-controlled electromagnetic valves alternately opened and closed the light beam (Fig. 13.1, Pi). When one beam was turned off, the other was

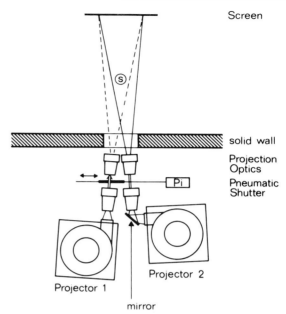

Fig. 13.1 *Setup of the stimulation equipment. Two carousel projectors were used to project the stimuli alternately, each for 2.5–4.2 s, onto a vertical reflecting screen placed at a distance of 2 m from the subject (S). By means of an automatically driven pneumatic shutter (Pi), one projector was turned off and the other turned on simultaneously within less than 6 ms. The shutter and the slide projectors were computer-controlled. The subject sat in another room. The size of the stimuli were about 4×6 degrees; i.e. they covered the foveal region and part of the parafoveal region.*

simultaneously turned on. Switching from one stimulus pattern to the next took less than 6 ms. During the change in stimulus patterns, the overall stimulus luminance remained constant. Shutter movement and slide change were controlled by computer signals. Each slide was classified by the computer into one of 4 stimulus categories, based on the signals generated by a small light source, two holes in the slide frame and two photocells. As a rule, a set of stimuli consisted of 160–180 slides belonging to 4 target categories, and of one additional set of slides forming the 'task category'. The respective tasks were selected in order to guarantee that the subject maintained a high degree of attention.

The different classes of stimulus categories are described in the sections below that deal with our findings. The subject was given a response key which allowed him to respond to the attention task. A recording session for about 180 slides, each seen on the average for 3.5 s, did not last longer than 11 minutes. This time was short enough to ensure that the subjects' attention remained at approximately the same high level. After a pause of 5 to 10 minutes, a second set of stimuli was normally tested for another 11 minutes (maximum).

Electroencephalographic and Electrooculographic Recordings

The electroencephalogram (EEG) was recorded by using Beckman Ag/AgCl electrodes attached with colodium to the skulls of the subjects. The skin was prepared beforehand with a cleaning paste. The electrode cups were filled with Beckman EEG electrode paste. After a few minutes, the electrode impedance was measured; it never exceeded 2 kΩ. The reference electrode consisted of 'linked earlobes' or 'linked mastoids'. We could record simultaneously from six sites at most. In the different studies, responses were evaluated from the following EEG electrodes: Oz, Pz, Cz, Fz, T3, T4, T5, T6, T8, F3, F4 (international 10–20 system; Jasper, 1958). The EEG signals were amplified by Grass P511A amplifiers (bandpass 0.1–1.0 Hz). At the same time, vertical and horizontal eye movements were recorded by a d.c. electronystagmogram whose amplifiers and optical insulation units operated at a bandpass frequency of 0–100 Hz. The EEG and the electrooculogram (EOG) signals were digitized (1:2048 for the amplitude) with a sampling rate of 200 to 400 Hz per channel; they were then stored on magnetic disks and evaluated off-line with an HP–1000 computer.

Data Evaluation

The digital computer programs allowed for backward and forward averaging of the EEG signals, which began the moment the slides changed. Signals containing large eye movements or blinks were not used in the averaging. As a rule, the EEG responses were averaged separately according to the stimulus categories for a period that began 100 ms before the stimulus change and that then continued for 700 or 800 ms after the stimulus change. Evoked potentials were averaged for each subject category and finally grand averages of the responses obtained for each question in a larger group of subjects (10 to 18 male and female subjects) were then computed. The respective standard deviations were also computed and plotted together with the grand average as a time function. The averaged EPs were further analysed by computing autocorrelation functions and cross-correlation functions between EPs obtained with different stimulus categories and recorded from the same electrodes. Cross-correlogram maxima were used for further evaluation. After transfer of the EPs that were averaged for the individual subjects to a SPS data file, selected grand averages obtained from 'monopolar' or 'bipolar' recordings underwent a further statistical test with regard to electrodes and stimulus categories. The

Wilcoxon test for dependent groups was computed for the EP data points with a sampling rate of 100 Hz for all possible category-related EP difference curves. To display these 'running' Wilcoxon test results, the P values were presented on a logarithmic scale (e.g. Fig. 13.4). For the graphical display of the EPs, a smoothing procedure of the amplitude data in the bins (which were sampled 200 or 400 per second) was performed according to the following equation: $a_{sj} = (2a_j + a_{j-1} + a_{j+1})/4$ where a_j, a_{j+1} and a_{j-1} were the respective amplitude values in the jth, $(j+1)$th and $(j-1)$th bin. This procedure led to an upper frequency limit of about 90 Hz.

Further computerized data analysis was performed by convolution of the individually averaged and grand averaged EPs with 'wavelets', i.e. second derivatives of Gaussian time functions of different widths. A few examples of this analysis are included in the following sections. Those interested in the details of this analysis are referred to Grüsser *et al.* (1991).

EEG Responses to Highly Schematic Faces

From the very simple schematic faces illustrated in Fig. 12.6, numbers 1, 6 and 12 were selected as stimuli. Figure 13.2 presents the grand averages obtained from 14 subjects (7 female and 7 male medical students) using 6 different recording electrodes. Small, category-specific differences were only obtained at electrodes T5, Cz and Oz, while the differences from the other electrodes remained within the noise level. Some data indicated that a slight gender-related difference in the EPs existed between the average responses of male and female subjects (Häussler, 1988). When 'bipolar recordings' (referred to Cz) were computed, the latency of peak N1 (about 100 ms) was significantly shorter for the 'good' face (1 in Fig. 12.6) than for the 'poor' face (6 in Fig. 12.6) or for the 'non-face' (12 in Fig. 12.6). These differences were more clearly visible at electrodes T5 and T7, located on the left side, than at the temporal electrodes T6 and T8, located on the right side (Bötzel *et al.*, 1989). In another test series in which simple schematic faces were applied (Fig. 13.3), the most significant stimulus category-specific differences (schematic face/scrambled face or schematic face/upside-down face) were also obtained at electrode Cz (Figs. 13.3, 13.4). As was the case with the first stimulus category (highly schematic faces), the differences between the grand averages of EPs recorded from male and female subjects were also most pronounced at the electrode Cz (Fig. 13.4).

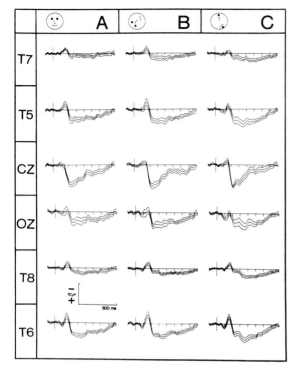

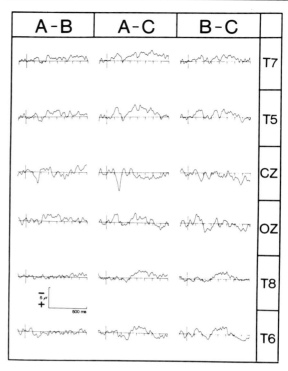

Fig. 13.2 Visual evoked potentials (EPs) obtained with highly schematic face or non-face stimuli (patterns 1, 6 and 12 from Fig. 12.6). Grand averages (± s.e.) of the EPs obtained in 14 subjects are displayed for 6 different recording electrodes, as indicated. Category-related difference curves are shown in the lower part of the figure. Electrode Cz led to significant differences in the categories face/poor face and face/non-face (from Bötzel et al., 1989).

EEG Responses to 'Realistic' Drawings of a Face, a Tree and a Chair

As illustrated by the data described in the preceding section, category-related differences in the EPs were rather small for schematic faces as opposed to non-faces. It seemed therefore meaningful in our search for face-responsive EP components to study the responses of subjects to realistic drawings of faces and non-faces. The stimulus sequence of this paradigm consisted of 160 slides of three different simple drawings (54 face, 53 tree and 53 chair, Fig. 13.5). The slides were presented in a semi-random order; direct repetition of one stimulus category was prevented, however. In the first series, black drawings on a white background were used (P-slides), and in the second series, negatives of the same drawings (N-slides). Figure 13.6 presents an example of grand averages of the responses obtained at electrode Cz. In contrast to the EPs evoked by the highly schematic faces in the study

described above, significantly more 'structured' EPs were obtained at the electrodes Cz, Oz as well as at the temporal electrodes. The differences between EPs obtained with N- and with P-stimuli were minimal. Fig. 13.7 shows mean latencies and mean amplitudes of the peaks measured relative to a pre-stimulus base line for all three stimulus categories. Data from the individual subjects and the grand averages are included. It is evident from Fig. 13.7 that a close correlation exists between these two types of data, and that with both types of data evaluation, the category-dependent differences were remarkable when EPs related to faces were compared with those related to non-faces. No significant difference was found, however, between the responses to the chair and those to the tree. This observation was confirmed by the category-related difference curves obtained using the respective grand average EPs. The recordings at electrode Cz are again used as examples in Fig. 13.8. The evoked potentials from the temporal electrodes (T5, T6) showed little variation with respect to the three categories of stimuli (Fig. 13.5); there were also no significant left–right differences. A detailed analysis of autocorrelation and cross-correlation

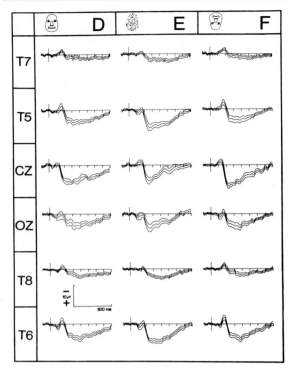

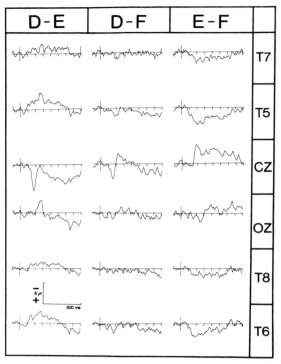

Fig. 13.3 *Grand averages of EPs computed from the responses to a schematic face (D), to the same stimulus 'scrambled' (increasing average spatial frequency content, E) and to the stimulus turned upside down (F). Grand averages of 14 subjects. Recording electrodes as indicated. The schematic faces were taken from Thornton and Pilowski (1982) (from Bötzel et al., 1989).*

Fig. 13.4 *Stimulus category-related difference curves of the recordings shown in Fig. 13.3. Note that the largest category-specific response differences were again recorded at the electrode Cz, but that significant category-related differences were also obtained at electrodes T5, T6 and Oz (only for category difference D–E) (from Bötzel et al., 1989).*

functions of the grand averages or of the category-dependent difference curves emphasized that the responses to faces stood out clearly when these simple drawings were used as stimuli.

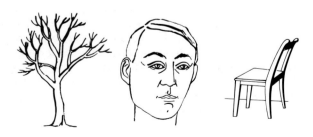

Fig. 13.5 *Simple drawings (black on white or white on black) used as stimuli.*

EEG Responses Evoked by Black and White Photographs of Faces and Non-faces

The experimental paradigm was again varied in order to obtain the new data described in this section. The stimuli consisted this time of 54 black-and-white photographs of different human faces of both sexes (frontal view, neutral expression, unknown to the subjects), 53 photos of differently decorated vases and 53 photos of different pairs of worn shoes photographed from above. Pairs of shoes and decorated vases ('*Jugendstil*') were chosen as comparison stimuli because they, like faces, have partial axial symmetry as well as structural complexity and individuality. In order to heighten the attention of the subjects, they were told to watch the slides carefully so that they would be able to recognize them later in a memory test. Up to six distinct peaks were identified in the EEG responses

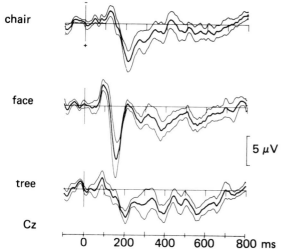

chair

face

5 μV

tree

Cz

0   200   400   600   800 ms

Fig. 13.6 *Grand average (± s.e.) of EPs recorded at electrode Cz in 5 female subjects. P-stimuli: black line drawings on a white background of a chair, a face and a tree (Fig. 13.5). Binocular stimulation was applied, as in all EP studies described in this chapter (Bötzel and Grüsser, 1988).*

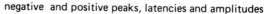

negative and positive peaks, latencies and amplitudes

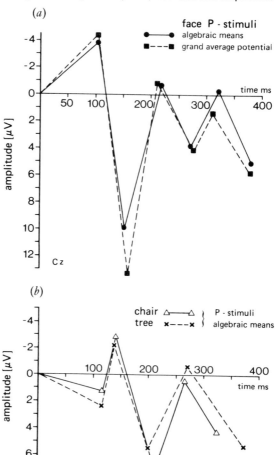

Fig. 13.7 *Amplitudes of negative and positive EP peaks (ordinate) plotted as a function of the respective peak latencies (abscissa). Data were from five female subjects. Stimulus patterns were as shown in Fig. 13.5. (a) Mean values of the individual EP responses to face stimuli (dots) and peak values of the corresponding grand average curve (squares). Data from electrode Cz. Note the similarity between the diagrams. (b) The mean values of the evoked responses to chair and tree P-stimuli are similar to one another (and also to the responses of the corresponding N-stimuli); they deviate considerably, however, from the algebraic means of the responses to face stimuli shown in (a) (Bötzel and Grüsser, 1989).*

evoked by the sudden change from one slide to the next; their latencies and amplitudes were measured. These values varied with the stimulus category and with the gender of the subjects. The face-responsive components were more pronounced in the EPs of female subjects than in those of males. This observation has been confirmed in most of the later studies on this topic. Figure 13.9 displays grand averages obtained in our own study: when the stimulus was a face, an early negative peak, occurring approximately 140–160 ms after the change in stimulus patterns, had the shortest latency and the highest amplitude at electrode Cz (algebraic mean of latencies for women/men: face 135/141 ms, vase 137/153 ms, shoes 148/154 ms). The category-dependent latency differences of the early negative peak were significant at the 99 per cent level at electrode Cz (Wilcoxon test for matched pairs). The amplitudes of the early negative peaks varied between -3 and $-10\,\mu V$, but did not differ significantly between the stimulus categories.

The first large positive peak was identified at 210–240 ms. The latency of this peak (measured at the temporal electrodes T5 and T6) was 12 ms longer than that measured at electrode Cz. Significantly shorter latencies were found at all three electrodes for the first positive peak in the EPs obtained with face stimuli, as compared to those obtained with the two other stimulus categories ($p < 0.01$, Wilcoxon test for matched pairs). The latencies of this peak were approximately the same for men and women; the amplitude did not change relative to the gender of the subjects or to the stimulus categories.

With face stimuli, a 'negative' peak appeared in most subjects at about 300 ms. This peak was either non-existent or small in the responses to non-face stimuli. For the EPs obtained in male subjects, the 'negative' peak at about 300 ms did not reach the baseline (upper part of Fig. 13.9). The lower part of Fig. 13.9 illustrates category-specific subtraction curves obtained from the EP grand averages

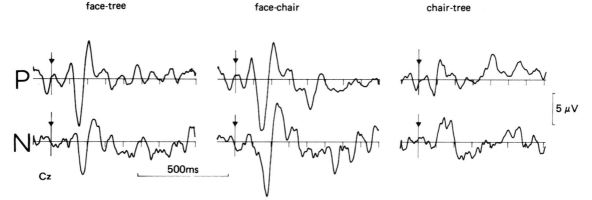

face-tree   face-chair   chair-tree

Fig. 13.8 *Subtraction curves of the EP grand averages, as presented in Fig. 13.6. Note the considerably larger differences when face stimuli were involved. Significant category-related response differences were restricted to the time period between 100 and 350 ms after the stimulus change (arrow). Data obtained with P-stimuli (black line drawings on a white background) are shown in the upper row, those obtained with N-stimuli (same drawings, but now white lines on a black background) in the lower row (Bötzel and Grüsser, 1989).*

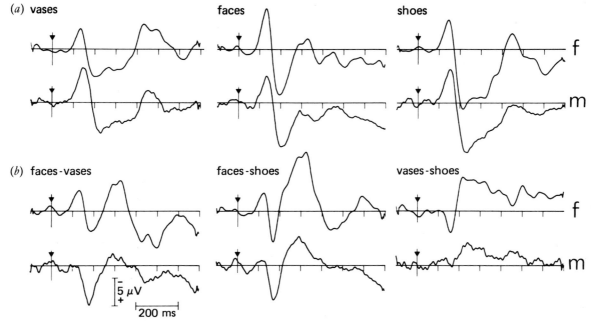

(a) vases   faces   shoes

(b) faces-vases   faces-shoes   vases-shoes

Fig. 13.9 *(a) Grand averages of evoked responses recorded at electrode Cz in 6 female (first row, f) and 5 male (second row, m) subjects. Stimuli were different black-and-white photographs of decorated vases, faces and pairs of worn shoes (from Bötzel and Grüsser, 1989). (b) Category-related subtraction curves of the EP grand averages presented in (a). The category-related differences are more pronounced in the averaged EPs of the 6 female subjects than in the averaged EPs of the 5 males (Bötzel and Grüsser, 1989).*

presented in the upper part of Fig. 13.9. Category-specific differences were more pronounced in female than in male subjects, and were most prominent when one of the two compared categories was face stimuli.

This study illustrated that when different photographs from one of the three categories were used, a face-responsive component was clearly hidden in the EPs, especially those recorded at electrode Cz. At this point in our investigation of face-responsive EP components, we investigated whether or not these components were modified by the fact that a face was known to the subject. This study will be dealt with in the following section.

Category-related Components in the Evoked Potentials Recorded During a Recognition Task – A First Approach

In the set of experiments described in the preceding section, the subjects directed their attention to the slide because they expected to take a memory test after the recording session. In the following set of experiments, in which 13 volunteers (4 male and 9 female students) were tested, the experimental paradigm was changed: the goal of this set of experiments was to find out whether or not evoked potentials might be altered by memory search processes that are followed by a decision process ('previously seen/not seen') related to the three different stimulus categories. These stimulus categories were the same as those used in the paradigm described in the last section. Before the recording session, the subjects were shown 9 slides of black-and-white photographs (10 seconds each slide). They were instructed to memorize each of these 9 slides (3 in each category) carefully in order to perform the 'flower task' correctly during the recording session (this is

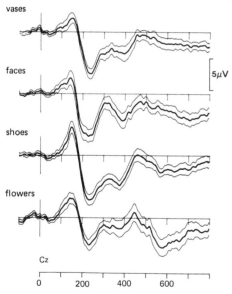

Fig. 13.10 *EPs (grand averages ± s.e.) obtained at electrode Cz in 13 subjects (4 males, 9 females). Stimuli were black-and-white photographs of vases, faces, shoes and flowers (not previously seen by the subjects). The subjects also had to perform a recognition task after the presentation of a flower. Responses to a fifth category, i.e. stimuli seen previously, were excluded from the averaging. The EPs evoked by the flowers exhibit a late positivity occurring between 500 and 700 ms, presumably related to the decision required after a flower appeared as a stimulus (from Bötzel and Grüsser, 1988).*

described below). These 9 slides appeared repeatedly during the recording session in random order within a set of 183 stimuli not known to the subjects (again photos of faces, decorated vases and worn pairs of shoes). A fourth category of photographs was added: a black-and-white slide of one or several flowers was shown every third to fifth slide. The subjects were asked to press a button whenever a flower slide appeared immediately after a face, vase or shoe slide that had been seen by them during the pre-test inspection period. The EEG responses obtained using the 9 slides that had been previously seen and that had repeatedly appeared during the recording session were excluded from averaging by the computer program.

The EPs obtained in this study showed peaks and troughs in latency ranges that were similar to those recorded during the tests described in the preceding section. A prominent 'negative' peak appeared again for the face stimuli at about 310 ms; a positive peak appeared at about 390 ms (Fig. 13.10). As in the two preceding paradigms, maximum category-specific response differences were again obtained in the recordings at electrode Cz. A very large positive wave, which did not appear in the other studies described above, appeared with a maximum at about 700 ms for faces, 792 ms for vases and 698 ms for pairs of shoes. This wave was most prominent in the EPs evoked by face photographs, and was better recognized in the recordings at electrode Fz than at electrode Cz. This late component was presumably caused by the experimental task, i.e. to compare the presented items with those previously memorized, and to store that information for a possible decision required in case a 'flower slide' was presented. The averaged EPs evoked by the flower stimuli exhibited a very pronounced positive wave peaking at 580 ms. This peak was probably caused by cerebral mechanisms responsible for the decision task that was required after the appearance of these stimuli. Category-specific difference curves similar to those shown in Fig. 13.10 showed the largest potentials for differences involving the following pairs: faces/shoes, faces/flowers, faces/vases.

EP Responses to Known and Unknown Faces

The investigation of whether or not memory processes had a measurable influence on the EPs was continued in two further series of experiments, in which stimuli were composed partly of known faces or non-faces and partly of unknown faces or non-faces. We normally recognize within less than a second whether an observed face is known or unknown to us. There are two large classes of known faces: (a) those known to us through personal acquaintance, and (b) faces of politicians, artists, entertainers, etc. who we know through the media ('public faces'). These two classes of faces were used in an extensive study involving 15 subjects (7 female and 8 male medical students). In order to get acquainted with formerly unknown faces, the subjects inspected eleven black-and-white photographs of faces for 6 seconds and then for 4 seconds approximately 10 minutes before the recording session started. During the inspection series, they were asked to judge the faces as 'friendly', 'unfriendly' or 'neutral'. In the second inspection series, they were asked to signal by pressing a bar whenever they recognized the faces that they had previously evaluated as 'neutral'. In the set of black-and-white photographs used during the recording session, about half the faces were known, i.e. the known faces appeared several times. The unknown faces were not repeatedly presented in the course of the recording experiment, however. Figure 13.11 shows grand averages of the responses obtained at electrodes T3, T4 and Cz for the two face categories. Although a left–right difference was present for electrodes T3–T4 under these stimulus conditions, the most prominent responses were again recorded at electrode Cz. With known faces, the maintained electrical negativity began about 400 ms after the stimulus change; it lasted longer than it did during responses to unknown faces (Grüsser and Naumann, 1988). This maintained negativity may have been caused by the 'preparation' of the required response: subjects (all right-handed) were asked to press a key with their right hand whenever the projected face was known to them. The early response components occurring between 100 and 350 ms did not differ significantly for the known faces as compared with the unknown, however.

The EPs evoked by 45 'famous' faces were studied using the same group of fifteen subjects. The photos of 'famous faces' were intermingled in a second set of experiments with unknown faces (slides of black-and-white photographs). The subjects were asked to press a key during the recording session whenever a famous face that was known to them appeared. EPs were only averaged when the subject correctly recognized the famous face. The average response time for this task was 730 ms, and the average of correct responses was about 75 per cent. Less than 6 per cent of the responses were 'false positive' responses, i.e. the subjects pressing the bar when unknown faces were projected. The EPs correlated with these responses were, of course, also not included in the averaging process. The responses to unknown faces did not differ significantly from those obtained during the known/unknown paradigm. The grand average EPs evoked by famous faces were very similar to those evoked by unknown faces (Fig. 13.11). In conclusion, the behaviourally tested fact that our subjects knew a face (either by getting recently acquainted with it prior to the test or by an earlier learning process with respect to public faces) did not lead to any measurably significant changes in the EPs. The face-responsive components appearing during the first 350 ms especially seem not to be affected by the fact that we know a face or that we see it for the first time. Thus the method of measuring averaged or grand averaged EPs seems to have reached a methodological limit in this task.

EEG Responses to Known and Unknown Flowers – A Control Experiment

The outcome of the experiments described in the preceding section was somewhat surprising to us, and led us to investigate whether or not the processes of learning visual patterns are generally not detectable in the evoked potentials of the human electroencephalogram. This question was tested using slides of black-and-white photographs of flowers. As with the faces, the subjects were asked to inspect a series of 11 black-and-white photographs of flowers, each for 6 seconds and then for 4 seconds. They then had to recognize the flowers during the recording session, and indicated their responses by pressing a bar. Figure 13.12 demonstrates grand averages obtained for the EPs at electrodes T3, T4 and Cz. We discovered a positive wave occurring between 200 and 400 ms; this was more pronounced and lasted longer with known flower stimuli than with unknown flower stimuli. When comparing the recordings obtained with known/unknown flowers with those in which known/unknown faces were used as stimuli, one recognizes typical face-responsive EP components, which normally reached a maximum at electrode Cz. The formal structural complexity of the face stimuli and of the flower stimuli were about the same for both categories. The most pronounced amplitude difference between flower and face stimuli was the negative peak occurring at about 280 ms with face stimuli. A comparison of Fig. 13.12 with Fig. 13.11 also supports the hypothesis that face-responsive components do indeed exist in the EPs.

Extending Face Stimuli to Person Stimuli: The Category-responsive Components in the Evoked Potentials Differ

Face-responsive components of the grand averaged EPs were demonstrated in the preceding sections. Some of these components have also been found in other studies

15 subjects (7 females, 8 males)   decision time paradigm

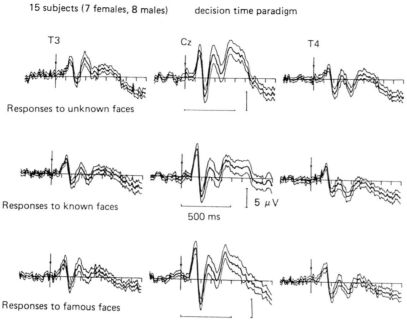

Fig. 13.11 *Grand averages (± s.e.) of EPs evoked by unknown, known and famous faces. Note the slight left–right difference for the EPs recorded at electrodes T3 and T4; the face-responsive components appearing between 180 and 350 ms do not differ for the three stimulus categories, however. Data from 15 male and female subjects (Grüsser et al., 1990).*

12 subjects (5 females, 7 males)   decision time paradigm

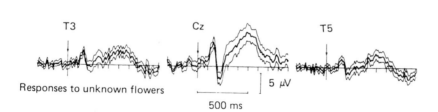

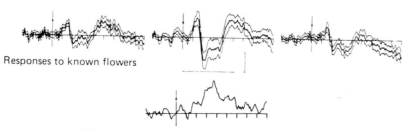

Difference curve at Cz. Unknown minus known flowers.

Fig. 13.12 *Grand averages (± s.e.) of EPs evoked by black-and-white photographs of known and unknown flowers. The most pronounced responses were obtained at electrode Cz, for which a significant difference between EPs evoked by unknown and known flowers was also found during the period between 200 and 500 ms. This is illustrated in the difference curve at the bottom of the figure (from Bötzel et al., 1989).*

(e.g. Jeffreys and Musslewhite, 1987; Jeffreys, 1989). Face-responsive components were hidden in the early sequence, in which a negative peak (80–110 ms) was followed by a large positive peak at about 150–200 ms and by rapid consecutive negativity. They reached a maximum amplitude when the EPs were recorded at electrode Cz. These face-responsive components became evident when the EPs were compared with those evoked by non-face stimuli of similar structural complexity. In several studies,

other face-specific responses have been reported: Small (1983) found a larger P300 wave over the right hemisphere when the EPs were evoked by face stimuli, as compared with those evoked by geometric patterns. Srebro (1985a, b), who computed spatial 'Laplacian' transformations using the responses across the recording sites above the temporal lobe, found small, category-specific differences that occurred 206 ms after the stimulus began. He compared EPs evoked by memorized faces with EPs evoked by

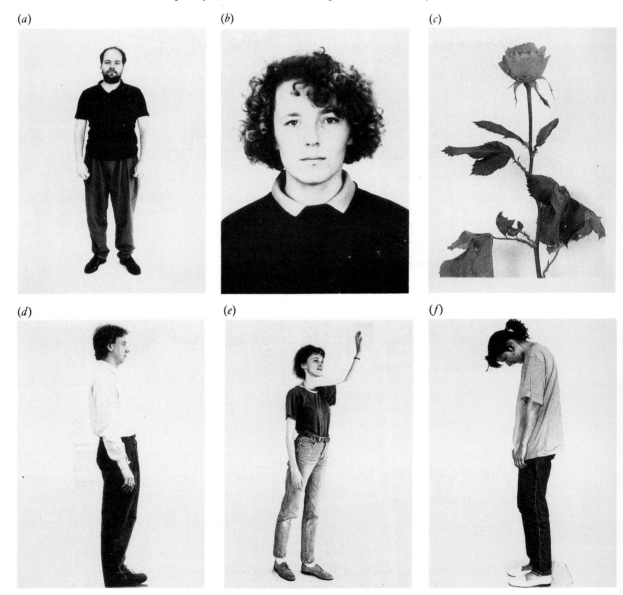

(a)   (b)   (c)

(d)   (e)   (f)

Fig. 13.13 *Examples of stimuli belonging to two sets of experiments in which full views of persons were used as separate stimulus categories. First set: (a) person, frontal view; (b) face; (c) flower (tool not shown). Second set: (d) neutral person, side view; (e) person greeting; (f) person in depressed mood (Seeck and Grüsser, 1991).*

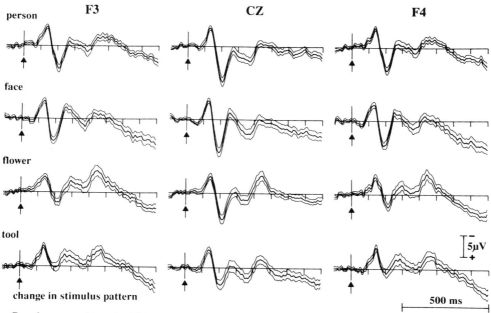

person F3 CZ F4

face

flower

tool

change in stimulus pattern

5μV

500 ms

Fig. 13.14. *Grand averages (± s.e.) of EPs obtained in 18 subjects. Stimuli were photographs of faces, persons, flowers and tools (Fig. 13.13). Data from 'monopolar' recordings at electrodes F3, F4 and Cz are shown (Seeck and Grüsser, 1991).*

memorized non-face stimuli. He did not detect significant differences between EPs evoked by unknown faces and by unknown non-face stimuli, however. Since he only used four subjects – which, based on our own experience, is much too small a sample – Srebro's data have to be considered with some caution.

The face can undoubtedly be considered as the most characteristic part of the human body. Nevertheless, the face-responsive components in the EPs described in the preceding sections and by the other authors just mentioned may not be specific signs for faces at all, but rather just response components related to body parts in general. To answer this question, we have performed several additional studies over the last years using other human body parts as stimuli. The responses evoked by faces were first compared to those evoked by photographs of complete persons. Photographs of tools and flowers were used as control stimuli (Seeck *et al.*, 1989; Seeck and Grüsser, 1991). In the first set of experiments, 160 slides of black-and-white photographs of the following stimulus categories were applied: (a) a person standing in a neutral, upright frontal position, (b) frontal views of faces with neutral expressions, (c) flowers, (d) tools (Fig. 13.13(a)–(c)).

Figure 13.14 presents the grand averages of monopolar EPs obtained with these 4 stimulus categories. The main category-selective differences were found in the EPs recorded at the frontal electrodes F3 and F4, and to a somewhat lesser degree in the EPs recorded at the central

electrode Cz. Neither with frontal nor with temporal electrodes were significant left–right differences found for any stimulus category. Category-related differences in the 'monopolar' recordings were detected by computing the corresponding difference curves, and by applying a statistical analysis to these curves. An example of this procedure is shown in Fig. 13.15 for electrode F4. The same results were essentially obtained for electrode F3 and to a lesser degree for electrode Cz: the most significant differences were found for the (face–flower) values, with peaks at about 185 ms and 460 ms. These peaks also appeared for the (face–tool) curves. The difference curves (person–tool) and (person–flower) peaked at 210 ms, while the other difference curves (person–face) and (flower–tool) hardly exceeded chance level between 100 and 600 ms. It is of interest that whenever faces were used as stimuli, a maintained potential difference appeared 350–800 ms after the change in stimulus pattern.

The computed category-specific difference curves of the EPs were also evaluated by computing the 'running' Wilcoxon test values. A comparison of the Wilcoxon test values with the amplitude values of the category-specific difference curves indicated high similarity. In the running Wilcoxon test values, a significance level of $p < 0.05$ normally occurred between 140 and 230 ms when EPs evoked by persons or faces were compared to those evoked by non-faces. A second period of highly significant differences appeared in the time range beyond 400 ms, provided that faces were one of the compared stimulus sets used

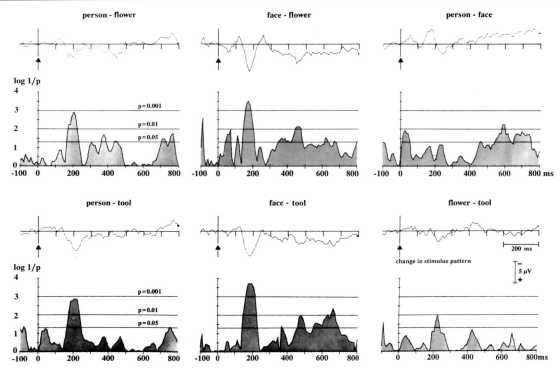

Fig. 13.15 *Category-dependent subtraction curves of the grand average EPs (18 subjects) recorded at electrode F4 and shown in Fig. 13.14. Category-related differences were prominent during the first 350 ms only when faces were involved. A late DC-shift occurring between 400 and 800 ms was only partially significant. It appeared when the EPs evoked by face stimuli were part of the subtraction curves. Similar responses were obtained for the EPs recorded at electrodes F3 and Cz (Fig. 13.14). The grey-shaded areas represent the values of the 'running' Wilcoxon test (Seeck and Grüsser, 1991).*

(Fig. 13.15). It is also evident from this figure that the difference curves obtained with the (face–tool) and (face–flower) pairs were larger than the difference curves obtained with the (face–person) pair. These two categories led to more similar EPs. This finding was also confirmed by the running Wilcoxon test.

It became evident from our recordings with the 'critical' electrodes (Cz, F3 and F4) that face-responsive components in the evoked potentials were, in general, more prominent than person-responsive components. This statement was corroborated by an analysis of the 'bipolar' recordings. The most interesting results were obtained in the EPs between the frontal and temporal electrodes or between the central and temporal electrodes (Fig. 13.16). In the light of the 8 grand averages presented in Fig. 13.16, one immediately realizes that faces and persons evoked one type of EP, while flowers and tools another type. These category-specific differences are quantitatively expressed by the maxima of the cross-correlograms, as indicated in the inset of Fig. 13.16. These maxima were higher for (person × face) EP correlograms and (flower × tool) EP correlograms than for any other combination. The most prominent variability in the EEG responses in the bipolar recordings (including the temporal electrodes) occurred during the first 300 ms; the overall variability of the EP amplitudes was higher for face stimuli than for person stimuli.

Figures 13.17 and 13.18 provide an example of another quantitative analysis that we performed in order to evaluate the significance of category-related subtraction curves. The EPs obtained with different subjects and stimulus categories were randomly shuffled, and the grand average EPs were computed for the four new, randomly shuffled response categories. Theoretically, these random averages should be identical for a given electrode, since subjects and categories were homogeneously mixed. Thus the subtraction curves from pairs of these randomly shuffled grand average EPs should fluctuate around zero, and the running Wilcoxon test between these randomly-shuffled subtraction curves should not exceed chance level. This is

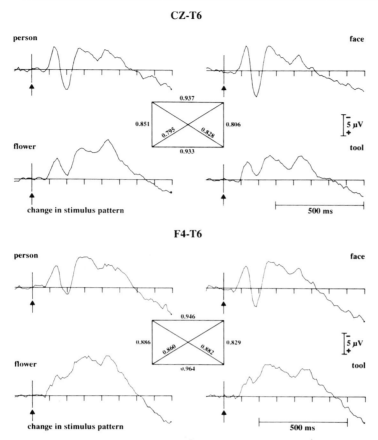

Fig. 13.16 *Grand average EPs obtained with 'bipolar' recordings (Cz–T6 and F4–T6) for four different classes of black-and-white photographs (persons, faces, flowers and tools). Note that the bipolar EPs are clearly grouped into two classes (persons and faces, flowers and tools). This grouping is also indicated by the maxima of the cross-correlation functions, as indicated in the in-set (from Seeck and Grüsser, 1991).*

illustrated in Fig. 13.17. Of the randomly-shuffled grand average subtraction curves, we always selected the one which, by chance, was furthest from zero, and computed the ±3-standard-error values around this curve (Fig. 13.18(c)). We then compared these statistical limits with the category-related grand average subtraction curve (Fig. 13.18(a)). The category-related difference curve exceeded the rather restrictive significance level of $p < 0.001$ whenever this curve exceeded the limits determined by the randomly shuffled subtraction curve ±3 s.e. When comparing Fig. 13.8(c) with Fig. 13.8(d), in which the running Wilcoxon test data are presented, one finds that both statistical methods led to very similar evaluations with respect to the significance of the category-related subtraction curves. In these combined tests, we finally reached a rather high degree of reliability in our search for the face-responsive components present in the evoked potentials.

Different Gestures Used as Stimulus Patterns Do not Lead to Different EPs

In this section we briefly present another example indicating the methodological limits involved in measuring evoked potentials. After it became evident in the study described in the last section that a 'person-responsive' component may exist in the EPs (a component certainly smaller than the 'face-responsive' component), we investigated whether the person-responsive components depended on the gestures made by the persons in the slides. Examples of the 4 stimulus categories applied in this set of experiments are illustrated in the lower part of Figs. 13.13(d)–(f). We used 160 black-and-white photographs of persons (side view) making 4 different gestures: standing neutrally, boxing, seeming depressed and greet-

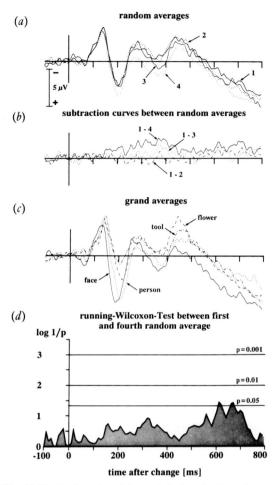

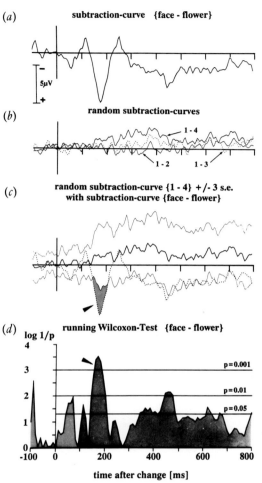

Fig. 13.17 *Explanation of the statistical evaluations of category-related EPs. (a) EPs recorded at electrode F4 for the four stimulus categories (faces, persons, tools and flowers) were randomly shuffled into four groups and grand averages were computed. Theoretically identical responses were expected. The differences characterize the statistical fluctuations in the data. (b) Subtraction curves were computed from these random averages. (c) Category-related grand averages (electrode F4). (d) Running Wilcoxon test for difference (1–4) of (b).*

Fig. 13.18 *(a) A category-related subtraction curve (face–flower) is presented. In the recordings from electrode F4, differences appear between 100 and 300 ms, while a late difference is present beyond 400 ms. (b) Three subtraction curves, as computed from random averages presented in Fig. 13.17(a). These subtraction curves should theoretically be near zero. (c) The largest random subtraction curve of (b) is plotted with its ± 3 s.e. limits. Superposed onto these curves is the subtraction curve (face–flower) from (a); it exceeds the ± 3 s.e. limits of the random curve in a range between 140 and 220 ms and marginally between 350 and 500 ms. (d) A running Wilcoxon test is computed for the substraction curves of the categories (face–flower) shown in (a). It exceeds the 99 per cent confidence level for the waves appearing between 160 and 210 ms. Note the statistical confirmation between the two tests (c) and (d) (arrows).*

ing with the hand. The 'person-responsive' components of the EPs appeared between 120 and 350 ms, as in the first paradigm, and were at a maximum in the bipolar recordings between the frontal and temporal electrodes or between the central and temporal electrodes. In all recording conditions (monopolar or bipolar), however, only very small category-related differences were found; these were at the limits of statistical significance. In monopolar recordings at electrodes Cz, F3 and F4, the negative peak at about 140 ms was larger for stimuli showing 'greeting',

'fighting' and 'depressed' gestures than for the stimuli in which a 'neutral' person was seen. This difference also appeared in the bipolar recordings between the central or

photographs of persons with different expressions

CZ-T6

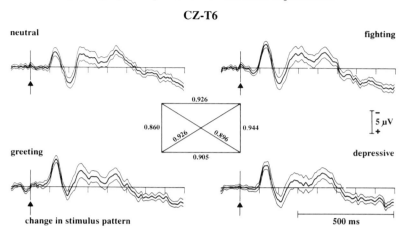

neutral

fighting

0.926

0.860   0.944

0.926   0.896

greeting   0.905   depressive

change in stimulus pattern

500 ms

5 µV

Fig. 13.19 *Grand averages ±3 s.e. of the EPs (bipolar recordings, electrodes Cz–T6 in 18 subjects – 9 male, 9 female). Stimuli were black-and-white photographs of persons making four different gestures (neutral, fighting, greeting and depressive, as indicated; see Fig. 13.13, lower row). Only small differences became visible in the EPs related to the four different stimulus classes. The lowest cross-correlogram maxima were obtained when the stimulus class 'neutral position' was used (Seeck and Grüsser, 1991).*

frontal electrodes and the temporal electrodes. One example is presented in Fig. 13.19. The negative–positive variation appearing between 100 and 230 ms was somewhat larger for the stimulus categories showing 'expressive' persons than for the stimuli showing neutral persons. The difference reached a significance level of $p < 0.05$ between 120 and 160 ms in the running Wilcoxon test. The time course and the amplitude of the EPs evoked by the 4 stimulus categories were otherwise very similar. This similarity was also expressed by the high maximum values of the cross-correlograms, as illustrated in the inset of Fig. 13.19.

Wavelet Analysis of the EPs Further Corroborates Face-responsive Components

The visual evoked potentials (individual ones or averaged ones) contain different temporal frequencies which are superposed on one another. To analyse the individual frequency components, it seemed meaningful to use suitable frequency filters. One such filter is the wavelet, the negative second derivative of a temporal Gaussian function, as illustrated in Fig. 13.20. For a quantitative evaluation the temporal width of the Gaussian, as characterized by the standard deviation, is systematically varied and the resulting second derivatives, i.e. the wavelets, are convoluted with the evoked potentials. As compared with other filter

functions, there are some advantages in using the wavelet for this purpose. In this respect, the fact that the temporal integral of a wavelet is zero and that the width of the wavelet is limited is extremely important (for further discussion see Grüsser *et al.*, 1991). By using wavelet analysis, the individual EP, the grand average EP or the category-related difference curves are converted into a three-dimensional graph, the extension of which is determined by the analysis time (*x*-axis) and by the temporal variability of the width of the wavelet functions used for convolution with the EPs (*z*-axis Fig. 13.20(a, b)). When this method was applied to category-related difference curves, the following question arose: what statistical measure could we use to determine the ranges of significance of the wavelet transformations (Fig. 13.20(c)). In order to answer this question, we used a method similar to the one described above: after random shuffling of the EPs recorded at a certain electrode or pair of electrodes, new, 'randomly-shuffled' grand average EPs and difference curves were computed and convoluted with the respective wavelet functions (Fig. 13.20(d)). The ±3 s.e.-fidelity limits were then computed and graphically displayed for this function. A significance was expected whenever the wavelet transformations of category-related difference curves exceeded these limits (Fig. 13.20(e)). In order to illustrate this significance range more clearly, the parts of the wavelet transformations that exceed the significance range have been specially marked in the graphical display (Fig. 13.20(f)). Finally, the lines were determined where the category-related and wavelet-transformed difference curves exceeded the corresponding ±3 s.e. significance

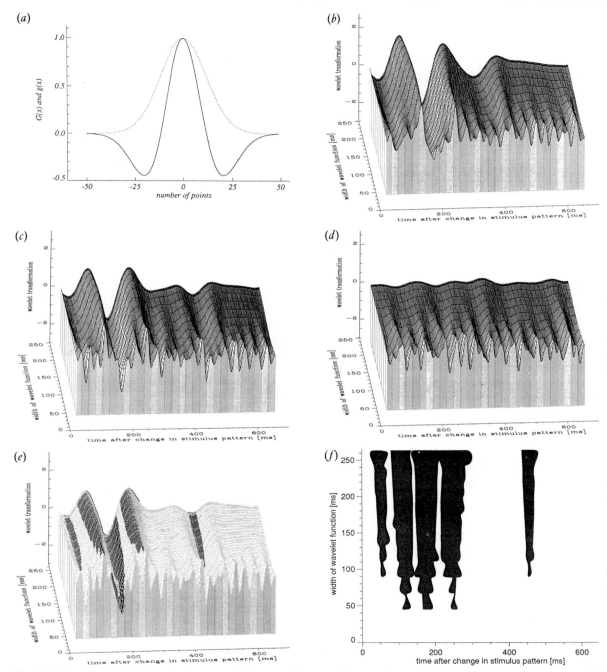

Fig. 13.20 *(a) Example of a wavelet function and the original Gaussian function. The wavelet function is the second derivative of the Gauss function multiplied by − 1. (b) Example of a W-diagram obtained by the convolution of a grand average EP (evoked by face stimuli, electrode F4) with wavelet functions of different width (± 2 s.e. of the Gaussian distribution). (c) W-diagram of category-related difference curves (face–flower, electrode F4). (d) W-diagram of the maximum difference obtained by subtraction of two random-shuffled grand averages (electrode F4). (e) W-diagram as in (c). All parts exceeding the ± 3 s.e. limits of curve (d) are marked in black. (f) Contour plots of the black-marked components of the W-diagram shown in (e). The blackened surface represents the time–frequency range of a significance of p < 0.001 in the category-related difference curves (face–flower, electrode F4) (Grüsser et al., 1991).*

level of the random shuffled curves; these were then plotted in a two-dimensional graph. With this method, the 'significance' profiles for category-related differences became easily visible in a plane defined by the time after the stimulus change and by the width of the wavelets used for convolution (Fig. 13.20(f)). Those interested in a more detailed explanation of this method are referred to Grüsser *et al.* (1991). The analysis that has been performed to date with this method has confirmed the simpler statistical analyses that had been applied in earlier studies to the visual evoked potentials of the human electroencephalogram recorded using faces and non-faces: there is good evidence which indicates that a face-responsive component in the EEG potentials is indeed evoked by a sudden change of visual patterns, from non-face to face stimuli.

Conclusions

In the different experimental studies described in this chapter, the main goal of our investigation was to test whether the behavioural 'uniqueness' of faces as visual stimuli leads to measurable signal differences in the EEG responses, as compared with those evoked potentials related to non-face stimuli. We believe that our analysis of EPs obtained with schematic faces, simple drawn faces and black-and-white photographs of faces of known and unknown persons indeed supports the hypothesis that face signals are processed in the human brain, as in the brains of other primates (cf. Chapter 7), as special events, as compared with those obtained with many other stimulus categories; they are presumably related to neuronal operations occurring in specialized neocortical and limbic brain structures. Based on the clinical studies described in the next chapter, it seems rather probable that face-related data processing occurs not only in certain parts of the visual association cortices which are located in man in the infracalcarine occipito–temporal region, but also in limbic structures such as the gyrus parahippocampalis, the amygdala, the hippocampus and perhaps also the gyrus cinguli. The maximum face-responsive components in the evoked potentials recorded in man were usually obtained at electrodes Cz, F3 and F4. These responses clearly differ from those obtained in monkeys (cf. Chapter 7). Several factors might account for this difference: (a) during hominid phylogenesis, the face-specific areas were considerably shifted from the inferior temporal to the basal occipito–temporal cortex, and/or (b) new face-responsive cortical neuronal data analysis developed during hominid evolution. From the data presented in this chapter, it is not at all possible to make any conclusion about where the face-responsive components recorded at electrodes Cz, T4, T5, F3 or F4 originate in the brain. More precise explanations are possible, however, with regard to the time involved in

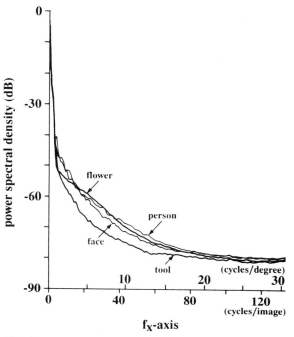

Fig. 13.21 *Average spatial frequency from the power spectra of all 116 slides of the four stimulus categories (faces, persons, flowers and tools) used in the experiments from which the data are presented in Figs. 13.13–13.18.). The example shows the power averages of spatial frequency across the x-axis. Note that very little difference exists between the four stimulus categories in the averaged spatial frequency distribution. All curves overlap in their ± 3 s.e. ranges. The same results were found for y-axis averaging and for 'circular' averaging. This example demonstrates that on the average, the four different stimulus classes contained approximately the same spatial frequency content (analysis performed by K. H. Dittberner and W. Seidler, 1991).*

face-related data processing: the formal structural analysis is evidently performed within 100 to 350 ms after the face stimulus appears. Emotional evaluations, memory processes (known/unknown faces) and name-searching presumably continue for another 200 to 500 ms; these processes can hardly be detected in the evoked potentials, however.

In light of our studies, it seems that the face-responsive components of EPs have three main properties:

1. The face-responsive components change little when realistically drawn face stimuli or photographs of faces are used.

2. The spatial frequency content of the stimuli in the different categories does not explain the category-related differences in the EPs. Figure 13.21 illustrates the averaged spatial frequency contents of the 4 stimulus categories used in the investigation described in the preceding

section. In light of such analyses, it became evident that the data of a spatial frequency analysis of the stimulus pattern does not at all explain the differences in EPs obtained from face and non-face stimuli.

3. The regularity with which the face-responsive components appeared between 100 and 350 ms after a change in the stimulus pattern slightly depended on the 'context', i.e. on the other three 'competing' stimulus categories chosen for comparison. It also marginally depended on the task that the subject was asked to perform during the recording session.

Finally, it should be emphasized that reliable and comparable findings in the grand average studies were obtained, as a rule, only when data from at least 10 to 15 subjects were averaged. We also want to emphasize once again the fact that differences in certain faces, in facial expression, and in the knowledge of the subject about the face (known/unknown) do not appear in the grand averaged EPs. The same is true for the person-related components in the evoked potentials. These EPs did not differ when neutral persons were used as stimulus patterns, as compared with EPs evoked by persons making expressive gestures. Evidently, the method used to measure pattern-generated visual evoked potentials imposes certain limits on the types of questions that can be answered.

Note

This chapter was written in collaboration with Dr Margitta Seeck of the Department of Physiology, Freie Universität Berlin.

14 Faces Lost: Prosopagnosia

Historical Introduction and Elementary Clinical Signs of Prosopagnosia

Prosopagnosia was defined by Hécaen (1962) as a failure 'To recognize people known to the patient on the basis of visual perception of their faces'. Benton (1985) added

When identification is achieved, it is based on the person's voice, size, clothes, gait, or even on an adventitious facial feature or accessory, such as a scar or blemish, a moustache, or eyeglasses. But the more essential features, such as facial structure, eyes, nose, and mouth, cannot be utilized for identification.

Patients who fail to recognize familiar people by their face have been noted for a long time. Bodamer (1947), who coined the term 'prosopagnosia', attributed the first clinical observation of this disturbance to Quaglino (1867). However, within the frame of a revival of Wigan's (1844) ideas on the interaction of the two cerebral hemispheres (Bogen, 1972), it became apparent that he had most likely been the first to report on a case of prosopagnosia. He stated:

Among the curious defects in the functions of the brain, is one which was brought to my notice a short time ago: A gentleman of middle age, or a little past that period, lamented to me his utter inability to remember faces. He would converse with a person for an hour, but after an interval of days could not recognize him again. Even friends, with whom he had been engaged in business transactions, he was unconscious of ever having seen. Being in an occupation in which it was essential to cultivate the good-will of the public, his life was made perfectly miserable by this unfortunate defect, and his time was passed in offending and apologizing. He was quite incapable of making a mental picture of anything, and it was not till he heard the voice, that he could recognize men with whom he had constant intercourse.

Other early descriptions of prosopagnosia were provided by Hughlings Jackson (1876), Charcot (1883) and Wilbrand (1887, 1892). Jackson described a patient who one day lost his way in the streets, didn't find his way home, didn't recognize familiar persons, but could identify and name objects correctly. Probably the most famous reports are those of Charcot (1883) and Wilbrand (1887, 1892). Charcot's case appeared under the title 'Abrupt and isolated suppression of the mental vision of signs and objects (forms and colours)'. The patient, a man who had been in possession of an extraordinary visual memory, had lost the ability to recognize as well as revisualize forms, places, colours and familiar persons like his wife and children. He was no longer able to visualize their faces or appearance, and when in their presence he thought he was seeing new traits and characteristics in their physiognomy. Once he even mistook his own mirror image for a stranger and begged his pardon for blocking his way. Charcot considered this man's disturbance as an unspecific loss of visual memory and mental imagery.

Wilbrand's (1887, 1892) patient was a 63-year-old woman who, after a loss of consciousness of several hours, remained in a dream-like state during which she was considered to be blind, although she knew she was not. She recalled having mistaken her physician for a dog and, on another occasion, her maid for a table. She also remembered that her field of vision was initially very restricted, but that the right half cleared after about 2 years. Upon examination 4 years after the event, an incomplete left homonymous hemianopsia and a small homonymous defect in the lower right quadrant were found. Like Charcot's patient, she was well-educated, spoke five languages and was known for her excellent visual memory and imagery; in contrast, she could evoke mental images, but when she was actually confronted with the real ones they appeared strange and unfamiliar to her. In her own words,

with my eyes closed I can easily walk through the streets of Hamburg [her native city] but if I am actually in one of those streets I don't know how to find my way,

or again,

entering my room I have the impression of being in a strange room which definitely belongs to someone else.

Concerning physiognomies she stated,

> *I look completely different in my mirror than I used to look. I do not see any similarity to my former image and I cannot understand that this face should be mine; or people I have met since my illness do not leave a visual memory, I cannot recognize them anymore, but easily identify them by the timbre of their voice.*

This intelligent woman concluded:

> *deducing from my own state, humans see more with their brain than with their eye. The eye is only a means for seeing, because I see everything clearly and precisely but frequently cannot recognize and don't know the meaning of what I see.*

One might keep in mind that this patient's discerning description of what later came to be known as 'visual agnosia' antedated Lissauer's (1890) famous case report by at least 5 years. Postmortem examination revealed a large inferior medial, occipito-temporal infarct in the territory of the right posterior cerebral artery and a small left occipital infarct.

Following these famous early descriptions, a number of similar observations were published in the late part of the last and early years of this century. Among the authors who reported disturbances in physiognomy recognition were: Wernicke (1881), Rheinhardt (1887), Freund (1889), Groenouw (1891), Probst (1901), Bonnhoeffer (1915), Poppelreuter (1917/18), Stauffenberg (1918), Reichhardt (1918), Heidenhain (1927), Jossmann (1929), Milian (1932), Beichl (1944), Feuchtwanger (1934), Frank (1934), Hoff und Pötzl (1937), Szatmari (1938), Donini (1939), Bengtsen *et al.* (1941), Pichler (1943). Reviews were presented by Pötzl (1928), Bodamer (1947), Gloning (1966), Benton (1979), and Hécaen (1981).

None the less, up to the 1930s a disturbance in face recognition was considered to be part of a complex visual agnosic disorder and not a specific agnosic syndrome. In 1937 Hoff and Pötzl published a report entitled '*On an Optic–Agnosic Disturbance of Memory for Physiognomies*'. Their patient recovered completely from alexia without agraphia, but could not identify familiar faces, including his own. Since the recognition of other visual stimuli was less impaired, the authors considered the inability to identify familiar faces for the first time as a specific form of visual agnosia, as well as rejecting the notion of this disturbance being a specific amnesia for physiognomies. Likewise, recognition of letters and words was considered for the first time in the history of visual agnosia to be specifically opposed to recognition of physiognomies. These two functions were viewed as complementary. Consequently face agnosia and pure alexia were interpreted as reciprocally linked symptoms. Bodamer (1947), following the suggestions of Hoff and Pötzl, isolated the failure to recognize familiar persons by their face from other disorders of visual recognition and gave this syndrome a new name – 'prosopagnosia'. In his seminal paper, after a short review of the literature on visual agnosia, he presented symptoms of three patients who, subsequent to Second World War brain injuries, suffered from an impaired processing of physiognomic information. In his attempt to show that prosopagnosia was a specific form of visual agnosia, he used the classical approach of double dissociation of function to make the contribution of different anatomical structures plausible. Only two of the three patients were prosopagnosic. The third suffered from severe distortions in face perception without having lost the capacity to recognize familiar faces.

In addition, Bodamer discussed another dissociation, namely that of face specificity in metamorphopsia. His second prosopagnosic patient occasionally suffered from severe visual metamorphopsias which spared only faces, while in his third patient metamorphopsias were restricted to faces. Bodamer considered the recognition of physiognomies to be a function of fundamental biological relevance. He based his assumption on studies of face perception in the newborn and infants (Bühler, 1934), face hallucinations caused by mescaline (Zador, 1930), and finally the often extraordinary auditory compensation of this defect, possible since auditory recognition is not impaired at all in prosopagnosia. Bodamer also speculated that prosopagnosia corresponded to a regression to an earlier state of primitive face perception, a view not shared by most succeeding authors. Although no autopsy was performed in the two prosopagnosic cases of Bodamer's, he maintained that both had considerable traumatic damage to both occipital lobes.

Questions in Prosopagnosia Research

Subsequent to Bodamer's (1947) publication, the interest in prosopagnosia and the number of publications centring around it continued to increase. Moreover, the advent of modern brain-imaging techniques, in particular computer tomography (CT) and magnetic resonance imaging (MRI), made it possible to localize *in vivo* the brain lesions subsequent to which prosopagnosia occurs. A number of articles have attempted to summarize the case material on prosopagnosia, with particular emphasis on the anatomical structures involved and the physiological processes disturbed (Hécaen und Angelergues, 1962; Gloning, 1966; Meadows, 1974b; Benton, 1979, 1985; Hécaen, 1981; Damasio *et al.*, 1982; De Renzi, 1986a, b; Landis *et al.*, 1986/88; Michel *et al.*, 1989) Most of the work has centred around five questions still discussed today:

1. Are face-specific visual stimuli distinctly different from other complex visual patterns and if so, is proso-

pagnosia a disorder affecting facial recognition in isolation or is it due to a failure of a more elementary and general ability to recognize familiarity of an item within a class of similar stimuli?

2. Is prosopagnosia due to a disorder of perception, memory, or both?

3. Do the two cerebral hemispheres have different specializations in the processing of facial information, in particular the recognition of familiar faces, and must bilateral lesions exist for prosopagnosia to occur or is a unilateral lesion sufficient?

4. Where is the crucial anatomical location for this defect to occur?

5. How do the two hemispheres interact with respect to the recognition of familiar faces? This question has been raised whenever the frequency of prosopagnosia following posterior cerebral lesions or the compensatory strategies used by prosopagnosic patients were considered.

During the last two decades interest in face recognition, its neurophysiological basis and its pathology has increased considerably and researchers outside the fields of behaviour neurology and clinical neuropsychology, such as visual neurophysiologists, psychophysicists and cognitive neuropsychologists, have become interested in prosopagnosia. This interdisciplinary approach is witnessed by topic issues in journals (e.g. Grüsser, 1984/85) and books (e.g. Davies *et al.*, 1981; Ellis *et al.*, 1986; Bruce, 1987; Bruyer, 1986).

Clinical Examination

Sometimes a patient will describe spontaneously his inability to recognize familiar persons or family members on the basis of their facial features alone and almost invariably add that he uses features such as hair-style, moustache, scars or glasses for identification and that he has no difficulty in recognizing the person by his voice or gait. Early in the course of their illness such patients have usually experienced a state in which recognition by such compensatory strategies was not possible – an often shock-like event – making them aware of their defect. On the other hand, many patients with prosopagnosia do not fully realize their difficulty, do not refer to it spontaneously, and sometimes even deny it.

Since prosopagnosia is a failure to recognize well-known persons on the basis of visual perception of their faces without the use of voice, stature, clothes, gait or facial 'paraphernalia' like glasses, earrings, beard, etc., the crucial test is to observe whether a patient can under such conditions identify a person familiar or even dear to him. This test is a purely clinical one and cannot be simulated reliably with photographic or drawn facial test material:

the patient should be confronted with several persons, uniformly dressed, one of whom ought to be familiar to him. All should be of the same sex and roughly the same stature and hair colouring, without beard or moustache, glasses or other paraphernalia. During the process of identification they should be completely silent and move as little as possible, since it is known that prosopagnosic patients may identify familiar persons on the basis of minimal cues such as coughing, smiling or body movements. If recognition fails, each of the persons should address the patient verbally, which, in the case of prosopagnosia, will lead to instant identification of the familiar person. In a hospital setting such a test is usually performed with familiar and unfamiliar nurses or physicians, wearing white coats and possibly surgeons' caps.

Although such a procedure sounds primitive in a time when all functions seem to be measurable by standardized tests, it may well be the only way of assessing prosopagnosia properly. The problem of relatives or close persons not believing a patient to be prosopagnosic and the insecurity of physicians as to whether the patient actually suffers from this defect is neither rare nor new. Even during the careful investigation of his famous cases Bodamer (1947) explicitly refers to this in his protocol:

January 17th, 1945. The head nurse seriously doubts that the patient suffers from a difficulty in recognizing faces because she is called and greeted by her name even from far away. Therefore it was necessary for the patient to recognize her by her face. To clear this point the head nurse and another nurse, both familiar to the patient, were presented to him, standing one beside the other, wearing the same dress, without moving or making a noise. They were both of similar size and stature, the one nurse was not wearing her usual glasses. However, the nurses were very dissimilar in facial appearance and they differed in age by about 20 years. The patient, who had been informed of this experiment, tried to identify the head nurse, and to his own dismay was completely incapable of doing so for a long time until the other nurse started to smile and he recognized her from her strikingly white and regular teeth.

Often prosopagnosic patients seem to have more difficulty in recognizing persons they have come to know well after the occurrence of prosopagnosia than persons known before, such as friends and family members. The crucial test therefore is to evaluate in a similar way if the patient recognizes people very close to him. Since this experiment may be quite distressing for a patient who denies suffering from prosopagnosia as well as for the close friends, such a test depends upon the circumstances. It can be important for a prosopagnosic patient for his friends to become aware of his disability. This may be exemplified by a passage from a photocopied letter one of our patients, a young veterinarian – prosopagnosic subsequent to hypoxia after resuscitation from a cardiac arrest – has sent to friends and acquaintances:

When I walk along the street, I never recognize anyone. If somebody looks at me, I always think "Who could that be? Do I know him or is he just looking at me incidentally?" If I look at somebody and this person looks back, maybe even starts to smile, I am completely perplexed .... "Should I meet you, don't recognize you and pass by, please don't think I am doing this on purpose, remember my inability to recognize faces, and please stop me and talk to me".

A careful assessment of prosopagnosia in the way described is mandatory and the frequent omission of this kind of examination in patients with posterior brain lesions may well explain the enormous differences in prosopagnosia incidence between different authors.

Frequency and Aetiology of Prosopagnosia

The estimation of the frequency of prosopagnosia in a clinical population is dependent upon a number of factors, such as a general awareness that this clinical entity exists, the way of assessing prosopagnosia, the time elapsed since the acute lesion (e.g. stroke), the aetiology of the lesion and whether only unilateral or bilateral posterior cerebral damage is considered. The awareness of prosopagnosia as a symptom to be considered in a clinical examination has grown in the last 10 to 15 years, witnessed by the increase in clinical reports of prosopagnosic patients. It appears that prosopagnosia, once considered to be exceedingly rare, is not that uncommon, at least as one symptom of other visual gnosic disorders subsequent to bilateral posterior cerebral lesions. The frequency of prosopagnosia reported in large series of patients with unilateral or bilateral posterior lesions depends highly upon whether the authors consider prosopagnosia as one symptom among other visual perceptive and visual gnosic defects or whether they report only 'pure' cases of an isolated defect in the recognition of familiar faces. Among 382 patients with uni- or bilateral posterior cerebral lesions Hécaen and Angelergues (1962, 1963) found 22 cases (6%) suffering from prosopagnosia together visual field defects, disturbances in object recognition, topographagnosia or problems in visual space exploration. Gloning *et al.* (1968), on the other hand, reported only one patient with a 'pure' prosopagnostic disturbance in a series of 241 patients with lesions of the occipital lobes and adjacent areas, and Zihl and von Cramon (1986) consider none of their 258 patients suffering from posterior brain lesions to have had an isolated prosopagnosia. The differences in these three studies are highly significant (chi-square test, $p < 0.01$), indicating a selection of patients or methods of investigation.

At the time when the existence of visual agnosia was denied (Bay, 1950) and the 'peripheral' nature of recog-

nition deficits stressed, attempts were made to explain prosopagnosia on the basis of visual disturbances, like those observed in glaucoma simplex. Thus Stollreiter-Butzon (1950) presented findings in four such patients. Only one of them had no difficulty identifying familiar persons by their faces, but all used voice, posture or gait as identification cues. This explanation loses some of its attraction, however, when one considers that prosopagnosic patients recognize everyday objects and printed material very well and a large number of patients suffering from severe peripheral as well as central primary visual disturbances never develop any signs of prosopagnosia.

The aetiology of the lesions in the large series mentioned above was very heterogeneous, comprising tumours, surgical lesions for epilepsy, encephalitis, haemorrhages and cerebral infarcts. In our own experience with patients – mostly during the acute stage – who have incurred ischaemic infarcts in the territory of the posterior cerebral arteries the frequency of prosopagnosia as a symptom among other perceptual and visual agnosic defects, especially when the lesions are bilateral, is considerably higher than 6%. We found prosopagnosia to be present in 7 out of 14 patients with unilateral posterior cerebral artery stroke in the acute stage (Landis and Regard, 1988). Since our group was preselected for the presence of visual agnosic symptoms and the lesions were mostly acute, this high percentage may not reflect the frequency of prosopagnosia subsequent to right posterior cerebral artery strokes. De Renzi (1986), who had reported on several patients with prosopagnosia subsequent to right posterior cerebral artery infarcts, has systematically investigated 12 patients with right posterior cerebral artery strokes and found no prosopagnosia in all 12 (personal communication).

Subdivision of Symptoms and Formal Testing of Prosopagnosic Patients

In an attempt to quantify prosopagnosia, or other defects in facial recognition, a number of investigators have developed more or less standardized tests such as facial matching or face recognition (Warrington and James, 1967; Benton and Van Allen, 1968; De Renzi *et al.*, 1968; Bornstein *et al.*, 1969; Tzavaras *et al.*, 1970; etc.). Tests aimed at investigating the patient's ability to recognize familiar faces usually employ faces of famous people and celebrities or are set up *ad hoc* with photographs of personal acquaintances of the patient. With regard to public figures such as politicians, artists, etc., one should keep in mind that many of these people have marked facial features or peculiarities in hairstyle, moustache, ears, nose or

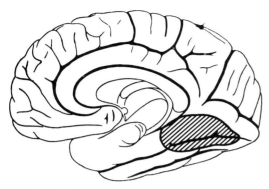

Fig. 14.1 *Schematic aspect of the mesial surface of a human brain. The region most frequently affected in prosopagnosia, either on the right hemisphere only or on both hemispheres, is cross-hatched.*

identifying accessories (headgear, glasses, cigars) often presented by caricaturists in an exaggerated form. Prosopagnosic patients almost invariably have trouble recognizing personal acquaintances in *post hoc* tests with photographs, provided paraphernalia including hairstyle are omitted. Frequently, but not always, prosopagnosic patients also have problems recognizing famous faces.

A disputed question is the prosopagnosic's ability to match unfamiliar faces. Investigating the facial matching performance of patients with right posterior lesions, Tzavaras *et al.* (1970) found an impairment in patients without prosopagnosia but none in two persons with prosopagnosia and comparable lesions. They were presented with two types of facial stimuli simultaneously (black/white photographs and stylized drawings) in order to minimize memory load and thus possibly favouring feature-by-feature analysis. Their unimpaired performance may reflect the observation that these patients are able to recognize the parts of a face (eyes, nose, mouth) and compensate their defect by using a feature-by-feature analysis, a perceptual strategy possibly associated with the left hemisphere. One of our prosopagnosic patients was able to perform the movie test on recognition of persons, facial expression and gestures, described below, without errors, but she required at least five times longer than normals for her detail analysis strategy (Grüsser *et al.*, unpubl., 1986).

The inverse observation, that most patients who are impaired in the discrimination of unfamiliar faces are not prosopagnosic, may be a reflection of the rarity of prosopagnosia (Rondot *et al.*, 1967; Assal, 1969; Benton and Van Allen, 1972; Tzavaras *et al.*, 1973; Mallone *et al.*, 1982), but also indicates that different cortical areas are dominant in these two tasks. Warrington and James (1967) found that the identification of well-known public figures and the discrimination of unfamiliar faces were impaired in patients with right hemisphere disease, but that the two

performances were not correlated with each other. It is now well established that recognition, matching and discrimination of facial material are far more frequently disturbed in patients with cerebral lesions in the posterior part of the right hemisphere than in patients with similar lesions in the left hemisphere. Failure in such tests, although pointing to right posterior cerebral damage, does not necessarily indicate the presence of prosopagnosia. Such tests serve as a screening measure but cannot positively establish a diagnosis of prosopagnosia.

Different Approaches to Cerebral Localization of the Lesions Crucial for Prosopagnosia

The classical approach of behaviour neurology, namely correlating a symptom or syndrome with the location and the anatomical extent of the cerebral lesion subsequent to which such a deficit occurs (Exner, 1881, 1894), has in a curious way failed to provide a clear answer as to the location of the crucial area for occurrence of prosopagnosia. Several anatomical, aetiological and clinical problems as well as some basic misconceptions of the explanatory power of clinico-pathological correlations may be at the root of the ongoing controversy over the anatomical basis of prosopagnosia. The majority of patients with prosopagnosia have suffered from lesions due to cerebrovascular disease. There is little doubt that most of these patients had bilateral lesions located in the infero-medial part of the occipito-temporal lobes in the gyrus fusiformis, the gyrus lingualis and the posterior part of the gyrus parahippocampalis, a brain region supplied by branches of the posterior cerebral arteries (Fig. 14.1). Since the two posterior cerebral arteries usually originate from a common trunk – the basilar artery – it is not unusual to find ischaemic infarcts in the brain regions supplied by both posterior cerebral arteries when the basilar artery is affected. Furthermore, it is well known that in the case of a unilateral posterior cerebral artery stroke, subsequent ischaemic attacks in the territory of the other posterior cerebral artery frequently occur. The inherent preponderance of bilaterality in any vascular disease concerning the vertebro-basilar system is of course no proof that bilateral lesions are necessary to produce prosopagnosia.

The second point concerns the absence of prosopagnosia in the presence of large unilateral or bilateral posterior cerebral artery lesions. Frequently the lack of prosopagnosia in the presence of a large right posterior cerebral artery lesion is taken as evidence against a crucial role of the right infero-medial occipito-temporal region in the recognition of familiar faces. Curiously, extensive infarcts in the territory of the left posterior cerebral artery not exhibiting alexia without agraphia raise no doubts about the importance of the left infero–medial occipito–temporal area for reading, nor does one question the dominance of the left hemisphere for language because of even larger infarcts in the territory of the left middle cerebral artery without aphasia. Since a clinico–pathological correlation does not tell us where a certain function is processed, but rather under what circumstances the remaining undamaged brain is not able to perform a certain function, it is a profound misunderstanding to associate the lack of a certain symptom with a specific function of a damaged area in the brain.

Establishing a clinico–anatomical correlation to prosopagnosia was performed in three ways. The first was a clinico–clinical approach; in the case of prosopagnosia, the extent and congruity of visual field defects were used as indicators (Faust, 1955; Hécaen and Angelergues, 1962; Gloning, 1966; De Renzi *et al.*, 1968; Meadows, 1974). This approach has been shown to be unreliable, however, since even in the presence of entirely unilateral neurological deficits, subsequent neuropathology or CT findings have shown the presence of bilateral lesions (Arseni and Botez, 1958; Bornstein, 1963; Benson *et al.*, 1974; for review see Meadows, 1974).

The second approach evaluates necropsy findings, but only a few cases of patients suffering from prosopagnosia have come for autopsy. These cases have been extensively reviewed several times (Gloning *et al.*, 1966; Meadows, 1974; Benton, 1979; Damasio *et al.*, 1982; Landis *et al.*, 1988; Michel *et al.*, 1989). One should keep in mind that between the onset of prosopagnosia and autopsy there is usually a long delay of several years during which subsequent infarcts in the territory of the vertebro–basilar system are not unlikely. This point is perhaps best illustrated by the second patient described by Cohn *et al.* (1977): '. . . following the first episode, there were several other insults that left him blind' (p. 180). In such cases, therefore, caution should be applied in establishing a causal connection between the bilateral posterior infarcts and prosopagnosia, since the bilaterality of lesions at autopsy cannot be taken as proof that bilateral lesions in the visual system are necessary for prosopagnosia to occur (Landis *et al.*, 1988).

The third approach is to apply modern neuroimaging techniques (CT or MRI) as early as possible, i.e. a few days after the onset of prosopagnosia and/or to rely upon intraoperative findings. Recent reviews of these results (De Renzi, 1986; Landis *et al.*, 1986; Michel *et al.*, 1989) support the crucial role of the right infero–medial occipito–temporal area, a view held long ago by Hécaen and his group primarily on the basis of clinical and surgical findings (Hécaen and Angelergues, 1962; for review see Hécaen, 1981).

Brain Neuropathology

Since the first necropsy report of Wilbrand (1892) only 13 patients with prosopagnosia have come under autopsy. Two of these cases suffered from tumours (Arseni and Botez, 1958; Hécaen and Angelergues, 1962) and 11 were vascular in origin (Wilbrand, 1892; Heidenhain, 1927; Pevzner *et al.*, 1962; Gloning *et al.*, 1970; Lhermitte *et al.*, 1972; Benson *et al.*, 1974; Cohn *et al.*, 1977; Cambier *et al.*, 1980; Nardelli *et al.*, 1982; Landis *et al.*, 1988). In all cases without exception a right medial occipito–temporal lesion was found. If anything consistent about the pathological cerebral involvement in prosopagnosia can be said, it is that an infero–medial occipito–temporal lesion in the right hemisphere seems to be a prerequisite. While this finding appears to be firmly established, there is a discordance of opinion concerning the necessity of a concomitant lesion in the left hemisphere, in particular a symmetrical lesion in the territory of the left posterior cerebral artery.

Only one of the anatomically verified cases with prosopagnosia had a lesion confined to the right posterior cerebral artery (Landis *et al.* 1988; Fig. 14.2). This patient, who became prosopagnosic subsequent to a stroke in the territory of the right posterior cerebral artery died 10 days after this event from pulmonary embolism. Autopsy revealed a recent, large, right-sided infero–medial temporo–occipital infarct and two older clinically silent lesions, a tiny cortical micro–infarct in the lateral left occipito–parietal area and a right frontal infarct. While this case may be considered the only pathologically verified case of a unilateral right posterior lesion having led to prosopagnosia, it remains an open question if prosopagnosia would have persisted, since the patient died shortly after the infarct. On the other hand the short delay between symptom and autopsy lends credit to the view that a right medial posterior cerebral lesion is sufficient for prosopagnosia to occur at least transiently.

The opinion that more or less symmetrical bilateral lesions in the visual system are conditio sine qua non for prosopagnosia can be further questioned by the fact that of the anatomically verified cases, those described by Hécaen and Angelergues (1962) and Pevzner *et al.* (1962) did not have left hemispheric lesions in the corresponding medio-basal posterior region. In particular the case described by Pevzner *et al.* showed at autopsy (4 years after the event), in addition to the typical right posterior medial infarct, a clinically silent left hemisphere posterio-lateral lesion including the middle of the infero-parietal lobule, angular gyrus and upper part of the superior temporal gyrus. The lesion consisted of a slight atrophy, gliosis and rarefaction of cells, which might have disconnected the left fusiform cortex and the temporal speech areas. A direct involvement of the angular gyrus cortex in prosopagnosia, however, seems rather improbable.

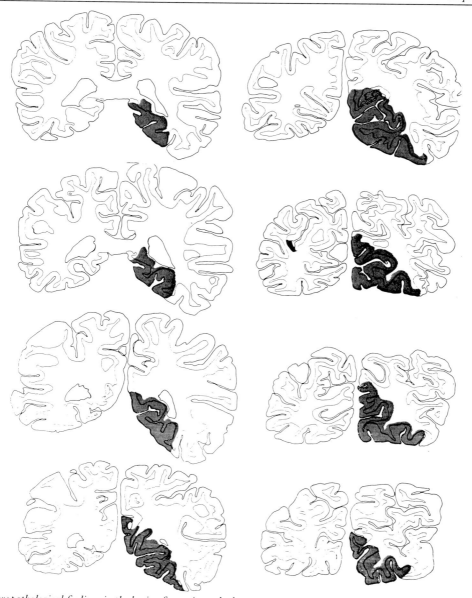

Fig. 14.2 *Neuropathological findings in the brain of a patient who became prosopagnosic owing to a large cerebral infarction in the territory of the right posterior cerebral artery. The patient died 10 days after the right-sided infarct. The cross-hatched areas illustrate the extent of the microscopically verified brain lesion. A small, old, clinically silent, cortical microinfarction was found in the left lateral occipito-parietal area (small black field, second row, right) (from Landis* et al., *1988).*

While a lesion in the posterior medial area of the right hemisphere seems to be uniformly present in all prosopagnosic patients, the lesions in the left hemisphere are not necessarily comprised of the symmetrically corresponding area and may in rare instances even be absent. This asymmetry in lesion distribution has led Meadows (1974) to express caution concerning the obligatory bilateral posterior lesions for prosopagnosia, while other authors

(Damasio *et al.*, 1982) took a stronger stance, claiming the necessity of functionally symmetrical medial occipito-temporal lesions in the visual system.

Although necropsy reports are undeniably important, their exclusivity in answering the question whether or not bilateral posterior lesions are necessary for prosopagnosia has probably been overemphasized. The recent advent of *intra-vitam* neuroimaging techniques such as CT scan and

MRI, which show structural cerebral damage in temporal correlation to the onset of prosopagnosia, may well alter our view about the cerebral localization of prosopagnosia.

Neuroimaging and Neurosurgical Reports

The increasing number of publications referring to the correlation of prosopagnosia with neuroimaging findings as well as the few reports on intraoperative findings have been subject to recent reviews (De Renzi, 1986; Landis *et al.*, 1986; Michel *et al.*, 1989). More than 13 cases of prosopagnosia have been reported in which CT scans show bilateral posterior cerebral lesions. In most of these patients prosopagnosia was only one symptom accompanied by other visual defects and visual agnosic signs such as achromatopsia, alexia or visual agnosia. Since these patients provided no additional information as to whether the crucial lesion in prosopagnosia is unilateral or bilateral, and where it is located, we just list the original reports: (Aptman *et al.*, 1977; Whiteley and Warrington, 1977; Levine, 1978; Kertesz, 1979; Mack and Boller, 1977; Ross, 1980; Dumont *et al.*, 1981; Damasio *et al.*, 1982; Bauer, 1982; Malone *et al.*, 1982; Nardelli *et al.*, 1982; Shuttleworth *et al.*, 1982; Bruyer *et al.*, 1983; Gomori and Hawryluk, 1984; Levine *et al.*, 1985; Habib, 1986; Riddoch and Humphreys, 1987).

Of more importance to the problem of cerebral localization are those cases of prosopagnosia in which neuroimaging or surgery has shown only unilateral lesions. As compared with necropsy, intraoperative findings and neuroimaging, in particular CT scans, are anatomically less precise and the existence of small undetected lesions in the apparently undamaged hemisphere cannot be excluded.

To our knowledge there are reports on 11 patients with prosopagnosia subsequent to right posterior cerebral lesions in whom neurosurgery was performed. Hécaen and colleagues (Hécaen and Angelergues, 1962) described two patients with prosopagnosia following surgery in the right posterior hemisphere for epilepsy. In one (Hécaen *et al.*, 1956, case 4) a right posterior temporal, parietal and occipital epileptic zone and in the other (Hécaen *et al.*, 1956, case 6) a right temporo–occipital epileptic zone was removed. The first patient developed prosopagnosia postoperatively, the second was prosopagnosic prior to surgery but this resolved within a few weeks. Assal (1969) reported on a patient who developed prosopagnosia subsequent to the evacuation of a right posterior intracerebral haematoma. The haematoma was parieto–temporal and the prosopagnosia lasted for at least several months.

In a patient of Meadows (1974), a haematoma caused by a small arteriovenous malformation in the posterior temporal region existed and the prosopagnosia was mild. Lhermitte and Pillon (1975) described a patient in whom prosopagnosia was documented one month after right occipital lobectomy for intractable seizures. This case is of particular importance, since 10 years later, while the hemianopic patient was still severely prosopagnosic, a CT scan and topographic distribution of cerebral glucose consumption (PET scan) could be obtained (Michel *et al.*, 1989). CT scan showed the right occipital lobectomy to be complete and no evidence of any lesion in the left hemisphere was obtained. Cerebral glucose consumption was absent in the operated right posterior part, but normal values were found across the left hemisphere. The absence of associated symptoms such as achromatopsia, colour agnosia, alexia, visual agnosia, visuo–spatial and mnestic problems makes this case a particularly pure example of prosopagnosia.

Sergent and Villemure (1988) reported on a 33-year-old lady in whom a right hemispherectomy had been necessary at the age of 13 and who 20 years later was still prosopagnosic. Although highly educated she was unaware of her deficits. Whitely and Warrington (1977) provided CT and surgical evidence for unilateral right posterior lesions in two of their three patients suffering from prosopagnosia. Case 2 developed prosopagnosia subsequent to a right occipital intracerebral hematoma, and case 3 developed transient prosopagnosia after an occipital lobectomy for the removal of a right posterior astrocytoma. During surgery, it was confirmed that the tumour did not cross into the left hemisphere. Similar CT and surgical evidence was presented in two of our own cases (Landis *et al.*, 1986, cases 5 and 6). One of the patients was operated for a right temporo-parieto-occipital glioblastoma, another for a right occipital oligodendroglioma. In the latter a follow-up study over 6 years revealed that he improved his recognition of familiar faces somewhat by the help of contextual cues.

Renault *et al.* (1989) presented the case of a prosopagnosic patient in whom they demonstrated covert knowledge of familiar faces by an ingenious experiment using visual evoked potentials. This patient developed prosopagnosia following a right occipito-temporal haematoma which was operated. This case is of particular importance since CT scan and PET scan as well as MRI have been performed. The MRI images (Michel *et al.*, 1989) demonstrate a purely unilateral right-sided, mainly subcortical lesion largely sparing the visual cortex and involving mostly the white matter of the fusiform gyrus (Fig. 14.3). PET scan shows that glucose metabolism was impaired in a larger area than demonstrated on MRI and included the lingual gyrus and the parahippocampal gyrus on the right side. Most important, no abnormalities in glucose metabolism were found in the entire left hemisphere.

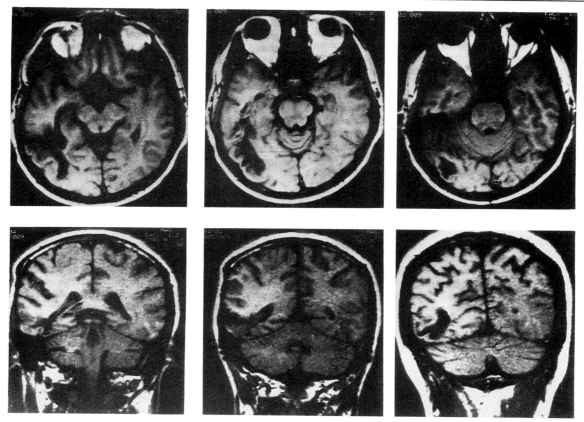

Fig. 14.3 *MRI scans of the brain of a prosopagnosic patient. The lesion (dark area) is restricted to the right occipital hemisphere and affects predominantly the subcortical region, sparing the visual cortex. The white matter of the fusiform gyrus is especially affected; for further explanation, see text. According to MRI convention, left/right are reversed (from Michel et al., 1989).*

In another group of 11 prosopagnosic patients the lesion site has been confirmed by CT scan. In all cases the lesion was in the posterior part of the right hemisphere and no sign of left posterior lesions was found. In the patients described by Michel *et al.* (1986) and Tiberghien and Clerc (1986) as well as in case 4 of our own study (Landis *et al.*, 1986), the lesion was due to a haematoma, while in the remaining cases (De Renzi, 1986b, cases 4 and 6 and cases 1, 2 and 3 of our own (Landis *et al.*, 1986)) the lesions were infarcts in the brain region supplied by the right posterior cerebral artery.

To summarize these findings, more than 20 cases have now been reported in which prosopagnosia occurred subsequent to unilateral posterior brain damage in the right hemisphere. These lesions were of different aetiologies but had a common location, confirmed intraoperatively and/or with neuroimaging techniques including MRI in one case and PET scan in two others. In many of these patients prosopagnosia has persisted for years.

A Possible Contribution of Left-Hemisphere Lesions to Prosopagnosia

Another question is whether patients have been observed who developed prosopagnosia following left posterior cerebral lesions. As far as we know, no case of prosopagnosia occurring subsequent to an isolated left posterior brain lesion in a right-hander has yet been published. De Renzi *et al.* (1987) report a series of unselected patients who had had strokes in the region of the left posterior cerebral artery. None of these patients was prosopagnosic. In our own series (Landis and Regard, 1988) covering 23 patients with unilateral strokes in the territory of either the left or the right posterior cerebral artery, none of the nine patients suffering from left posterior cerebral artery strokes was prosopagnosic. Thus, unilateral left occipital lesions in right-handers do not seem to produce either permanent or transient prosopagnosia.

Conclusions on Specificity in Prosopagnosia and Correlated Cerebral Lesions

1. Most reported cases with prosopagnosia have shown bilateral posterior infero–medial occipito–temporal lesions, as would be expected by the frequency of bilateral lesions in this vascular territory.

2. In each of the cases with bilateral lesions the posterior medial occipito–temporal area of the right hemisphere was involved but the left hemispheric lesion was located in some cases outside this region.

3. There exists one autopsied case and an increasing number of patients with neuro–imaging findings showing evidence of right posterior medial occipito–temporal lesions alone being sufficient to produce prosopagnosia under certain conditions.

4. In rare instances right occipital lobectomies and right hemispherectomies have produced persistent prosopagnosia. However, in the majority of such patients no prosopagnosia was noted.

5. Prosopagnosia has never been reported subsequent to unilateral left posterior medial lesions.

6. Bilateral posterior cerebral infarcts and even large right posterior medial lesions can be present without prosopagnosia.

There is little doubt that the right infero–medial temporo–occipital area is the crucial area for prosopagnosia (Fig.14.1). However, a number of questions still remain open:

1. Are concomitant lesions in the left hemisphere, especially the posterior medial part, necessary or do they modify the symptoms of agnosia?

2. Why in the presence of apparently similar lesions do some individuals develop prosopagnosia and others not?

3. What is the role of compensatory strategies and learning?

It may be meaningful to look at other symptoms succeeding right-sided medial temporo–occipital lesions. If one holds the view that prosopagnosia is a disturbance occurring in a cascade-like projection system concerned primarily with colour, contours and form information (cf. Chapters 4 and 5), which projects in a highly bi-directionally interconnected fashion from the striate cortex into the inferior medial-temporal lobe and from there to the limbic system, lesions at different stages of this cascade may lead to variations in face recognition distur-bances and the associated symptoms. Considering that the most frequent aetiology, namely vascular lesions, produces cortical as well as subcortical damage in discrete vascular territories which are not necessarily identical with the neurophysiological sites processing visual submodalities, it is not surprising that it has been difficult to find really 'pure' prosopagnosia. Therefore problems in assessing the specificity of prosopagnosia occur at different levels.

1. Lesions may extend into the medial temporal lobes and prosopagnosia be associated with memory disturbances.

2. Lesions could extend into striate areas and prosopagnosia be associated much more elementarily with visual disturbances.

3. Lesions may extend into other peristriate areas and prosopagnosia coexist with other types of visual agnosias.

Associated Memory Disturbances in Prosopagnosia

Prosopagnosia, an inability to recognize faces learned before the cerebral lesion and to learn new faces, even those of persons to whom one was or is constantly exposed, has been described repeatedly within the framework of a more widespread memory disturbance and discussed as an amnesic syndrome. This may be exemplified by a patient one of us (O.-J. G.) examined some years ago. This 52-year-old lady suffered from severe amnesia following an alcoholic Korsakoff psychosis. This patient also exhibited signs of prosopagnosia. She did not recognize her husband or old friends nor photographs of well-known politicians in the newspaper, but could recount stories about them when told their names. She was also not able to learn the faces of hospital personnel. When her physician, who visited her two to three times a day, entered her room in a white coat, she addressed him as 'Herr Doktor'; when he appeared in normal dress, however, she could not recognize him. Her verbal memory was reduced to a '*Sekundengedächtnis*' (Conrad and Uhl, 1958), but her ability in spatial learning was well preserved. In contrast to pure prosopagnosia, she had also lost the ability to recognize people by their voices but could differentiate voices very well, as well as other complex sounds like music. Reading, colour perception, colour naming and language functions were well preserved. In the context of a severe amnesic syndrome, face and person memory seemed to be particularly impaired in this patient. In such a frame of reference, prosopagnosia is of course not 'pure', since the memory deficit usually includes sensory modalities other than visual (e.g. voice identification), and if it is predominantly visual it concerns not only faces but other visual objects as well. Although amnesic syndromes are frequently seen after closed head injury, toxic and metabolic disorders or strokes with bilateral diencephalic involvement, three of the four patients in whom the issue of prosopagnosia due to amnesia has been raised had suffered focal lesions or encephalitis comprising predominantly the temporal lobes (Damasio *et al.*, 1985; De Renzi *et al.*, 1987; Sergent and Poncet, 1990). An exception to this aetiology is the patient HM who became amnesic subsequent to bilateral medial temporal lobectomy (for review see Corkin, 1984). All four cases are untypical examples of prosopagnosia, as all had disturbed recognition of familiar voices and person recognition in some was not facilitated by the typical contextual cues. This somewhat unusual pattern of deficits, in particular the differences in type of amnesias and extent of lesions, may shed some light upon the border zone between prosopagnosia and prosopamnesia as well as between prosopagnosia and a general deficit in recognizing 'personal familiarity' in objects. In all four cases temporal lobe lesions were dominant:

1. In the patient HM the ablations of the temporal lobes extended about 8 cm bilaterally on the medial side from the temporal pole in the occipital direction. Thus the amygdala and the hippocampal formation as well as the parahippocampal gyrus were excised bilaterally. Primary sensory cortices as well as their projections into the limbic system were left intact (Scoville and Milner, 1957). Since his operation this patient had, with the exception of some perceptuo–motor tasks, been unable to learn new information, regardless of the sensory modality of input (Milner, 1966). Thus he could also not commit new faces to memory and was not able to recognize people with whom he had come in contact since the operation. His amnesia for contextual or biographical information and general events was equally severe. However, there was little amnesia, if at all, for items including faces related to the pre-operative period.

2. The patient described by Damasio *et al.* (1985) suffered from extensive bilateral damage of the medial and lateral temporal lobes and of the basal forebrain structures due to *Herpes simplex* encephalitis, being much more marked in the right hemisphere. In the CT scan damage is visible to the splenial fibres in the right hemisphere and to the medial occipital–temporal junction including the parahippocampal gyrus as well. This patient had incurred a complete anterograde amnesia, equally so for generic (semantic) and contextual (episodic, autobiographical) information, whereas the retrograde amnesia, which spanned five decades of his life, was less pronounced for generic (semantic) information. Although this dissociation did not really extend to faces, except that a face was recognized as a face, Damasio and Damasio (1986) advocated the view that

Prosopagnosia is not confined to human faces but rather encompasses any stimulus that, as human faces, (a) requires specific and context-related recognition (as opposed to non-specific, generic recognition only), and (b) is visually ambiguous, (i.e. a stimulus that is part of a group that has numerous different members with similar visual structure)....

If one considers prosopagnosia to be due to a more or less specific memory disorder confined to the visual modality but reflecting the dissociation in memory processes into semantic and episodic memory, as proposed by Tulving (1983), it would be inconceivable to find prosopagnosia associated with an inverse pattern of memory disturbance as that described by Damasio *et al.* (1985). However, De Renzi (1986b) and De Renzi *et al.* (1987) described a patient who following a probable herpetic encephalitis developed an inverse pattern of amnesia with severe impairment in semantic (generic) memory, but a relatively well-preserved autobiographic (episodic, contextual) memory. This striking double dissociation of functional impairment in two patients with virtually identical aetiology may be resolved by considering the differences in structural anatomical damage in these two cases. Both had bilateral lesions in the temporal lobes, but as to the hemisphere concerned, the damage was very asymmetric. In the case of Damasio *et al.* (1985) the damage was much more marked in the right hemisphere, while in the case of De Renzi *et al.* (1987) it was far more extensive in the left, spreading from the temporal pole to the parahippocampal gyrus and the anterior part of the fusiform gyrus. In the right hemisphere De Renzi's patient showed minimal signs of pathology in the white matter of the inferior temporal lobe.

It is of course tempting to attribute the semantic versus episodic memory dissociation to different degrees of hemispheric specialization in the encoding of new information. The pathology and clinical symptoms in the two cases of De Renzi and Damasio *et al.* fit the well-known specialization of the left hemisphere for language and semantic information and that of the right hemisphere for contextual information (for review see Cook, 1986). With regard to face recognition, however, both cases did not entirely follow the recognition defects found for other visual stimuli. The patient reported by Damasio *et al.* (1985) suffered from defective face recognition abilities which encompassed all of his friends and relatives as well as all of the persons that had come in contact with him since the onset of the illness, while in the case of De Renzi *et al.* (1987) the patient did not recognize any of the famous faces but did recognize some of her 'old' very close personal acquaintances by their face. The striking dissociation of face recognition or face memory, as compared with episodic autobiographic information, may be exemplified in this patient by the following event:

On a Sunday the psychologist who had repeatedly tested her came to the wards with her child and waved to the patient when she met her. The patient did not recognize her and anxiously asked who she was. The next day, the patient remembered the event perfectly, but again failed to recognize the psychologist.

(De Renzi, 1986b)

The last patient to be considered in the frame of atypical, non-vascular lesions, located largely outside the classical areas of the vascular distribution of the posterior cerebral arteries reported in most cases of prosopagnosia, is the patient described by Boudouresques *et al.* (1979) and again by Sergent and Poncet (1990). This patient suffered from an encephalitis, probably herpetic in origin, which destroyed most of the right temporal lobe, as evidenced by a CT scan performed in 1975. A second CT scan, published in 1989 (Michel *et al.*, 1989), demonstrated that the inferior part of the left temporal lobe had also been involved. Unfortunately the two CT scan images published do not permit a definite decision as to whether or not the crucial structures of the parahippocampal gyrus and the anterior part of the fusiform and lingual gyrus have been damaged on the right side. This patient had a severe impairment in the recognition of not only familiar faces but also familiar places, familiar handwriting (a symptom first reported by Niessl von Maiendorf, 1935), familiar paintings and also personal objects. The impairment included the auditory modality; the patient had difficulty in recognizing familiar voices. An extensive analysis of the facial aspect of her recognition difficulty for familiarity was carried out by Sergent and Poncet (1990), showing that in the absence of 'contextual memory' or 'memory for familiarity', semantic knowledge about unrecognized faces was preserved. Considering the striking asymmetry of the lesion, with the damage involving mostly the right temporal lobe, this case again points to a hemispheric dichotomy with respect to encoding and storing information according to their semantic or contextual content.

Since prosopagnosia, referring to the recognition of familiar faces, by definition implies dealing with stored information, the mnesic part of this peculiar syndrome may well be explained along the line of a particular deficit of contextual or episodic memory preferentially in the visual modality. In the evaluation of 'purity' of prosopagnosia one has therefore to consider:

1. How pure the memory disorder is with respect to the semantic/episodic dichotomy.
2. How pure the memory disorder is with respect to the sensory modality involved.
3. And finally, concerning the visual modality alone, how far the loss of familiarity is restricted to faces or whether other visual stimulus categories are involved as well.

In the patient of Sergent and Poncet (1990), the loss of contextual memory appears quite striking as opposed to semantic memory; however it was restricted neither to the visual modality nor to faces but extended to a whole variety of visual object classes. While the memory deficit was overwhelming in these four atypical cases of failure to recognize familiar faces, it should also be mentioned that in most cases of prosopagnosia caused by more restricted lesions in the medial temporal–occipital junction memory disturbances more restricted to figural than verbal information have also been noted.

Primary Visual Disturbances Frequently Associated with Prosopagnosia

Most prosopagnosic patients also had visual field defects. The reason for this concurrence can easily be seen. Most lesions in the territory of the posterior cerebral arteries, and especially the vascular ones, were not restricted to the associative visual areas inferior to area V1 but also damaged striate areas or involved parts of the optic radiation. If one accepts prosopagnosia as being 'pure' only in the absence of primary visual disturbances, no single case of 'pure' prosopagnosia probably exists.

The area of the visual fields most frequently involved is the left upper quadrant. This visual field is associated with a lesion in the right infero–calcarine part of area V1. The frequent association of homonymous left upper quadranopsia with prosopagnosia has already been noted by Faust (1955) and Gloning (1966a), and extensively reviewed by Meadows (1974). Only a few cases have been reported in which prosopagnosia was not associated with visual field defects as detected by normal light perimetry (i.e. with a Goldmann perimeter, Faust, 1955; Macrae and Trolle, 1956; Hécaen *et al.*, 1957; Benton and Van Allen, 1972; Michel *et al.*, 1986). But even in these cases, there was no guarantee that primary visual qualities were completely intact, since a perimetric evaluation of colour, form, depth, and movement on flicker fusion was usually not performed (for review see Zihl and von Cramon, 1986). Moreover, a high proportion of patients with lesions in the territory of both posterior cerebral arteries suffered from transient visual symptoms in the early stages of the disease, described as 'dimness', 'blurring' or, on the contrary, as 'discomforting light reflexions or photophobia', sometimes combined with simple visual illusions. These disturbances have been described and discussed by various authors (Poppelreuter, 1917; Wilbrand and Saenger, 1917; Horrax, 1923; Poetzl, 1928; Bender and Furlow, 1945; Critchley, 1965; Gloning *et al.*, 1968); they have been called 'cerebral obscurations' or 'cerebral asthenopia' and have been attributed by some to an impairment in dark- or light-adaptation.

Complex Visual Disturbances Associated with Prosopagnosia

The most frequent damage leading to prosopagnosia – bilateral cerebral infarctions of cortical areas supplied by the posterior cerebral arteries – extends into visual associative areas of the medial occipito-temporal brain associated with the higher-order processing of form and colour. It is therefore not surprising to find prosopagnosia associated with disturbances in the recognition of form and colours. In an analysis of 22 patients with face agnosia, compared with 395 patients with unilateral retro-rolandic lesions without prosopagnosia, Hécaen and Angelergues (1962) found prosopagnosia to be associated with spatial dyslexia, spatial dyscalculia, dressing apraxia and distortions in visual coordinates, while they found no correlation with aphasia and acalculia. If the lesion in the left hemisphere was large in the case of bilateral posterior lesions, prosopagnosia might be associated with pure alexia or associative visual object agnosia. In cases where prosopagnosia was due to an apparently unilateral right posterior lesion, pure alexia or associative visual object agnosia was never observed. The association of achromatopsia with prosopagnosia in bilateral posterior lesions has been reviewed by Meadows (1974b).

It is not surprising, of course, that bilateral lesions, destroying large parts of the visual system of both hemispheres, may give rise to complex visual disturbances, extending over a broad spectrum of visual stimulus classes. Of particular interest, however, is the frequent association of prosopagnosia with spatial agnosias, especially with the loss of topographic memory (Hécaen and Angelergues, 1962). Analysing a large series of cases with unilateral hemispheric lesions, these authors found prosopagnosia and topographagnosia to be highly correlated, but with different mutual probabilities: in prosopagnosic patients they found topographic memory loss in 38%, but in patients with topographic memory loss, prosopagnosia was present in 77% (Hécaen and Angelergues,1963). Thus in the case of topographic memory loss, also referred to as 'topographagnosia' (see Chapter 21), it is much more likely to find concomitant prosopagnosia than the reverse. We have recently reported on 16 patients with a loss of topographic familiarity (Landis *et al.*, 1986) and found prosopagnosia to be present in seven. Of these 16 patients all had right posterior medial cerebral lesions and in only three of them was an involvement of the left medial posterior area found as well.

The similarity in anatomical localization between loss of topographic familiarity and prosopagnosia is indeed striking and indicates that both abilities may share common functions. Common to both symptoms is the inability to experience familiarity, in the sense of an emotionally toned recognition of a complex visual pattern which had been personally very close to the patient and with which the patient had experienced behavioural interaction before the brain lesion. Other complex visual pattern recognition remained intact. That this loss of a feeling of personal familiarity is not restricted to long-known surroundings or human faces is suggested by patients in whom the recognition of familiar birds (Bornstein, 1963) or familiar cows (Assal *et al.*, 1984) has been selectively disturbed with or without persistent prosopagnosia. The differences in the association of topographical memory loss and prosopagnosia observed by Hécaen and Angelergues (1963) suggest a gradient in impairment severity of a system designed to be triggered by an emotional component of personal familiarity and experience, i.e. the memory components referred to as contextual, episodic or autobiographic. The differences in frequency of occurrence between the two symptoms could then well be explained by the fact that the topographic environment contains many more semantic or verbalizable cues than does a personally and emotionally familiar face. A patient with damage to a system concerned with visual familiarity would be much more likely to be able to compensate for the loss of topographic familiarity than facial familiarity. This was indeed the case with several of our patients in the acute and subacute stages subsequent to right posterior cerebral artery strokes. During the first weeks after the cerebral lesion prosopagnosia was invariably associated with some degree of loss of topographic familiarity, which improved over time, while prosopagnosia did not.

Prosopagnosia and the 'Specificity of Faces'

If a prosopagnosic patient's difficulty appears on first sight to be restricted to the recognition of familiar faces, several overlapping questions arise:

1. Are unfamiliar faces handled in a normal way?

2. Is the recognition of one item within a class of similarly appearing items (e.g. faces) restricted to faces, or does it extend to other classes of similarly looking items?

3. Is the deficit primarily a deficit in recognition of familiarity of an item, i.e. a personal emotionally acquired link to the item, not necessarily restricted to faces (e.g. one's own belongings among similar items belonging to others)?

4. What is the role of awareness in prosopagnosia and how does 'covert' recognition of familiar faces fit into models of hemispheric specialization?

Recognition of Familiar and Unfamiliar Faces

Of practical and also theoretical importance are the few prosopagnosic patients who have been reported to score normally on facial discrimination tests with unfamiliar faces (Assal, 1969; Tzavaras *et al.*, 1970; Benton and van Allen, 1972; Malone *et al.*, 1982; Bauer, 1984; Christen *et al.*, 1985; De Haan *et al.*, 1987). This dissociated performance between the recognition of familiar and unfamiliar faces has been taken as evidence for a specificity of the functional defect in prosopagnosia for the processing of facial familiarity and hitherto for a disturbance in face memory as opposed to face perception. Two points argue against this view.

Firstly, when prosopagnosics give a normal performance in face discrimination tests, they usually score in the very lowest ranks of normals. Secondly, prosopagnosic patients are extremely slow in such tests, master them only with an enormous amount of effort, and rely heavily on learned compensation strategies (e.g. Shuttleworth, 1982). Bauer (1984), who reported on a prosopagnosic patient with an unconscious awareness of faces, described his patient's performance on the Benton test of facial recognition (Benton *et al.*, 1975) as done 'in a piecemeal fashion that greatly compromised speed and accuracy'. This opinion corroborates our personal experience with all prosopagnosic patients we have seen. It seems that while matching or discriminating unfamiliar faces can be quantitatively in the low range of normals, it definitely differs qualitatively.

This view is reinforced by the striking performance failure of prosopagnosic patients in tests with unfamiliar faces when there is the slightest time constraint. We have investigated this phenomenon experimentally and found a double dissociation of function in patients with right posterior cerebral lesions with prosopagnosia versus those without prosopagnosia concerning matching unfamiliar faces given unlimited time as opposed to a restricted viewing time of one second in a tachistoscope (Christen *et al.*, 1985; Fig. 14.4). Given an unlimited period of time, prosopagnosic patients performed flawlessly, while patients with right posterior cerebral damage without prosopagnosia were moderately impaired. However, the impairment of patients without prosopagnosia was not influenced by reducing viewing time to one second, while the performance of prosopagnosic patients completely collapsed.

Yet another indication of a general deficit in processing visual information, not restricted to familiar faces (nor even to faces) comes from four experiments carried out on a few selected prosopagnosic patients and compared to the performance of normals (Davidoff and Landis, 1990). In particular it was investigated whether prosopagnosic patients would profit from the well known '*face superiority*

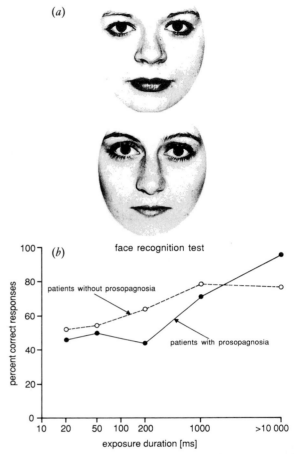

Fig. 14.4 *(a) Example of a stimulus pair of pure faces (i.e. the inner parts of faces) applied in a tachistoscopic test in which patients had to decide whether the two faces were identical or not. Different exposure times were applied. (b) The score of correct responses (ordinate) in the recognition test on face pairs as illustrated in (a) is plotted as a function of exposure time (log, abscissa). Averages of three patients suffering from prosopagnosia (solid circles) and three right-hemisphere, posterior, brain-lesioned patients without prosopagnosia (hollow circles) are shown. At unlimited exposure durations, prosopagnosic patients performed as normals while non-prosopagnosic patients showed some impairment in this test. With a reduction of exposure duration to 1000 ms or 200 ms, the performance of the prosopagnosic patients was greatly reduced, while that of the non-prosopagnosic patients was less strongly affected (from Christen* et al., *1985, modified).*

effect' (Homa *et al.*, 1976; Van Santen and Jonides, 1978) and the newly introduced '*object superiority effect*' (Davidoff and Donnelly, 1990). Both of these superiority effects are critically dependent on the spatial relationship between the internal feature parts (Davidoff, 1986). The critical stimulus for obtaining face or object superiority is an outline in which parts are placed in critical positions. The idea behind these experiments was that if prosopagnosic patients have a disorder specific to the recognition of *familiar faces*, the face superiority effect should not be lost for *unfamiliar faces* and also not for objects. However, the results of the experiments show that no difference in the pattern of recognition performance was found between normal and unusual arrangements of unfamiliar faces and objects in prosopagnosic patients, but that their performance pattern differed from both unilateral brain-damaged patients and normal controls. The results of these studies indicate that these prosopagnosic patients were impaired for the recognition of unfamiliar faces, and that their problem was not even specific to faces.

These arguments suggest that the underlying defect in prosopagnosia is on a general visual precognition or cognition level. However, it is undeniable that while prosopagnosic patients may display a relatively good performance in matching faces, they usually are severely impaired when it comes to recognizing faces they had to learn previously. This point would not necessarily favour a mnemonic defect as the origin of prosopagnosia. It could be due to an impairment in integrating the parts of a face, a function which could be essential in identifying whole faces in the matching tests. This interpretation is corroborated by introspective reports of prosopagnosic patients that all subjects look alike or even alter their physiognomies in a similar manner ('all subjects look Chinese').

Recognition of Items within a Class of Similarly Looking Items

That prosopagnosic patients can have difficulty not only in distinguishing between faces, but also between members of a class of similarly looking visual items, has been known for a long time. Therefore Faust (1955) considered prosopagnosia to be neither a primary sensory deficit nor a disorder limited to the specific visual category of the human face. He thought that the major problem of these patients was to appreciate the structural signs in any figure that confers individuality. This view was shared by several subsequent authors (Lhermitte and Pillon, 1975; Damasio *et al.*, 1982; Blanc-Garin, 1986), primarily on the basis of a number of prosopagnosic patients who had difficulty distinguishing between items of the same class, provided they had a similar shape. A patient of Faust (1955), for example, could not distinguish the picture of a chair from that of an armchair. As mentioned previously, a patient of Bornstein *et al.* (1969), who was an experienced bird-watcher, had lost his ability to differentiate visually between birds and another patient of these authors, a farmer, could no longer recognize his cows. The same difficulty in recognizing and identifying his cows happened to another farmer seen by

Assal *et al.* (1984). This patient was transiently prosopagnosic but recovered his ability to recognize familiar persons although his inability to recognize previously familiar cows persisted. De Renzi *et al.* (1968) reported on a prosopagnosic patient who had problems distinguishing different fruits, playing cards or housefronts. Yet another class of objects in which prosopagnosic patients appear to have difficulty in extracting individuality is automobiles. This particular weakness has been noted by Macrae and Trolle (1956), Gloning *et al.* (1966), Rondot *et al.* (1967), Lhermitte *et al.* (1972), Lhermitte and Pillon (1975) and Damasio *et al.* (1982). Three patients described by Damasio *et al.* (1982) found it particularly confusing to locate their own car in a parking lot. No signs of prosopagnosia were reported.

The patient described by Boudouresques *et al.* (1979) was handicapped in recognizing her own handwriting as well as distinguishing between the painting styles of famous painters well known to her or personal objects among other objects of the same class. One of our own prosopagnosic patients (Landis and Regard, 1988a, b) complained about an inability to recognize her own handwriting and on formal testing was unable to learn to discriminate the handwriting of different persons, nor was she able to recognize handwriting familiar to her prior to a right posterior cerebral artery stroke. However, she had no difficulty distinguishing between cars, animals or fruits. Yet another class reported is the predicament of such patients when they must choose between national and foreign coins (Blanc-Garin *et al.*, 1984).

While the ability to discriminate between similarly appearing items of the same class may be impaired in prosopagnosic patients, it is certainly premature to conclude that prosopagnosia is due to a general inability to detect individuality within a given item class, since there are patients in whom this defect does not extend beyond faces (e.g. De Renzi, 1986). Furthermore, experimental investigations comparing the recognition scores for similar items of a given category and those for facial recognition have failed to correlate (De Renzi and Spinnler, 1966; Tzavaras *et al.*, 1970).

Recognition of Items with a Personal Emotional Familiarity

Clinically it has frequently been noted that prosopagnosic patients fail to visually recognize objects or surroundings to which they had a personal emotional link. Some of these, such as familiar places – in particular one's own house, the street or village where one was born and raised – one's own handwriting, car, glasses or other personal belongings such as one's own pets, have been mentioned earlier in this chapter. This has been taken as evidence that prosopagnosia is only one aspect of a memory disorder concerning mainly the evocation of the autobiographic context in which a stimulus has been perceived and learned, making its specific recognition impossible, while the recognition of the class to which this stimulus belongs remains unimpaired (Damasio *et al.*, 1982). When it comes to recognizing faces in daily life, the question is 'whose face?'; for the majority of objects it is sufficient to recognize the class to which they belong. Therefore Damasio *et al.* (1982) stated:

> But it has not been noted that if instead of being asked to identify, say, a "book" or "chair" the patient is asked "whose book?" or "whose chair?" it is, the patient will fail to answer. He will be just as incapable of evoking the history of a familiar object as he will be of evoking the history of a familiar face.

Three difficulties with such a generalization come to mind:

1. A general difficulty in recognizing one's own belongings would almost certainly give rise to problems in daily life, which have not been noted as a frequent symptom in prosopagnosic patients (Blanc-Garin, 1986; De Renzi, 1989).

2. There is at least one carefully investigated patient with prosopagnosia who did not show such a difficulty, either in daily life or on formal testing (De Renzi, 1986).

3. This concept, which resembles the distinction between semantic and episodic memory proposed by Tulving (1983), is unfortunately often used very loosely, referring both to the distinction of the particular item in a class of similarly looking items and to the detection of an object of personal emotional familiarity among other similar objects. This controversy has been recently discussed in detail by De Renzi (1989).

Prosopo-metamorphopsia

As Bodamer had pointed out, in order to consider an agnosia specific for faces, simple perceptual facial distortion, so-called metamorphopsias, had to be excluded. To strengthen his point he argued that two types of patient should be found: those with prosopagnosia but no facial metamorphopsia on the one hand, and, on the other, patients with facial metamorphopsias but without prosopagnosia. In fact, the last of his three cases experienced face-specific metamorphopsias but had no difficulty identifying persons by their face, despite the distortions. Moreover, he described a double dissociation with respect to metamorphopsias concerning faces versus all other visual stimuli, since his first case, a severely prosopagnosic patient, experienced distortions of his visual world in which the only stable, undistorted visual images were faces.

We shall reconsider visual distortions and pseudohallucinations specific to faces, a condition termed 'prosopo-metamorphopsia' by Critchley (1953), on the basis of the few cases reported thus far in the literature and the experience of three of our own patients (Landis *et al.*, unpublished) to be described first.

The first patient, a 62-year-old, right-handed laboratory technician, was on a walk with her husband when she became suddenly aware that the left half of his face was distorted, the left part of his nose being swollen, the left eye and left corner of the mouth swollen and tilted downwards. She was also struck by the fact that his left hand looked enlarged and distorted. Because of the drooping of the mouth, she told her husband that he must have suffered a stroke. Since he denied having felt anything, they hurried home and both looked at themselves in a mirror. To her own surprise and dismay she found that her own face looked distorted on one side in a manner identical to that of her husband. All left halves of faces of living people, and also those of photographs of faces, were distorted in a similar manner, and for about two weeks the same was true for left hands. She initially also had difficulties in reading, albeit not in writing. ('Left' means real left on the body of the person concerned, i.e. this person's left hand, i.e. a part related to the right field of gaze of the *patient*.)

By the time the patient came to our attention, three weeks after the onset of the symptoms, neurological examination was normal except for visual extinction in the right visual field on bilateral simultaneous stimulation. She complained about photophobia and left hemifacial distortions and, to a much lesser extent, distortions of left hands. According to her, these distortions were far less pronounced than at the time of onset. The initial alexia without agraphia had disappeared. She read fluently and understood written text. There was no aphasia, anomia, apraxia or agnosia. In particular, she had no difficulty naming colours or correctly identifying the pictures of famous people or people well known to her. However, the left half of the faces on these photographs looked distorted in the above-mentioned manner. When facial photographs or real faces were presented mirror-imaged, it was still the left side of the faces which looked distorted, indicating that this face- and hand-specific distortion was related to the right visual field (i.e. the left hemisphere) of the patient and not to any particular side of the face observed. When shown a variety of visual stimuli, real or in photographs, such as everyday objects, tools, faces of animals, plants and cars, she experienced no metamorphopsias, nor was there distortion of background non-facial features. This patient was not prosopagnosic at all. This was quite strikingly demonstrated on admission, when she immediately recognized one of us (T.L.) whom she had not seen for 10 years.

Also, in a more formal clinical examination, she had no difficulty in choosing familiar persons from a group, all of whom were disguised with white coats and had removed or hidden distinctive facial features such as hair and glasses. She had no trouble recognizing and matching famous faces, unknown faces, facial expressions, animal faces, bird silhouettes, hands, letters, and symmetrical as well as asymmetrical objects. Only in matching snowflake pictures was she slower than normal subjects. Except for facial stimuli, no metamorphopsias occurred with these stimuli. All facial material, famous faces, unknown faces, stylized drawings of facial expressions and even 'jumbled up faces' (Davidoff and Landis, 1990) appeared distorted on the left side, with the left eye and nose swollen, and the left half of the face tilted downwards. The distortion, however, was much stronger in real faces than in jumbled up faces.

Magnetic resonance images taken 2 months after the event showed two tiny infarcts placed on either side of the splenium of the corpus callosum, the one on the left side being somewhat larger and impinging upon the region of the parahippocampal gyrus (Fig. 14.5). The latter infarct

showed a streaked structure towards the occipital pole, corresponding to early axonal degeneration (Danek *et al.*, 1990), suggesting that this infarct lay at the origin of the symptomatology. Within months of the onset the hemifacial metamorphopsia disappeared, but the patient noted that some distortion of faces was still present under stress and that a mild photophobia also persisted.

The second patient, a 53-year-old, right-handed civil engineer, suffered from a sudden onset of right frontal headaches. He was found to be topographically disoriented and a left homonymous hemianopia was noted. Within 24 hours, the severity of the headache increased, he complained of dysaesthesias in the left arm, and a mild left hemiparesis became apparent. On neurological examination there was minimal nuchal rigidity, a homonymous left hemianopia, more dense in the upper quadrants, and a discrete left facio-brachial sensorimotor hemisyndrome. Mental status examination showed the patient to be slow and topographically disoriented. There were no signs of aphasia, alexia, anomia or apraxia, nor disturbances in object recognition. He had some problems recognizing famous faces, but had no difficulty recognizing persons

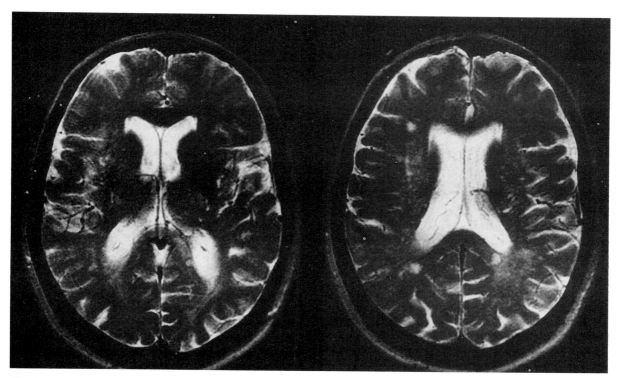

Fig. 14.5 *MRI-scans of the brain of a patient suffering from metamorphopsias afflicting the left half of human faces seen by her (real faces or face photographs). Two tiny infarcts are visible on either side of the splenium corporis callosi, the one on the left side being somewhat larger and impinging upon the region of the parahippocampal gyrus. A somewhat scattered region of higher signal intensity extends from the small dense lesion toward the occipital pole on the left half of the brain (axonal degeneration). Note that following MRI convention, left/right is reversed (from unpublished observations of T. Landis, H. Vogt and M. Regard, 1986).*

well known to him by their faces. CT scan showed a hypodense area in the vascular territory of the right posterior cerebral artery.

The patient came to our attention 8 months later because of disturbing metamorphopsias and pseudohallucinations which had appeared shortly after the initial event. He complained about visual distortions on the left side of faces of people he encountered. Faces were swollen on the left side, and the mouths were grotesquely distorted in a frightening way. Occasionally he also experienced brief visual sensations in the form of little men or rotating swastikas, which he realized were unreal. Sometimes he experienced flashes of bright light. Fast-moving objects and bright light caused discomfort. Neurological examination was normal except for the upper left quadranopic field defect. Mental status examination was normal – in particular, there were no signs of prosopagnosia.

During tachistoscopic investigation, face-specific hallucinations could be repeatedly and reliably induced. Only when presented with face stimuli did he experience face hallucinations, and never with other stimuli such as words, nonsense words, letters, colours, or photographed or drawn objects. The hallucinations always covered the whole visual field and consisted of grotesquely distorted faces or parts of faces. The visual sensations usually increased in size and lasted for a few seconds to minutes. They occurred at different exposure durations and usually bore no resemblance to the face stimulus shown. Only once did he experience a gradually enlarging and frighteningly grotesque distortion of a tachistoscopically presented face. Such brief face pseudo-hallucinations could be induced by a wide variety of stimuli such as famous faces, half-faces (Young *et al.*, 1990), faces showing strong emotion (Landis *et al.*, 1979) and 'pure' faces devoid of distinctive expressive features (Regard and Landis, 1986). These face-specific hallucinations, occurring uniquely following the short presentation of facial stimuli, were elicited during several test sessions in the course of one week. The patient was not available for follow-up studies.

The third patient, a 62-year-old, right-handed secretary, suffered from a stroke in the region of the right posterior cerebral artery (Landis *et al.*, 1986). The infarct left her with a persistent left upper quadranopsia impinging into part of the lower quadrant and with prosopagnosia. Two types of face-specific visual perseverations occurred 9 months after the stroke, without any apparent change in her clinical state. Both lasted for approximately half an hour and happened within a few days of each other. The first episode occurred while she was riding a bus. She was looking at a fellow passenger holding a poodle in her lap. When she looked at the passenger's face she saw the poodle's face instead of a human face. Frightened by this illusion, she looked at other passengers in the bus and realized that all had poodle faces (Fig. 14.6). She left the

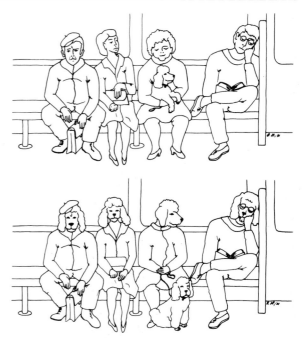

Fig. 14.6 *Schematic drawing of the experiences reported by a 62-year-old prosopagnosic lady while riding in a bus. She looked for some time at the poodle on the lap of a passenger on the other side of the bus and then at the other passengers. What she then perceived is shown on the lower part of the figure (drawing by D. Starke).*

bus and for another half hour all people she encountered had poodle faces, until the illusion faded. The poodle face illusion appeared on no other visual background than on human faces. The second episode happened at work in her office. She suddenly noticed that when the other secretaries moved their heads, they appeared to have multiple eyes or noses in the direction of the head movement, as if eyes or noses were placed around the head. In the absence of head movement this phenomenon did not occur. Other body parts, such as the hand, did not show multiplications, even when moving. Neurological examination between these two episodes was unchanged, the EEG did not show any signs of seizure activity, and a CT scan showed no new lesion beside the old right posterior cerebral artery infarction. The patient has been followed closely for the last 4 years and no similar episodes have occurred.

All three patients exhibited different types of visual metamorphopsic phenomena, all due to vascular lesions in the territory of the posterior cerebral arteries. The common denominator among these phenomena was the restriction to faces. The first patient experienced visual distortion of the left halves of faces and to a lesser extent also of left hands.

Of the 12 cases of prosopo-metamorphopsias reported in the literature (Szatmari, 1938; Pichler, 1943; Bodamer, 1947; De Ajuriaguerra and Hécaen, 1949; Faust, 1951; Hécaen *et al.*, 1957; Gloning *et al.*, 1968; Brust and Behrens, 1977; Young *et al.*, 1989), four experienced hemiface distortions contralateral to the side of the lesion, as described in our first and second patients (Gloning *et al.* 1968; Brust and Behrens 1977; Young *et al.*, 1989). Moreover, a case anecdotally reported by Hécaen *et al.* (1957) experienced diplopia restricted to faces and hands. This combination, also experienced by our first patient, is of particular importance, since single cells in the infero-temporal cortex in the monkey have been shown to respond selectively to faces as well as to hands (Gross *et al.*, 1972). Distortions of the specific configuration of a face but preserving the ability to recognize its identity suggest that different anatomical structures may be involved with the encoding of the typical configuration of a face, on the one hand, and, on the other, the encoding of features characteristic to a person's identity. Moreover, hemiface distortions are observed opposite the site of the lesion, irrespective of whether the lesion is located in the left or right occipito-temporal area. On the other hand, for prosopagnosia to occur, the crucial area is damage to the right occipito-temporal region, suggesting that hemispheric specialization is introduced between these two levels of facial encoding.

'Covert Knowledge' in Prosopagnosia

In recent years a small number of prosopagnosic patients were studied for their ability to possess an access to some knowledge about the faces of persons who are either famous or of personal relevance, without being consciously aware of having this information. These patients were unable to use this 'covert knowledge' to recognize familiar persons by their faces alone. The differences in experimental procedure used to uncover covert knowledge, in the experimental paradigms and tests used, and in localization, aetiology and extent of lesions in patients in whom covert knowledge has been demonstrated, are quite striking. Therefore each of these patients will be described separately.

To our knowledge the first to indicate covert remembrance of familiar faces in prosopagnosia were Bruyer *et al.* (1983). Their patient became prosopagnosic a year prior to testing, subsequent to an infarction of both posterior cerebral arteries: on CT scans the lesion on the left side was restricted to the occipital pole, while the lesion on the right also extended into the area of the occipito-temporal junction. Neurological examination was reported to be

normal and no visual field defects were mentioned. Neuropsychological examination revealed a particularly 'pure' prosopagnosia restricted to famous and familiar faces. This patient had also lost a feeling of familiarity for conscious experience. When asked, however, to sort facial photographs in a forced-choice paradigm according to the critera 'already seen' and 'never seen', he correctly discriminated between personally familiar and unfamiliar faces but not between famous faces and unfamiliar faces. While he could not associate country or profession to famous faces, he was above chance in associating the correct names to famous faces in a multiple-choice task. Moreover, he was above chance in correctly choosing contextual cues to famous faces and showed a negative interference in pair learning when an incorrect name was included for the pair [famous face–name]. This study clearly demonstrated covert knowledge, since the patient had access to primarily semantic information about familiar or famous faces who subjectively evoked no feeling of familiarity and who were never consciously recognized.

A somewhat different approach to 'covert recognition' was taken by Bauer (1984). His patient suffered from bilateral intracerebral haematomas subsequent to a motorcycle accident. Both haematomas were occipito-temporal and predominantly lateral as compared with the usual lesions occurring with infarcts. The left-sided lesion was much smaller than the right-sided, which extended into the posterior temporal and medial temporal lobe. There was a bilateral upper quadranopia and a left homonymous inferior quadranopia as well. In psychophysiological testing using electrodermal responses ('Galvanic skin reflex') to emotional versus non-emotional visual and auditory material, the patient showed a hypoarousal to visually presented emotional material, but a hyperarousal to auditory emotional material. Bauer viewed this symptom of visual hypoemotionality as a 'visual-limbic disconnection syndrome'. In a later paper (1984) he extended the study of electrodermal responses to face stimuli, and covert recognition of famous faces and those of family members could be demonstrated by electrodermal responses to the correct name associated with these faces in the absence of any correct spontaneous naming and chance-performance on conscious multiple-choice name selection.

The same consciously unaware access to semantic knowledge about faces was demonstrated in another patient with bilateral infarcts in the region of the posterior cerebral arteries. Circumscribed lesions of the brain were again very asymmetric, leaving the medial occipito-temporal region on one side relatively spared. In another patient, suffering from bilateral medial occipito-temporal infarctions more marked on the right side (Ross, 1980), Bauer (1986) could not demonstrate covert face recognition. Tranel and Damasio (1985, 1988) took up Bauer's experimental procedure of using electrodermal responses and applied the idea of Bruyer *et al.* (1983) to classify faces into familiar or non-familiar. They found evidence of covert knowledge about the familiarity of faces in four patients with bilateral medial occipito-temporal lesions (for review see Tranel and Damasio, 1988) in the absence of any recognition of familiarity by verbal rating. It is important to mention that of the seven patients in whom electrodermal responses were measured in the presence of prosopagnosia, six who showed an effect of covert recognition were not alexic, while the one who did not was.

De Haan *et al.* (1987a, b) and Young and de Haan (1988) demonstrated covert face recognition in a single prosopagnosic patient by analysing patterns of semantic facilitation and interference in learning and priming tasks along similar lines to those used by Bruyer *et al.* (1983). This patient had suffered a severe closed head injury about 5 years before, at which time he had been unconscious for at least 12 days; CT scan showed generalized cerebral oedema. Again this patient was not reported as being alexic. Another patient reported by Newcombe *et al.* (1989) suffering from prosopagnosia and object agnosia has been examined for the presence of covert face recognition. This patient had incurred meningoencephalitis in 1970, and a CT scan carried out in 1980 (Ratcliff and Newcombe, 1982) showed extensive bilateral infarctions of the posterior part of the brain, mainly occipital but extending forward into the parietal and temporal lobes, particularly in the right hemisphere where the lesion was most extensive. In this patient no covert knowledge could be demonstrated, although reading (word naming) was reported to be normal, but other aspects of visual naming were impaired (Ratcliff and Newcombe, 1982).

Yet another interesting approach to demonstrating covert knowledge has been applied by Renault *et al.* (1989) in a patient in whom there was every reason to believe that the occipito-temporal haematoma causing prosopagnosia was restricted to one side (the patient is referred to in the section on cerebral localization, p. 266). The authors used an 'odd-ball paradigm', the P300 component of visual evoked potentials with two classes of facial stimuli – familiar and unfamiliar ones. In showing an inverse function of probability for each category of faces despite the patient's inability to consciously recognize the familiarity of these faces, covert knowledge of familiar faces could be demonstrated. The patient had no difficulty reading or using a visual–verbal route in language.

Sergent and Poncet (1990) recently reported covert recognition of faces in a patient with a large right-temporal and small left-temporal lesion following encephalitis, who again had no difficulty reading or accessing a visual–verbal route of language (this case is referred to earlier).

Two further examples of covert knowledge in prosopagnosia stem from two of our own patients, both having

suffered from unilateral right temporo-occipital infarctions in the territory of the right posterior cerebral artery, one proven by autopsy (Landis and Regard 1988), the other demonstrated on CT scan (Landis *et al.*, 1986). Both patients could read and had no apparent problems accessing a visual–verbal route of language. The first patient could not recognize any familiar or famous faces, but occasionally she showed a 'negative' approach. For example, when seeing the picture of J. F. Kennedy, she said 'I don't know who this person is, but it is certainly not Kennedy.' We called this phenomenon 'paradoxical knowledge'. It denotes access to covert semantic information, leading to an active denial. The second patient had been subjected to a tachistoscopic 'go–no-go' experiment with random presentation of famous and unfamiliar faces. These stimuli (150 ms exposure duration) were presented twice, giving a total of 96 stimulations. In the first part the patient had to press response keys as quickly as possible whenever she thought that a face was familiar and in a second experiment when the face was unfamiliar. She could not name or recognize any of the famous faces presented and her performance in judging these faces as being familiar or unfamiliar was at the chance level. However, her response latencies in a curious way indicated that she must have been able to differentiate somehow between the two classes of faces: in both tasks, whether responding to familiar or unfamiliar faces, the response latencies were significantly shorter whenever the response was wrong, i.e. a false alarm. Moreover, this effect was only significant for stimuli presented to the left visual field.

In yet another approach to demonstrating covert knowledge in prosopagnosia, Greve and Bauer (1989) showed implicit learning of faces in the prosopagnosic patient described earlier by Bauer (1982, 1984), using the 'mere-exposure' paradigm (Moreland and Zajonc, 1977). They could give evidence that their prosopagnosic patient had a normal preference for newly learned target faces despite poor recognition of these faces as targets.

Thus in altogether 14 patients with prosopagnosia, covert knowledge has been explored in various ways. Twelve of these patients had unconscious access to some semantic knowledge about familiar faces or displayed some indication of class discrimination between familiar and unfamiliar faces. In two patients, experimental investigation failed to disclose covert knowledge.

In all prosopagnosic patients with covert knowledge about familiar faces from whom neuroimaging findings were published or described, the lesion appeared either to be unilateral right-sided, including the crucial infero-medial occipito-temporal junction, or to be asymmetrically bilateral with the right hemispheric lesion more extended. The two patients in whom no covert knowledge could be demonstrated had extensive bilateral occipito-temporal lesions. It is interesting to note that the 12 patients in whom covert knowledge could be shown were not alexic, while the two in whom it could not be demonstrated were either alexic or showed signs of a visual–verbal disconnection.

Bauer (1986), influenced by the view that lesions in prosopagnosia have to be bilateral infero-medial-occipito-temporal (Damasio *et al.*, 1982), thus disconnecting the visual system functionally from the memory stores (Benson *et al.*, 1974), considered his findings in the frame of a selective 'hypoemotionality' restricted to the visual domain. Prosopagnosia and visual hypoemotionality would both result from a bilateral interruption of the ventral visual–limbic pathway (Bear, 1983). Since his patients showed electrodermal responses to semantic knowledge of familiar faces, however, it was evident that some information about the personal relevance of familiar faces must have reached their limbic system. Bauer (1986) proposed the dorsal visual–limbic pathway (Bear, 1983), which projects via the superior temporal sulcus region and the inferior parietal lobule into the cingulate gyrus as an alternative access to the limbic system responsible for the covert facial knowledge. A similar, though less firm stand has been taken by Habib (1986). His prosopagnosic patient was not tested for the presence of covert knowledge, but she displayed a striking visual hypoemotionality as well as profound prosopagnosia and a dense left homonymous hemianopsia. CT scan showed a huge right posterior infarction virtually covering the whole territory of the right posterior cerebral artery and a small infarct in the subcortical white matter of the left occipital lobe.

The ventral visual–limbic pathway uses similar, if not identical, cerebral structures to those shown to be instrumental in the higher-order processing of form and colour, while the dorsal visual–limbic pathway is predominantly associated with structures concerned with the processing of movement and orientation in space. Bilateral lesions interrupting the ventral visual–limbic pathway would thus lead to an agnosic performance across all classes of visual stimuli, including objects and reading. In none of the patients in whom covert knowledge could be demonstrated was this the case. Moreover, in the frame of a general visual hypoemotionality syndrome, the dorsal visual–limbic pathway would carry a weak emotional or attentional trigger of some familiarity detection gained from an earlier non-damaged form and colour analysis. However, in the experiments of Bauer (1984, 1986) electrodermal responses were elicited by semantic associates to familiar or famous faces, such as to the presentation of their names, which demands a quite precise, though not completed or verbally accessible analysis of facial identity. Also one would expect electrodermal responses to visual stimuli to be evenly reduced across classes and certainly never more pronounced than in normal controls. While Bauer (1986) could demonstrate a reduction in electrodermal responses to erotic visual stimuli, this was much less evident for electrodermal responses to famous faces. His second prosopagnosic even displayed stronger electrodermal responses than controls matched for age and education.

In the light of these twelve cases we propose a somewhat different explanation: clinically there are many reasons to believe that beyond the level of elementary sensory processing visual stimuli are analysed differently by the respective visual systems of the left and right hemispheres. Moreover, it is evident from the clinical literature that in the case of damage to the associative visual areas in one hemisphere, the remaining intact visual system of the other frequently fails to compensate for the loss of higher-order visual analysis (Landis *et al.*, 1988). We conjecture that in terms of face processing in normal individuals, part of the visual system in the right hemisphere is concerned with a variety of facial features in an emotional and contextual domain, enhanced by the increased personal relevance of a face, which remains largely non-verbal. Correspondingly, the learning process regarding face identity remains unrecognized by the individual. The left-hemispheric visual association system, on the other hand, consciously extracts salient features of the stimulus by means of a verbalizable domain and shifts the information into the semantic domain. Thus, well-known people can be described verbally.

In the case of interruption in the right-hemispheric medial occipito-temporal visual pathway, the patients can only compare prior facial representations with facial percepts analysed by the left-hemispheric visual system alone. This means that faces will be devoid of a specific right-hemispheric visual analysis concerning emotions, context and personal relevance. Such faces remain faces and may keep semantic facial information, which in a very typical way enables the prosopagnosic patient to recognize a face as a face and even familiar persons by salient verbalizable facial features or paraphernalia. But this percept is sufficiently estranged from the stored facial representation, in which a complete left and right hemispheric visual analysis has been integrated, to evoke a vague feeling of familiarity only without leading to precise recognition. Since even a 'left-hemispheric-filtered' facial percept is more 'similar' to a stored representation than an unfamiliar one, we conjecture that the degree of similarity in this estranged percept, reaching the limbic system via the left ventral visual–limbic pathway, is far more capable of evoking an autonomous response than an equally filtered percept for which a stored representation is completely lacking. Since some prosopagnosics describe especially familiar faces as strange and altered, a sufficiently high degree of similarity between percept and stored representation may lead, in the absence of overt recognition, to reactions ranging from vague discomfort to active denial of the identity of the percept in question, which we have called 'paradoxical knowledge'.

Childhood Prosopagnosia

This term refers to children who, subsequent to cerebral damage, have lost their ability to recognize familiar persons by their face. It also implies that these children had been able to perform this task in a normal way prior to their cerebral injury; otherwise the defect would be called developmental prosopagnosia. To our knowledge there is only one case in the literature which meets these criteria and only a few patients reported as 'developmental prosopagnosics'. We will briefly summarize these cases:

1. Sergent and Villemure (1989) describe a girl with normal birth history and normal psychomotor development up to 5 years of age. She was not formally tested, but considering the approximate age when the recognition of very familiar faces becomes a specialized procedure, one can assume this patient to have acquired 'normal' familiar face recognitions skills. After the age of 5 she developed Jacksonian epilepsy with twitching in the left leg, which progressed to the left arm and the left half of the face as well. At the age of 7 brain surgery was performed and 'epileptogenic tissue' was removed from the right frontal–parietal parasagittal, and right central and parietal opercular regions of the brain. At age 10 the seizures reoccurred and at age 13 a complete right hemispherectomy, sparing the basal ganglia, was performed. At the time of extensive neuropsychological work at age 33, neurological examination showed a dense left hemianopia and sensorimotor hemisyndrome. The patient was not aware of and did not complain about her prosopagnosia, which had been picked up incidentally when the patient mistook the examiner's identity just because the examiner had changed clothes. Extensive examination revealed her to be prosopagnosic but to have no difficulty discriminating between gender and age using face cues, whereby she relied heavily on contextual and extra visual cues to identify familiar persons. Although in our experience (Landis *et al.*, 1986) unawareness of prosopagnosia is not rare, at least in the acute stages of the illness, this patient's inability to even imagine that facial identity could be detected in another way than she was doing is unique. This raises the question whether she was ever able to identify faces in the way non-prosopagnosic patients do. It is difficult to decide whether this patient had acquired childhood prosopagnosia or developmental prosopagnosia; she is none the less the first described case of prosopagnosia subsequent to right hemispherectomy in childhood and an important example for the crucial role of the right hemisphere in the recognition of familiar faces.

2. Young and Ellis (1989) presented a patient, who at the age of 14 months suffered a severe meningococcal meningoencephalitis with coma and general convulsions. She developed bilateral hydrocephalus, became blind for a few weeks and was hemiparetic on her left side. By the age of 4 she had suffered a number of medical complications including six operations for cerebral ventricular shunt revisions. Extensive neuropsychological testing carried out between 8 and 12 years of age revealed a number of visual gnosic problems including prosopagnosia. The wide variety of visual–perceptual and agnosic problems in this patient makes an interpretation of the results from the extensive investigation of facial information processing difficult. However, in this case in which cerebral damage occurred at the early age of 14 months, it is even more questionable than in the case above of Sergent and Villemure (1989) whether the patient ever acquired 'normal' recognition of familiar faces.

3. Another patient, described by Lewis (1987) and thought to be a possible example of childhood prosopagnosia by Young and Ellis (1989), suffered from Capgras's syndrome, a kind of reduplicative paramnesia for persons (Capgras and Raboul-Lachaux, 1923) as well as reduplicative phenomena for places and animals, but not from prosopagnosia.

4. The last case is that of a woman reported by MacConachie (1976) and later by Campbell *et al.* (1990). She had never been able to recognize famous or familiar people by sight alone. Her mother was also found to experience the same difficulty. This patient must, of course, be considered a developmental prosopagnosic.

A summary of all cases published so far does not reveal unequivocal evidence for the existence of a childhood prosopagnosia showing other symptoms than those mentioned in adult patients.

Impairment of Face and Person Recognition in Non-prosopagnosic Patients Suffering From Brain Lesions Outside the Medial Occipito-temporal Region

Recognition of a person's identity in daily life comprises a complex cognitive operation based on visual cues beyond the actual face surface. Individual paraphernalia (e.g. glasses, beard), characteristic movements and gestures, physical stature and clothing form a detailed set of signals for person recognition. It is fairly improbable that only the 'face-specific' medial occipito-temporal area of the brain is involved in this task; more likely, extended regions of both

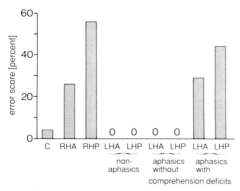

Fig. 14.7 *Error score (per cent, ordinate) in the Benton–Van Allen test of face identification in controls (C), patients suffering from anterior right-hemisphere lesions (RHA), posterior right hemisphere lesions (RHP), and corresponding anterior or posterior left-hemisphere lesions (LHA, LHP). Aphasics without comprehension deficits made no errors, while left-hemisphere-lesioned patients (LHA and LHP) suffering from aphasia had about the same error scores as right-hemisphere-lesioned patients (from Hamsher et al., 1979, modified).*

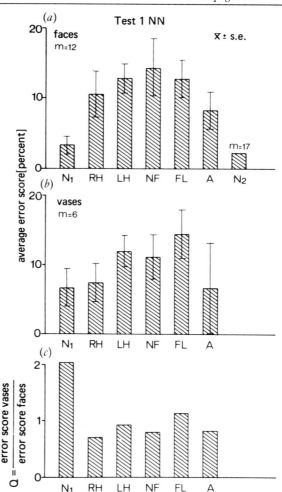

Fig. 14.8 *Distribution of the error scores for recognition of upright faces (a) or vases (b) one hour after inspection. Data from 15 normal subjects (N1, matched to the patients) and 126 normal subjects (N2, students), 18 patients with right-hemisphere lesions (RH) and 35 patients with left-hemisphere lesions (LH). All LH patients were aphasics, 15 suffering from non-fluent Broca aphasia (NF), 15 from fluent Wernicke aphasia (FL) and 5 from amnesic aphasia (A). The relationship of error scores for recognition of vases and faces is displayed in (c). In normals, faces were better recognized than vases, whereas brain-lesioned patients lost this 'face-bonus' (from Grüsser et al., 1990).*

hemispheres contribute to this accomplishment. Indeed, careful investigations of patients suffering from hemispheric lesions without clear signs of prosopagnosia revealed that a rather large and disseminated system of the brain seems to participate in face and person recognition. This assumption is also supported by the fact that patients suffering from 'pure' prosopagnosia learn to use other visual, person-specific 'markers' for person-identification.

Like Tsavaras *et al.* (1970), Hamsher *et al.* (1979) tested facial recognition in 145 patients suffering from unilateral focal cerebral lesions, but not from prosopagnosia. This group of subjects was divided into four classes according to the lesion categories left/right and anterior/posterior, whereby the postcentral gyrus was defined as the border between 'anterior' and 'posterior'. The left-hemispheric-lesioned patients (LH) were divided into non-aphasic subjects and those suffering from aphasia. As Fig. 14.7 illustrates, the Benton–van Allen test score was significantly subnormal in all patients suffering from right-hemispheric lesions (RH), whereby posterior lesions (RHP) affected the face identification ability, as required by this test, more than anterior lesions of the right hemisphere (RHA). In the patients afflicted with left-hemisphere lesions another dichotomy became evident: non-aphasics and aphasics without comprehension deficits performed without error, while the group of aphasics with comprehension deficits were considerably impaired when they had to match frontal-view with three-quarter-view face photographs (Fig. 14.7). This was indeed a finding which also corresponded to the conclusions of Tsavaras *et al.* (1970).

Lewis *et al.*, (1977) also applied the Benton–van Allen

test in patients suffering from closed head injuries of varying severity, grouped into three categories: (a) patients without lengthy coma and without neurological symptoms; (b) those with neurological deficits, indicating in particular brain stem lesions and duration of coma shorter than 24 hours; (c) subjects who remained in coma longer

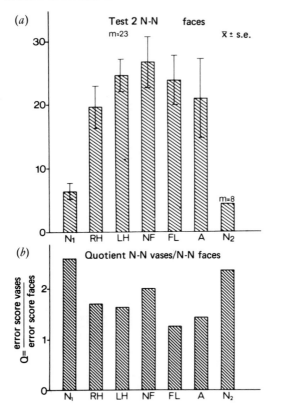

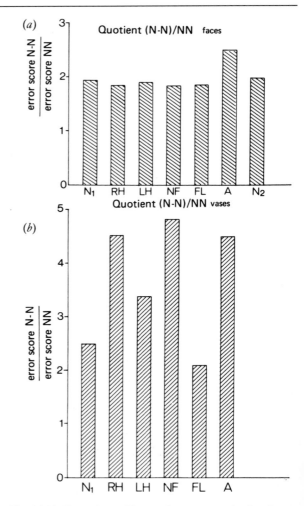

Fig. 14.9 *Face-recognition test after a delay of one week. Same subjects as in Fig. 14.8. (a) Error score for recognition of faces seen in the inspection series one week before. (b) Quotient for error scores for vase recognition and face recognition. Note the higher 'face bonus' in the two group of normals (from Grüsser et al., 1990).*

Fig. 14.10 *Recognition of faces and vases one week after the inspection series. Same subjects as Figs 14.8 and 14.9. The quotient of error scores in the test performed after one hour (NN) or after one week (N-N) was computed for faces (a) and vases (b). Time had the same relative effect on the error score of normals and patients in the face-recognition tests but different effects on the error score in vase recognition (from O.-J. Grüsser and N. Kirchhoff, unpublished, 1985).*

than 24 hours and experienced lasting neurological deficits including pupillary abnormalities, oculomotor palsy and vestibular disturbances. Duration of coma and the severity of neurological signs, indicating brain stem afflictions, were inversely related to accuracy of performance in the Benton–van Allen test. Impairment in facial identification was specifically associated with neurological signs of concomitant hemispheric and brain stem injury.

Krickl *et al.* (1987) tested the ability of normal controls, right- and left-hemisphere-lesioned patients to recognize meaningless drawings and face photographs 5 minutes after the first presentation. During the initial inspection either the full-size figure or the face was seen for 2.5 seconds or a sequential presentation was made, whereby the stimuli were given in three stages of completeness. The first face stimulus was about the upper half of the head with forehead, eyes and bridge of the nose, the second exhibited the top three quarters of the head and the

last the complete face (stimuli duration altogether 2.1 seconds). In a third test the face photographs and the meaningless figures were presented in a 'fragmentary' mode; only the upper half was shown for 2.1 seconds, while for testing the complete face or figure had to be identified among distractor items. The performance of both right- and left-hemisphere-damaged patients was inferior to normals in all tasks. Somewhat surprisingly, the RH patients were less impaired in recognition after sequential presentation of the items than after 2.1-second

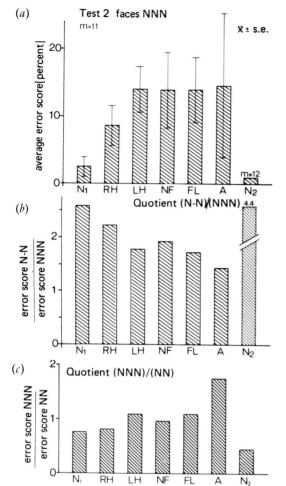

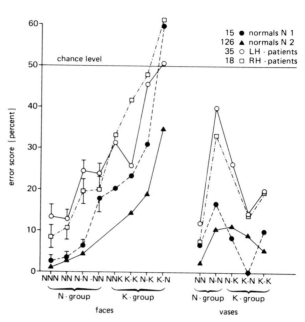

Fig. 14.12 *Summary of data obtained in the recognition tests of faces and vases in normals and brain-lesioned patients as described in Fig. 14.8. Different stimulus conditions as indicated. N: items seen in upright position; K: items seen upside-down. Patients suffering from right-hemispheric lesions (squares) have a lower error score when the faces were shown in the normal position compared with the heft-hemisphere-lesioned patients (circles). For all tests in which the face was turned upside-down, RH patients performed with a higher error score than the LH patients (from Grüsser et al., 1990).*

Fig. 14.11 *(a) Error score in recognizing faces one week after they were presented for six seconds in the inspection series and six seconds during the first test. (b) The quotient of the error scores for the condition N-N and the condition NNN demonstrates the advantage in recognizing items seen twice one week before the recognition test. (c) In contrast, the quotient for face recognition for the condition NNN and the condition NN demonstrates that in normals and in brain-lesioned patients, with the exception of amnesic aphasics, seeing the face twice compensated the time effect of one week on memory and recall (from O.-J. Grüsser and N. Kirchhoff, unpublished, 1985).*

presentation of the full face during which at least four saccades were performed.

In our own studies (Grüsser and Kirchhoff, 1985; Grüsser *et al.*, 1990) 53 patients and 15 age-matched normal adults and a second 'supernormal' group of 191 normals (students) were investigated with a slide projection test. From the patients, 18 suffered from a right hemisphere lesion (RH), 35 from a left hemisphere lesion (LH). The latter group was composed of 15 patients with typical

signs of non-fluent Broca aphasia (NF), 15 of fluent Wernicke aphasia (FL) and 5 of amnesic aphasia (A). Three patients suffered from bilateral frontal lobe lesions without aphasia, where the left frontal lobe was more impaired than the right. Black-and-white photographs of faces and vases of about 14×11 degrees visual angle (average luminance 8.5 cd m^{-2}) were projected onto a screen. The investigation consisted of three series: the initial inspection series, the first forced-choice test (T1) performed one hour after the inspection series, and the second test (T2) performed one week later. During the inspection series, 60 slides were projected, 21 with a female, 23 with a male face in frontal view and 16 art nouveau vases with ornaments. Ten of the items were shown upside down (condition 'K'), the other items in the normal upright position ('N'). Three response categories were possible: 'sympathetic' (aesthetically pleasing), 'not sympathetic' (not pleasing) and 'neutral'. Each slide was shown for 6 seconds. The subjects then had another 6 seconds to make their decision, followed by the next slide, etc. The subjects did not know

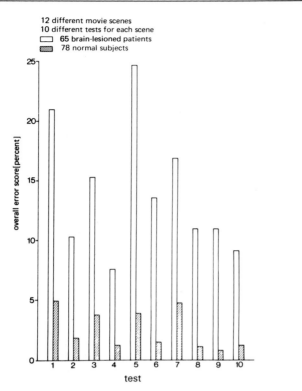
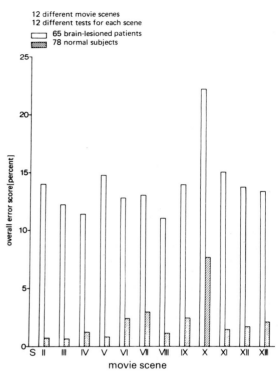

Fig. 14.13 *The ability to recognize facial expression, gestures and the persons seen in short movie scenes was investigated in 65 brain-lesioned patients (31 RH, 30 LH and 4 bilateral lesions) and for comparison in 78 matched normals. (a) Distribution of the error score obtained in 10 different tests. Tests 1–5 and 10 were averbal; tests 6, 8 and 9 were verbal. (b) Same study. Error score is averaged from the 10 subtests for each of the 10 movie scenes separately (from Grüsser et al., 1985, published in Grüsser et al., 1990).*

that successive tests on their ability to recognize faces would be performed. In the hour following, one of the investigators spoke with the patient, a Token test was performed with most, and tea and cookies were served.

One hour after the inspection series, the subjects were informed that their ability to recognize the items seen during the inspection series would now be tested: 18 items (6 female faces, 6 male faces, 6 vases) were presented with an unknown 'partner' ('NN') for 6 seconds. One week later, the subjects were tested again. Now the test set consisted of 66 items, 27 pairs of female faces, 29 pairs of male faces and 10 pairs of vases. An item seen in the inspection series but not in the first test had the notation 'N–N', one seen in the inspection series, the first test, and the second test 'NNN'. With the notation '–NN', items were characterized which had been seen as partners in the test 1, but as targets in test 2 with another partner. Correspondingly, items shown upside down are noted as 'K' (e.g. 'N–K', 'K–N' etc.).

In the inspection series we noted that brain-lesioned patients responded (more pronounced in LH than in RH patients) with a higher percentage of positive emotional or

aesthetic evaluations for faces and vases than the group of normals. Item recognition after one hour is shown in Fig. 14.8. The quotient of the error scores for vases and faces, which was about 2 in normals, decreased to below 1 in patients. Compared to normals, the increase in error score for faces in all patient groups was significant, while no major differences in error scores were found between RH and LH patients and between the different groups of LH patients. A significant increase in the error score for vases was found for NF- and FL-aphasic patients.

The second recognition test, performed one week after the inspection series, showed a stronger impairment due to the brain lesions, as expected (Fig. 14.9). With respect to upright stimuli, three classes of conditions were investigated: 'N–N', 'NNN' and '–NN'. Compared with normals, the increased error scores in all groups of brain-lesioned patients were statistically significant. In all groups, male faces were recognized better than female (1.88 times in normals, 1.47 in RH, 1.38 in LH, 1.33 in NF, 1.43 in FL, 1.54 in A). Comparing the data of test 1 (NN) and test 2 (N–N) led to an estimate of the time effect on memory for faces. The quotient of the corresponding error scores (Fig. 14.10(a)) was between 1.9 and 2 in all experimental groups, except for the patients suffering from amnesic aphasia, where it increased to 2.5 (Fig. 14.10(a)). This finding indicates that the relative effect of time on face memory was not essentially changed by the brain lesions.

Faces of the category 'NNN' were seen during the inspection series, during test 1 one hour later and during test 2 one week later. A comparison of the 'N–N' and 'NNN' results allows an estimate of the effect of repeated presentation. The increase in the patient error scores for condition 'NNN' was significantly higher than that in normals (Fig. 14.11). The performance of LH patients (all aphasics) was inferior to RH patients (14.0 ± 3.34 errors in LH, 8.6 ± 2.98 errors in RH, t-test $p < 0.05$). The quotient of the error score 'N–N' and the error score 'NNN' gave an estimate of the relative efficiency for the fact that the face was seen twice. In normals, face recognition improved by a factor of 2.6, while in RH (2.28) and in LH (1.76) it was less. With the exception of amnesic aphasics, seeing the face twice compensated in all groups for the decrease in face recognition due to time in test 2 (Fig. 14.11(c)).

Recognition of faces from the group '–NN' was recognition of an item which had been shown as a 'less important' partner in the first recognition test T1. Therefore the error scores were expected to be significantly above those with 'N–N' faces. This was only the case however in normals (quotient –NN/N–N = 2.8). In brain-lesioned patients the differences were negligible (quotient –NN/N–N in RH 1.02, LH 0.98, NF 0.87, FL 1.00, A 1.28). Perhaps this was due to the fact that during test 1 the patients spent more time looking at the partner item than the normals did.

In normals, face recognition in test 1 was about twice as good as recognition of vases. This 'face advantage' was absent in all brain-lesioned patients (Fig. 14.8(c)). In the test after one week, the corresponding error score (N–N vases)/(N–N faces) increased in normals to 2.59. In long-term recognition, however, brain-lesioned patients also performed somewhat better with faces than vases; thus, some advantage for face recognition was still preserved.

Figure 14.12 displays a summary of all data, including the test with the rotated ('K') items, ranked according to test category difficulty as found in the control group of matched normals. It is evident that rotation of the items increased the error scores more in the RH than the LH patients. In all groups, rotation or inversion affected vase recognition considerably less than face recognition.

In 31 of the 35 aphasic patients, Token-test data were obtained and correlated with the error scores found in tests 1 and 2. Token-test and face recognition scores were only loosely correlated with each other ($r = 0.49$).

The computer tomograms of patients were evaluated and the extent of the brain lesion was estimated by a plani-

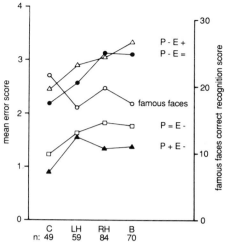

Fig. 14.14 *The Carey–Diamond face discrimination test (after Grafman* et al., *1986). $P - E +$, paraphernalia changed, expression same; $P - E =$, paraphernalia changed, expression neutral; $P = E -$, paraphernalia same, expression changed; $P + E -$, paraphernalia same, expression same.*

metric method obtained in three standardized CT planes. A clear effect of brain lesion size on error score existed, which was more pronounced for recognition of faces ($r = 0.67$) than vases ($r = 0.58$). This correlation seemed to be fairly independent of the site of the lesion, provided it was outside the medial temporo–occipital part of the brain, and was valid for lesions of the right and left hemispheres.

Finally, another study performed in LH and RH patients supported the view that brain structures outside the classical 'prosopagnosia area' contribute to recognition of faces and gestures (Grüsser, Kiefer and Landis, unpubl., 1985). The movie test described in Chapter 15 was applied in RH and LH patients (with and without aphasia) and in a matched control group. In order to keep stress at a minimum, we decided to test the patients without a response time-limit. This condition, of course, improved the overall performance of the patients considerably. If time constraints had been applied, the error scores would have increased by at least a factor of 2; in normals performance would not have been affected at all.

Figure 14.13 summarizes the data obtained in this test. It clearly indicates that brain lesions outside the medial occipito-temporal region affected the recognition of a person, gestures and facial expression. On the average RH and LH patients were similarly impaired, but the highest error scores were found in patients suffering from lesions of the right posterior hemisphere.

In an extensive study in 213 brain-injured Vietnam war veterans and 49 normal controls, Grafman *et al.* (1986) studied the effects of penetrating head injury upon face discrimination and face memory in non-prosopagnosic patients. Brain lesions were determined by CT scans and three large experimental groups were investigated (LH, RH and bilateral brain-lesioned patients). In a thorough statistical analysis other subgroups were formed according to the cortical regions lesioned. Face discrimination and memory were examined with a method similar to that applied by Milner (1968). In the immediate identification task, i.e. face discrimination, the subjects had to find a matching face in a closed array as quickly as possible and compare it with the target face. When the choice was wrong, another choice had to be made. For delayed identification the subjects were presented with two sets of photographed faces. They were told to study them carefully so as to be able to recognize them when presented a second time together with faces not already seen. Face discrimination was tested with a method developed by Carey and Diamond (1977). In this test facial expression and paraphernalia (hats, shirts, scarves, necklaces, eyeglasses and wigs) were manipulated to make the recognition task easier or more difficult. On each trial the subject was shown a card with three photographs of faces, one at the top (the target face) and two at the bottom (comparison faces). The subjects were asked to indicate which of the two comparison faces was the same as the one at the top. Responses to several conditions as indicated in the caption of Fig. 14.14 were studied. Errors were higher on the average when 'fooling' paraphernalia or expressions to help recognition were used than with the reverse condition (Fig. 14.14). In general, Grafman *et al.* came to the following conclusions:

1. Lesions of the temporal lobe, in particular the right one, had a detrimental effect on memory for unfamiliar faces.
2. Lesions of the left temporal lobe impaired memory for 'famous' faces more than lesions of the right temporal lobe.
3. RH lesions in general had a stronger effect upon discrimination of facial features than LH lesions.
4. Bilateral hemisphere lesions in general impaired face memory and face recognition more than unilateral lesions. The performance on these 'face tasks' was independent of other visual–spatial or verbal tasks.

In summary, the work reported here indicates not unexpectedly that brain lesions outside the area lesioned in typical prosopagnosic patients also affect memory, recognition and perception of faces. Moreover, the lack of correlation with other visual and visuo–spatial tasks, as found in the study of Grafman *et al.* (1986), leads to the conclusion that face signals are also treated as a special set of visual information in neuronal networks outside the occipito–temporal 'face areas' of the brain.

15 Impairment of Perception and Recognition of Faces, Facial Expression and Gestures in Schizophrenic Patients

Schizophrenia and the Phylogenetic Development of the Human Brain

The research work on schizophrenic patients described in this chapter is interpreted in the light of three hypotheses:

1. Schizophrenia is a disease caused by transmitter–receptor interaction disturbances in extended nerve cell nets and/or by structural deficits in the neuronal networks located in man-specific cerebral areas, i.e. those areas that developed during hominid evolution from *Homo habilis* to *Homo sapiens sapiens*.

2. The process underlying schizophrenia is not restricted to circumscribed brain regions such as parts of the hippocampus, the area entorhinalis, the hypothalamus or the frontal lobe areas. It affects extended man-specific cortical functions, including the cortico–limbic and cortico–thalamic neuronal circuits.

3. The variability of clinical symptoms indicates that the role played by different limbic, neocortical and sub-cortical regions in schizophrenia must differ somewhat from patient to patient (cf. Grüsser, 1991).

With regard to these hypotheses, it is not of importance whether the disturbance is primarily affected by genetic or epigenetic (e.g. viral or environmental) factors, since internal and external mechanisms act within cerebral structures on a common terminal path, having influence on the signal processing by synaptic structures and nerve cell membranes.

As the size of the hominid brain increased during the last 2.5 million years, phylogenetically old cortical areas also increased; moreover, new man-specific cytoarchitectonic cortical regions evolved, establishing the basis for the development of the 'higher' brain functions necessary for the foundation of Palaeolithic culture. One may define three phylogenetic growth zones in the human brain con-

taining extended man-specific cortical integration areas: the orbital and part of the dorso–lateral, prefrontal cortex, parts of the parietal association areas and the upper temporal regions located in the first and second temporal gyrus. The temporal integration cortex provides the neuronal machinery necessary for the elementary language functions that take place in the 'dominant' left hemisphere, while musicality and prosody of speech functions are correlated with 'subdominant' right cerebral hemisphere functions (Fig. 15.1). The parietal phylogenetic growth zone provides the man-specific mechanisms associated with manual skill, constructive ability, object recog-

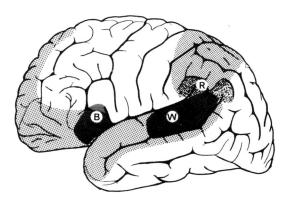

Fig. 15.1 *Schematic drawing of the left hemisphere of a human brain, indicating the neocortical brain structures which have developed during hominid phylogenesis of the last 2.5 million years. In addition, those regions which are especially relevant for language functions and for reading and writing (Chapters 17, 18) are indicated. B: Broca's speech area. W: Wernicke's sensory speech area extends into the planum temporale of the first temporal lobe convolution. The planum temporale is not visible at the outer surface of the brain. R: Regions of the gyrus supramarginalis (circumflexus) and gyrus angularis which participate in reading and writing.*

nition and manipulation, spatial planning and spatial thought. The frontal cortex contains Broca's motor speech area on the left side, a corresponding region on the right hemisphere necessary for the metaphorical use of language, and the regions essential in man for long-range planning, reflective thought, social creativity and constructive motivation. In general, the thalamo–cortical connections of these man-specific cortical association and integration areas are characterized by late axonal myelinization during postnatal brain development, a fact which Paul Flechsig (1896a, b) and Cécile and Oskar Vogt (1919) had recognized and systematically explored. Myelinization of the prefrontal integration cortex connections, for example, continues through late adolescence. Similarly, the formation of dendritic spines, which function as loci of synaptic contacts between neurones, continues into adulthood. These morphological signs of postnatal maturation take place much earlier in life for nerve cells found in the elementary sensory and motor fields.

In the light of cytoarchitectonic evidence as well as the cognitive and precognitive sensory functions in man and other primates, it is evident that in man the phylogenetic differentiation of a large part of the higher-order visual association cortices has not advanced excessively in comparison with that of other higher primates (cf. Chapters 5–7); the opposite is true with regard to the integrative auditory areas. This difference is reflected in the wide gap between man's linguistic and musical behaviour and that of all other primates. Visual functions that have developed further during hominid evolution include social signals such as elaborate face recognition, perception and understanding of gestures, learned facial expression or other averbal communication signals, constructive visual abilities regarding individual objects or larger spatial structures, spatial planning and visual 'pars-pro-toto functions' which are used, for example, for reading (Chapter 17).

When one analyses the dominant psychopathological symptoms of schizophrenia, both productive and defective, one has the impression that the pathological process affects some higher brain functions and elementary 'limbic' functions related to man-specific behavioural patterns simultaneously (e.g. Eggers, 1981). This observation is not surprising considering the fact that phylogenetic development of new neocortical integration areas automatically required a reorganization of the neocortical–limbic connections, providing a phylogenetic adaptation of 'old' limbic structures to new neocortical integration areas as well as the development of man-specific limbic structures (e.g. in the entorhinal area). In addition, some phylogenetic adaptations of the intrinsic dopaminergic system of the forebrain became necessary. This system is presumably involved in schizophrenia. It extends from brain stem regions to the hypothalamus, several limbic structures and the prefrontal cortex (including the orbital,

man-specific areas). New connections became necessary within this system whenever new neocortical integration areas had developed during phylogenesis. Similar considerations are probably valid for the noradrenergic and serotonergic systems of the brain.

If the hypothesis is correct that schizophrenia is a disease affecting predominantly man-specific neocortical integration areas, including their limbic connections, this fact should be reflected in the psychopathology of this disease and a 'hierarchical order' of productive schizophrenic symptoms would become predictable: complex auditory hallucinations (e.g. hearing 'voices') should occur much more frequently than all other types of hallucinations. Complex visual hallucinations, for example, should be fairly rare events and restricted to the above-mentioned man-specific abilities of the visual domain: faces, facial expressions and persons acting in social communication. According to our hypothesis, the second most frequent sensory domain involved in schizophrenic hallucinations should be the somatosensory modality, since its representation in the parietal lobes required considerable reorganization and expansion during hominid evolution. The development of upright gait, complex tongue, mouth, eye and head mobility, and hand motor skills led not only to a reorganization of the cortical somatosensory maps but also to an enlargement of parietal somatosensory association areas. Olfactory and gustatory hallucinations occur relatively infrequently in schizophrenics, for the neocortical representations of these sensory modalities diminished considerably during hominid evolution, while parts of the central olfactory and gustatory system in man have acquired new functions and connections. The occurrence of schizophrenic vestibular hallucinations should also be rare, since the cortical vestibular fields (area 2v, area 3a neck region and the parieto-insular vestibular cortex, PIVC) exhibit a close homology in man and other higher primates; furthermore, the reorganization necessary during the phylogenetic development of upright gait involved mainly the brain stem vestibular system. The frequent symptoms of dizziness and vertigo in normals indicate the narrow limits of this phylogenetic adaptation.

Provided that the Kielmeyer–Haeckel rule, i.e. that 'ontogeny recapitulates phylogeny', is applicable for man-specific psychopathological symptoms, the relative frequency of hallucinations related to the different sensory modalities should be age-dependent in schizophrenics. This is indeed the case. As schizophrenic children and adolescents grow older, visual hallucinations occur less frequently (Eggers, 1973). This phenomenon, however, is also observed in non-schizophrenic, exogenic psychotic states in children (Eggers, 1975).

Based on these general assumptions, we do not believe that schizophrenia is caused by a general or diffuse impairment of cognitive functions of varying strengths, nor by selective malfunctions of certain brain structures like the frontal lobe (Crockett *et al.*, 1986; Weinberger *et al.*, 1988; Heinrichs, 1990). We feel, rather, that it is a disease which selectively affects with variable intensity of those neocortical functions that have developed only 'recently', i.e. during the last 2.5 million years. In our investigation of visual cognitive function in schizophrenics, we concentrated, therefore, on those man-specific visual cognitive abilities. Several new tests were applied; two of these dealt with the perception and recognition of faces, facial expression and gestures. The results of these tests are described in the following section, since they indicate a surprisingly strong impairment of the processing of face signals and averbal communication in schizophrenic patients.

Paraprosopia in Schizophrenic Patients

Paraprosopia is a term used to describe a productive symptom appearing in schizophrenic patients that is closely related to the perception of faces and facial expression. Patients report that a face considered to be 'normal' or 'friendly' by other observers transforms within a few seconds into a 'monster', 'werewolf', 'vampire' or 'devil' having large fangs, huge threatening eyes, bushy eyebrows and hair 'standing up on end'. These alterations in facial perception are not simple geometrical dysmorphopsias of the faces and are observed by patients in both real faces and photographs of faces (Fig. 15.2). Dewdney (1973) published several impressive drawings of schizophrenic children which depicted the facial changes that they perceived in others. Less dramatic changes were also described by schizophrenics who either mistook one person for someone else (Kahlbaum–Capgras Syndrome, Chapter 16), simultaneously saw the same face in

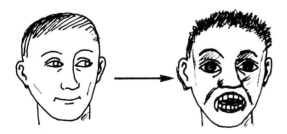

Fig. 15.2 *Scheme of alterations seen by some schizophrenic patients when viewing faces or face photographs (paraprosopia). As a rule, it takes several seconds for the 'dracula-face' to appear. When the face is removed and reshown after several seconds, it is seen firstly as normal again and a few seconds later paraprosopia reappears (Berndl and Grüsser, 1987).*

two persons, or perceived in one face the mixture of two or more individual faces (cf. Enoch *et al.*, 1967). The Kahlbaum–Capgras syndrome was also observed in patients suffering from prefrontal cerebral lesions (Kahlbaum, 1861; Capgras and Reboul-Lachaux, 1923; Merrin and Silberfarb, 1976; Morrison and Tarter, 1984; Benson and Stuss, 1986; cf. Chapter 16).

The following report of a female student illustrates a case of paraprosopia. When one of the authors (O.-J. G.) saw her for the first time several years ago, she was 23 years old and had already been suffering from a fairly severe schizophrenia of the paranoic-hallucinatory type for several months. She reported that the faces of strangers changed within a couple of seconds into 'dracula faces' with large canines, a threatening grin and a 'hypnotic gaze'. She frequently saw 'beams' coming out of the 'menacing' eyes and heard 'hissing sounds' associated with the beams. She believed that the beams were pointed at her body, where she could feel them (*coenaesthetic* hallucinations).

At the same time, she believed that she possessed a 'new power' by which she could force the people at whom she was looking to take on her own facial expression. She believed that with this 'power' she could make television anchormen imitate her own facial expressions. With the exception of those of friends and family members, the patient often responded to neutral or pleasant facial expressions or gestures with fear and sometimes even with terror. Periodically, she also felt an emotional distance from all averbal communicative signs in her surroundings. The faces of all other persons then appeared 'empty and dead'.

During this acute psychotic state, she repeatedly misinterpreted the intentions and/or the social roles of others. For example, she mistook her court hearing concerning compulsory psychiatric hospitalization for a 'religious ceremony'. When she falsely recognized or perceived illusory changes in faces and facial expression, her own facial expressions were markedly reduced: she expressed no emotion and made fewer gestures. All of these changes, which were observed before the patient had been treated, slowly diminished over the weeks following commencement of neuroleptic administration.

Although paraprosopia has been observed in schizophrenic adults, it seems to occur more frequently in schizophrenic children and adolescents. This corresponds to observations that eidetic pseudohallucinations – the '*phantastische Gesichtserscheinungen*' of Johannes Müller (1826) – occur more frequently in normal children than in adults; in addition, these sensations are related mainly to face, person and animal perception. This fact was well known to Greek scientists (cf. Chapter 23; Aristotle: *On dreams*).

An example of a Kahlbaum–Capgras syndrome and of

adult schizophrenic paraprosopia is found in Daniel Paul Schreber's (1842–1911) personal account of his own psychotic experiences, *Denkwürdigkeiten eines Nervenkranken.* In this book, the former president of Dresden's *Oberlandesgericht* (Court of Appeal) describes his repeated observations of changes in the faces and facial expressions of other patients in a psychiatric hospital:

> They [the other patients] *appeared absolutely silent when they entered the salon, one after the other. They also left the salon quietly, one after the other, apparently not taking notice of each other. I have repeatedly seen that individual patients exchanged heads while in the salon, i.e. without leaving the room, and suddenly walked around with another head during the period of my own observations* . . . .(Schreber, 1903/ 1973, p. 75).

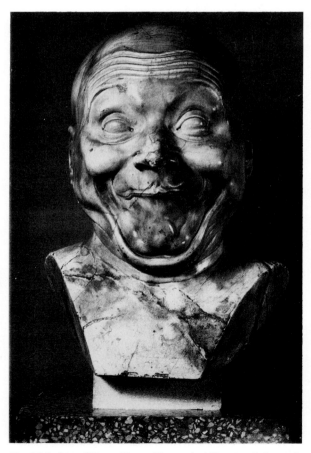

Fig. 15.3 *One of Franz Xaver Messerschmidt's portrait busts of grimacing people (*'Charakterköpfe'*) with the title* 'Ein absichtlicher Schalksnarr' *(*'wilful foolish jester'*). It is one of more than 50 portrait busts showing excessive facial expression. It was sculptured about 1780. (Vienna: Österreichische Galerie; Pötzl-Malikova, 1984).*

This high-court judge, who suffered from chronic schizophrenia, also reported that he once perceived two gentlemen whom he had met at the spa in Warnemünde 'as devils with particularly red faces and red hands', and that he once observed Geheimrat W. as the Oberteufel (chief devil, Schreber 1903/1972, p. 16). A much older biographical report of a chronic psychotic patient, which described more than 50 years of psychotic experiences, contains repeated accounts of paraprosopia and illusionary facial perception (Krauss, 1852, 1867).

Paintings by schizophrenic patients may also tell us something about changes in their perception of faces. Faces with eye-, nose-, and mouth-region deformations are typical examples of this phenomenon, as one can see in many paintings belonging to the Prinzhorn Collection (Prinzhorn, 1968), in Adolf Wölfflin's paintings as reported by Spoerri and Glaesemer (1976), in the paintings of schizophrenic patients published by Hofer and Wiechert (1970), and also in August Walla's paintings and those of other patients at the psychiatric hospital in Gugging (Austria) as described by Navratil (1983, 1989). A glance at the works often found in a museum of modern art reminds us, of course, that paintings with deformed faces or facial expression are by no means a sign of individual psychopathological problems or disease. When, however, the oeuvre of a painter or sculptor is dominated by massive distortions in facial expression, deformation of the facial structures or expressions of 'emptiness', terror or fear, one may wonder whether the artist's creativity was indeed influenced by psychotic experiences. Many of James Ensor's (1860–1949) paintings as well as the many masks he produced, some of which are exhibited in the Ensor Museum in Ostende, as well as Franz Xaver Messerschmidt's (1736–1783) sculptures ('*Charakterköpfe*'), are examples of such distortions (Fig. 15.3; Kris, 1979; PötzlMalikova, 1984; Krauss, 1986; Bücherl, 1989; Schoonbart *et al.*, 1989).

Neuropsychological Investigations of the Recognition of Faces, Facial Expression and Gestures in Schizophrenic Patients

Tests with Slides or Photographs

Formal studies have confirmed clinical observations that schizophrenic patients differ from normal patients in their ability to encode and decode facial expression and body language (see Izard, 1959; Levy *et al.*, 1960; Iscoe and Veldman, 1963; Pishkin, 1966; Dougherty *et al.*, 1974; Muzekari and Bates, 1977; Neal, 1978; Pilowsky and

(a)

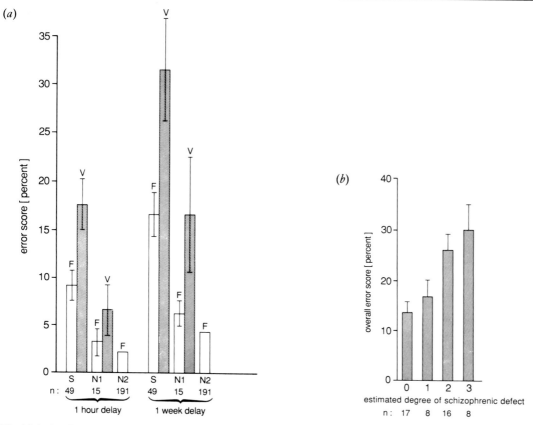

(b)

Fig. 15.4 *(a) Error score (ordinate per cent) for recognition of upright face photographs 1 hour and 1 week after the set of faces was inspected for 6 seconds each. Data were from schizophrenic patients (S), age and educationally matched to normals (N1) and from a supernormal group (medical students, N2). Control items were ornamented vases of art nouveau style. In both normals and schizophrenics face recognition is better than recognition of vases. Error scores increased significantly for both items in schizophrenia (49 patients) as compared with normals. (b) Overall error score for recognition of upright and inverted face photographs 1 week after inspection (6 seconds for each item) related to the degree of schizophrenic defect categorized into four groups (0 = no sign of schizophrenic defect, 3 = severe schizophrenic defect). Algebraic mean ± s.e. (O.-J. Grüsser and H. Kremer, unpublished, 1985).*

Bassett, 1980; Cutting, 1981; Walker *et al.*, 1980; 1984; Novic *et al.*, 1984; Mandal and Palchoudhury, 1985; Feinberg *et al.*, 1986; Grüsser and Kremer, 1985; Kremer-Zech, 1987; Grüsser *et al.*, 1990). Most of these studies were carried out using photographs or slides. Some examples of the results obtained in such studies are shown in Figs 15.4(a, b) and 15.5. According to extensive patient data obtained in our own studies on degree of psychosis, schizophrenic defect, duration of illness, duration of hospitalization, age, school education, duration of psychopharmacological therapy, amount of psychopharmaceuticals taken, type of schizophrenia and gender, only the first two factors influenced the test results (Fig. 15.4(b)).

Since faces, facial expressions and gestures made under 'natural' conditions are in part dynamic signals, a test using short movie scenes seemed more appropriate for

investigating the perceptual abilities of normal subjects and schizophrenic patients (Berndl *et al.*, 1986a). In extensive studies of adult and adolescent schizophrenics (Berndl *et al.*, 1983, 1986a, b, c; Berndl and Grüsser, 1987), severe impairment of face recognition and facial expression and gesture perception was found. Evaluation of the data indicated that the duration of illness, type of schizophrenia, medication, duration of hospitalization and gender had no significant effect on the degree of overall impairment of the above-mentioned cognitive abilities. Again, the degree of psychosis and schizophrenic defect were correlated with the error score.

The Movie Test

This test, which investigated the ability of subjects to perceive and recognize faces, facial expressions and body lan-

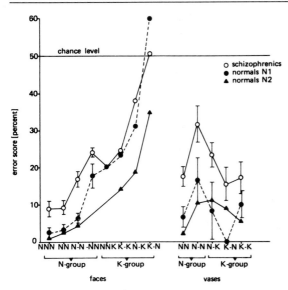

Fig. 15.5 *Summary of error scores in the face and vase recognition test (as in Fig. 15.4) performed in normals (●, N1; ▲, N2) and 49 adult schizophrenic patients (○). NN: recognition of items in normal position after 1 hour delay. N–N: same after 1-week delay. NNN: items in normal position but seen in the inspection series, in test 1 after 1-hour and in test 2 after 1-week delay; error score for this test. K: items seen upside down. During the inspection series the subject saw each item for 6 seconds and had to make an 'emotional' decision on the item. (From Grüsser and Kremer, 1985, in Grüsser et al., 1990.)*

guage, has already been described in detail by Berndl *et al.* (1986a). It consisted of 13 colour silent movie scenes, each lasting 10 seconds. In each scene, an actor or actress dressed in black performed, using facial expressions and gestures, a short pantomime depicting a simple situation: SI – nausea, SII – silence, SIII – fear, SIV – farewell, SV – physical effort, SVI – offensive smell, SVII – noise, SVIII – ignorance and perplexity, SIX – quiet grief (helplessness), SX – pain, SXI – fatigue, SXII – anger and SXIII – laughter (Fig. 15.6). The first movie scene (SI) was used for instruction purposes, while the other 12 scenes were scored using 5 non-verbal multiple-choice tests (T1–T5, 1 correct answer out of 5 choices). Five cards with 5 colour photographs each were used to measure the subjects' ability to recognize the person, the gesture and the facial expression shown in the preceding movie scene (Fig. 15.6). Following the last movie scene (SXIII), a 10- to 15-minute break was taken, during which the patients were served coffee and cookies. Afterwards, the 13 movie scenes were shown again, but this time in reversed order (SI, SXIII, SXII, . . ., SII). Following each scene, 5 new multiple-choice tests were given: 3 verbal, 2 non-verbal. Of the non-verbal tests, the last one (T10) was identical to T3 (of the first test sequence). T6

required a short verbal description of the movie scene. In T7, the subjects had to select 1 of 5 simple drawings that best fitted the pantomime seen in the preceding movie (Fig. 15.7). In T8, the patients had to select 1 of 5 written words which best fitted the movie scene, and in T9, one of five words read aloud. All patients and normal subjects had been informed that the test was being conducted for scientific purposes and that their participation was voluntary.

Figure 15.8 summarizes the scores obtained for 81 schizophrenic patients and in a second study for two different age groups based on the results of 10 different tests (T1–T10) averaged for the 12 movie scenes (SII–SXIII), or averaged over all 10 tests for each of the 12 different movie scenes. As one can see from these figures, the 12 scored movie scenes (SII–SXIII) produced, on the average, fairly homogenous results. Error scores varied similarly for the two different age groups and were fairly consistent for a given group of subjects watching the same movie scenes. Thus, the test had a more or less regular structure and coherence with respect to the data obtained in the different movie scenes. When the error scores for the 10 different subtests were compared with those obtained by the two age-groups comprised of normal subjects and schizophrenic patients, a positive linear correlation coefficient of $r = 0.60$ and $r = 0.63$ was found. Thus, when a subtest was relatively more difficult than average for normal subjects, the same was also true for schizophrenic patients. Further statistical evaluations of the data are described by Berndl *et al.* (1986c). In all 10 tests (T1–T10), the middle-aged group of normal subjects and schizophrenic patients made more errors than the corresponding adolescent groups (Fig. 15.8(b)). This difference was significant for most pairs of tests at $p < 0.01$ or $p < 0.05$ (*t*-test) and was about the same percentage-wise for normal and schizophrenic patients. This confirmed the earlier data report obtained for 81 schizophrenic patients and 78 normals, which indicated that the error score for adult subjects increased slightly with age (Berndl *et al.*, 1986b).

As Fig. 15.8 demonstrates, schizophrenic patients made considerably more test errors than normal subjects. Adolescent patients (YP in Fig. 15.8(b)) had an average error score of 14.2 per cent, the control group (YN) only 1.0 per cent. For middle-aged patients, an error score increase of up to 20.5 per cent was found, while the control group had an error score of 2.9 per cent. The error score differences obtained for patients and normal subjects were somewhat smaller for tests measuring recognition of persons, facial expressions and gestures (T1–T5, T10) than for the more complex test in which movie scenes had to be related to an appropriate sketch. The same was true for the verbal tests (T7–T9). All of the patients' error scores differed at a significance level $p < 0.001$ from the error scores of the

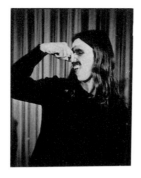
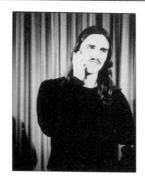
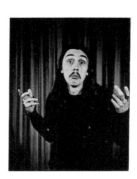
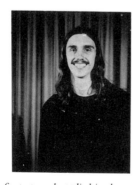
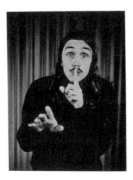

Fig. 15.6 *Example of a test card applied in the movie test (subtest 2). Five colour photographs were presented. The actor seen in the preceding movie scene was displayed in the colour photographs miming five different expressions. The subject had to decide which photograph depicted the action displayed in the preceding movie scene (from Berndl et al., 1986).*

corresponding group of normal subjects (age, education and social status matched). Significant differences between the performance of adolescent and middle-aged patients were observed in tests T7 ($p < 0.05$), T8 ($p < 0.05$) and T9 ($p < 0.05$; t-test). In all these tests, the older patients had higher error scores than the younger ones.

In conclusion, the movie test indicated that recognition of faces, facial expression and gestures as well as the understanding of body language were impaired in both adolescent and middle-aged schizophrenic patients. In addition, the relative deficit, i.e. the error scores related to the error scores of the corresponding normal control groups (errors patients/errors normals), was significantly larger for the younger patients than for the adults. This finding indicates that impairment of the neuropsychological functions tested was present at, or even predated, the onset of the disease and that it was at least as strong in the

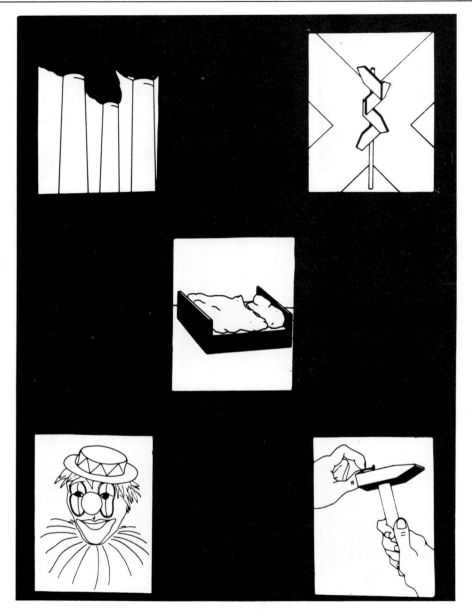

Fig. 15.7 *Example of a card used in subtest 7 of the movie test. Five simple drawings depicted different events or situations. The subject had to decide which picture fitted best the action seen in the preceding movie scene (Berndl et al., 1986).*

early stages as in later years. The decrease in these man-specific precognitive and cognitive abilities is, as a rule, accompanied by disabilities related to motor control of facial expression and gestures, which lead either to 'para-mimic' and 'paragestural' expressive movements in schizophrenics or to reduced facial expression. These symptoms can be interpreted as 'paraphasia' or 'dyspha-sia' of the body language, corresponding to the changes in verbal language of some schizophrenics ('schizophasia'). In the movie test data, from all psychopathological abnor-malities explored, only the degree of schizophrenic defect evaluated as the sum of negative symptoms had a disease-

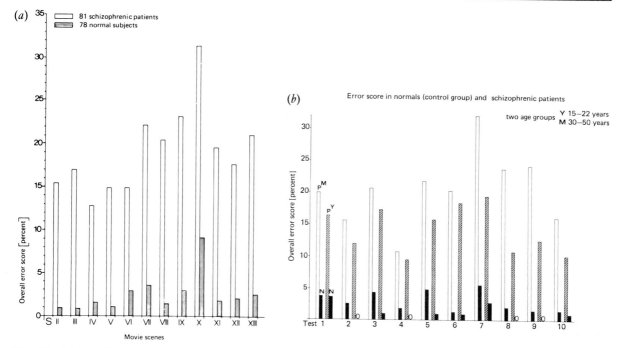

Fig. 15.8 *(a) Overall error score from the 12 different movie scenes (SII–SXIII). Errors averaged for all 10 subtests. Data were from 81 male and female schizophrenic patients of all age groups and 78 normal subjects matched for gender, age and educational level to the patient group. For all movie scenes the error score differences are significant at the p < 0.001 level. (From Berndl et al., 1986.) (b) Error score in the movie test obtained in normals (N, black bars) and schizophrenic patients (P) from adolescent (15–22 years) subjects (Y) and middle-aged (30–50 years) subjects (M). Data were from 38 middle-aged schizophrenic patients (PM, white bars, 40.0 ± 0.9 s.e. years), from 28 adolescent schizophrenic patients (PY, hatched bars, 19.0 ± 0.4 s.e. years). In several subtests a group of young adolescent normals had no errors; this is marked by '0'. The data of 33 middle-aged normals (MN, 39.4 ± 1.1 s.e. years) are given in black bars, that of 9 adolescent normals (YN, 18.2 ± 0.9 s.e. years) in dark grey bars. Data were from 10 different subtests as described in the text (Berndl et al., 1986b).*

specific impact on error scores for both adult and adolescent schizophrenic patients.

Problems and Conclusions

Both traditional clinical descriptions and modern neuropsychological investigations agree that the process leading to schizophrenia affects the basic cognitive abilities of most patients (e.g. Kasanin, 1946; Yates, 1966; Dussik, 1968; Tucker *et al.*, 1969; Weiner, 1970; Reed, 1970; De Wolfe *et al.*, 1971; Alpert and Martz, 1977, Matthysse *et al.*, 1979; Abrams *et al.*, 1981; Hemsley, 1982; Taylor and Abrams, 1984; Hatta *et al.*, 1984; Donelly, 1984). Clinical studies have indicated that these cognitive impairments increase, at least in some patients, with the duration of the illness (Aarkrog 1975, Aarkrog and Mortensen 1985); the effects associated with ageing, however, occur parallel to the schizophrenic process and are presumably similar in normal people and schizophrenic patients. The strong

impairment in recognition of faces, facial expressions and gestures found in adult and adolescent schizophrenics (cf. also Frith *et al.*, 1983) could be interpreted as one of many signs of deterioration in cognitive abilities caused by the disease, which also affects the mechanisms of attentive interaction with the external world as well as the memory functions necessary for normal cognitive behaviour. This interpretation is not very probable, however, since recognition of faces, facial expression and gestures seems to be significantly more impaired in cases of schizophrenia than any other visual cognitive function. No experimental or clinical data suggest, for example, serious disturbances in elementary space recognition, general visual orientation or even more elementary visual functions. Clinical experience indicates, however, that schizophrenics are frequently misled by animate or inanimate structures having some physiognomic components, for example animals, houses, automobiles, trees of a certain shape, etc., and develop a delusionary fear when confronted with these stimuli. Repeatedly we have seen patients suffering from schizophrenia who reported perceiving very strong physiognomic signals from inanimate objects which in normal observers generated only mild features of this type, if at all. Also the physiognomic quality of animal faces may change in the course of a schizophrenic disease. As in fairy tales, animals can become more human. One of the authors (O.-J. G.) once observed a 34-year-old lady suffering from acute paranoic–hallucinatory schizophrenia, who reported that horses grazing on a pasture had 'mixed facial expressions, man-like and horse-like', and spoke to her with human voices, so sending messages from a non-existent lover.

Together with the results of the formal tests discussed above, paraprosopia, the Kahlbaum–Capgras syndrome, and impaired facial expression and body language perception, all support the idea that man-specific averbal visual functions which guide social interaction are selectively more impaired than the other visual or non-visual abilities of schizophrenic patients. It seems probable that impairment of the ability to recognize faces, facial expressions and gestures is a basic psychopathological sign of schizophrenia, and explains, at least in part, the difficulties that schizophrenic patients have in everyday social communication. These findings also contradict the assumption that the primary defect of schizophrenia is an attentional deficit related particularly to the left hemisphere (for discussion, see Goldstein, 1990), since signal processing of faces, facial expressions and gestures is a right-hemisphere-dominant ability (cf. Chapter 14).

It was argued above that perception of faces and facial expression as well as the recognition of body language is a man-specific ability in which parts of the medial occipito-temporal and limbic regions of the right cerebral hemisphere play a larger role than do any other associative brain structures. Provided that this explanation is correct, it is not surprising that studies analysing the brain structure of schizophrenic patients *in vivo* by means of multiplanar magnetic resonance imaging techniques showed a significant reduction of brain tissue in the temporal lobes in comparison with normal control subjects, matched for age, gender and educational level (Rossi *et al.*, 1990). From the observations made in patients suffering from prosopagnosia caused by circumscribed brain lesions, one can deduce the possible impairment of brain structures in schizophrenic patients which may be responsible for the difficulties they experience in recognizing faces and facial expression. A malfunction of the neuronal structures and connections ranging from the infracalcarine right mesial occipito-temporal cortex to the gyrus parahippocampalis and from there into other structures of the limbic system may be responsible for the peculiar disabilities of schizophrenic patients described in this chapter.

16 The Splitting of 'I' and 'Me': Heautoscopy and Related Phenomena

Introduction

During hominid phylogenesis an elaborate neuronal system developed, which is used by man to recognize his fellows and their facial expressions (Chapter 12). Understanding gestures and facial expressions leads to liminal innervation of the receiver's own expressive system and therefore under certain conditions to a more or less 'mirror' play of features, as one can observe in the audience at an emotionally moving play or film or in the participants at political rallies. The hysterical phenomena seen in religious or political demonstrations are more dramatic events based on the same neuronal mechanisms of 'mirror emotions' and their corresponding motor expressions. Motor components interacting with visual signals are also present when we see ourselves in the mirror. Under 'natural' conditions man's mirror image was restricted to the plain water surfaces of ponds or mud-holes. After the Palaeolithic invention of pottery, bowls filled with water also provided reflecting surfaces. Until the use of polished metal surfaces as mirrors in the Bronze Age and the invention of glass mirrors about 3000 years ago, man was rarely confronted with his own image.

It is interesting that only man and the great apes recognize themselves as 'selves' in a mirror, and children learn at the age of about 2.5 years to correctly identify their own mirror image (Chapter 12). Once they have accomplished this self-identification, children enjoy playing with their mirror images and learn to correlate their emotional expressions with the motor commands leading to facial and gestural movements (cf. Chapter 12). As adults we still know our facial expressions in a rather limited manner by sensing somatosensory and proprioceptive input together with feedback signals of motor innervation patterns. An actor may still use the mirror as a feedback device when learning to control a certain facial expression or gesture.

The coordination of somatomotor and somatosensory signals with the expressive visual signals of our face and gestures is a learned accomplishment. These mechanisms of visual–somatosensory integration are activated every time when one looks at one's own face or person in a mirror, and our knowledge about our own face is being continuously updated. Furthermore, most of the time when looking into a mirror, the average human makes some adjustment to his appearance (combing the hair, brushing teeth, washing the face, applying make-up etc.), i.e. relates his visual perception of the self with some motor activity.

Persons standing in the public eye in modern societies have in addition the questionable privilege of seeing themselves repeatedly in the movies or on television. This technical heautoscopy, however, is not the topic of this chapter (cf. Michel, 1978). Nothing is known of how people who see themselves frequently on television experience pathological heautoscopy.

In the light of these ideas, it seems probable that visual hallucinations concerning one's own body image are related to the neuronal correlates integrating the visual signals of one's own person with the probably genetically determined and epigenetically modified somatosensory body image, which relies heavily on the internal feedback of motor commands for movements. In the following we will present a short review on the phenomenon of heautoscopy and then discuss some peculiar disturbances in the processing of face and gesture signals related to our social partners.

Seeing a 'Doppelgänger'

Symptomatology

Heautoscopy ('autoscopy', 'double', 'Doppelgänger') is a not very frequent but consistent peculiar change in the experience of the self, which can be divided into four main categories (types a–d) and is also associated with two further types (e and f) of psycho-pathological phenomena:

(a) Visual hallucinations of the inner organs of one's own body (inner heautoscopy, Kerner, 1824, 1829; Comar, 1901; Sollier, 1903; Lannois, 1904).

(b) Visual hallucinations of one's own body or of the self perceived like an external mirror image a few metres away at the most. As a rule the double appears in the true size and is frequently copying the body movements of the observer (outer heautoscopy).

(c) Visual hallucinations as in (b), but associated with vestibular sensations related to 'I' or to 'me' (visuo-vestibular splitting of the somatosensory body image).

(d) Partial heautoscopy in which parts of one's own body, especially the limbs, are seen in different places than their 'real' position.

(e) Related to hallucinatory heautoscopy is a kind of illusionary heautoscopy: the patient meets another person and sees in him his own double (Leonhard, 1957; 'syndrome of subjective doubles', Christodoulou, 1978).

(f) Also related to heautoscopy but involving somatosensory and (rarely) vestibular functions rather than visual hallucinations is the 'somaesthetic *doppelgänger*', a doubling phenomenon in which the subject perceives half of his body double or senses a doubling of his whole body without seeing it.

Inner Heautoscopy (a-Type Heautoscopy)
This rare symptom appears in dreamy states of hysteric and perhaps of epileptic origin. The patients report seeing their inner organs and frequently also changes within their bodies caused by a disease. Sometimes they claim to perceive simultaneously the organs of other persons, for example of their doctor (Kerner, 1824). Reports on inner heautoscopy have been extremely rare during the last 80 years (Leischner, 1961).

Outer Heautoscopy (b-Type Heautoscopy)
Arieti and Bemporad (1974) provided a short, clear definition of the b-type autoscopic syndrome: 'The patient sees a person nearby, who looks exactly like himself, talks, dresses and acts as he does.' Critchley (1953) characterized b-type heautoscopy by a 'delusional dislocation of the body-image in the visual sphere'. Menninger-Lerchenthal (1946) gave a more detailed description:

Suddenly one perceives one's own person in front of oneself. This vision resembles the observer more or less and is perceived in every case as being identical with the observer, even when certain differences to the real person exist. The observer is intensely frightened, stays under the impression of the heautoscopy for a long time and is not able to remain indifferent to this vision...

Dress, age and even size of the double are not necessarily identical with that of the observer, who is nevertheless directly and deeply convinced that he sees his own double. As a rule this double copies the observer's position and movements. In one of the oldest reports on b-type heautoscopy, the double was described as a shadow image walking with the observer, and the author, Aristotle, preferred a physicalistic interpretation of the phenomenon:

... because of a disease, the reflection [of the visual rays] also appears without any increase in density of the air. This happened once to a man with weak eyes. While looking straight ahead; whenever he walked about, he gained the impression that his shadow image was walking in front of him gazing at him. The reason was that his visual impressions were reflected because of the disease of his eyes ...
(Aristotle, *Meteorology*, 373b).

Visual-vestibular Heautoscopy (c-Type Heautoscopy)
This is b-type autoscopy associated in addition with vestibular sensations. In the following, we quote with the permission of the author, a well-known American neuroscientist, his account of a c-type heautoscopy to provide the reader with a realistic description of what one perceives during this strange phenomenon:

An 'Out-of-Body Experience'. I have once in my life had a brief out-of-body experience, and it made a strong impression in me. The incident occurred more than 35 years ago, but I remember it in great detail. I was standing before a small audience, not more than ten people, in a well lit college classroom, delivering a speech which was so well prepared that I could nearly recite it like a memorized poem. Without prior warning, I suddenly had the clear impression of observing myself from the outside, from a position more than a metre above my head and somewhat to the side: near the ceiling of the room. This impression probably did not persist for more than 15 seconds, but for that time, it was as though my "body" was down below the real "me", continuing to deliver the prepared speech, while "I" watched from above. The experience ended as suddenly as it began, and I continued with the speech, with no known aftereffects. None of the audience, including several friends, commented afterward on noticing anything unusual in my behaviour.

I was, at the time, 19 years old; I had taken no drugs, and had drunk no alcohol for at least the preceding 24 hours. I had never previously experienced anything which conflicted with my natural-scientist view of the world, nor have I ever since had any experience even remotely similar, under any circumstances whatever. I do not consider myself to be someone with an unusually graphic imagination; most of my dreams, for example, when I recall them, tend to be vague, and more emotional than pictorial in content. Previous to this experience, I had read a very modest amount about Eastern religions, spiritualism and parapsychology. I had certainly heard of out-of-body experiences, but I considered them then, as I do now, to be hallucinations, when not outright fraud. I did not then, nor do I now, believe in the existence of a non-material soul, or any "essence" of person which might be separable from the physical, flesh-and-blood-and-nervous-system persona. For all these reasons, associated with my prevailing belief system, I was unprepared for this experience. I was not frightened nor was I "converted" to any alternative belief system. I was simply intrigued.

I have since then read a modest amount about the experiences which sometimes occur under the influence of hallucinogenic drugs. It is my tentative hypothesis that this experience may have been triggered by some sort of endogenous biochemical effect, perhaps related in mechanism to drug-induced hallucinations.

In this report two characteristics of c-type heautoscopy are described, the vestibular sensation of being elevated outside one's own body and the splitting of 'I' and 'me'. In heautoscopy associated with vestibular sensations, as a rule, 'I' looks down on 'me', while in mirror image b-type heautoscopy 'I' looks at the double outside or at 'someone' who 'mimicks me and my activity'.

Partial Heautoscopy (d-Type Heautoscopy)

This is usually restricted to a double perception of one's own limbs. Such a pseudo-hallucinatory perception is described in the following report of another neuroscientist, quoted with permission:

Once in my life I had a partial heautoscopic experience. I woke up from a dream, in which during folk dancing an unknown girl turned me about by holding me by my feet and swinging me around fairly quickly. On awaking I saw feet and legs suspended in the space above the bedspread at about an angle of 45 degrees. I thought "Oh, a hypnagogic hallucination" and realized that I could not move my real legs voluntarily. This partial cataplexic state persisted for about 30 seconds, during which I saw my legs slowly moving down through the bedspread to the place where my "real" legs were. Otherwise I was fully awake during this surprising experience, which never happened again. During the hypnopomp hallucination I could discern typical noises in the house and concluded therefore that I was not dreaming. I could also move my arms and head without difficulty, but the legs remained completely immobilized till the end of this hallucination and I could "feel" this paresis of my legs, while I saw the "other" legs moving slowly downwards...

Somaesthetic Doppelgänger Heautoscopy (e-Type Heautoscopy)

This is not visual, hence the '-scopy' is somewhat misleading. Two classes of somaesthetic heautoscopy have been reported:

1. Doubling of the body half contralateral to the brain lesion, occurring most frequently with right-sided parietal cortex lesions (Chapter 22). Fairly seldom patients report seeing the doubled half.

2. Doubling of the whole body with a perceived spatial distance between 'I' and the double, which is not seen at all, but nevertheless convincingly experienced ('*Anwesenheit*' phenomenon, 'somatoparaphrenia'; Nightingale, 1982). This symptom is rarely associated with vestibular sensations, and the *alter ego*, or the presence of another subject, is felt to be on the same level of the extra-personal space as the self. Temporal lobe epilepsy, exogenic psychoses and narcolepsias are the most frequent diseases in which this e-type double appears (Jaspers, 1914; Giljarowsky, 1923; Menninger-Lerchenthal, 1935; Thompson, 1982). It is evoked fairly frequently in high-altitude mountain climbers (above 6000 metres; Brugger et al., 1989).

History

Heautoscopic hallucinations were repeatedly reported in medieval and Renaissance medical texts (Hamanaka, 1991) and with Wigan (1844), Griesinger (1867, 1868) and Féré (1891, 1898) they reached the status of a psychiatric diagnostic category: 'self-vision' or 'hallucination autoscopique ou speculaire'. Heautoscopic phenomena were reported in religious visions and fairy tales and are vivid still today in folklore (Brierre de Boismont, 1852; Crawley, 1911; Schmeing, 1937, 1943; Todd and Dewhurst, 1957, 1962). The transcultural coincidence of *doppelgänger* descriptions is very high. Sheils (1978) investigated 70 non-Western cultures and in 95% found fairly uniform reports on the phenomenon. A few cases of heautoscopy were described in the medical literature of the eighteenth century (e.g. Bonnet, 1760; Gmelin, 1791). Heautoscopy attracted the attention of physicians and poets during the period of Romanticism. The German poet Jean Paul in his novel *Siebenkäs* (1796/1797) introduced the term *doppelgänger*. The *doppelgänger* phenomenon became a very popular topic in Romantic poetry (e.g. E. T. A. Hoffmann '*Elixiere des Teufels*', 1815/1816; Heinrich Kleist '*Amphitryon*', 1807; E. A. Poe '*William Wilson*', 1843), an indication of the impact of psychology and medicine of that time. Of course the ideas of those physicians believing in occultism and parapsychological phenomena, such as Schubert (1814), Justinus Kerner (1824, 1829) or Hagen (1837), had particularly easy access to poetry. This was enhanced when the physician, such as Kerner, was also a Romantic poet (Grüsser, 1987a). Even the 'anti-Romantic' Heinrich Heine took up the topic and in his *Buch der Lieder* devoted a short poem to this peculiar phenomenon (*Die Heimkehr*, 1823/1824, Nr. 20). Franz Schubert composed one of his songs to this text:

> *Still ist die Nacht, es ruhen die Gassen,*
> *In diesem Hause wohnt mein Schatz;*
> *Sie hat schon längst die Stadt verlassen,*
> *Doch steht noch das Haus auf demselben Platz.*

Da steht auch ein Mensch und starrt in die Höhe,
Und ringt die Hände, vor Schmerzensgewalt;
Mir graust es, wenn ich sein Antlitz sehe —
Der Mond zeigt mir meine eigne Gestalt.

Du Doppelgänger! du bleicher Geselle!
Was äffst du nach mein Liebesleid,
Das mich gequält auf dieser Stelle,
So manche Nacht, in alter Zeit?

Doppelgänger phenomena were also described in nineteenth century Russian literature (e.g. Gogol), and Dostoevsky dedicated a whole novel to this phenomenon (*The Double*, 1847). Since luetic paralysis and epilepsy are neurological conditions in which *doppelgänger* hallucinations are relatively frequent, it is not surprising that poets suffering from one or the other described these phenomena in novels or even experienced them personally. Guy de Maupassant, afflicted with a luetic dementia, was the most famous patient to report a continuously hallucinated double during the last years of his life (Munthe, 1931; Todd and Dewhurst, 1957, 1962). People believing in parapsychic phenomena often argue that the *doppelgänger* experience (and other experiences in epileptic dreamy states) 'proves' their belief-system. Du Prel (1886, 1888), for example, argued that by heautoscopy the existence of an 'astral body' is directly demonstrated (for a critical discussion see Menninger-Lerchenthal, 1946; Lhermitte, 1951; Brügger, 1979).

Neuropathology and Pathophysiology of Heautoscopy

In reviewing the published cases of the four types of 'visual' heautoscopy (a–d), one does not find clear indications of circumscribed brain diseases, but temporal lobe afflictions, more frequently of the right side than the left, seem to be predominantly involved in the phenomenon. This also explains the frequent association of heautoscopic experiences with vestibular sensations: in c-type heautoscopy the pathological activation spreads most likely from the posterior part of the insula to the retroinsular regions, thus affecting the parieto-insular vestibular cortex (PIVC) located deep in the insula and the retroinsular region of the Sylvian fissure (Grüsser *et al.*, 1982, 1990a, b; Akbarian *et al.*, 1988). The epileptic activity also invades the retroinsular and parietal visual areas, thus connecting body sensations in epileptic aura with pathologic vestibular and visual activity. Skworzoff (1931) considered c-type heautoscopy as a neuropsychological 'vestibular' syndrome. The not very frequently observed size-changes of the *doppelgänger* who is seen unnaturally small or large,

could also be attributed to pathological involvement of cerebral mechanisms of vestibular sensations or space percepts. Jantz and Behringer (1944) observed several soldiers who immediately after a left or right temporal or parieto-temporal brain lesion (gun-shots or shell fragments) experienced long sensations of elevation and free-floating above the battlefield. This vestibular percept was frequently associated with the hallucination of auditory noise followed by a pleasant feeling of quietness. These abnormal sensations indicated involvement of the auditory and vestibular cortex together with complex visual activity, which led to the percept of the battlefield seen from a bird's-eye view. One of the authors (O.-J. G.) observed a patient with such a brain lesion from the Second World War who suffered from rare epileptic seizures beginning with an aura of floating in the air and a corresponding change in visual perspective. These findings also support the interpretation that c-type heautoscopy is a combination of visual and vestibular hallucinations involving the posterior insular and retroinsular cortex. B-type and c-type heautoscopy seem to be a pathological activation of the insular representation of the body image together with limbic or temporal visual memory field (Chapters 5–7).

With regard to aetiology, in looking through the pathology of the published cases of *doppelgänger* hallucinations, one can classify the different diseases associated with heautoscopy into three large groups:

1. Diffuse brain diseases caused by intoxication, infection, fever, drugs or meningoencephalitis.
2. Temporal lobe seizures of differing aetiologies.
3. Highly emotional affective states in normal subjects.

These conditions are listed in the following in more detail:

1. Drug abuse including marihuana, opium, heroin or other 'hard' drugs like mescaline or LSD (Sollier, 1903; Menninger-Lerchenthal, 1935; Schmitt, 1948; Sengoku *et al.*, 1981; Salama, 1981; Aizenberg and Modai, 1985).
2. High fever including typhoid fever (Reil, 1803; Leuret, 1834; Leuret and Gratiolet, 1837/1857; Giljarowsky, 1922, 1923; Hirschberg, 1932; Sivadon, 1937; Faguet, 1979).
3. Alcoholic delirium tremens (Lasegue, 1884; Sollier, 1902, 1903; Naudascher, 1910; Galant, 1929) or other exogenic or traumatic psychoses (Heintel, 1965; Hamanaka, 1991).
4. Luetic paralysis (Gurewitsch, 1933).
5. Hemianopia due to visual cortex lesions, whereby the double appears in the blind hemifield (Engerth *et al.*, 1935; Dewhurst and Pearson, 1955; cf. Chapter 9).
6. General brain lesions due to carbon monoxide intoxication, diffuse meningo-encephalitis (Sivadon, 1937; Lhermitte, 1956; Mize, 1980), CS_2 intoxication (Rosen-

stein and Rawkin, 1929) or multiple tumour metastases (Hamanaka, 1991). Cerebral hypoxia, beginning cerebral oedema, isolation and extreme stress occurring together explain the high incidence of heautoscopy in high-altitude mountaineers, especially as many mountain climbers on the basis of irrational arguments reject the use of an additional oxygen supply. Therefore above an altitude of 6500 metres heautoscopy or seeing a companion doing the same ('heteroscopy') is almost a 'normal' event (cf. Brugger *et al.*, 1989). Smythe (1934) reported his experience during an attempted ascent on Mount Everest:

> *All the time that I was climbing alone I had a strong feeling that I was accompanied by a second person. This feeling was so strong that it completely eliminated all loneliness I might otherwise have felt. It even seemed that I was tied to my "companion" by a rope, and that if I slipped "he" would hold me. I remember constantly glancing back over my shoulder, and once, when, after reaching my highest point, I stopped to try to eat some mint cake, I carefully divided it and turned round with one half in my hand. It was almost a shock to find no one to whom to give it. It seemed to me that this "presence" was a strong, helpful and friendly one, and it was not until camp VI was sighted that the link connecting me, as it seemed at the time to the beyond, was snapped, and although Shipton and the camp were but a few yards away, I felt suddenly alone.*

In these hallucinations of high-altitude mountaineers it is not always clear whether the companion is an *alter ego* or someone else. As Oelz and Largiadèr (1987) reported, the person hallucinated under such conditions could be someone else, another climber, who, however, looks rather similar to the hallucinating subject. Such a hallucinated companion can give rather absurd and dangerous recommendations regarding the path the hallucinating subject should take:

> *A tall, German-speaking fellow, whom I had never seen before, walked beside me and told me to leave the track and take a short-cut straight down a steeper route. I was by no means surprised to meet this gentleman here and followed his reasonable advice. It got darker and darker and my route became steeper and steeper. My new friend disappeared...*

After bivouacking overnight, the author hallucinated the other members of his group whom he had left on the 7193-metre-high summit:

> *Suddenly, my expedition friends appeared and I welcomed them with deep relief; but they did not talk to me nor greet me; they started to build a cable car. As soon as they had finished it, they played with it. I implored them to take me down, but they did not answer. It was now around noon and I slept for about an hour in the warm sun...*
> (Oelz and Largiadèr, 1987).

This report demonstrates that in addition to an unknown 'companion' doing the same things as oneself, in this dan-gerous state of impaired brain function, the lonely mountaineer also hallucinates other persons in a complex scenario.

7. Schizophrenia is also a disease in which heautoscopy can appear (Galant, 1935; Glück, 1946; Reda and Anderson, 1953; Trelles *et al.*, 1962; Damas Mora *et al.*, 1980). Self-reports are at hand of *doppelgänger* hallucinations in schizophrenic patients (Krauss, 1852, 1867; Staudenmaier, 1912). McConnel (1965) described a pregnant patient who also saw a *doppelgänger*. Since she suffered from a schizoaffective psychosis, the latter was presumably the cause of heautoscopy. A male patient of Letailleur *et al.*, (1958) perceived a heterosexual *doppelgänger* who induced sexual phantasies.

8. Epilepsia, or in the modern literature more specifically temporal lobe epilepsia, is the most frequent disease in which heautoscopy was reported (Nasse, 1834; Griesinger, 1868; Féré, 1890; Nouet, 1923; Marchand and Ajuriaguerra, 1940; Genner, 1947; Lhermitte, 1951a, b; Constantinidis, 1954; Russell and Whitty, 1955; Hécaen and Ajuriaguerra, 1952; Zutt, 1953; Dewhurst and Pearson, 1955; Todd, 1955; Vizioli and Severini, 1955; Lukianowicz, 1957; Gloning *et al.*, 1963; Vizioli and Liberati, 1964; Heintel, 1965; Silva, 1965; Lunn, 1970; Maximov, 1973; Hécaen and Green, 1987; Devinsky *et al.*, 1989). In rare cases the double is multiplied and seen five to twelve times simultaneously (Pick, 1901).

9. An extensive brain tumour (glioblastoma) in the left parieto-occipital and temporal lobe region led to occasional perception of a 'double' (Pearson and Dewhurst, 1954 (case 2); Gloning *et al.*, 1963). The patient of Gloning *et al.* (1963) also suffered from a disturbance in the visual orientation of his own body. In one patient a large pituitary tumour, which led to blindness and probably affected the hypothalamic-limbic connections, evoked a chronic heautoscopy (Conrad, 1953).

10. Migraine is reported to be associated with heautoscopy (Schilder, 1914; Lippman, 1951, 1953).

11. The same is true for bipolar depression (Schumann, 1943).

12. Emotionally stressful situations in normals can also lead to heautoscopy (Grotstein, 1983). The most famous description of a heautoscopic experience of this type was published by Johann Wolfgang von Goethe: It occurred while he was a student at Strasbourg. After saying farewell to his dear friend Friederike Brion of Sesenheim, he saw himself dressed in grey returning on horseback to Sesenheim, while he was in actual fact riding from Sesenheim to Strasbourg ('*Dichtung und Wahrheit*'; Menninger-Lerchenthal, 1932). The physiologist Johannes Müller (1826a, b) attributed self-vision in normals to the class of abnormal ecstatic states, related to the 'popular vision of ghosts'. He explained these phenomena by spontaneous internal activation of brain mechanisms responsible for

visual signal processing, whereby, as in all subjective visual phenomena, the percept is 'projected' into the extra-personal space. Near-death experiences are sometimes also associated with heautoscopy (Müller-Erzbach, 1951; Gabbard *et al.*, 1981).

13. *Doppelgänger* perception can be purposely induced by hypnosis (Schubert, 1814, 1818; Féré, 1891).

14. Sometimes hypnopomp or hypnagogic hallucinations contain a *doppelgänger* (Menninger-Lerchenthal, 1935, 1954, 1961). Partial persistence of dreams can lead to partial heautoscopy (d-type heautoscopy) correlated with limb cataplexy, as mentioned above.

15. Hysteria, which in the medicine of past generations could, of course, not be separated from dreamy states or other abnormal changes in consciousness caused by temporal lobe epilepsia, also led to heautoscopic phenomena in some patients (e.g. Kerner, 1824, 1829; Comar, 1901; Burat, 1902; Sollier, 1902; Bain, 1903; Bahia, 1911; Schilder, 1914).

Reviewing all published cases, one can say as a tentative conclusion that most heautoscopic phenomena are presumably associated with temporal lobe abnormal activity, which must not necessarily reach the disease stage. It seems probable that the right temporal lobe is more important for this phenomenon than the left, but considering the connections between both structures, abnormal activation of both sites could be present.

Negative Heautoscopy

Negative heautoscopy is an illusion in which the subject no longer recognizes himself in the mirror (Sollier, 1903; Anderson and Semerari, 1954). Such phenomena can occur in normals, as in the absent-minded scientist, as well as in different brain diseases. Ernst Mach reported in his *Die Analyse der Empfindungen* (1906) on two negative heautoscopic episodes experienced by himself:

> *As a young man I suddenly saw on the street a rather unpleasant annoying face in profile view. I was startled considerably before I realized that it was my own face which I saw through two reflecting mirrors while passing by a mirror shop. Another time, very tired after a rather stressful night-long railway trip, I got into a bus just as a man entered from the other side. I thought: what a lousy schoolmaster that is boarding the bus. It was, however, myself since opposite me was a large mirror. The habitus of my social class was closer to my percept than my particular appearance* (p. 3).

Negative heautoscopy has been observed in schizophrenia (Sollier, 1902, 1903), in endogenous depression (Anderson and Semerari, 1954), in general brain diseases (Hecaen and Ajuriaguerra, 1952) and in epileptic patients (Magri

and Mocchetti, 1967). Patients suffering from visual hemineglect, not to be confused with negative heautoscopy, cannot recognize the left half of their face in the mirror, a phenomenon representing a general neglect of the left half of the extra-personal space and objects (cf. Chapter 22). Negative heautoscopy also occurs regularly in prosopagnosia (cf. Chapter 14; Charcot, 1883).

Alienation with Faces

In addition to heautoscopy a large variety of illusionary or hallucinatory transformations of face or person perception has been reported in the psychiatric literature (e.g. Christodoulou, 1986; Koehler and Ebel, 1990). We will mention some of these pathological deformations in face and person signal processing, which frequently lead to secondary behavioural disturbances especially when patients interact socially.

Kahlbaum–Capgras Syndrome

Related to heautoscopy is an illusory change in the perception of faces and persons, which was described by Kahlbaum (1866) and later by Capgras and Reboul-Lachaux (1923): the patient observes changes in the faces of relatives or other people well-known to him. The faces are more or less dominated by alienating features, strange in appearance, and no longer look as they did days or weeks ago. A delusionary interpretation is the consequence: the family members or friends have been replaced by impersonators. This syndrome is observed mainly in schizophrenia and temporal lobe epilepsia, but can be seen as well in patients suffering from severe head injury (Stern and McNaughton, 1945; Dietrich, 1962; Weston and Whitlock, 1971; Klempel, 1973; Vogel, 1974; Merrin and Silberfarb, 1976; Christodoulou, 1977; Alexander, Stuss and Benson, 1979; Lehmann, 1980; Gensicke, 1982; Berson, 1983; Morrison and Tarter, 1984; Koehler and Ebel, 1990).

Fregoli Syndrome

Patients suffering from schizophrenia or organic psychoses may report that they perceive family members as strangers without the slightest physical resemblance to their former selves; nevertheless these persons are still categorized by the patient as 'known relatives'. A Fregoli syndrome has also been observed in the course of an epileptic psychosis (Courbon and Fail, 1927; Christodoulou, 1976, 1978). Koehler and Ebel (1990) associated a similar illusion to the Fregoli syndrome: unknown faces are perceived as neighbours or family members: A patient identified the Queen of England seen on television as her neighbour Mrs Schultz.

The Syndrome of Intermetamorphosis

This syndrome is related to the Kahlbaum–Capgras phenomenon. The patient reports that persons unknown to him are transformed psychologically and physically into other unknown persons (Snell, 1860; Schreber, 1903 (self-report); Courbon and Tusques, 1932; Bick, 1984). Intermetamorphosis is the delusionary impression that unknown social partners have changed their faces. It is predominantly reported by schizophrenic patients.

Paraprosopia

This is a transient illusion described in schizophrenic patients which occurs more frequently in children and adolescents than in older schizophrenics. The patient perceives characteristic changes in faces, predominantly in strangers. Paraprosopia is described in more detail in Chapter 15.

Face- and Person-generating Visual Illusions

These are pareidolias in which the structure of an object seen is transformed into a face or person. Such an imaginary transformation is required in a well-known psychological test: the ink-spots of the Rorschach-test tables (or the Z-test) are perceived in part as faces or persons. Leonardo da Vinci once recommended to his less imaginative pupils to sit in front of a randomly structured rock wall and just to stare at the rocks. He guaranteed that they would soon see faces, persons, landscapes, and entire scenes, all products of the imagination (Chapter 2). The perception of persons or animals in dense fog belongs to the same class of illusory visual percepts.

Face- and person-generating illusions can also appear as symptoms of brain disease. One of the authors (O.-J. G.) observed an intelligent 60-year-old woman suffering from multiple mamillary carcinoma metastases located bilaterally in the occipito-temporal region of the brain. She reported that the flowers in a large pretty bunch of chrysanthemums were transformed into moving and smiling heads of small children. She recognized this as an illusory percept, but was still annoyed by it and asked that the chrysanthemums be removed from her view. She also suffered from visual pseudo-hallucinations, which are described in Chapter 23. Face pareidolias also appear together with other hallucinatory or illusionary percepts in alcoholic Korsakoff psychoses. Face and person hallucinations, predominantly those with terrifying expressions or menacing gestures, are frequent symptoms of all those psychiatric states correlated with general changes in consciousness (cf. Parish, 1894) and appear in organic brain diseases, drug intoxication and cerebral dysfunctions including states of cortical blindness (Chapter 9).

Acknowledgement

We thank Dr P. Brugger, Zurich, for providing his reprint collection on heautoscopy and for his comments on the manuscript of this chapter.

17 Reading and Script: Historical, Statistical and Neuropsychological Observations

Spoken words are symbols of intellectual experience and written words are symbols of spoken words
(Aristotle, *De interpretatione*)

Introduction

Before describing reading impairments caused by lesions in visual association areas of the brain ('pure alexia'), we first present some facts and ideas about reading and script necessary for a deeper understanding of the clinical symptoms affecting the ability to read and write. Neither the ontogenetic developmental aspects of reading nor developmental dyslexia (legasthenia) are discussed, since they are dealt with in Volume 13 of this series.

The History of Script

Reading and writing are man-specific visuo–motor and visual cognitive abilities associated with man's linguistic competence, which is based on a phoneme–grapheme transcoding system that has developed during the last 5200 years. In English as in many other languages, the word 'write' is etymologically deduced from a much older root meaning scratch, the Old Norse word '*ríta*', which suggests the origins of script several thousand years ago (Gelb, 1952). Much older than script, however, is human verbal communication using phonation and the complex auditory apperceptive system ('cortical speech areas') necessary for understanding speech. Human speech evolved during early hominid phylogenesis and was presumably used by *Homo habilis* hunting groups about 2 million years ago, despite the fact that tongue motility, the labial muscles and the oral-pharyngeal resonance space

were far less well developed than in *Homo sapiens sapiens*. Anatomical reconstructions from palaeoanthropological records indicate, however, that *Homo habilis*'s articulatory abilities were sufficient to enable him to create a set of elementary phonetic signs; these were used to organize group activity and allowed for interaction between individuals.

Half a million years ago, the articulatory abilities of *Homo erectus*, who had a considerably larger and better developed brain than *Homo habilis*, were none the less far below those of present-day man; the same was also true for *Homo praesapiens*, who lived up to 100000 years ago (cf. Laitman, *et al.*, 1977; Laitman and Heimbuch, 1982; Lieberman, 1984, 1985; Laitman, 1985). Verbal communication by means of speech developed slowly enough during human phylogenesis to allow for the phylogenetic growth of the specific neocortical areas controlling the related sensory and motor functions. In right-handers and about half of all left-handers, the sensory and motor speech areas are located in the temporal, temporo–parietal and orbito–frontal cortices of the dominant left hemisphere (Fig. 15.1).

The short history of script poses considerable problems for neuroscientists, who have discovered from clinical observation of alexia and agraphia occurring together or separately that specialized cortical areas exist which are predominantly used for reading and writing. How could such areas have developed for functions not more than 6000 years old, and what purpose do these areas serve for the inhabitants of illiterate societies? Before discussing these questions, we shall first comment on the cultural development of script, which is of course still in progress

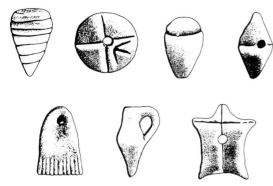

Fig. 17.1 *Simple small clay tokens which were used to register delivered or stored goods in the warehouses of Mesopotamia more than 5000 years ago. These small tokens were also used as elementary pictorial logograms to control the correct delivery of merchandise. For this purpose they were put into clay balls which, after being fired, accompanied the transport of goods. Redrawn from a large collection published by Schmandt-Besserat (1988). Early Sumerian cuneiform script used these symbols.*

since complete global literacy has not yet been achieved. According to a UNESCO report published in 1974, 7 per cent of the adult world population is illiterate. This estimate is certainly much too low: a more realistic figure lies somewhere between 20 and 35 per cent. Weigl (1981) has even suggested that the global illiteracy rate is more than 50 per cent. In Germany, the percentage of adult illiterates was estimated in 1988 to be about 5 per cent.

The history of script was a topic widely addressed during the period of the European Enlightenment, especially during discussions focusing on the historical development of different languages (e.g. Tetens, 1796; Herder, 1772). According to modern research, the oldest set of characters used for script in the modern sense of the word was the proto-cuneiform script of the Sumerians, which was first used about 3200 BC in Mesopotamia. Early Egyptian script developed about 250 years later. Cuneiform script developed within a fairly short period of time covering several generations; it was based on a somewhat older pictorial script that had been used by Sumerian merchants living mainly in the region around the city of Uruk in southern Babylonia. Because of favourable changes in climate and a sophisticated irrigation system, the lower part of Mesopotamia had become very fertile, which resulted in crop overproduction. Excess crops were stored in large warehouses for later transport to other cities located in less fertile regions. Since around 8000 BC, records of stored goods were kept in Mesopotamia by means of fired clay tokens (Schmandt-Besserat, 1977, 1988). Around 3500 BC, storehouse supervisors developed another system consisting of small clay tokens hung on strings or rods which were used to indicate quality and quantity (Fig. 17.1). This

method allowed for rapid inventory checks of all available goods. For long-distance trade, the merchants invented a 'safe-trade' control mechanism: about 3200 BC, sets of small clay tokens were used to control the correct delivery of merchandise. One set was kept by a merchant at the warehouse; the other set, representing the actual contents of the delivery, was put into a clay ball ('bulla'), which, after being fired, was sent with the transport. It served as a sort of fraud-proof receipt. The person receiving the agricultural products broke open the 'bulla' and compared the delivered goods with the description provided inside by the clay tokens. Within a generation or two, the contents of the bulla were also represented by engravings on the outer surface of the clay ball which depicted the figurines inside. These engravings were produced in part by roll-seals. In this way a back-up system was created. Within another two to three generations, this 'way bill' system evolved further: instead of using clay balls and tokens, symbols indicating the amount of delivered goods were inscribed on clay tablets. This invention made the bulla system superfluous and marked the beginning of protocuneiform script, which was predominantly composed of pictorial logograms. Soon, storehouse records written on clay tablets were also used to describe property, the distribution of agricultural products, administrative organization, etc. Within a few more generations, a fairly sophisticated system of elementary script had evolved; it was composed of about 1200 pictograms, which included 60 signs representing numbers which were arranged in a sexagesimal system. The rather abstract elementary pictograms used for cuneiform script were soon partly transformed into phonograms and signs having syntactic meaning ('determinatives', Gaur, 1984). Cuneiform script was eventually taught in special schools.

The invention of early cuneiform script (which has in the meantime been deciphered) seems to have considerably facilitated trade, market conditions and political organization in Mesopotamia. All systems of script used by mankind today can be traced back to cuneiform script, which means that an amazingly large variety of systems serving verbal–visual communication has been created within the last 5000 years (e.g. Falkenstein, 1936; Gelb, 1952; Schmandt-Besserat, 1977, 1985, 1986a, b; 1988; Klengel, 1983; Gaur, 1984; Damerow et al., 1988; Nissen, 1988; Kruckenburg, 1989; Nissen et al., 1990).

A few generations after Sumerian cuneiform script had been invented, Egyptian script developed a rather sophisticated logographic–syllabic system. Egyptian script, used by the administrative echelons of the different dynasties that ruled Egypt during the third millenium BC, certainly contributed to the highly self-reflective and self-assured theo-political system of the Pharaonic empire (Kees, 1973). 'Scribe' was one of the highest ranks in the administration. With the invention of script, schools were created in Egypt (as in Mesopotamia) in which children and adolescents – but not adults – were taught to read and write. Since Egyptian script was more pictorial than cuneiform, graphomotor abilities and artistic skill were required in order to become an expert scribe in the empire of the Pharaohs.

Before the invention of gramophones and tape recorders, speaking and listening were ephemeral events in verbal communication requiring a dialogue between speaker and listener. Communication by script made information transfer independent of time and space. In contrast to speaking, writing is a sort of monologue preserved on 'paper' which can be read later by someone else or by the writer himself. It is for this reason also a powerful mnemonic device. Cuneiform script was presumably the first human invention allowing for a systematic and quantitative recording of material facts and thoughts (e.g. the contents of a warehouse, personal property such as land and livestock, the sequence of historical events, astronomical observations, records of climate, descriptions of family matters, socially important information and religious ideas). This innovation was invented by merchants living in a prosperous society that had developed a remarkably complex social structure as well as high cultural standards. Written material, even a clay tablet used as 'paper', could be reproduced, thus becoming available to different people at different times and places. Sending off clay tablets inscribed with cuneiform script did indeed extend the breadth of verbal communication. In addition, written information recorded on a tablet was less subject to modification than was information sent by word of mouth; in other words, script increased the reliability of verbal communication. However, the invention of communication by reading and writing reduced some of the emotional aspects associated with spoken dialogue. Script lacks not only the prosody of language but also the non-verbal signs such as facial expressions and gestures which usually accompany verbal communication. Through rhyme, rhythm and the metaphoric use of words, written poetry tries in part to recreate the emotional components of communication lost in script.

For many generations, learning script and having access to information transfer through script was a social privilege reserved only for certain groups. In Western society, competence in reading and writing was for hundreds of years reserved for specially trained persons who, surprisingly, were frequently not members of the upper, ruling class. This was not only true in Egyptian, Greek and Roman societies, but also in large parts of Europe up until the seventeenth century. Not only were the lower classes in a feudalistic society illiterate, but also most of the ruling sovereigns as well. The latter group had to rely on the penmanship of secretaries who, until the Renaissance, were predominantly clerics. Modern literacy in Western society developed hand in hand with the spread of Enlightenment ideas during the second half of the eighteenth century and with the process of political democratization during the nineteenth century.

Reading and writing by means of modern script are just one way of communicating by means of visual signals. Several other communication techniques also use the visual channel for verbal or behavioural information transfer. Man's visual communicative abilities can be divided into two categories: static signals, to which script belongs, and dynamic signals. The formal type of information content contained in such signals can in turn also be classified: pictorial-prelinguistic and verbal. In illiterate societies, elementary mnemonic devices serving as precursors of script improved the reliability of messages sent by persons from one place to another: message sticks, marked beans, certain sequences of shells fixed on a string, nodes of different types ordered in certain sequences on a string, etc. are examples of different devices that were used to improve memory; each individual symbol stood for a certain fact, event or action. Rosary beads used by the members of the Roman Catholic Church, for example, are a preliterate mnemonic device indicating prayer sequence. Table 17.1 summarizes the major techniques used by man for visual communication.

The most important of several requirements necessary for effective script is a close and reversible correlation between the characters and the verbal signals or content that they represent (grapheme–phoneme correlation). Scripts that fulfil this requirement use rather different methods: pictorial, syllabic or alphabetic.

Pictorial Script

This represents objects, facts and circumstances either with symbols directly derived from nature or with more or less abstract drawings. There are several levels of abstraction in this process: pictograms, logograms and ideograms. Pictograms are simplified drawings; logograms represent spoken words. Ideograms, on the other hand, can be highly complex symbols, expressing with a single sign a linguistic piece of information that can be translated into Western script only with a long sentence. Gelb (1952) has separated logograms into different classes:

1. Primary logograms, such as a circle representing the sun.

2. Associative logograms: e.g. the sign for sun means 'bright day'.

3. Diagrammatic logograms with artificial grapheme–word correlation: e.g. a circle represents the number ten.

4. Combined logograms with a 'semantic' indicator: e.g. combining the signs for 'plough' and 'man' produces 'ploughman'.

Table 17.1 *Communication by means of visual signals.*

	Non-verbal	Verbal
Static signs	(a) objects with symbolic character known by sender and receiver, e.g. 'flower language', 'object writing'	(a) written word or other signs of written language
	(b) picture letters	(b) mathematical signs and those of some 'higher' programming languages
	(c) colour code	(c) musical notes $\flat$, $\natural$
	(d) traffic signs	(d) binary code of elementary computer language
	(e) musical notes ♩, ♫, ♩	
	(f) pictograms	
	(g) maps	
	(h) construction plans, wiring diagrams	
	(i) comics	
	(k) technical railway timetables (graphic displays)	
Dynamic signs	(a) facial expression	(a) sign language of deaf-mutes
	(b) gestures	(b) lip reading
	(c) pantomime	(c) flag salute
	(d) smoke and fire signals	(d) semaphore
	(e) ritualized gestures of a policeman, referee or a priest	(e) moving letters and words in advertisement
	(f) ritualized body movements e.g. when greeting people	(f) silent movies used for instruction
	(g) expressive dancing, especially ritual dances	
	(h) cartoons	
	(i) event transmitted by movies or television	

5. Phonetic transformation of logograms: i.e. the logogram is associated with another homophone.

6. Phonetic indicators added to a logogram to indicate correct pronounciation.

These classes were derived from an analysis of Chinese script and its development. The first three classes were regular precursors of the syllabic or alphabetic script which has developed during the last 3000 years.

Linguistic competence is necessary for reading ideographic script aloud in order to correlate the script with the phonation. Examples of this are the ancient Egyptian pictorial script as well as parts of Chinese and Japanese Kanji script (the historical development of Kanji can be traced to Chinese ideograms). Because of the many homophones in the Chinese language, some of the originally ideographic characters also acquired phonetic meaning (cf. Gelb, 1952, 1958; Karlgren, 1962, 1975). In order to lessen ambiguity, some of these characters also acquired additional signs indicating correct pronounciation. A competent reader transfers visual signals into phonetic speech based on his knowledge of the language. The advantage of ideographic script is that the same set of characters (logograms) can be used to represent the same objects, ideas, actions and complex facts in completely different languages, as in the case of Japanese Kanji and Chinese characters. A literate Japanese who does not understand Chinese can, however, communicate with a literate Chinese reader by writing in Kanji symbols. Traditionally, Chinese script and old Kanji were written in vertical columns. In modern Japanese, Kanji is combined with Kana signs and written horizontally from left to right.

Numbers and mathematical symbols form a universally understood logographic sign system. Each symbol represents a well-defined mathematical operation or has a well-defined mathematical meaning (e.g. 3149, $+$, Σ, $\int$, etc.) which usually has a different name in different languages. Mathematicians can communicate using this ideographic system without understanding their respective mother tongues.

Syllabic Script

The second and third classes of script deviate considerably from the principles of ideographic script in that a close correlation is developed between the sounds of the spoken language (phonemes) and the character sequences of the script (graphemes). Although this correlation is fixed by the correspondence rules of a given language, ambiguities have nevertheless developed in many languages.

The syllabic script system selects individual characters representing distinct syllables in a spoken language. In Japanese Hirakana and Katakana script, for example, 63 of the 68 characters represent a distinct syllable and 5 represent vowels. In addition, some of the Chinese and Japanese Kanji characters have acquired phonetic meaning, especially when used for phonetic transcription of words from foreign languages. A transitional stage between syllabic and alphabetic script is found in ancient Hebrew, which is composed of consonants and only 3 vowel signs. The correct vowels or diphthongs are interposed by the competent reader when reading aloud. One can easily demonstrate that it is

n.t n.c.ss.ry t. wr.t. all v.w.l.s wh.n a m..n.ngf.l m.ss.g. .s r..d b. a c.mp.t.nt r..d.r.

Alphabetic Script

This script, i.e. the typical Western script system, is composed of consonants and signs for vowels, including vowel mutations (e.g. *umlauts*) and diphthongs. Western alphabetic script developed from Greek script, which in turn can be traced back to Phoenician syllabic script. The direction of early Greek script, which was rectilinear, was presumably right to left because it was easier for right-handed individuals hammering letters into stone to proceed from right to left (Paschinger, 1990). The right–left direction is still used today in Hebrew and Arabic script. Before left–right linearity evolved, a short boustrophedon period appeared in Greek script, i.e. regularly alternating left–right and right–left lines were used, whereby the right–left lines were frequently written with upside-down letters. 'Boustrophedon' means 'the way an ox-drawn plough is turned'. In other ancient script systems, linear vertical (up–down or down–up), circular or spiral letter and word-sequence orders were used (Gaur, 1984).

As every reader knows, a considerable ambiguity has emerged in most Western languages which use traditional Latin, Greek or cyrillic alphabets. In English, for example, many homophones are written differently (e.g. you, crew) and many homographs are pronounced differently (e.g. rough, dough). For this reason, correct reading and writing requires a level of language competence beyond the knowledge of the grapheme–phoneme correlation. In some Western scripts, capitalization of first letters follows a complex system of rules (e.g. as is the case in German), which, once learned, greatly facilitate reading speed and comprehension.

To understand the neurobiological mechanisms of reading and writing, it is important to understand first the differences between logographic (or ideographic) and syllabic-alphabetic script systems. The various correlations between phonemes and graphemes in these two systems led researchers to expect effects of brain lesions affecting the linguistic ability to read and write to vary accordingly (Chapter 18). Investigations of Japanese patients suffering from alexia or dyslexia caused by brain

lesions have helped to better understand the different mechanisms related to a dominant phonetic or a dominant logographic script. All educated Japanese are competent in both script systems, the logographically dominated Kanji and the phonematic–syllabic Kana. Although symbols from both systems are normally mixed in newspaper texts etc., traditional poetic Japanese is written solely in Kanji. While the Kanji logograms, as a rule, denote lexical units as substantives, Kana characters are more frequently used for words representing grammatical structures. Although it is possible, on the other hand, to express all Japanese words in Kana, this is by convention not done in daily script and print. In the contemporary Japanese school system, instruction in reading and writing begins with the Kana system and then proceeds to Kanji.

Precursors of Script and Some Phylogenetic Considerations

Five thousand years of modern script is certainly much too short a period of time for the development of any specialized brain structures responsible for this remarkable ability in modern man. Therefore one has to look for other reasons to explain why circumscribed lesions in the neocortical grey matter produce the symptom of pure alexia, as if a specialized part of the brain existed for reading or, more generally, for visuo-verbal communication. Before we present our explanation of this apparently paradoxical situation, we shall first comment on the historical precursors of modern script. No palaeoanthropological records of script-like graphic signs are reported for *Homo erectus* or for *Homo presapiens*, who lived up to about 100000 years ago, nor for *Homo sapiens neanderthalensis*, who preceded *Homo sapiens sapiens*. It seems probable that indeed none existed before the appearance of *Homo sapiens sapiens* 60000 years ago. Antecedents of script such as geometrical symbols, repetitive dots, or abstract figures are found, however, in between the beautiful pictorial drawings and paintings produced by early *Homo sapiens sapiens* in many caves in western Europe. Abstract, script-type signs can also be seen on petroglyphs, natural or carved pieces of bone, ivory or stones dating from the Upper Palaeolithic periods known as the Aurignacian (35000–28000 BC, Figs. 17.2, 17.3) and Gravettian (27000–20000 BC). Liberally estimated, however, all of these precursors of script are not more than 30000 years old; most of them are considerably younger (Sethe, 1939; Gelb, 1952; Földes-Papp, 1966; Müller-Beck and Albrecht, 1987 fig. 17.3). These observations imply that the phylogenetic time was too short to allow for the development of new brain regions associated with modern systems of 'real' script or with any

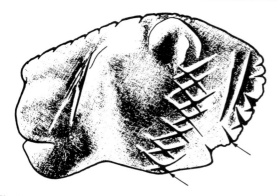

Fig. 17.2 *Head of a lion (2.5 × 1.8 × 0.6 cm) in ivory with linear and cross-shaped engravings, which possibly had a symbolic meaning. Dating: about 30,000 BC from the Vogelherd cave, south Germany. Redrawn from a photograph of Müller-Beck and Albrecht (1987) (Württembergisches Landesmuseum Stuttgart Nr. V 72,38).*

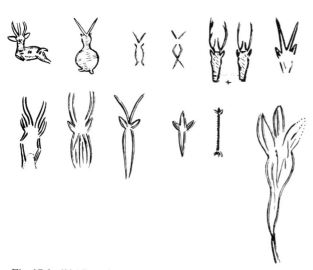

Fig. 17.3 *Abbé Breuil's explanation of an abstraction progression in depicting animals. He composed this figure from findings (mainly bone engravings) which originated over several thousands of years from the period of Aurignacian (about 30 000 BC) to the late Magdalénien (about 12 000 BC) (from Obermaier, 1912, and Földes-Papp, 1966).*

possible precursors of script lacking grapheme-phoneme correlation.

In light of this fact, the cultural ability to read and write evidently relies on brain regions which must have developed during hominid phylogenesis for other visual cognitive purposes. When looking for such phylogenetically old visual cognitive abilities in man, tracking, an ability required by all groups of *Homo* that lived from hunting, comes to mind. We think that reading and writing is a special cultural adaptation of the hunting *Homo's* ability (which existed perhaps even as early as *Homo habilis*) to read game tracks, and to determine from these visual signposts the number of animals, the species, the speed and the direction of movement, as well as the time elapsed since the tracks were made (Grüsser, 1988). This track reading ability, as also the ability to read script, constitutes an example of a more general visual cognitive ability which might be called 'visual *pars-pro-toto* perception', a process in which one identifies a whole object from one of its smaller parts, e.g. seeing a hand and recognizing a person, seeing the tail of a cow and concluding that the entire cow is present, seeing smoke and assuming fire, etc. It is interesting that in today's Neolithic societies, which have been studied by anthropologists over the last hundred years, track reading is taught by a combination of tactile and verbal instructions at exactly the same age as the first reading instruction takes place in literate societies. Moreover, it seems to be very difficult for someone 'illiterate' in track reading to learn this ability as an adult. Similarly, learning to read and write script becomes very difficult beyond adolescence. Presumably, the ability for visual *pars-pro-toto* recognition is based on bilateral brain functions. Reading and writing are lateralized, since the grapheme–phoneme correlation process formed during the reading and writing learning process associates a visual function with an auditory–verbal function. Therefore, the left side of the cortical hemisphere is selected during the learning period for reading and writing script, as is the case for most other human verbal functions (Chapter 18) .

A Flow Diagram of Reading

Reading and writing are indeed possible without visual signals. A blind child learns to read Braille script and is later able to generate text using a Braille typewriter which he, other blind people or people with normal vision who have learned Braille script can read. A normal child who has learned to read and write is able, without further training, to read letters or numbers drawn on his skin in the dark. Competence in reading is thus a linguistic ability extending beyond the visual domain. In the flow diagram of Fig. 17.4, we have included only the visual and cognitive functions related to reading. The neuronal mechanisms of visual cognition and prelinguistic visual character perception are distributed rather symmetrically throughout both hemispheres. For this reason, the diagram is symmetrically organized up to this level. Because of the linear and horizontal organization of Western script, a functional asymmetry is induced. The part of the text just read is in the left visual hemifield, while the part still to be read is in the right visual hemifield. Since the text is

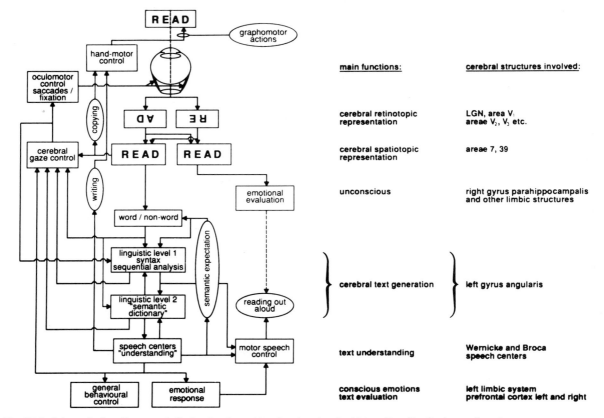

Fig. 17.4 *Schematic flow diagram of all visual and cognitive functions involved in reading. For further explanation, see text.*

sampled during short fixation periods in between saccadic eye movements, however, the actual uptake of information within the 'new' segments seen by the fovea is about equally distributed in the left and right hemifoveae during the process of reading. The elementary linguistic functions are lateralized in the speech-dominant left hemisphere in most right-handers and in about 50 per cent of left-handers. Therefore visual text processing, which is beyond elementary visual perception and is associated with an understanding of the meaning of the text, is also lateralized. Interestingly, lateralization of written verbal material prefers the left hemisphere only when a given script's dominant property is a grapheme–phoneme structure, as in the case of alphabetic and syllabic script. Clinical evidence has shown that in shorthand reading, an opposite lateralization occurs with right hemisphere dominance (Chapter 18).

Correct reading not only requires linguistic competence and an intact afferent visual signal flow but also a complex interaction of these signals with the motor control mechanisms required for reading and for speaking while reading aloud, i.e. a coordinated sequence of saccadic eye movements and fixation periods (Fig. 17.5). Reading is a mechanism controlled by meshed sensorimotor loops; even in silent reading, subliminal motor speech action can be present. Although this fact is most likely a specialized manifestation of the close correlation between thinking and speaking (Wygotski, 1934/1974), it should not be overemphasized, since one can read silently as much as two to three times more quickly than one can read aloud. Because of the thematic restriction of this volume to visual cognitive functions, we shall not elaborate upon the transformation of read script (grapheme sequences) into internal speech signals (sememes), or into the corresponding subliminal phoneme sequences which are produced when reading silently, or into audible phoneme sequences when reading aloud. A similar transformation occurs in writing when the writer reads his own script. For the sake of simplicity, these motor mechanisms have been greatly reduced in Fig. 17.4.

Statistics of Script

In the following section, we shall deal only with Western script. Together with the umlauts (ä, ö, ü) and even when

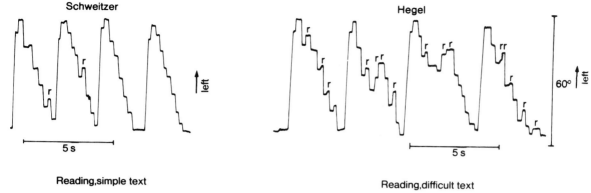

Fig. 17.5 *Horizontal eye movements recorded by means of an electro-oculogram during reading. The horizontal lines of the text are sampled by a sequence of short saccades and fixation periods. Shifting to the next line is achieved by one large right–left backward saccade. For recording purposes, the text was enlarged considerably over normal size. The subject read two different types of German texts: (a) a paragraph of Albert Schweitzer's autobiography* Aus meiner Kindheit und Jugendzeit, *which is written in a clear and easily understandable German style, and (b) a simply written text with difficult content (G. F. Hegel:* Einführung in die Philosophie*). The subject was asked to try to understand the texts during silent reading. When reading the conceptually more difficult text of Hegel, regression saccades (r) from right to left occurred much more frequently than for the Schweitzer text, the total number of saccades per line increased and the speed of reading declined (modified from H. Ghazarian and O.-J. Grüsser, unpublished 1977, from Grüsser, 1982).*

separating i and j, the maximum number of letters used in most Western languages is not greater than 30. The maximum number of words, W_{max}, composed of one to n letters with a maximum string of m letters, is (homographs excluded) given by:

$$W_{max} = n^m \qquad (17.1)$$

Of course, the actual lexicon of a language is far below W_{max}, where for everyday purposes in Western languages $m < 26$; that is,

$$W_{max} \ll 30^m \qquad (17.2)$$

Because of the statistical structure of phoneme sequences in spoken language, a similar but not identical structure of sequential dependencies appears in written language. To prevent too many errors resulting from graphical similarity, the number of different letter strings existing in a real written language is considerably smaller than W_{max}. The letter sequence within the words is determined by Markov chain properties of higher orders; the sixth order is approximately computable (Fig. 17.6). The Markov chain properties vary from language to language; with artificial words corresponding to third- or fourth-order Markov chains, one recognizes in most cases to which language the artificial word belongs. In a Markov chain, the probability that a certain letter will be followed by another one, or that a certain letter string will be followed by another selected letter, is expressed as conditioned probability. For example, the probability in English that the letter 'r' as the first letter in a word will be followed by

'e' is much higher than the probability that it will be followed by a 't' (no such word appears in the *Oxford English Dictionary*). The probability that 're' is followed by 'd' ('red') is higher than the probability that it will be followed by 'h' ('reh', as in 'rehearsal'), etc. In every real language, the probability, $p(1, 2, 3, \ldots, j)$ that a certain sequence of letters will occur in a word consisting of j letters is considerably larger than the product of the probabilities of occurrence p_j of these letters in that language. In addition to Markov chain properties of letter strings in real words, the probability of letter occurrence is unequally distributed.

Different languages have different Markov chain properties, as illustrated in Fig. 17.6 for words generated from first- to fourth-order Markov chains in English or German (Shannon, 1951; Küpfmüller, 1954). Similarly one can compute the Markov chain properties of word sequences in a language, and can generate from the data an artificial text which resembles real language but remains nevertheless nonsensical (Fig. 17.6).

The statistical structure of letter sequences in words (or of word sequences in sentences) for different languages is determined by other general laws applicable in a similar manner, at least for Western languages of Greek, Latin, Germanic or Slavonic origin. One of the rules is expressed by the so-called harmonic law of Zipf (1935, 1949), which relates the rank order, r, of a word, i.e. its position in the frequency dictionary of a given language, with the frequency or probability, p_r, that that word will occur:

$$p_r = k/r \qquad (17.3)$$

Markov chain order	German letters
0th order	ITVWDGAKNAJTSQOSRMOIAQVFWTKHXD
1st order	EME GKNEET ERS TITBL BTZENFNDBGD EAI E LASZ BETEATR IASMIRCH EGEOM
2nd order	AUSZ KEINU WONDINGLIN DUFRN ISAR STEISBERER ITEHM ANORER
3rd order	PLANZEUNDGES PHIN INE UNDEN ÜBBEICHT GES AUF ES SO UNG GAN DICH WANDERSO
4th order	ICH FOLGEMÄSZIG BIS STEHEN DISPONIN SEELE NAMEN

	English letters
0th order	AMNDALOEQCESHFIVTRTSUE
1st order	OCRO HLI RGWR NMIELWIS EU LL NBNESEBYA TH EEI ALHENHTTPA OOBTTVA NAH
2nd order	ON IE ANTSOUTINYS ARE T INCTORE ST BE S DEAMY ACHIN D ILONASIVE TUCOOWE
3rd order	IN NO IST LAT WHEY CRATICT FROURE BIRS GROCID PONDENOME OF DEMONSTRURES
4th order	IT HIFT TO AND ON TSING HERSE HALL VERTH TORY LY IN GOT BECHE WORLD SKED MUSTUBLE PHIL WILL ROFEAME SHE

	German words
Markov chain order	
1st order	DENKEN ES ENTSAGEN ICH ZU WENN AUS DIESE VERANSTALTET ZEIT
2nd order	WEIL JEDER ANLAGE HAT NACH DEM PFERDE NICHT ALLEIN DER HERR WILL ALS OB ICH FAST JEDES HAUS ZU SITZEN

	English words
1st order	REPRESENTING AND SPEEDILY IS AN GOOD APT OR COME CAN DIFFERENT
2nd order	THE HEAD AND IN FRONTAL ATTACK ON AN ENGLISH WRITER THAT THE CHARACTER OF THIS

Fig. 17.6 *Artificial German and English texts generated from the statistics of printed language. Markov chain properties of different orders of letter or word sequences were used for text generation as indicated (from Küpfmüller, 1954).*

This relationship is not trivial since it predicts a 'smooth' and homogeneous decline of p_r. A straight line with an inclination of -45 degrees is expected from equation 17.3, when p_r and r are plotted on a logarithmic scale (Fig. 17.7; for further discussion of Zipf's law, see Rapoport, 1982; Orlov, 1982a, b; Guiter and Arapov, 1982; Andersen, 1985):

$$\log p_r = \log k - \log r \qquad (17.4)$$

Above rank order 8, this law is fulfilled in German and English up to a rank order of approximately 8.500. Since the sum of all p_r should be 1, equations 17.3 and 17.4 have a validity limit which is reached at $r = 8727$ (Shannon, 1951). From Zipf's law, one can estimate the information content, C_w, in bits, of an average word in a given language as follows:

$$C_w = -p_r \, \mathrm{ld} \, p_r = 11.82 \qquad (17.5)$$

where ld stands for the duadic logarithm. Since average word length varies between 5 and 6 letters, the average information content, C_l, of a letter in English, in bits per letter, is given as follows:

$$C_l > 11.82/6 = 1.97 \qquad (17.6)$$

Maximum information content of a set of 30 characters is ld $30 \approx 4.9$ bits per character. Because of the unequal distribution of characters, this value in real Western languages is about 4.1 to 4.2 bits per character, from which the average redundancy, R_w, in bits per letter, of coding letters into words follows:

$$R_w = 4.1 - 1.97 = 2.13 \qquad (17.7)$$

As an alternative to the harmonic law of Zipf, Mandelbrot (1954) suggested another relationship between p_r and r. This is called the canonic law, and has been successfully tested in several languages:

$$p_r = c/(r + r_0)^{\beta} \qquad (17.8)$$

where c, r_0 and β are constants. The constant β has an empirical value approaching 1. At low numbers of rank order r equation 17.8 describes the empirical data somewhat better than Zipf's law (equation 17.3). Above rank order 20, both equations provide very similar results.

The relationship expressed by the harmonic law of Zipf or by the canonic law of Mandelbrot is not only a description of the statistical properties of words used in a written language, but also forms part of the statistics of a given language unconsciously used by the average speaker or reader. Since most people rarely utilize more than 2000 different words for written or verbal communication, statistical properties must play an important role not only in their active linguistic ability but also in their ability to correctly recognize written words. These statistical properties have not always been taken into consideration

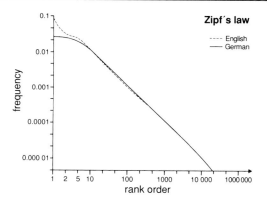

Fig. 17.7 *Graphical representation of the harmonic law of Zipf which relates the rank order (abscissa) of a word with its frequency or probability of occurrence (ordinate). For the English language, the empirical data deviate from this law only for high-frequency short words.*

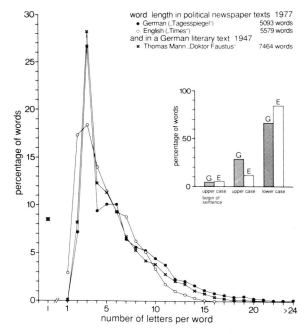

Fig. 17.8 *Quantitative relationship between the frequency of words in German and English newspaper texts (ordinate in percentage of occurrence) and the length of the words expressed by the number of letters per word (abscissa). The inset shows the percentage of words beginning with upper-case letters either at the beginning of a sentence or within a sentence. Significant differences between English and German owing to the grammatical rule that all substantives must be written with upper-case letters in German (from J. Dames and O.-J. Grüsser, unpublished 1977).*

when investigating alexic patients, or in studies in which word recognition was tested by means of tachistoscopic stimulation. In those studies in which word frequency was taken into consideration, it was found that recognition threshold decreased with the logarithm of word frequency (e.g. King-Ellison and Jenkins, 1954).

In addition to the two laws mentioned above, other factors determine word frequency, F_w, and word length, L_w. Figures 17.8 and 17.9 demonstrate that the frequency of words used in a written text and the length of words (as expressed by the number of letters or the number of syllables) follow a non-trivial monotonic rule with the exception of words composed of one or two letters: the larger the number of letters in a word, the less frequently the word will be used on average. When word length is expressed by the number of syllables, a monotonic decaying function is also valid for word frequency with increasing word length. Such statistical dependencies are determined on the one hand by the increasing need for words with increasing sophistication of the language, and on the other hand by daily economizing in everyday speech: the greater the number of words in a language, the greater the need to use long words; the more frequently a word is used, the greater the pressure to shorten the word. The latter tendency is easily recognizable in the common abbreviations used for many long words. The probability that a long word will develop is determined by at least two opposing factors: a 'word growth factor' facilitating word length caused by an increase in linguistic volume of a language, and the need for a reasonable phonetic and graphic dissimilarity between words in order to prevent confusion. Growth in word length is controlled by an 'inhibiting factor' which helps maintain fluency of speech. Both factors are dependent on the functions of neuronal networks in individual brains as well as on the acceptance of new words by the 'collective brain' of society. It seems meaningful, therefore, to use a function for the growth of word length which combines excitation (facilitation) and inhibition as in neuronal networks. We therefore define the probability, p_z, that a word in a real written language consists of z or less characters by

$$p_z = az/(1+bz) \qquad (17.9a)$$

or by

$$P_z = k(1 - e^{-k'(z-1)}) \qquad (17.9b)$$

Similarly the probability that a word consists of n_s or less syllables is defined by

$$P_w = a^* n_s (1 + b^* n_s) \qquad (17.10a)$$

or by

$$P_w = k^*(1 - e^{-k_1 n_s}) \qquad (17.10b)$$

The relationship expressed by equations 17.9 and 17.10

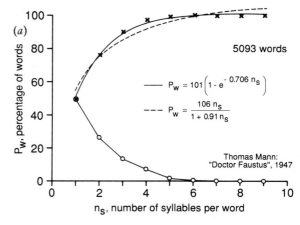

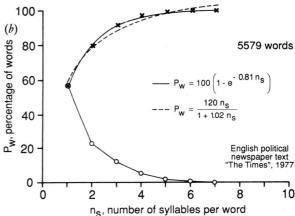

Fig. 17.9 *Relationship between the frequency of words (ordinate) and word length expressed by the number of syllables per word (abscissa, lower curve). In the upper curves the cumulative values and the curve fitting this value according to Equations 17.10a and 17.10b are plotted. (a) German literary text (Doctor Faustus by Thomas Mann, 1947) and (b) English political newspaper text 1977 (J. Dames and O.-J. Grüsser, unpublished, 1977).*

can be tested by computing the cumulative curves of word frequency composed of certain numbers of letters or syllables. The correlation between empirical data and prediction is very good (better for the exponential than for the hyperbolic function; Figs. 17.9, 17.10; equations 17.9a, 17.10a). It is interesting that neologisms (new words) that developed in order to describe new facts are, as a rule, rather long words which are usually abbreviated when used daily (this is especially true for the technical and natural sciences). Neologisms created by schizophrenic patients are frequently characterized not only by the strange combinations and thoughts expressed, but also by their length.

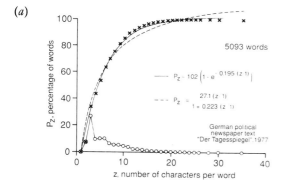

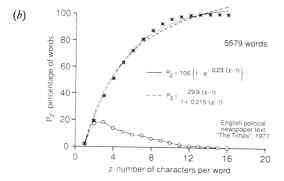

Fig. 17.10 *Simple (circles) and cumulative curves (crosses) of frequency of occurrence for words consisting of different numbers of letters in (a) German and (b) English newspaper texts. The curves represent functions computed according to Equations 17.9a and 17.9b (J. Dames and O.-J. Grüsser, unpublished, 1977).*

To summarize, the statistics gathered on written language indicate that letter sequence, word length, rank order and the probability that a word will appear in a written text depend not only on the semantic content expressed by the writer, but also on the statistical properties of word formation in the particular language. When analysing a text, the competent reader unconsciously relies upon these statistical language properties and on the Markov chain properties of the letter strings forming words and also on certain Markov chain properties in the sequence of words. Because of these structural rules for written language and language redundancy, there is no need to perceive every single letter or word when reading; the text is nevertheless well understood. This conclusion is important in order to understand the strategies of signal sampling used during reading.

The formal structure of a text using paragraphs, punctuation marks and upper-case/lower-case letters facilitates reading. In German, for example, one can guess with good approximation the contents of a text just by glancing at all the words written with upper-case first letters; this is not possible when only words written in lower case are used (J. Dembler and O.-J. Grüsser, unpublished, 1978). In addition, the formal graphical structure of the printed text does not convey an equal amount of information. Since Hoey's study (1908), it has been repeatedly confirmed that the upper half of the letter strings contains more information about the text than does the lower half (Gibson and Levin, 1975).

Handwriting and Printed Words

When reading the handwriting of earlier generations, one realizes that:

1. Handwriting is dependent upon the individuality of the writer and that documents illustrating graphomotor behaviour could perhaps express parts of his personality.
2. Handwriting reflects stylistic properties of the period and the writer's region of origin, as well as the type of handwriting taught at his school.

The first idea led to the not very successful but still practised 'art' of graphology, which claims to be able to tell the personality of a writer based from his handwriting. What is visible in most handwriting, however, is a certain personal flair expressed graphically. It is therefore not surprising that the personal character of handwriting can also be perceived by an alexic patient, who can correctly attribute a given handwriting to a certain person – despite the fact that the patient can no longer read handwriting. On the other hand, prosopagnosic patients can lose the ability to recognize individual handwriting although they have no difficulty reading it (cf. Chapter 18).

The ability to read handwriting requires a somewhat different ability from that required to read printed type; none the less, printed letters also have considerable 'individuality', and the kind of printed characters used certainly changes from one generation to the next. In testing patients for alexia, therefore, one also has to consider the kind of print which was common at the time the patient learned to read in school. In testing the reading abilities of alexic patients, upper-case and lower-case letters should be used as separate stimuli for both print and handwriting.

Furthermore, the size of print plays a considerable role in correct recognition, especially in the elderly and in patients suffering from lesions in the visual system associated with foveal function (Chapter 18).

In testing alexia it also seems useful to ask a patient to place a set of characters into alphabetical sequence, to discriminate between characters and meaningless visual signs of a similar complexity, and to discern pairs of upper-case and lower-case characters as well as pairs of printed and handwritten characters, or pairs of printed characters of different size or print.

Shorthand is a special type of handwriting. The abbreviations used, which may include individual symbols created by a particular writer, place shorthand into both the logogram and the ideogram categories. It is therefore interesting to study the ability to read and write shorthand of patients with brain lesions who are competent in shorthand, and then to compare their performance when confronted with normal script (Chapter 18).

Reading Competence and Eye Movements during Reading

When one asks a reader of average experience how he moves his eyes when reading, the most common answer is: the eyes move continuously from left to right and then jump back to the left in order to start anew on the next line. This report corresponds to the perceived temporal continuity of information uptake during reading. More careful observations and measurements of eye movements during reading indicate, however, that the uptake of visual signals occurs in short fixation periods after which the centre of gaze jumps with a fast saccade to the next fixation point (Valentin, 1844; Fig. 17.5). Since the first recordings of such eye movements (Erdmann and Dodge, 1898), it is known that a text is sequentially sampled during successively displaced fixation periods. Erdmann and Dodge found in their subjects 5 to 7 fixation periods per line, whereby the number increased with text difficulty and, of course, with the length of the line.

The duration of saccades in between fixation periods varies between 20 and 45 ms depending on the angular size of the saccades. The saccadic eye movements shift the image of the read page very quickly across the retina (up to $450 \, \text{deg s}^{-1}$). Because of the limited temporal upper frequency of the retina and the central visual system, the stimulus during such a saccade corresponds to a short, more or less homogeneous grey which is not consciously perceived. Similarly, the reader is also not aware of the blinking of his eyelids, which are correlated with saccades. For a skilled reader, the fixation periods between saccades last between 180 and approximately 500 ms. The average duration of the fixation period depends on the individual characteristics of the reader, on his reading training and on the difficulty of the text. When the latter is greater, the frequency of backward saccades increases. In most cases, the reader is not aware of these backward saccades. Whenever the lines of a text are very long, eye movements are accompanied by head movements which accompany the shift of gaze. Since the discontinuous uptake of information is below the conscious threshold for average reading,

one must conclude that the time of the neuronal processing of the information transmitted by the text is much longer than the average interval between successive saccades. Understanding of the text lags considerably behind the moment it is read, at least 1 to 2 seconds for easily understandable texts. This time increases with text difficulty.

To gain a first impression of an individual's reading competence, the average reading speed (words read out loud per minute) for a standardized text should be measured. Reading speed is, of course, greatly diminished in patients suffering from alexia or from non-fluent aphasia. A second measurement is average reading error, which should be below 1 per cent for not very difficult texts and for the average reader. When eye movements are recorded during reading (using either an electrooculogram, the infrared reflexion technique or the electromagnetic search coil technique), duration of fixation periods, number of fixations per word or per line, size of forward saccades measured in degrees or in number of characters, frequency and size of backward saccades (regression saccades) and eventually the exact target of fixation can all be measured. Since Walker's (1933) and Taylor's (1966) extensive studies, it has been repeatedly confirmed that an improvement in reading skills during the first years of schooling is characterized by a reduction in the number of fixations per word or line, by an increase in the size of foreward saccades and by a decrease in the number of regression saccades as well as in the duration of fixation (Fig. 17.11). American college students, for example, needed on the average 90 saccades to read a 100-word text, i.e. the lexic span of a fixation period was about 1.1 words and the average duration of fixation periods was 0.24 seconds. At normal reading distance and speed, although not all the letters of a single word are seen with the acuity necessary for individual perception, most of them are still correctly perceived (Aubert, 1865). As mentioned above, because of the redundancy of letters in words and of words in sentences, individual letter recognition is not at all necessary for text comprehension. Correspondingly, when a text is read in search of printing errors, reading speed decreases by a factor of 3 or 4 as compared with normal reading speed (Erdmann and Dodge, 1898). Context information influences reading speed, eye movements and eye–voice span. Artificial words generated by 0th- to 6th-order Markov chains of the English language were, not surprisingly, read better and faster the closer the approximation to real English (Morton, 1964).

The decrease in correct word and letter recognition is a function of retinal eccentricity (Fig. 17.12). Similar results were obtained in experiments conducted by Bouma (1973): typewriter characters with upper-case letters having a vertical size of 2 mm and lower case letters of 1.5 mm were presented at a reading distance of 50 cm to

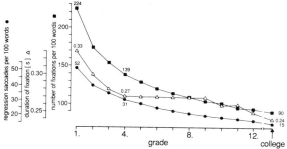

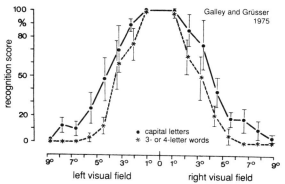

Fig. 17.11 *Quantitative studies on eye movements during reading. The data were collected in about 10,000 US-American pupils of different age. Three values are plotted in the diagram: number of regression saccades per 100 words (solid circles), duration of fixation (triangles) and number of fixations per 100 words (squares). All of these values decrease with age, i.e. years in elementary and high school, and in college (abscissa). Redrawn according to the data published by Taylor (1966).*

Fig. 17.12 *Correct recognition percentage of a letter or a word (three- or four-letter words) as a function of retinal eccentricity (abscissa). The subjects had to fixate carefully a small central target. Upper-case letters appeared randomly distributed horizontally left or right of the fixation target and were tachistoscopically projected for 500 ms. Monocular experiments, right eye, four subjects; algebraic means ± s.e. of the data are plotted as a function of retinal eccentricity. Solid circles: data with upper-case letters. Asterisks: three- or four-letter words (from Galley and Grüsser, 1975).*

subjects who fixated carefully on a small central target: single letters or words consisting of 3 or 4 letter strings, which were horizontally projected tachistoscopically onto the visual field to the left or right of the fixation target for 0.5 seconds (monocular observation). Single letters were significantly better perceived outside a region of 2 degrees from the fovea centre than were letters within short words, a fact which was presumably a result of mutual masking effects (see below).

Curves like those shown in Fig. 17.12 allow for an estimate of reliable word recognition as a function of saccade size. Since an average line on a standard page contains 10 to 12 words and since the width of a line in an average book (having one column per page) is 8 to 12 cm (corresponding at a 50 cm reading distance to about 9 to 14 degrees), 7 to 9 saccades per line are, as a rule, sufficient in order to understand the text. When column width is smaller and letter size is as a result diminished, as in the case of this book's text (chosen by the publisher and not by the authors), reading at a distance of 50 cm may be somewhat difficult even with normal visual acuity. The necessary reduction in reading distance demands an increased effort in refractive power (accommodation) of the lense, resulting in fatigue. By lessening reading distance, however, the reader can again optimize his reading strategies with 7 to 8 saccades per line. It is not surprising that the subjective 'readability' determined by typography correlates fairly well with the values obtained by eye movement recordings (Tinker, 1958, 1963; Tinker and Patterson, 1955, 1958, 1963).

Eye movements during reading depend not only on the graphical structure of the printed or handwritten text, but also on the word structure, the syntax of the text and the

semantic difficulties involved in understanding the text. Reading speed for artificial words increased for native English readers the more similar the text was to correct English. The eye–voice span for reading aloud varied between 615 and 708 ms and did not depend systematically on the similarity of the text to written English (Morton, 1964). Intuitively, one agrees with Morton's arguments (1969) that in reading, the perception of a word depends on word frequency and on the position of the word in a sentence, since the subject compares his 'internal information' about the language and about the statistics of that language with the text actually read. Therefore, knowledge of syntactic and semantic rules and statistics facilitates reading speed. The difficulty involved in understanding the content of the read text also affects reading speed. This is illustrated schematically in Fig. 17.13: three different German prose texts were read by native German speakers. Albert Schweitzer's *Aus meiner Kindheit und Jugendzeit* is written in a clear and simple German which is easy to understand. Günter Grass's text from *Der Butt*, a novel published in 1978, has a somewhat complex syntactic structure but simple, easy to understand content, while Hegel's text *Einführung in die Philosophie* is characterized by a simple syntax, but a content which is rather difficult to understand. Reading speed decreased from Schweitzer to Grass and from Grass to Hegel and was also progressively slower for reading aloud than for reading quietly; under both conditions, it was somewhat slower for left-handed individuals as compared with right-handed

(a)

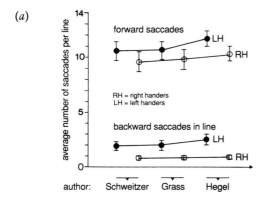

(b)

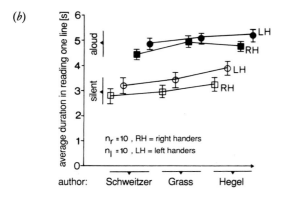

Fig. 17.13 *Ten right-handed (RH) and 10 left-handed (LH) adult male and female subjects read paragraphs of 3 different types of text: Albert Schweitzer's* Aus meiner Kindheit und Jugendzeit, *the novel* Der Butt *by Günter Grass and* Einführung in die Philosophie *by G. F. Hegel. The Schweitzer text was simple in style and content, the Grass text complex in style but simple in content and the Hegel text simple in style but difficult to understand. (a) Average number of forward and backward saccades per line while reading the three different texts without any pressure to understand the text. Data for silent reading and reading out loud. The number of backward saccades increased considerably for the Hegel text (Fig. 17.5) when the subjects were asked to try to understand the text. (b) Same subjects and texts. The average time needed to read one line was, as the number of saccades in (a), longer in left-handed than in right-handed subjects (H. Ghazarian and O.-J. Grüsser, unpublished 1977).*

ones (Fig. 17.13). The number of backward saccades increased with text difficulty, as was also true for the number of forward saccades. The latter phenomenon was a result of the increased frequency of backward saccades, since the forward saccades which followed a backward saccade were, on the average, not considerably increased in size. As a rule, although the readers did not consciously perceive the increased number of forward and backward

saccades in connection with the Hegel text, they reported having greater difficulty understanding this text. In general, however, the differences in eye sampling strategies with these three types of text were rather small, and the interindividual variability was high. The reader's backward saccades increased by a factor of 4 to 6 only when he really tried to understand the Hegel text, as was the case for the recordings shown in Fig. 17.5 (cf. also Walker, 1933; Morton, 1964). Eye–voice span for reading aloud was on the average 0.67 ± 0.06 (s.e.) seconds (cf. Buswell, 1930).

The average duration of the fixation periods for the easy text (Schweitzer) was 295.8 ± 11.1 ms for reading aloud and 262.1 ± 6.8 ms for reading quietly to oneself; while for the difficult text (Hegel) the respective values were 334.4 ± 1.7 ms and 280.7 ± 7.1 ms. Most of the subjects, however, hardly understood the Hegel text – either when reading aloud or when reading silently. Correct pronunciation and prosodic style had no relation to text comprehension. Hence, the Austrian poet Thomas Bernhard (1931–89) was correct when he wrote in the 'Prélude' to his play *Ein Fest für Boris*:

> *I have repeatedly observed that people who have not the slightest idea what they are reading aloud recite the text excellently.*

Which parts of the text are preferably fixated on by the centre of the fovea? First letters, words with a letter in upper case and words at the beginning of a line or new section are above average fixation targets. Duration of fixation does not depend on word length. The probability that a letter within a word was fixated on depended not only on its position, but also on word length. With long words consisting of more than 8 to 12 letters, even experienced readers might perform a saccade within the word. Although fixation on the first letter was more frequent than on the last letter, the last letter was more frequently fixated on than was any letter in the middle of the word (cf. Mehler *et al.*, 1967). The probability of fixating on the empty space between words was considerably lower than was fixating on the words themselves. This was true whether or not the empty space contained punctuation marks. All of these observations indicate that the text structure itself also has some influence on which part of the text is precisely projected to the centre of the fovea during the fixation periods. This observation indicates an interaction between deeper text comprehension and gaze movement control during reading.

Because reading saccades are sequentially determined, small but significant positive correlations were found for reading saccades that followed each other (correlation coefficient between 0.09 and 0.18 for the amplitude and duration of the saccades). The 'preprogramming' of saccadic eye movements across the text can also be demon-

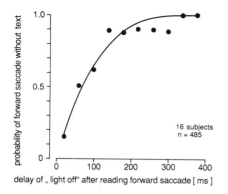

16 subjects
n = 485

Fig. 17.14 *Data obtained in 16 adult female and male subjects reading aloud the text of Albert Schweitzer (see Figs 17.5 and 17.13). The light illuminating the text was turned off at random at different times after a forward reading saccade. The probability that another forward saccade occurred without text (ordinate) is plotted as a function of time. This curve demonstrates the 'preprogramming' of reading saccades (H. Ghazarian and O.-J. Grüsser, unpublished, 1977).*

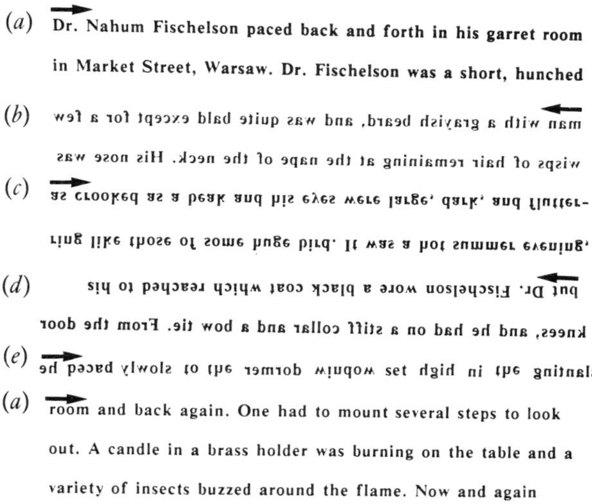

(a) Dr. Nahum Fischelson paced back and forth in his garret room in Market Street, Warsaw. Dr. Fischelson was a short, hunched

(b) man with a grayish beard, and was quite bald except for a few wisps of hair remaining at the nape of the neck. His nose was

(c) as crooked as a beak and his eyes were large, dark and fluttering like those of some huge bird. It was a hot summer evening,

(d) but Dr. Fischelson wore a black coat which reached to his knees, and he had on a stiff collar and a bow tie. From the door

(e) slanting in the high set window of the dormer and to slowly paced he

(a) room and back again. One had to mount several steps to look out. A candle in a brass holder was burning on the table and a variety of insects buzzed around the flame. Now and again

Fig. 17.15 *Increasing difficulties in reading text when the letters are rotated. The text is taken from I. B. Singer's* The Spinoza of Market Street, *opening paragraph. (a) Normal text, (b) mirror text, (c) text upside down, (d) mirror text upside down, (e) text composed of words treated as in (a) to (d). Most readers will experience some difficulty in reading the lines (b) to (e), which may illustrate to the normal reader the difficulties encountered by dyslexic or alexic patients when reading.*

strated by a simple experiment: if the text is turned off later than 50 ms after the beginning of the fixation period after a saccade occurs, another saccade will inevitably be performed in the 'empty' field. This 'meaningless' saccade is sometimes followed by a second one after another delay of 300 to 400 ms (Fig. 17.14).

For mirror-image text or for text composed of inverted letters, the number of fixations per line increase by a factor of two or three; as a result, more time is necessary for reading. The reader can study his own ability to read text composed of transformed letters by using Fig. 17.15. Reading becomes even more difficult when every letter is individually rotated along the vertical axis (for details see Kolers, 1970). The reader might experience the same reading difficulties experienced by an alexic patient when trying to read the texts in Fig. 17.15, in which only the graphic structure of the print is changed by rotation through different axes. The linguistic aspect of the text is not at all changed. From Kolers's observations (1970), it became evident that the recognition of single letters depends significantly on transformations such as those performed in Fig. 17.15. Letter recognition was more difficult when the letters formed pseudo-words having 0th-order Markov chain properties than when each letter was separated from its neighbour by an interspace (Kolers and Perkins, 1969).

Retinal information uptake during reading is normally performed by the fovea. It is therefore interesting to explore reading in the absence of foveal function, or reading with a restricted field of foveal and parafoveal vision. Reading without the fovea can be achieved by producing a strong foveal afterimage which leads to temporary foveal blinding, by reading under scotopic adaptation conditions or, more elegantly, by generating a visual mask which obliterates foveal vision and moves in synchrony with the eye movements along a text appearing on an oscilloscope screen. Since visual acuity decreases as the distance away from the fovea increases, identification of words or letters decreased markedly in the presence of such a visual mask as the distance from the centre of the fovea increased.

McConkie and Rayner (1975) varied the size of the window around the fovea by 'illuminating on a cathode ray tube a certain field around the fixation target'. This window moved synchronously with the eye movements. Similar studies were reported by Rayner and Bertera (1979). They varied the amount of characters visible in the window from one character to a full line of text ($>$ 29 character space). The field of useful vision during a fixation period was about 12 to 15 characters. As the window size shrank below these values, reading speed decreased considerably; the same was true for saccade amplitude. Furthermore, the duration of the fixation periods and the number of fixations necessary to read the text also increased (Fig. 17.16).

Masking the fovea resulted in a more dramatic reading impairment (Fig. 17.16a–d). Masking was achieved by dimming the text on the cathode ray tube around the point

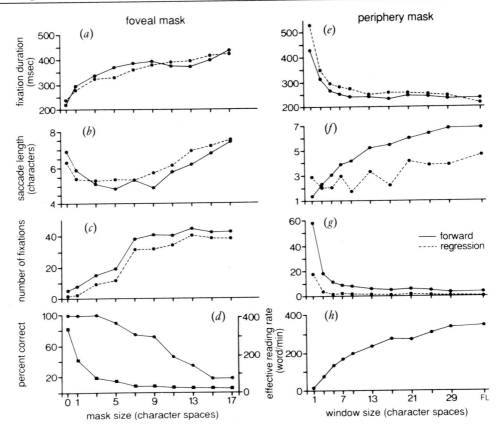

Fig. 17.16 *Analysis of reading performance when a foveal mask (a–d) or a peripheral mask (e–h) coupled to the eye movements was applied. (a, e) The duration of fixation periods, (b, f), saccade amplitude measured in number of characters, (c, g), the number of fixations and (d, h) the percentage of correct recognition of the words are plotted as a function of mask size (character spaces). Data related to forward and regression saccades are separately plotted. For further explanation, see text (from Rayner and Bertera, 1979, redrawn).*

of fixation. Effective reading rate (words per minute) decreased from about 300 to 160 words per minute when the mask covered only the central letter. When 6 letters were covered, reading rate was reduced to about 10 per cent. Correspondingly, the duration of fixation increased with the size of the foveal mask; the amplitude of saccades formed a U-shaped curve, and the number of fixations increased with mask size (Fig. 17.16c). As mask size increased, the percentage of correctly read words in the sentence diminished. When the mask covered 13 or 14 characters, the subjects could report nothing about the text in 18 per cent of the trials. They saw words in the parafovea and visual field periphery, but could not correctly report the words even by guessing.

These important findings should be considered when testing the reading ability of patients suffering from lesions found either in the afferent visual pathways or in the primary visual cortex which affect foveal projection (Chap-

ter 9). It is always necessary in an evaluation of alexia to compare the ability of the patient to read normal-sized texts as compared with texts composed of considerably oversized, clearly printed letters (cf. Chapter 18). Otherwise, it is difficult to discriminate between a perceptual defect and a cognitive defect of alexia (for further discussion, see Bay, 1950).

Reading without Eye Movement: Tachistoscopic Projection of Letters or Words

As already mentioned above, reading is a discontinuous foveal sampling process which occurs during the fixation periods in between the fast saccades performed when reading along a line of text. Eye movement, however, is a motor strategy which is not necessary for reading. It is a visuo-motor adaptation to the graphical structure of the text. With unmoved eyes, letters, words or short pieces of text projected successively into the centre of the visual field can also be read, provided that the temporal sequence is properly selected and that letter size is adapted to the visual acuity of the part of the visual field explored. Although tachistoscopic projection of verbal material is, of course, a rather artificial way in which to test reading or letter recognition abilities, it provides an interesting tool for gaining knowledge about the function of the left or right hemispheres in the process of reading, and has offered some insight into the cerebral mechanisms of reading which could not have been obtained solely using normal visuo-motor reading strategies.

Historical Remarks

Tachistoscopic projection of letters or words was first used during the last decades of the nineteenth century. The investigators were, as a rule, especially interested in measuring the temporal properties of visual perception and visual cognition in order to distinguish between the mechanisms of perception and apperception (e.g. Donders, 1868; Catell, 1885, 1886; Erdmann and Dodge, 1898; Zeitler, 1900; Wundt, 1904, 1911). According to Wundt (1911), G. W. Leibniz was the first to separate conceptually the process of perception and apperception. Tachistoscopic studies attracted greater interest after Erdmann and Dodge's discovery (1898) of the visuo-motor sampling strategies used for reading (see above). A new momentum in tachistoscopic reading studies set in when neuropsychologists discovered the differences in perception and recognition of verbal material projected either into the left or right visual hemifield; they believed that the contribution of the right or left cerebral hemisphere could be systematically explored using this method (Mishkin and Forgays, 1951; Orbach, 1952). During the last 40 years, an overwhelming number of papers have been published on tachistoscopic recognition of verbal material. In the following section, we shall deal only with a few selected papers on this topic in order to introduce the problem of tachistoscopic reading, a method which can also be applied to studies of alexia.

Experimental Paradigms

When either the letter 'A' or 'B' or a word is projected somewhere into the field of vision, three main response criteria can be applied:

1. The frequency of correct recognition at preset stimulus properties (contrast, stimulus duration, level of adaptation).

2. The duration or intensity of tachistoscopic presentation needed to reach response criteria.

3. The psychomotor response time (RT) to suprathreshold stimuli.

Frequency of correct recognition or of correct discrimination in a 'same' or a 'different' task is taken as an indication of the probability that the given task was correctly performed. One has to keep in mind, however, that reaction times depend on the task: 'same' responses in perceptual matches are, as a rule, faster than 'different' responses (Krueger, 1978). The investigators have to be careful when interpreting the frequency of correct responses. Goldiamond and Hawkins (1958) performed an intriguing '*Vexierversuch*': their subjects had first to learn nonsense words (with different training periods for different words). The subjects were then asked to recognize subthreshold stimuli; the investigators pretended that by each presentation, one of the learned nonsense words was projected by the tachistoscope. The subjects had to guess the projected word. In fact, nothing was projected at all, but a power function was found between the frequency of training time for a certain word and the frequency that this word was selected as a response.

With respect to tachistoscopic reading, three types of verbal material were used for Western script: letters, words or sentences. With respect to letter perception or letter recognition, the main experimental variables were the following: angular size of the stimulus, position in the visual field, orientation when deviating from the usual upright position, upper- or lower-case letters, printed or hand-written letters. In matching tasks, physical identity (A/A) or letter identity (A/a) were the two main criteria used when two or more letters were projected simultaneously into the visual field. To separate the process specific to letter recognition as compared with recognition of graphically similar structures, letter/non-letter discrimination tasks were used.

Similar criteria were used to test word recognition: size, orientation and position in the visual field, inverted or upright letters, mirror stimuli, rotated letters. In matching tasks, the most frequently used variables were as follows: discrimination between real words and non-words (bear/brea), physical identity (red/red), name identity (RED/red), identical or non-identical categories (red/blue), synonyms or similar meanings (large/big), graphical symmetry (plug/gulp), word length (red/read/reader/reading), pronounceability of nonsense words (BRIP/RBPI), visual versus phonological similarity (house/mouse, bee/key), concrete or abstract words, frequent or rare words, ambiguous or unambiguous words, words related to each other in a categorical hierarchy (apple/fruit) and spatial organization of letter sequence.

Recognition of sentences is usually tested in tachistoscopic experiments by using a sequence of words projected either into the same or into different parts of the visual field; the time intervals between the text segments are the most critical parameters, provided that the recognition of single words is above a defined experimental threshold. Catell (1885, 1886) found that short sentences composed of 2, 3 or 4 simultaneously projected short words can also be used in tachistoscopic experiments.

Single Letter Recognition

Reaction time and recognition probability for a letter depends on the typography of the letter (Catell, 1885; Sanford, 1888), and, consequently, also on the rank order of legibility produced by the graphical structures, a fact which has been carefully explored by Bouma (1971). Probability of correct letter recognition is, of course, also determined by letter size and by the position of the stimulus within the visual field, since visual acuity decreases monotonically moving from the centre of the fovea into the visual field periphery (Fig. 17.12). Speed of letter recognition decreased when degraded characters were used (Sternberg, 1967). Discrimination between letters and non-letters of similar structure added an additional 50 to 70 ms to the simple psychomotor reaction time. Evidently, the process of constituting the invariant configuration of a letter depends also on the orientation of the letter (Cooper and Shepard, 1973; Tilgner, 1978; Tilgner and Hauske, 1979; Fig. 17.17). Not unexpectedly, the fastest recognition time was obtained when the letters were in a normal, upright position; 20 to 30 ms have to be added to the RT for this task when the letter is rotated by 60 to 90 degrees to the left or right.

As one would expect, letters projected into the right visual field (RVF) were, under certain conditions, better and more quickly recognized than were letters projected into the left visual field (LVF; Kimura, 1961, 1966). Cor-

rect letter recognition decreased with retinal eccentricity and was in both the LVF and RVF better in the upper than in the lower quadrant (Heron, 1957). Schmuller (1979) found in adults an RVF advantage for letter recognition; this advantage increased with the complexity of the task, i.e. as the numbers of letters increased from which the target letter had to be selected (cf. also Egeth and Epstein, 1972; Cohen, 1973; Krueger, 1975). Cohen (1973) reported only for the RVF an increase in RT as the number of letters in a word increased; RT for words projected into the LVF depended little on word length. In contrast, nonsense shapes produced similar reaction times in both hemifields. Egeth and Epstein (1972) concluded from their experiments using letter pairs that while the detection of 'sameness' is easier for stimuli projected into the LVF, the detection of 'difference' is facilitated for RVF stimuli. Thus RVF superiority for letter recognition has to be modified according to the difficulty of the task involved in recognizing the letter. During one set of experiments, for example, the subjects investigated by Jonides (1979) had to discriminate graphically similar upper-case letters (E, F) or graphically dissimilar upper-case letters (C, E) in the parafoveal LVH or RVH. Discriminating graphically dissimilar letters (E, F positive; C, G negative) was easier than was discriminating letters grouped in mixed categories (C, E positive, F, G negative; date for C, E and E, F are given in Fig. 17.18). In the latter case, LVF superiority was observed. Expectedly, although RT increased for the more difficult condition, the effect of training was clearly evident for both paradigms. Jonides

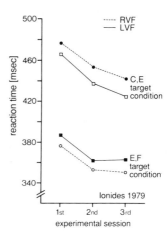

Fig. 17.18 *Reaction time (ordinate) in discriminating graphically similar (E, F) and graphically dissimilar (C, E) upper-case letters in the parafoveal left visual hemifield (LVF) and the parafoveal right visual hemifield (RVF). Reaction times decrease with experience of subjects. For further explanation, see text (redrawn from Jonides, 1979).*

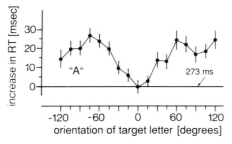

Fig. 17.17 *Dependency of reaction time (ordinate) in recognizing a target letter as a function of the orientation of that letter. The mean differences ± s.e. are given relative to the reaction time for recognizing the letter A in the normal upright position (redrawn from Tilgner, 1978).*

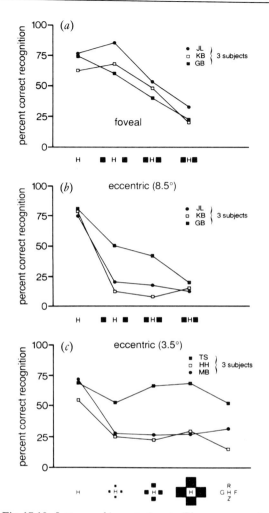

Fig. 17.19 *Letter-masking experiments. The percentage of correct letter recognition in tachistoscopic tests depends on the distance, but very little on the size, of the masking stimuli surrounding the target letter. Data from Loomis (1978, redrawn).*

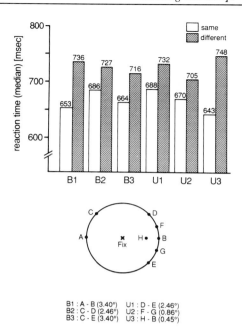

Fig. 17.20 *Medians of reaction time (ordinate) obtained in a same/different task for different pairs of letters projected into the left or right visual hemifield, as indicated by the inset. For further explanation, see text (from Schmitz-Gielsdorf et al., 1988, redrawn).*

also found that when an easy discriminating task (C/F) was incorporated into a difficult discrimination task (F/E or F/T), LVH superiority was found for all tasks.

Geffen *et al.* (1972), Cohen (1973) and Davis and Schmit (1973) found a RVH superiority with a reaction time advantage of 30 to 40 ms in letter-matching tasks (upper case/lower case, name identity); no significant visual field effects on physical identity were observed. The RVH advantage did not depend on the subject's gender (Segalowitz and Stewart, 1979).

Interference or 'lateral masking' has been observed with letters or non-letters used as lateral masks when more than

one letter were projected simultaneously into the visual field (Bouma, 1970, 1973; Eriksen and Rohrbaugh, 1970; Shaw and Weigel, 1973; Anstis, 1974; Eriksen and Eriksen, 1974b; Estes *et al.*, 1976). As expected, the masking effect depended on the distance of the masking stimulus from the target letter for both foveal and parafoveal vision. This is illustrated in Fig. 17.19 (Loomis, 1978). Elementary lateral inhibiting mechanisms in the afferent visual system and in the primary visual cortex are presumably the main factors accounting for this effect (Chapters 3 and 4).

The interaction of right and left hemisphere stimulation involved in letter recognition was studied by projecting letters either bilaterally into symmetric parts of the two visual hemifields, or unilaterally into one hemifield. The task was to judge 'sameness' and 'difference'. Early studies, such as those performed by Davis and Schmit (1971, 1973), indicated a faster response for bilateral, as compared with unilateral, stimulation (cf. Dimond and Beaumont, 1972). In Davis and Schmit's studies, bilateral stimulation was performed, however, with horizontal letter arrangement, and unilateral stimulation with vertical letter arrangement. To compensate for this condition, Schmitz-Gielsdorf *et al.* (1988) tried to eliminate this factor by systematically varying letter position for unilateral or bilateral presentation (Fig. 17.20). They formed pairs of upper-case letters (A, B, C, D, E, F, G, H) with either the same or different lower-case letters (e.g. D, d or D, h, etc.). Thus the decision of 'same' or 'different' had to be made based on 'name identity'. Although RTs for 'same' responses were expectedly shorter than for 'different' responses, no significant differences between bilateral and unilateral presentations were found when the spatial arrangement of the letters was balanced (Fig. 17.20).

Not unexpectedly, the RVF advantage for letter matching develops during the early years when children first learn to read. In Davidoff and Done's study (1984) of 4-year-old children, an LVF advantage was observed for boys, while an RVF advantage was found for 5- to 7-year-old boys and girls. The authors interpreted this finding to indicate not only a left hemisphere advantage for language processing that presumably existed already before reading begins, but also an integration of the visual–verbal material into this left bias occurring at the time a child learns to read.

Word Recognition

While an RVF advantage also existed for recognition of high- or low-frequency words, none of the visual fields indicated better responses for non-words or nonsense forms (Terrace, 1959). This finding was independent of or only slightly dependent on the statistical approximation of the non-words to actual English words (Bryden, 1966, 1970; Lieber, 1976). It also did not depend on synchrony or on the degree of asynchrony of the stimuli (McKeever, 1971). Similarly, Bradshaw and Gates (1978) and Bradshaw *et al.*, (1979) found shorter RT values for English words projected into the RVF than those projected into the LVF; the difference was greater for words than for homophonic non-words, and relatively small for non-homophonic non-words. Cohen (1973), confirming the RVF advantage, found an increase in reaction time only for the RVF as the number of letters in a word increased; he wrote the well-known statement that the semantic signals in the RVF are sequentially processed by the left hemisphere, the LVF signals holistically by the right cerebral hemisphere. Egeth and Epstein (1972) confirmed an RVF advantage for word recognition in their tests of word 'sameness'. An LVF advantage was noticed, however, when the subject's decision was based on 'difference' criteria.

Pierce (1960) considered the slightly better recognition of subliminal words to be a function of word frequency, attributing this not to perceptual advantages but rather to 'better guessing abilities' for high-frequency words. This interpretation is in accordance with an idea put forth by Solomon and Postman (1952), who found that when a word is presented only in fragments, the letters serve as constraints on the guessing process: patients select the

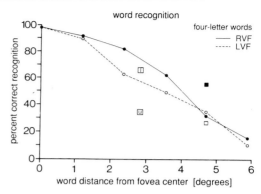

Fig. 17.21 *Recognition score (ordinate) for four-letter words tachistoscopically projected into the right (RVF) or left (LVF) visual hemifield decreases with horizontal stimulus eccentricity. 'l' in a square: recognition score for eight-letter words projected into the lower visual hemifield; u in a square: same for the upper visual hemifield; filled square: same for the right visual hemifield; open square: same for the left visual hemifield (data from Mishkin and Forgays, 1951, redrawn).*

word based on the statistical structure of the language. This view is supported by the results of Goldiamond and Hawkins's above-mentioned '*Vexierversuch*' (1958). According to Orenstein and Meighen (1976), the position of a word on the 'abstract–concrete scale' did not influence the RVF advantage in word recognition.

In general, the same RVF advantage for words as compared with non-words was also found for Hebrew trigrams (Babkoff and Ben-Uriah, 1983; cf. also Carmon *et al.*, 1976). This finding, which corresponds to results published earlier by Barton *et al.*, 1965), was based on experiments which had used vertically printed Hebrew and English trigrams; it indicated that letter sequence from left to right (English) or from right to left (as is the case in Hebrew) was not a major cause of RVF advantage in such experiments. Boles (1984), who relied on his own studies as well as on an analysis of published data on 'meta-analysis', confirmed that for lexical decisions, RVF advantage is not essentially dependent on the gender of the subjects. When applying recognition thresholds by manipulating the duration of tachistoscopic stimuli, Goodglass and Barton (1963) found not only an RVF advantage for both right-handers and left-handers tested with vertically printed English trigrams projected at 2.6 degrees lateral from the fovea centre, but also confirmed an RVF advantage for monocular stimulation of the left or right eye.

Mishkin and Forgays (1951) investigated responses to 4- and 8-letter words tachistoscopically projected into the LVF or the RVF. Recognition scores were determined for words presented above and below as well as left and right of the fixation target. The right and lower visual half-fields were significantly superior to the left and upper visual half-fields. Although the recognition curves for 4-letter words appearing at different retinal eccentricities from 0 to 6 degrees decreased as the distance increased from the fixation point, RVF superiority was found only for eccentricities between 1 and 4 degrees (Fig. 17.21). A non-significant LVF advantage was found for Yiddish 8-letter words written in Hebrew letters; since the subjects had considerably less practice reading Yiddish, however, recognition scores were more than 50 per cent better for English than for Yiddish words presented under the same stimulus conditions (cf. also White, 1969). These findings do not contradict the data mentioned below, which indicate that an RVF advantage also exists for native Hebrew speakers reading Hebrew words.

Riegel and Riegel (1961) also determined thresholds of stimulus duration for recognition of large lists of words selected according to word frequency. The threshold increased with word length as measured in number of letters (linear correlation coefficient $r = 0.42$), with the number of different letters ($r = 0.28$), with letter repetition and symmetry ($r = 0.36$), with letter frequency ($r = 0.39$) and with the number of syllables ($r = 0.38$). The lower the word frequency, the lower the probability of correct recognition ($r = -0.50$ with logarithm of word frequency). The semantic content of the word played an important role: concrete nouns were much better recognized than were abstract nouns. Orenstein and Meighen (1976) confirmed an RVF advantage for abstract words, but not for concrete words.

An increase in statistical approximation of letter strings to words of the written English language (using 0th- to 4th-order Markov chain properties of 8-letter words) facilitated, of course, correct recognition (Miller *et al.*, 1954). Statistical frequency of a word in everyday language also influenced recognition probability. High-frequency words were recognized after a shorter exposure time than were low-frequency words, presumably because of better guessing chances for high-frequency words (Pierce, 1960). Several authors (Heron, 1957; White, 1969) have argued that RVF advantage for word recognition is caused by asymmetric attentional scanning. McKeever (1971) and McKeever and Huling (1971) questioned this interpretation, however, pointing to results obtained in a rather intriguing experiment: their subjects were asked to fixate and simultaneously recognize a fixation digit while words were presented in both hemifields. RVF superiority was increased in these experiments from 1.5:1 to a surprising 5:1. McKeever and Gill (1972), who varied letter and word position in the RVF and LVF, confirmed the RVF advantage. In addition, recognition scores for vertically spelled words were less than those for horizontally spelled words. Thus reading habits might also influence recognition probability.

Another argument against RVF advantage in tachistoscopic word recognition was put forward by Eriksen and Eriksen (1974a). These authors argued that in the RVF, the first letter of the word is closer to the fixation point than is the first letter of the word projected into the LVF. This argument, however, is not supported by the findings published by Barton *et al.* (1965), Bryden (1970) and McKeever and Gill (1972), who presented vertically written words in the RVF or LVF and still reported RVF superiority. Tomlinson-Keasey *et al.*'s work (1983) has also contributed to this problem. These authors shifted horizontally written four-letter words within the RVF and LVF so that the position of the first letter was always an equal distance from the fixation target (a digit). In another test condition, they placed the last letter at equal distance from the fixation target. Responses to vertically written 4-letter words placed equally distant from the fixation target were also measured. Finally, horizontally written words were placed equally distant from the middle of the word to the fixation target. In all experiments a group of high-frequency and low-frequency English 4-letter words, balanced for 'concreteness', were used. The subjects had to identify first the fixation digit, and then the words that they saw in the LVF and RVF. After naming the fixation digits, the subjects usually first reported the word perceived (or guessed) in the LVF and then the one in the RVF. Thus they used a spatial scanning strategy similar to the one used in normal reading. Considering the different stimulus conditions, RVF advantage was confirmed (Fig. 17.22). No visual field advantage was found, however, for recognition of first letters of words. This suggests that when a first letter is embedded in a word, and word recognition is an experimental task, the RVF advantage in recognizing letters will disappear; this factor had, however, only a small effect on recognition. Thus the first letter of a word serving as a cue for word recognition was not extremely important in these experiments. RVF advantage in word recognition disappeared and even shifted to LVF advantage when, in comparable experiments, the mirror images of the words were projected (White, 1969).

In their early work, Wispé and Drabarean (1953) tested whether emotional factors had any impact on the recognition of tachistoscopically projected words. They investigated three groups of subjects deprived of food and water for 0, 10 and 24 hours respectively, and matched the stimulus words for commonness and food/water relevance. In measuring the duration thresholds of tachistoscopic presentation for correct recognition, the data indicated that word commonness was the most important factor, but that need-related words were also more rapidly recognized as need increased. Word commonness was not a significant interacting factor. These findings indicate that limbic con-

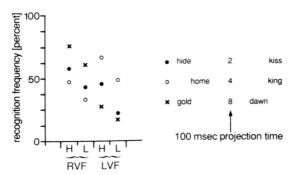

Fig. 17.22 *Recognition score (ordinate) for words projected tachistoscopically (100 ms) into different parts of the visual field. The positioning of English four-letter words presented bilaterally from a fixation target was varied, as shown on the right side of the graph. The subjects had to report the fixation digit (arrow) first, then the words they had seen. Subjects typically reported after the fixation digit the LVH word first. The distance of the words left and right of the fixation target was varied as indicated. From the results (left half of the graph), it is evident that the position of the first letter of a word relative to the fixation target had some impact on recognition score in the RVF and LVF (from Tomlinson-Keasey et al., 1983, redrawn).*

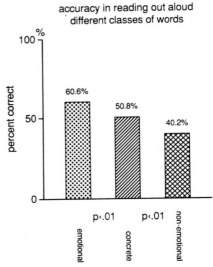

Fig. 17.23 *Thirty-four aphasic patients were tested in reading aloud 12 emotional abstract nouns, 12 non-emotional abstract nouns and 12 concrete nouns. Twenty-two of these patients could read at least one, but not all, of these words. The percentage of correct reading out loud is plotted on the ordinate axis. Emotional words were read aloud correctly with the highest percentage (from Landis et al., 1982).*

nections affect cognitive operations in the visual–verbal domain.

Clinicians have long noted that some severely aphasic patients continue to curse with precision and that their speech improves when emotionally aroused. These observations became a part of neurological literature more than a century ago and led Hughlings Jackson (1874) to suggest that while 'automatic' speech, including emotional phrases, could come from the right hemisphere, propositional speech is formed in the left hemisphere. To investigate whether or not aphasic patients possess a particular capacity to read 'emotional' words, we tested their ability to read emotional, concrete and non-emotional words aloud. Three lists of 4-letter nouns matched for frequency were made up (Thorndike-Lorge, 1944; Kucera-Francis, 1967). One consisted of twelve emotional abstract nouns (e.g. love), one of 12 non-emotional abstract nouns (e.g. fact) and one of 12 concrete nouns (e.g. coat). Thirty-four aphasic patients were tested. The analysis of the data obtained from those 22 patients who could correctly read at least one, but not all the words, is shown in Fig. 17.23. Aphasic patients could read the emotional abstract words significantly better than either concrete or non-emotional abstract words. These results suggest that in the presence of aphasia, the emotional tone of 'abstract' words has a facilitating effect for reading aloud (Goodglass et al., 1980; Landis, et al., 1982).

The emotional and non-emotional abstract noun word-

lists were also used in a tachistoscopic experiment involving normal subjects who were simultaneously presented with two words for 150 ms, one to the right and one to the left of the fixation target. Either both words were nonsense words that could be pronounced in English, or one of the two was a real English word (either an emotional or a non-emotional abstract noun). They were asked to press the response keys only when they saw a real English word ('go–no-go' lexical decision; Graves et al., 1981). The results shown in Fig. 17.24 illustrate that the subjects were generally more accurate in detecting a real word when it was presented to the RVF, which reflects the advantage of the left hemisphere when dealing with written language. No difference in accuracy was found between 'emotional' and 'non-emotional' words, suggesting that for left hemisphere data processing the 'emotional' tone of words is irrelevant. A very different pattern emerged for words projected to the LVF. Although the detection of real words was at chance rate for 'non-emotional' words, 'emotional' words could be detected. These results suggest that the right hemisphere's special affinity for processing emotional information also applies to language; furthermore, it indicates that two different reading or word detection processes are at work, depending on the visual field stimulated.

Since we presented the same words to aphasic patients

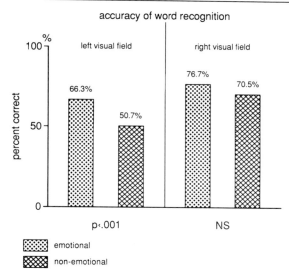

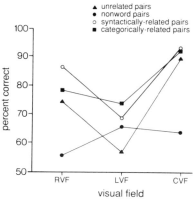

Fig. 17.25 *Semantic priming effects for word recognition. Stimuli were presented to the right (RVF), left (LVF) and central (CVF) visual fields. The recognition score is plotted on the ordinate axis (per cent correct recognition). Stimuli were three- or four-letter words falling in the middle range in word frequency. Four types of word pairs were applied: unrelated pairs (e.g. dog/rain), pairs with one non-word (ant/trem), syntactically related pairs (dog/bark) and categorically related pairs (rain/snow). 100 ms tachistoscopic projection time; visual angle of words 3.5 × 3 degrees; horizontal eccentricity 2.5 degrees. The subject had to press a 'yes' key when both stimuli were actual words and a 'no' key when one of the stimuli was a non-word (redrawn from Walker and Ceci, 1985).*

Fig. 17.24 *Tachistoscopic tests in 24 normal subjects with the same emotional and non-emotional abstract nouns used in Fig. 17.23. The accuracy of correct word recognition (ordinate axis, percentage) obtained with 150 ms presentation time is plotted on the ordinate axis. This lexical decision task was tested in the left and right visual fields, as indicated. Correct recognition for emotional words was significantly higher in the left visual field than for non-emotional words. No difference in the recognition scores was found for the right visual field (from Graves et al., 1981).*

and lateralized tachistoscopically to the LVF and RVF of normal subjects, we could correlate the number of times each word was correctly read by aphasic patients with the number of times it was correctly recognized in the LVF or RVF by normal subjects (Goodglass *et al.*, 1980; Landis, 1987). Although there was no correlation between the performance of aphasic patients and the recognition of words projected to the RVF of normal subjects ($r = + 0.119$, $p > 0.05$), a significant correlation was found for LVF word recognition ($r = + 0.56$, $p < 0.003$). These results suggest that the same process allowing aphasic patients to succeed with some words and not with others also operated with LVF tachistoscopic presentation of words in normal subjects. Since the aphasic patients had an intact right but a damaged left hemisphere, and since the LVF projects directly to the right hemisphere, the anatomical substrate responsible for this 'alternative' reading process, which is facilitated by the emotional quality of words, is most likely to be located in the right hemisphere.

Several studies have investigated the effects of 'semantic priming' on word recognition and reaction time. For example, Meyer and Schvaneveldt (1971) and Schvaneveldt (1973) had patients perform a task in which they had to decide between English words and non-words.

They found that the RT for words was significantly shorter whenever a semantically related word preceded the critical stimulus. When the subjects had to decide on two pairs of letter strings and were asked to respond only when both strings were words, the RT was shorter when the words were semantically related to each other than when the word pairs were unrelated. Thus semantic 'fields' activated by a priming stimulus facilitate lexical decision for tachistoscopically presented words (cf. also Winnick and Daniel, 1970; Neely, 1977; Ceci, 1982a, b; Howard *et al.*, 1980). Walker and Ceci (1985) tested response accuracy and RT for four types of word pairs: syntactically related pairs (dog/bark), categorically related pairs (rain/snow), unrelated pairs (dog/rain) and pairs of words and non-words (ant/trem). The word pairs were projected into the right, left or central part of the visual field for 100 ms. The subjects were asked to press a 'yes' or 'no' key corresponding to the above-mentioned categories. While a clear RVF advantage was found for both values (percentage correct responses and RT) for word pairs, LVF was slightly better than RVF for correct responses when a non-word was part of a pair (Fig. 17.25). The authors concluded from their data that response speed is facilitated by the 'relatedness' of word pairs, regardless of whether the relationship is syntactical or categorical. Despite the RVF advantage, this also occurred in the LVF and, of course, for words projected into the foveal region.

Interestingly, words presented in the periphery of the LVF or RVF with just subliminal stimulus conditions (and therefore not reported) may bias the perceived meaning of a semantically ambiguous word (homograph) projected onto the foveal retina (Bradshaw, 1974). The same author used a homograph paradigm in a second experiment (Bradshaw, 1974). A word having two different meanings typed in upper-case letters was flanked on both sides by lower-case words projected into the parafoveal region. One of the two meanings of the homographs was always 'dominant'. The flanking words, equated for letter and syllable length as well as for word frequency, contained either in the LVF or in the RVF a word semantically related to one meaning of the homograph; the other was not related (e.g. join/MINT/coin). In a control experiment the homograph was flanked by two non-related words (e.g. laugh/MINT/drip). The subjects were asked to generate rapid associates to the homograph, i.e. the upper-case central word. The data led the author to conclude that during 'unconscious semantic processing of disambiguating words, the flanking words can influence the interpretation of the homographs'. But this effect, which was of course related to linguistic competence, was clearly independent of the half of the visual field to which the 'disambiguating' word was projected.

Morton (1969) tried to explain the effect of word frequency and word position in a sentence on word recognition (e.g. Solomon and Postman, 1956; Tulving and Gold, 1963); he assumed that in order to recognize the verbal stimuli, the subject combines internal information about statistics and the syntactic structure of the language with the perceptual process.

Semantic Paralexias

These are incorrect but meaningfully related reading errors (e.g. 'daisy' instead of 'rose', 'father' instead of 'brother', etc.). It has been suggested that they result from a loss of grapho–phonemic decoding capacity (Marshall and Newcombe, 1973) and from a reliance on non-phonemic decoding in the right hemisphere (Coltheart, 1980). Aphasic patients who make an unusually high number of such semantic paralexias are called 'deep dyslexics' (Coltheart et al., 1980). A large and still unsettled controversy arose over the suggestion that this particular type of reading impairment may illustrate 'right-hemisphere reading' (for review see: Coltheart et al., 1980; Benson, 1982; Marshall and Patterson, 1983, 1985; Coltheart, 1985; Patterson and Besner, 1984; Jones and Martin, 1985; Code, 1987).

An analysis of the reading errors made by an unselected group of aphasic patients showed that semantic paralexias occur significantly more frequently with 'emotional' words than with 'concrete' or 'non-emotional' words

Ranked lesion size

With	Without
20	
19	
18	
	17
16	
15	
14	
13	
12	
11	
10	
	9
	8
	7
	6
	5
	4
3	
	2
	1

With	Without

Semantic paralexia

Fig. 17.26 *The reading ability of 22 aphasic patients was tested with the 36 emotional, concrete and non-emotional words used in Fig. 17.23. Lesion size was assessed from CT scans and the patients were grouped in rank order of lesion size. The appearance of semantic paralexia while reading the 36 words is applied as a second category of grouping. Note that lesion size is closely correlated with the appearance of semantic paralexias. For further explanation, see text.*

(Landis et al., 1982). Since most of the 'deep dyslexic' patients were severely aphasic and had very large lesions (detected by CT scanning; Marin, 1980), one could consider 'deep dyslexia' to be a form of rudimentary reading with the right hemisphere. This view was contested, however (Patterson and Besner, 1984; Marshall and Patterson, 1983). We believe that the larger the left hemisphere lesion, the more likely the involvement of right-hemisphere reading and, consequently, a higher probability of semantic paralexia. To test this hypothesis we compared lesion size (as measured by CT scans) to the occurrence of semantic paralexias previously obtained from data on the reading ability of aphasic patients (Landis et al., 1983). The data shown in Fig. 17.26 support our interpretation: 9 out of 10 patients suffering from large lesions made at least one semantic paralexia, while only 1 out of 10 patients suffering from smaller lesions made such errors.

Our argument for a close correlation of semantic paralexias and 'right-hemisphere reading' is supported by the results of another study which compared errors in word

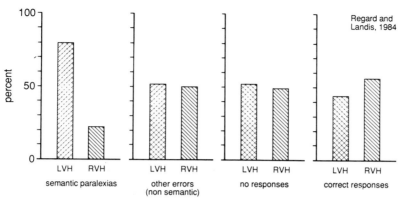

distribution of errors, no responses and correct responses
for stimuli projected to the RVH and the LVH

Regard and
Landis, 1984

Fig. 17.27 *Tachistoscopic test with four-letter nouns projected to the right (RVH) or the left (LVH) visual hemifield. Experiments performed in 20 normal subjects. The subjects were required to read the words out loud. The exposure duration was reduced to an average of 9 ms, leading to 25 per cent correct responses. All four response classes (no responses, semantic paralexias, non-semantic errors and correct responses) occurred with about the same frequency. The percentage of occurrence in the left (LVH) and right (RVH) visual hemifields is plotted on the ordinate. Note that nearly four times as many semantic paralexias appeared when the words were projected to the left visual field. The distribution of the other possible response classes (correct responses, no responses, non-semantic errors) was approximately equal over the LVH and RVH (Regard and Landis, 1984, modified).*

recognition of four-letter nouns projected to the RVF and LVF of normal subjects. The exposure times were reduced to a mean of 9 ms. As a consequence, only 25 per cent of the words were read correctly (Regard and Landis, 1984).

Under these conditions, as illustrated in Fig. 17.27, normal subjects made almost four times as many semantic paralexias when the four-letter nouns were flashed to the LVF as when flashed to the RVF. Other errors and average correct word recognition did not differ significantly between the two visual half-fields. This result is directly connected to our observations of the generation of frequent semantic paralexias in deep dyslexic aphasic patients.

A qualitative analysis of the semantic paralexias (Landis, 1987) for words projected into the LVF led us to assume that a wider semantic distance between target and response must exist than for semantic paralexias found for words projected to the RVF. To test this, we created two sets of noun pairs matched for frequency and length. One set consisted of pairs with a small semantic difference in meaning (e.g. salary/work), the other set with a more distant semantic relationship (e.g. autumn/age). These latter pairs also had poetic connotations. The pairs of words were presented tachistoscopically for 100 ms to either the LVF or the RVF. Forty-six normal, right-handed subjects were investigated. They were asked to press response keys whenever they felt that the two words were related to each other in meaning. The results of this experiment are pre-

sented in Fig. 17.28 (Rodel, 1989; Rodel *et al.*, 1989; Landis and Regard, 1989). A significant ($p < 0.001$) interaction between the hemispheres was involved and a semantic difference was found. This result indicates that the two hemispheres appreciate word meanings differently and also implies the presence of two different types of reading strategies in each hemisphere.

Recognition of Kanji Signs and Kana Words

Hatta (1977a, b) found LVF superiority for normal Japanese subjects who were asked to identify single Kanji signs. This superiority was greater for 'concrete' words than for 'abstract' ones. In comparing the recognition of words composed of Kanji or of Kana signs, an LVF advantage was also found for Kanji, while the reverse was true for Kana (Hatta, 1981). A similar LVF superiority was found for Chinese subjects who were asked to read Chinese characters (Tzeng *et al.*, 1979). It was suggested that the contribution of the left and right hemispheres in reading and understanding Kanji signs depended on the levels of processing, shifting from right hemisphere advantage to left hemisphere superiority when a shift from elementary perception to verbal recognition occurred. In accordance with this interpretation, Hatta (1981) reported an LVF advantage for physical identity matching of Kanji signs, and an RVF advantage for semantic congruency decisions. These differences were confirmed by Hatta *et al.*, (1983), indica-

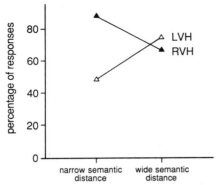

Fig. 17.28 *Tachistoscopic test in 46 right-handed normals. Pairs of words were projected to the centre of the visual field and to the parafoveal region shifted horizontally to the right or left side of the fovea centralis (2–4 degrees). The subject had to press the key whenever two words seemed to be related to each other in meaning. Words with a narrow semantic distance led to a higher correct recognition when projected into the right visual field than to the left. When the semantic distance was wide, however, the right-visual-field advantage disappeared and a small left-visual-field advantage appeared (Landis and Regard, 1989).*

ting shorter RT values for responses to two physically identical Kanji signs when projected to the LVF rather than to the RVF (730 ms/740 ms). Decision time for semantic classification (recognition of an identical category, such as plant or animal) was more than 100 ms longer; such a classification showed RVF advantage (860/825 ms). Hartje *et al.* (1986) compared the reponses of German subjects who had had no prior knowledge of the Japanese language. They had to discriminate 20 Kana characters, 20 'simple' Kanji characters composed of 3 to 5 strokes, and 20 'complex' Kanji characters composed of 10 to 15 strokes. The same stimuli were used by Hojo, Willmes and Hartje (unpublished) for Japanese subjects. First, a stimulus was projected for 100 ms into the foveal region, which was subsequently masked by a random dot disc; thereafter, either different or identical Kanji or Kana characters were projected approximately 3 degrees eccentrically to the LVF or RVF. The subjects were asked to respond if they thought the two stimuli were identical. Although reaction time increased in the German subjects from Kana to simple Kanji and from simple Kanji to complex Kanji (435 to 505 ms), no significant difference between LVF and RVF RTs were observed. The response differences to Kana and Kanji signs in the LVF and RVF are thus not caused by different structural complexities, but rather by learned linguistic competence.

Reading Shorthand

As discussed above and in more detail in Chapter 18,

Western shorthand stenography may under certain circumstances serve as an analogue to Kanji reading. The differences in reading normal script and shorthand are believed to correspond to the differences in reading Kana and Kanji. We tested by means of tachistoscopy whether differences between the ability to read print and stenography in patients suffering from pure alexia is also present in normal subjects (Regard *et al.*, 1985). Two identical conditions were used in the experiment, with the exception that in one condition, the words and non-words were written in regular upper-case print, in the other, in German 'Stolze-Schrey' stenography. Two four-letter strings were presented, one in the LVF and the other in the RVF. These letter strings formed either a German word or a pronounceable 'German' non-word. In another set of measurements, two pronounceable German non-words were projected, one into the LVF, the other into the RVF. The subjects had to press a response key whenever they thought they saw a real German word. The experiments were run at three different exposure times: 150, 100 and 50 ms. As illustrated in Fig. 17.29, lexical decisions on printed words resulted in RVF advantage, independent of exposure time. When the same words were written in shorthand stenography, however, the visual field advantage shifted to an LVF superiority at short exposure times. From these results, one can derive a hierarchy of stimulus factors determining the left- or right-hemisphere contribution to word recognition. Under certain conditions, stimulus form (writing system) can become a stronger deciding factor than stimulus duration (exposure time).

'Reading' and 'Writing' in Apes

In 1748, Julien Offray de la Mettrie (1709–51) published *L'homme machine*, in which

> *he put on paper some vigorous thoughts about materialism . . . . This work, which was bound to displease men who, by their position, are declared enemies of the progress of human reason, roused also the priests of Leyden against its author . . .*
> (Frederick II of Prussia, 1752)

In this book, LaMettrie not only presented a mechanistic–materialistic interpretation of brain function, but also suggested that great apes might be intelligent enough to learn language by means of training methods which had been introduced at that time by the Swiss teacher Johann Konrad Ammann (1669–1730), who had taught deaf-mutes to speak by having them imitate the motion of his lips, tongue and larynx. Since Ammann was also able to teach deaf-mutes to read and write using this method, la Mettrie thought that visual training could be used to develop language abilities in apes. He did not consider using abstract symbols or gestures to allow for

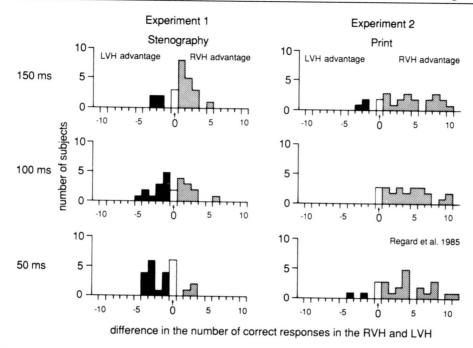

Fig. 17.29 *Experiments performed in 24 normal subjects, all proficient in short-hand stenography. In Experiment 1, a pair of stenographically written words was projected into the visual fields, one to the left visual hemifield (LVH), the other to the right visual hemifield (RVH). Three exposure times were as indicated on the left side of the figure. In Experiment 2, the same tachistoscopic test was performed with strings of printed letters. The subjects had to discriminate between words and non-words. The recognition of stenographically written words or non-words necessary in a lexical decision led to a left-visual-field advantage for short exposure times, while for 150 ms exposure time, a right-visual-field advantage was present. In contrast, the same lexical decision required for printed words led to a right-visual-field advantage for all exposure times. For further explanation see text (Regard et al., 1985, modified).*

communication between apes and humans, methods which have been first applied only during the last 30 years. In the nineteenth century and in the first half of the twentieth century, repeated attempts were made in vain to teach young chimpanzees a human language. W. and L. Kellog trained a female chimpanzee raised in their home to understand about 100 words, but she was not able to pronounce a single one. K. and C. Hayes have reported a similar experience. This failure was finally recognized as a problem connected with the animals' phonation abilities.

The American psychologists A. and B. Gardner (1971) taught the female chimpanzee Washoe American sign language. Washoe managed to learn a fairly impressive set of different gestures made with fingers and hands and used these signs to communicate with the investigators. A. J. and D. Premack taught a young chimpanzee Sarah to read and 'write' using tokens of different shapes and colours, whereby each token represented a word. Sarah acquired a 'vocabulary' which allowed her to express elementary wishes and needs. The combination of different tokens led to short logographic or pictographic sentences. The

investigators taught the animal conditional relations, class concept of colour and negations. The ability of these apes to use symbols arranged in a certain sequence in order to express desire or 'opinions' is now accepted by most investigators (for discussion see Premack and Premack, 1972; Rumbaugh, 1977; Gardner and Gardner, 1984; Savage-Rumbaugh *et al.*, 1985, 1986). It seems that this ability varies considerably in different species of hominoids; the most 'intelligent' subjects were pygmy chimpanzees (*Pan paniscus*). One of these animals even spontaneously began to use symbols to communicate; he learned without being directly taught, and could use graphic symbols which he had learned by imitating human behaviour. This animal also understood many spoken English words, and 'wrote' in multi-word utterances. This case (Savage-Rumbaugh, 1986) provided a new argument against the generally sceptical attitude in regard to whether or not apes can really produce meaningfully structured sentences (Terrace *et al.*, 1979).

Under natural conditions, the pygmy chimpanzee (*Pan paniscus*) uses a richer and more varied repertoire of gestures and vocal signs than do common chimpanzees *(Pan troglodytes)* (Savage and Wilkerson, 1978). In comparison with other apes, the pygmy chimpanzee is considered by some researchers to be more similar to the australopithecines than the other great apes (Zihlman *et al.*, 1978; Zihlman, 1984). Savage-Rumbaugh *et al.* (1985) reported on a young male pygmy chimpanzee who could use the communication system designed by Rumbaugh (1977); it consisted of non-iconic graphic symbols placed on touch-sensitive plates. A computer recorded each time a symbol was touched. At 6 months of age, the subject Kanzi learned to use graphic symbols by observing his mother Matata, who was at the time being trained at the Yerkes language research centre to use these symbols to request different kinds of food, outdoor trips, grooming etc. Kanzi was not trained at all, but could observe his mother. When Kanzi was one and a half years old, he spontaneously showed interest in the symbols his mother was learning and started to interfere with his mother's activity, 'slapping haphazardly at the keys' (Savage-Rumbaugh *et al.*, 1985). When Kanzi was two and a half years old, his mother was separated from him for breeding purposes. Kanzi subsequently became strongly bound to his human caretaker. During his mother's absence, he began to use the keyboard, selecting goal-directed specific symbols; he also gestured to his caretaker to show what he meant after pressing a key. Thus he asked for food by pressing the appropriate keys, and was able to select the one that he had requested when several types of food were presented by using the correct key. Further research was done in order to see whether or not Kanzi could learn by observing others using the keyboard. During this 'verbal' learning period, it was evident that Kanzi very carefully observed the human caretaker who wandered about with him through the rather large 55-acre habitat in search of food, etc. Kanzi used the correct symbols to request walks in the habitat to different places where different types of food were stored. Within the first week of his mother's absence, Kanzi was able to use the eight symbols which the investigators had tried to teach his mother during the previous year. Unlike other chimpanzees, Kanzi used symbols for absent objects, i.e. for food available only some distance away somewhere in the habitat. Since he did not like to walk alone in the woods, he 'convinced' his care-

taker to take him to those places by using abstract signs indicating the specific food available at a given place. When approaching this spot, Kanzi was able to lead the caretaker to the correct place, i.e. he had associated the place, the specific food available at that place and the abstract sign indicating that food. Savage-Rumbaugh *et al.*'s other observations (1985) were equally remarkable:

> *In the evening when Kanzi is getting ready for bed, he uses his keyboard to ask for various items that are not present and that he does not wish to get for himself . . . . He often asked for more 'blankets', which he uses to build a large sleeping nest and for his 'ball' which he likes to sleep with . . . . He frequently also asks for something cold to drink at night such as water, ice, ice water, Coke, etc . . . .*

Kanzi also used the panel symbols for social interaction, such as tickling or chasing; when tired, he asked to be 'hugged'. Kanzi's vocabulary growth and combinatorial utterances increased with age. The list published by Savage-Rumbaugh *et al.* (1985) indicates that most of his vocabulary was related to food. By using the keyboard, Kanzi also asked people to perform certain operations using requests such as 'chase person', 'chase Kanzi', 'apple me eat', etc. The investigators realized that the verbal use of English words in Kanzi's presence helped him to find the symbols on his keyboards; they also noted that Kanzi responded to conversations not concerning him. For example, when he heard another chimpanzee's name, e.g. 'Austin', he immediately came down to the keyboard and pressed the key with the symbol for Austin and simultaneously gestured to go towards Austin's cage.

These observations indicate that under optimal conditions, chimpanzees are able to use man-made symbols rather than gestures for visual communication; in this way, they can express wishes and needs to the caretaker or investigator.

In summary, these and other studies on the 'reading' ability of great apes indicate that at least the more intelligent ones are able to use visual symbols in an abstract way, correlate these symbols with behavioural goals or actions and combine symbols to create very short meaningful strings of information, which can be interpreted as the most elementary type of 'sentence'.

18 Lost Letters: Pure Alexia

Definition

Summarizing nearly a century of research, Benson and Geschwind (1969) defined alexia as 'an incapacity in the comprehension of written or printed words produced by a cerebral lesion, referring only to acquired defects in contrast to dyslexia (Critchley, 1967), a term designating an innate or constitutional inability to learn to read.' Alexia is most frequently reported in the frame of aphasia, i.e. an acquired language disorder, where written language may be affected as well. In the context of visual agnosia, we will deal only with 'pure alexia', a 'visual' disorder or a disorder of impaired visual–verbal integration. In this primarily visual variety of alexia the core feature is the loss of the ability to read printed or handwritten material with a retained ability to write both from dictation and spontaneously. This peculiar condition has been given a number of different names such as 'occipital alexia', 'alexia without agraphia', 'posterior alexia', 'sensory alexia', 'agnosic alexia', 'optic alexia', 'pure word blindness', 'verbal alexia', 'primary alexia', 'receptive alexia' and 'pure alexia' (Benson, 1979). The different terms used by various authors show the differences in weight which have been put upon either the purity of alexia with respect to the absence of aphasia and especially agraphia, the exclusive sensory, receptive or agnosic nature of this syndrome, or the anatomical location of the lesion leading to this syndrome. An exception is made by the term 'verbal alexia', which refers to the inability of such patients to read words, while frequently, but not always, they are able to read letters. 'Literal alexia' or 'letter blindness' is an inability to recognize letters; it appears usually in the frame of a non-fluent aphasia, which will not be discussed here. Throughout this chapter we will use the term pure alexia ('*Reine Wortblindheit*'), well knowing that in the past the term 'pure' has been disputed because virtually always some other neurological or neuropsychological accompanying signs can be found (Beringer and Stein, 1930; De Massary, 1932/1933). As with other neurological behaviour disturbances, we feel that the word 'pure' does not stand for an isolated symptom but rather for a symptom which dominates the clinical picture. Thus the term pure alexia is used in the following to describe an alexia without significant agraphia or aphasia.

Historical Review and Clinical Signs of Pure Alexia

Literacy is of course the prerequisite for alexia to be reported. In past times when literacy was the exception, alexia must have been rare compared with aphasia. However, the striking phenomenon of a person perfectly capable of writing spontaneously, but no longer being able to read his own written production, impressed people even in antiquity to the point of their leaving testimony. No reports on alexia have been found so far on the clay tablets of cuneiform script (H. J. Nissen, personal communication, 1989), while the earliest report in the Latin tradition, cited by Benton (1964) in his paper on aphasia before the time of Broca, dates from 30 AD. Valerius Maximus described a man who lost his memory for letters subsequent to a head injury and who appeared to have no other defects. Benton (1964) cites other early reports of alexia, namely by Mercuriale in 1588 of a patient, who subsequent to a generalized seizure could write but could not read what he had written. Johann Schmidt in 1673 reported on two alexic patients, one of whom improved in reading with retraining and Johann Gessner described in 1770 a patient in whom the alexia was more pronounced in his native German than in Latin (cf. Chapter 2).

In the nineteenth century and especially around the time of Broca a small number of reports on patients with pure alexia were published, in some of which for the first time findings now commonly associated with this syndrome were described. As early examples of pure alexia in the French literature, Charcot (1887) mentioned Genderin, who in 1838 reported patients who could not read but could write letters, and Trousseau who in 1865 described a patient who was not aphasic but could not read newspaper headlines and could not read what he had written correctly (for review see also De Massary, 1933).

Between 1870 and 1890 there was a growing interest in the anatomical and functional disorders leading to alexia, and a good number of patients with more or less pure alexia, some with associated clinical findings, as well as the first postmortem study were reported. Broadbent (1872) in his paper on 'Cerebral mechanism of speech and thought' described a patient (case 8) who, following an acute cerebral ischaemic attack, could no longer read printed or written words, while he wrote correctly from dictation and composed and wrote letters with a little prompting. He said: 'I can see them' pointing to words, 'but cannot understand'. The only exception to his reading inability was his own name, which he recognized whether printed or written but could not be sure whether the initials or full Christian names were given. This observation is the first, to our knowledge, pointing to what nowadays is called 'covert knowledge', namely an instance in which meaning was conveyed without the awareness of detailed recognition. Whatever aspect, emotional connotation or shape (perhaps the overlearned appearance of his own name) triggered correct detection remains in this case an open question, but this peculiar phenomenon has been described repeatedly and received increasing attention in recent years. Broadbent's (1872) case suffered from a relatively pure alexia with respect to the absence of agraphia and aphasia, but displayed a severe naming disorder. This patient was tested on a variety of visually presented stimuli including colours, which he failed to name. Broadbent thus described one of the frequent deficits associated with pure alexia, namely colour anomia and anomic amnesic aphasia, indicating an involvement of left inferior parietal lobe structures.

Broadbent's patient was the first case of pure alexia which came to autopsy. He died about two months after the first stroke from a massive haemorrhage involving large parts of the left hemisphere, which did not permit a definite anatomo–clinical correlation. Broadbent, however, drew particular attention to an old infarction which he found in addition to the fresh haemorrhage in the white matter below the left parieto–occipital junction. He suggested that this earlier infarction, which was localized at a crucial carrefour of fibre tracts necessary for visuo–verbal information transfer and also impinging upon callosal fibres, could be responsible for the alexia.

Westphal (1874) described an actor (case 3) who became mildly anomic, paretic on the right side and could not read what he had easily written from dictation a few moments earlier. Westphal reported to our knowledge for the first time the phenomenon that his patient, though not able to read, managed to recognize single letters by tracing them with his finger and thus, by using proprioceptive input and possibly motor efference copying, was able to read a few words in a letter-by-letter sequence while virtually rewriting them (see below). Only a few years later, Charcot (1887), who was fascinated by this phenomenon, presented the first experimental analysis of a patient with pure alexia, who also showed some reading ability by tracing letters – in this case, however, in the air with his right hand. Even when he traced the letters behind his back, he could recognize them in the same way. Using this special ability, Charcot documented a steady improvement in letter-by-letter reading over the days of training, as measured by the time used for reading a single line. Charcot's patient could recognize words even when one moved his hand holding a pen over the letters. He apparently relied upon the recognition of sensorimotor engrams and had a greater facility to recognize his own writing by motor tracings than printed material. Charcot also demonstrated the importance of the word meaning by measuring the speed of recognition. Highly overlearned words with some emotional connotation, such as '*république*' took his patient only a few seconds to decipher, while other quite familiar words such as '*indépendance*' were read only after a delay of one minute.

Another important defect recognized relatively early as being associated with pure alexia is a right homonymous hemianopia. This finding was first reported to our knowledge by Westphal (1874), although he did not consider this visual field defect as being responsible for the inability to read. By 1890 the association of a right hemianopia with the syndrome of pure alexia was already common knowledge among those interested in aphasia and related disorders. The first to have clearly outlined pure alexia as a distinct entity and given it a name, namely '*Wortblindheit*', generally is considered to be Kussmaul in his book *Die Störungen der Sprache* (1877). By 1890 the syndrome of pure alexia (*Wortblindheit, cécité verbale*) as a clinical entity was well established, documented by some 20 published cases reviewed beautifully by Charcot (1887; also citing the cases of Guéneau de Mussy, 1879; Bertholle, 1881; Chauffard, 1881; Skwortzoff, 1881; Armaignac, 1882; D'Heilly and Chantenesse, 1883).

Major progress in the understanding of pure alexia was achieved through two papers published by Dejerine in 1891 and 1892. In the first (1891) he presented a patient who 8 months before his death suddenly realized that he could no longer read and write, other than his own name. There was no visual field defect or aphasia except for a mild verbal paraphasia, which subsequently disappeared, while reading and writing remained impossible. At autopsy an old infarct involving the major part of the cortex of the angular gyrus with an extension to the occipital horn of the lateral ventricle on the left side was found.

In the second paper Dejerine (1892) presented the clinical and autopsy findings of a patient referred to him by the ophthalmologist Landolt (1888a, b), who had already detected alexia, right partial hemianopia and complete right hemiachromatopsia. Dejerine followed this patient closely for over 4 years until his death subsequent to a second stroke, which left him severely aphasic for the last 10 days. After the first stroke this patient had become suddenly alexic for letters and words without having lost the ability to write. His language, auditory comprehension, naming and general intelligence were reported to have remained entirely normal. Writing was somewhat easier when done with the eyes closed than when looking at what he had written. Objects placed in the right visual half field appeared 'dimmer and less clear' than in the left visual field. In addition a complete and dense right hemiachromatopsia existed, but colour naming in free vision was not impaired. While writing from dictation was normal and fluent, copying written information was slow, impaired and performed as in 'slavish' drawing. Dejerine's detailed case analysis contained a number of new associated symptoms, which later became known to frequently accompany pure alexia: his patient had no difficulty in reading numbers, even long ones, and performing written arithmetic operations. He also could not read musical scores any more, but could write them. He had, however, not lost his sense of music, continued to sing correctly and had even learned by ear the scores of new operas composed during the years after his stroke. At autopsy two lesions were found in the left hemisphere. There was a fresh infarct involving most of the left angular gyrus, an old infarction covering the territory of the left posterior cerebral artery entirely and involving posterior and inferomedial aspects of the occipital lobe and the occipitotemporal junction, as well as a small infarction of the posterior end of the splenium of the corpus callosum.

Dejerine's first patient became alexic and agraphic due to a lesion in the left angular gyrus, while his second patient with pure alexia had a left infero-medial occipitotemporal as well as a small splenial lesion. The latter later became aphasic and agraphic, however, following a second infarct in the left angular gyrus. Dejerine thus conjectured that the angular gyrus of the language dominant hemisphere was a centre for the optic images necessary for written language. Since in his second patient with pure alexia, this centre of optic images for letter and words was initially intact, it was clear for Dejerine that language, and writing, as well as writing on dictation, had to be normal. Dejerine specifically referred to the two varieties of alexia proposed on theoretical grounds by Wernicke (1874; 1881; 1886) – namely cortical and subcortical alexia. While the former was viewed as being due to a lesion in the centre of the visual images for written language, in the latter this centre was thought to be intact, but disconnected from its visual input. The two cases presented by Dejerine provided the most beautiful anatomical verification of these theoretical predictions. Much controversy, however, arose from the fact that Dejerine did not consider the small lesion in the posterior part of the splenium of the corpus callosum to be of much importance in the clinical syndrome of subcortical – or pure alexia. He stated:

The lesion in the white matter underlying the left occipital lobe, considering its extension towards the ventricular ependyma, was sufficiently large to interrupt the fibres which connect the two occipital lobes with the left angular gyrus, without having to have recourse to explain the disconnection by the small lesion at the end of the splenium of the corpus callosum. There is too little known about the effects of callosal lesions to insist upon their importance.

Both Dejerine and Wernicke viewed pure alexia as a syndrome of disconnection. While Dejerine postulated a centre for the optic images necessary for written language in the area of the inferior parietal lobule, Wernicke did not consider letters to be sufficiently different from other visual information, such as objects, symbols, etc., to merit a special centre. In his view (Wernicke, 1903) the optic images necessary for written language are generated in the visual system of both hemispheres, while visual–linguistic recognition is elaborated in the left hemisphere. The disconnection is thus situated between the language area in the left dominant hemisphere and the visual letter images (in particular their auditory component), which are generated bilaterally. Thus, for Wernicke, a callosal lesion or a lesion disrupting callosal fibres was mandatory, while for Dejerine only disruption of those callosal fibres reaching the left gyrus angularis region was relevant. Out of this theoretical argument has grown a controversy about the importance of the additional splenial lesion, frequently present in posterior cerebral artery strokes. In particular the influence of size, location and aetiology of splenial lesions upon the occurrence of pure alexia and associated symptoms has been investigated. This controversy, reviewed by Hécaen and Kremin (1976) and Greenblatt (1977), is documented by a series of papers extending over a period of 80 years (Redlich, 1895; Hinshelwood, 1900; Brissaud, 1900; Wernicke, 1903; Souques, 1907; Bonvicini and Pötzl, 1907; Foix, 1925; Foix and Hillemand, 1925; Quensel, 1927; Hoff and Pötzl, 1937; Trescher and Ford, 1937; Péron and Goutner, 1944; Nilson, 1946; Maspes, 1948; Hécaen *et al.*, 1952; Alajouanine *et al.*, 1960; Kinsbourne and Warrington, 1963; Ajax, 1964, 1967; Hécaen and Angelergues, 1963; Geschwind and Fusillo, 1966; Oxbury *et al.*, 1969; Cumming *et al.*, 1970; Goldstein *et al.*, 1971; Wechsler *et al.*, 1972; Greenblatt, 1973; Iwata *et al.*, 1974; Greenblatt, 1976; Hécaen and Gruner 1974).

By the turn of the century the two varieties of alexia – alexia with agraphia, and alexia without agraphia (pure alexia) – were well established entities, widely recognized, and the localization of the lesions leading to this syndrome was common knowledge among the neurologists and ophthalmologists of that time. Dejerine's and Wernicke's theories concerning the origin of alexia were generally accepted and used to explain these acquired reading disturbances. Outside the strictly neurological field the interest in the different varieties of reading disturbances is documented by a number of case reports on pure alexia around 1900 in leading ophthalmology journals, for example *Graefes's Archiv für Opthalmologie*, or internal-medicine-oriented journals such as *The Lancet*. Subsequent to a number of papers in the *The Lancet*, Hinshelwood (1900) published a first monograph on *Letter-, Word- and Mind-blindness* referring to a series of 28 cases of 'mind blindness', including 6 of his own patients. Further reviews in English on pure alexia include that by Weisenburg and McBride (1935/1964), Holmes (1950) and more recently Benson and Geschwind (1969), updated by Benson (1985). In French, subsequent to Charcot's (1887) early review, a comprehensive review is provided by de Massary (1932/1933) and more recently by Hécaen and co-workers in a series of monographs (Dubois-Charlier, 1976; Hécaen and Kremin, 1976). In German, Lange (1936) reviewed the German contributions in Bumke and Foerster's *Handbook of Neurology*, and more recently Leischner (1957) wrote a book on this topic. Anatomical perspectives of alexia were stressed in the papers by Greenblatt (1977), Damasio and Damasio (1983) and De Renzi *et al.* (1987).

While connectionist ideas about brain functioning persisted in the European writings on alexia, they were virtually absent in American medical publications until the early 1960s. At this point Geschwind's paper on the 'Disconnection syndromes in animals and men' (1965) and the studies in split-brain patients (Sperry *et al.*, 1969) revived clinical interest in pure alexia, especially among American behavioural neurologists. It may be a historical curiosity that the first described case of pure alexia due to a brain tumour was presented at the Tuesday conference of the neurological Institute of New York in March 1913 by Casamajor: a 35-year-old patient with a right homonymous hemianopia and bilateral papilloedema suffered from a severe alexia without agraphia and a very slight sensory aphasia caused by a tumour in the mesial wall of the posterior part of the left lateral ventricle. What is remarkable about Casamajor's case presentation is the quotation of Wernicke's original work, of Liepmann's views about alexia and agraphia and of Dejerine's hypothesis about a centre of visual word memory. Casamajor presented a diagram from Liepmann implying full understanding of the current views of interhemispheric as well as intrahemispheric disconnection, apparently assuming his audience to be familiar with these ideas, only recently rediscovered by American neurologists.

By now, well over 200 cases of pure alexia have been

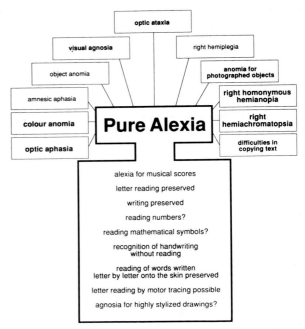

Fig. 18.1 *Scheme of other symptoms related most frequently to pure alexia. The print size of this figure is loosely correlated with the frequency of the symptom association with pure alexia. In the lower part the main symptoms of pure alexia are listed; those associated only casually with alexia are indicated by a question mark.*

published – the syndrome and its anatomical correlates are well established – but variations in pure alexia, associated symptoms, incongruencies and its frequent absence in spite of the classical lesions continue to make pure alexia a phenomenon worthy of research investigations and reports.

Symptoms Frequently Associated with Pure Alexia

Many findings associated with pure alexia have been mentioned in the first studies on alexia (Fig. 18.1). Thus Broadbent described knowledge about the meaning of a specific letter configuration, such as the patient's own name, without the ability to read it, Westphal and Charcot the preservation of single-letter reading improved especially by tracing, Westphal the presence of a concomitant right homonymous hemianopia, Broadbent the frequent association with anomia, Charcot the importance of the meaning of the word in relation to the recognition by speed of tracing. Dejerine emphasized the difficulty in copying written material, and Landolt and Dejerine emphasized the association with hemiachromatopsia. Another important finding associated with pure alexia is the inability to name colours (cf. Chapter 20), when patients can recognize colours by matching or pointing but are unable to name them correctly, and are able to name other visual information without problems. This important association has been emphasized by Pötzl (1928) and in the German literature has been called Pötzl's syndrome ever since. Pötzl (1928) in his seminal work *Die optisch-agnostischen Störungen*, quoted Wilbrand (1887) as the first to have recognized the frequent association of the inability to recognize written symbols with the impairment of colour naming. Although Pötzl considered this combination to be a syndrome, he felt

that this syndrome is best understood if one considers that pure alexia and colour agnosia represent two different optic–agnosic varieties, whose clinical concomitance is best explained by the spatial neighbourhood of the cerebral areas which, when lesioned, produce these two different kinds of optic agnosias regularly.

He considered amnesic aphasia restricted to colours (colour anomia) as a 'special variety of an optic aphasia', in contrast to the view of earlier authors including Wilbrand, who considered colour anomia to be a primary disturbance in naming. Subsequently other members of the Viennese school of neurology (Gloning *et al.*, 1966b; 1968) as well as French authors such as Hécaen *et al.* (1957) have extensively studied the association of pure alexia and colour anomia and have also found that this combination is frequent, but by no means compulsory, and that both pure alexia and colour anomia may be present alone. This long-known association of the inability to name letters and words as well as colours has been revived in the English literature by Geschwind and Fusillo (1966) and Geschwind (1965) in the 'neo-disconnectionistic' approach to higher cortical focal disturbances, an approach which around the turn of the century had also been taken by Liepmann, not only for the apraxic syndrome, for which he is well known, but also for agnosic symptoms in his paper '*Über die agnostischen Störungen*' (1908).

The inability to recognize letters and words as well as colours while preserving the ability to recognize numbers has been explained by Geschwind by the fact that letters and colours are learned exclusively through the visual modality, unlike numbers which are learned by tactile counting, therefore opening multimodal visuo–tactile associations transferred through extrasplenial callosal fibres. Yet another complex of visual disturbances frequently associated with pure alexia is 'optic aphasia' and 'visual object agnosia'. This association was noted very early (Freund, 1889; Henschen, 1890, 1892; Lissauer, 1890; Bruns and Stölting, 1894) and throughout the history of pure alexia it has been a controversal topic, complicated by differences in the conceptualization of the visual agnosias and in lesion localization and aetiologies. Pure

alexia has been described as a part of a general visual agnosic syndrome, frequently accompanied also by topographical disorientation (Dide and Botcazo, 1902; Adler, 1944; Holmes, 1950). In a similar manner widespread visual agnosic symptoms during recovery from cortical blindness, usually due to bilateral occipital infarcts or general hypoxia, may be accompanied by alexia without agraphia, a form called by Pötzl (1928) 'asthenopic alexia'. Alexia has also been viewed in the frame of the so-called simultanagnosia (Wolpert, 1924) (Chapter 11). Along this line a number of authors (Davidenkov, 1956a, b; Luria, 1959; Kinsbourne and Warrington, 1962) have viewed alexic disturbances. The patient described in Chapter 19 suffering from movement agnosia, for example, was not able to read normal newspaper text, since she felt 'totally disturbed by the many different letters', interfering with each other and preventing word recognition. Thus she prepared a mask by means of a sheet of paper and moved the window of this mask along the headlines of the newspaper text. She reported that by this measure reading speed was greatly reduced, of course, but she became able again to grasp what was going on in the world (Grüsser, unpubl. 1985).

Major theoretical problems arose with optic aphasia, however, and with the associative form of object agnosia, both syndromes in which lesions identical to those associated with pure alexia are regularly found. Such cases, although rare, also suffer as a rule from pure alexia (Freund, 1889; Lissauer, 1890; Mueller, 1892; Souques, 1907; Niessl von Mayendorff, 1935; Scheller, 1966; Lhermitte and Beauvois, 1973; Caplan and Hedley-White, 1974; Hécaen *et al.*, 1974; Pillon *et al.*, 1981; Morin *et al.*, 1984; Ferro and Santos, 1984; Larrabee *et al.*, 1985; for review see Benson and Geschwind, 1969; De Renzi *et al.*, 1987). The general question as to whether pure alexia is just a subform of optic aphasia or associative visual agnosia, or a disturbance related to impaired access to a necessary centre for generating the optic images of written language, or a peripheral 'perceptual' form of written language disturbance, remains unresolved and has been the subject of intensive investigations over the last 50 years, and in particular during the last 15. As argued in Chapter 17, pure alexia can also be considered a 'visual *pars-pro-toto* defect' of the speech-dominant hemisphere and the prediction is made that patients suffering from pure alexia should also have some impairment in recognizing objects from their parts. Pure alexia, optic aphasia and associative visual agnosia, although occurring with similarly placed lesions, do not necessarily occur together. A number of patients have been reported in whom these three entities were found in isolation (e.g. Davidenkov, 1956; Gloning *et al.*, 1955; Hécaen *et al.*, 1957; Gomori and Hawryluk, 1984).

Subsequently the approach to visual agnosia and associated symptoms was two-fold: some authors (Hécaen *et al.*, 1952; Hécaen *et al.*, 1957; Alajouanine *et al.*, 1960; Hécaen and Angelergues, 1963; Hécaen and Angelergues, 1965; Hécaen *et al.*, 1967; Gloning *et al.*, 1968; Damasio and Damasio, 1983; De Renzi *et al.*, 1987) have analysed large series of patients with similarly placed posterior lesions of various aetiologies with a standardized set of experimental tests including careful clinical investigations. Such an approach permitted an outline of the frequency distribution of pure alexia and its associated symptoms with respect to the anatomical correlate. Other authors, especially in the last 20 years, have analysed single cases of pure alexia with experimental tests designed to investigate the functional nature of the reading disturbance. From the mid-1960s on, neurolinguists and cognitive neuropsychologists became increasingly interested in alexia in general but also in pure alexia.

Alexia and Neurolinguistic Models

With the application of linguistic and statistical analysis of error types and frequencies to the study of aphasia by Howes (1962) and Goodglass *et al.* (1966, 1969, 1970) a new chapter in the history of language disorders along with that of the alexias began. Two different disciplines, neuro- or psycholinguistics and cognitive psychology or cognitive neuropsychology entered the field of acquired language and reading disturbances by analysing the performances of patients having suffered from cerebral lesions in the dominant hemisphere.

These approaches, for the most part without concern for cerebral localization, lesion size, or neurophysiological mechanisms, have given new insight into the nature of language and reading disturbances. By analysing the language performances of single cases within the framework of different linguistic theories or theories of information processing, an increasing number of constantly reshaped models of language or reading processing have been developed. The success and popularity of this approach in recent years is witnessed by an explosive increase in publications, the foundation of new journals in neurolinguistics and cognitive neuropsychology and also a number of books or review chapters (Coltheart *et al.*, 1980; Patterson *et al.*, 1985; Friedman and Albert, 1985; Roeltgen, 1985; Margolin, 1984; Huber, 1977; Caramazza and Berndt, 1978; de Bleser *et al.*, 1987; Patterson, 1981; Frith, 1986; Dubois-Charlier, 1971; Weigl and Bierwisch, 1976; Marshall and Newcombe, 1973; Richardson, 1975; Shallice and Warrington, 1975; Warrington and Shallice, 1979, 1980; Hécaen and Kremin, 1976, Temple, 1987).

Concerning pure alexia, surprisingly few neurolinguistic or cognitive neuropsychology reports deal with this syndrome. In their psychological descriptions of letter-by-letter readers, a syndrome which may be considered a synonym of pure verbal alexia, Patterson and Kay (1982) attempt to explain the paucity of cognitive psychology reports on this syndrome. They also stated:

Nonetheless it is slightly puzzling that cognitive psychologists have largely ignored this syndrome, at least until very recently (for exceptions see Gardner and Zurif, 1975; Staller et al., 1978; Warrington and Shallice, 1980). After all, the existence of a possible neurological account does not preclude accounts at other levels of description. Indeed it has been argued that neurological data such as lesion site place no constraints whatsoever on psychological or functional descriptions. One reason for contributing to the relative neglect of this syndrome within cognitive psychology may be this: letter-by-letter reading is not, in the terminology of Shallice and Warrington (1980), a form of central dyslexia but is rather one of the peripheral dyslexias. The function locus of the deficit in letter-by-letter reading is probably 'prelinguistic', i.e. relatively 'early' in an information processing sense. Questions about reading likely to be of interest to many cognitive psychologists, such as the organization of the internal lexicon or the semantic system, may be addressed more clearly by syndromes of central dyslexias (deep dyslexia, phonological dyslexia and surface dyslexia) than by peripheral dyslexias (attentional dyslexia, dyslexia involving neglect, and letter-by-letter reading).

On theoretical grounds Patterson and Kay (1982) even questioned whether cognitive psychologists should be interested at all in pure alexia, since a disruption of function at a relatively early stage of signal processing might mean that the rest of the system was normal. They analysed four patients with pure alexia (letter-by-letter readers) and found no evidence that comprehension of a word could occur prior to or in the absence of the letter-by-letter analysis required for oral reading. In two of their patients, an additional lexical deficit often prevented a correctly identified sequence of letters from achieving recognition as the correct word.

At this point it may be worth recalling that Charcot (1887) was the first to use an experimental neurolinguistic approach to pure alexia. He attempted to study the influence of word length and meaning in a pure alexic who was helped by tracing letters by measuring the time the patient needed for recognition.

Two recent topics of interest in the research on pure alexia – namely, alexia in Far-East languages, and access to the meaning of letters and words not recognized – both have historical roots. Reading disturbances different from those observed in Western languages have been reported for a long time in single case studies of Japanese and Chinese patients (Assayama, 1914; Lyman *et al.*, 1938; Panse and Shimoyama, 1955; Sasanuma and Fujimura, 1971; Yamadori, 1975; Hatta, 1977; Sasanuma *et al.*, 1977; Yamadori, 1980; for review see Benson, 1985). In particular the association of alexia for Kanji, an ideographic writing system (Chapter 17), subsequent to lesions in the non-dominant right cerebral hemisphere has triggered conjectures about the non-dominant hemisphere ability to read. Studies with patients proficient in stenography, i.e. in the use of any Western shorthand writing system with many ideographic components, who became alexic led to the same question (Gloning *et al.*, 1955; Regard *et al.*, 1985a, b; for review see Landis, 1987).

Indications that the meaning of words or letters can be accessed without the patient being able to read in the traditional sense were made quite early. As mentioned above, Broadbent's (1872) patient was able to recognize his own name, despite his inability to recognize the initials or the full Christian name; Charcot's (1887) patient recognized the word '*république*' much faster than other words of equal length, and a patient described by Dejerine (1912) showed visual pattern context facilitation: He could not read the letters 'R' and 'F' until they were inscribed on a typical medallion, in which case they corresponded to the initials of '*République Française*' and were immediately recognized. A number of recent papers concerned with similar observations at different levels of word comprehension in pure alexia will be described later in detail (Kreindler and Ionescu, 1961; Caplan and Hedley-Whyte, 1974; Stachowiak and Poeck, 1976; Assal and Regli, 1980; Landis *et al.*, 1980; Warrington and Shallice, 1979, 1980; Grossi *et al.*, 1984; Shallice and Saffran, 1986; Coslett and Saffran, 1989; Landis, 1987; Landis and Regard, 1988).

Clinical Examination of Alexic Patients

The vast majority of patients with a pure alexia have suffered a stroke in the territory of the left posterior cerebral artery. As a rule, they are aware of their inability to read and it is usually this deficit which leads them to seek medical help. They may be unaware of their capacity to write, or of some preserved comprehension of written material (Regard *et al.*, 1985b), or of their hemianopia, but as far as we know, they never deny alexia. This is in contrast to patients who have suffered infarctions in the territory of the right posterior cerebral artery. Quite frequently alexic patients initially put the blame, as do illiterates in our society, on eye problems such as poor sight and ever since the famous patient of Dejerine (1892) the ophthalmologist is often the first medical person they see (Landolt, 1888a, b).

Since it is well known that reading disturbances may be due exclusively to peripheral visual problems or to primary visual sensory disturbances, it is mandatory in cases of pure alexia that a careful examination of visual function

be performed. Depending upon the clinical situation and the technical possibilities, a test for visual acuity (using Landolt rings or other, non-letter-like symbols), a light and colour perimetry and tests for visual neglect should at least be carried out (Chapters 9 and 22). If technical means are available, more extensive visual testing including measurement of spatial frequencies, form perimetry and visuo-motor tracking tasks should be conducted (for review see Zihl and von Cramon, 1986).

The clinical examination is directed on the one hand towards detecting perceptual factors and on the other to excluding concomitant agnosia or aphasia, which could easily account for the occurrence of alexia. Moreover, one has to define the reading disturbance itself. Besides the above-mentioned visuo-perceptual testing, a patient with pure alexia requires a complete aphasia workup, as outlined in many comprehensive texts on clinical aphasiology (e.g. Goodglass and Kaplan, 1972; Huber *et al.*, 1983; Benson, 1979; etc.), and special attention should be given to the examination of associative visual object agnosia, colour and object naming and matching, and verbal memory. De Renzi *et al.* (1987) in their examination of 16 consecutive patients with left posterior cerebral artery infarcts – the lesion typically found in pure alexia – have shown pure alexia to be present in 75 per cent; however, most also had some degree of colour anomia, object anomia and photograph anomia and all showed some degree of verbal memory impairment. Thus alexic patients should be confronted with a large variety of colours, objects, photographs of objects, stylized drawings of objects, unusual views of objects, and facial photographs. They should be asked to name these items, point to them, and match them on visual presentation. Naming should also be tested in the auditory and tactile modality, as De Renzi *et al.* (1987) have also shown deficits in naming with sensory input outside the visual modality. Verbal memory can be tested using standardized procedures such as those described by Wechsler (1945) or Rey (1964). Of special importance is De Renzi *et al.*'s finding (1987) of a particular deficit in naming photographs of objects.

Analysing 23 patients with unilateral posterior cerebral artery lesions, 9 of whom were left-sided, we found pure alexia to be present in 5 of these 9 patients (Landis and Regard, 1988a, b). In two of them a peculiar inability to name highly stylized drawings of objects was present but no difficulty in naming real or photographed objects. Stylized drawings, even more than photographs as compared with real objects, contain a symbolic component and may be considered the opposite of unusual views in terms of accessibility to the object name. Accordingly, in the examination of pure alexics we recommend not only the naming of typical or untypical object views (Warrington and Taylor, 1973), but also that of stylized drawings and partial drawings of objects.

In order to look for simultanagnosia pure alexics should also be confronted with complex scenes and asked to grasp the meaning of the whole scene rather than single items (see Wolpert, 1924; Kinsbourne and Warrington, 1962). More elaborate tests, usually confined to the research situation, include eye-movement monitoring, testing for the 'pop-out' phenomenon in various arrays of texture (Julesz, 1981; Treisman, 1982; Chapter 1) or the short-exposure presentation of the above-mentioned items in a tachistoscope (Kinsbourne and Warrington, 1962; Landis *et al.*, 1980; Patterson and Kay, 1982). In particular the tachistoscopic presentation of stimuli is of importance, since pure alexia might occur in one visual half-field only (Castro-Caldas and Salgado, 1984), while isolated naming defects, e.g. of colours, may occur only on short exposure (Landis *et al.*, 1980).

Tests for writing include the spelling of letters and words and the writing of single upper- and lower-case letters from dictation, single words of different lengths and degrees of concreteness and emotional connotation as well as function words, and sentences. Of importance is the writing of nonsense words. The patient should write in print as well as cursive and the spatial arrangement of written sentences has to be considered.

Copying letters, words, sentences, numbers, mathematical symbols, nonsense signs and drawings as well as the transformation of upper- to lower-case letters should be investigated.

Reading is separated into reading aloud and comprehension of written or spelled information. In reading aloud the patient is asked to read letters, numbers, words and sentences audibly. For the reading of words of different classes, emotional connotations, imaging abilities, and lengths, it is worth measuring the time of the performance, since the so-called letter-by-letter readers may not always display their spelling behaviour overtly, but will take an unduly long time to perform. Tachistoscopic presentation of words of increasing length, as done by several investigators (Kinsbourne and Warrington 1962; Patterson and Kay, 1982), may help to reveal this difficulty. The patient may also be asked to spell the word as quickly as possible and attention should be given to the speed of comprehension, whether it is faster by rapid spelling or by silent reading. The patient should also be asked to read whole sentences out loud. Moreover, and mainly for research purposes, letters as well as letter combinations and words should be presented tachistoscopically in each visual field at different exposure durations in order to assess the time the patient needs in each field to name one or more letters.

Tests for comprehension of printed or cursively written material are usually modified from examiner to examiner. In free vision the comprehension of single letters may be tested by having the patient match upper- to lower-case letters or printed letters to script. Moreover, letters may be

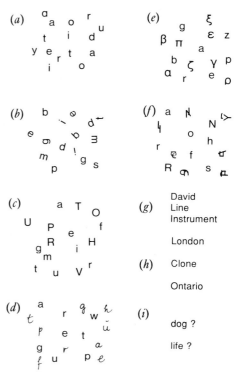

Fig. 18.2 *Simple tests applicable in investigating alexic patients. (a) Finding pairs of letters. (b) Finding pairs of letters written in different orientations. (c) Finding pairs of letters written in upper and lower case. (d) Matching pairs of letters presented in print and in handwriting. (e) Matching pairs of letters in the Latin and Greek alphabets. (f) Discriminating between letters and non-letters. (g) Finding the same letter (i) in three words. (h) Finding a two-letter combination (on) in several words. (i) Finding the three- or four-letter word which consists of the same letters as the word presented.*

matched to spatially rotated letters, or to letters altered in their graphemic components or to 'neographemes' (Huber, 1989; cf. Fig. 18.2). The comprehension of single letters and words may be tested by crosshatching the letters or words (Goldstein and Gelb, 1918; cf. Fig. 18.3) or by presenting these letters in shadow writing or interrupted lines (cf. Fig. 18.4). If recognition after crosshatching fails, the strokes of the letters may be enhanced until recognition takes place despite the now less pronounced crosshatchings. In some patients small movements of the reading target may enhance reading comprehension (Botez *et al.*, 1964). Thus, if the patient fails to comprehend the static information, letters as well as words should be moved in front of him. The same procedure should be done with numbers. An important test in pure alexia is to see whether words spelled out loud are understood. Words

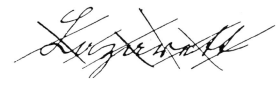

Fig. 18.3 *Cross-hatching of hand-written or printed words can impair reading recognition by alexic patients (from Goldstein and Gelb, 1918). Here the word is 'Lazarett'.*

(a)

(b)

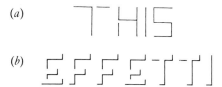

Fig. 18.4 *(a) A broken-line figure which is frequently read by alexic patients as 7415 (Landis et al., 1982). (b) Word composed of shadow letters (from Kanizsa, 1979).*

of different lengths or degrees of complexity may be used (e.g.   U-S/U-S-E/H-O-U-S-E/H-O-U-S-E-W-I-F-E; B-A-L-L/Y-A-C-H-T).

The patient should be tested for the detection of incorrect letters, signs or symbols within otherwise correctly written words and real words of his native language within a group foreign words or non-words (lexical decision). For these real words the degree of word length, word frequency, word class (e.g. function words, nouns, etc.), personal familiarity, imageability, emotionality, or concreteness may be varied. The patient should be asked to sort the words according to semantic classes (e.g. colours vs. furniture, etc.). Words, in particular object names, should be matched with line drawings or photographs of the corresponding object or with the object itself. In this setting distractor pictures representing semantically or graphemically similar items should be presented as well. The patient should be asked to point to the corresponding objects or body parts when shown the written word. He should also execute simple and more complex written commands, in particular those related to whole body movements, such as 'stand up', 'turn round', etc. The patient should also read entire sentences and attempt to indicate their meaning by choosing pictures of corresponding scenes. This list of possible tests for reading comprehension is, of course, incomplete and additional testing would have to be tailored to individual clinical symptoms.

Considering the relative rarity of pure alexia, each of these patients is a potential candidate for more elaborate research investigation. In the frame of alexia research, in

particular when the patient is a letter-by-letter reader, most of the above-mentioned comprehension tests can be adapted to tachistoscopic use. This is of particular importance, since the two visual fields can be tested separately, i.e. the information can be projected into the damaged as well as the non-damaged hemisphere. When employing tachistoscopic techniques, different exposure durations, above and below the patient's ability to read single letters, should be used. Moreover, when the patient fails to give correct answers, he should be encouraged to guess. It has repeatedly been shown that pure alexic patients may display guessing well above chance in situations where they are not consciously aware of being able to gather the meaning of written information. Some of the cueing or guessing techniques used in pure alexic patients to uncover hidden comprehension will be described and discussed below.

Pseudoalexia: Reading Difficulties Due to Spatial Hemineglect and Hemi-inattention

Parietal lobe lesions of the right side and sometimes also frontal eyefield lesions lead to an abolition or reduction of gaze movements goaled towards the contralateral hemifield. This gaze disturbance also affects reading. With right parietal lobe lesions, for example, the patients frequently disregard the left half of a page or column when the print is organized into two or three columns on a page. When asked to read, the patients do so correctly for the right side of the page or column. Intelligent patients confabulate text to achieve meaningful combinations of consecutive lines. They are not aware of having passed over part of the text and, when questioned, they insist, as a rule, that they have read all of the text that is there. When the investigator asks the patient to underline what he is reading with his right index finger, he moves the finger only one-half to two-thirds of the way to the left of the page or column. When the investigator moves the patient's finger to the beginning of the line, the patient starts to read this line correctly, but then disregards the first words on the left on the next line. These patients usually have no difficulty reading single letters or words. Their impairment in reading is caused entirely by hemi-inattention or hemineglect. They read single lines completely when requested to do so in a 'vertical' direction, but have difficulty with this technique in shifting to the next line, which in Western script is inevitably on the left side. Therefore patients with a left spatial hemineglect, even when highly literate, rarely read and sometimes come to the conclusion that what is written is rather 'sketchy' or nonsensical, as reported to one of us (O.-J. G.) by a German poet who incurred a left-sided spatial neglect (cf. Chapter 22).

Cerebral Lesion Localization and Aetiologies in Alexia

Unlike in prosopagnosia, in pure alexia there is little disagreement as to the side and site of lesion. Well over 20 autopsied cases of pure alexia in the last 100 years and a continuously increasing number of modern cases documented by neuroimaging techniques like CT scans or MRI confirm Dejerine's (1892) finding of a lesion in the territory of the left posterior cerebral artery. The published cases of pure alexia who came for autopsy up to 1969 have been extensively reviewed by Benson and Geschwind (1969). They refer to 17 cases (Landolt, 1888; Lissauer, 1890; Dejerine, 1892; Hahn, 1895; Redlich, 1895; Brissaud, 1900; Dide and Botcazo, 1902; Hinshelwood and MacPhail 1904; Paterson and Bramwell, 1905; Bonvicini and Pötzl, 1907; Pötzl, 1928; Ehrenwald, 1930; Kleist, 1934; Niessl von Mayendorf, 1935; Gloning *et al.*, 1955; Geschwind and Fusillo, 1966; Gloning *et al.* 1966). Two additional cases of pure alexia, one whose autopsy report revealed a vascular lesion in the left lingual gyrus and a second small vascular lesion close to the right occipital pole (Hoff *et al.*, 1954), and another by Gloning *et al.* (1966) recently came to our attention. We will first discuss the atypical neuropathological findings, namely lesions in the right occipital lobe.

The patient of Gloning *et al.* (1966, case 3), a 71-year-old, ambidextrous lady, though described only briefly without much clinical detail, is interesting with respect to aetiology and the question of cerebral dominance. She was found to have a complete left homonymous hemianopia and a pure alexia with spared reading of numbers. There was a marked colour agnosia and a mild anomic aphasia. At autopsy a large glioblastoma in the basal part of the right occipital and temporal lobes was found. This tumour extended into the white matter of the lingual gyrus, involving the splenial fibres and the lower angular gyrus as well. In view of the ambidexterity, the classical picture of pure alexia and colour agnosia, the anatomical involvement and the anomic aphasia, one has to assume that in this patient the right hemisphere was language dominant. With the exception of this and one other case (Gloning *et al.*, 1955; Gloning *et al.*, 1966), all patients suffering from pure alexia had pathological involvement of the left occipital lobe. In all but the cases of Dide and Botcazo (1902), Kleist (1934) and Hoff *et al.* (1954), the lesion was unilateral left-sided. In one case (Bonvicini and Pötzl, 1907) the left calcarine cortex itself was reported as being intact, but surrounded by infarcted cortex. In all other cases, although the area involved was somewhat variable, the lingual gyrus and part or all of the fusiform gyrus, i.e. the inner and under surface of the left occipital lobe, were lesioned. In 9 cases involvement of the corpus callosum or the connection between the right and left visual areas was described.

The first case of a presumed right-hander suffering from alexia caused by an autopsically verified lesion in the territory of the right posterior cerebral artery was described by Gloning *et al.* (1955). This 54-year-old lady, employed at the post office, presented a number of unusual clinical features worth mentioning in more detail. In August 1953 she became aware of visual disturbances and frequently ran into objects located on her left side. Ophthalmological examination revealed a left lower homonymous quadranopia. In early October 1953 she realized that she could no longer read her own stenography (a syllabic German shorthand in which she had previously been fluent) although writing it presented no difficulty. She had problems copying her own stenogram as well. The patient also failed to read the 'ideographic' abbreviations of shorthand script with the exception of the word 'but'. At this time the patient had few problems reading print, but made numerous typing errors. Her competence in typing was always limited as she needed visual feedback. In mid-October 1953 she experienced visual pseudohallucinations, suddenly seeing letters and signs for a few seconds where none existed. Neurological examination at the end of November 1953 revealed a complete left homonymous hemianopia. There was no aphasia, spontaneous writing was flawless and writing to dictation unimpaired, but copying was markedly disturbed, including spatial rotations of letters by 90 degrees or mirror copies. There was no difficulty reading letters but the reading of words fluctuated considerably: sometimes she could read headlines without difficulty, on other days no word could be identified. The patient complained that she had lost her competence to grasp the meaning of whole words and sentences. Reading of stenography remained completely impossible but writing it spontaneously or on dictation was unimpaired. Unlike 'normal' pure alexic patients, but very typical for patients with lesions in the territory of the right posterior cerebral artery, the patient had a severe topographical disorientation. She could not find her way around the ward, her inner imaging of the city topography was severely disturbed and her orientation with a map disastrous. In December 1953 she died subsequent to another stroke in the territory of the left middle cerebral artery. Autopsy revealed a large infarct in the territory of the right posterior cerebral artery, destroying the infero-medial surface of the occipital lobe including the occipito-temporal junction, the anterior two-thirds of the calcarina and the cuneus. There was a softening in the splenium of the corpus callosum on the right side and a small right-sided thalamic infarction.

To summarize, this patient suffered from a stroke in the territory of the right posterior cerebral artery, which left her with a homonymous lower left-sided quadranopia, a pure alexia for stenography with only minor reading disturbances for print. Subsequent to a second stroke in the vascular territory of the same artery visual pseudohallucinations, a complete left-sided hemianopia, pure alexia for print but less marked than for stenography, and a severe topographical agnosia were noted.

Since the review of Benson and Geschwind (1969) a number of additional autopsically verified cases of pure alexia have been published (e.g. Cumming *et al.*, 1970; Greenblatt, 1973; Boucher *et al.*, 1974; Fincham *et al.*, 1975; Caplan and Hedley-Whyte, 1974; Ajax *et al.*, 1977; Landis *et al.*, 1980; Cambier *et al.*, 1980; Damasio and Damasio, 1983; Guard *et al.*, 1985; Landis and Regard, 1988). Of these 12 cases, two were bilateral and in the others, with one exception, the crucial localization of the inner- and lower-surface of the left occipital lobe in pure alexia was confirmed. In the bilateral cases (Cambier *et al.*, 1980; Fincham *et al.*, 1975) the pathology in the first was a bilateral infarct in the territory of both posterior cerebral arteries with a global agnosic picture including prosopagnosia and visual agnosia and in the second, multiple metastases. The latter case (Fincham *et al.*, 1975) is of particular interest in that this case together with the two cases of Gloning *et al.* (1955/66) appear to be the only ones in which the left-sided infero-medial-occipital area was not damaged. At autopsy large metastases involving virtually the whole right occipital and right parietal lobe were found, as well as a left superior parietal metastasis with a subcortical extension in the vicinity of the ventricular trigone. Moreover, areas of oedema and demyelination in the anterior part of the splenium of the corpus callosum as well as in the left-sided parietal white matter were noted. Whether the multiplicity of lesions at different sites and/or oedema and demyelination, undercutting the angular gyrus, were responsible in this case for the pure alexia remains conjectural. Since this patient had a dense left homonymous hemianopia resulting from the extensive right posterior metastases, it is not necessary, of course, to invoke an additional splenial lesion to compromise visual transfer, because visual information reached the intact left hemispheric visual cortex directly. In 7 of these additional pathologically proven cases various degrees of damage to the splenium of the corpus callosum or damage to the connection between the visual areas of the two hemispheres was reported.

Although the aetiology of cerebral damage in most cases of pure alexia has been vascular, primarily ischaemic infarcts, other aetiologies have been reported. While ischaemic infarcts in the territory of the left posterior cerebral artery produce relatively uniform clinical syndromes, other aetiologies produce lesions at non-typical sites, which may help to enhance our understanding of the clinico-pathological correlation in pure alexia. Such aetiologies are arteriovenous malformations (Casey and Ettlinger, 1960; Ajax, 1967; Sroka *et al.*, 1973; Greenblatt, 1976), haemorrhages (e.g. Ajax, 1964, 1967; Wechsler *et al.*, 1972; Assal and Hadj-Djilani, 1976) abscesses (e.g. Warrington and Shallice, 1979), subdural haematoma (e.g. Papadakis, 1974), surgical removal of the left occipital lobe (e.g. David *et al.*, 1955; Hécaen *et al.*, 1952), strokes in the course of a syphilitic disease (Higier, 1896; Kreindler and Ionasescu, 1961), multiple sclerosis (Shiota *et al.*, 1989), toxoplasma-encephalitis associated with AIDS (Lüscher and Horber, 1991), closed or open head injury (Heilmann *et al.*, 1971; Abe *et al.*, 1986), migraine headache (Bigley and Sharp, 1983; Fleischman *et al.*, 1983) and brain tumours (Casamajor, 1913; Hoff and Poetzl, 1937; Warrington and Zangwill 1957; Gloning *et al.*, 1966, 2 cases; Walsh and Hoyt, 1969; Greenblatt, 1973; Fincham *et al.*, 1975; Cohen *et al.*, 1976; Vincent *et al.*, 1977; Landis *et al.*, 1980; Warrington and Shallice, 1980; McCormick and Levine, 1983; Larrabee *et al.*, 1985; Regard *et al.*, 1985b; Landis and Regard, 1988).

By virtue of their non-ischaemic aetiologies, many of the above-mentioned lesions can be localized outside the territory of the left posterior cerebral artery and frequently involving only part of this territory. In particular, the splenium of the corpus callosum was often spared. Thus, while pure alexia is the hallmark of the clinical symptomatology, associated clinical findings such as right visual field defects, hemiachromatopsia, colour anomia, visual agnosia or memory deficits are frequently lacking. This can be of great theoretical importance, when it comes to judging the importance of the role of the splenial lesion, or the value of the association of colour anomia with alexia. Both of these questions will be discussed later. Before concentrating upon the unusual cases of pure alexia, we will consider the question of whether pure alexia due to the 'classical' ischaemic lesion in the territory of the left posterior cerebral artery represents a uniform clinical syndrome.

Left Posterior Cerebral Artery Strokes, Neuroimaging of the Lesion and Correlations with the Different Syndromes Associated with Pure Alexia

With the advent of modern neuroimaging techniques it has become possible to correlate clinical symptomes *intra vitam* with cerebral pathology. This method, though not as precise as autopsic macro- and microanatomy, has also been applied to pure alexia. Two recent studies will be discussed here, one attempting to outline clinical syndromes of patients with strokes in the territory of the left posterior cerebral artery selected on the basis of the presence of pure alexia (Damasio and Damasio, 1983), the other outlining the general scope of clinical signs and symptoms in an unselected group of patients suffering from strokes in the territory of the left posterior cerebral artery (De Renzi *et al.*, 1987). Both studies report on 16 right-handed patients and both used primarily CT scans as the basis of their anatomical considerations. From 23 patients with pure alexia, Damasio and Damasio (1983) selected 16 showing a focal vascular lesion. All patients had CT scans and 2 of them came to autopsy. In 1 of these 2 patients the autopsy findings are reported, in the other the lesion is dealt with in a much the same way as the CT scan findings. These lesions are transcribed upon standardized anatomical brain slices, which could give the somewhat misleading impression that computer-tomographic density findings correspond to real anatomy. On the basis of associated symptoms Damasio and Damasio distinguished three different syndromes of pure alexia (Fig. 18.1), as follows.

Type I Alexia

This consisted of six patients with pure alexia who also had a complete right homonymous hemianopia, colour anomia and unilateral optic ataxia. Two of these patients had also suffered from memory deficits, one from visual agnosia. In addition they had the most extensive cortical and subcortical white matter involvement. The most discriminative anatomical involvement with respect to the other two groups was the cortical involvement of the mesial occipito-temporal junction. This type of infarct apparently corresponds to the classical and most extensive syndrome where anatomically there is an massive infarction of the posterior cerebral artery territory including calcarine, splenial and mesial temporal branches.

Type II Alexia

This was found in six patients who suffered only from pure alexia together with right homonymous hemianopia, but did not have colour anomia, memory deficits, optic ataxia or visual agnosia. The correlation with the CT lesion revealed cortical involvement of the mesial occipital lobe in all but one case and of the lateral occipital lobe as well in three, but in no instance was the mesial occipito-temporal junction affected. In none of these cases was there a lesion of the splenium of the corpus callosum but in all of them callosal fibres in the forceps major were affected and also the paraventricular white matter in all but one. Of

particular interest is case number 13 in whom there was only a small lateral occipital lesion which extended towards the left occipital horn and into the peritrigonal region. In the lesions leading to this second pure alexia syndrome type the disconnection was apparently more intra- than interhemispheric. Owing to a complete right homonymous hemianopia, conscious visual input was confined to the right hemisphere visual system, and the interhemispheric visual transfer of colour information was intact.

Type III Alexia

Distinguished by Damasio and Damasio (1983), this was observed in four of their patients. This type differed clinically from type II in that there was only a right superior homonymous quadranopia, e.g. no complete right homonymous hemianopia, but the patients were achromatopsic in the intact right lower quadrant. As in type II there was no colour anomia, memory deficit, optic ataxia or visual agnosia. In these cases the lesion involved the inferior compartment of the optic radiation, the occipital paraventricular white matter and the infero-calcarine visual association cortex. The major difference between type II and type III was the lack of forceps major involvement. The crucial difference between the three syndromes is therefore the involvement or sparing of the left mesial occipito-temporal junction and the forceps major. The distinction made by these authors into mesial occipital and mesial occipito-temporal cortex, which in their series well separates patients with pure alexia from those with pure alexia and associated colour anomia, is an arbitrary one, springing from the difficulty of outlining precise anatomy on CT scan slices. Therefore it is not trivial to compare the Damasio findings with the many earlier attempts at clinical pathological correlation in pure alexia, which were primarily based on autopsy and expressed in terms of precise anatomical structure. By 'mesial occipital cortical involvement' Damasio and Damasio (1983) understand the occipital pole and the posterior half of all cortex behind the splenium, while by 'mesial occipito-temporal cortical involvement' is meant the anterior half of all cortex behind the splenium and the mesial temporal cortex. In terms of anatomical landmarks this implies, on the one hand, an artificial separation into a posterior and anterior part of the lingual gyrus and the adjacent fusiform gyrus, but there is no indication, on the other hand, to what extent the anteriorly contingent structures of the hippocampus and parahippocampus were involved.

This is of some importance, as Viennese authors like Pötzl, Hoff or Gloning and collaborators since the mid-1920s have maintained the position that the left lingual gyrus is the crucial structure for pure alexia in combination with colour anomia. They found this structure to be spared in cases of pure alexia not associated with a colour anomia (e.g. Hoff and Pötzl, 1937). Moreover, they considered variations in the involvement of the forceps major to play a role whenever 'atypical' cases were found in the literature. They also believed the dissociation between alexia for letters and numbers to be of importance in correlation with the extent of the lesion. They found that whenever an alexia for numbers and musical notes was present in addition to one for letters, the pathological process extended more dorsally into the area of the lower horn roof (Henschen, 1920–1922; Pötzl, 1928). The analysis of CT scans by Damasio and Damasio (1983), though not distinguishing the lingual and the fusiform gyrus, seem to confirm, nevertheless, this long-known importance of mesial occipito-temporal cortical structures for the symptoms associated with alexia.

A somewhat different approach to the clinical picture of lesions in the territory of the left posterior cerebral artery has been taken by De Renzi *et al.* (1987). This group investigated 16 consecutive patients with CT scan evidence of an infarct confined to this territory with a test battery assessing reading and writing, naming and pointing to colours, naming objects and coloured photographs of objects and verbal memory. They analysed the location and extent of the lesions on CT scans with respect to the clinical symptomatology and found various degrees of verbal memory deficit in all of these patients. In almost 75 per cent, alexia without agraphia (pure alexia) was accompanied by some degree of disturbance in colour naming and in object naming, particularly when the objects were photographed. Moreover, the naming deficit was found to be not restricted to the visual modality but to be also present in the tactile modality, in spite of the integrity of the traditional language areas. De Renzi *et al.* (1987) described a far more widespread impairment of visual and even extra-visual functions than just pure alexia with or without colour naming disturbances. This interpretation was corroborated by the reviews of Michel *et al.* (1979) and Morin *et al.* (1984), who came to the conclusion that object naming difficulties are almost as frequent as colour naming deficits associated with pure alexia, and that extra-visual naming difficulties have been found in cases of visual agnosia or optic aphasia.

De Renzi *et al.*'s analysis of the CT scans revealed that the area most frequently damaged in patients who had become purely alexic was the lingual gyrus. Moreover, an inferior or superior extension of the lesion to the CT scan cut representing the lingual gyrus seems to aggravate the picture of alexia. In particular the role of the fusiform gyrus (Hoff *et al.*, 1962) and the cuneus (Foix and Masson, 1923; Kurachi *et al.*, 1979) were discussed and De Renzi *et al.* surmise 'that its damage concurs to make alexia worse, though being probably insufficient to disrupt reading, if

the lingual gyrus is spared (Marie and Crouzon, 1900)'. However, De Renzi *et al.* emphasized '. . .that more data are needed to definitely settle the issue'.

To summarize, it appears that in ischaemic infarctions in the territory of the left posterior cerebral artery in right-handers, there is concordant evidence that the mesial occipital and occipito-temporal structures, e.g. the lingual and the fusiform gyrus, are crucial for the occurrence of pure alexia. The heterogeneity of testing procedures, anatomical analysis and differences in theoretical viewpoints render a finer clinical anatomical correlation to associated symptoms difficult. It appears, however, that an involvement of more anterior parts of the lingual gyrus and maybe the fusiform gyrus will lead to some degree of colour agnosia or anomia and possibly to minor forms of associative visual agnosia or optic aphasia. The advent of MRI imaging with its much greater anatomical approximation of cortical and subcortical structures may, in the future, clarify this point. Brain imaging in right hemifield pure alexia contributed also to the question of where a visual association area necessary for word perception might be located. Castro-Caldas and Salgado (1984) reported on a 54-year-old office clerk who suffered from a stroke which led to a temporary right hemianopia, clearing within a few days. On returning to work the patient realized that his reading speed had decreased considerably, with words and letters missed. Owing to a previous trauma he had been blind in the right eye for about 20 years. Tachistoscopic stimuli projected for 100 ms into the left and right visual fields of his good left eye revealed a reduction in the correct naming of colours, letters, single digits and arithmetic symbols and diminished reading of single words in the right visual hemifield. The reduction in colour naming was less in the left than in the right hemifield. Colour matching was fairly good in both hemifields, while that of letters, words, digits or arithmetic symbols not recognized in the right visual hemifield was also not correct. Selection and matching of meaningless drawings, however, were unimpaired in both hemifields.

The CT scan showed that a hypodense area in the left inferior rostral occipital lobe, i.e. parts of gyrus lingualis and gyrus fusiformis was impaired, while the area striata and forceps major were spared. Also the splenium of the corpus callosum was not affected. Castro-Caldas and Salgado discussed the various pathways possible between the right visual association cortices and the left parieto-temporal area necessary for correct reading (cf. Fig. 18.7).

Before discussing individual cases of preserved reading in pure alexia we would like to briefly address two questions which, though linked, have preoccupied many clinicians and researchers in pure alexia, namely: Visual naming, in particular that of colours and objects; and the role of the lesion in the splenium of the corpus callosum in pure alexia.

Visual Naming in Pure Alexia

Anyone who views pure alexia as a syndrome of visual disconnection, as has tradionally been done ever since Dejerine (1892) and Wernicke (1874), is confronted with the questions: 'Why does this visual disconnection concern only words, but not letters?' 'Why only letters and not numbers?' 'Why sometimes words and colours but not objects?' 'Why sometimes all visual stimuli?' And, even more difficult to answer: 'Why sometimes only colours but not words?' or 'Why objects but not words?' The problem is further complicated by the fact that our brain has two hemispheres and therefore two perceptive visual systems which, as far as we know from the monkey, are anatomically and physiologically very similar. The above mentioned considerations lead to further questions such as: 'Is the non-dominant hemisphere not capable of analysing all visual signals?' 'Is there a problem in transferring this information to the language centres of the dominant hemisphere?' And if so, 'At what level of transfer does interruption occur?'

Let us consider these questions for the example of colour anomia/agnosia. In the literature the problem has been approached in three different ways:

1. By regarding discrete cortical areas in a cortical processing chain of visual information as being specialized for the processing of different types of information.
2. By alotting the responsibility for carrying of different visual information to different fibre bundles within fibre tracts.
3. By considering fibre tracts as channels with a finite capacity for information transfer which when impaired would lead to a faster overload of information transfer, whereby the more complex information is affected first.

The first approach was taken by Pötzl (1928) while investigating the syndromatic nature of the combination of pure alexia and colour agnosia and subsequently pursued by his younger associates in Vienna. It has also been taken up in a modern, neurophysiologically oriented frame by Damasio and Damasio (1983). The second approach has been taken by many authors trying to detect specific fibre connections, especially those for colour, running through the dorsal splenium (e.g. Cumming *et al.*, 1970; Greenblatt, 1973; Ajax, 1977; Vincent *et al.*, 1977). The third approach is that of Oxbury *et al.* (1969) and Damasio *et al.* (1979). The third model, suggesting a limited information-carrying capacity of the information transfer, implies clinically a gradient ranging from 'letters' to 'letters and colours' to 'letters, colours and objects'.

All three models have their limitations. The third model cannot account for cases in which colour naming has been impaired but reading spared (Mohr *et al.*, 1971) or those in which the naming of objects was impaired but not reading (Albert *et al.*, 1975; Newcombe and Ratcliff, 1974). The second model, in which differences among the splenial fibres are involved, can be discounted on the basis of the numerous cases with full visual fields in which there is no doubt that the visual information has reached the left hemisphere's visual zones (e.g. Hinshelwood, 1900; Hoff and Pötzl 1937; Adler, 1944; Peron and Goutner, 1944; Alajouanine *et al.*, 1960; Ajax, 1967; Goldstein *et al.*, 1971; Heilmann *et al.*, 1971; Greenblatt, 1973; Assal and Hadj-Djilani, 1976; Greenblatt, 1976; Cambier *et al.*, 1980; Castro-Caldas and Salgado, 1984).

The model most difficult to discount is the first one which implies discrete cortical areas specialized for the treatment of different visual information or, of course, their connections within the left hemisphere to the language zones. A point which has to be raised concerning this model is the fact that many cases exist (e.g. De Renzi *et al.*, 1987) in which there are extensive lesions affecting these crucial areas but neither alexia, colour anomia nor object agnosia has been found. In favour of this first hypothesis speaks the fact that in the cases with full visual fields, in which at least intact primary visual sensory areas as well as some further processing to assure awareness of the full field must be postulated, associated defects of colour or object naming are much rarer than in cases with impairment of visual fields.

An elegant approach to the question why colour naming and word naming seem to be more afflicted by a disconnecting lesion than object or number naming has been taken by Geschwind (1965). He pointed out differences in learning these various stimuli. Thus objects in addition to numbers which one learns by digit counting are experienced by several sensory modalities, which may allow this information to use intrahemispheric multimodal association areas of the right hemisphere and to pass directly via parietal callosal fibres to the language-dominant zones, circumventing the visual block in the splenium. As pointed out by De Renzi *et al.* (1987), there is a problem with this interpretation, in that

letters and colours are not the only instances of stimuli, which we uniquely know through vision. There are many other things we never experience with senses other than the visual one, e.g. whatever exists in the sky (the sun, the moon, the stars, the clouds), trees, mountains, lakes, buildings, monuments, etc.

Moreover, it is difficult to explain cases of object agnosia without alexia, or colour anomia without alexia.

We have recently seen a patient whose case weakens this hypothesis in yet another way. This patient, a 51-year-old, right-handed businesswoman, suffered from slowly progressive difficulties in reading, calculation and word finding, without any problem in writing. Subsequent to severe left-sided headaches and generalized seizures she came to our attention. A complete right homonymous hemianopia was found but no other sensory or motor defects. Her spontaneous speech was fluent with occasional word finding problems and circumlocutions. Auditory comprehension was only minimally impaired, while there was a severe disturbance in verbal learning and recall. Writing was normal, except for a downward tilt of the baseline at the end of the sentences. Reading was completely impossible with the exception of a few letters, while orally spelled words were well understood. Tactile presentation of letters presented no problem and whole words could be integrated by this means. Reading was greatly facilitated when the patient was allowed to trace the letters with her fingers, a strategy which she spontaneously used. There was no apraxia, no prosopagnosia, no object agnosia nor topographical disorientation. Nonetheless, besides this complete alexia without agraphia, there was a peculiarly dissociated visual anomia. The patient was unable to name any familiar or famous faces or most visually presented objects, but had absolutely no difficulty naming colours. Computer tomography revealed a large mesial temporal tumour, reaching into the left trigone. There was some midline displacement but little oedema. At operation the tumour was found to involve the mesial parts of the entire left temporal lobe reaching from the pole to the occipitotemporal junction, infiltrating completely the amygdala, the hippocampal formation, the para-hippocampal gyrus and into the latero-basal area of the trigone. The tumour was extirpated almost completely; the histological finding was an astrocytoma grade III. The patient also showed some evidence of preserved reading capacity, e.g. the ability to make lexical decisions on tachistoscopic presentation in her intact left visual field, which will be referred to below.

This case of pure alexia with the typical improvement in letter reading by tracing as well as the retained capacity to make lexical decisions exhibited a pronounced anomia for all kinds of visual stimuli including faces and objects, but a quite remarkable sparing of colour naming.

It is apparent that the anatomo–clinical correlation of visual naming in pure alexia has not yet been solved satisfactorily. Nonetheless, cases of isolated colour anomia without alexia (Mohr *et al.*, 1971), the many cases of pure alexia without colour naming and our case of pure alexia with spared colour naming but impaired naming of object and faces would imply a double dissociation of function, which is indicative of different anatomical substrates for each function.

Pure Alexia and Hemialexia Subsequent to Splenial Lesions

Isolated lesions in the splenium of the corpus callosum are extremely rare. Of the few reported cases (Trescher and Ford, 1937; Maspes, 1948; Akelaitis, 1941, 1944; Bogen

and Gazzaniga, 1965; Damasio *et al.*, 1980; Wechsler, 1972; Iwata *et al.*, 1973; Gazzaniga and Freedman, 1973; Sugishita *et al.*, 1978; Levine and Calvanio, 1980; Sidtis *et al.*, 1981; Abe *et al.*, 1986; Sperry *et al.*, 1969), most had either sections of the corpus callosum extending much further than just the splenium and/or the lesion in the splenium was accompanied by sizable extra-callosal damage and/or the reason for surgically splitting the splenium was intractable epileptic seizures. The extent of the splenial lesion in some of these patients was confirmed by operation, by CT scan and, in a few, by MRI scan (Sugishita *et al.*, 1986; Bogen *et al.*, 1988). Moreover, the testing for reading in these patients was performed in very dissimilar ways, using different kinds of stimuli, tachistoscopic exposure duration and tasks. Some of the patients were tested pre- and postoperatively, some only many years after the onset of the splenial pathology. Although it is difficult to compare these situations, all patients had left visual field hemialexia.

In the following we will discuss one of these patients. In 1937 Trescher and Ford presented the case of a 37-year-old woman who with certain head positions developed severe headaches and signs of increased intracranial pressure. Together with an increasing frequency of these episodes she was also transiently unconscious. A ventriculography provided the diagnosis of a colloid cyst of the third ventricle and the tumour was surgically removed by a posterior approach during which the posterior half of the corpus callosum was dissected. Prior to the operation neurological and ophthalmological examination had been entirely normal. After the operation she was disoriented for many days and subsequent to this period her husband noted that she had lost her memory for localities, while her memory for persons had remained intact. She got lost in her own house, didn't recognize streets and lost her way while driving her car. 20 days after the operation she was re-examined:

The visual fields were first tested. The outlines of the fields on the right were normal, but on the left the patient sometimes failed to notice the test object. She would be conscious of something to her left but would not recognize it. After many tests it was determined that the outlines of the left fields were normal and that the colour fields were unaltered, but that the patient's powers of attention were diminished and that she could not recognize objects on that side. For example, when a large wooden letter was held just to the right of the fixation point, she always recognized it, but when it was held on the left, she had no idea of its nature. However, she could touch objects in the left fields accurately. There seemed to be no real difficulty in naming objects fixed in central vision, for she named 10 familiar objects without error in rapid succession. She could read and write fluently and understood what she had read.

That this difficulty in recognizing objects and letters in her left visual field, despite her ability to detect that something was there, was not simply the consequence of a hemispatial neglect is demonstrated by the following sentence: 'She could count small objects scattered over her bed'. While the patient had no hemisensory loss and no loss of position sense in her left hand, she was unable to recognize wooden letters placed in her left hand, but she had no difficulty identifying objects placed in this hand. According to the patient's husband, all these symptoms persisted, though somewhat improved, over several years.

To summarize, subsequent to the surgical section of the posterior part of the corpus callosum, this patient had not only become the first case of left visual field hemialexia, but had also suffered from left visual field hemiagnosia for objects and not for colours. Moreover, she displayed a left tactile alexia, but not a left tactile agnosia. Although the examination was not performed tachistoscopically, it appears that the splenial or posterior callosal lesion prevented letters and objects, but not colours, from being named. This finding would speak against a crucial role of the splenium of the corpus callosum in the colour naming difficulties of some pure alexic patients.

The above case of Trescher and Ford (1937) is a remarkably distinct example of a posterior callosal lesion. Most of the subsequent cases with left hemialexia had some additional damage, compromising interpretation. Moreover, there appear to be some patients who subsequent to the section of the whole or posterior part of the corpus callosum did not develop hemialexia (Akelaitis, 1941, 1943; Sperry and Gazzaniga, 1967), indicating that individual differences in the developmental organization of the right hemisphere may in some instances be sufficient to support at least the reading of tachistoscopically presented letters and words.

Kanji and Kana Alexia in Patients with Lesions of the Posterior Corpus Callosum

Two recently published cases of hemialexia in Japanese patients, both suffering from quite pure posterior callosal lesions, will be discussed in the following. The special interest in Japanese patients for the study of reading is derived from the fact that they use two different reading systems, Kanji, an ideographic script, and Kana, a phonological syllabic script (Chapter 17). The study of aphasic Japanese patients (for review see Sasanuma, 1980) has shown dissociated deficits in the reading impairment of these two scripts, and the right hemisphere in particular was thought to play an important role in the decoding of the Kanji logograms.

The first case was published twice, 3 and 11 years after the operation (Sugishita *et al.*, 1978; Sugishita *et al.*, 1986).

The patient was a right-handed man who subsequent to the diagnosis of a pineal tumour was operated on via the right occipital route with a transection of the splenium. Neurological examination displayed a right third nerve palsy and an upward gaze paralysis, both of which disappeared within a few days after the operation. There was no visual field defect and visual acuity was normal. The neurological examinations 2 and 11 years postoperatively were within normal limits. Language examination one year after the operation showed severe left hemialexia for both Kana and Kanji words. However, 3 years postoperatively hemialexia for ideographic Kanji words had recovered to some degree (Sugishita *et al.*, 1978). 11 years after the operation Sugishita and co-workers (1986) attempted to uncover the nature of the partial recovery of Kanji word reading by using a tachistoscopic interfield same/different judgement paradigm. The patient had to decide whether two words, one presented to the left visual field the other to the right, were the same or different. The task was performed with pairs of Kanji as well as Kana words. The authors conjecture that when the task was correctly performed, the recovery from hemialexia resulted from a transfer of visual word information from the right hemisphere to the left via extrasplenial fibres and, in contrast, if the task was impossible, recovery was due to the development of an ability to read aloud or to comprehend reading in the right hemisphere. The complete absence of the splenium in their case was confirmed by MR imaging. When single visual hemifield presentation was used, reading Kana phonograms aloud was significantly impaired in the left visual hemifield (only 50 per cent of the words could be read), while there was no significant difference between the visual fields for Kanji ideogram words. Reading compre-hension of Kana words, tested by pointing to a picture match, was still impaired in the left visual field, though less markedly (63 per cent correct comprehension).

When testing for intra- and interfield same/different judgements, Sugishita *et al.* (1986) found that intrafield-same as well as intrafield-different judgements could be performed by either visual field remarkably well. Interfield judgements for the same comparison, however, were at chance level with ideograms as well with phonograms, but different judgements were significantly above chance level for both types of words. In a second study with more words the same pattern emerged but this time all decisions were above chance level. The authors interpreted the results as evidence for the postoperative development of an alternative crosscallosal pathway and against the development of some right hemispheric reading capacity. We think, however, that this question has not yet been settled, since in the first experiment no transfer capacity for same judgements could be demonstrated for ideograms and for phonograms, in spite of almost 100 per cent correct same judgements in the intrafield experiment of each hemisphere. This is even more astonishing in as much as intrahemispheric same judgements are more difficult, as a rule, than interhemispheric same judgements for words in normal subjects. Thus, for this specific task at least, one could well defend the hypothesis that the right hemisphere has somehow learned to match words for their graphical similarity.

Another Japanese patient (Abe *et al.*, 1986), a 25-year-old, right-handed businessman, suffered from a stab wound with an icepick penetrating through the midline of the whole brain and dissecting the inferior third of the splenium of the corpus callosum. Neurological examination including visual field testing was normal and the patient underwent tachistoscopic hemifield testing with Kana and Kanji words one year after the operation following the accident. As with the above-mentioned patient of Sugishita *et al.* (1978, 1986), reading aloud of both ideograms and phonograms was impaired in the left visual field, more pronounced for phonograms. Reading comprehension as tested by word/picture matching was the same in both hemifields for Kanji ideograms but impaired in the left visual field for Kana phonograms.

Both studies suggest that in the case of a relatively pure disruption of the splenium of the corpus callosum, Kanji sign comprehension is barely impaired, if at all, in the disconnected right hemisphere's visual system, while Kana sign comprehension and the reading aloud of both phonograms and ideograms is impaired. These findings may mean that the right hemisphere's visual system is able to gather the meaning of ideograms, and that the transfer of the probably preprocessed ideogram information to the left hemispheric oral language centres could use extrasplenial callosal pathways. Another possible explanation is that the right hemisphere deciphers the shape of the ideograms (but not of the Kana signs) and transfers this signal via anterior corpus callosum connections to the speech centres of the left hemisphere (Fig. 18.7).

Tachistoscopic Studies in Hemialexia

In 1976 we had the opportunity to investigate six patients tachistoscopically prior to and after surgery for arteriovenous malformations (AVM) in the posterior part and the splenium of the corpus callosum. One of these patients showed some unusual findings, sufficiently interesting to be reported here. This 27-year-old, right-handed sculptor had an uneventful medical history until age 12 when she suffered an episode of acute headache and transient neck stiffness. During the next 15 years she experienced about once a year an identical episode, accompanied on one occasion by a short loss of consciousness. She never had any focal neurological deficits or a history of seizures. Neurological examination on admission was entirely normal, including visual fields and colour perimetry. Angiographically there was an arteriovenous malformation in the posterior part of the corpus callosum and the splenium with some parasplenial extension on the right side. During neurosurgery the splenial and parasplenial AVM could be radically extirpated (Professor Yasargil, Zürich), as evidenced by a completely normal control angiography. The patient recovered rapidly from the operation, the only remaining neurological deficit being a brief impairment of position sense in the left hand. Formal mental status examinations before and after operation revealed no deficit; in particular the patient was able to read and write normally.

Tachistoscopic hemifield testing took place the day before operation and two weeks and two years postoperatively. Tachistoscopic testing was accompanied by extensive testing for any difficulties in auditory and tactile transfer, which were all completely normal before and after operation; in particular there was no left ear suppression in dichotic listening experiments. The tachistoscopic experiments using words, numbers, colours and faces were identical pre- and postoperatively, but differed for the last examination 2 years after the operation. Visual stimuli were presented at different exposure durations ranging from 20 to 100 ms and answers were given either verbally or by pointing to the identical stimulus in a multiple-choice setting for each hand separately.

For the first two examinations we will consider only the verbal report. Before and after the operation the patient had no problems naming colours in either visual field. The naming of digits was equally good (80 per cent) in the right visual field pre- and postoperatively, while digit naming in the left visual field fell from 50 per cent preoperatively to 20 per cent postoperatively. The most striking result by far was that of word reading. Before the operation the patient was completely hemialexic for words presented to her left visual field, while there was a normal performance in her right visual field. Postoperatively, however, the patient could read words at the same exposure durations equally well in both visual fields. It thus appears that the extirpation of the splenium had 'cured' this patient from a previous left hemialexia due to a splenial angioma. 2 years later colour naming was still intact in both visual fields and digit naming was still impaired, though somewhat improved in the left visual field only. She still had no difficulty reading short concrete nouns in both visual fields. None the less, when presented with abstract emotional and abstract non-emotional nouns (Landis *et al.*, 1982) unilaterally, she could read all of them in her right visual field, but only 67 per cent of the emotional and 40 per cent of the non-emotional abstract words in her left visual field. An additional experiment using a bilateral lexical decision paradigm (Graves *et al.*, 1981), during which she only had to press a button with her hand ipsilateral to the visual field in which she felt there was a real word, showed the left visual field to be incapable of performing this task in the presence of a simultaneously presented letter string to the right visual field. The performance of the right visual field was completely normal.

Callosal AVM provides another model for testing interhemispheric information transfer. In contrast to longstanding epilepsy and callosal surgery as well as vascular disease or tumours, it has the property of being a congenital anomaly which grows slowly without producing pathology except, perhaps, to lead to differences in the development of interhemispheric connections.

In our case there was a complete left hemialexia prior to operation. This implies either complete block of visual splenial transfer or, as we believe, sufficiently impaired splenial transfer to inhibit the function of alternative interhemispheric visual pathways. Subsequent to the operation the patient could read words equally well in both visual fields, which we interpret as a consequence of the disappearance of transcallosal inhibition by the extirpation of the splenium. If the right hemisphere, freed from left hemispheric inhibition, discovered its own way of accessing meaning from written symbols or if extrasplenial pathways became functional remains an open question, but the time of only two weeks which elapsed between the two examinations would not have allowed an efficient relearning process to have taken place. In fact, the interference of right visual field stimulation upon the lexical decision in the left visual field 2 years later does speak rather in favour of an opening of predeveloped alternative extrasplenial pathways subsequent to the interruption of a misfunctioning but dominant splenial connection.

To summarize, the evidence from relatively pure splenial lesions or complete dissection of the corpus callosum with or without the commissures cannot completely resolve the question of whether there is a visual centre for word images in the right hemisphere or not. However, it appears that the posterior part of the right hemisphere is able to access the meaning of words, possibly in its own way, but not the oral naming of these words. In fact, what we know from hemialexia due to splenial lesions would rather favour Wernicke's as opposed to Dejerine's view about a specific left hemispheric reading centre.

Preserved Access to Written Information in Pure Alexia

By preserved reading we understand a preserved access to the meaning of written symbols despite an apparent inability to read. This retention of access to meaning may appear at different levels of symbol recognition and in different experimental situation, a fact that was discovered very early in alexia research. Broadbent's report (1872) on a patient who could not read a single word but recognized his own name without knowing if it consisted of the initials alone or of the whole name and Dejerine's description of the patient who recognized the initials of the French Republic only when inscribed on a medallion (Dejerine, 1912; see above) indicated that alexic patients have access to otherwise hidden meaning. The question is whether such access represents the ability of the right hemispheric visual system to decode parts of the meaning of written symbols.

In recent years a number of studies have shown preserved access to lexical meaning to exist in cases of pure alexia. Kreindler and Ionasescu (1961) reported a patient who subsequent to a left posterior stroke with a right homonymous hemianopia became purely alexic. Although he recognized only about 50 per cent of single letters, he had no difficulty in sorting letters, numbers and punctuation marks, but could not match printed and cursively written letters. He failed when shown a written word and asked to point to the correct picture, but when he was shown a picture and asked to designate the adequate word he was almost always correct. Moreover, when he was shown a written word and asked to identify it from several spoken words, he was equally correct in almost all instances. Stachowiak and Poeck (1976) used similar 'deblocking' methods (Weigl, 1968) in another patient with a left posterior stroke and a right-sided hemianopia. This patient could not read words but identified about 70 per cent of individual letters correctly. He showed correct word identification in a multiple-choice setup when the word was presented auditorily and also when the word was represented in a pictorial form.

Caplan and Hedley-Whyte (1974) reported a patient who according to the autopsy records had suffered from an infarct involving the medial aspect of the left occipital and posterior left temporal lobe, and showed a right hemianopia, pure alexia and a severe verbal memory deficit. She also had difficulties in colour and object naming, and exhibited every sign of a Gerstmann syndrome without agraphia. Although unable to read a single word or letters or numbers, she would place letters upright in the correct position whenever they were in the incorrect order. She was able to place letters in alphabetical order without recognizing them, recognize incorrect signs in words or incorrectly arranged letters integrated into words and discover additional incorrect letters at the end or beginning of a real word. Moreover, cueing questions, restricting the possible categories, helped her recognise the word, and as in the two previous cases she was able to select the correct word in about two-thirds of the instances when they were presented in a spoken list. A similar access to word meaning has been reported by Grossi *et al.* (1984) in a patient who became purely alexic subsequent to a large left posterior cerebral artery stroke with a right homonymous hemianopia. Though the patient had limited success in recognizing some single letters, he was not able to match printed words to printed words in a list but was almost always correct in matching verbally presented words to printed words, and pictures and objects to written words in a multiple choice setting. A similarly almost perfect matching performance of objects and words as well as words to objects has previously been reported by Assal and Regli (1980) in a pure alexic patient with two left posterior strokes, a temporo–occipital and a second parietal one with a right homonymous hemianopia.

The observation of Caplan and Hedley-Whyte (1974), that their patient could distinguish real words from non-word letter strings, despite the inability to comprehend or read the real word, has been pursued by Shallice and Saffran (1986) and Coslett and Saffran (1989). They report five patients with pure verbal alexia (letter-by-letter readers) who were unable to explicitly identify stimuli presented briefly but could distinguish words from non-words. Moreover they performed better than chance on forced-choice word categorization tasks.

We have recently observed a similar patient operated for a left posterior glioblastoma who suffered from a severe pure alexia for words and letters and was hemianopic to the right side. She could distinguish between words and non-words presented tachistoscopically to her left visual field but had no idea what the real words meant, not even when she was asked to point to the corresponding images in a multiple-choice task. In a therapeutic approach over several months we found that by varying the degree of familiarity of such words presented in a tachistoscopic lexical decision paradigm, her ability to extract meaning by pointing greatly improved, but not her oral reading. Above-chance semantic categorization has also been found by Warrington and Shallice (1979) in a patient who became more alexic than agraphic subsequent to a left parietal intracerebral abscess with mild hemiparesis and complete right homonymous hemianopia.

Yet another approach to show preserved unconscious reading in pure alexia was initiated by Charcot (1887), who demonstrated unusually fast word recognition during tracing of emotionally familiar or high frequency words (see above). This approach has been pursued by Bub *et al.* (1983) and Bub (1986). In patients with pure verbal alexia (letter-by-letter readers) these authors found that the speed at which high-frequency words were recognized and pronounced was much higher than with low-frequency or nonsense words and independent of word length. Bub *et al.* suggested two different processing mechanisms for these two types of reading.

As outlined above, there is increasing and ample evidence for certain types of preserved reading abilities in patients suffering from pure alexia due to left posterior lesions with right hemianopia; however, this is not found in all pure alexic patients who have been tested in a similar manner (Staller *et al.*, 1978; Warrington and Shallice, 1980; Patterson and Kay, 1982; Prior and McCorriston, 1983; Friedman and Alexander, 1984). Many letter-by-letter readers have no rapid unaware access to lexical semantics.

In the last few years we have examined a number of patients with left posterior lesions due to various causes who displayed varying degrees of reading disturbances. It was not possible in all of these patients to demonstrate access to lexical meaning without awareness or without using a slow letter-by-letter strategy, although we examined most of them tachistoscopically with a wide variety of stimuli including words and letters. A major obstacle was the reluctance of some to guess, because they were not aware of having seen anything. Another difficulty was the large variation in performance between different patients at different exposure durations. If one believes that right hemisphere access to lexical meaning is dependent on diminished control by the dominant left hemisphere, one can expect to find access to lexical meaning to be dependent upon exposure duration, since short exposure duration in combination with a partial anatomical disconnection may add up to a complete functional disconnection in pure alexia. Two of our own observations and experimental results in pure alexic patients may exemplify this last point.

The first patient (Landis *et al.*, 1980), a typical letter-by-letter reader with a complete homonymous hemianopia, was tested tachistoscopically subsequent to the removal of a left occipito-temporal glioblastoma. He was asked to fixate a central dot, and stimuli were flashed in his left visual field, projecting to the healthy right hemisphere. Only at exposure durations which permitted letter-by-letter reading, generally well above 1000 ms, was he able to read whole words of 4 or 5 letters. In order to read single letters he required exposure durations of 50 ms. When 8 names of familiar objects were presented at 30 ms each, i.e. below the exposure he needed to recognize individual letters, he instantly read the first one correctly, but for the remaining 7 he said: 'I don't see anything, it's just a flash of light.' From a display of 20 familiar objects (including an object sharing the same initial letter as each target word) we asked him to point 'intuitively' to the objects the names of which he had not been able to see or read aloud. To his great astonishment he pointed to the correct object in 5 of 7 instances. When he was verbally unaware of written information, this patient could extract meaning (shown by correct word–object matching) only at very short exposure durations. Stimulus presentation amounted here to subliminal stimulation (for review see Dixon, 1971; 1981;

Holender, 1986). Since the same unawareness of written information is the rule in split-brain patients (Sperry *et al.*, 1969), one may conjecture that verbal unawareness of lexical information may be the prerequisite for using the right hemisphere's reading capacity. Verbal awareness, even of minimal lexical information such as individual letters, would activate analytic, left-hemispheric reading, which in turn would inhibit right-hemisphere reading.

On a later retesting of our patient, with identical experimental conditions, his alexia was clinically unchanged but he could read single letters at exposures as short as 10 ms and was thus able to name some individual letters of words presented at 20 and 30 ms. When presented again with the 8 names of familiar objects exposed for 20 ms, he instantly read 2 correctly, recognized individual letters in 5 of them and denied having seen a word or even a single letter in the remaining 1. However, only in the latter case could he point correctly to the corresponding object, while he mismatched the 5 words from which he had been able to read the individual letters.

This performance suggests that right-hemisphere reading is best or maybe exclusively demonstrated in a condition where verbal awareness is missing, i.e., in a total functional disconnection from verbalization, as is the case in split-brain patients. Since our patient was able to verbalize letters (letter-by-letter reading), the anatomical disconnection was incomplete, but we suggest that the short exposure duration induced a complete functional disconnection. We conjecture that the presence of a significant degree of left-hemisphere (letter-by-letter) conscious verbal reading inhibits alternative right-hemisphere reading comprehension. As has been pointed out by Patterson and Kay (1982), Patterson and Besner (1984a, b) and more recently by Shallice and Saffran (1986), our theoretical speculations from this case are based on a limited number of observations. Nevertheless, the correct choice of 1 object out of 20 is already a significant performance at the $p = 0.05$ level. 5 correct choices out of 7, as in our patient, is a highly significant performance and can hardly be dismissed or considered fragmentary.

Five months after testing the patient died from a recurrence of the glioblastoma and an autopsy was performed. The right hemisphere was shown to be free of a tumour (Landis *et al.*, 1980). This case probably represents the first experimental investigation of what nowadays would be called 'covert knowledge in alexia'.

Our second case (Landis and Regard, 1988) may enhance the above considerations. This 62-year-old, right-handed man had been operated for a left occipito-temporal glioblastoma. He had a right homonymous hemianopia, a pure verbal alexia (letter-by-letter reading) and mild naming difficulties for the faces of famous persons but no colour anomia and his writing was fluent. He was tested in his intact left visual field tachistoscopically with a whole array of stimuli, including single letters, concrete nouns, colour patches, pictures of objects, and signs and symbols at five different exposure durations (unlimited exposure, 500, 100, 50 and 20 ms).

As shown in Fig. 18.5, the patient read or named all stimuli except signs and symbols when they were exposed for longer than 5 s. To read concrete 4- and 5-letter nouns he used a letter-by-letter strategy. Thus his performance dropped dramatically when exposure duration was reduced (Fig. 18.5). Single letters were read much better. At exposures as short as 20 ms he could still read 2 out of 10 single letters and, like the above-mentioned patient (Landis *et al.*, 1980), could not match nouns to objects when he was verbally aware of individual letters (Fig. 18.5). While colours were named and matched equally poorly, pictures of objects were matched at exposure durations much shorter than those they were named at (complete object anomia at 50 ms, but 10 out of 12 correct picture-to-picture matchings at 20 ms and even 7 out of 12 correct at 10 ms). This latter performance shows comprehension of complex visual information in the absence of precise verbal/lexical knowledge, since at such short exposures the patient could neither read object names, match objects with pictures, nor name pictures of objects.

In this particular patient we failed to demonstrate word–object matching even at short exposure durations. A peculiar observation during experimentation, however, led us to test his ability for categorization of nouns projected for different durations (Fig. 18.6). When we presented abstract and concrete German nouns of high emotional content (i.e. *Liebe* (love), *Hass* (hatred), *Kuss* (kiss), *Mord* (murder), etc.), he could not read them at reduced exposure durations, but spontaneously produced approving or disapproving grunts, as if he had some knowledge of the meaning of these words.

To investigate if he had sufficient semantic knowledge for the word categorization at exposure durations at which reading and even word–picture matching was impossible, we presented lists of words tachistoscopically at different exposure durations (unlimited exposure, 100, 50 and 20 ms). Each word list was made up of words from two categories and was presented in random order several times at each exposure duration. The patient was forced to choose between the two categories after each presentation, even when unable to read the word or even when claiming not to have seen anything. There were 4 word lists, each with 12 German nouns 3 to 5 letters long and with 6 words in each category. The categories were: (1) emotionally positive, pleasant (e.g. love, kiss)/emotionally negative, unpleasant (e.g. hate, murder); (2) cars/colours (e.g. Volvo/green); (3) animals/clothing (e.g. dog/hat); (4) natural environment/body parts (e.g. lake/nose) (Fig. 18.6).

As can be seen in Fig. 18.6, the patient could read and

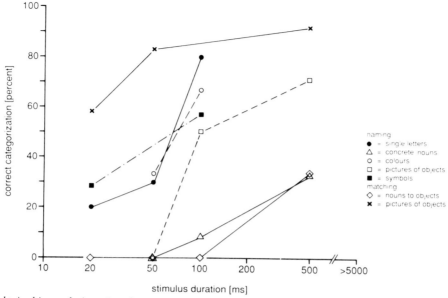

Fig. 18.5 *Data obtained in an alexic patient. Responses to stimuli projected to the left visual hemifield. On the abscissa stimulus duration, on the ordinate correct responses are plotted for the following tasks: naming of single letters (dots), concrete nouns (triangles), colours (circles), pictures of objects (open squares) or symbols (filled squares). Matching of nouns to objects (diamonds) and pictures of objects (crosses) was also tested (from Landis and Regard, 1988, redrawn).*

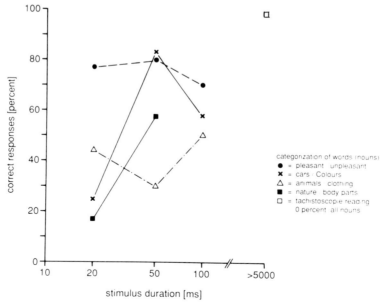

Fig. 18.6 *Results of a test performed in an alexic patient who had to categorize nouns projected to the left visual hemifield. The percentage of correct categorization is plotted on the ordinate, the stimulus duration on the abscissa. The patient had to group nouns according to the following categories: pleasant/unpleasant (dots), cars/colours (crosses), animals/clothing (triangles), nature/body parts (filled squares). Data from separate sessions. Tachistoscopic reading (open squares) was 0 per cent correct for all nouns. All tasks were correctly performed for presentation times above 5 s (from Landis and Regard, 1988, redrawn).*

categorize these words only at unlimited exposures. There was, however, one exception: his reliable emotional categorization of pleasant or unpleasant nouns. He correctly indicated the emotional category to which these words belonged at very short exposures (70 per cent at 100 ms, 80 per cent at 50 ms, 77 per cent at 20 ms) where even single letter recognition was impaired. This demonstrates that some aspects of semantic knowledge about a written word can be maintained in the absence of correct reading aloud, single letter recognition, or verbal awareness.

The patient died 5 months after testing from a recurrence of the glioblastoma. At autopsy, the pathology was a diffuse infiltration of nearly the entire left hemisphere, but no pathological process involving the right hemisphere.

Again we suggest that in this patient with a clinically incomplete posterior anatomical disconnection syndrome, the difficulty produced by decreased exposure duration led to a complete functional disconnection. Knowledge of emotional meaning of written words could represent another facet of right-hemisphere reading comprehension. Moreover, the patient's failure to categorize other concepts reliably argues in favour of specific reading comprehension for emotional lexical information, possibly mediated by the right hemisphere.

According to the hypothesis of interhemispheric inhibition and release of function, a functional impairment of the dominant hemisphere for a certain task should at one point or another uncover a coexisting, but inhibited, capacity of the opposite hemisphere to process the same task. In the patients tested we believe that the dominant function had been impaired by a combination of the lesion and the additional difficulty induced by reduced exposure time.

We have recently taken a completely different approach in the search for covert knowledge in three patients with pure alexia without a significant degree of writing disturbance (Brugger *et al.*, 1990, unpubl.). Two of them showed the classical vascular lesion in the territory of the left posterior cerebral artery and had some degree of colour naming difficulty, while in the third patient the cause was a left-sided occipito-temporal tumour and alexia was not accompanied by colour anomia. All three patients had right homonymous hemianopias. The clinical histories are briefly as follows.

Case I
This was a 52-year-old, right-handed man, who was operated on for a left occipito-temporal, peritrigonal tumour (histologically an oligoastrocytoma grade II) four years ago. Postoperatively there was a right upper quadranopia. A few weeks before testing the patient developed a complete right homonymous hemianopia and alexia without agraphia. There was some difficulty with verbal memory and calculation and minimal word-finding difficulties, but no colour naming disturbances. Visual acuity

was normal and neurological examination except for the right hemianopia and a discreet right hemihypaesthesia was normal. MRI showed a recurrence of the tumour.

Case II
A 79-year-old, right-handed woman, this patient had an uneventful medical history until 2 weeks prior to testing, when she suddenly had a brief episode of vertigo subsequent to which she had a right homonymous hemianopia and a pure alexia. Neurological examination was normal except for the right hemianopia and on mental status examination there was a severe alexia, a mild anomic aphasia and no agraphia. Computer tomography showed an occipito-temporal infarction in the territory of the left posterior cerebral artery.

Case III
The history of this 65-year-old, right-handed woman has been described elsewhere in more detail (Campbell *et al.*, 1986). After an uneventful medical history the patient became purely alexic and hemianopic to the right side subsequent to a stroke in the territory of the left posterior cerebral artery. Her reading difficulties in follow-up examinations during the last 6 years have not improved.

Besides extensive neuropsychological testing, a tachistoscopic experimental investigation was carried out, designed to uncover reading comprehension by means of a word–colour interference. The three patients were shown cards tachistoscopically for 50 ms exposure duration and asked to fixate a central dot. In the centre of each card there was a greyish dot of 1.2 degrees visual angle in diameter; 2–4 degrees off-centre, either in the left or the right visual field, a printed word was presented together with the central greyish dot, the colour of which remained constant. Patients were told that the dot would appear more 'reddish' on some trials and more 'greenish' on others. It was stated that the incidence of each colour was 'about 50 per cent'. The patients were explicitly encouraged to consider the exercise as a 'guessing task' since the difference in colour would be very faint. No mention was made about the words which would appear lateral to the dot and no exercise trials were given. The experiment consisted of two runs alternating between patients, whereby in the first run they had to press a button with each hand whenever they felt that the central dot was more 'reddish' and in the second run when the dot was more 'greenish' and vice versa. The 'pseudorandom order' of the stimuli was identical for both runs. The patients received a total of 192 stimulations each. The words which were presented lateral to the dot can be grouped into three classes. They consisted of either colour words (*rot* (red)/*grün* (green)), semantic cues (*Blut* (blood)/*Gras* (grass)) or 'neutral' words (*Ort* (place)).

The results of the three patients are concordant and quite striking. The dimension we looked at was the time patients needed to decide whether the dot was rather 'reddish' or 'greenish' respectively. The hypothesis was that whenever some unaware comprehension of the written word was present, the colour word 'green' or the semantic cue 'grass' would facilitate the decision that the central dot appeared 'greenish' but interfere with the decision that the central grey dot was rather 'reddish', and vice versa for the colour word 'red' and the semantic cue 'blood'. Neutral words should show neither facilitation nor interference. We found this to be the case in colour words and to a lesser degree in the semantic colour cues as well. The most striking and yet unexplained result, however, is that this word–colour interference was significantly more pronounced whenever the words fell within the right visual field, i.e. the hemianopic field.

The results described in this section indicate that the type of covert knowledge demonstrated in prosopagnosia can also be found in alexia. Thus covert knowledge is rather precise, more than just a lexical decision or semantic categorization. It consists of a category-item-specific interference and, more important still, interference by semantic associates. The result of a much greater interference in the right visual field projecting to the language dominant but hemianopic hemisphere is unexpected and difficult to interpret.

For two reasons it is hard to dismiss these results just on the basis of an inaccurate fixation, i.e. that the subject would consistently look to the right of the fixation dot as well as to the right of the greyish target. The patients were not told that words would appear in the left or the right visual field and their task was simply to judge the reddishness or greenishness of the central dot. Since the results are consistent for all three patients, a deviation of fixation is also highly improbable. Moreover, the lateralized covert knowledge in prosopagnosia (cf. Chapter 14) which we report in a patient with a left homonymous hemianopia is significant only for her hemianopic left visual field and thus indicates an inverse pattern for a stimulus, namely faces, associated with dominant processing of the right hemisphere's visual system. If one dismisses incorrect fixation, these results would mean that the dominant hemisphere for a certain stimulus type is also the one which 'knows without knowing' when its area V1 input is damaged. These results, though premature, might also be interpreted as an example of 'semantic blindsight'. Moreover, as opposed to our previous interpretation of preserved reading in alexia, these results would lend credit to the concept that in actual fact the passage of information through the dominant but damaged left hemispheric visual system is necessary to achieve reading in whatever form, and the same is also true for face identification and the right hemisphere's visual system.

Alexia and Shorthand (Stenography)

On p. 341 we mentioned a patient suffering from infarction in the territory of the right posterior artery who lost her ability to read stenographic script but could write it fluently and had only minor difficulties in reading printed text. In the following we present further observations on the capability of the right hemisphere in meaningful visuo-verbal operations or written signals. As described previously, Japanese patients suffering from lesions in the left occipito-temporal inferior cortex with or without splenial involvement were shown to exhibit pure alexia primarily in Kana but not in Kanji and Japanese patients with lesions in the left angular gyrus displayed alexia with agraphia for Kana but not necessarily alexia for Kanji (Iwata *et al.*, 1981; Iwata, 1984, 1985; Torii and Enokaida 1979; Yamadori, 1982; Yamadori *et al.*, 1985; Oka *et al.*, 1985; Mochizuki and Ohtomo, 1988). Such patients may be able to read and understand Kanji texts relatively fluently, while they are incapable of reading single words in Kana. Usually these findings have been interpreted as a capacity of the right hemisphere to recognize and analyse ideograms and transfer the preprocessed information by extrasplenial pathways to the left hemisphere for oral pronunciation and understanding.

The interpretation that the right hemisphere may deal generally with ideograms but not at all with a syllabic script is questioned, however, by observations made in a central European patient a few years ago (Regard *et al.*, 1985). This 84-year-old, right-handed architect had become purely alexic for German, French and English written in regular print, subsequent to a metastasis in the left temporo-occipital area from a rectosigmoid carcinoma. He was hemianopic to the right and had a mild paresis of the right arm which did not prevent him from writing correctly without major difficulty. The peculiarity in this patient was that he had been a proficient stenographer all his life using a syllabic shorthand system (Stolze-Schrey stenography) as well as parliament stenography. Stolze-Schrey stenography is a non-orthographic shorthand system that is syllabic to a large extent, has signs for consonants and expresses vowels by spatial displacement and shading of the consonants. Parliament stenography is an almost purely ideographic writing system consisting of a large number of individual signs for whole stereotyped sentences and abbreviations. It appeared that this patient, while being completely unable to read printed words or letters, was normally fluent in reading stenography of both types, the syllabic as well as the ideographic one. The patient, a former member of the editorial board of the *Swiss Stenography Journal*, continued to read and write stenographic texts of considerable length with ease, while he was unable to read without difficulty a single word which he himself had written in normal script or cursive writing.

If breakdown in performance with respect to the hemispheres involved depended upon the ideographic nature of the script, this patient would have failed to read syllabic stenography but would have retained reading of parliament stenography, which was not the case, however. It seems therefore plausible that in persons who have learned Western script, a more complex syllabic system like the Stolze-Schrey stenographic system involves right hemisphere functions, because the corresponding left hemisphere regions are 'occupied' by visual processing of Western script.

The last example of the preservation of complex graphical analysis in pure alexia is the recognition of familiar handwriting. On several occasions it has been observed that patients with pure alexia were able to identify specimens of individual handwriting, despite their inability to recognize words or even single letters (e.g. Alajouanine *et al.*, 1960; Landis and Regard, 1988). In our patient described above, this ability was not restricted to previously familiar handwriting, such as her own or that of close family members, but she was able to learn to recognize new handwritings in spite of her inability to read at all. This capability corresponds to that of healthy persons for recognizing the author of an autograph without having read a single word. Another prediction from this observation is possible: a specialist in art styles, especially someone competent in graphics, who had become alexic, would be still be able to recognize the creator of a certain drawing, etching or lithograph.

That tasks of this type are probably performed by the non-dominant right hemisphere's visual system is suggested not only by the occurrence of pure alexia for stenography, but also by the reports on patients who have lost their ability to recognize familiar handwriting in the presence of unimpaired reading subsequent to lesions in the posterior right hemisphere (e.g. Niessl von Mayendorf, 1935; Bouduresque *et al.*, 1979; Landis and Regard, 1988).

Although agreement has existed on the crucial anatomical structure for the occurrence of pure alexia ever since Dejerine (1892), this syndrome continues to be a riddle, inspite of the increasing number of cases and experimental investigations and the theoretical considerations outlined in this chapter.

Neuronal Circuits for Reading: A Proposed Model

Figure 18.7 depicts a diagram of proposed neuronal connections within the visual brain in which we have tried to

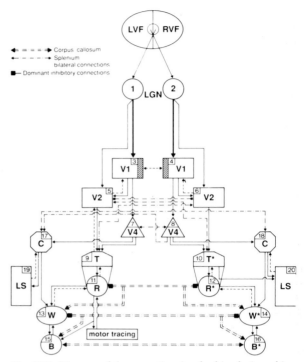

Fig. 18.7 *Diagram of the connections involved in alexia and in cerebral disturbance of colour vision. The connections marked with filled squares are dominant inhibitory ones (homotopic connections through the corpus callosum). LVF = left visual hemifield, RVF = right visual hemifield, LGN = left (1) and right (2) lateral geniculate nucleus. V1 = area V1, i.e. area striata of the occipital cortex. V2 = area V2 (peristriate visual cortex). V4 = area V4 containing many colour-specific nerve cells. C = 'colour category processor' located in the left and right angular gyrus. T = 'structural text processor' located presumably in the vicinity of the left angular gyrus. R = sensory reading area of the left angular gyrus. W = Wernicke's sensory speech area of the upper gyrus of the left temporal lobe. B = Broca's motor speech area in the left orbito-frontal lobe. LS = part of the limbic system connected with the colour processing region of the gyrus angularis. This part of the limbic system (the gyrus parahippocampalis?) mediates emotional aspects of colours. For further explanation, see the text. Note that the connections through the splenium are drawn differently to the other callosal connections.*

summarize clinical and anatomical evidence for the pathways between the hemispheres, the speech centres and the limbic structures relevant for reading. Despite the speculative aspects of such 'wiring diagrams', schematic drawings of this type have the advantage over lengthy verbal descriptions of leading more easily to testable hypotheses, the falsification of which forces a revision of theoretical interpretation and a subsequent correction of the wiring diagram (cf. Greenblatt, 1976, Castro-Caldas and Salgado, 1984; Geschwind, 1965). Figure 18.7 is simplified and reduces the afferent visual system to two binocular hemifields connected via the left or the right lateral geniculate nucleus (LGN) with area V1 of each hemisphere. It also disregards reading difficulties due to gaze movement problems and hemi-inattention mentioned earlier. For the projection of the LGN to the visual cortex, it contains the still questioned 'direct' connection of some LGN cells to area V2 (Chapter 3). We have included an area 'T' in the scheme responsible for structural text processing, the cerebral location of which still remains unclear: temporo–occipital areas or part of the gyrus angularis region. This area seems to be a necessary relay between area V1 and V2 counterprocessing and a linguistic transfer of the text by the left gyrus angularis region R. Area T fulfils the pre-reading operation of the 'visual *pars-pro-toto* function' mentioned above. The function of area T in reading is letter combinations to words and graphical classification of words/non-words without lexical association. The right area T* is required for covert knowledge of the meaning of words in alexic patients or split-brain patients reading in the LVF. Callosal connections through the splenium are characterized in Fig. 18.7 by symbols other than connections through the main corpus callosum. Homotopic callosal connections are presumed to be predominantly inhibitory ('squares' at the endings of the connections in Fig. 18.7 indicate this inhibitory function). In heterotopic callosal connections the excitatory functions dominate. Included in the scheme are pathways relevant for colour vision, which are discussed in detail in Chapter 20.

Using this diagram we will discuss several possible lesions or disconnections leading to alexic symptoms. The numbers refer to those used in Fig. 18.7. Two numbers (e.g. 1–2) indicate the connection between the numbered areas.

1. When the left LGN or the left visual radiation (1, 1–3) is destroyed, a hemianopia of the right visual field (RVF) is the result, while reading and vision through the left visual field (LVF) are still possible.

2. When a RVF hemianopia is caused by a lesion of the left area V1, poor residual vision may still be available in the RVF, transmitted by the connections from the left LGN to area V2 (1–5) or through the left tecto-pulvinar-cortical pathway not illustrated in Fig. 18.7. To test this residual reading ability, one should use single words in large print. Reading in the LVF should not be impaired by such lesions.

3. An isolated lesion of area V2 in the left occipital brain should lead to hemialexia and hemiagnosia in the RVF without hemianopia and permit normal reading in the left visual hemifield.

4. A lesion of the connections between area V2 and the 'structural' text processor T and reading area R, located in the region of the left angular gyrus, produces hemialexia (5–9).

5. When simultaneously the splenium of the corpus callosum is lesioned and the connections (6–9) and (10–9) are interrupted, a pure alexia is the consequence. Since the connections between area V4 (8) and the 'colour category processor' C in the left angular gyrus region are frequently interrupted (connections 8–17) under these conditions, the alexia is accompanied by hemiachromatopsia of the LVF. If a break in the the connections of area V4 on the left side with the colour category processor also occurs (7–17), alexia is accompanied by achromatopsia, whereby some emotional colour information processing is still possible through the connections (8–18–20) of the right hemisphere.

6. The contribution of splenium lesions to alexia has been disputed since Dejerine (1892) dismissed them as not being relevant to his interpretation of pure alexia. Wernicke (1903), Liepmann (1908), Geschwind (1965) and Geschwind and Fusillo (1966) attributed to splenium lesions, however, a prime role in the development of alexia (cf. also Foix and Hillmand, 1925b; Hécaen and Gruner, 1974; Hécaen and Kremin, 1976). An isolated lesion of the splenium would interrupt the connections (8–17), (8–7), (7–18); the consequence would be hemialexia and hemiachromatopsia in the left visual hemifield with some residual knowledge of the emotional effects of colours and judgement of emotional words. In Japanese patients, Kana hemialexia could be the consequence, while some Kanji recognition would be preserved in the LVF. In patients with hemialexia from Western cultures, reading stenography should still be possible in the LVF. Emotional processing of recognized colours and words read in the RVF should be impaired, but the discovery of this defect would require very careful hemifield testing.

7. A lesion of the 'structural' text processor T would lead to a pure alexia (including reduction in recognition of letters written on the skin) without affecting colour vision or writing, and the same should be true for a disconnection (9–11) between T and the angular gyrus reading area R.

8. When the connections between area V2 and T are interrupted but the structural processor T is intact, pure alexia should result but does not involve the reading of words or letters written on the skin or motor tracing of the letters as a tool in slow letter-by-letter reading.

9. When reading area R, localized presumably in the left angular gyrus, is destroyed, alexia with agraphia results. Some averbal understanding of the text is still possible through the connections 6–10–12–14–16. When the patient is forced to guess, a limited correct output might be transferred for concrete, highly imaginable and emotional words through the connections 14–13 or 16–15 from the right to the left half of the brain.

10. When the connections in the right hemisphere

between area V2 and area T* are interrupted, no impairment in text comprehension should be observed. We predict, however, that under these conditions the patients will have difficulty finding rhymes to written words or appreciating the melodies of lyrics read, while lyrics heard should still be well received. Through T* and R*, we think that visual signals have an input to W*, the corollary of the Wernicke speech area on the dominant side of the brain. It is thus presumed that with lesions at 10, 12 or (10–12), lyrics read out loud will be linguistically correct, but with a monotonous intonation.

11. In the light of the general hypothesis on brain mechanisms and reading mentioned in Chapter 17, lesions in T and R should also affect track reading, the visual *pars-pro-toto* function and 'reading' of figural symbols. Lesions in T* and R* should affect rapid behavioural responses to track reading and give rise to a negligence of emotionally alarming visual signs.

12. Since it is assumed that the areas T and R and especially the areas T* and R* have an input to the limbic system, which also receives direct inputs from area V2 and V4, some emotional effects of frequent and overtrained words related to more or less stereotyped and overlearned emotional responses could be present in pure alexia, except in those patients in which the output of V2 and V4 is interrupted or these visual association cortices are destroyed on both sides. This seems to be the case in general visual agnosia (*Seelenblindheit*, Chapter 11).

19 Visual Movement Agnosia, or Motion Blindness: A Rare Clinical Symptom

Introduction

As already discussed in Chapter 6, extended neuronal systems exist in the posterior part of the primate brain which are involved in movement perception. It is rather likely that similar systems, specialized for either the perception of small moving objects or large field visual motion, are also present in the human brain. There are, however, only a few clinical reports on patients suffering from a rather selective impairment of visual movement perception caused by circumscribed brain lesions. Extended bilateral lesions of the parietal or parieto-occipital regions, which lead to Balint–Holmes syndrome (Chapter 22), also impair man's ability to detect local or global movement; not only are thresholds for movement detection increased, but the ability to recognize movement direction correctly is also frequently lost. These defects in visual movement recognition are combined, however, with other visuo-spatial and visuo-motor deficiencies that interfere with one another. As a result, only indefinite conclusions about cortical mechanisms specifically related to movement perception may be drawn from observation of these patients (Pötzl, 1928; Kleist, 1934). The same is true when spatial orientation and object recognition are impaired because of extended occipito-parietal lesions. One also finds in such patients severe defects in visual movement perception, which is just one of many other symptoms (e.g. Pötzl and Redlich, 1911; Pötzl, 1928). To date, clinical observations of 'pure' visual movement agnosia consist of only a few case reports in which rather circumscribed bilateral lesions of the parieto-occipital part of the brain are described. Before we discuss these observations, we shall first deal with some general neurobiological aspects of movement perception. This summary should serve not only to introduce the reader to the field of visual movement research: it is also intended as a basis for further studies on movement agnosic patients.

Different Types of Movement Perception and Their Biological Relevance

Visual movement perception is a 'submodality' or 'quality' of the visual modality, just as colour, brightness, size, etc. are sensory qualities related to the perception of the visual world (Exner, 1875). In an extensive review article, Nakayama (1985) called movement perception a 'dimension' of vision. Neuronal systems detecting visual movement and movement direction are most likely present in the nervous system of all animals that respond to visual signals more complex than simple light–dark gradients. In analysing these systems one may differentiate between responses to 'local' and 'global' visual motion. An example of local movement is the translatory movements of prey and enemies across an animal's habitat. The ability to detect this local movement is very important for most animals. In the visual world of modern man, the most dangerous local movements are those occurring in traffic. In a natural environment, local visual movement is also evoked when the wind blows through trees and bushes, moving leaves and twigs back and forth without causing general positional changes. The movement of an image of the stationary world across the retina by voluntary and involuntary movements of the eyes, head or body is an example of global movement stimulation, since a large part of the visual world changes its position on the retina. 'Passive' global visual movement, i.e. visual motion seen with a large part of the retina, occurs rather seldom under natural conditions, e.g. when one looks at a flowing river, observes a large waterfall from close up or gazes at low, fast-moving clouds. In our technical world, however, large-field, 'passive' movement stimulation is an everyday event. This is the case, for example, when we drive a car or ride in a train moving at constant speed (which cannot be detected by vestibular receptors). These types of locomotion through the environment generate characteristic visual 'flow fields' which serve as input signals for both eyes (e.g. Koenderink, 1989).

A special type of local movement can be discriminated from all other types of translatory movement: movement in which the stimulus remains within a rather narrow local range, and returns more or less periodically to its original position. Technical rotatory, spiral or back-and-forth movements (without additional translation of the equipment in space) are such types of local, non-translatory movement. Local, non-translatory, more or less periodic movements may be combined with translatory movement, e.g. someone seen waving a handkerchief from a moving train, or a crow moving its wings up and down while flying across the observer's visual world.

The phylogenetic development of movement-sensitive neuronal systems, a phenomenon which is widespread throughout the animal kingdom, was evidently necessary for several reasons, as follows:

1. Detection of local visual movement against a stationary visual background.
2. Local visual movement detection by the foveal and parafoveal retina controlling gaze pursuit of small moving objects.
3. Detection of large-field (global) visual movement, which, as an isolated stimulus, may evoke a feeling of apparent self-movement in the observer ('vection'). This type of movement detection is mainly used by the organism for visual–vestibular coordination during head and body movement caused by locomotion.
4. Detection of relative visual movement of objects in a three-dimensional world when the organism moves through that world (parallax movement). Parallax movement within a flow field also allows for the detection of objects ('shape by movement', Chapter 1); it also facilitates figure–ground separation as well as the perception of depth in the extra-personal space. The amount of time before the observer collides with an object may also be estimated from the flow field (Lee, 1976).

Visual detection of movement is a sensory as well as a motor capability. As is discussed below, one can discriminate between 'afferent' (sensory) and 'efferent' (motor) movement perception. This discrimination is somewhat artificial when natural conditions for visual movement perception are taken into consideration, since both mechanisms frequently work together in order to create uniform perception. Researchers interested in movement detection divide movement sensation into two other classes: the perception of 'real' visual movement, which is evoked by a change in the position of objects located in the three-dimensional extra-personal space; and the perception of apparent motion, which occurs in a great variety of natural or laboratory conditions.

Visual motion is perceived when an object changes its position in the visual world relative to a background perceived as stationary. Visual movement is detected when the change in position is above the threshold for minimal dislocation and minimum angular velocity (Aubert, 1886, 1887; Basler, 1906; Koffka, 1931; Graham, 1966). For a quantitative analysis of visual movement perception, the following parameters of a stimulus moving through the extra-personal space have to be considered: metrical velocity [m s^{-1}] or angular velocity [deg s^{-1}], size, contrast, position and distance of the moving object, duration of motion, and change in angular size when the object is moving along the z-axis of the extra-personal space towards or away from the observer. The general level of light and colour adaptation has some impact on movement perception; thresholds for movement detection are higher for scotopic than for photopic vision.

With regard to the perception of curvilinear movements through the extra-personal space, the range of movement velocity can be divided into four regions, as follows:

1. Very low stimulus velocities V_s, at which neither movement nor direction can be directly perceived; through intermittent observation, however, the observer is convinced of movement by changes in position. The sun disappearing behind the horizon is a natural example of this type of subthreshold visual movement ($V_s < 0.004$ deg s^{-1}).
2. Above a minimum angular velocity and displacement, there is a large range of stimulus velocities at which movement and direction of motion are correctly perceived. The Weber fraction $\Delta V_s/V_s$ was found to be about 5 per cent within a wide range of visual movement (Nakayama, 1981; McKee, 1981). Like the Weber fraction, the precision involved in discovering changes in movement direction depends on stimulus size, contrast and luminance, and amounts to about 1–2 degrees for movement in a fronto-parallel plane.
3. Only movement can be detected above a certain angular velocity (450–600 deg s^{-1}), which depends on the size and contrast of the moving stimulus; the ability to discriminate the direction of the moving stimulus is no longer possible.
4. At very high speeds, neither movement nor movement direction can be recognized; one perceives only a short change in the visual stimulus.

The angular velocities separating these four different perceptual stages depend on the parameters mentioned above. The most important factor seems to be the temporal frequency of the pattern stimulating the single photoreceptor (Foster, 1969).

As already mentioned above, global or local movement in the extra-personal space can be detected in two different 'modes', conveniently designated as afferent and efferent visual movement perception. The terms sensory and motor visual movement are also used (Grüsser and Grüsser-Cornehls, 1969, 1973; Dichgans *et al.*, 1969). In afferent visual movement perception, the eye is stationary and the visual world moves across the retina. In 'pure' efferent movement perception, however, the visual stimulus is attentively pursued by gaze movements; consequently, the stimulus image remains stationary on the retina. This state is approached when the gaze angular velocity and direction approximately corresponds to that of the object ('gain 1'). This occurs under optimal attentive pursuit. 'Gain 1' is precisely reached when a perfectly stabilized parafoveal retinal image is pursued by voluntary eye movements. This is the case, for example, when one tries to pursue a parafoveal afterimage (see below).

Under natural conditions, of course, the perception of local or global movement is usually caused by both the efferent and afferent mechanisms of visual movement recognition. The perceived visual movement is then the result of a cerebral integration of sensory and gaze motor signals.

In psychophysical experiments involving human observers, a power function with an exponent having a value somewhere between 0.79 and 0.81 was found to describe the relationship between the perceived velocity V_p and the angular velocity V_s of a small moving object (Mashhour, 1964) in units of movement perception:

$$V_p = k_v V_s^{0.8} \qquad (19.1)$$

where k_v is a constant that depends on stimulus size and contrast. A large, moving pattern composed of either black-and-white stripes or random dots (as used in an optokinetic drum), however, leads to an approximately linear relationship between angular velocity and the perceived speed of motion (Dichgans *et al.*, 1969; Körner, 1969). Interestingly, the speed of a moving object is estimated to be about 1.6–1.8 times higher when the eyes are fixed on a stationary target, as compared with when they attentively pursue a moving object; in the latter case, the image is more or less 'stabilized' on the retina (Aubert, 1887; Filehne, 1922; Brown, 1931; Kornmüller, 1931; Körner and Dichgans, 1967).

Movement of an object against a stationary background facilitates object recognition, since all points belonging to the moving object move coherently: this evidently contributes to 2-D- or 3-D-shape vision. A simple shape such as a disc, cross or letter cut out from random dot paper and placed on a random dot background having the same statistical structure is completely camouflaged. The figure immediately becomes visible, however, when it is moved against the background, since the spatio-temporal correlation of coherent movement leads not only to movement

detection, but can evidently also be used by the central visual system to generate the outlines of the moving figure. These mechanisms also operate with stroboscopic illumination (e.g. van Doorn *et al.*, 1985; Koenderink *et al.*, 1985). This is not surprising, for it is well known that even in simple movement detecting systems, such as in frog retinal ganglion cells (as well as in the visual cortex movement detecting nerve cells of mammals), stroboscopically illuminated moving stimuli evoke strong neuronal responses (Grüsser-Cornehls *et al.*, 1963; Grüsser-Cornehls, 1968; Grüsser and Grüsser-Cornehls, 1973).

Within certain limits, human observers are not able to discriminate between sequentially displaced stationary stimuli (phi-movement) and continuous visual movement. Therefore, a memory device must operate somewhere within the visual system that integrates successive retinal signals. Such a short-term memory device is also required in order to detect movement direction by means of delayed autocorrelation (Reichardt, 1961). Depending on the time constant of these mechanisms, one can predict that discovery of movement direction by visual neurones will break down when stroboscopic illumination of a certain frequency is combined with selected stimulus speeds. This leads to a displacement velocity which is faster than the spread of directional selective lateral inhibition within the neuronal system in question. Examples of such a breakdown in directional selectivity of neurones located in the visual association cortices are discussed in Chapter 5. From this observation, one may conclude that movement and movement direction recognition may be impaired in patients suffering from brain lesions if the temporal data processing is slowed down. The most frequent effect on movement perception reported by patients with occipitoparietal brain lesions is indeed their difficulty in detecting the direction of a moving object. Short-time memory processes for movement and shape detection can be easily demonstrated with a stroboscopically lit, moving random dot pattern. One perceives apparent motion in such a pattern at flash frequencies above 1 flash s^{-1}. Above 9 flashes s^{-1}, one also discovers a vertical striation oriented perpendicularly to the direction of movement (α-stripes; Adler and Grüsser, 1979; Adler *et al.*, 1981). The period P_α (degrees) of this striation depends on the angular velocity V_s of the random dot pattern and the flash frequency f_s:

$$P_\alpha = V_s/f_s \qquad (19.2)$$

Evidently a short-term visual memory is necessary to generate the α-striation from a pattern which does not contain any spatial periodicity. We think that essentially the same short-term visual memory enables the observer to detect shapes from motion as illustrated by random dot figures moving on a random dot background (for further discussion see Adler *et al.*, 1981).

Apparent Visual Movement

As phi-movement illustrates, visual movement is sometimes also perceived even in the absence of physical movement, i.e. movement sensation is caused by special properties of the neuronal structures that detect 'real' visual movement. There is a large variety of movement illusions which all support the hypothesis that visual movement is a primary quality of vision:

1. A small, stationary object seems to move in a direction opposite to that of the large, surrounding background ('induced movement'). The moon seen 'wandering' behind apparently motionless clouds in a darkened sky is a well-known example of just such an illusion, which leads to a rather paradoxical phenomenon: one sees the movement, but simultaneously realizes that the moon does not change its position.

2. When a large visual field is moving, the moving stimulus may be perceived as stationary, while the observer experiences a sensation of being 'moved' through the extra-personal space ('circular' or 'linear' vection; Mach, 1875; Fischer and Kornmüller, 1930). This phenomenon can easily be demonstrated by placing a subject in a large, horizontally rotating drum covered with vertical, black-and-white stripes (this device is normally used to measure optokinetic nystagmus (OKN)). Vection is stronger when the subject's optokinetic eye movements are suppressed for a longer period of time (e.g. by fixating on a small, stationary target) than is the case during attentive OKN (Bötzel *et al.*, 1981). During circular vection, the observer experiences the illusion of being rotated in the direction opposite to that of the moving drum; the induced circular vection depends on the angular velocity of the optokinetic pattern and on the duration of stimulation, as illustrated in Figs. 19.1(a) and (b). Vection also depends on the observer's head position relative to the rotating optokinetic field and to the field of gravity. When a vertically rotating field moves around an observer sitting or standing in an upright position, he experiences a body inclination in the direction opposite to that of the visual movement (Figs. 19.2(a),(b)); he does not experience continuous self-rotation. When the subject lies horizontally, however, the same visual stimulus ('vertical' optokinetic stimulation relative to the subject's head) causes circular vection: the rotation axis of vection corresponds approximately to the rotation axis of the optokinetic field (Figs. 19.3(a)–(c)). Circular or linear vection is much more effectively induced when apparent 'three-dimensional' visual patterns are applied which exhibit correct parallax movement of the objects within the visual flow field during rotation and/or linear motion. Patterns that simulate a 3-D space perceived when one turns oneself around or moves across a natural environment create an illusion of self-

movement within less than 0.3 s. The slow 'buildup' of circular vection (as illustrated in Fig. 19.1(b)) is shortened to a fraction of a second. Such stimulus patterns are effectively applied in flight simulators used to train aircraft pilots.

3. Passive movement of the eyeball allows for the perception of visual movement of the whole visual world. Objects in the central part of the visual field seem to make larger movements than do objects located in the periphery

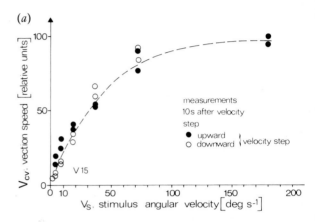

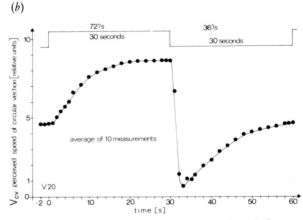

Fig. 19.1 *(a) Relationship between the perceived speed of horizontal circular vection* V_{cv} *(ordinate) and stimulus angular velocity* V_s *(abscissa). Data for steady-state conditions are plotted. Measurements were made 10 s after the onset of movement stimulation. (b) Time course of perceived circular vection* V_{cv} *after a positive and a negative velocity step. The subject sat in a cylinder 280 cm in diameter and 197 cm high. Moving random dots of light were projected using a planetarium projector onto the inner white wall. The horizontal movement velocity was changed for 30 seconds from 36 deg s^{-1} to 72 deg s^{-1}. Note the slow increase in circular vection and the abrupt reduction when movement velocity was reduced (from Bötzel et al., 1981).*

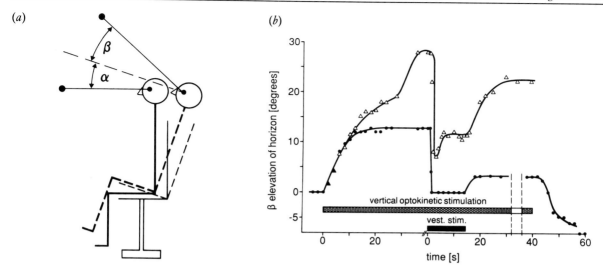

Fig. 19.2 *(a) A subject sat in an upright position in a chair. A random light spot pattern moving in a vertical direction downwards at 30 deg s^{-1} was projected onto the wall of a cylindrical room. The subject fixated on a stationary, light-emitting diode that was placed on the wall in front of him at eye level. The optokinetic downward stimulation led to two illusionary perceptions: the subject had a feeling of backward inclination at an angle α and his subjective horizon, i.e. the apparent height of the fixation target, was elevated but exceeded α by an additional angle β. Both phenomena were considerably reduced when an attentive optokinetic downward nystagmus (following the stars of the optokinetic field) was performed. Horizontal sinewave rotation of the subject (0.5–1 Hz, 10–20 degrees amplitude) considerably reduced α and β. (b) The apparent elevation $\alpha + \beta$ of the horizon slowly increased with the duration of the vertical, optokinetic downward stimulation. Sinewave horizontal rotation of the subject, which leads to activation of the semicircular canal receptors ('vest. stim.'), abolished or reduced the apparent inclination of the horizon. Data from two measurements (from Grüsser and Guldin, 1991).*

of the visual field. Paradoxically, one does not see any relative movement between the objects within the visual field (MacKay, 1970). Similarly, visual movement is perceived in the presence of involuntary eye movements, as is the case with vestibular nystagmus or pathological nystagmus caused by cerebral lesions.

4. As already mentioned above, when a long-lasting afterimage is imprinted on the retina, voluntary eye movements (saccades or pursuit eye movements) cause the observer to perceive afterimage motion. Pure efferent visual movement perception is present under such conditions, since the afterimage is absolutely 'stabilized' on the retina. Passive eye movements in the dark do not shift the perceived position of the afterimage, however, and do not induce any afterimage movement (Bell, 1823; Purkinje, 1825; Fig. 19.4). When a human observer tries to fixate on an afterimage shifted by 0.2–1 degrees off the fovea centre, smooth-pursuit eye movements are induced. The subject perceives smooth movement of the afterimage in the direction of the eye movements; this movement increases in angular velocity the longer the afterimage is pursued. This acceleration is caused by a continuous temporal summation of efferent movement signals, as explained in the caption to Fig. 19.5. When the afterimage is placed at

eccentricities larger than 1.5–2 degrees, the intention to shift the centre of gaze towards the afterimage produces a sequence of saccades (Fig. 19.5(b)). As a result, the subject perceives jerky afterimage movements. Alternating spatially directed attention towards two parafoveal afterimages (one on the left, the other on the right side of the fovea) leads to sinewave eye movements and to a corresponding perception of pendular movements for the two afterimages (Fig. 19.5(c)).

5. The movement of an afterimage seen during voluntary eye movements is pure efferent movement perception, i.e. movement perception caused by efference copy mechanisms, which is discussed in detail below. Similarly, sigma movement and sigma optokinetic nystagmus are efferent movement perception phenomena that are dominantly controlled by efference copy mechanisms. The sigma paradigm (Stoper, 1967; Lamontagne, 1973; Behrens and Grüsser, 1978, 1979, Adler *et al.*, 1981) is explained in Fig. 19.6: a long row of equidistant dots or stripes (period P_s) is stroboscopically illuminated at a flash frequency f_s. When the centre of gaze performs pursuit movements across this pattern at an angular speed V_g, identical retinal images are generated 'flash by flash' and sigma movement appears when the constant $k > 1$ is an

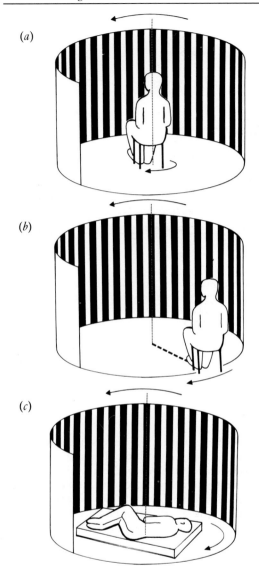

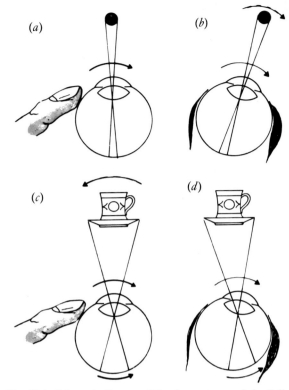

Fig. 19.4 *Schematic diagram of the observations made by Bell (1823) and Purkinje (1825) during investigations of the apparent motion of a long-lasting foveal afterimage or of an object located in the extra-personal space. (a) The subject observed a stationary foveal afterimage in complete darkness. No afterimage movement was perceived when the eyeball was passively moved. (b) The subject perceived afterimage movement in the direction of the eye movement during active, saccadic eye movements, however. By daylight, the subject fixated on an object located in the extra-personal space by using foveal vision. Passive eye movement led to apparent motion of the stationary visual object in the direction opposite to the eye displacement. (d) When the image of the object was moved across the retina during a saccade, the object was perceived as remaining stationary in space, despite the fact that its image moved on the retina during the saccade (from Grüsser, 1986).*

Fig. 19.3 *Illustration of the phenomena related to circular vection. (a) The subject sat in the centre of a large, horizontally rotating optokinetic field. Movement of the optokinetic field towards the left produced in the subject a feeling of self-rotation (circular vection) towards the right. (b) Circular vection was also experienced when the subject sat eccentrically to the rotation axis of the optokinetic field, as if the platform were rotating around the cylinder axis. In addition to this feeling of apparent rotation, the subject also experienced pseudo-centrifugal forces. (c) The subject lay horizontally within the rotating visual field and turned his head sidewards. The optokinetic stimulation was therefore in a vertical, downward direction relative to the subject's head coordinates. The subject experienced a feeling of self-rotation (as in (a)) around an axis that corresponded to the cylinder axis. The speed of perceived circular vection corresponded to that experienced in (a) (Fig. 19.1(a)).*

integer in the following equation (degrees s^{-1}):

$$V_g = k\,P_s f_s \tag{19.3}$$

As in the afterimage experiment involving sigma movement, the quasi-stabilized retinal pattern is also seen moving in the direction of the gaze pursuit movements. The perceived sigma movement perpetuates the sigma pursuit movements of the eyes or the gaze, and evokes an optokinetic nystagmus (sigma OKN), which in turn maintains the kinetic illusion *ad libitum*. According to Equation

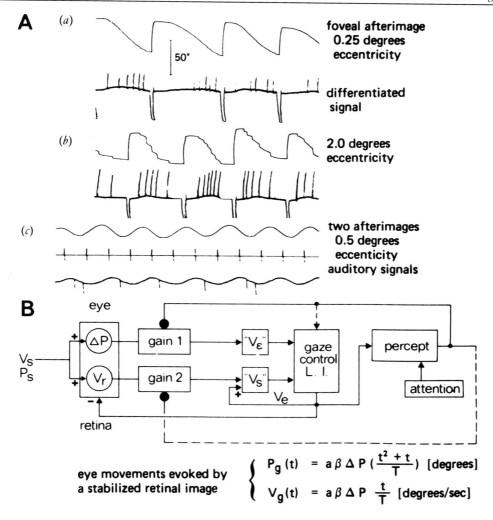

$$P_g(t) = a\,\beta\,\Delta P \left(\frac{t^2 + t}{T}\right) \text{ [degrees]}$$

$$V_g(t) = a\,\beta\,\Delta P \;\frac{t}{T}\; \text{ [degrees/sec]}$$

Fig. 19.5 *A(a) Intentional fixation on a small foveal afterimage placed at 0.25 degrees eccentricity from the foveal centre led to smooth pursuit eye movements. The subject perceived smooth movement of the afterimage, which increased at an angular velocity parallel to the increase in eye velocity. The voluntary backward saccades led to a shift of the afterimage in the direction of the saccades. The perceived velocity of the afterimage corresponded approximately to the angular speed of the smooth eye pursuit movements. (b) A sequence of saccades resulted when a long-lasting afterimage was placed at 2.0 degrees eccentricity from the fovea centre and the subject tried to pursue the afterimage. As a result, the subject perceived jerky afterimage movements in the direction of the eye movements. (c) In this experiment, two afterimages were horizontally placed at 0.5 degrees eccentricity to the left and right sides of the fovea centre. Auditory signals (vertical impulses in the middle recording) were applied at regular intervals. The subject shifted his attention to the left or right afterimages respectively when the auditory signal was applied. This procedure led to horizontal, pendular eye movements and, correspondingly, to an apparent horizontal sinewave motion for the afterimage. In (a)–(c) the upper signal represents eye position, the lower eye velocity. Eye position recordings by means of the electromagnetic search coil technique (Collewijn and Grüsser, 1982; from Grüsser, 1986). (B) Block diagram and a corresponding mathematical model that predicts the non-linear time course of smooth-pursuit eye movements and movement perception evoked by a stabilized extrafoveal stimulus (towards which the subject directs his visual attention). This model assumes that the initial speed of the eye pursuit movements depends on the distance ΔP of the pursuit stimulus from the fovea centre (up to about 1.5 degrees eccentricity), and on the retinal angular velocity V_r of the pursued moving stimulus. V_r was zero in the afterimage experiment. The 'efference copy' signal is added to V_r in a feedback loop, resulting in V_s, the velocity signal fed into the gaze-motor control system. The perceived velocity corresponds to V_e, but also depends on attention. The equations illustrate the eye position ($P_g(t)$) as a function of both time t and the distance ΔP of the retinal afterimage from the fovea centre. The gaze velocity $V_g(t)$ or $V_e(t)$ respectively increases with time when a subject intends to pursue the parafoveal afterimage.*

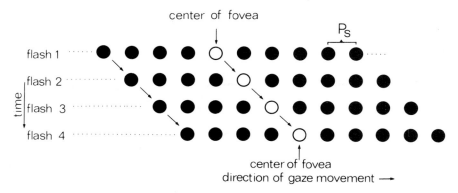

Fig. 19.6 *Explanation of the sigma paradigm for optokinetic nystagmus or pursuit eye movements. A row of regularly spaced dots or stripes is stroboscopically illuminated by short flashes of light (< 1 ms duration). During the intervals between successive flashes, the centre of gaze moves one dot to the right. Thus identical, 'flash-by-flash' retinal images are generated. This leads to apparent motion of the dot row in the direction of the eye movements (sigma movement), since no movement signals are generated on the retina. In turn, sigma movement perpetuates the eye movements, etc. The sigma paradigm is also fulfilled when the eyes move 2, 3 or 4 dots ('mode' 2, 3 or 4) during a flash interval.*

19.2, the gaze pursuit velocity increases with flash frequency f_s and with the period P_s of the periodic pattern (Fig. 19.7(a), 19.10(a)). Sigma movement and sigma OKN may also be evoked by stroboscopically illuminated random dot patterns, which generate periodic stripes on the 'cyclopean eye' (Figs. 19.7(b), 19.10(c)). Under such conditions, the perception of periodic stripes is allowed for by brain functions beyond area V1 (Julesz and Payne, 1968). The same is true for the interaction of efference copy signals and for the visual pattern leading to sigma movement of these stereostripes and sigma OKN (Adler and Grüsser, 1979; Adler *et al.*, 1981). Equation 19.3 was also found to be valid for sigma OKN evoked using such stroboscopically generated stereostripes (Fig. 19.10(c)).

Sigma pursuit movements may also be evoked when, instead of linear periodic patterns, a circle or any other closed figure composed of intermittently illuminated equidistant dots on a two–dimensional plane (or identical objects in a three–dimensional space) are used as stimulus patterns (Figs. 19.8–19.11). Sigma OKN is easily evoked in primates other than man and obeys then the same rules as expressed by Equation 19.3 (Fig. 19.10(b)).

6. Apparent motion is perceived as an after-effect of real visual movement. When one looks for a sufficient length of time at a rotating disc (e.g. a rotating record disc) or any other visual pattern continuously moving in one direction (e.g. a waterfall), one will eventually perceive the stationary objects to be moving in the direction opposite to that of the conditioning stimuli. This movement after-effect was first described by Aristotle (*On Dreams*, 459b). It was rediscovered by Purkinje (1825) and later described as the 'waterfall illusion' by Adams (1834). It is best seen

with a moving random dot pattern. The movement after-effect is strongly reduced when one eye is conditioned by the moving stimulus, and the stationary test stimulus is then observed by the other eye. This observation suggests that the movement adaptation responsible for the movement after-effect is a result of properties of the neuronal systems located peripheral to binocular fusion. Directional selective neuronal networks evidently adapt when continuously stimulated in one direction (cf. Chapter 5). Movement after-effect is a phenomenon that has been repeatedly studied by several generations of visual scientists (e.g. Wohlgemuth, 1911; Sekuler and Ganz, 1963; Pantle, 1978).

7. Apparent motion is also perceived after a certain temporal delay when two stationary visual stimuli are briefly projected onto different parts of the visual field (phi movement; Exner, 1875; Wertheimer, 1912; for reviews see: Aarons, 1964; Anstis, 1978). In modern psychophysical studies of movement perception, a 'short-range' process (<0.5 degrees) is discriminated from a 'long-range' movement perception process that operates across a retinal distance of 15 degrees or more (Braddick, 1974, 1980; Anstis, 1980). Classical phi movement is considered to belong to 'long-range' motion perception. Phi movement is also induced when the two stationary stimuli have different shapes. In this case, the moving stimulus changes its shape during the apparent motion. Phi movement can, of course, be perpetuated when a stationary stimulus shifts its position periodically and is illuminated stroboscopically (Fig. 19.8). Movement perceived in a movie or on a TV screen is an example of phi movement involving both short-range and long-range processes.

(a)

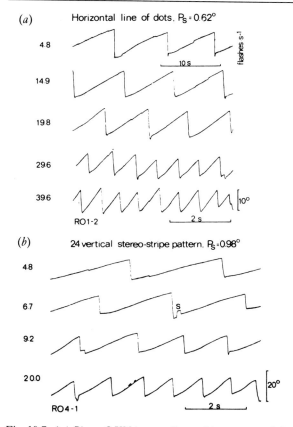

(b)

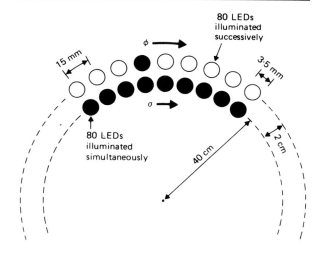

Fig. 19.8 *Schematic design of a simple device used to evoke circular sigma movement or phi movement. Two sets of 80 equally spaced light-emitting diodes (LEDs) are placed in two concentric circles with respective diameters of 40 and 42 cm. By switching the short current pulses (8–25 ms duration) at a temporal frequency* f_s *from one LED to the next (outer circle), a single spot is seen moving along the circle (phi movement). The speed of this phi movement can be varied by changing* f_s. *Smooth, circular eye movements result when the subject fixates on the apparently moving light stimulus. When, in addition to the phi stimulus located in the outer circle, all LEDs in the inner circle are simultaneously flashed at flash frequency* f_s, *the circle is perceived as rotating in the direction of the slow eye pursuit movements (sigma movement). The single stimulus in the outer LED circle can be switched off as soon as sigma movement is perceived. The sigma movement of the inner circle continues at a 'circular' frequency* $f_e = f_s/n$ *(Hz), where n is the number of LED's in the circle. The speed of sigma movement and sigma pursuit eye movements can be varied by changing* f_s. *In order to measure linear phi and sigma movements, a double horizontal row of 40 LEDs was used in the same manner as for the concentric circles (Grüsser and Rickmeyer, 1981).*

Fig. 19.7 *(a) Sigma OKN in man. Eye position was recorded using the electromagnetic search coil technique. A horizontal line of dots located 0.62 degrees apart was stroboscopically illuminated at different flash frequencies, as indicated. Note the increase in the slow pursuit component of the sigma OKN, as predicted by Equation 19.2. (b) Sigma OKN evoked by a vertical stereostripe pattern. The stereostripes generated on the cyclopean retina were separated by 0.98 degrees. Different flash frequencies were as indicated (from Adler* et al., *1981).*

This discrimination between short-range and long-range movement processes seems to us somewhat artificial. Van de Grind *et al.* (1983) explored the detection of coherent motion in stroboscopically illuminated, moving random dot patterns projected at different visual field eccentricities. They found the motion–detection performance to be invariant up to 48 degrees eccentricity, provided that the stimuli were scaled according to the retino–cortical magnification factor (cf. Chapter 4). This finding makes 'near' and 'far' distant movement processes dependent on the location of the moving stimuli in the visual field. A complete structural invariance in terms of eccentricity-scaled movement detecting neuronal systems was sug-

gested instead (van de Grind *et al.*, 1986). This movement recognition mechanism was found to be widely independent of the black–white contrast in the moving pattern (van de Grind *et al.*, 1987; for further discussion see van de Grind, 1988, 1990).

One class of experiments, however, does seem to indicate two different movement mechanisms: phi movement seen with one eye, and binocular phi movement seen when the stimuli are alternately perceived through the left and right eyes. A simple experiment may serve to demonstrate the binocular phi phenomenon: when one reaches out one's arm and monocularly fixates on the thumb first with one, then with the other eye, the thumb and hand

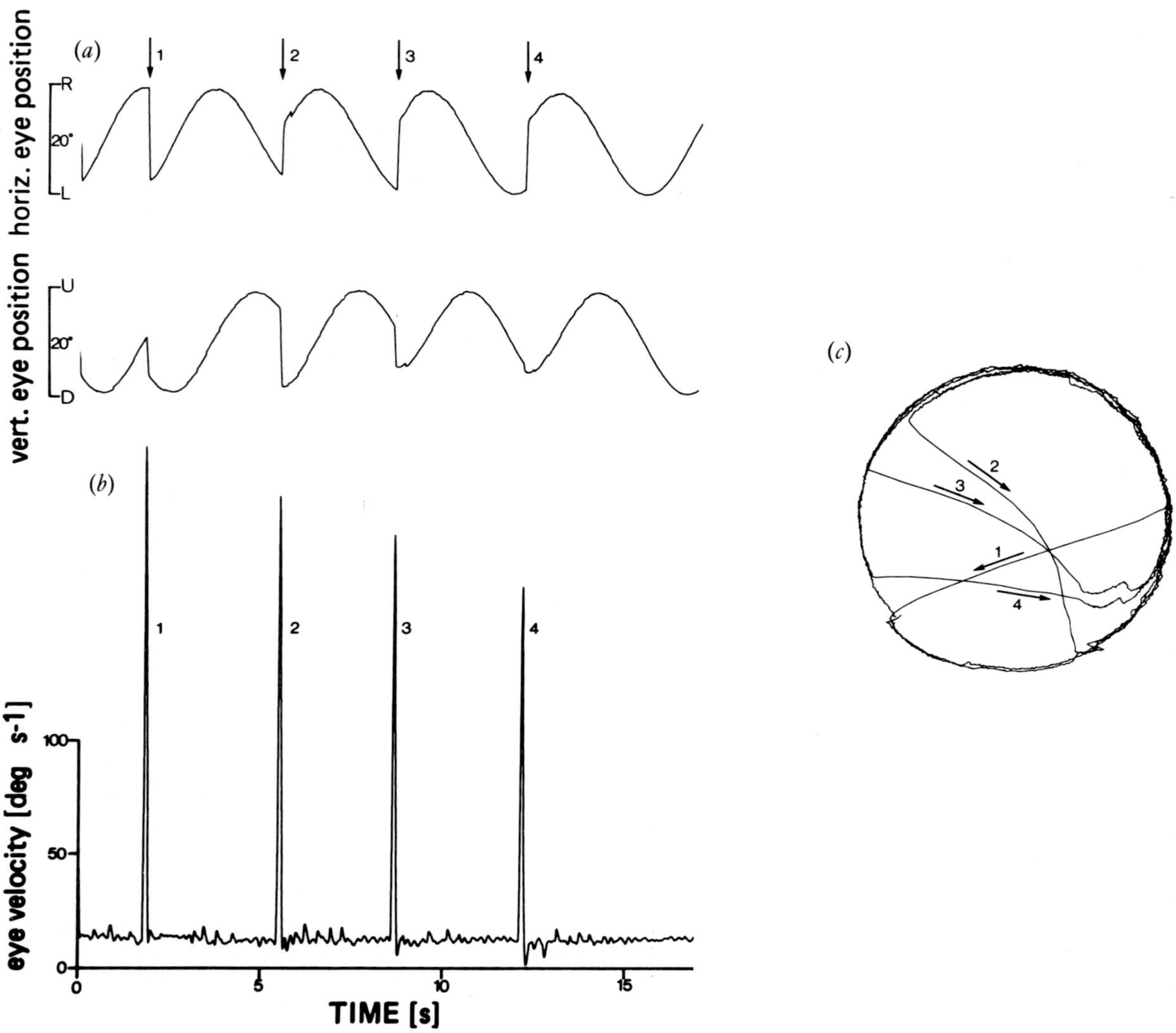

Fig. 19.9 *Sigma pursuit movement across a stroboscopically lit dot circle. The smooth eye pursuit movements were interrupted by voluntary saccades which the subject performed in order to gaze about the apparently moving circle. These saccades did not interrupt the perception of smooth rotation by the circle. The horizontal and vertical eye position are presented in (a), eye velocity along the circular path in (b). Eye position is represented on a two-dimensional plane in (c). The numbers refer to the saccades seen in (a) and (b) (Behrens and Grüsser, 1979).*

seem to move relative to the background. From this experiment, one can deduce that this type of movement perception has to rely on 'binocular' neuronal networks beyond area V1 (existing in addition to other neuronal systems sensitive to 'monocular' movement).

8. Another type of apparent motion is evoked by stationary visual stimulus patterns which change their luminance. A simple lecture hall experiment demonstrates this illusion: a ring of light surrounding a spot of light is pro-

jected onto a screen. The luminance of the ring is varied sinusoidally in time at 0.5–3 Hz. The stationary spot, which is not as bright as the ring, apparently expands and contracts synchronously with the sinusoidal change in ring luminance. The apparent movement of the borders of the spot of light is probably caused by lateral inhibition, evoked by the change in ring luminance.

9. Apparent motion of a visual stimulus is also seen when one fixates on a small visual target in total darkness

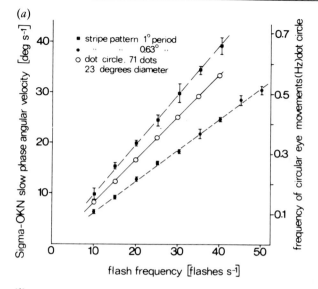

(a)

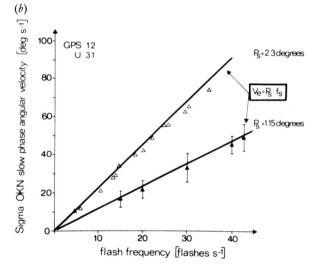

(b)

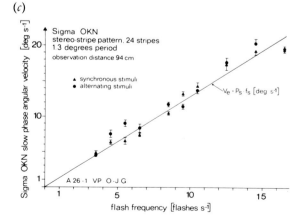

(c)

without performing any other voluntary eye movements. After several seconds of fixation, rather large and irregular target movements are perceived. It is assumed that this 'autokinesis' is caused by small, involuntary eye 'drifts', which shift the stimulus image from the fovea to adjacent parafoveal areas; this leads to an activation of movement-sensitive neurones. Because the degree of the drifts and the extension of the stimulus's apparent movement do not correspond to each other, Crone and Verduyn-Lunel (1969) attributed this illusion of movement to the activation of a highly sensitive class of 'movement-detecting neurones', which have their receptive fields near the fovea. These neurones are normally used to control slow pursuit eye movements when the eyes follow a slow moving object.

10. A special class of apparent motion is that related to motion in depth. When the size of an object suddenly increases, it is automatically perceived as moving towards the observer; when it decreases in size, it is perceived as moving away.

11. Abnormal vestibular stimulation, cerebral intoxication or acute diseases may cause pathological nystagmus, which leads to the perception of motion in the stationary visual world. Involuntary eye movements evidently do not evoke efference copy signals, which compensate for the visual movement perception induced by the shift of the image across the retina. Interestingly, no apparent motion of the visual world is perceived by subjects who suffer from congenital nystagmus. Such patients

Fig. 19.10 *(a) Relationship between flash frequency (abscissa) and the angular velocity of horizontal sigma OKN slow phase obtained using two different vertical stripe patterns (squares 1 degree period, dots 0.63 degree period). The open circles represent the relationship between flash frequency and the frequency of circular eye movements (right side ordinate) obtained using a dot circle having 71 dots and a diameter of 23 degrees (Behrens and Grüsser, 1979). (b) Data from sigma OKN evoked in a Java monkey. According to Equation 19.3, the sigma OKN slow-phase angular velocity (ordinate) depends on flash frequency (abscissa). The open triangles represent data obtained using a stripe period of 2.3 degrees, the filled triangles those with a stripe period of 1.25 degrees. Note that the experimental data very closely approximate the predictions obtained using Equation 19.2 (from Grüsser et al., 1979). (c) Sigma pursuit eye movements evoked by a stroboscopically illuminated stereostripe pattern with 24 stripes at a period of 1.3 degrees. The sigma OKN slow-phase angular velocity (ordinate) increases with flash frequency (abscissa), as predicted by Equation 19.3. The apparent motion and the stereostripes were generated by using synchronous binocular stimuli (triangles) and by alternatively stimulating the left and right eyes (dots) (from Adler and Grüsser, 1981).*

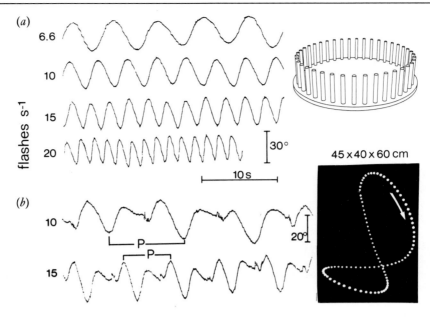

Fig. 19.11 *(a) Sigma pursuit movement recorded in man by means of a horizontal electrooculogram. The sigma movement was evoked by using a stroboscopically illuminated rod circle (inset) with a diameter of 65 cm. Flash frequencies were as indicated. The inspection angle was 52 degrees. The distance between eyes and the centre of the rod circle was 136 cm. (b) Complex sigma pursuit movements evoked by a three-dimensional object composed of 100 balls equally spaced (inset). Flash frequencies were as indicated. Complex pursuit eye movements were evoked in the horizontal EOG. P indicates the overall period of the eye movements evoked by the stroboscopically lit three-dimensional stimulus. The average observation distance was 110 cm (from Adler et al., 1981).*

frequently perform compensatory head movements in the direction opposite to that of the pendular nystagmic eye movements.

12. Perception during and after voluntary saccades depends not only on efference copy mechanisms, but also on the structure of the stimuli seen during the saccadic eye movements. During a saccade, the retinal image is shifted at a rather high speed (up to $600 \deg s^{-1}$) across the retina. The visual world is nevertheless perceived as stationary. It was formerly assumed that a general suppression of visual perception occurs during voluntary saccadic eye movements. This was believed to be caused by central inhibitory mechanisms (Holt, 1903; Jung, 1953). In our opinion, however, general visual inhibitory mechanisms are rather marginal during saccades. They are also unnecessary: the fast shift of the structured visual world across the retina does not lead to disturbing visual percepts, since the per-saccadic stimulus corresponds to a 'grey interval'. Owing to the high speed of the eyes, the image of the spatially structured visual world while shifting across the retina leads to high-frequency, intermittent stimulation of the photoreceptors far above flicker fusion frequency. Thus during a saccade, the response of the receptor output level approximately corresponds to that elicited by a short medium-grey stimulus, which does not

last long enough to disturb Gestalt perception. A dark interval has to last at least 60–80 ms in order to attain the perception threshold (Basler, 1906). It is also well known that blinks of the eye are normally correlated with saccades (Adams, 1957; Haberich and Fischer, 1958). Short blinks also produce grey stimuli which are too short to evoke a conscious interruption of the perceived complex visual signals.

A simple experiment demonstrates that visual perception is not suppressed during eye saccades: when a small, stationary spot of light is stroboscopically illuminated, and a subject performs a saccade across this spot of light, he sees several spots of light placed alongside one another. While working in von Helmholtz's laboratory in Heidelberg, Lamansky (1868) used this method in order to determine the angular speed of the eyes during voluntary saccades (cf. Chapter 1). All phenomena of apparent visual movement illustrated above are evoked in normal human observers and are frequently characterized by quantitative rules, describing the relationship between certain stimulus parameters (as angular velocity or duration of movement) and the movement illusion. Testing these illusionary visual movement percepts is strongly recommmended in patients suffering from brain lesions affecting movement perception.

Visual Movement Perception and Efference Copy Mechanisms

The image of the visual world is shifted by every saccade across the retinotopic representation of the extra-personal space in the brain. It is therefore necessary to update the relationship between retinotopic and spatiotopic coordinates continuously; 'efference copy' mechanisms are necessary for this purpose in order to 'stabilize' the spatiotopic coordinate system. The evaluation of the motor commands leading to saccadic shifts in gaze begins shortly before a saccade; it is maintained during and after a saccade with the goal of 'recalibrating' the relationship between the retinal and spatial coordinates (further discussed in Chapter 22). In this section, we shall only add a few comments related to the concept of efference copy mechanisms, which, in our opinion, are necessary in order to update the relationship between retinotopic and spatiotopic coordinates.

The following observation has puzzled many generations of scientists: although the image of the world shifts on the retina during active voluntary eye movements, it is nevertheless perceived as stationary. Nicolaus Cusanus (cf. Chapter 2) interpreted this problem by assuming that the spiritus visibilis necessary for seeing was emitted from the eye only when the gaze was shifted from one place in the visual world to the next by attentional mechanisms. This idea suggested a sampling of the visual signals related to attention and to eye movements. As already mentioned in Chapter 2, Franciscus Aquilonius was presumably the first to discriminate between afferent and efferent movement perception; he postulated that when one pursues a moving target with precise eye movements (which leads to a quasi-stabilization of the image on the retina), internal motor commands guiding the eye pursuit movements are evaluated in order to perceive the visual movement of the object pursued by the gaze movements. The interpretations of afterimage movements observed by Erasmus Darwin (1796), Bell (1823) and Purkinje (1825; Fig. 19.4) were rather similar. Purkinje was the first to postulate *expressis verbis* that movement perception, which should occur because of the shift of the retinal image during voluntary eye movements, is prevented by a central, active inhibitory mechanism. He assumed that the source of this 'cancellation' was the same cerebral structure that controlled the movement of the eyes or gaze (Purkinje, 1825). The idea of an internal feedback system preventing motion perception during voluntary eye movements was repeatedly discussed in the second half of the nineteenth century (e.g. Mach, 1885/1906). After Mach had published the first block diagram of this idea, another, more generalized version was published by von Uexküll (1920) which illustrated the inhibitory sensori motor interaction

that had been suggested by Purkinje (Fig. 19.12; cf. Henn, 1970). This tradition led to the concepts of 'reafference principle' and 'efference copy', which were developed by von Holst and Mittelstaedt (1950): all active (voluntary) gaze movements performed by either saccades or pursuit commands generate an 'efference copy' of these motor acts within the central nervous system. The efference copy signals interact with the afferent visual movement signals found reaching the visual centres responsible for visual

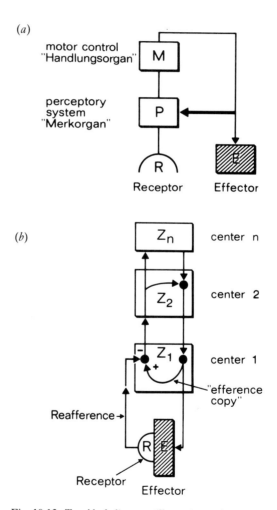

Fig. 19.12 *Two block diagrams illustrating an interpretation of the interaction between gaze motor signals and visual movement signals (published by von Uexküll (1920) (a) and von Holst and Mittelstaedt (1950) (b)). Von Holst and Mittelstaedt coined the term 'reafference principle' to denote the cerebral interaction of efference copy signals related to the motor commands and the afferent retinal movement signals (reafference).*

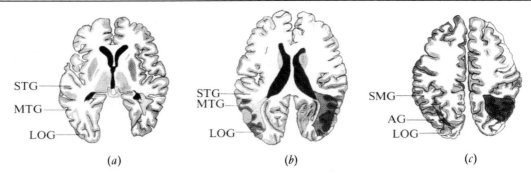

STG
MTG
LOG

(a)

STG
MTG
LOG

(b)

SMG
AG
LOG

(c)

Fig. 19.13 *Computer tomography results in patient L. M. The diagrams are arranged in the following sequence: from (a) (low ventricular level) through (b) (high ventricular level) to (c) (supraventricular level). High-density lesions are marked in different shades of grey. The lesions affecting the right hemisphere in the occipital region are more severe than in the left hemisphere. AG = gyrus angularis, LOG = gyrus occipitalis lateralis, MTG = gyrus temporalis medialis, SMG = gyrus supramarginalis, STG = gyrus temporalis superior (from Zihl et al., 1983; by permission of Macmillan Journals Ltd).*

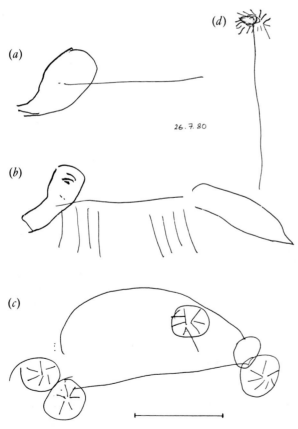

(a)

(b)

(c)

(d)

26.7.80

Fig. 19.14 *Drawings made by patient L. M. (July 1980). (a) 'Dog' – first trial. (b) 'Dog' – second trial. (c) 'Automobile'. All 3 were attempts to draw from memory. (d) 'Daisy'. The patient was given a flower and asked to copy it. Scale at the bottom: 5 cm.*

movement perception. The efference copy signal 'cancels' the movement component of the afferent visual signal, as Purkinje had assumed (see Fig. 19.4). This general idea of interaction between an efference copy and an afferent visual signal flow ('reafference') seems to be of some use in interpreting certain of the visual movement illusions described in the preceding paragraph. In order to explain sigma movement, for example, one assumes that a movement illusion must result whenever (a) efference copy signals are sent to the neuronal structures of the visual movement system, and (b) no adequate visual movement signal from the retina arrives in these structures. The same interpretation is applicable to the experiments illustrated in Fig. 19.5.

On the other hand, a movement sensation should be evoked whenever the retinal image is shifted because of involuntary eye movements, since only voluntary goal-directed gaze movements seem to be included in the efference copy mechanism. Therefore, pathological nystagmus caused by brain stem lesions or peripheral labyrinth disease, for example, are inevitably accompanied by an apparent rotation of the visual world, which leads to a state of vertigo in the patient.

Cerebral Impairment of Complex Movement Perception: A Case Report

This section describes the case of a patient suffering from bilateral posterior brain damage, which led to serious impairment of complex movement perception. At the age of 43, Mrs L. M. was admitted to a hospital in a stuporous

(a)

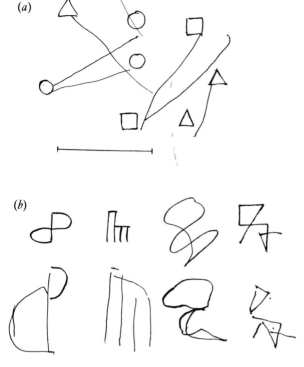

(b)

Fig. 19.15 *(a) Mrs L. M. was asked to draw straight lines to connect symbols of identical shapes: 3 triangles, 3 circles, 2 squares, all drawn by the investigator. (b) Mrs L. M. was asked to copy 4 nonsense figures drawn by the investigator. Her attempts to copy these figures are shown in the bottom row (performed on the same day as those in Fig. 19.14). Scale: 5 cm.*

state: she suffered from severe headaches, vertigo, nausea and repeated vomiting. A superior sagittal sinus thrombosis was diagnosed based on neurological symptoms and angiographic findings. Approximately 19 months after the onset of her illness, the patient was admitted in the Spring of 1980 to the neurology section of the Max Planck Institute for Psychiatry in Munich, where she was carefully examined and repeatedly tested over the next several years by Dr J. Zihl and his colleagues. Dr Zihl kindly offered one of us (O.-J. G.) the opportunity to investigate the patient for two days in July 1980 approximately two months after she had been admitted to the institute for the first time. Fig. 19.13 depicts schematic diagrams of her bilateral brain lesions (Zihl *et al.*, 1983). It is evident from this figure that the right-sided lesion in the outer occipito-temporal region was more severe than the left-sided lesion. A slightly hypodense patch was observed in the cortical surface of the posterior middle temporal gyrus. Furthermore, bilateral hypodense zones were found in the CT

in the retrorolandic area; bilateral symmetrical lesions were present in the periventricular segment of the temporo–parietal and occipital white matter, partly extending into the posterior segment of the middle temporal and lateral occipital gyri. The gyrus angularis was partially lesioned on the right side; only a small lesion was found on the left side in the subangular white matter of this brain region. Ten years later, the extent of the brain lesions was further determined by magnetic resonance scanning: small spots of high signal intensity were found in the middle of the right optic radiation. The middle temporal gyrus and the adjacent portion of the occipital gyri seemed to be severely damaged on both sides in the area surrounding the widened posterior horns of the lateral ventricles. A large zone of high signal intensity indicated impairment of the lateral occipital and occipito–parietal white matter on both sides. This confirmed the earlier diagnosis that the bilateral lesions were caused by a venous thrombosis in the territory of the occipital branches of the superior cerebral venes (Zihl *et al.*, 1991).

With regard to Mrs L. M.'s visual performance, Zihl *et al.* reported the following in 1983: elementary visual function tests revealed visual acuity of 0.8 minutes of arc^{-1} in both eyes, normal binocular vision, binocular fusion, vergence and accommodation, normal colour vision (as tested by the Farnsworth–Munsell 100–hue test), and a near normal recognition of visual objects and words (determined using a tachistoscopic test). Visual evoked potentials measured with an alternating checkerboard stimulus were in the range found for normal subjects tested under similar conditions. Visual fields (measured with a Tübingen perimeter) were within the normal range for achromatic and chromatic stimuli; the same was true for the distribution of sensitivity to flickering stimuli projected to different parts of the visual field (determined by critical flicker fusion frequency, CFF). Detection of two spots presented simultaneously within the left and right visual fields was within normal range, i.e. no signs of unilateral visual neglect were discovered using competitive bilateral stimulation in order to search for an extinction phenomenon (Chapter 22). Eye movements directed towards eccentrically presented targets were normal for both the left and right visual fields.

During our investigation of Mrs L. M. in July 1980, we made the following observations: mild signs of constructional apraxia (Fig. 19.14(a)–(b)), some difficulties copying figures mirror-symmetrically on an axis and some difficulties copying simple, meaningless figures (Fig. 19.15(b)). The patient also had difficulty reading: she was 'disturbed' by the many letters that were simultaneously present in the text. There was no sign of true alexia with regard to single words or simple sentences, however. In order to compensate for the graphical–structural difficulties that she experienced when reading, the patient

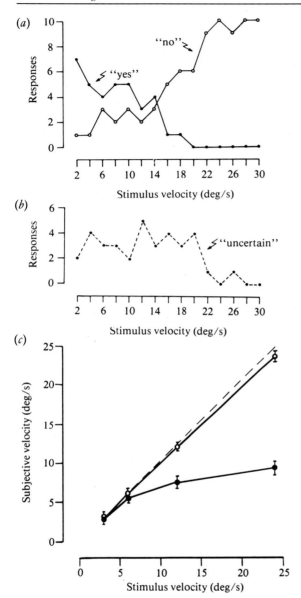

Fig. 19.16 *Test of visual movement detection for L. M. (a) and (b) The patient had to detect visual movement of a 2.4-degree round spot of light moving horizontally through an amplitude of 30 degrees. (a) The frequency of detection decreased with stimulus speed. (b) The frequency of 'uncertain' responses is plotted as a function of stimulus velocity. (c) In another experiment, the patient had to estimate the velocity of a target moving horizontally at different angular velocities along a path having a width of 10 degrees. The subjective velocity was determined by estimating the time that the target would need to reach a target 20 degrees away horizontally from the endpoint of movement. The dots are data obtained from the patient, the circles from a control subject (from Zihl et al., 1983, by permission of Macmillan Journals, Ltd).*

adopted the following strategy during the first weeks after the onset of her disease: she took a sheet of white paper, cut out a small window, and moved this 'gadget' along the newspaper headlines. This reading technique allowed her to obtain some information about what was going on in the world. When tested in July 1980, she still reported that the simultaneous presence of many complex visual stimuli made it difficult for her to discriminate between the different visual objects. As Fig. 19.15(a) illustrates, the patient did indeed have difficulties drawing lines between signs having the same shape when different signs were jumbled together. We also tested her ability to perceive α stripes (Adler and Grüsser, 1979, cf. p. 361), which are striations seen in a stroboscopically lit, moving random dot pattern. The temporal properties of the 'iconic memory' operating in normal form perception generate these striations. Although Mrs L. M. was not able to discover any α-striation, she was very much disturbed by the 'many flickering dots' seen during this test, a rather unpleasant experience for her.

When tested for her ability to estimate distance and determine object position in a garden, she made no errors in the grasping space but some errors in the near-distant action space (Chapter 21). Her ability to estimate the distances of objects located more than 8 to 10 metres away was severely impaired. L. M. had great difficulty trying to estimate distances between different trees and a house in the background, or between different houses. She also had difficulties estimating distance along the street. When asked if an object A was in front of or behind another object B, she typically concluded that A must be nearer than B when A partly covered B. She said that this was a logical conclusion, but that she was not actually able to perceive the spatial distance. This distance estimation impairment was about the same for both monocular and binocular observation. When walking across the garden or along the street, she reported that she had the impression that the objects in her extra-personal space were moving up and down. This was especially annoying for her when walking through a crowd of people. She reported that the heads always moved up and down. Besides the difficulties she experienced in perceiving many simultaneously presented objects correctly in space, she was evidently also not able to use information about parallax movement, which is normally helpful for estimating depth in the extra-personal space. This was the reason why she performed so poorly when estimating distance in the free field. She had great difficulty walking downstairs without tactile guidance, for she had serious difficulties perceiving the depths of the stairs. She once sneezed, for example, while walking down the stairs, and held her right hand, which she normally used to guide herself by grasping the handrail, in front of her mouth. Upon opening her eyes, which she had closed while sneezing, she immediately lost her balance and fell down the stairs.

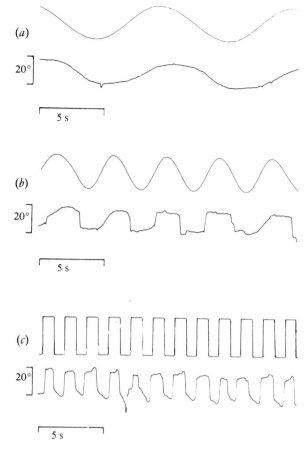

Fig. 19.17 *(a) and (b): Electro-oculographic recordings of horizontal pursuit eye movement with a target moving sinusoidally in horizontal directions to and fro at about 10 degrees amplitude and 0.1 Hz (a) or 0.24 Hz (b). In (c) saccadic responses to a target 'jumping' about 20 degrees horizontally to and fro at a rate of 1 s⁻¹ are shown (from Zihl et al., 1983 by permission of Macmillan Journals Ltd).*

Movement Perception

The patient reported that she had great difficulties perceiving movement under 'natural' stimulus conditions, i.e. discriminating between moving and stationary objects in a complex visual scene, or estimating the speed and direction of cars or bicycles in traffic. When walking through Munich, for example, she did not see individual car movement, but concluded that there must have been car movement, since the cars had changed their position with time. On the other hand, she often saw stationary objects 'move'. As already mentioned above, this apparent motion was evidently related to her own body movements while

walking. She especially noted these apparent shifts by objects located at eye level, and consequently experienced serious difficulties when walking through crowds. All movement perception became especially poor when she walked. We had the impression that under these conditions the perception of individual motion was masked by parallax motion. One and a half years after the acute brain lesion had occurred she still preferred to be accompanied by a friend when walking downtown. It was evidently not only the apparent motion of stationary objects, but also the simultaneous presence of many stationary as well as moving visual patterns that caused her perceptual problems.

Zihl and his co-workers used several methods in order to test Mrs L. M.'s movement perception experimentally, as follows:

1. Figures 19.16(a) and (b) illustrate some of her responses during a simple movement-detection task. A 2.4-degree round spot of light moved horizontally back and forth at constant speed through an amplitude of 20 degrees. The patient had to determine its speed. The higher the speed of the stimulus, the less correct the estimation of movement. 'Afferent' movement perception was explored in this test, in which the patient was asked to fixate on a stationary target. Data similar to those presented in Fig. 19.16(a) and (b) were obtained for vertical movement detection.

2. Perception of motion in depth was tested with a wooden cube moved on a table, and was found to be seriously impaired.

3. In addition to the threshold for the detection of a stationary target located in the periphery of the visual field, thresholds for the detection of target movement were tested by using a Tübingen perimeter. The time she needed in order to detect motion was nearly twice the amount of time required by normal subjects; the time required by the patient to detect movement direction correctly was more than three times that required by normal subjects. Her performance was very poor when estimating the velocity of a target moving horizontally in front of her over a path of 10 degrees visual angle. In order to quantify her ability to estimate movement velocity in this task, she was asked to estimate the time the moving stimulus would have needed to reach a stationary target placed 20 degrees of visual angle from the end point of stimulus movement. For normal control subjects, the perceived velocity of the stimulus increased linearly with respect to its actual velocity, and corresponded very closely to the actual speed between 2 and 25 deg s⁻¹. Mrs L. M. perceived only a slight increase in stimulus speed when the angular velocity of the stimulus was increased (Fig. 19.16(c)).

4. Motion after-effects were tested using either horizontally moving striped patterns or the rotating spiral of Archimedes (Holland, 1957). The conditioning lasted 30

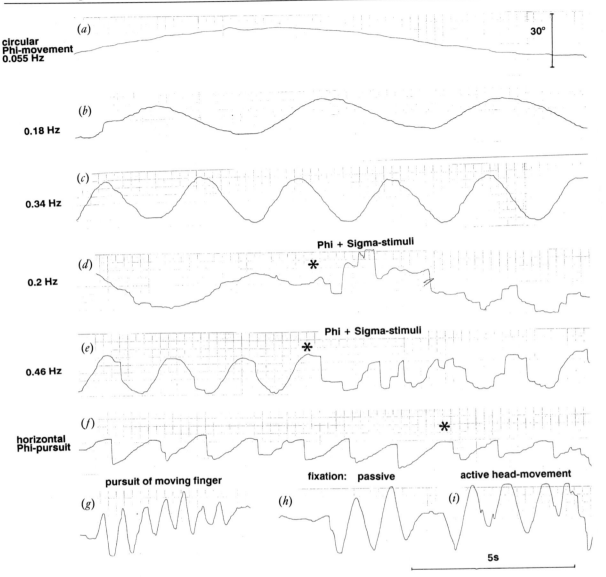

Fig. 19.18 *Electro-oculographic eye movement recordings in L. M. (a)–(e) Circular phi movement evoked by using the machine illustrated in Fig. 19.8. A dot moves at different speeds around a circle having a diameter of 26 degrees, as illustrated (0.055–0.46 Hz). The patient perceived the phi movement, and could also perform corresponding eye pursuit movements. In addition to the phi stimulus, the inner stimulus circle (Fig. 19.8) was turned on in (d) and (e) (asterisk) in order to evoke sigma movement perception in the patient. The phi pursuit movements were interrupted as soon as the flashing dot circle appeared. The patient reported that she was 'disturbed' by the flickering dots. (f) Horizontal phi pursuit. (g) Pursuit of the investigator's finger, which was moved at a distance of about 50 cm. (h) The patient fixated a stationary target; her head was moved passively during fixation. (i) She moved her head actively while fixating the target. Time scale for (a)–(e), 5 s; for (g)–(i), 10 s (O.-J. Grüsser and J. Zihl, unpublished, 1980).*

seconds for the horizontally moving optokinetic patterns. The patient was asked to report motion after-effects after the optokinetic pattern had stopped. She observed a very short motion after-effect, lasting 1.2–2.1 s, only 3 times out

of 10 trials. On the same test, normal observers saw, on the average, movement after-effects lasting 6.7 s, even though their conditioning time was only 5 s. With the rotating spiral of Archimedes, the patient could not see any movement after-effects or any apparent changes in the size of the spiral phenomena that are experienced by all normal observers.

5. Mrs L. M.'s eye pursuit movements were studied while recording her eye position with an electro-oculogram. As Fig. 19.17 illustrates, the patient could pursue horizontal, sinusoidal movement of targets when the frequency was below 0.2 Hz (5–15 degrees amplitude). Above this value, pursuit of a horizontally moving target was characterized by many saccades. Fixation on a stationary target during passive or active head movements led to smooth pursuit eye movements (Fig. 19.18(h),(i)). As is also the case for normal subjects, the vestibulo-ocular reflex (VOR) faciliated the precision of smooth eye pursuit for Mrs L. M.

6. Phi movement was tested under different conditions:

(a) Two circular spots of light were presented at different positions for 500 ms. The distance between the spots was varied between 2.5 and 15 degrees visual angle, and the interstimulus interval was varied between 0 and 200 ms. The patient did not report any apparent movement under conditions in which normal subjects saw clear phi movement, but rather saw only two distinct spots (Zihl *et al.*, 1983).

(b) In our own investigation of Mrs L. M. we used a test involving sequential phi movement. The stimulus pattern consisted of a single spot of light (light diode), which sequentially changed its position along the circumference of a circle, as illustrated in the pattern drawn in Fig. 19.8. When horizontal as well as circular phi movements were tested, the patient not only reported having seen phi movement, but also could pursue the apparently moving spot of light with her eyes. Several electrooculographic recordings of horizontal eye position, made during two experimental sessions with Mrs L. M., are presented in Fig. 19.18. In an angular velocity range of 0.1 to 20 deg s^{-1}, the patient's performance was about the same as that of a normal subject. When the velocity was increased, the patient's performance was less precise than that of normal subjects. Eye pursuit movements evoked by horizontal phi movement above 15 deg s^{-1} were more easily performed towards the left than towards the right side. Circular phi movement led to circular eye pursuit movements up to approximately 0.4 Hz (Fig. 19.18). When the stationary flickering dot circle was turned on simultaneously to the single dot during circular phi pursuit eye movements (Fig. 19.8), the patient had great problems pursuing the individual dot and reported that the many flickering dots of light seriously impaired her ability to direct her spatial attention on the single dot seen during phi motion (Fig. 19.18(d), (e)). Thus it was not possible to test sigma movement in this

patient. She reported, however, that when the flickering circle was turned on initially, she perceived it for a fraction of a second as rotating. Horizontal pursuit of a single dot was similarly impaired when a second row of forty simultaneously flickering dots was turned on at the same time (Fig. 19.18(f)).

7. By using drifting light–dark gratings, Hess *et al.* (1989) measured the patient's perception of different spatial frequencies, contrast sensitivity and temporal resolution abilities. They found her spatial and temporal response properties to be impaired; temporal frequency resolution and velocity discrimination were more seriously reduced, however, than was detection of fine spatial gratings. They found no measurable temporal frequency discrimination above 6 Hz, and no velocity discrimination above 6 deg s^{-1}. The ability to detect the direction of the moving pattern was also lost above 6 deg s^{-1}.

8. McLeod *et al.* (1989) examined Mrs L. M.'s ability to search for a target intermingled with stationary or moving non-targets (the number of non-target stimuli present in the test field was systematically varied). Two types of responses were investigated: discrimination of a moving target (an *X*) from many non-moving ones, and detection of a stationary *X* located in between many stationary, horizontal dashes. Mrs L. M.'s performance was slower than that of normal subjects for the first task; there was little effect, however, on her ability to respond correctly when the number of masking non-targets was increased, which was also the case for normal subjects. Similarly, she could quite easily detect a static *X* among a field of static dashes.

A combination of the two tasks was applied in two further experiments: the patient was asked to detect a single *X* moving together with horizontal dashes; many *X*s formed the stationary background in one type of stimulus display. In the other type of stimulus display, horizontal dashes and one *X* moved, while another set of horizontal dashes formed the stationary background. With the second type of stimulus pattern, the moving *X* was discovered, while, when many *X*s formed the stationary visual background and the target *X* was moved together with dashes, detection time considerably increased with set size and the percentage of correct responses decreased. In normal subjects, set size in these experiments had no effect on detection time or on the percentage of correct detections. The authors concluded that Mrs L. M. could not restrict her visual attention to the moving items, and therefore was not able to separate the moving dashes from the single moving *X* when other *X*'s formed the stationary background.

Twelve Years of Movement Agnosia

Recently, Zihl *et al.* (1991) performed an extensive follow-up study of Mrs L. M. In general, the examination did not reveal any significant changes in the patient's clinical state, which suggests that her movement perception disorder was irreversible. After 12 years of impairment, the patient had developed certain 'detour' strategies in order to compensate for the difficulties she experienced seeing movement. When many objects moved simultaneously, for example, she tried to ignore the visual motion signals. She had adopted behavioural strategies which prevented her from seeing complex visual motion with foveal vision. For example, when listening to a person speak, she usually looked away from the speaker's face and concentrated on what he was saying; in this way, she was not disturbed by the movement of the speaker's mouth. Several objects, e.g. people, moving simultaneously in different directions still greatly disturbed her visual perception. She still had difficulties walking through crowded places and streets: 'The more people walk, the more difficult and unpleasant it is.' Similarly, her difficulties judging road traffic did not improve. She was still unable to estimate the speed of a car.

Additional tests of Mrs L. M.'s visual space perception were performed in the follow-up study: Zihl *et al.* (1991) measured the patient's ability to estimate distances along the horizontal perimeter at a viewing distance of 100 cm. The patient performed very well during this task; the same was true for her ability to estimate depth with respect to target position within the grasping range (maximum distance 130 cm). In order to test the direction of the vertical and horizontal axes of her visual space, she was asked to adjust a 1 degree × 18 degree bar of light into a vertical or horizontal position. The bar appeared against a dark background on a high-resolution screen (25 degrees × 19 degrees) at a distance of 60 cm. Her performance in this test (Bender and Jung, 1948) was normal. The same was true for a line bisection task (Chapter 22), as well as for discrimination of individual line orientations. Similarly, the patient's performance in face and object recognition tasks was found to be within normal range.

The times required for detecting target movements were tested for different target velocities, and were found to be about four times the normal values for targets moving between 10 and 30 deg s^{-1}. For low velocities, the latencies increased up to 20 times the values found for normal subjects. Mrs L. M.'s simple visual reaction times to stationary targets deviated only slightly, however, from the values obtained in normal control subjects. Another test examined the minimal displacement required for movement perception of a small target. This value slightly increased in normal subjects with increase in displacement speed from 0.16 to 20 deg s^{-1}, but remained below 10 seconds of arc. For Mrs L. M., displacement thresholds increased at very low angular velocities up to about 95 seconds of arc at a stimulus velocity of 0.16 deg s^{-1}, and

up to 24 seconds of arc at a stimulus velocity of 0.32 deg s^{-1}. At a stimulus velocity of 20 deg s^{-1}, miminal displacement required for movement detection was still about twice that of a normal control subject.

From the results of CT and MRI scans, Zihl *et al.* (1991) concluded that the main impairment of this patient's ability to detect movement was caused by bilateral lesions of a brain region corresponding to area MT (or area V5) in primates (Chapter 5). The interesting experimental, psychophysical data already discussed explored only part of the patient's difficulties in perceiving moving objects, however. Although she mainly complained of difficulties with regard to the perception of object movement in the extra-personal space when different stationary objects and/or different moving objects were simultaneously present, we feel that her other difficulties, i.e. perceiving motion in depth in the near-distant action space and her failure to use parallax motion for depth perception, should also be tested experimentally. Furthermore, part of this patient's problems seem to be caused by a mismatch between afferent movement signals and efference copy signals. This mismatch may result from an incompatibility between the two signals in time, and not from a loss of efference copy signals. This suggestion is supported by the findings of Paulus and Zihl (1989), who investigated Mrs L. M.'s postural performance by performing posturographic measurements on a platform. She looked at a half-cylindrical white background covered with randomly arranged coloured dots (placed at a distance of 1 m). As compared to normal subjects, her swaypath in this test was considerably increased (open and closed eyes). Interestingly, her visual stabilization of posture decreased under stroboscopic illumination of the cylinder wall when the flash frequency was increased from 1 to about 10 flashes s^{-1}, and improved slightly between 10 and 20 flashes s^{-1}. In normal subjects, increasing flash frequency above 1 flash s^{-1} considerably improves the visual stabilization of posture. In light of the fact that the visual stabilization of posture in Mrs L. M. was significantly worse at flash frequencies between 1 and 20 flashes s^{-1}, as compared to the stabilizing effect of steady illumination, a temporal mismatch between visual signals and motor control seems indeed to be present in this patient.

Further tests should be developed in order to understand Mrs L. M.'s problems with respect to everyday movement perception: a test of multiple movement as well as tests of parallax movement detection and depth perception caused by parallax movement could shed some light on the subject's impairments. Baker *et al.* (1991) have taken a first step in this direction. In their investigation of the patient, these investigators used a smoothly drifting field of randomly distributed dots as a stimulus. The coherent movement of these dots could be disturbed by non-coherent noise; the signal–noise ratio could be varied until a 'snowstorm' appeared on the experimental screen (at zero coherence). The patient was able to discover correctly the direction in which a 100 per cent coherent dot pattern moved; when incoherent noise was added, her performance rapidly declined. Her responses were at chance level with 40 per cent coherence. In normal observers, a coherence of 2 to 4 per cent allows for correct movement detection. Baker *et al.* reported that they were 'most surprised' by the fact that the presence of a very small percentage of stationary 'noise' was sufficient to destroy her ability to detect the direction of the coherently moving dots. In our opinion, however, this finding closely corresponds to the patient's own remarks quoted above and indicates that she suffered from Type (b) simultanagnosia (see Chapter 11).

Other Case Reports of Movement Agnosia and Related Disorders

Mrs L. M. is certainly the most thoroughly investigated patient suffering from movement perception impairment brought about by a cerebral lesion. There are several other reports in the literature which also indicate the existence of visual movement perception disorders caused by brain lesions. Redlich and Pötzl (1911) reported a dissociation of visual movement and space perception with regard to the recovery of visual functions in a patient suffering from bilateral occipital lobe lesions. Pötzl (1928) reported that some of his patients with occipital lesions perceived disturbing, apparent visual object motions, a symptom also mentioned by Beichl (1944). These apparent visual motion sensations are seen during gaze movements and are presumably caused by a temporal mismatch between the afferent visual movement signals and efference copy signals of gaze motor or locomotion commands. From the dissociations of visual functions observed in patients suffering from occipital brain lesions, Riddoch (1917) concluded in another early report that 'movement may be recognized as a special visual perception', an idea that had already been proposed by Exner in 1875.

Riddoch's main argument rested on the observation that after cortical blindness had occurred, visual movement perception recovered before shape perception. The patients could see visual movement without recognizing the moving object. In his study Riddoch also noted a dissociation in recovery of visual movement perception and form perception in patients suffering from homonymous hemianopia. We shall describe one of his patients in order to illustrate these observations: the patient suffered from a right occipital brain lesion caused by a bullet wound. His skull was trephined, and the bullet removed. Six and a half months after this injury, Riddoch found a left homonymous hemianopia and complete absence of object vision.

In contrast, movement detection was present in the blind hemifield; moreover, good movement perception had recovered in a large part of the retinal periphery. A central scotoma for movement perception did not recover, however. The isolated recovery of peripheral movement perception caused some difficulties in the patient's visual orientation responses. Riddoch especially noted in such patients that 'the disparity between the stimuli received from the two halves of the retina is frequently sufficient to affect equilibrium when walking. They usually sway to the partially blind side . . .' In addition, 'The inequality of the sensations received by the brain is often a source of considerable annoyance for the patient.' The patient mentioned above reported unpleasant visual experiences especially when riding in a train. He was disturbed by movement perception, even though he did not see the moving objects in his left visual field. He perceived the 'moving things' having no distinct shape or colour as 'shadowy grey' events.

This dissociation in recovery of movement perception and form perception after occipital brain lesions, now called the 'Riddoch phenomenon', may also be interpreted as an early investigation of 'blindsight' (Chapter 9). In his extensive study Riddoch observed another group of patients suffering from homonymous visual field defects. Form and movement vision showed a parallel deterioration and recovery. Riddoch's postulate 'that movement should be given a place among the stimuli which are recognized as originating visual perceptions' is fully appreciated today. The Riddoch phenomenon might partly be caused by the fact that afferent visual movement signals may reach the neocortex along extrageniculate pathways, as already discussed in Chapter 9.

While movement perception recovered first in Riddoch's patients, visual movement perception remained seriously impaired in Goldstein and Gelb's (1923) famous patient Schn., who had suffered from a diffuse occipital or occipito-parietal brain lesion. Some of the results of their thorough investigation of movement perception are worth mentioning in detail:

To answer the question whether and how the perception of movement was impaired in our patient, we investigated the patient (1) with moving real objects and (2) with apparent movement stimuli.

(1) Real movement
(a) Experiments under daylight conditions
If a fast top-down movement of the hand is performed in front of the patient at about a distance of 1 m, he always reported seeing the hand either at the top or at the bottom position. Asked whether he could see anything between these two positions, he always replied that he could not, and said that the hand first appeared at the top and then at the bottom. If the movement was performed more slowly, and the patient was asked to fixate continuously on the moving hand, one observed

continuous eye pursuit; nevertheless, the patient still replied that he could not see any hand movement. What he apparently saw between the top and bottom positions were single, isolated hand positions.

When the hand movement was performed extremely slowly and the patient was asked whether or not there was movement, he replied that the hand was not moving after having observed it for 2 to 3 seconds. When the hand movement continued, subsequent to a movement of about 10 degrees, the patient usually declared, frequently with an exclamation of astonishment, that the hand was now in a new position, which led him to say that movement must have occurred, although he did not actually see it.

When he was asked to look at the seconds hand of a clock, and was asked to follow the hand with his index finger or with a pencil, he declared every 5 to 10 seconds that the hand was 'here' and then 'here'. He did not follow the moving hand, but jumped with his finger from one position to the other. The positions that he indicated were visually distinct, i.e. they were larger marks, such as dots or numbers, which became partially covered by the moving hand.

(b) Experiments in the dark
A light was moved in a range of about 0.5 m at a distance of about 2 m. The results of these experiments were similar to those performed under conditions of general illumination. With fast movement, the patient indicated the start and end positions of the light, while with slow movement the patient indicated several positions along the path, without actually having seen the movement.

Goldstein and Gelb also investigated this patient's ability to see phi movement: they attempted to create an impression of movement by successively presenting two spatially separated red dots or vertical lines (separations of 11, 18, 15 and 30 cm, with a viewing distance of 2 m). The time interval between the presentation of the 2 stimuli was systematically varied. The patient did not experience movement at any interval (i.e. the time between one spot of light being extinguished and the other turned on), but sometimes reported phenomena that the investigators had trouble understanding. At the smallest distance (11 cm), for example, he reported that both dots appeared and disappeared simultaneously; at distances of 25 and 30 cm he reported that the left dot remained stable, while the right dot appeared and disappeared. Tactile movement, on the other hand, was immediately perceived; he could easily determine the different speeds at which the object moved on the skin.

After these experiments, Mr Schn. became aware of his disability and suddenly reported real-life experiences that he had considered to be strange and inexplicable prior to the investigation. With regard to real, moving objects, for example, he reported the following: 'When the streetcar arrives, I recognize it at about a distance of 5 metres. Thereafter I usually do not see anything, and then suddenly it is standing directly in front of me.' Mr Schn. also

wondered why he could not perceive the movement of a train, which he realized must be moving because of the noise. His movement perception was also disturbed when it involved movement in depth in a three-dimensional space. He reported, for example, that he had once gone out walking with his sister-in-law. She left the house before him, and he followed her at a distance of about 20 m. He was surprised that although his sister-in-law suddenly stood still, he did not seem to approach her and had the impression that the distance between them did not become less.

Thus, like Mrs L. M., Mr Schn. was unable to see car and train movement, even though he saw changes in the position of the objects and could therefore logically infer that the objects must have moved. Further defects related to this patient's visual agnosia are discussed in Chapter 11. Landis *et al.* (1982) observed a case very similar to that of Mr Schn. Their patient did not complain about a loss of movement sensation, and could follow small moving targets rather precisely with his centre of gaze. However, he was not able to detect movement of an individual object moving across a complex visual scene. He also failed to perceive any apparent movement in a tachistoscopic test using phi movement.

Pötzl (1928) emphasized the double dissociation in recovery of movement perception and form perception after brain lesions. In the light of modern studies of shape discrimination, it seems to be important that in further studies with brain-lesioned patients impairments in the perception of local, single dot movements, global movement and parallax movement should be separated. Furthermore, the effects of visual movement signals to 2-D or 3-D-shape perception should be studied in patients suffering from brain lesions similar to those observed in Mrs L.M.

A fresh approach to movement agnosia was taken by Vaina *et al.* (1990), who reported on a 60-year-old left-handed man, A. F., who suffered from repeated cerebral haemorrhages that finally led to bilateral lesions involving the temporo-parieto-occipital junction of the brain. The lesion was found to be larger in the right hemisphere than in the left. Both lesions extended along the lateral margins of the lateral ventricles, through the white matter into the posterior parietal lobe. The visual radiation was impaired, leading to a congruous loss of the left, lower visual hemifield and part of the left, upper visual hemifield. Besides impairment of movement perception, this patient suffered from constructional apraxia and difficulties in binocular stereopsis, as determined using Julesz's (1971) random-dot stereograms. He also had difficulties with depth perception within the grasping range. His verbal IQ (measured by the Wechsler Adult Intelligence Scale) was 104, while his performance IQ was only 68. Object recognition from a non-canonical view (Warrington and Taylor,

1973b) was severely impaired; in contrast, his performance on tasks requiring recognition of simple shapes, colour and contrast discrimination was normal. He deviated pathologically, however, in the line bisection test, had difficulties estimating the length of lines and made many errors on formal and informal tests of spatial localization using visual cues.

According to the CT scans and the MRI findings, Mr A. F. had bilateral damage of the posterior parietal cortex. Therefore the authors assumed (as had Zihl *et al.* (1991) regarding Mrs L. M.) that Mr A. F. suffered from bilateral lesions in the cortical area MT. Consequently, different tests were used in order to investigate the patient's movement perception ability, as follows:

1. Since Julesz's study (1971), it has been well known that coherent movement of a part of a random dot pattern creates 'shapes from motion' (Chapter 1). Mr A. F.'s ability in two-dimensional form discrimination was not seriously impaired. It seemed therefore meaningful to test his ability to detect 'shape from motion' systematically. He performed well: his results were statistically within the range of six control subjects matched for age.

2. When part of a random dot pattern moves in one direction on a computer screen and the other part in another direction, a boundary generated by shearing

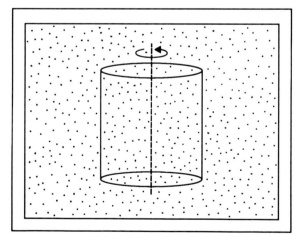

Fig. 19.19 *Explanation of the generation of three-dimensional shapes by coherent motion of random dots. Some of the random dots move on the screen as if they were part of the rotating cylinder's surface; the others move at random. The cylinder was only visible whenever this surface rotation was simulated. The cylinder disappeared in the random dot background whenever the coherent movement stopped. Incoherently moving dots masked the perception of a 3-D cylinder only when 90 per cent of the dots in the region of the cylinder were moving randomly and unrelated to the cylinder rotation.*

motion is seen (cf. Nakayama, 1985). The shape of this boundary was correctly recognized by the patient.

3. While shape from motion was correctly recognized in the simple test described in (1), the patient exhibited serious impairments when asked to perform a more complex task. In this task, two-dimensional forms of a random dot pattern had to be recognized only from the difference forming the target shape moved at a different speed from that of the random dots forming the background. Six different shapes were tested. While the average recognition score for normal control subjects was 95 per cent, the patient correctly recognized only 17 per cent of the patterns, i.e. his performance was near chance level.

4. A. F.'s ability to discriminate local speed was significantly below that of normal control subjects.

5. Like Mrs L. M., Vaina's patient also had a considerable threshold increase for detecting coherent motion. From his inability to use speed differences in order to extract two-dimensional shapes from motion, his inability to differentiate between different speeds of visual motion and his poor motion coherence performance, the authors concluded that A. F. 'had a deficit either in local motion or in integrating the output of the local motor system, particularly in the presence of noise'.

6. Another experiment using coherently moving random dot patterns tested Mr A. F.'s ability to use local motion information in order to generate form vision. In normal subjects, such patterns generate a three-dimensional shape from a two-dimensional display. This is illustrated in Fig. 19.19: when many of the random dots move on the screen as if they were part of the surface of a rotating cylinder and the other background dots move at random, the cylinder is indeed seen by a normal observer as soon as the motion begins. This 3-D perception is amazingly robust against additional incoherent noise stimuli. Normal subjects detected the rotating cylinder more than 90 per cent of the time when less than 10 per cent of the individual dots in the field of the cylinder were moving coherently. Vaina *et al.* (1990) were suprised to discover that A. F.'s performance on this task was within the range of normal values up to a noise level of 60 per cent, and that he still achieved a 75 per cent correct recognition rate with 90 per cent noise (50 per cent is chance level).

As already mentioned above, Mr A. F. performed very poorly on tasks designed to test elementary motion mechanisms. Nevertheless, he was evidently still able to use local motion information for 3-D visual perception. In our opinion, this indicates that the motion information used for 'shape for motion' detection is 'branched off' immediately beyond area V1, and does not rely on the neuronal mechanisms which elaborate global motion within areas MT and MST, regardless of whether or not it is used to generate shapes in the 2D or 3-D domains.

This view is supported by the results of a final test

reported on by Vaina *et al.* (1990). They used Johansson's (1973) test in a movie: Johansson placed small sources of light at the head and main joints of one or two actors, and made a movie in which only these light sources were visible. When a human actor stood quietly, the twelve dots of light went unrecognized as being part of a meaningful shape. However, when the actor performed prototypical actions (e.g. walking, dancing, riding on a bicycle, climbing stairs, etc.) or when two actors shook hands, walked together, danced or hugged, the scene was immediately recognized correctly by normal observers. Mr A. F. also had no difficulties performing this task correctly: 'In all of the trials, he quickly recognized that the display portrayed a human actor performing a series of specific activities.' For example, he correctly identified the direction of movement of a man walking in different directions in Johansson's movie; he also recognized other, more complex movements.

Neuronal Circuits for Local and Global Movement Perception

As discussed in Chapters 3–7, many visual neurones are movement sensitive, i.e. respond better to moving than stationary stimuli. In some of the neurones, this movement sensitivity is nothing more than an adaptation to the shift of the visual image of the retina occurring every 0.18–0.6 s because of eye saccades and/or head movements. In addition to this temporal frequency adaptation, however, 'true' movement-sensitive visual neuronal systems exist in selected regions of the cerebral hemispheres which process either local or global movement (Chapter 5). Intensive anatomical studies in connection with microelectrode recordings have revealed several important connections of the extrastriate visual areas, serving as a pathway for visual motion analysis (Chapter 5; Boussaoud *et al.*, 1991). These pathways for visual motion analysis support different classes of visual movement detection, which are in part related to object recognition, and in part to visual movement perception necessary during locomotion.

The main movement pathway seems to be characterized by the connections of the 'magnocellular' components (Chapter 5) of the striate and peristriate visual areas to areas MT, MST, FST and the regions located deep in the supratemporal sulcus (STS) cortex anterior to area FST (summarized as anterior supratemporal sulcus, area AST, in Fig. 5.10). Some of the properties of signal processing by MT, MST and FST neurones have been determined by single unit recordings. For these cortical areas, located along the posterior part of the STS, the same functional principles as for the inferior temporal lobe areas apply:

1. The size of the visual receptive fields increases considerably with the level an area attains in the hierarchy MT-MST-FST-AST.

2. The concommitant retinotopic organization characterizing the cerebral representation of the contralateral half of the visual field becomes less precise and disappears in the areas FST and AST (IPa) where the receptive field sizes of individual neurones may extend across a considerable part of the visual hemifield.

3. The receptive fields extend beyond the vertical meridian into the ipsilateral visual hemifield, especially for the nerve cells of area MST and FST. This fact is presumably caused by the callosal connections from the homotopic areas of the other cortical hemisphere.

4. The further up a movement processing area in the hierarchy the more the visual movement signals are modified by those related to gaze movements.

The neurophysiological results obtained so far from these visual-movement related areas allow some speculations, which lead to experimentally falsifiable hypotheses and which may also be helpful in understanding and interpreting the different symptoms observed in patients suffering from visual movement agnosia (akinetopsia). From various neurophysiological studies (Gattass and Gross, 1981; Baker *et al.*, 1981; Maunsell and Van Essen, 1983a,b; Albright *et al.*, 1984; Felleman and Kaas, 1984; Burkhalter *et al.*, 1986; Desimone and Ungerleider, 1986; Saito *et al.*, 1986) and the anatomical connections published so far (reviews: Van Essen, 1985; Maunsell and Newsome, 1987; Boussaoud *et al.*, 1991), we deduced the following hypotheses on different classes of visual movement perception and their cerebral representations (Fig. 19.20):

1. Local movement, e.g. movement of an animal in a natural habitat, is perceived through the connections V1-V2-MT-IP, but also through an extrastriate pathway. Signals concerning local visual movement may reach the area MT via the superior colliculi and the pulvinar.

2. The regions MST and FST are connected with the supratemporal polysensory area STP. In addition, area FST is connected to the infero-temporal regions TEO and the different areas of TE (see Chapter 7). The neuronal connections of movement-sensitive areas to the inferotemporal visual areas operate object recognition by transmitting object-related movement signals. Two types of object-related movement signals must be considered: local movements, typical for individual objects, such as eye movements in a face or the movements for facial expression; and object recognition by discrimination between the moving object and the stationary background (contour recognition by evaluating the coherent displacement of the visual components of an object).

3. As mentioned above, global visual movement under non-technical, 'natural' conditions is predominantly the

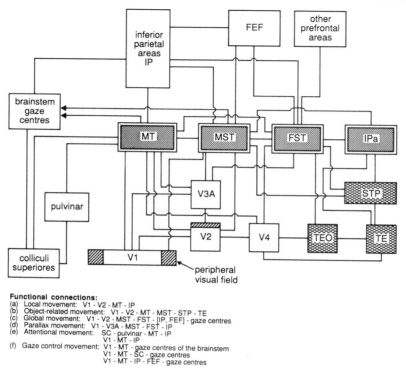

Functional connections:
(a) Local movement: V1 - V2 - MT - IP
(b) Object-related movement: V1 - V2 - MT - MST - STP - TE
(c) Global movement: V1 - V2 - MST - FST - [IP, FEF] - gaze centres
(d) Parallax movement: V1 - V3A - MST - FST - IP
(e) Attentional movement: SC - pulvinar - MT - IP
           V1 - MT - IP
(f) Gaze control movement: V1 - MT - gaze centres of the brainstem
           V1 - MT - SC - gaze centres
           V1 - MT - IP - FEF - gaze centres

Fig. 19.20 *Scheme of the neuronal connections supposedly involved in the different types of movement perception. The cortical areas of the inferior parietal lobe and the inferior temporal lobe are not displayed in detail. For further explanations see text. Abbreviations: FEF = frontal eye field; FST = fundal part of the supratemporal sulcus region; IP = inferior parietal areas combined together; IPa = inferior part of the supratemporal sulcus region; MST = medial supratemporal area; MT = medial temporal area; STP = supratemporal polysensory area; TE = areas of the middle and anterior part of the inferior temporal lobe; TEO = occipital part of the area TE.*

movement of the retinal image by gaze movements or locomotor activity. These movement signals involve the pathway V1-V2-MST-FST, i.e. visual movement regions in which not only retinal signals, but also efference copy signals seem to modify the neuronal activity. The nerve cells of MST and FST have large or very large visual receptive fields and their axons transmit, in part, information to inferior parietal areas (IP). These areas are important for the general orientation in the extrapersonal space (Chapter 7).

4. Akin to the space-related global movement signals are visual operations evaluating parallax movement perceived when objects are present in a three-dimensional space. Parallax movement is generated whenever head movements or general locomotion are executed. These parallax movement signals are supposed to reach the inferotemporal region along the pathway V1-V3a-MST-FST-IT. They provide essential information about the depth of the extra-personal space perceived and about the distances between objects.

5. A further important component of movement processing in cerebral structures is 'attentional movement'. By this we mean the fact that sudden movements in the extra-personal space lead to a goal-directed shift in visual attention, which usually is accompanied by corresponding gaze movements. Part of these attentional movement responses are involuntary reflexes involving the pathway from the retina to the superior colliculi and from there to the brainstem gaze control centres. However, a cortical loop via the pulvinar and area MT, and another loop via V1-V2-MT are involved in controlling space-related visual attention (Fig. 19.20). Spatially directed attention, of course, is also changed by 'internal' factors through limbic and prefrontal activities using the pathways between the frontal eye fields (FEF) and the inferior parietal lobule (Chapter 6).

6. Finally, visual movement systems serve to control voluntary gaze movements, either the smooth pursuit movements or the saccades. Goal-directed visual pursuit, as performed when one observes a bird flying across the

sky, seems to utilize the pathway V1–MT–brainstem gaze centres, while the exploratory gaze movements, using eye saccades and head movements, operate via the connections of areas V1 and MT with the superior colliculi or via the inferior parietal areas and the frontal eye fields as illustrated in Fig. 19.20.

From Fig. 19.20, one can deduce some arguments regarding the lesions of patients suffering from akinetopsia. Mrs L. M., for example, was well able to perceive and to pursue single targets moving through an empty visual space, i.e. the lesion did not abolish the function of MT. She was, however, seriously impaired when several stimuli moved together and she had to concentrate on a single one. When she was asked to pursue a single small object, moving across a complex stationary world, she experienced great difficulties. Also her visual perception of complex stationary structures was impaired whenever she was walking. Her perceptual difficulties, appearing under these conditions, indicated that she presumably suffered from a lesion involving the connections and/or the structures of areas MST and FST.

In contrast to Mrs L. M., Mr A. F. was able to recognize shapes by motion, but he failed to judge local speed correctly. He also had difficulties in detecting the speed of coherent motion and failed in more elementary tasks of local motion detection. We think that in this patient, the area MT and perhaps part of the area MST were involved, while area FST and area IPa (Fig. 19.20) were still functioning. Since the structures of areas V1 and V2, representing the peripheral visual field, project directly into MST and also area V4 has a direct input to FST, global movement detection can still operate when area MT is seriously disturbed.

Of course, our functional interpretation of the anatomical connections included in Fig. 19.20 is wide open to criticism, but at least it provides a starting point for the design of experiments in which the enigma of the primate cerebral movement areas may slowly disappear.

20 The World Turns Grey: Achromatopsia, Colour Agnosia and Other Impairments of Colour Vision Caused by Cerebral Lesions

Introduction

Colour perception helps one to recognize objects and to perceive object–background separation. For example, colour vision certainly allows for quick recognition of red, yellow or orange fruits against a background of green leaves. Furthermore, colour perception evokes emotional responses. The delicate distribution and changes of colours in a human face play an important role in social interaction; blood seen streaming across a wounded face or across other body parts leads in most people to empathic emotional reactions expressed in the form of immediate aid, flight or psychic shock. The setting produced by horticulture, the hues of the rooms in which we live, the colours of buildings, furniture, carpets, flowers, paintings and, more recently, chromatic light sources illuminating rooms and places in colours other than the warm red of an old-fashioned open fireplace, all affect the emotional well-being of modern man. The brilliant colours of the woods in New Hampshire on an Indian Summer day or of a spring sunset in the Sierra Nevada arouse other emotional feelings than do the unsaturated, mild coloration of a misty autumn morning on Dartmoor or the bluish glare of the Morteratsch glacier field seen against grey rocks and a deep-blue summer sky. The colour of clothing contributes to the aesthetics of everyday life as do, though in a more limited way, the different colours used by women who wear make-up. If the balance of colours chosen for a dress or for make-up is seriously disturbed, this results in a rather peculiar appearance, as occurs fairly frequently with patients suffering from manic or schizo-affective psychoses. In some special groups of our society, colours are symbols of a social hierarchical order, e.g. the different garments which signify the clerical hierarchy of the Roman Catholic church or military ranks. The colours of flags help to identify certain social entities such as nations, political parties, cities or soccer clubs. The chroma of light produced by stained glass windows contributes to the magnificent setting inside gothic cathedrals. Certain coloured signals control our behaviour: warning signs, traffic signs, the tail lights of an automobile, etc. Some psychologists use coloured tokens to determine the choice preference of their subjects; they believe that in doing so, they can correctly recognize a subject's character traits. Finally, colourful fireworks express joy and hope; pyrotechnics has developed into an exercise involving the sophisticated creation of short-lived form–colour paintings possessing a certain grandeur.

Colour constancy is another aspect of colour vision. The perceived colours of natural objects change little, although the spectral composition of daylight varies considerably. When the sun is near the horizon, long-wavelength light dominates; when the sun is near zenith, daylight spectral composition in the short-wavelength range is at a maximum. Not only average luminance but also the spectral composition of daylight depends heavily on the types of clouds in the sky (cf. Henderson, 1977). Colour constancy is achieved (within certain limits) by physiological mechanisms related to retinal and cerebral signal processing: the spectral composition of the light originating from a certain object surface that reaches the retina is not only evaluated by three different types of cones operating locally, but also by computation of the fraction of these three colour signals relative to the average chromatic stimulation of a large retinal area. By computing quotients of local and global colour parameters, the chromatic signals generated within the retina and the central visual system convey information about the spectral reflectance of the object surfaces, but not about the light reaching the retina. For each point in space, the latter corresponds to the product of spectral reflectance and spectral illumination. This colour constancy mechanism was proposed by Hering (1864, 1920) and elaborated upon more recently by Land (1977, 'retinex theory'; cf. also

Brou *et al.*, 1986). Corresponding to colour constancy is the ability to remember the colours of objects. Hering's '*Gedächtnisfarben*' are constant. This constancy is schematized by labelling certain objects with colour names (grass = green, tomato = red), whereby the different hues of a certain colour are not taken into consideration.

To begin with, in early Greek theories of vision, colour was treated as a separate quality of the visual modality. Colour perception was soon considered to be caused not only by an object's material properties, but also by the physiological events that follow light stimulation of the eye. Aristotle's description of the changes in hues of a long-lasting afterimage suggests this interpretation:

> *And if, after looking at the sun or some other bright object, we shut our eyes, then, if we watch carefully, light appears wherever the sight is directed, first in its own proper colour; then it changes to red, and then to purple, until it fades to black and disappears.* (On Dreams, 459 a).

According to ancient Greek, Scholastic and Renaissance colour theories, the perceived world of colours was organized according to three principles (cf. Chapter 2):

1. There are three or more primary colours.
2. The perceived world of colours (the colour space) is structured according to a natural sequence of 'neighbouring' colours, which are also visible, in part, in the colour sequence of the rainbow.
3. Colour perception is characterized by contrasting hues, such as green/red or black/white. Leonardo da Vinci (1519), for example, defined red, yellow, green and blue as the basic colours of a contrastingly organized colour space (*Trattato della pittura*, Donders, 1881; Ludwig, 1882; Steinitz, 1958).

These rather vague ideas on colour vision clearly dominated the colour theories of the eighteenth and nineteenth centuries from which our present conception has evolved:

1. Three different types of cones, so-called retinal photoreceptors, each characterized by the different spectral sensitivities of their photopigments (Bowmaker and Dartnall, 1980; Bowmaker *et al.*, 1980), are distributed in unequal numbers within the receptor layer of the foveal and parafoveal retina. They form the first level of colour vision, the 'sensor space' described quantitatively by the Young–Helmholtz trichromatic colour theory (Young, 1802; Helmholtz, 1860, 1896; Stiles, 1978; Boynton, 1979; Wyszecki and Stiles, 1982). Because of the sensitivity of the cones, colour vision is restricted in man and other primates to the stimulus conditions of photopic vision, i.e. to the luminance levels above the twilight conditions present before sunrise or after sunset. The scotopic vision of an eye adapted to the dark is performed by means of the 'colour-blind' rod system, which operates best in moonlight (duplicity theory, Schultze, 1866; Chapter 3).

2. There are different X-chromosome-linked genetic deviations in man that affect both the cone system and retinal colour processing, producing different types of colour vision anomalies (anomalous trichromacies) or dichromacies (protanopia, deuteranopia, tritanopia). In the rare symptom of congenital total colour blindness (monochromacy), one finds only the rod pigment rhodopsin in all photoreceptors of the eye (reviews: Donders, 1881; Jaeger, 1972).

3. The 'sensor space', the first physiological level of colour representation, is transformed by a multi-step neuronal operation (which takes place in the retina, the lateral geniculate nucleus and the primary visual cortex) into a second-order colour space characterized by opposing colour mechanisms: red–green, blue–yellow, black–white (Hering, 1868, 1920, 1964). These three mechanisms represent a homogeneous and three-dimensional abstract 'colour space' in which the hues perceived by man are represented in a regular order, as Tobias Mayer (1752; Chapter 3) and P. O. Runge (1810) had anticipated. This representation is realized in a subset of neurones distributed across the primary visual cortex according to a fixed retinotopic map (Chapter 3). At this level mechanisms for colour and form vision are separated. As a consequence, dissociation of the two mechanisms is observable, as is the case in strabismic amblyopics. In some of these patients the sensitivity to achromatic gratings is greatly reduced, and equiluminant chromatic grating patterns at comparable spatial frequencies are detected (Hilz and Rentschler, 1989). As discussed in Chapter 3, the separation of chromatic and achromatic 'channels' occurs in steps: while beyond area V1 some of the visual cortical areas seem to process dominantly shape, colour or movement information, the separation is related to different columns and layers within area 17 (V1), which are of course interconnected.

4. From the neuronal representation of the perceptual colour space, a third level of colour categorization is derived by mechanisms which finally place 'labels' of different behavioural categories or names on certain substructures found in the colour space. This colour categorization includes the phenomenon of 'colour constancy' mentioned above: within certain limits, the perceived chroma of a given object's surfaces remain constant despite changes in the spectral distribution of the illuminating light. Colour constancy of the 'surface colours of objects' (Katz, 1911) is also elaborated upon at the preceding level of opposing colour mechanisms (Boynton, 1988; Jameson and Hurvich, 1989). Colour categorization might take several steps. The first step seems to depend essentially on the activity of a subset of area V4 neurones in primates. Colour responses from area V4 are transmitted to the infero-temporal cortex, where perceptual colours and remembered colour mechanisms may interact (Desi-

mone *et al.*, 1980; Fuster and Jervey, 1982; Braitman, 1984). Colour categorization corresponds at the uppermost level to the ecological needs of primates. In man, the cultural habits of the observer certainly have an important impact on colour cognition, which depends heavily on learning as well as on the observer's education and social position. Although the grouping of hues by certain colour names may be different in languages used by remote human cultures, comparative studies have shown that there are generally eleven colour names which most frequently appear in many languages: black, white, grey, red, orange, brown, yellow, green, blue, purple, pink (Berlin and Kay, 1969; Zollinger, 1973, 1984, 1988). Colour naming competence also varies considerably in our own society.

5. As mentioned above, certain emotional changes are associated with colour perception – simultaneously to and, in part, independently of the process in which colours are labelled with names and assigned behavioural meanings. Based on this fact, we presume that cerebral colour perception mechanisms feed signals into the limbic system (Fig. 18.7). As for other human limbic system operations, the cultural background, i.e. behavioural patterns of the individual acquired in early childhood and adolescence, has a strong impact on these emotional responses. Nevertheless, one cannot exclude that a few universals also exist in man, i.e. inborn mechanisms which control the emotional components of colour perception. The colour 'red' along with its different shades, for example, is not only the first colour name to appear in most languages, but is also considered universally to be the colour of heightened emotion. Because of its association with fire, it is usually perceived to be a 'warm' colour. It seems probable that this emotional response to red is present universally and determined by genetically pre-programmed connections between area V4 and the limbic structures, in particular connections with the gyrus parahippocampalis. The majority of emotional responses evoked by colours or colour patterns, however, is apparently learned during childhood and adolescence, indicating the high plasticity of the interplay between the neocortical and limbic mechanisms performing this function.

A remarkable temporal dissociation of colour discrimination and colour naming has been reported repeatedly during ontogenetic development (review: Bornstein, 1985). Bornstein *et al.*, (1976) reported, for example, that 4-month-old infants were able to discern spectral wavelengths according to the four basic colour qualities, red, yellow, green and blue. Correct and consistent colour naming, however, occurs rather late, and develops earlier in girls than in boys. In colour naming, many children first use a single term for all colours. Later, when more than one colour term is used, colour naming is frequently random. The names of colours first assume a constant and

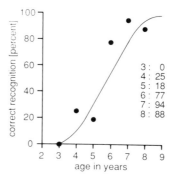

Fig. 20.1 *The ability to name eight basic colours correctly develops slowly between the ages of 4 and 8 years. The correct recognition score (percentage, ordinate) is plotted as a function of age in girls and boys (abscissa). (Redrawn from Synolds and Pronko, 1949.)*

accurate meaning between ages 5 and 7, despite the fact that 3- or 4-year-old children can use colour competently to recognize objects (Fig. 20.1; Synolds and Pronko, 1949). By measuring the recognition time in children of different ages for the four basic colour words, Schiller (1966) found a considerable decrease in reaction time between first and second graders. This remarkably late development of a constant correlation between the names of colours and their behavioural use is perhaps caused by the fact that the application of colours to recognize objects is predominantly a non-linguistic function of the right hemisphere and the knowledge of proper colour names is behaviourally irrelevant. Although photographs of objects in which the colours were accurately reproduced had no effect on the precision of object recognition in adults, it facilitated object naming. Such a facilitatory effect was not found for abstract shapes. Not unexpectedly, naming the colour of an accurately coloured object was about 100 ms faster than naming the correct colour of an object seen in a black-and-white photograph. Correct naming of objects in colour photographs (806 ms average latency) was faster than naming objects in black-and-white photographs (844 ms). Finally, colour naming was slower (852 ms) than object naming (806 ms) in colour photographs (Ostergaard and Davidoff, 1985).

The frequent association of colour naming deficits in patients suffering from pure alexia (Chapter 18) has raised the question of whether or not the colour-naming ability is especially disturbed in dyslexic children. Critchley (1970) reported that none of his 125 patients suffering from 'developmental dyslexia' had colour naming difficulties. He noted, however, that Warburg (1911) had mentioned several such cases. Based on these observations, Denckla (1972a, b) performed two studies, one designed to assess the colour naming abilities of normal kindergarten children and children between ages 7 and 11, the other to detect delayed or impaired competence for colour naming in children with reading disabilities. Both groups were given the same tasks: tracing pseudoisochromatic plates (Dvorine), sorting and matching pairs of pieces of yarn having difficult-to-name hues, pointing to certain coloured pieces of yarn in response to hearing the examiner say the name of the colour of these pieces of yarn, without time pressure, and timed naming of the colours red, green, yellow, blue and black. Finally, questions such as 'what colour is grass?' also had to be answered. Denckla found a clearly better performance in colour naming in her normative group of kindergarten children (average age of 6) than that reported by the Gsell Institute, which found that at age 5, only 61% of the children could reliably name red, blue, green and yellow, despite their good performance naming objects (Castner, 1940). Moreover, in this group of 154 kindergarten children Denckla found only one child, a boy aged 5 years 5 months, who showed a severe bidirectional (naming and pointing) impairment restricted to colours.

On the other hand, out of 56 children aged 7 to 11 who had been referred to her because of reading difficulties, the same author found 5 boys aged 7.5 to 10.7 years who suffered from a syndrome of severe dyslexia and colour naming difficulty; they exhibited no comparable difficulty in object or picture naming, nor any conspicuous neurological signs indicating brain damage. These observations also support the idea that the correlation between colours and colour names uses neuronal operations distinct from the correlation of objects and object names. It would be interesting to know whether or not these 'colour dyslexics' also have difficulties describing the appearance of surface textures (smooth, rough, etc.).

The History of Achromatopsia up to the End of the Nineteenth Century

Acquired 'cerebral' achromatopsia is a term used to designate the loss of colour vision caused by cerebral lesions in a subject who had possessed trichromatic or dichromatic colour vision before occurrence of the brain lesion. Achromatopsia affects either the whole visual field or only part of it; it appears in 'retinotopic' coordinates. When achromatopsia is restricted to the left or right half of the visual field, it is called hemiachromatopsia. Incomplete states of this defect have been described: the patient does not report a complete loss of colour vision, but rather describes all colours as either 'pale' or 'washed out' (dyschromatopsia).

This state is also observed during recovery from a complete cerebral achromatopsia. Nothing is known about achromatopsia in dichromates or anomalous trichromates. One may assume, however, that the symptoms are similar to those present in normal trichromates. This prediction is based on Critchley's observation (1965) of a migrainous red–green dichromatic student whose colour perception faded temporarily during migraine attacks.

Acquired colour defects are observed not only after the development of cortical or white matter lesions, but also in special cases of retinopathy (e.g. chloroquine intoxication, diabetes, hypertension) as well as in the presence of certain optic nerve diseases (Leber's optic nerve atrophy, retrobulbar neuritis, optic nerve trauma, tumours exerting pressure on optic nerve fibres, e.g. pituitary adenomas) or intoxication (e.g. xanthochromacy with digitalis overdoses, Purkinje, 1825). These conditions of 'peripheral achromatopsias' will not be discussed in this chapter (cf. Grützner, 1966, 1972; Travis and Thompson, 1989): we shall restrict our discussion to 'central' achromatopsias and other cerebral colour deficiencies caused by lesions proximal to the lateral geniculate body.

It is not clear when the first Western observations of cerebral achromatopsia took place. Although Albertus Magnus wrote in the thirteenth century about subjects unable to recognize any colours, he did not indicate whether this symptom was congenital or acquired after birth. Since Albertus Magnus described photophobia as a symptom of colour blindness, it seems rather probable that he knew about and perhaps even observed monochromats (i.e. subjects who suffered from congenital total colour blindness), for photophobia is a symptom frequently associated with total 'peripheral' colour blindness.

In 1688, Robert Boyle published a pamphlet entitled *Some Uncommon Observations About Vitiated Sight*. In 'Observation XI' of the publication he described a young woman suffering from acquired colour blindness (Mollon *et al.*, 1980; Mollon, 1989). This was presumably the same patient mentioned by D. Turberville, a celebrated oculist of his time, in a report published in 1684 in the *Philosophical Transactions of the Royal Society in London*. Turberville mentioned 'a maid, two or three and twenty years old . . . . who could see very well, but no colour beside black and white...'. Boyle (1688) reported his observations on this patient in more detail. The young lady, after suffering most likely from meningo-encephalitis, recovered slowly from cortical blindness with the typical stages of recovery as described in the following. The only symptoms present when Boyle examined her were achromatopsia and easy visual fatigue:

> *The gentlewoman I saw to day, seems to be about eighteen or twenty years old, and is of a fine complexion, accompanied with good features. Looking into her eyes, which are grey, I could not discern any thing that was unusual or amiss; though*

her eye-lids were somewhat red, whether from heat, or which seemed more likely, from her precedent weeping. During the very little time that the company allowed me to speak with her, the questions I proposed to her were answered to this effect:

That about five years ago, having been upon a certain occasion immoderately tormented with blisters, applied to her neck and other parts, she was quite deprived of her sight.

That some time after she began to perceive the light, but nothing by the help of it: than then she could see a window, without discerning the panes or the bars: that afterwards she grew able to distinguish the shapes of bodies, and some of their colours: and at last she came to be able to see the minutest object; which when I seemed to doubt of, and presented her a book, she not only without hesitancy read in it a line or two, (for her eyes are quickly weary) but having pointed with my finger at a part of the margin, near which there was the part of a very little speck, that might almost be covered with the point of a pin, she not only readily enough found it out, but shewed me, at some distance off, another speck, that was yet more minute, and required a sharp sight to discern it. And yet, whereas this was done about noon, she told me, that she could see much better in the evening, than in any lighter time of the day.

While she was looking upon the printed paper I shewed her, I asked her, whether it did not appear white to her, and the letters black? to which she answered, that they did so; but that she saw, as it were, a white glass laid over both the objects. But the things, that were most particular and odd in this woman's case, were these two. The first is, that she is not unfrequently troubled with flashes of lightning, that seem to issue out like flames about the external angle of her eye, which often make her start, and put her into frights and melancholy thoughts. But the other, which is more strange and singular, is this, that she can distinguish some colours, as black and white; but is not able to distinguish others, especially red and green; and when I brought her a bag of a fine and glossy red, with tufts of sky-coloured silk, she looked attentively upon it, but told me, that to her it did not seem red, but of another colour, which one would guess by her description to be a dark or dirty one: and the tufts of silk, that were finely coloured, she took in her hand, and told me they seemed to be a light colour, but could not tell me which; only she compared it to the colour of the silken stuff of the laced petticoat of a lady, that brought her to me; and indeed the blues were very much alike. And when I asked her whether in the evenings when she went abroad to walk in the fields, which she much delighted to do, the meadows did not appear to her clothed in green? she told me they did not, but seemed to be of an odd darkish colour; and added, that when she had a mind to gather violets, though she kneeled in that place where they grew, she was not able to distinguish them by the colour from the neighbouring grass, but only by the shape or by feeling them. And the lady that was with her, took thence occasion to tell me, that when she looks upon a Turkey carpet, she cannot distinguish the colours, unless of those parts that are white or black . . . . (pp. 450–451).

In this report, Boyle summarized the characteristic

properties of pure achromatopsia in the absence of any serious impairment of other visual functions except for the easy visual fatigue. In 'Observation XII' of the same publication Boyle added an observation on partial colour blindness and reported on a case 'not so odd' but having 'yet an affinity with the newly recited case' of 'Observation XI'. This patient, a 'mathematician, eminent for his skill in optics, and therefore a very competent relator of phenomena belonging to that science' had normal visual acuity and light–dark adaptation, since he made 'excellent use [of his eyes] in astronomical observation and optical experiments'. He reported to Boyle that 'there are some colours, that he constantly sees amiss'. Presumably this mathematician was a dichromat, since he described some colours as being of a 'darkish sort of cloth' colours, which to Boyle and 'other men appeared of quite differing colour'. It is interesting that this report preceded by nearly one century another description of congenital colour anomalies and dichromacies. In a letter written in 1777 to Joseph Priestley, J. Huddart, a country clergyman, described that 'Harris the shoemaker' and several of his brothers suffered from red–green blindness of the type nowadays referred to as protanopia. The letter was subsequently published in the *Philosophical Transactions of the Royal Society*. As Walls (1956) had discovered, G. Palmer, presumably an English chemist, had developed a trichromatic 'theory of colours and vision' in 1777 and in a 1786 pamphlet, written to encourage sales of a special lamp, described not only his trichromatic colour theory but also mentioned people, e.g. a '*poète Colardeau*,' who suffered from reduced colour vision. To explain this condition, Palmer pointed out that this man possessed only two of the three classes of retinal 'fibres' necessary for full colour vision. John Dalton's (1798) description of his own red–green colour blindness (Donders, 1881) became more familiar to vision scientists. Congenital colour blindness came to be known in the English literature as Daltonism.

Towards the end of the eighteenth century, these two principally different classes of colour perception defects were accepted by physicians and mentioned in a number of nosological books. For example, achromatopsia caused by brain lesions was included in the *System der Nosologie*, published in 1797 by the Tübingen professor of medicine, W. G. Ploucquet. In the section entitled 'Diseases of the external senses', disturbances of vision and colour perception ('*Gesichtstäuschungen*', '*Farbentäuschungen*') are mentioned as separate entities which were attributed not only to peripheral diseases but also to lesions of the central nervous system – despite the fact that at that time visual diseases were believed to be caused mainly by peripheral pathology of the eye. Some physicians recognized that 'cerebral apoplexy' or '*hydrocephalus*' (Ploucquet, 1797) could also cause visual defects. Ploucquet divided disturbances of colour vision ('*colour illusion*', '*Farbentäuschung*') into two subgroups: one type in which the patient could no longer discriminate colours, and another type in which the patient could not clearly distinguish between different colours (colour anomia?). The state in which colour vision was no longer possible was further subdivided into two different subcategories, one accompanied by an abnormal increase in sensitivity to light, the other characterized by 'some darkening of visual perception'. The first type of colour blindness presumably corresponded to congenital monochromacy; the 'increased sensitivity' to light was most likely a description of photophobia, a common symptom appearing in most monochromats. The other type of colour blindness which appeared together with 'some darkening' of vision was presumably acquired achromatopsia; the darkening of vision was an allusion either to visual field defects or to accompanying cortical amblyopia. Since no generally accepted concept of visual field defects existed at the end of the eighteenth century, we can only speculate about Ploucquet's remark.

After neurologists and ophthalmologists had recognized certain rules governing the correlation of visual field defects and brain pathology and introduced the use of more systematic clinical perimetry (including colour perimetry), a more distinct concept of achromatopsia was developed during the second half of the nineteenth century. Achromatopsia, a sudden loss of colour vision affecting either the entire visual field or only one hemifield (hemiachromatopsia), was often carefully described during the 1870s and 1880s. For example, Treitel (1879), who emphasized the value of exact colour perimetry in diagnosing cerebral vision deficiencies, considered hemiachromatopsia to be 'partial hemianopia'. Steffan (1881) mentioned in a report several earlier observations of achromatopsia; Quaglino (1867) reported on a patient who, after having developed severe apoplexy, suffered from left hemiplegia, left incomplete homonymous hemianopia, object agnosia and complete achromatopsia. Cohn (1874) described the recovery from cortical blindness of a patient who, after a post-traumatic, two-week coma, regained a visual acuity of a tenth of the normal value, but remained totally colour blind. Steffan (1881) described in detail the symptoms of a professional colour printer who still had normal visual fields and visual acuity (15/20) following a stroke, but suffered from achromatopsia from which he did not recover within the next 5 years. Steffan used papers of different colours to investigate this patient's colour discrimination abilities. Using small tokens, the patient could perform this task only according to brightness levels. With very large sheets of well-illuminated coloured paper, however, correct rudimentary responses to red, yellow and blue, but not to green, were observed. Coloured yarn could not be discriminated, and Stilling's pseudoisochromatic plates (first issued in 1877) were recognized only in the yellow–blue range. The colours of

the sunlight spectrum were perceived as 'red, yellow and dark'. Steffan's patient reported to have 'seen all colours beforehand as well as any of his co-workers and never had mixed up any colours'. Thus Steffan assumed 'that there is no other conclusion left than that the patient became suddenly colourblind due to cerebral apoplexy, without any reduction in visual acuity'.

Although no brain pathology was available to Steffan, he nevertheless concluded from his observations that there is 'in our central organ a special centre for colour vision' located somewhere in the brain outside the region responsible for light–dark vision, which was normal in his patient. This opinion was also put forth by Samelsohn (1881) and von Seggern (1881), who described a similar phenomenon in patients suffering from hemianopia who had full visual acuity in the remaining visual hemifield, which was nevertheless totally colour blind.

Brill (1882) reported on a patient who had suffered from severe impairment of colour perception following a cerebrovascular infarction in the territory of the left cerebral posterior artery. He claimed that his patient had no impairment of visual acuity, nor any visual field defects. Based on the neuropathological records, Brill could demonstrate that the patient had suffered from an extended lesion within the posterior part of the gyrus lingualis (Fig. 20.2). He concluded that colour vision and light–dark vision were located in cortical regions adjacent to each other. The findings in another patient observed by Swanzy (1883) confirmed colour perception impairments in parts of the visual field which exhibited no changes in light–dark perception.

Reinhard (1887a) also observed a patient suffering from a right homonymous hemianopia which later improved considerably. In the part of the visual hemifield where no disturbance of light–dark vision was later observed, a 'partial' visual agnosia and hemiachromatopsia remained. The patient, an alcoholic, suffered from an infarction of the left

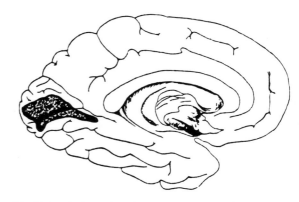

Fig. 20.2 *The lesion found in a patient suffering from cerebral achromatopsia (Brill, 1882).*

gyrus fusiformis and the upper parietal lobule, and, in addition, had an extended sclerosis of the hippocampus. In another case, Reinhard (1886) described incomplete homonymous defects in both hemifields and emphasized the close congruence of field defects for light–dark vision and colour perception. Visual field defects were caused in this patient mainly by lesions in the white matter; the mesial part of the occipital cortex was spared. A comparison of the two cases led Reinhard to suggest the existence of a separate 'colour centre' located in the lower part of the medial occipito-temporal cortex. Reinhard (1887b) concluded that although defects in conscious colour and space perception might be related to 'mind blindness,' they lack all signs of visual memory defects characteristic of the complete mind-blindness syndrome.

Wilbrand (1884, 1887) wrote a systematic summary of these early cases, which were clearly different from peripheral colour blindness (Schoeler and Uhthoff, 1884). Wilbrand suggested three separate 'centres' in the occipital brain, the first for light–dark vision, the second for colour vision and the third for form vision. He believed that afferent optic nerve fibres reach these centres directly. Thus, Wilbrand assumed three separate 'channels' in the afferent visual pathway, one for the light sense, one for the colour sense and one for visual form perception. This idea of separate cerebral 'centres', located by Wilbrand in the different layers of the visual cortex, each responsible for different aspects of the visual modality, was soon included in neurological textbooks. For example, Gowers (1888) also discussed the idea of a separate centre for colour vision; in contrast to Wilbrand, however, he thought that 'all impressions go first to the region of the apex of the occipital lobe, since disease here causes absolute hemianopia, and that a spatial half-vision centre for colours lies in front of this' (Gowers, 1887).

Verrey (1888) also contributed significantly to the question of a separate cortical colour centre. Based on the necropsy findings of a patient suffering from a right-sided hemiachromatopsia, he concluded that a cerebral colour centre existed in the region of the gyrus lingualis and the gyrus fusiformis, i.e. outside the area striata, which was considered by Henschen to be the 'cortical retina', the cerebral centre of vision (cf. Fig. 20.3). Förster (1890) described a patient suffering from extended bilateral hemianopia with small achromatic islands of vision. Dejerine (1892) investigated a patient suffering from a pure hemiachromatopsia in the right visual field. Later, Vialet (1893) published the neuropathology of this patient's brain and described a circumscribed lesion in the mesial occipital region below the area calcarina (which was spared), including the gyrus lingualis, gyrus fusiformis and some white matter below these structures.

Not all ophthalmologists or neurologists, however, were convinced by these observations. They refuted the notion

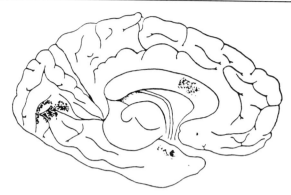

Fig. 20.3 *Lesions found in a patient suffering from right-sided hemiachromatopsia (Verrey, 1888).*

of a distinct cerebral colour-processing mechanism supposedly located in the occipital mesial cortex separate from the area striata. Because the presumed 'colour centre' in the fusiform and lingual gyri was located in the immediate surroundings of the striate area, hemiachromatopsia not accompanied by large homonymous visual field defects occurred rather seldom. As a result, many clinicians did not personally observe patients suffering from pure achromatopsia or hemiachromatopsia, and therefore did not accept the conclusions advanced by Steffan, Reinhard or Verrey until they themselves had observed such a patient. Zeki (1990) illustrated this using the example of MacKay, who had originally attacked Verrey's conclusions in 1888, but then accepted them 11 years later (MacKay and Dunlop, 1899) after having personally observed a 'remarkable case': a patient with 'a total acquired colour blindness from a cerebral lesion', who also suffered briefly from alexia. This patient's lesion was located predominantly in the grey matter of the fusiform gyrus.

Siemerling (1890) reported on a patient suffering from visual object agnosia, hemianopia of the right visual field and complete achromatopsia in the remaining visual field, where everything appeared as different shades of grey. This patient's object agnosia and achromatopsia both recovered. Lissauer (1890) described a patient suffering from visual agnosia ('mind blindness') and homonymous hemianopia of the right visual field who had also had difficulties naming colours. Lissauer could clearly demonstrate that the 'ability to perceive and to discriminate colours was indeed well preserved [in this patient] and [that] errors appeared only when the patient had to connect certain colour percepts with verbal or other complex abstract ideas'. Wilbrand (1884) called this condition 'amnesic colour blindness'. It is nowadays referred to as 'colour anomia' (cf. p. 402). This observation indicated a clear dissociation between visual object agnosia and achromatopsia.

The idea of a separate cerebral representation of colour vision outside the area striata was not fully appreciated by Wilbrand and Saenger (1917) in their competent review of visual field defects. Other researchers, however, had accepted the anatomical 'separation of colour perception' ('*Abspaltung des Farbensinnes*') from form vision, as postulated by Lewandowsky (1908), who had demonstrated categorical deficiencies in object–colour correlation without achromatopsia in patients suffering from left occipito-temporal brain lesions, a defect he differentiated from 'amnesic colour blindness'. The majority of neurologists and ophthalmologists working during the first decade of the twentieth century recognized three stages of colour vision cortical impairment:

1. achromatopsia or hemiachromatopsia;
2. colour agnosia, i.e. disturbances in object–colour relation (Lewandowsky, 1908);
3. colour anomia (amnesic colour blindness, Wilbrand, 1896).

A minority of neurologists even questioned the existence of selective cortical impairment of colour vision (e.g. Holmes, 1918a), an idea which was upheld even against anatomical evidence in two postmortem cases (Lenz, 1921) and has been periodically discussed up until the present (review: see Zeki, 1990).

A Case Report Introducing the Main Symptoms of Cortical Colour Blindness: A Painter Suffering from Achromatopsia

In 1987, Sacks and Wasserman reported extensively on the symptoms and self-observations of a 65-year-old 'rather successful artist', Jonathan I., who realized after a car accident that he could no longer discern colours or letters. He also suffered from a temporary reduction in visual acuity. Although alexia and amblyopia evidently recovered, absolute colour blindness did not. This descriptive essay presented by Sacks and Wasserman depicted not only the perceptual but also the emotional consequences of achromatopsia. It was the result of cooperation between a precise, self-observing patient, a painter who had previously had extensive professional experience working with colours, and a neurologist well known for his literary accounts of neurological diseases (Sacks, 1985). In this section, we shall quote a number of passages from this well-written report in order to illustrate the characteristic symptoms of acquired achromatopsia.

In March 1986, the painter described in a letter to one of his physicians the incident which led to achromatopsia:

I am a rather successful artist just past sixty-five years of age. On January 2nd of this year I was driving my car and was hit by a small truck on the passenger side of my vehicle.

When visiting the emergency room of a local hospital, I was told I had a concussion. While taking an eye examination, it was discovered that I was unable to distinguish letters or colors. The letters appeared to be Greek letters. My vision was such that everything appeared to me as viewing a black and white television screen.

Within days, I could distinguish letters and my vision became that of an eagle – I can see a worm wiggling a block away. The sharpness of focus is incredible.

But – I am absolutely colourblind ...

Sacks and Wasserman saw the patient for first time about 3 months after the accident. They noted that he had suffered from an anterograde amnesia for several hours following the accident and exhibited signs of depression. The initial alexia and reduced visual acuity had evidently soon recovered, but achromatopsia remained a problem:

'You might think', Mr I. said, 'loss of colour vision, what's the big deal? Some of my friends said this, my wife sometimes thought this, but to me at least it was awful, disgusting.' It was not just that colours were missing, but that what he could see had a distasteful, dirty look, the whites glaring, yet discoloured and off-white, the blacks cavernous – everything wrong, unnatural and impure ...

To Mr I., people looked 'like animated grey statues'. He could hardly stand his own changed appearance in the mirror – 'flesh-coloured' now seemed 'rat-coloured'. His previously well-developed eidetic abilities were similarly changed, as was his real visual perception: all images seen by means of visual imagery were colourless. There were also behavioural consequences: he avoided social interaction and found sexual intercourse impossible. Because of its grey, dead appearance, food became disgusting to him. Verbal association of colours with objects and the colours of paintings known to him were not disturbed, however. 'He knew all the colours, but could no longer see them, either when he looked or in his mind's eye, his imagination or memory.'

Loss of colour vision affected his emotional interaction with the world; in particular, he missed the brilliant colours of spring. In bright sunlight, contrasts were in part enhanced, in part reduced; faces were often unidentifiable to him until seen from up close. Sacks and Wasserman believed this defect not to be caused by prosopagnosia, but rather by a loss of 'colour and tonal contrast'.

After Mr I. recovered from the initial shock of having lost his colour vision, he started once again to paint. The black-and-white paintings which he produced during the first months following the incident 'gave a feeling of violent forces – rage, fear, dispair, excitement', and indicated the emotional problems caused by the achromatopsia. The content of the paintings changed within months, however, returning to 'living themes he had not touched in thirty years, back to representational paintings of dancers and race-horses. These paintings, even though still in black and white, were full of movement, vitality and sensuousness' and characterized 'the beginnings of a renewed social and sexual life, a lessening of his fears and depressions and a turning back to life'. Later, he painted a 'grey room' in which he tried to express what he felt, namely, life 'in a world moulded in lead'.

Interestingly, his appreciation of music was also impaired. Before the accident, Jonathan I. had experienced intensive synaesthesias and saw vivid coloured pictures in his mind's eye when listening to music. These experiences vanished after the accident. Even the chromaticity of migraine phosphenes, which he had previously experienced, disappeared after the accident. The same was true for the colours in his dreams: 'Now his dreams were washed-out and pale, or violent and contrasty, lacking both colour and delicate tonal gradients'. The loss of colours in dreams is not always reported by cerebral achromatopic patients. This symptom perhaps indicates an interruption of the connections between the visual system and the limbic structures.

Using coloured objects, photographs and yarns (the Holmgren test) comprised of thirty-three distinct colours which the patient could precisely sort according to grey-scale tonal values (but not by chroma), Sacks and Wasserman performed an extensive examination of colour vision in this patient. Although Mr I. was unable to place the colour tokens used for the Farnsworth–Munsell test into any chromatic order, he perceived the blue tokens to be 'paler' than the others. A printed colour spectrum appeared to him in varying shades of grey. In light of his description of the 'spectrum' (unfortunately, no real spectral light but rather a printed 'spectrum' was used for comparative testing), the authors thought that the patient's photopic luminosity curve had reached a peak at around 560 nm, corresponding to maximum sensitivity of photopic vision. None of the Ishihara pseudoisochromatic plates was recognized correctly.

Form vision, form memory and drawing from memory were all perfect. One year after the accident, the authors, together with S. Zeki, checked for colour constancy using 'Mondrian' patterns (McCann *et al.*, 1976; Land and McCann, 1971; Land, 1977). Mr I. could distinguish most of the rectangular components of the Mondrian pattern, but 'only as consisting of different shades of grey, and he instantly ranked them on a one-to-four grey scale, although he could not distinguish some colour boundaries' (Sacks *et al.*, 1988). The grey-scale values of the shapes changed when the chromaticity of the illuminating light was switched. As for everyday observations, colours which appeared to normal observers as blue were predominantly described by the patient as 'pale'.

Sacks and Wasserman concluded that while 'the visual association cortex ... had been damaged' in their patient, the primary visual cortex had remained intact. Although significant changes in these regions are often the case subsequent to closed head injury, CT and MRI scans did not indicate any nor, for that matter, were they indicated anywhere else in Mr I's brain. Since the symptoms described were typical for achromatopsia caused by cerebral mesial occipital lesions, the authors' conclusions seem justified. What is especially remarkable about this case is the careful analysis of the patient's emotional reaction to his world turning grey. In other patients, such consequences have not been experienced at all, or not as dramatically, or have not been as carefully evaluated. Perhaps the lesion in this patient extended beyond area V4 (Chapter 5) into the posterior part of the limbic system, in particular into the gyrus parahippocampalis, which would account for the change in the patient's emotional state. Interestingly, a further emotional and behavioural adaptation occurred in the achromatopsia of the patient within a year. This fact is mentioned by Sacks and Wasserman in a postscript written in October 1987: 'The intense sorrow that was so characteristic at first, as he sat for hours before his (to him) black lawn, desperately trying to perceive or imagine it as green, has disappeared as has the revulsion (he no longer sees his wife or himself as having "rat-coloured" flesh)'. Mr I. changed his habits and became a 'night-person': 'he has taken to roving about a great deal, exploring other cities, other places, but only at night ... then wandering about the streets for half the night.' Jonathan I. began to love the night time, experiencing it as 'a whole new world'. He also developed increased sensitivity to scotopic vision.

Testing for Colour Vision, and Typical Responses of Patients Suffering from Achromatopsia

In addition to conventional neurological and neuropsychological examinations, the following tests are recommended whenever achromatopsia is suspected.

1. Perimetry should be performed in a Goldman or Tübingen perimeter using conventional as well as adequately sized red, green and blue spots of light (Chapter 9). In addition to monocular perimetry, binocular perimetry may be performed (e.g. Zihl and Mayer, 1981). Two examples of chromatic visual fields for red, green and blue perception, and for light–dark perception are shown in Fig. 20.4 (Zihl and von Cramon, 1986).

2. Before measuring the additive colour mixture (Raleigh equation) in the Nagel anomaloscope (red + green = yellow), it is especially important to ask male

(a)

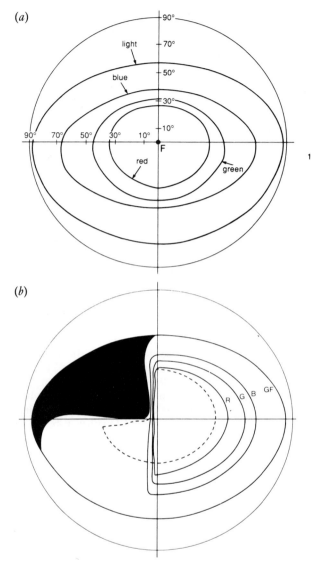

(b)

(c)

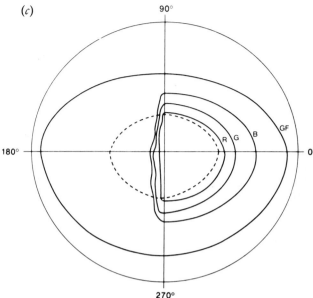

Fig. 20.4 *(a) Binocular achromatic and chromatic visual field borders as considered to be normal in the studies of Zihl and his coworkers (modified from Zihl and von Cramon, 1986). (b) Chromatic and achromatic visual field defects in a 44-year-old patient suffering from an infarction of the right posterior cerebral artery. Note the upper-left quadranopia. (c) Same from a 24-year-old patient: left homonymous hemiachromatopsia without visual field defects for light detection and form vision (dashed line; modified from Zihl and von Cramon, 1986).*

patients whether a congenital colour anomaly had been present before the cerebral lesion occurred. In most countries, professional as well as military service examinations include tests of colour vision. Patients with a typical achromatopsia accept any red-green mixture as possible on the Nagel anomaloscope, and can equilibrate it in brightness to the yellow light. Figure 20.5 shows the results obtained using the Nagel anomaloscope on a patient observed by Jaeger *et al.* (1989), and in our own patient, Mr W. M., who could match any red-green mixture in brightness to the yellow half-field, but could not detect differences between these hues. In addition, both patients suffered from bilateral upper quadrantanopia, pure alexia and

prosopagnosia as well as some topographagnosia caused by bilateral infarctions in the territory of the posterior cerebral arteries.

Jaeger *et al.*, (1989) also used the colour mixture of the tritanomaloscope (470 nm + 517 nm = 470 nm + white light; Jaeger, 1981) and discovered that their patient was less capable of discriminating between blue and green as compared with normal subjects. Colour mixtures in large test fields up to 35 degrees in diameter were investigated using a projection anomaloscope and the Raleigh equation, which corresponds to that of the Nagel anomaloscope (545 nm + 670 nm = 584 nm). The larger the test field, the smaller the range of colour mixtures perceived by the patient to be of equal hue. Thus, large colour fields led to some colour discrimination in the red-green range.

3. Although Stilling or Ishihara's pseudoisochromatic plates are usually not recognized by achromatic patients, guessing is often above chance (e.g. Green and Lessell, 1977). The performance of some patients using the Ishihara plates was, in fact, remarkably good (e.g. Mohr *et al.*,

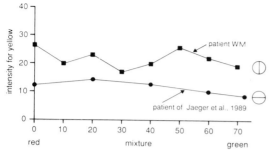

Fig. 20.5 *Results of matching tasks in additive colour mixture of the Raleigh equation in the Nagel anomaloscope in two patients suffering from cerebral achromatopsia. On the abscissa the relative components of green in the additive colour mixture of spectral green and red presented to the patient is given; on the ordinate is the intensity by which the patient equated the spectral yellow to the red/green mixture for equal brightness and hue. Data from Jaeger* et al. *(1989), and from patient W. M. Since W. M. suffered from an upper visual field hemianopia, the anomaloscope was turned by 90 degrees. Both patients accepted all mixtures on the red/green axis as being of the same hue, i.e. they were completely colour blind in the red–yellow–green range.*

1971). Since literal alexia might be associated with achromatopsia, one should also use averbal Ishihara plates. Our patient's recognition of the Ishihara plates improved when we allowed him to move the plates back and forth on the table. In doing so he presumably generated slight brightness differences along the chromatic borders, since shifting the image across the retina results in intermittent activation of the three cone channels (each having different temporal transfer frequency properties). Although Mr W. M.'s decision was correct in 6 out of 15 Ishihara plates in the first examination (4 weeks later he was correct in only 2 plates), he needed up to a minute to decide for each single plate. His performance with the averbal plates was comparable. When Ishihara plates are placed at a distance greater than 2 metres away from the patient, achromatic patients may also be able to read the numbers correctly, although they fail to do so from a normal reading distance (Mollon *et al.*, 1980). This effect could not be found in Mr W. M. It is produced by an additive colour mixture occurring within individual retinal cones, since the size of the individual spots of the retinal image on the Ishihara plate are then less than the diameter of a single cone.

4. Sorting of coloured wool strings (the Holmgreen test) is a traditional test used since the nineteenth century to diagnose achromatopsia and other colour deficiencies. It is still used by clinicians as a test which is relatively easy to evaluate. Like all 'direct' colour tests, it has one shortcoming, namely the usually not standardized conditions of white light illumination of the scene.

5. Patients taking the Farnsworth–Munsell 100-hue

test (Farnsworth, 1943; Han and Thompson, 1983; Zihl and Meyer, 1983; Victor, 1988) are asked to sort eighty-five tokens of different hues into different colour continua. When correctly illuminated, the different hues have approximately the same brightness and saturation. Typically, the patients suffering from cortical achromatopsia deviate rather significantly from the values obtained by normal patients across a wide range of the colour space (Lhermitte *et al.*, 1965; Pearlman *et al.*, 1978; Scarpatetti *et al.*, 1983; Jaeger *et al.*, 1989). Results of an achromatic patient's performance on the FM 100-hue test are shown in Fig. 20.6 (Zihl and von Cramon, 1986). The Farnsworth panel–15 test (saturated or non-saturated colour tokens) may be used (Jaeger *et al.*, 1988) instead of the Farnsworth–Munsell test. It was repeatedly reported that patients without achromatopsia who suffer from left- or right-hemisphere lesions also have higher error scores on the FM 100 test (De Renzi and Spinnler, 1967; Assal *et al.*, 1969). In an investigation conducted by Scotti and Spinnler (1970), patients suffering from right-hemisphere lesions with additional left-visual-hemifield defects had significantly higher error scores in comparison with the control group and with patients suffering from right-hemisphere lesions without hemianopia, as well as in comparison with patients suffering from left-hemisphere lesions. Capitani *et al.*, (1978) also reported increased error scores in the FM 100 test in patients suffering from right frontal brain lesions, but the highest error score was found in patients suffering from right-parietal brain lesions.

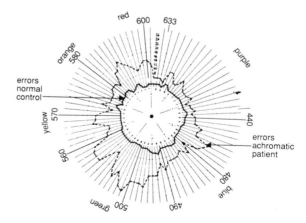

Fig. 20.6 *Results from the 100-hue Farnsworth–Munsell test in a 60-year-old patient suffering from cerebral achromatopsia (dashed line). For comparison, the data from a normal subject of about the same age are presented (continuous line). The results indicate a considerable reduction in the patient's hue discrimination in the entire range of the colour space. The largest deviations were found in the green and the orange–red (arrows; from Zihl and von Cramon, 1986, modified).*

6. The photopic spectral sensitivity curve is measured by determining the threshold values (ΔI) for a barely noticable increase in stimulus intensity I, whereby the wavelength of the stimulus is varied across the visible spectrum. Defining sensitivity as $I/\Delta I$ and plotting these values as a function of wavelength , maximum sensitivity is reached at about 560 nm, as expected from the normal photopic sensitivity curve. Using large test fields, Jaeger *et al.*, (1989; Fig. 20.7) demonstrated a blue, green and orange peak in a patient suffering from achromatopsia. Large-field spectral adaptation using yellow, purple or blue light showed that the three different cone mechanisms were separable in this patient; the spectral sensitivity curves changed correspondingly. This demonstrated the 'peripheral' function of the three different cone mechanisms. In a case of hemianopia and 'dyschromatopsia' of the other visual half-field, Victor *et al.* (1989) also found normal chromatic contrast sensitivity. The visual-evoked

potentials to isoluminant colour gratings or chequerboards were present in the electroencephalogram of this patient and were therefore attributed to area V1 functions (Fig. 20.8). The finding that the region of the right area V1 (related to the left dyschromatopic visual half-field) was preserved, as revealed by the MRI-scan, corroborated this observation. From these findings one can conclude that $\Delta I/I$ values specific for monochromatic stimuli of different wavelengths are obtainable when area V1 function is preserved.

7. Davidoff *et al.* (1991) also investigated the above-mentioned patient W. M., who not only completely failed the Farnsworth 100-hue test, but also could not discriminate the colour of the spots of light in a Tübingen perimeter used for colour perimetry. Davidoff *et al.* tried to prove normal peripheral trichromatic cone vision by demonstrating the 'survival of chromatic boundaries' in achromatopsia. They divided a computer-controlled colour TV screen into four quadrants and used different chromatic stimuli:

(*a*) Green or red quadrants having the same hue but different luminance ('monochromatic stimuli').

(*b*) 3 green and 3 red quadrants having either no luminance contrast between the 2 colours ('equiluminant' conditions) or having clear luminance differences in addition to the colour contrast.

(*c*) Each quadrant consisted of many equiprobable red and green pixels of 0.4 degrees^2; the luminance in 1 quadrant was higher than that of the other 3 quadrants. The dependable variable was the reaction time needed to press the correct key from 4 possible choices, each corresponding to the 4 quadrants of the stimulus field. The achromatic patient's responses clearly signified colour contrast; consequently, the patient obtained a rather low error score.

8. Mollon *et al.* (1980) applied colour specificity of the movement after effect (Chapter 19) to an achromatic patient. Lovegrove *et al.*, (1972) had previously demonstrated that the movement after effect is strongest when adapting and test stimuli are the same colour. Although this effect was questioned by Day and Wade (1979), Mollon *et al.* (1980) emphasized that at a low angular velocity of the conditioning stimulus, colour specificity in the movement aftereffect is present. These authors could demonstrate that colour specificity of the movement aftereffect still existed in their patient, even when no colours were seen because of achromatopsia.

9. The measurement of the *photopic critical flicker fusion frequency* (CFF) is a simple method used to demonstrate the operation of cone function. The photopic CFF values of our patient W. M. did not deviate from those of the investigators. It is predictable that when photopic CFF values are measured with monochromatic flicker sti-

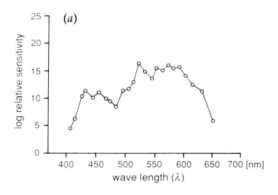

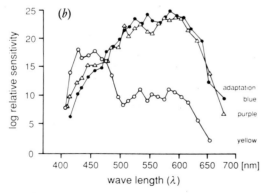

Fig. 20.7 (a) Relative sensitivity ($I/\Delta I$; ordinate, logarithmic scale) in a patient suffering from cortical achromatopsia. Peaks in the blue (440 nm), green (530 nm) and orange (590 nm) appeared. (b) These peaks were more prominent when large-field, chromatic adaptation was applied. From these measurements the normal function of 'peripheral' colour mechanisms is deducible (from Jaeger et al., 1989, redrawn).

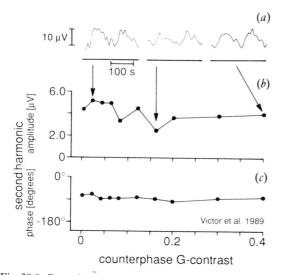

Fig. 20.8 *Data obtained in a patient suffering from cerebral dyschromatopsia. Visual-evoked potentials (a) were measured with alternating isoluminant colour gratings. Recording examples were selected for three different counterface brightness contrast values, as indicated by the arrows. In (b) and (c), the amplitude (b) and phase (c) of the second harmonic of the evoked potential is plotted as a function of the luminance contrast of the colour grating (abscissa). This value does not change essentially and thus indicates the presence of a luminance-invariant colour contrast mechanism in this patient suffering from hemianopia and cerebral dyschromatopsia of the seeing visual hemifield (modified from Victor* et al., *1989).*

muli of equal energy, the CFF should be a function of the wavelength of the flickering light similar to that of normal observers, i.e. CFF should change parallel to the photopic spectral sensitivity curve.

10. When rotated at an adequate speed, the Fechner–Benham disc (Fig. 20.9(a)) induces apparent colour perception in normal subjects. We tested this method on our patient W. M.: whenever normal observers perceived characteristic flicker colours, he reported only differences in brightness.

11. As emphasized by Hering (1864), not only the 'chromatic colours' but also the local shades of grey from black to white are colours in the colour space (cf. Mayer, 1751; Chapter 2). Hering, who named these 'achromatic colours', recognized that achromatic colours determine one axis of the three-dimensional colour space as well as the different levels of saturation of a certain chroma. In light of this, it is not surprising that patients suffering from cortical achromatopsia also exhibit reduced sensitivity across the black–grey–white scale. In experienced observers such as Jonathan I., whom we have already encountered above, these changes are consciously perceived to be alterations in the grey-tone scale (cf. also the patient of Körner *et al.*, 1967). Heywood *et al.*, (1987) also reported a distinct impairment in an achromatic patient in discriminating different shades of grey. We used a black–white multiple sector disc rotating at a speed above CFF: 12 different shades of grey were generated by different light–dark ratios and were easily visible to the normal observer (Fig. 20.9(b)). In addition, a clear brightness

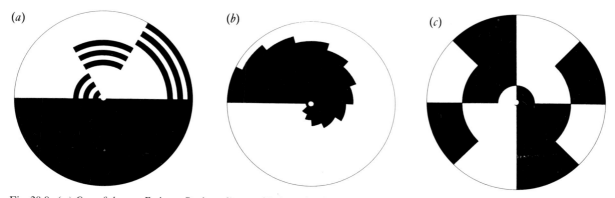

Fig. 20.9 *(a) One of the two Fechner–Benham discs used in investigating patient W. M. When this disc is rotated at a certain speed (3–8 Hz), the normal subject perceives the nine different circles in different colours, which change according to the speed of rotation. In normals, a considerable variability in the optimum rotation speed for seeing Fechner–Benham colours is found. Patient W. M. saw only brightness differences changing with rotation frequency and no colours whatsoever. (b) When this disc is rotated above flicker fusion frequency, 12 different shades of grey are seen and a border contrast enhancement is detectable. Patient W. M. could only discriminate 8 different shades of grey and did not see the border contrast. (c) Rotating the disc below flicker fusion frequency leads to different flicker rates (1:2) for the stimuli produced by the inner and outer ring. Below flicker fusion frequency of both rings, the perceived brightness of the inner and outer rings is different, a fact due to the Brücke–Bartley brightness enhancement effect. The achromatopsic patient W. M. reported changes in brightness along the grey-tone scale corresponding to those observed by the two investigators. His flicker fusion frequency under photopic stimulus conditions also corresponded to that of the investigators.*

enhancement along the contrast borders became visible to normal observers (Mach's simultaneous border contrast; Chapter 1). The 12 levels of grey were far below the limits of normal discrimination on a grey scale. At least 40 levels of grey can be discriminated under such stimulus conditions. Our patient W. M. could see only 8 different shades of grey; he did not see the border contrast at all. A reduced sensitivity to white-light stimuli was frequently reported for the achromatopic visual field (e.g. Eperon, 1884; Wilbrand and Saenger, 1917; Hecaen *et al.*, 1952). To our knowledge, however, no $\Delta I/I$ measurements extending over a wide range of I were performed in achromatopic patients or in different parts of the achromatopic visual field. Mr W. M. exhibited increased $\Delta I/I$ thresholds for vertical gratings of different spatial frequency.

12. A special illusion in the grey tone scale is the Craik–Cornsweet illusion, which is not a retinal phenomenon (Grüsser, 1976). Our patient W. M. did see the Craik–Cornsweet illusion as printed in the book by Schober and Rentschler (1986) and on the corresponding fast-rotating disc. Surprisingly he did not see the illusions of darkening on the crossings of the Hermann grid, while he could perceive the Ehrenstein illusion. In contrast to the Hermann grid illusion, the Craik–Cornsweet illusion develops owing to long-range cortical mechanisms, subserving perception of large-field shades of grey. This mechanism is evidently not correlated with the colour vision mechanisms disturbed in achromatopsia.

13. At sufficient speed, the rotation of a black-and-white multiple-sector disc with different numbers of black-and-white sectors (Fig. 20.9(c)) leads to simultaneous flicker stimulation at different frequencies below CFF. With photopic flicker stimuli, the normal observer perceives brightness enhancement at flicker frequencies between 6 and 12 Hz (Brücke–Bartley effect), a phenomenon caused mainly by retinal mechanisms (Grüsser and Creutzfeldt, 1957; Grüsser and Reidemeister, 1958). Our achromatic patient reported the same brightness enhancement perceived by two normal observers. The photopic CFF and the Brücke–Bartley brightness enhancement indicates that cerebral achromatopic patients use their retinal cones and the cerebral projection of the cone system, since rod vision (scotopic) CFF does not exceed 28 Hz (Schaternikoff, 1902) and no brightness enhancement is perceived by normal subjects or achromats with flicker stimuli when scotopic stimulus conditions are applied (Hess and Nordby, 1986a, b).

14. When a normal observer fixates for one minute on a red square against a green background, and then looks at a white sheet of paper, he sees an afterimage of complementary colours. Achromatic patients do not report any colour in the afterimage; they also have difficulties discriminating between different levels of brightness in afterimages (based on our observations of patient W. M.).

15. Colour flicker is the dynamic change in hue produced by shifting the stimulus along the wavelength axis between two selected wavelengths, λ_1 and λ_2, or by alternating between isoluminant monochromatic stimuli λ_1 and λ_2. In contrast to brightness flicker, colour flicker sensitivity is at a maximum at low stimulus frequencies ($>$ 1.5 Hz, e.g. Jameson *et al.*, 1982; Varner *et al.*, 1984). A variation in the colour flicker can be applied by changing the colour mixture (red and green, for example) as a function of time. At 1-Hz colour flicker, a normal observer can typically see without difficulty the change from red to green or any other selected λ-values. For a red–green colour change at about 0.5–1 Hz, our patient W. M. perceived only changes in brightness.

16. Colour matching and colour naming tests are used to discriminate between achromatopsia and higher-order colour perception disturbances as follows:

(*a*) Matching one colour to the same colour in a set of tokens displayed simultaneously or delayed, is disturbed, as a rule, in patients suffering from cortical achromatopsia. The same is true for naming the different colours of the tokens or a selection of colours named by the investigator. The responses of our patient W. M. fitted into this scheme.

(*b*) The selection of a token from several others, the colour of which is appropriate for an object in a drawing or a black-and-white photograph, may be disturbed in both cortical achromatopsia and higher-order colour deficiencies. Mr W. M. failed in this task.

(*c*) Although naming the typical colour of a drawn object or an object seen in a black-and-white photograph or naming the colour of an object named by the investigator is not disturbed in pure achromatopsia, it is in the presence of higher-order colour deficiencies. Mr W. M. had no difficulty in finding colours for objects mentioned to him and in naming objects for colours mentioned to him by the investigator. He also had no trouble imagining different hues (Hering's '*Gedächtnisfarben*'). This ability may be lost in other patients suffering from cortical achromatopsia.

(*d*) Although the ability to construct a 'colour circle' from a set of pure colour tokens is impaired in achromatopsic patients, it may be preserved in patients suffering from pure colour anomia.

(*e*) Grouping differently coloured tokens into three or more groups with colours 'related to each other' is disturbed in achromatopsia and colour agnosia but not in pure colour anomia.

(*f*) Selecting from colour drawings of objects the one incorrectly coloured or recognizing absurd colours in a drawing (e.g. a red elephant or the Swiss national flag with a green cross on a yellow background) is impaired in achromatopsia, may be impaired in colour agnosia and is frequently preserved in colour anomia and colour aphasia.

Table 20.1 *Schematic overview of the outcome of different tests in cerebral disturbances of colour vision (cerebral achromatopsia, colour agnosia, colour anomia and colour aphasia).*

Tests	Central achromatopsia	Colour agnosia	Colour anomia	Colour aphasia
Visual – visual				
Nagel anomalscope	3	0	0	0
Colour perimetry	3	1	0	0
Stilling or Ishihara plates	2	0	0	0
Photopic achromatic flicker stimuli	0	0	0	0
Isoluminant chromatic flicker	2	1	0	0
Farnsworth–Munsell 100 hue test	3	1	0	0
Colour matching	2	1	0	0
Hue sorting	2	1	0	0
Colour border contrast	3	1	1	0
Fechner–Benham flicker colours	3	2	0	0
Grey scale	1	0	0	0
Craik–Cornsweet illusion	2	0	0	0
Colouring line drawings of objects	2	2	1	1
Pointing to colour tokens for objects seen	2	2	1	0
Recognition of absurd colours of objects	2	3	1	0
Pointing to objects for a colour token	2	2	1	1
Visual – verbal				
Object: naming colour	0/1	2	1	3
Colour: naming object	2	2	1	0
Naming colour of colour tokens	2	2	3	3
Verbal – visual				
Pointing to named colour tokens	2	2	1	3
Pointing to named objects	0	0	0	1
Token test	2	2	2	3
Verbal – verbal				
Naming colours from memory	0	0	1	3
Naming colour for named object	0	1	3	3
Naming object for named colour	0	1	2	3
Naming colours for objects selected from memory	0	0	2	3
Others or spontaneous				
Eidetic colours	0/1	1	1	0
Imaging colours named	0	2	2	2
Imaging colours of named objects	0	1	1	3
Colour of dreams	0/1	2	0	0

0 = no impairment
1 = mild impairment
2 = impaired
3 = function practically lost

17. Several tests have been invented to measure whether or not an impairment of the categorial order of colour perception is present. For example, De Renzi *et al.* (1972a) investigated the association of colour with form by presenting line drawings of objects to the patients and asking them to colour these drawings appropriately. For this task, the patient could select one of thirty different coloured pencils. Especially when using very typical items such as bananas, tomatoes, apples, oranges, certain animals or the national flag, this 'colour pencil test' allows for easy recognition of the impairment. Of course, achromatic patients perform near random on such a test. Interestingly, in non-achromatic patients suffering from left- or right-hemisphere brain lesions, De Renzi *et al.* (1972) found that a left-hemisphere lesion in the presence of aphasia led to a stronger impairment in the ability to perform this test than did any other form of brain damage. This finding was attributed to an impairment of 'object

conceptualization' in aphasics (cf. Sittig, 1921).

18. Spatial colour contrast easily seen by normal observers is not perceived by achromatopic patients. Our patient W. M. was tested, for example, with the red–purple hue of a plate published by Schober and Rentschler (1986). When this colour appears on an orange background, it is seen by normal trichromatic observers as dark purple, on a violet background, red. Mr M. did perceive lightness differences in the simultaneous presentation of the two conditions, but no colour or chroma changes.

19. Binocular stereoscopic vision, as tested with Julesz patterns for example, may be preserved in cerebral achromatopsia, thus offering the chance to investigate the contribution of colour vision to stereopsis. It was originally believed that isoluminant colour contrast was not suitable for stereopsis (Lu and Fender, 1972; Gregory, 1977). Later experimental evidence showed that colour signals can serve as a source of information in binocular stereopsis (e.g. Comerford, 1974; De Weert, 1979; Grinberg and Williams, 1985; Jordan *et al.*, 1990). Cerebral achromatopic patients should also be able to utilize colour signals for binocular depth perception. To our knowledge, no experimental evidence is available so far on this subject.

Table 20.1 summarizes the results of tests of patients suffering from central achromatopsia and provides a schematic overview of the outcome of such tests in colour agnosia, colour anomia and colour aphasia.

Residual Colour Vision in Achromatopsia

Some patients suffering from achromatopsia have reported that before chromaticity of the visual world disappears totally, colours lose their brightness and look pale or washed out. When the full symptoms of achromatopsia have developed, everything appears in different shades of grey to most patients; sometimes, unusual light–dark contrasts and glare are also experienced. Frequently, 'white' looks 'dirty' to the patients. The emotional responses to the loss of colour vision vary considerably in different patients: not all patients become aware of their defect, thinking at first that the colour pattern of their surroundings has changed, or, for example, that people suddenly prefer to dress in black and white or in pale colours.

Although some achromatopsic patients can match colours fairly well, most are rather lost when asked to perform this task. The Farnsworth–Munsell colour sorting test mentioned above nearly always pointed to problems in colour sorting across a relatively wide part of the colour space. As described above in the case of the painter Jonathan I., the sorting of coloured wool strings performed in the Holmgren test produced categories determined by

perceived brightness. In other patients, some of the coloured yarn selections are correct whenever saturated colours are seen.

As Meadows (1974) has pointed out, traditional colour vision tests are not very suitable for differentiating cortical achromatopsia. When a patient who claims not to recognize any colours has to choose colour names in a forced-choice experiment, certain parts of the colour space are sometimes recognized correctly. There is residual colour vision, even when the patient believes that everything is a different shade of grey. In our patient W. M., forced colour guessing suggested a rather well-preserved ability to recognize saturated red and yellow colours; other hues of the colour space were named at random. In contrast to the painter J. I., our patient felt blue to be always darker than red, and, in turn, red always darker than light green. He correctly matched only yellow colours – presumably because of a judgement based on lightness. While he could correctly place an orange token between dark red and yellow in the sequence green–red–yellow, he could not find any place for a blue or a white token between green, red and yellow. Similarly, he correctly placed a light-green token between green and yellow, and realized that orange did not fit between the three colours blue–green–yellow, which he referred to as different shades of grey. He described colour tokens (small squares of the Pfister–Heiss 'Farbpyramidentest') to be different shades of grey, but correctly named red in a forced-choice test; he always called green 'brighter'.

Because little is known about the emotional effects of colour in achromatopsic patients, and measurement of galvanic skin reflexes to brightly coloured stimuli of equal energy has not been performed, to our knowledge, in these patients, such investigations are recommended for further research. We would not be surprised that, as in other cognitive defects caused by cortical lesions, an input to the limbic system also exists for colour vision which uses a different pathway from the one closely associated with the cognitive properties of conscious colour perception.

Symptoms Associated with Achromatopsia

General Visual Field Defects

Although any type of visual field defect may be associated with achromatopsia, upper-quadrant visual field defects are the most typical ones. In several patients, both upper quadrants are affected; in addition, a complete achromatopsia has been observed in both lower quadrants of the visual field (e.g. Lenz, 1921; Kleist, 1923, 1934; Bodamer, 1947; Beyn and Knyazeva, 1962; Cole and Perez-Cruet, 1964; Critchley, 1965; Rondot *et al.*, 1967; Körner *et al.*,

1967; Meadows, 1974; Brazis *et al.*, 1981; Scarpetti *et al.*, 1983; Jaeger *et al.*, 1985; our patient W. M.). Hemianopia of the left or the right visual field can be associated with achromatopsia of the other hemifield, in which form vision and light–dark vision appear to be normal. Finally, there are reports of patients suffering from hemiachromatopsia in which both visual fields were normal when tested with achromatic light stimuli; in very few cases (e.g. the colour-blind painter mentioned above), achromatopsia of the whole visual field was observed without any other visual field impairment.

Prosopagnosia

Prosopagnosia associated with achromatopsia or hemi-achromatopsia of the left visual field has been reported frequently (Heidenhain, 1927; Bodamer, 1947; Duensing, 1952; Hécaen *et al.*, 1952; Pötzl, 1953; Alajuanine *et al.*, 1953; Pallis, 1955; Beyn and Knyazeva, 1962; Cole and Perez-Cruet, 1964; Critchley, 1965; Ruddoch *et al.*, 1967; Körner *et al.*, 1967; Meadows, 1974; Beck *et al.*, 1978; Brazis *et al.*, 1981; Scarpetti *et al.*, 1983; Jaeger *et al.*, 1989; our patient W. M.). This correlation is discussed in detail in Chapter 14.

Topographagnosia

This has also been found frequently in the presence of achromatopsia (Lenz, 1912, 1921; Hecaen *et al.*, 1952; Pallis, 1955; Beyn and Knyazeva, 1962; Cole and Perez-Cruet, 1964; Critchley, 1965; Ruddoch *et al.*, 1967; Körner *et al.*, 1967; Meadows, 1974; our patient W. M.). This association is also discussed in Chapter 21.

Pure Alexia

This may be associated with hemiachromatopsia of the right visual field. This correlation is discussed further in Chapter 18.

Object Agnosia

This has been reported repeatedly in achromatopic patients (e.g. Lissauer, 1890; Siemerling, 1890; Liepmann, 1902; Heidenhain, 1927; Körner *et al.*, 1967; Duensing, 1952; Pallis, 1956). These patients, as a rule, suffered from rather extended occipito-temporal bilateral lesions.

Pure Homonymous Hemiachromatopsia

Considering the location of colour-specific areas in the mesial inferior occipito-temporal cortex, cases of pure homonymous hemiachromatopsia are of special interest. Bjerrum (1881) reported on a patient suffering from a brain abscess in the temporo-basal region who exhibited signs of left homonymous hemiachromatopsia. This patient, however, had normal visual fields for light–dark perception. Careful investigations of sensitivity to light stimuli in the achromatopic half-field frequently reveal a reduction in sensitivity to white light (e.g. Axenfeld, 1915). Samelsohn (1881) described a patient suffering from a left homonymous hemiachromatopsia caused by a stroke occurring in the territory of the posterior cerebral artery who also had normal visual fields for light targets. The medial border of the hemiachromatopic field crossed the fovea centre, as was also observed by Dejerine in a hemiachromatopic patient (1892). In one of their patients, Bender and Kanzer (1939) found an incomplete hemi-achromatopsia to be the only symptom remaining in a 23-year-old woman who had suffered from a subarach-noid haemorrhage. Two patients suffering from pure homonymous achromatopsia in an upper quadrant of the visual field were reported by Kölmel (1988), who was also able to obtain CT and MRI tomography of his patients. The first patient, a 34-year-old radiologist, had a history of migraine. He observed one morning a right homonymous hemianopia accompanied by mild paraesthesia in the right arm and a somewhat unsteady gait. These neurological symptoms disappeared within a few weeks, except for a homonymous hemiachromatopsia of the right visual hemifield, which slowly reduced to a homonymous achro-matopsia of the right upper quadrant. Magnetic resonance tomography revealed a lesion in the left mesial occipito-temporal gyrus (= gyrus fusiformis) extending into the gyrus parahippocampalis. Xenon clearance studies using single photon emission tomography suggested a reduced perfusion in the left occipito-temporal region. This and another similar case reported by Kölmel (achromatopsia of the left upper quadrant) support the old notion that a separate cortical area existing in the infracalcarine region of the mesial occipital cortex is responsible for the colour processing leading to conscious recognition of different hues. It is not surprising that in Kölmel's patient suffering from achromatopsia of one quadrant of the visual field, no impairment was found in colour tests using Ishihara plates; the FM100 test was also nearly normal. In such cases, colour vision has to be explored by tachistoscopic stimuli restricted to the achromatic parts of the visual field, as, for example, Albert *et al.*, have done (1975).

The dynamics and interplay of perception and recognition of light and colour with respect to awareness of a disturbance is illustrated by the pattern of recovery of one of our patients. The initial clinical history of this patient has briefly been reported (Christen *et al.*, 1985): this 60-year-old ambidextrous saleswoman suddenly suffered one day an acute onset of right frontal headaches, ataxia and vertigo. Twenty-four hours later she suddenly became blind for an undetermined period of time (at most 1 hour). Although she could subsequently distinguish movement, everything appeared blurred and dimmer. She was also incapable of finding her way in familiar surroundings and got lost in her own neighbourhood. She had no difficulties recognizing relatives, did not spontaneously complain about colour disturbances and could voluntarily recall visual images. Although there was no indication of alexia, she had difficulties finding the beginning of lines. She had a complete left homonymous hemianopia and a discrete lesion in the territory of the right posterior cerebral artery (found using a CT scan); the lesion reached from the occipital pole to the medial aspect of the occipital horn, sparing the anterior part of the occipito-temporal junction. Four months after the stroke, she underwent extensive tachistoscopic testing with a variety of stimuli; however, her colour vision was not tested.

Her complaints during the first 6 months of illness were centred on an annoying 'dimness of vision', blurred and clouded movements, without any awareness of the left hemianopia or loss of colour sensations. One year after the event, she suddenly realized that the world had once again become coloured. After this experience, she mentioned to us for the first time that colours had been lost earlier. Within a few months she noted that she could detect movement in her left visual field and that the dimness had also disappeared. From the time her vision became brighter, the uneasiness caused by her visual impairment increased enormously. She describes the world as strange, as if seen 'through moving water', has difficulty recognizing objects when they are in motion, and an inability to grasp a whole pattern all at once. There is a wall in her shop full of regularly arranged tobacco pipes. Prior to the event, she could see at a glance if a pipe was missing whenever a customer left the shop. She has not yet recovered this ability and has to check each row to see if all the pipes are still there.

Perimetric testing 18 months after the stroke revealed full visual fields for light detection, but a complete left homonymous hemiachromatopsia of which the patient was not aware.

This case demonstrates that even complete achromatopsia may not be reported spontaneously, and that the subjective experience of losing colour vision can be less dramatic than in the case of the above-mentioned painter J. I. Similarly, our patient W. M. was not emotionally affected by loss of colour vision. Because achromatopsia restricted to parts of the visual field is frequently not noticed by patients, clinicians should perform colour perimetry in any case involving cerebral visual disturbance (e.g. Zihl and Mayer, 1986). Moreover, a dissociated recovery of light- and movement-detection function and that of colour vision is often observed in patients suffering

from occipital brain lesions.

Other cases of homonymous hemiachromatopsia have been described by Treitel (1879), Samelsohn (1881), Verrey (1888), Behr (1909), Poppelreuter (1917), Wilbrand and Saenger (1917), Albert *et al.*, (1975), Damasio *et al.* (1980), Zihl and Mayer (1981), and Henderson (1982). Lenz (1905, 1909) reported that 76 out of 81 patients observed suffered from a homonymous visual field defect for all visual qualities, the other 5 from a selective homonymous achromatopsia without impairment of light–dark vision.

Of special interest are, of course, the few cases described by Steffan (1881), Young *et al.* (1980) and Sacks and Wasserman (1988) in which a complete achromatopsia was observed without any accompanying changes in the visual fields. Uhthoff (1916) reported on a soldier who suffered from bilateral occipital brain lesions. After recovering from cortical blindness, he showed signs of complete achromatopsia, although his light–dark vision was present; adequate testing required rather extended stimuli. One has to assume that patients with complete achromatopsia suffer from bilateral infracalcarine mesial occipital lesions or from a unilateral left lesion of this region and a complete interruption of the fibres reaching the left half of the brain via the splenium corporis callosi. From the pathological data and the CT scan, lesions of the infracalcarine regions of the mesial occipito-temporal region, i.e. of the gyrus lingualis and gyrus fusiformis, lead to retinotopically organized achromatopsias. This localization corresponds to the 'colour centre' in the cerebral cortex of man, as found using positron emission tomography which measured local changes in cerebral blood flow when multi-coloured patterns (as compared with black-and-white displays) were used as stimuli (Lueck *et al.*, 1989).

Colour Agnosia

As illustrated in the preceding sections, central achromatopsia, a disturbance in colour vision caused by a localized cerebral lesion, is strictly related to the visual fields, i.e. the neuronal mechanisms disturbed in achromatopsia still possess a gross retinotopic organization. This condition suggests that achromatopsia appears whenever the homologue to the primate area V4 in the human brain is lesioned (cf. Zeki, 1990; Chapter 5). This region seems to be located in the anterior infero-calcarine region of the gyrus fusiformis of the human brain. CT and MRI scans support this interpretation and form a sound basis for further research on the different types of achromatopsia. Since the 1960s the existence of cerebral achromatopsia has been accepted by most neurologists interested in this field, despite opposing views from leading authorities such as Holmes (1918), Teuber *et al.* (1960) or Critchley (1965) (review: Meadows, 1974). In contrast, colour agnosia is still a debated topic, rather variable in its clinical symptoms and even questioned by competent researchers. For example, Zihl and von Cramon (1986) considered the existence of a colour-specific agnosia to be an open question. This uncertainty is due in part to methodological problems and weaknesses in the research done so far on this issue. It is also related, however, to the paucity of pure colour agnosia not covered over by other visual or language defects. For further research two steps appear necessary:

1. To apply a scheme of cerebral functions involved in colour vision.
2. To design a wiring diagram of cerebral structures responsible for the different operations of normal colour perception.

From such schematic diagrams falsifiable predictions on the effect of cerebral lesions on colour vision can be derived and methodologically stringent tests can be designed which might be useful in confirming or falsifying the concepts invested in such diagrams. A remarkable example of such a procedure is the recent work of Fukuzawa *et al.* (1988).

Figure 20.10 illustrates a preliminary function diagram which we will use to define symptoms on colour agnosia,

colour anomia and colour aphasia as described in the literature. It is not a detailed neuronal circuit diagram, as Fig. 5.9: the connections between the retina (1) and the elementary visual centres of the brain can be divided into two classes: a retinotopic representation with a mixed chromatic and achromatic input (2) and several retinotopic representations with achromatic inputs (3). Regarding colour vision, the mixed input is important. It is finally mapped into the primary visual cortex (2, cf. Chapter 3). From area V1 functionally separate outputs reach different cortical visual centres, where signals for the surface colours (4), the contours and borders of objects (5), texture of object surfaces (6), three-dimensional depth (7), and movement and movement direction (8) are processed. At this level, the signal processing is still characterized by retinotopically organized neuronal circuits; retinotopy may be rather 'loose' owing to a considerable increase in the receptive field size of cortical nerve cells as compared to area V1 neurones. The next step in neuronal data processing 'abstracts' signals on objects or events *in space*, i.e. it has a spatiotopic organization. This can be seen in neurophysiological experiments by the fact that the neuronal responses become invariant on gaze position. Colour signals at that level are integrated to functions like object recognition and symbol recognition (11, 12). For this purpose, contour and texture information is correlated with colour categories (11). Furthermore, colour information is behaviourally grouped into 'colour categories', hues are

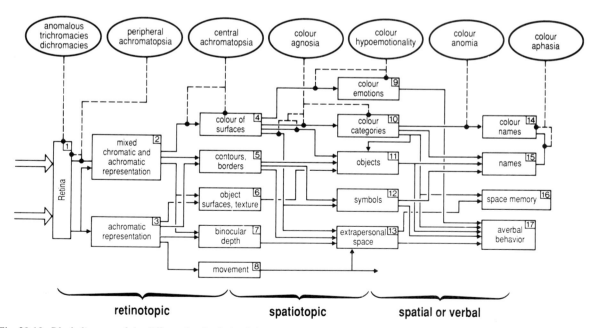

Fig. 20.10 *Block diagram of the different levels of visual data processing involving colour vision and possible sites of lesions producing the different symptoms of colour vision impairments. For further explanation, see text.*

'related' to each other (10), and the emotional aspects of the colours perceived are separated at this level (9). Colour signals also contribute to the perceived depth of extra-personal space (13), but their importance for this function is certainly not dominant. Engerth (1934) reported on a patient who suffered from a left parietal lesion which led to a Gerstmann syndrome, spatial disorders, difficulties in depth perception and a curious neglect for the colour blue.

For the perception of objects and symbols a correlated interaction of colour, texture and contour signals is impor-tant. Any disturbance in this interaction leads to a separ-ation of colour and contour percepts and the behavioural correlation between the two is either loosened or no longer possible at all. For example, a patient of Gelb (1918, 1921) reported that he perceived the colours as separating from the object surfaces and being transformed into indepen-dent transparent colour layers of a certain thickness (cf. Goldstein, 1927). This loosening between contour and colour signals is sometimes described by the patient as 'colour spread' (Critchley, 1965). Pötzl (1928) called this phenomenon 'colour irradiation'. For a normal observer this percept is difficult to imagine, but it could be similar to what one perceives in a theatre when coloured spot-lights are moved randomly across achromatic black, white and grey objects on the stage and changed simultaneously in size. The reduced close correlation of colours and object surfaces is only one possible symptom of colour agnosia. A loosening of colour and object is also present when a patient no longer recognizes absurd hues in a drawing (e.g. a red elephant), despite colour discrimination possibly being preserved.

To exemplify this controversial point we will here briefly present a patient who may be as close as possible to what could be called colour agnosia (Schnider, Regard and Landis, 1991, unpublished data). The patient, a 66-year old mechanic, was a heavy hypertensive smoker who had suffered two myocardial infarctions and had received three aorto-coronary bypasses a few years ago. Within a three-day interval he suffered first from a left-sided, then from a right-sided stroke in the territory of the posterior cerebral arteries. On the left side the infarct involved the posterior two-thirds of the parahippocampal gyrus, the whole fusi-form gyrus and the anterior third of the inferior temporal gyrus, and on the right side the inferior temporal gyrus, parts of the anterior parahippocampal gyrus and the anter-ior half of the fusiform gyrus. He appeared thus, as evi-denced by MRI-scan, to have extensive damage to both medial temporal lobes with an involvement of the left occipito-temporal junction as well. The patient was densely amnesic and severely anomic and had a right hom-onymous upper quadranopia. However, he could read and write flawlessly and had no problems in recognizing real or drawn objects as evidenced by correct gesturing of its use or correct matching. With respect to colours he could correctly match colours of different hues and showed a flawless performance on the Farnsworth 16-hue test Moreover, while the naming of virtually every item was severely impaired, the naming of colours was selectively spared. Not only could he name colours but could also select the correct colour when the name was verbally given. If, however, asked to imagine the colour of typical objects, such as 'banana', 'cloudless sky', 'strawberry' etc, he consistently chose the wrong colour name and chose the wrong colour out of an array of colour chips. Moreover, when asked to colour line drawings of objects with colour pencils, he consistently chose the wrong colour and did not appear to be disturbed by pictures of a yellow sky or a brown strawberry. This peculiar difficulty to associate col-ours and objects in the presence of flawless colour match-ing and colour recognition as well as good colour naming and colour selection from colour names disappeared within three months after the stroke.

Colour signals are also processed independently of con-tours, shapes, objects and spatial position. This is easily illustrated by the fact that we can judge whether two objects of a different shape and size presented simultan-eously or successively at two different places in the extra-personal space have the same hue or a surface colour belonging to the same general class (e.g. 'red', 'green', etc.). Hereby, verbal factors (14) do not necessarily play an important role, since one can also group colour categories behaviourally without using colour names (10).

As mentioned below, colour categorization seems to be impaired in colour agnosia, whereby the abstract space of colour categories shrinks and becomes more closely related to surface colours of concrete objects. Only those who believe that naming is a necessary condition for such a categorization attribute this defect to colour anomia.

The emotional aspects of colours are also represented independently of the retinotopic and spatiotopic coordi-nates (9). Our scheme predicts a loss of emotional quality when the input to neuronal operations, presumably located within the limbic system of the right hemisphere and dealing with colours at a non-verbal level, is inter-rupted.

Finally there exists a level of colour representation totally devoid of any retinotopic or spatiotopic properties, but related to extra-personal space. Colours may appear in 'landmarks' included in topographic memory (16) when-ever a specific chromatic property of a landmark is pre-sent: 'the tree with the blue blossoms', 'the balcony with the golden roof'. Retinotopic or spatiotopic relations are also lost when colour categories are represented by colour names (14), as objects are designated by proper names (15). Destruction of the input from the system represent-ing colour categories into that representing colour names leads to colour anomia. The patient has lost the correlation between apperception of colours (10) and their names. He can no longer tell the name of a colour seen, but he still associates colour names with object names ('What colour is a banana?' 'Tell me an object which is red'). When the neuronal circuitries necessary for colour naming are destroyed, the 'mental' correlation between object names and colour names is no longer possible and colour aphasia appears. The same is true when presumed connections between the neuronal functions of colour naming and object naming are interrupted (14/15). Verbal associations of colours and objects are then no longer possible, but behavioural colour categories are not necessarily affected. Of course, combining colour names metaphorically with objects or as a kind of proper name ('rire jaune', 'yellow submarine') is also no longer possible in colour aphasia, as is the case for the conventional association of object names and colour names (tomato–red, grass–green, sky–blue).

By means of Fig. 20.10 different symptoms of colour agnosia reported in the literature can be classified but not yet explained. Since some authors do not separate colour agnosia from colour anomia, the symptoms categorized in our scheme as belonging to colour agnosia are frequently reported in the literature under the heading 'colour anomia'. Furthermore, with regard to Fig. 20.10, it should be emphasized that this scheme does not represent a network of neuronal connections. As we know from recent neurophysiological studies, the visual brain centres beyond the retina are characterized by strong backward projections, which are at least as strong as the afferent signal flow from the retina to the primary visual centres and from there to the higher-order visual cortices (Chapters 4–7). Thus functions displayed and numbered in Fig. 20.10 may be the result of 'crosstalk' between different cortical visual areas including efferent signals fed back from higher visual centres to area V1.

Kleist (1934), who attributed hemiachromatopsia or complete cerebral achromatopsia to a partial lesion of area striata or the visual radiation and not to an impairment of cortical functions beyond the primary visual cortex, accepted the symptom of visual agnosia as being caused by lesions of the lower parietal (gyrus angularis) or parieto-occipital cortex outer surface of the left hemisphere and three, not necessarily associated, symptoms as belonging to colour agnosia: separation of object surfaces and surface colours as mentioned above, loss of general colour categories and impairment of colour imagination. He considered this amnesia for colours as a symptom due to changes in colour categories. Kleist wrote:

A patient who has lost the general concept of colours behaves to colour stimuli as a normal subject behaves to certain odours. We can discriminate a large number of odours, but we do not have general concepts for related types of smells and no names . . . .

We have summarized in Table 20.1 the main symptoms of colour agnosics and the experimental findings when certain tests were applied. Pure colour agnosia should not be affected by any disturbance in elementary colour sensation and colour perception: the different types of colour mixture equations (the most common one is the Raleigh equation used in the Nagel anomaloscope) should be within normal limits. Colour-agnosic patients should recognize the Ishihara pseudoisochromatic plates correctly and their error score in the Farnsworth Munsell 100-hue test should be within or not far beyond the normal limits. Also, no defects in visual colour fields as explored with perimetry should be present. The patients are not able to associate colours correctly with objects; they do not reject absurd object colouring (a 'green elephant', a 'yellow poodle') or symbols (the Union Jack with green stripes on a red background). They cannot group colours into appropriate categories and therefore may produce errors when asked to name the colours of tokens or objects presented to them. Lissauer (1890) characterized the impairment as either verbal or averbal:

The ability to discriminate and to perceive colours is preserved. Errors occur only when the patients are asked to associate certain colour impressions with words or other complex conceptual mental images.

Patients suffering from colour agnosia can name by memory the colours of objects told to them and they also can select appropriate object names for colours said to them. They may, however, display difficulties perceiving stable relations between objects seen and the surface colours of those objects.

With regard to the localization of colour agnosia, either a disconnection of the left-sided 'cognitive colour centre' located in the parieto-temporal region of the gyrus angularis has occurred or part of the gyrus angularis region itself has been destroyed. Colour agnosia should also appear when area V4 on the left side and splenial connections from the right side are destroyed. Under these conditions colour agnosia is associated with hemiachromatopsia of the right visual field. With corresponding lesions in the right half of the brain we postulate the appearance of colour hypoemotionality.

The symptoms most frequently associated with colour agnosia are pure alexia, alexia with agraphia, acalculia and components of the Gerstmann syndrome. Duensing (1952) described a 47-year-old male patient, who recovered from cortical blindness following a second cerebral vascular insult and showed symptoms of 'partial visual object agnosia', prosopagnosia, homonymous bilateral restrictions of the visual fields, topographic disorientation and also colour agnosia. The patient had some difficulty recognizing numbers and letters on the pseudoisochromatic plates of Stilling and could only sort coloured yarns according to the main colour categories. He had serious problems in finding the appropriate objects for colour tokens. He also suffered from a reduced memory for colours and his colour imagination was impaired.

Colour agnosia seems to be a rare event, but when associated with hemiachromatopsia or hemianopia restricted to one half of the visual field it cannot be explained by disturbances in retinotopic colour processing mechanisms. Of course, a complete achromatopsia or hemianopia associated with hemiachromatopsia of the other half of the visual field leads necessarily to functional colour agnosia as well as colour anomia (cf. p. 392). The symptoms mentioned for colour agnosia have been described in the literature repeatedly, but in hardly any case was the investigation advanced to the level where, on the basis of the results, a clear separation of the different tasks was possible, as required by the scheme of Fig. 20.10 (Wilbrand, 1884, 1892; Lissauer, 1890; Levandowsky, 1908; Sittig, 1921; Gelb, 1921; Gelb and Goldstein, 1925; Goldstein,1927; Pötzl, 1928; Stengel, 1948; Hécaen and Angelergues, 1963; Kinsbourne and Warrington, 1964; Gloning *et al.*, 1968; Bauer and Rubens, 1985).

Colour Anomia and Colour Aphasia

The core symptom of colour anomia, i.e. Wilbrand's 'amnesic colour blindness', is the inability to 'match seen colours by their spoken names' (Geschwind and Fusillo, 1966). The naming inability affects the colours of items seen, like colour tokens, the colours of object surfaces, the different components of spectral colours as seen in the rainbow or in another light spectrum. The association of a colour name to the name of an object, however, is preserved in both directions (Table 20.1). Colour anomia is frequently associated with reading disturbances (pure alexia or alexia with agraphia), mild amnesic aphasia and left–right orientation difficulties in the extra-personal or personal space. Colour anomia can be separated from amnesic aphasia, provided that object naming is much better preserved than colour naming. Frequently colour anomia is associated with some of the symptoms of colour agnosia. It is then difficult to separate the two complexes. As a rule patients with colour anomia make more errors when naming the colours of tokens or objects, while they may be less impaired when asked to point to a named colour. When the purely verbal task, i.e. giving a name to the colour of an object mentioned or naming an object for a mentioned colour, is impaired, the term colour aphasia is correct. Oxbury *et al.*, (1969), however, included this symptom in colour anomia and, henceforth, divided colour anomia into two varieties.

While investigating patients suffering from common aphasia, the naming of colours and comprehension of colour names has struck clinicians as being often dissociated from the naming and understanding names of items belonging to other categories (e.g. Goodglass *et al.*, 1966; Yamadori and Albert, 1973). Goodglass *et al.* (1966) investigated this observation formally in two separate experiments. In the first study 24 aphasic patients with an excellent comprehension of the names of 128 pictures of 16 classes (i.e. body parts, letters, colours, household items, animals, occupations, vehicles, tools, famous faces, birds, musical instruments, cartoon characters, insects, fish, plants and landmarks) were asked to name these items seen on photographs. Goodglass *et al.* found a deviantly high or low naming score to occur only in the classes body parts, colours and letters. In the second experiment the naming and recognition performance of 117 unselected aphasic patients with the pictures belonging to the classes objects, colours, letters, numbers, activities and body parts were analysed. Of particular interest were those patients who, inversely to the usual pattern in aphasia, could understand item names but not correctly recognize the items. Again, the most deviant classes were letters, colours and body parts. The functional dissociation in naming these classes in aphasia suggests differences in the perceptory access to the semantic representation, which for colours is exclusively visual.

In the following we will illustrate colour anomia by describing a case observed by one of the authors (O. J. Grüsser and H. Schöll, unpublished, 1954): This 54-year-old lady, who suffered from ischaemic insults in the region of the left gyrus angularis and gyrus circumflexus, also showed some symptoms characteristic of colour agnosia, as described above. She exhibited signs of a mild alexia for words, more pronounced when the printed letters were in 'Latin' print than in the old-fashioned German 'Gothic' print. The alexia was also more obvious when sentences or words were handwritten in Latin than in the old 'Sütterlin' script which the patient had learned first in school and used in everyday writing. Some paragraphias and mild object anomia were present. Difficulties with the abstract interpretation of numbers and a corresponding impairment in simple algebraic operations were observed; verbal paraphasias, some problems in understanding verbal abstract words and a Gerstmann syndrome completed the list of symptoms in our patient.

With regards to colour naming, her performance was rather poor when naming of the tokens of the Pfister–Heiss 'colour pyramid test' or of wool strings was required. However, when asked, she put the different hues of the test tokens in the correct order and could discriminate between minor differences in hue. Naming the colours of flowers shown to her was somewhat better than that of colour tokens. When asked to put together 'all red', 'all brown', 'all yellow' and 'all green' tokens from the set of 45 different tokens of the Pfister–Heiss colour pyramid test, she generated categories deviating from those applied by normals. She combined blue tokens and different hues of green into one category, orange, violet and red into a second group, red, brown, dark green and dark violet into a group called 'brown', while the category 'yellow' included different shades of yellow as well as light green. This alteration in her colour categories was a constant phenomenon. She had no trouble in putting the colour tokens into a 'natural' order, however. Her emotional response to colours was present. She could separate the same hues consistently into the classes 'ugly' or 'pleasant' colours. When asked to build 3 'pretty' colour pyramids (15 tokens for every pyramid) from the colour tokens available, all 3 looked rather similar and the same was true when she produced three 'ugly' colour pyramids. There was, however, a distinct difference between the ugly and the pretty colour pyramids, in that saturated colours were preferred for the 'pretty' colour pyramids and unsaturated for the 'ugly'. She also had no difficulty in associating colours correctly to objects named for her (oral or written). Here she selected hues very carefully which were fitting for the objects. For example, when asked to select a colour token for the sun, she took a light yellow and a light orange, pointing out that the latter is the colour of the sun in the evening. Similarly, when asked to select colours looking like the sky, she selected light blues and light yellows. Brown and a dark purple were chosen as a colour 'like blood'. She did not pick the more abstract token 'red' for blood. This selection corresponded precisely to her own experience of the colour of blood, as someone living and working in a farming area where certain sausages ('*Blutwürste*') were produced at home. Like the patient of Gelb and Goldstein (1921), her handling of colour categories had shifted from an abstract level to a more 'concrete' object-related categorization.

This patient did not show any sign of visual object agnosia. When difficulties arose in naming concrete objects, she could immediately explain with pantomime or using other words how such an object can be used.

The symptoms of this patient with respect to her colour anomia, her 'new' and less differentiated classification of colours and her more realistic selection of hues related to certain objects resembled those of a patient described by Gelb and Goldstein (1925). Since she was able to name the colour of characteristic objects mentioned to her (banana = yellow, blood = red, etc.), she had no signs of colour aphasia. When asked to select appropriate colours for an object, she always chose 'realistic' hues (blood = dark brown, dark purple) and not colours traditionally used for these objects. This behaviour corresponded to a reduction in abstract handling of the concept of colours, which was also observed by Gelb and Goldstein (1925) in the patient, who showed signs of difficulties in naming colours. One can, of course, take the transformation of the more

abstract, symbolic, object–colour relation into a more concrete colour–object association as a sign that a verbal factor is impaired. With this interpretation the less abstract, colour–object correlations become part of colour anomia and not of colour agnosia. Since no empirical data are available, to our knowledge, to settle this question, the separation of the symptoms into pure colour agnosia and those of colour anomia remains open for further investigations.

Geschwind and Fusillo (1964, 1966) observed a patient with pure alexia, right homonymous hemianopia and colour anomia who also had spatial orientation problems. He could not identify the colours of sheets of paper or object surfaces, but could name the colours of unusual objects mentioned to him. He could not point to the appropriate sheet of paper when the colour was spoken out loud. When the colour of an object was named and he was asked 'is this red?', his answers were haphazard. When told the correct colour of the object, he did not correct his response but said: 'It may look red to you, Doctor, but it looks grey to me'. His ability to match colour tokens to each other and to the colours of objects seen was nearly normal as was his recognition with the pseudoisochromatic Ishihara plates. The sorting of colours was all right, with the exception of some red–green confusion.

The postmortem examination of this patient's brain showed extended lesions in the left hemisphere from the thalamus to the visual cortex, which was completely destroyed. Geschwind and Fusillo (1964, 1966) explained the colour naming difficulties of this patient by a disconnection between the colour centres of the right-hemisphere and the left-hemisphere speech regions due to an infarction of the splenium of the corpus callosum.

As mentioned, colour anomia may be associated with signs of colour agnosia. Bleuler (1893) described a patient suffering from extended left-sided lesions of the insula, the parieto-temporal cortex and the frontal white matter who exhibited a right hemiplegia, right homonymous hemianopia, alexia, amnesic aphasia and also Wilbrand's amnesic colour blindness. This patient no longer understood the words to describe colours. Moreover, he also failed to recognize absurd coloration in drawings of objects or persons that he could name without difficulty. We think that the inability to detect wrong surface colours is one of the symptoms of colour agnosia frequently associated with colour anomia.

The patient of Lhermitte and Beauvois (1973), suffering from 'optic aphasia', pure alexia, topographagnosia, some memory problems and colour anomia also showed signs of colour agnosia: he made errors in colouring sketches with coloured pencils and had difficulty detecting absurd colours of objects or selecting the correctly coloured object in a multiple-choice test. Association of colour names to names of objects, however, was not impaired.

The disconnection hypothesis for colour anomia of Geschwind and Fusillo (1964, 1966) is supported by findings in a patient reported by Zihl and von Cramon (1980). This patient had a lesion of the right occipital lobe including the splenium of the corpus callosum and suffered from a left homonymous achromatopsia of the upper quadrant in addition to a colour anomia for the complete left hemifield beyond 2 degrees eccentricity. The colour anomia was explained as a disconnection of the colour centres in the right hemisphere from the language areas of the left hemisphere. Evidently no such disconnection existed for the signals representing visual objects in the left visual hemifield.

Patients suffering from colour aphasia exhibit all signs of pure colour anomia and, as pure colour anomics, perform correctly in elementary perceptual tasks for colour vision, as mentioned above. In addition to the defects in colour naming, they are not able to associate the correct colour name by memory to objects named to them or presented to them in black-and-white photographs. These colour aphasic patients also have difficulties in colouring drawings of objects correctly, but may still be able to recognize absurd coloration of objects ('red elephants' etc.). Kinsbourne and Warrington (1984) reported on such a patient, but included this defect in 'colour agnosia'. Colour aphasia also appears as a symptom of general amnesic or sensory aphasia, of course, and, not infrequently, general aphasics also have problems in handling colour categories. In all four groups of aphasic patients (global, sensory, motor or amnesic aphasics) Poeck and Stachowiak (1975) found about the same impairments in naming the colours of tokens. Colour naming errors were correlated in this group of patients with errors in object naming. In patients suffering from right hemisphere lesions, colour naming was always less impaired than in the left-hemisphere lesioned aphasics. In analysing the data it became evident in the study of Poeck and Stachowiak that the basic colour names white, black, red, green, blue and yellow were less impaired than the others (Fig. 20.11).

Neuronal Circuits Involved in Cerebral Colour Deficiencies

From the preceding descriptions of cerebral achromatopsia, colour agnosia, colour anomia and colour aphasia, the reader will have become aware of the uncertainty in evaluating the reports on these disturbances as soon as 'higher-order colour processing' is involved, i.e. mechanisms beyond the retinotopic colour processing disturbed in cortical achromatopsia. The localization of brain

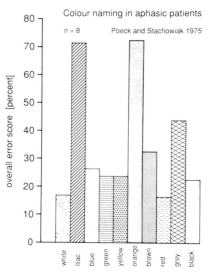

Fig. 20.11 *Distribution of the overall error score (ordinate) as found in eight aphasic patients when required to find the name of 10 different colour tokens. As can be easily seen, the names of the elementary basic colours (black, red, yellow, green, blue, white) lead to fewer errors than lilac, orange, brown and grey (from Poeck and Stachowiak, 1975, redrawn).*

lesions leading to colour agnosia or colour anomia eventually centres around the region of the gyrus angularis and the gyrus circumflexus of the dominant hemisphere. Comparable lesions in the non-dominant hemisphere, in our opinion, should lead to a colour hypoemotionality. On this rather shaky neuropsychological and clinical basis, we have tried to construct in Fig. 20.12 neuronal circuits possibly involved in cerebral colour signal processing.

Nowadays neurophysiologists agree that colour signals are transmitted from the retina to the primary visual cortex via the parvocellular system of the lateral geniculate nucleus, i.e. via medium-sized retinal ganglion cells and LGN nerve cells (latency class II system). Since this system may be more vulnerable to certain intoxications or to local oedema, one could imagine that lesions of the optic tract of the visual radiation affect the parvocellular system fibres more than the larger magnocellular system fibres. Thus a different degree of impairment in the chromatic and achromatic afferent systems is possible and could also lead to mild symptoms of hemiachromatopsia owing to visual radiation lesions, as assumed, for example, by Kleist (1935). Whether nerve cells of area V1 transmitting colour signals into higher-order visual cortices are selectively disturbed, is an open question. These nerve cells are preferably located in regions ('blobs'; Chapter 4) characterized by a high cytochrome oxidase content, indicating a higher

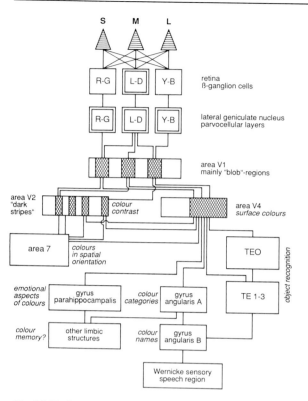

Fig. 20.12 *Scheme of neuronal pathways involved in colour vision. Beyond area V4, the connections are highly hypothetical. For further explanation, see text.*

metabolism than the nerve cells of the 'interblob' regions of area V1. This difference might consist of diverse sensitivities to ischaemia and a dissimilar vulnerability of the chromatic and the achromatic system nerve cells of area V1. To our knowledge, however, no histological evidence for such a selective impairment of the chromatic system distributed across area V1 has been reported so far. Perhaps animal experiments can settle this question. On the other hand, clinical experience indicates that recovery from cortical blindness (Chapter 9) may go through a state in which the patient can discriminate colour but not shapes of objects (Pötzl, 1928; Faust, 1955; Hecaen and Albert, 1978). This recovery state is usually attributed to a recovery dissociation for different cortical visual areas. One cannot exclude, however, that different sensitivities of area V1 nerve cells to ischaemia also contribute to this dissociation.

In most cases cerebral achromatopsia (hemiachromatopsia or bilateral achromatopsia) seems to be caused by the interruption of the input from area V1 and area V2

to area V4 or by a destruction of area V4, located presumably in man in the anterior part of the gyrus fusiformis. In primates, however, neurones of area V2 also process colour signals; consequently the assumption of a total restriction of conscious cerebral colour processing to area V4 seems unjustifiable. To date it is not clear which part of Brodman's cytoarchitectonic area 18 of the human brain (Fig. 2.27) corresponds to area V2 of the primate brain. Therefore the contribution of area V2 in the human brain to colour perception has still to be clarified. Perhaps the colour signals in area V2 are transmitted to those parts of the human brain involved in space perception and topographic memory (Chapter 21), thereby contributing to the perception of depth and structure in the extrapersonal space, including the coloured landmarks for topographic orientation. This hypothesis is included in the scheme of Fig. 20.12.

Our opinion on colour processing beyond the retinotopic areas V2 and V4 is also illustrated in Fig. 20.12. In contrast to other authors (e.g. Geschwind and Fusillo, 1966), but in the tradition of Gelb and Goldstein, we assume the existence of a brain structure, correlating object shape and surface colours, plus another area responsible for the averbal behavioural categorization of colours. Due to the close association of colour anomia and colour agnosia, the assumed 'parieto-temporal colour centre' is located in the region of the gyrus angularis near the regions where colour signals are processed further, resulting in names as labels for colours and colour categories. An interruption in the input to this latter region leads to colour anomia, a destruction to colour aphasia. A relatively selective impairment or selective sparing of naming surface colours or colours of liquids or tokens in aphasic patients also points to the circumstance that colour naming is a function differing, at least partially, from object naming. Colours, like faces, belong to the categories of visual items in the object world which cannot be recognized by touch, as compared with objects in man's daily surroundings.

The averbal association of surface colours to objects is also elaborated most likely in the 'parieto-temporal colour centre' of the right hemisphere and related to the emotional aspects of colour perception, which are developed further in the limbic structures of the right hemisphere. Rudimentary colour matching and even colour naming abilities in right-hemisphere functions tested in split-brain patients support this interpretation (Levy and Trevarthen, 1981).

The frequent association of pure alexia and colour agnosia or colour anomia is not accidental in our opinion. As mentioned above, when reading and writing, man uses an essential function in object recognition, which we have called the *'pars-pro-toto'* function. This function operates beyond a retinotopic representation of the objects and has to interact with a memory storage representing the objects. This seems to be a prerequisite of man's ability to recognize an object seen only in part. For reading, this function is especially trained and interacts for word recognition with a storage of word images. With regards to colour processing, surface colours have to be integrated with the shapes of objects which are also stored in a specialized memory not necessarily related to any verbal function. The association of visual impressions with names (colour names, object names) represents a step beyond these averbal operations, as is the case in the association of a word's graphic signs with the item represented in language. Thus similar brain mechanisms related to association cortices in the left gyrus angularis and circumflexus are involved in colour naming and in reading. In normal subjects both functions depend essentially on visual perception and are related not at all (colours) or only rudimentarily (reading) to kinaesthetic sensations.

Finally, we have to point out that, as mentioned in Chapters 3, 4 and 5, the strong, efferent 'top-down' connections of all cortical regions involved in visual perception and recognition and the interpretation of disconnections between cortical areas must always take into consideration the signal transmission from 'lower' to 'higher' centres and vice versa. Therefore some of the symptoms of colour agnosia and colour anomia may be due to a missing backward activation of area V4 functions. In particular, the changes in colour categorization, as described above are very likely caused by a change in the cognitive control of perceptual input.

21 Getting Lost in the World: Topographical Disorientation and Topographical Agnosia

Introduction: Perception and Orientation in the Extra-personal Space

The space directly perceived by man can be divided into two major parts: the personal space and the extra-personal space. The personal space consists of the space of the self (ego-space); it is perceived by the 'inner senses' and is normally located within the limits of the body space. Ego-space, however, is not identical with body space. One can perceive parts of one's own body just as one perceives objects in the extra-personal space. For example, a person may analyse the shape and structure of one of his fingers much as he would examine an object held in his hand. However, personal space can also be experienced even when no body parts are actually present, such as in cases of 'phantom' limbs or in cases in which one half of the body is perceived as doubled by patients suffering from parietal lobe lesions (Chapter 22). As discussed in Chapter 16, there are illusionary phenomena in which the subject experiences his ego-space in a very ambiguous manner (heautoscopy). In an awake and attentive subject, the subjective localization of the ego normally remains within the limits of the body space; within these limits, however, it is vague and not well defined (Kant, 1796).

The extra-personal space is perceived by the 'outer senses' and may be subdivided phenomenologically into four different compartments: the grasping space (which is further divided into the intraoral, perioral, manual and general grasping spaces), the near-distant action space, the far-distant action space and the visual background (Fig. 21.1; Grüsser, 1973, 1978). The perceived coordinates of the extra-personal space are closely related to the coordinates of the ego-space ('egocentric' coordinate system), or as von Kries (1923) wrote, 'the concept of our own body

participates in all spatial percepts'. The perceived coordinates of the extra-personal space depend not only on visual signals, but also on vestibular, somatosensory and proprioceptive information. For example, when the head of the whole body is inclined, the subjective vertical is tilted. With small head inclinations, the subjective vertical is tilted in the same direction, with larger inclinations opposite to the direction in which the head is inclined (Aubert, 1861; Mulder, 1888; Müller, 1916; Schöne, 1964; Day and Wade, 1969). Similarly, the perceived coordinates 'forward/backward' depend on head in space position and on head on trunk position (Fischer and Kornmüller, 1930). More recent quantitative studies on visual, vestibular, somatosensory and proprioceptive interaction have provided important insight into the brain mechanisms generating the egocentric and allocentric ('spatiocentric') coordinates (Mittelstaedt, 1982, 1989). It is of some interest that with respect to the perception of vertical and horizontal direction, otolith signals do not play the essential role frequently attributed to them in physiology textbooks. When experienced underwater swimmers and divers were immersed in water approximately 6 m deep and were rotated several times blindfolded, errors of up to 180 degrees between subjective and objective verticality were found. The errors still depended on head position, however, and were greatest with the head held downward or backward. Because gravitational signals along the body were minimal in these experiments while otolith signals were not changed (as compared with normal conditions), it seems that the contribution of the latter to the perceived vertical/horizontal coordinates is rather limited (Brown, 1961). In outer space, where neither otolith nor pressure gradient signals across the body are available, the egocentric coordinate system has to rely on visual cues, joint receptors and proprioceptive signals. Severe states of dizziness may be experienced by astronauts during the period of adaptation to weightlessness, which are caused by losing

(a)   (b)

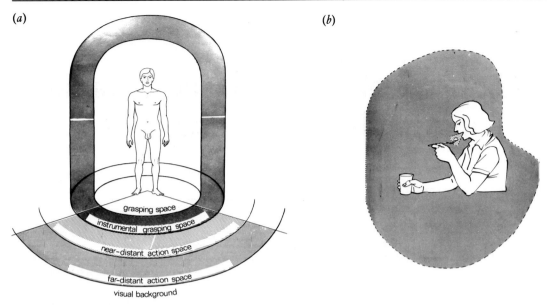

Fig. 21.1 *The three major parts of the extrapersonal space. (a) The outer borders of the near-distant action space are about 6–8 metres away from the subject. The grasping space can be extended by using instruments. (b) The grasping space is subdivided into subcompartments: the general (whole body), manual (dark raster), perioral and intraoral grasping space are illustrated in this figure (Grüsser, 1978, 1983).*

otolith and pressure gradient information, which normally contributes to the multimodal function of space perception.

Under normal conditions, the coordinates of the different compartments of the extra-personal space are aligned with one another. In patients with parietal lobe lesions, this alignment, essential for correct orientation and action in space, may be disturbed. Mislocation concerning up/down or left/right and large errors in estimating distances may develop, leading to micropsia, macropsia, dysmorphopsia or an apparent tilt of the extra-personal space.

Grasping Space

The area immediately surrounding our body is called the 'grasping space' (Fig. 21.1). Objects located in the grasping space have multimodal properties. They are perceived as largely invariant even when the intensity or the modality of the signals from a given object changes. Object properties are directly derived from the sensory signals of the different modalities. A cup of tea on a given subject's desk, for example, is not only invariant with respect to the perceptual modalities and their intensities (seeing, touching with the hand or lips, smelling, etc.), but is also experienced as the same object by the observer, who knows or assumes that it remains in the same place even when it is

temporarily outside his sensory field. In other words, one may turn away from the table and no longer see or touch the cup; nevertheless, one can reach towards the cup. Thus space-related short-term memory plays a fundamental role in the perception of objects located in the extra-personal space.

Observations of the ontogenetic development of object perception in the grasping space led to a physiological subdivision of the grasping space: oral grasping, which plays quite an important role in object recognition during the first six months of life, is guided by visual, olfactory and tactile signals. Later, during the last months of the first year, hands and fingers become more and more specialized, allowing for object recognition by manual grasping; eye–hand coordination also begins to develop at this time. This development continues during the second year of life (Spitz, 1965). Coordinated visual perception as well as manual and oral grasping are used by all primates when eating. It is therefore not surprising that in primates, prefrontal cortical neurones have been found which have both tactile and visual receptive fields related to the hand, finger and mouth regions. Neuronal networks composed of such nerve cells may guide hand–mouth interaction as a special behavioural pattern related to the grasping range (Rizzolatti *et al.*, 1981 a, b).

The manual grasping range can be extended by using instruments. It is important to note that when using instruments for grasping, objects perceived by means of instruments are located in the 'correct' or at least 'visually correct' position in the extra-personal space, and not at the points where the instruments transmit the signals to the mechanoreceptors located in the skin, muscles or tendons (Fig. 21.2). Visual signals largely determine the perception of the object manipulated in the grasping space. Although

an object seen within the grasping space produces a certain expectation with regard to its tactile shape and structure, tactile signals in combination with active hand and finger movement may lead to object recognition through manipulation of an invisible object, i.e. a mental image is derived from the tactile signals. In order to demonstrate this phenomenon, one of the members of our graphics department was blindfolded and asked to handle bimanually an object unknown to him for a period of 20 seconds (Fig. 21.3(a)). The object was then taken away, the blindfold was removed, and he was given 20 seconds to draw it (Fig. 21.3(b)). He was then permitted to see the object for 20 seconds and could make a second drawing of the object during this time period (Fig. 21.3(c)). He was then blindfolded a second time and asked to draw the object once again (Fig. 21.3(d)). It is evident from Fig. 21.3(a–d) that an artist is indeed able to draw a realistic picture of an object that he has not seen but merely explored with his fingers, and that he can draw a previously seen object even when blindfolded. It is important to note that inner ('mental') visualization derived from tactile cues depends on active touching. When an object is passively pressed into the hand of a blindfolded observer, he is not able to perceive its shape (Steinbuch, 1812; Sechenov, 1878; Gibson, 1950). The construction of a mental image and the inner visualization of an object perceived by tactile signals is impaired when subjects grasp the object bimanually with crossed hands. The experiment shown in Fig. 21.4 is a somewhat more complex variant of 'Aristotle's pea': touching a pea with crossed fingers creates the impression of two peas at two different places (Fig. 21.5). Not only can one correctly perceive certain properties of the surface texture of an object through tactile signals, but one can also imagine the visual

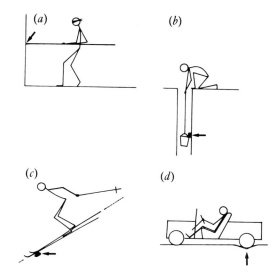

Fig. 21.2 *Cartoon of 'instrumental' experiences in the extrapersonal space. The subject perceives sensory information not at the site of the sensory receptors stimulated under these four conditions: the wall is correctly perceived at the tip of the stick (a), the resistance in elevating the pail out of the pit (b), the stone on the tip of the ski (c) and the pot-hole under the rear wheel of the car (d).*

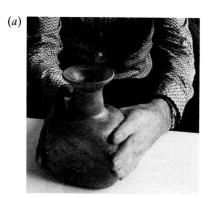
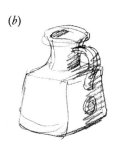
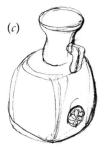
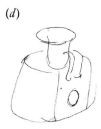

Fig. 21.3 *(a) The blindfolded subject touches an object, a copy of an Etruscan vase, for 20 seconds. (b) Drawing of the object made after blindfolded inspection. (c) Drawing made while seeing the object for 20 seconds. (d) Drawing made while blindfolded for 20 seconds after having touched and seen the object and after having made drawings (b) and (c). Note that the shape of the blindfolded drawing (d) resembles drawing (b) more than drawing (c). (From Grüsser, 1983, modified.)*

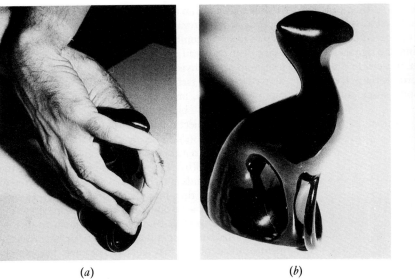
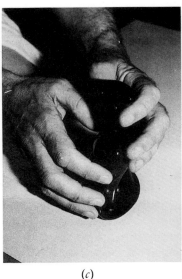

(a)   (b)   (c)

Fig. 21.4 *(a) A subject touches an object, a somewhat abstract sculpture of a cat (b), with crossed hands. Of fifteen blindfolded subjects who performed this task, none could recognize the object within 20 seconds. (c) When touching was allowed using normal hand position, object recognition occurred, as a rule, in less than 5 seconds ('a cat' or 'an elongated animal'; O.-J. Grüsser, unpubl. 1978).*

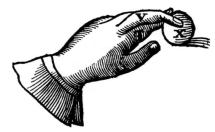

Fig. 21.5 *Illustration of the tactile illusion of 'Aristotle's pea' by Descartes (1664). One perceives two distinct small objects.*

appearance of the texture. There are, however, some remarkable limits on mental imagery derived from tactile information: when blindfolded subjects touch the faces of different persons, for example, they can hardly construct a mental image of the individual face. Face signals are dominantly based on visual cues, as are colours and percepts in the far-distant extra-personal space. In order to understand the pathological mechanisms leading to visual agnosia, it is of some importance to divide visually perceived objects into two categories: purely visual ones, i.e. items that cannot be touched, and items which are also perceivable by somatosensory and/or kinaesthetic neuronal signals.

Our mental images of objects perceived within the grasping space are generated by visual, tactile and motor perceptions: olfactory, gustatory or auditory signals may

be included, depending on the type of object in question and the way in which it is handled. When an object of certain complexity is visually perceived in the extra-personal space, eye movements scan the object surface by means of saccades occurring every 0.18 to approximately 0.6 seconds. Relevant signal uptake is restricted to the fixation periods in between saccades. The direction of the saccades is not random but rather follows certain prominent contours or characteristic components of the object (Yarbus, 1966; see Chapter 12 for an example). This sampling strategy indicates that recognition of complex objects also involves short-term visual memory. Since different, sequentially sampled retinal images have to be combined with each other in order to produce detailed object perception, object recognition requires neuronal mapping of the signals from a retinotopic space to a spatial percept characterized by spatiotopic (egocentric) coordinates.

The relation of near-distant objects to each other determines the perceived Euclidean structure of the grasping space: binocular stereoscopic cues, parallax movement of objects caused by head movements, perspective size changes and partial covering of more distant objects by nearer objects all provide the visual signals necessary for perception of the three-dimensional grasping space. These visual signals are further modified during grasping by tactile, proprioceptive and efference copy signals.

Disturbances related to interaction with the grasping space can occur on the perceptual, conceptual or motor levels. With regard to perception, the most prominent disturbances are observed in connection with visual hemineglect, which is discussed in Chapter 22. With respect to conceptual defects, the different types of constructive apraxia (not discussed in detail in this book), ideational apraxia and some object agnosias are caused by disturbances in signal processing related to the grasping space. Motor control relevant to perception in the grasping space is disturbed in the presence of ideomotor apraxias.

Near-distant Action Space

Beyond the grasping space is the near-distant action space (Fig. 21.1), which may be perceived by visual, auditory, kinaesthetic, vestibular and sometimes olfactory signals. The extent of this space depends on body size and walking speed. Its radius can be estimated by performing a simple experiment: the subject, standing in a large area, is asked to inspect carefully his immediate surroundings. He is then blindfolded (or the lights in the room are turned off) and asked to walk in a certain direction straight ahead. After eight to fifteen steps, he becomes more and more unsure about his position in space. Any sensory stimulus within the grasping range, such as a touched piece of furniture or a short flash of light illuminating part of the room (when the experiment is performed in a completely dark room), immediately improves the spatial behaviour of the subject, allowing him to proceed with renewed confidence. As anyone who has ever walked blindfolded across a large empty area knows, the feeling of uncertainty which indicates the limits of the near-distant action space has nothing to do with the fear of bumping into obstacles. Even when the subject knows that no objects are in the way, uncertainty arises after a few steps. For normal subjects, 'updating' visual cues are necessary in order to guide locomotion within the near-distant action space. The distance before which uncertainty develops when walking or running blindfolded can be extended to 20–50 metres by training 20 to 30 minutes daily for 8 days (Grüsser, unpublished observations, 1974). For the blind, the auditory domain assumes the task of general orientation in the near-distant action space. When acoustic reflection is greatly diminished, as in the case of an open area covered by a heavy snowfall, the blind experience the same uncertainties within the near-distant action space as the blindfolded, normal sighted subject ('snow is the blind man's fog').

Far-distant Space

Beyond a distance of 6–8 m, the near-distant action space gradually becomes the far-distant action space. This is essentially a visually perceived space whose egocentric coordinates also depend on vestibular signals as well as on mechanoreceptor signals produced by the body's pressure gradient. Some auditory cues contribute to the perceived structure of this space, although usually with rather imprecise spatial location. The far-distant visual space is the outer part of the far-distant space.

While the grasping and near-distant action spaces have a phenomenologically Euclidean structure, the far-distant space is perceived as non-Euclidean. In a normal environment, 100 metres horizontal distance seems shorter than 100 metres vertical distance. This non-linear scaling of the extra-personal space is also demonstrated by the 'moon illusion', which was first described by Aristotle (*Meteorologica*, Book 3, Chapter 4), and later correctly interpreted by Alhazen in his *Optics* (Chapter 2) as a subjective, psychological illusion: the moon (or any other object) on the horizon appears much larger than when at the zenith. The illusion disappears when one looks at the moon on the horizon with the head held upside down, e.g. while standing on one's head. The perceived non-Euclidean structure of the far-distant space changes with certain training; for example, the horizontal–vertical inhomogeneities seem to be less for experienced mountaineers, aeroplane pilots or construction workers who regularly work on top of high buildings.

Visual Background

The far-distant space is limited at its outer border by the visual background. As one can see in the sky on a clear night, the visual background appears to be a non-spherical shell surrounding the perceived extra-personal space. The borders between the far-distant action space and the visual background depend on the condition of general visibility and, of course, on the speed of the observer: for example, because visual depth depends on parallactic movement, different mountains apparently forming the planar visual background of a landscape are seen three-dimensionally as soon as the observer moves at high speed (e.g. in a fast aeroplane) along the mountain chain.

Coordinates of the Extra-personal Space and Modes of Visuo-spatial Orientation

Perception of the extra-personal space coordinates depends on visual, vestibular, somatosensory and motor efference copy signals. Visual cues indicating verticality are mainly trees, houses and walls; water planes indicate horizontality. In most cases, floors and ceilings of rooms are also horizontal. When we enter a room with oblique walls and look out of a window, the buildings outside appear to be tilted in the direction opposite to that of the room (For example, the University of Bochum's main lecture hall building has oblique walls and horizontal floors, while the walls and floors are both oblique in the leaning tower of Pisa. The illusion regarding the tilt of other buildings seen from inside these structures appears under both conditions.) Vestibular cues for verticality include otolith signals generated in the sacculus and utriculus receptors of the inner ear. As mentioned above, these signals are not dominant for the outcome of the perceived space coordinates, but are evaluated in conjunction with neck receptor signals (which monitor the head-on-body position) and with signals indicating the pressure gradients in the body (which are measured by mechanoreceptors found in the joints and tendons). In addition, signals from skin mechanoreceptors located in all those body parts touching the ground constitute non-visual cues which may modify the perceived coordinates of the extra-personal space. The elementary egocentric coordinate directions (forward–backward, up–down and left–right) are all modified by these signals. It seems that our 'body image' is continuously integrated into the perception of the extra-personal space coordinates; in turn, the perceived extra-personal space depends on the body-related 'egocentric' coordinates.

Navigation

Vertebrates, which need the ability to navigate in order to move through their environment, have several ways of transforming the egocentric (spatiotopic) coordinate system into an allocentric navigational system, a task necessary for safe locomotion. Goal-directed movement through the environment can be achieved in four different ways:

1. The organism follows a certain gradient perceived in the habitat leading to the goal (luminance gradient, chemical gradients, etc.).

2. As a rule, each living higher organism, like mammals or birds, possesses a learned, highly abstract mental map of its daily environment. When the organism is in motion, its position is continuously adapted to this map, whereby certain landmarks serve as updating or adjusting points. In man, this ability allows for 'topographic familiarity'. When we move through our environment, topographic relations are automatically stored and used to generate a rough map of the space we have 'experienced'. This process usually takes place unconsciously and allows for the remarkable ability of 'home finding': when we want to return to the starting point after a walk through an unknown region, the 'inner map' is correctly read and left and right are now reversed.

3. Goal-directed movement, however, can also be guided by stable orientation markers used for navigation. Astronomical indicators or distant, highly visible landmarks can be used for this purpose. This is illustrated in the case of path finding in many migrating birds. In humans a motor command routine is used to approach a certain goal under such conditions: 'Walk 800 steps towards the sun, then turn 45 degrees right, proceed another 80 steps, then turn 20 degrees left and after another 220 steps you will have reached your goal.'

4. The fourth possibility in goal-directed movement is orientation by means of sequentially perceived prominent local landmarks: 'Walk up to the red house, turn until you see the church tower, then walk towards the church tower. At the church, turn towards the traffic lights, go towards them and from there you will see your goal, the old farmhouse in the large orchard.' One usually uses this type of approach, i.e. finding typical local landmarks (crossings, street names, houses, etc.) on a map, when one walks or drives through a completely unknown region and knows one's own position and the location of the goal (e.g. by looking at a printed map).

In our everyday environment, we usually control our locomotion using the second method, i.e. relying on unconsciously acquired topographic familiarity. It is this topographic familiarity which, when impaired, leads to topographic agnosia, which is discussed below.

The Coordinates of the Extra-personal Space and Prism Adaptation

When a subject places specially designed prisms or mirrors in front of his eyes, visual signals are artificially and systematically reversed or displaced with respect to up–down or right–left. Under these conditions, perceptual adaptation slowly takes place. After several hours or days of wearing such reversing prisms or mirrors, objects in the extra-personal space are again perceived in their correct position, despite the fact that the retinal image is inverted 180 degrees with respect to its normal condition (Erismann and Kohler, 1948; Kohler, 1951). Active movement is required for this adaptation (Held and Hein, 1958; Held and Bossom, 1961; review: Gyr *et al.*, 1979). During the adaptation period, apparent motion in the extra-personal space, which is associated with head and body movements, is observed. When left–right reversing prisms are worn, subjects also experience apparent motion in the extra-personal space, and initially even experience disturbances in left–right orientation related to their own body (Stratton, 1887; O. Bock, personal communication, 1980). When subjects try to grasp an object while still going through the adaptation period, they often report that the left or right arm feels as if it were connected to the contralateral shoulder. This observation indicates that visual perception related to the personal space might overrule proprioceptive signals, since the visual percepts of the personal and extra-personal space are not totally independent of each other.

In the prism experiments mentioned above, one also observed disturbances in visually guided hand–mouth interaction. The same was true for observations made during an acute palsy of the extraocular eye muscles. One of us (O.-J. G.) was the subject of several experiments in which one eye was immobilized by means of a local anaesthetic injected into the orbit (Kornmüller, 1931; Grüsser *et al.*, 1981). Provided that the visual world was *monocularly* observed with the immobilized eye, all voluntarily intended eye movements led to an apparent shift of the visual space in the direction of the intended movements (cf. von Graefe, 1864). During the recovery period, the subject experienced 'tilting and shifting' of the extra-personal space for about 2 hours; this was caused by a palsy of the medial rectus and the inferior oblique muscle of the left eye (the right eye was covered during the experiment). This apparent tilting of the extra-personal space was accompanied by disturbances experienced when walking, which were a result of the fact that visual, vestibular, motor and somatosensory signals were not precisely adapted to each other. Perceptual and motor difficulties were greatly reduced when a wall was present which the subject was allowed to touch with one finger at most every 2 seconds. Coordination between personal and extra-personal grasping space was also affected, as illustrated by the following monocular observation: while eating with a fork, the subject quickly learned to find the plate (which appeared to be shifted). After adaptation of hand movements and visual signals, however, he repeatedly missed his mouth because his hand moved the fork too much towards the left. This coordination error immediately disappeared when the eyes were closed. Impairment of hand–mouth coordination decreased when the subject intentionally compensated for the false hand–mouth coordination; it disappeared entirely only after the eighth trial. This observation indicates that the visual coordinates determining the perception of the extra-personal space and the interaction of the subject with objects in this space can be complemented by non-visual somatosensory signals and by efference copy signals of the motor action related to hand–object or hand–mouth interaction.

Emotional Aspects of the Extra-personal Space

Under certain conditions, the perception of the extra-personal space may lead to conscious or unconscious emotional responses. Standing on top of a high cliff or tower can lead to height vertigo, which may induce fear and vegetative responses. Walking through a narrow gorge or entering an unknown cave might also be accompanied by negative emotions. On the other hand, familiarity with places in one's town and the surrounding countryside, or familiarity with one's own home or garden, is frequently accompanied by positive emotions, especially when the familiarity (*Vertrautheit*) is connected with childhood memories and has developed as a result of space exploration during childhood and/or adolescence. These positive emotional responses are not only related to pleasant memories, but also evidently develop as a result of familiarity with the space, which in turn induces a feeling of safety (*Geborgenheit*).

The size and proportion of the rooms in which we live, furniture, accoutrements, colour and window views all contribute to our feeling of well-being. Some people suffer from claustrophobia in a room whose small size poses no problem for most other people. Others experience agoraphobia when crossing a large, empty place or even when walking along an unknown street. Our feeling of personal safety depends essentially on a familiarity with our surroundings. Fairly large, well-proportioned halls might induce feelings of grandeur and tranquillity, as one might experience when sitting in a Gothic cathedral, for example. Similar feelings may be aroused by a well-designed park. Most readers will remember their fascination with the views that they saw when they first stood on top of a high mountain peak or flew in an aeroplane at high altitude across land or sea for the first time.

Space 'occupied' by man is also a symbol of social or political power or wealth. In our industrialized society, office size is frequently considered to be an indication of social rank. The same was also true in relation to the size of the 'family towers' that were built in some Italian Renaissance cities. In San Gimignano, for example, these towers are still an attraction for visitors. Wars were fought over literally useless desert countries as well as over space which had gained mere symbolic value. Space as a symbol of power is also demonstrated by monumental buildings or other structures built by megalomanic dictators or religious organizations wishing to express their political or social power.

These few examples indicate that perception of extra-personal space is closely related to several emotional components, a fact which has not yet been thoroughly investigated in patients with brain lesions suffering from disturbances in space perception or topographical orientation.

Different Types of Topographical Disorientation

Topographical orientation depends essentially on three sets of signals: the generation of a stable and adequate percept of the extra-personal space, the 'fitting' correlation between space perception and the actions of the organism within the extra-personal space, and the accompanying interaction between the spatial percept and the mental map of that space stored in memory. This mental map of the extra-personal space may be considered to be a special type of visual memory to which non-visual sensory signals and the efference copy signals of an organism's motor acts have access. Topographical disorientation or failure in route finding may have rather different causes, which may be correlated with different cerebral lesion sites. With respect to the extra-personal space outside the grasping range, four classes of serious topographic orientation disorders can be schematically discerned:

Type A: Perceptive Topographagnosia

Spatial neglect subsequent to the formation of right parietal lesions, which is discussed in Chapter 22, is not necessarily associated with topographical disorientation. In many patients suffering from hemineglect, however, topographical difficulties result initially from the perceptual deficit; they are later compensated for behaviourally by means of longer and slower spatial orientation activities. No real topographic disorientation is then present. There are, however, other patients suffering from neglect who clearly suffer chronically from perceptive topographagnosia. This is especially the case when bilateral parietal lobe lesions are present (Balint or Holmes syndrome). In these patients, a mismatch between the stored spatial memory of a certain environment and the 'wrong' or incomplete percept of that habitat leads to topographic disorientation, which, however, is correctable when recognized. In addition, these patients have difficulties creating new spatial maps. Those spatial maps that are created, however, are preserved and, as a consequence, familiarity with the environment is not lost. With regard to the test of spatial mental imagination performed by Bisiach and his co-workers (1979), two subgroups of patients with perceptive topographical disorders were present: those suffering from unilateral neglect with unimpaired spatial mental imagination, and those in whom the mental image also exhibited hemispatial neglect (for details see Chapter 1).

Type B: Apperceptive Topographagnosia

This type of topographic agnosia is caused by lesions in the lateral temporo-parieto-occipital lobe. The clinical symptoms are presumably somewhat different for right-sided and left-sided lesions. These patients lose their way when moving through their environment. Although they are soon aware of this error, they have little success in correcting it, which means that they rarely find their goal without additional help. They have difficulties with eye pursuit movements and/or fixation, and may show signs of unilateral optic ataxia (Chapter 22); in addition, they may

have difficulties perceiving the depth of the three-dimensional extra-personal space correctly. Although the inner representation of spatial maps is not impaired, they have difficulties matching the perceived spatial structure with the inner maps of that structure and therefore easily become puzzled when performing complex spatial tasks in locomotion. They may have difficulties with movement perception (Chapter 19) and when interpreting parallax movement. They orient themselves well with respect to landmarks, but do make detail errors and experience their difficulties in spatial orientation as an inability to combine the different structures located in the extra-personal space in the right order. Patients with left-sided brain lesions fail when travelling through the extra-personal space predominantly because of incorrect 'local' decisions. Patients with right-sided, lateral, temporo-occipito-parietal lesions, however, correctly recognize local details, but fail to put these details together into a larger frame for the perceived extra-personal space. One could call this subtype of type B topographagnosia 'constructive topographic agnosia'.

Type C: Associative Topographagnosia

This type refers to patients suffering from mesial inferior occipito-temporal lesions. They have no neglect, suffer predominantly from right-hemisphere or bilateral lesions, get lost when travelling through their environment and recognize this fact. They develop rather complicated detour strategies (discussed below) and might reach their goals, although with some delay. As a rule, their inner representation of the extra-personal space is maintained for non-visual modalities, they suffer from an inability to match the visual percept with the inner representation. They acquire a feeling of unfamiliarity or 'strangeness' from this mismatch.

Type D: Cognitive–Emotional Topographagnosia, Environmental Agnosia

These patients, like those in type C, have no neglect, get lost regularly when walking through their environment, and become aware of the fact that they are lost but cannot use any landmarks in order to reconstruct a spatial concept. They can also develop verbal compensating strategies, but, despite a maximum of effort, the inner representation of the mental maps is lost and cannot be regained; the same is true for their familiarity with their daily habitat. Type D is caused by lesions in the mesial infero-calcarine occipito-temporal cortex extending into the region of the gyrus parahippocampalis.

The different symptoms of topographical disorientation which are caused by these four conditions are discussed in the following sections.

Six Early Cases of Topographical Disorientation

In 1874, Hughlings Jackson discussed the 'duality' of the cerebral hemispheres and suggested that unique functions might be ascribed to the right hemisphere. He believed that the left hemisphere was responsible for the automatic revival of images, and that the right hemisphere performed volitional revival of images. Jackson stated that 'the posterior lobe – or let us speak more generally – the hinter part of the brain on the right side is the chief seat of the revival of images in the recognition of objects, places, persons, etc.' He also suggested that a defect in this area would so upset the processing of visual information that 'the patient could not preconceive his way'. In support of this hypothesis, he described the case of a 59-year-old woman suffering from a glioma in the right posterior temporal lobe (Jackson, 1876). Her illness began with headaches that lasted about two months; soon thereafter, she suddenly became unable to find her way in familiar surroundings. Jackson wrote,

> *She was going from her own house to Victoria Park, a short distance and over roads that she knows quite well, as she has lived in the same house for thirty years, and has had frequent occasion to go to the park; on this occasion, however, she could not find her way there, and after making several mistakes she had to ask her way, although the park-gates were just in front of her. When she wished to return she was utterly unable to find her way, and had to be taken home by a country relation whom she was showing the park for the first time. When she got home she seemed as usual, but from that point on she began to alter, and during the next three or four weeks she seemed to age rapidly, got weaker and more feeble. Now and then too she would do odd things: she would put sugar in the tea two or three times over, she made mistakes in dressing herself; put her things on wrong side first, and did little things of that kind.*

The patient's condition deteriorated rapidly. She became hemiparetic on the left side and apathic. Although the visual fields could not be tested, an autopsy revealed a large glioma in the posterior part of the inferior right tempero-occipital area (especially in the entire area beneath the posterior horn of the right lateral ventricle) and some smaller extensions near and in the right hippocampus.

Hughlings Jackson, one of the most famous neurologists of his time, considered this case to be very important, writing,

> *There was what I would call 'imperception', a defect as special as aphasia.* [He added:] *I think, as Bastian does, that the posterior lobes are the seat of the most intellectual processes. This is in effect saying that they are the seat of visual ideation, for most of our mental operations are carried on in visual ideas. I think too that the right posterior lobe is the 'leading' side, the left the more automatic.*

This patient's brain had revealed a circumscribed lesion restricted to the right inferior posterior part. The case did not receive much attention from other neurologists, however. As De Renzi has suggested (1982), this can perhaps be explained by the fact that the patient's condition deteriorated rapidly, thus preventing Jackson from writing more than an anecdotal case description. This case presumably characterizes topographic disorientation of unilateral type B.

Another early reported case of severe topographical disorientation received just as little attention: Badal (1888) described a 31-year-old woman who had become comatose subsequent to an onset of eclampsia. Upon recovery, her intelligence appeared to be the same as prior to the illness; although her memory was unchanged, she responded more slowly to sensory stimuli. She suffered, however, from a peculiar and persistent 'visual' disorder affecting her 'sense of space'. Her visual acuity was normal, as was her colour vision. Nevertheless, she was unable to fix her gaze, to direct her attention voluntarily towards a target, to judge distances or the size of visual stimuli, or to locate visual stimuli. When walking, she collided with objects in her way, and could often not even correctly reach for these objects. She had a severe dressing apraxia, a constructional apraxia, a severe alexia with agraphia, all the conditions of a Gerstmann syndrome as well as a lower hemianopia (bilateral inferior quadranopia). This case was probably the first description of what later came to be known as Holmes's syndrome (Holmes, 1918) and Gerstmann's syndrome (Gerstmann, 1924; finger agnosia, left–right problems, acalculia, agraphia) (for review, see: Benton and Meyers, 1956; De Renzi, 1982; cf. Chapter 22). Although no neuropathological evidence about the size and location of the lesion became available in this case, severe biparietal damage must be inferred based on the clinical evidence. For the purposes of this chapter, another aspect of this patient's disability deserves mention: she suffered from a complete loss of topographical orientation. She could not remember the topography of Bordeaux, although she had lived there for 10 years, and could neither remember nor relearn the short way from her apartment to the hospital. As Badal (1888) wrote, '. . . on leaving the hospital, it would be completely impossible for her to tell if she had to turn right or left to go home'. Unlike the case reported on by Jackson (1876), topographical disorientation in Badal's case occurred in connection with a severe spatial perceptual disorientation, and, also unlike Jackson's case, was caused by bilateral cerebral disease. Although Badal beautifully described and disentangled this difficult patient's multiple signs and symptoms and even recognized the spatial nature of the main symptomatology, he was uncertain about the organic nature of the disease, advancing the idea that this patient might have suffered from a 'neuropsychosis'. This may be one of the reasons why the case did not receive the attention from other neurologists that it deserved. This lady suffered from bilateral topographic disorientation of type A.

In 1890, Förster presented the first detailed clinical description of a patient who had lost the ability to find his way in a previously familiar environment. Förster's patient, a 44-year-old postal clerk, had suffered from a sudden onset of right homonymous hemianopia with macular sparing and reduced visual acuity. Although visual acuity subsequently normalized, the right hemianopia persisted. While on a mountain tour 5 years later, he developed within 3 days a new visual disturbance that had been preceded by memory problems. By the third day, visual dysfunction was so severe that the patient had to be guided like a blind man. The first examination 6 weeks later showed that an extremely small central visual field had remained intact in this apparently 'blind' individual. Although the patient could not see colours in the remaining field, there were no signs of visual object agnosia, of aphasia or of alexia; fundus examination was completely normal. He had lost, however, the ability to imagine the relative position of things in space. He was much more disoriented than ordinary blind people usually are. Without guidance, for example, he could not find the ward bathroom located only 2 m away from his room – even after 3 weeks of daily use. When blindfolded and brought towards a familiar piece of furniture and asked to find his way by tactile exploration to another piece of furniture nearby, he was completely lost. He had no idea where to move, and when asked to guess the way, he usually guessed incorrectly. He was not able to create a mental image of his extra-personal space, nor was he able to rely behaviourally on the experience of space that he had had before the brain lesion. In other words, his mental imagination could not recall the topography of his room. This severe topographical disorientation could not be explained solely as a consequence of a restricted visual field, for such a phenomenon had not been observed in other patients with tunnel vision. He oriented himself by randomly moving his eyes in all directions until a familiar object such as a 'dark door' or 'white bedcover' fell within his intact visual field, and then directed himself toward that target. Thus his orientation was guided by directly visible 'local landmarks'.

Not only could he not learn new topographies, but the topographical knowledge that he had acquired during the

time prior to the second vascular infarction was also largely lost. Consequently, he could neither describe the office in which he had worked for 4 years, nor indicate the relative position of the window, tables, etc. The same was true for his own apartment: he knew only that he had to climb upstairs to reach it. He did not know where the door was, or even to which side he had to turn. He was unable to make a sketch of his apartment. Although raised for 9 years in Breslau, he was unable to tell the way from his old school to the central market place, or even whether he had to turn first left or right to get there. He understood the meaning of 'left' and 'right' under normal circumstances, however. He could not remember even the most familiar paths. Although he knew some street names, he did not know whether to take the first, second or third street to the right or left.

As a postal clerk, he had learned the shapes of European countries as appearing on a map of Europe. When asked to draw the outline of Spain, he hesitated, then drew a square, but was unable to indicate the relative positions of the Pyrenees, or the borders with France and Portugal. However, when asked to draw the shape of Italy, he smiled, said 'a boot' and immediately started drawing – not the shape of Italy, but a real boot. He was completely confused when asked to indicate the itinerary from Königsberg to Breslau, but knew the itinerary from Berlin to Vienna, immediately responding, 'This is the well-known Berlin–Breslau, Breslau–Vienna line'. He apparently did not need the inner image of a map; his memory of names was sufficient. When the patient died 5 years later, Sachs (1895) published the autopsy findings, which indicated extended bilateral temporo–occipital infarctions. This case of topographical disorientation is a well-described example of type D bilateral topographagnosia.

Wilbrand (1887, 1892) also studied patients suffering from topographical disorientation. In his authoritative *Handbuch der Neurologie des Augen* written together with Saenger (1917), he summarized topographical disorientation symptoms ('Orientierungsstörungen') with respect to visual field defects. Of particular importance was Wilbrand's famous patient, a 63-year-old, highly educated lady suffering from an incomplete left hemianopia and a right lower quadranopia (described in more detail in Chapter 14). Initially, she had had difficulties recognizing objects, a symptom which subsequently disappeared. Visual acuity and colour vision were normal. Although her visual agnosia normalized, prosopagnosia and a profound topographical disorientation of type C persisted. Wilbrand emphasized two aspects of this case:

1. A loss of visual familiarity in the extra-personal space: all that she saw, including familiar surroundings, was devoid of any feeling of personal, emotional familiarity and appeared therefore somewhat strange to her.

2. She was nevertheless able to visualize and imagine familiar surroundings and to experience a sense of personal, emotional familiarity with these 'inner' mental images: 'With closed eyes, she has no difficulty evoking in her imagination the streets of Hamburg, her home city, but when she finds herself actually in these once familiar streets, she is completely lost topographically'.

An autopsy was later performed which revealed a large, right-sided mesial occipito-temporal lesion, and a smaller, left-sided, more lateral occipital infarction. Wilbrand noted the 'verbal' compensatory strategies that this patient had used to overcome the deficit: she oriented herself using landmark sequences in order to find her way. When Wilbrand told her that she had already found the way from her apartment to that of her friend without any assistance, she replied,

I know that from here, from my apartment, I have to turn left. Then I come to the 'Steindamm', where I only have to take a few steps to reach the house of a friend whom I frequently visited in the past. Once there, I continue straight ahead, because I know I'm on the right track. I continue until ... Oh my goodness, I reach that place with the many buses painted red and white. From there I have no idea what to do and every few steps I have to ask so that I don't get lost. People laugh at me because when I've finished asking one person the way, I right away ask another.

In his monograph on visual agnosia (*Die Seelenblindheit als Herderscheinung*, 1887), Wilbrand described another patient suffering from an acute onset of topographical disorientation (bilateral lesion, topographagnosia type D). This 59-year-old man suffered from an incomplete left-sided hemianopia. He was able to see everything well, and even recognized and knew the names of his surroundings. Nevertheless, he considered them to be somehow changed, strange and different from the way they were prior to the event. He gave up all attempts to reach his neighbours because although he could see the road and different paths, he was unable to select the correct one. The city in which he had lived for 17 years had taken on such a strange appearance that he found himself unable to find his way. It was again this loss of spatial and emotional familiarity with the environment which had impressed Wilbrand.

Dunn (1895) reported a case in which a 'loss of sense of locality' occurred simultaneously with an abrupt onset of a left homonymous hemianopia in a patient who had already suffered from a right homonymous hemianopia. The first stroke had produced a right hemianopia without any signs of topographical disorientation. A second stroke 2 years later produced complete blindness and a left transient hemisyndrome. Eight days later, however, macular vision recovered to the point that his visual acuity had once again become good enough for him to read short words. At this

point it became apparent that the patient had completely lost his orientation in familiar surroundings, a problem which persisted for over 2 years. Although Dunn concluded that bilateral lesions were necessary to produce this syndrome, he drew a distinction between centres of visual images associated with locations and those associated with the visual configuration of persons; moreover, he implied that the destruction of a 'geographical centre' possibly located in the right hemisphere was necessary in order for topographical disorientation to occur.

Clinical Examination of Patients Suffering from Topographical Disorientation

In order to understand loss of topographical or environmental familiarity, we have to keep in mind how we originally learn to get around in our environment. As already mentioned in the introduction, a person brought for the first time to another place knowing that he has to find his way the next time on his own will attempt to store the route information much as he has learned to read maps or to orient himself on a map. He will look for clear and simple verbalizable landmarks, for the number of turns to the right or left and will note crossings and distances. This is not the way we usually become acquainted with the topography of our everyday environment. Having passed the same way several times without paying particular attention, we will decide to take a right turn simply on intuition, even years later ('it looks right,' or 'it must be this turn because it looks familiar'). We will just as easily recognize a familiar room as familiar, or be struck by a feeling of unfamiliarity when things have been moved or the appearance of a room has somehow changed. We apparently learn topographical or environmental information in a non-verbal, 'automatic' fashion, a way we would not even consider to be active learning. In 'environmental agnosia', i.e. type C or D topographagnosia, it is the access to the storage of this spatial information which is no longer possible or the storage of spatial information is completely lost.

Only rarely is it possible in a neuropsychological test to simulate a situation in which a patient's estimation of environmental familiarity can be tested. As with prosopagnosia testing, only a confrontation with a real life situation devoid of easy verbalizable cues would constitute conclusive evidence. While this is to some extent possible for faces, it is usually more difficult for places. Consequently, a number of only partly adequate tests for topographical orientation have been developed. While it is mandatory to use such tests in order to assess topographical disorientation, both careful investigation of the subjective experience of the patient and a thorough and critical evaluation of the reports of relatives or friends about the patient's spatial behaviour in real situations are both equally important.

The following is a small sample of spatial and constructional tests developed and used by neuropsychologists. To assess the spatial abilities of patients, the Corsi block taping test (Milner, 1971) is used to test spatial short-term memory, while maze-learning tests are preferred for testing spatial long-term memory (e.g. Elithorn, 1955; Milner, 1965) The use of different kinds of landmarks is explored in order to test spatial orientation (e.g. Hécaen *et al.*, 1972). The following tests may also be useful: tests designed for map reading, road map tests (e.g. Semmes *et al.*'s map reading test, 1963; Money *et al.*'s road map test, 1965), tests of body part position (e.g. Ratcliff's 'manikin test', 1979), tests of constructional abilities, e.g. copying the complex figure of Rey (Osterriet, 1944), Kohs's block design (Wechsler, 1955) or Benton's three-dimensional block constructions, and tests for memory of spatial locations (Smith and Milner, 1981). It should be noted, however, that most of these tests measure spatial performance within the grasping space (cf. also Critchley, 1953).

An examination of the patient's capacity for inner spatial transformations, such as those tested by presenting unusual views of objects (Warrington and Taylor, 1972) or by measuring the patient's ability to discriminate between rotated and mirror-image figures, is of some value as well. It is equally important to test the patient's ability to visualize topographic memory mentally. This can be done by asking for a verbal description of well-known places or buildings, e.g. asking Milanese patients to describe the Piazza della Duomo in Milan as seen from different viewpoints (Bisiach *et al.*, 1979; cf. Chapter 22).

As a rule, these tests should be adapted to the patient's actual situation. One also has to distinguish between the patient's topographical orientation while learning new routes in the hospital or its immediate surroundings, as opposed to the patient's ability to find his way in surroundings familiar to him prior to the onset of the illness (anterograde/retrograde topographical amnesia). It is of prime importance to monitor how the patient manages to find the correct route. The patient should also be asked which cues he used to orient himself (e.g. the number of steps he had to take, room numbers, verbalizable landmarks, etc.).

The patient should be asked to give a verbal description of routes known to him prior to the onset of the illness (e.g. 'what do you see when leaving the rail road station of your home town?' or 'imagine you drive a car up the main road of your home town – what do you see?'), or to give precise descriptions of how to go from one place in his home town to another, with details about turning points and alterna-

tive routes or about what is seen at the end of a given route. One can also show the patient photographs taken from different or unusual angles of buildings and other places with which he is familiar. His performance should be contrasted with his ability to recognize unfamiliar buildings seen only recently for the first time (Whiteley and Warrington, 1978). The patient should also be asked to draw maps of certain routes with which he is familiar, to draw a plan of his apartment and, of course, to locate the main cities on blank maps of his country (cf. Chapter 22). Finally, we found it helpful to evaluate a patient's impairments by going for a walk with him in the neighbourhood surrounding the hospital. During this walk, we usually ask the patient to perform simple tasks such as guessing distances of objects in the near-distant or far-distant extrapersonal space, estimating the speed of cars passing by, or telling us which of two buildings is further away, etc.

Are Unilateral Occipital Lesions Sufficient Cause for Topographical Agnosia?

Because of the variable brain pathology described in the early cases of topographagnosia mentioned above, the question arose whether right-sided unilateral occipitotemporal brain lesions are sufficient or whether additional bilateral posterior cerebral damage is necessary in order for topographical disorientation (types C, D) or topographical amnesia to occur.

The importance of a right posterior cerebral lesion in type C and D topographagnosia was emphasized in two cases described by Peters (1896) in which topographical disorientation was accompanied by a left homonymous hemianopia. In one of these patients, autopsy data were obtained after death resulting from a second stroke in the territory of the left posterior cerebral artery (this stroke had not worsened his topographical disorientation). Although the autopsy showed bilateral medial occipital infarctions as well as a right thalamic infarction, Peters emphasized that only the first unilateral lesion in the right hemisphere was responsible for topographical disorientation.

Meyer (1900) presented three cases of topographical disorientation in a paper entitled 'Ein- und doppelseitige homonyme Hemianopsie mit Orientierungsstörungen.' The first and also the most extensively studied of Meyer's patients was a 49-year-old man who, after suddenly becoming blind for several hours, completely recovered vision in his right visual field; a left homonymous hemianopia persisted, however, for 1 year. This patient showed no signs of aphasia, alexia or agraphia, and was able to name and draw common objects. He could recognize his wife during her visits to the hospital, but only when she started talking, i.e. he was prosopagnosic. His most profound deficit was his poor topographical orientation. Although his verbal knowledge of town views along a well-known route or of well-known buildings in his native city, Breslau, was fairly good, he was not able to imagine or describe the way leading from one place to another except for the name of the very first street. His orientation within the ward depended entirely upon 'verbalizable' landmarks such as the presence of a man with a beard (his room mate), which helped him to identify his room, or the position of the bedpan, which helped him to identify the head or foot of his bed. When walking through Breslau, he relied heavily on landmarks such as street signs, restaurant signs, and names of well-known shops in order to orient himself. After some time, he had learned to a certain degree to use this information in order to find his way alone in previously well-known surroundings; but even after 2 years he had not recovered his confidence, and in less familiar surroundings frequently lost his way.

Meyer's second patient was a 64-year-old mail office employee who suffered from a right homonymous hemianopia and a mild right-arm paresis; he showed no signs of topographical disorientation, however. Eight years later the patient suddenly became blind. The visual field recovered partially within 5 days: he had tunnel vision of 3 degrees diameter, which allowed the patient to read single letters with probably normal acuity. The most pronounced defect in this patient was a loss of topographical orientation. The fact that he was unable even after many weeks to find his way from his bed to the armchair or table a few feet away – a task blind people usually master without difficulty – may serve as a telling example. Moreover, this patient had completely lost knowledge of the relative positions of cities and states on maps, an ability which he had possessed prior to the incident. Autopsy in this case of type D topographagnosia revealed bilateral occipital softenings.

The third of Meyer's patients, a 26-year-old woman, suffered from a right-sided homonymous hemianopia in conjunction with postpartal fever which probably led to an embolization of the left posterior cerebral artery. Although there was apparently no aphasia, she had a severe verbal memory deficit. The patient easily forgot what she had just said and often repeated herself. The most pronounced deficit, however, was her inability to find her way around her apartment or around the village where she lived.

Touche (1900) published findings on another patient suffering from a loss of topographical orientation from whom autopsy data later became available. This patient was initially cortically blind, but later recovered vision in his right visual field to some extent. Touche emphasized the dissociation of visual memory in this case. Thus this patient could, during the period of complete blindness,

precisely describe the colours and to some extent also the shapes of his personal belongings, but was completely unable to describe topographical relations. While colour memory remained intact and memory of shapes improved enormously, topographical amnesia persisted. An autopsy revealed extensive bilateral posterior damage with an extensive infarction in the territory of the posterior cerebral artery on the left as well as equally extensive damage on the right side, but with an extension into the lateral occipito-temporo-parietal areas.

In 1909, Wendenburg presented another well-documented case of topographical disorientation based on autopsy findings that verified a unilateral lesion in the right hemisphere. His patient, a 41-year-old man, suffered from a gradually increasing inability to find his way in familiar surroundings. A left homonymous hemianopia and an astereognosis of the left hand were the only two other neurological defects from which he suffered. Although a right occipital tumour had been clinically diagnosed, the patient refused an operation. The patient died with signs of increased intercranial pressure. At autopsy, a right occipital endothelioma of the dura mater with a marked compression of the right occipital lobe was found; no other macro-pathological alterations were discovered.

During the first decade of this century, topographical disorientation received extensive attention, especially in German neurological studies. Lenz (1905) reported on 8 patients suffering from topographical difficulties and unilateral homonymous hemianopia which, in 7 of these patients, affected the left visual hemifield. While reviewing topographical disturbances ('*Orientierungsstörungen*') in the presence of homonymous hemianopia, Wilbrand and Saenger (1917) collected 5 reports of topographical disorientation in patients also suffering from bilateral homonymous hemianopia (Anton, 1896; von Monakow, 1900; Benöhr, 1905; Kutzinski, 1910; Redlich and Bonvicini, 1911). In addition to these 5 patients, Wilbrand and Saenger reported on another 3 suffering from bilateral homonymous hemianopia and sparing of a central visual field (Anton, 1899; Lunz, 1897), and referred to 15 other cases of topographic disorientation with similar symptomatology (Freund, 1889; Förster, 1890; Köppen, 1893; Magnus, 1894; Peters, 1896; Laqueur, 1898; Gaupp, 1899; Meyer, 1900; Touche, 1900; Wilbrand and Saenger, 1917, pp. 137–139; for a review of the cases by Larsen and Neukirchen; Grüger; and Reyher, see Wilbrand and Saenger, 1917, pp. 384ff.). In addition, Wilbrand and Saenger mentioned 6 more patients suffering from topographagnosia in which various combinations of bilateral visual field defects were found, where the combination of a complete or partial homonymous hemianopia with incomplete field defects on the other side dominated (Groenouw, 1892; Vorster, 1893; Küstermann, 1897;

Pourtscher, 1900; Wilbrand and Saenger, 1917, p. 123; Endelmann, 1972). In 5 patients suffering from persistent topographical disorientation, right homonymous hemianopia was the only other defect present (Gelpke, 1899; Meyer, 1900; for a review of the cases reported by Hosch, Grüger, and Pauly see Wilbrand and Saenger, 1917, pp. 384 ff.). Only 1 left homonymous heminanopia was found in another 13 cases (Wilbrand, 1887; Müller, 1892; Peters, 1896 (two cases); Lunz, 1897; Uhthoff, 1899; Meyer, 1900; Hartmann, 1902; Preobrashensky, 1902; Wilbrand and Saenger, 1917, p. 69; for a review of the cases reported by Bernheim, Laehr, and Voster see Wilbrand and Saenger, 1917, pp 384 ff).

To summarize, cerebral localization may be based either on purely clinical findings, on clinical findings and neuroimaging measures, or on autopsy reports. With regard to particular vascular lesions in the region of the posterior cerebral arteries, localization based solely on the clinical deficit, in particular on the visual field defects, can be misleading. The optic radiation and the primary visual cortex may remain intact in spite of damage in the visual association cortex leading to profoundly greater visual disturbances. Thus a homonymous visual field defect will be indicative of damage in contralateral visual brain structures; its absence, however, does not exclude such damage. With this point in mind, the localizing clinical evidence outlined in detail in this chapter reveals in the majority of cases a left-sided homonymous visual field defect, in other

cases a bilateral homonymous field defect and in a few cases a right-sided homonymous field defect. Visual field defects were found to be mostly of the hemianopic type, but all kinds of inferior and superior quadrantic defect combinations have been reported (Wilbrand and Saenger, 1917). Thus, from the clinical evidence alone, a lesion in the posterior part of the right hemisphere appears to be especially important, though not always crucial, for the occurrence of topographical disorientation of type C or D.

Further Considerations on Cerebral Localization and Aetiology of Topographagnosia (Types C and D)

As a rule, the most reliable source of information with respect to cerebral localization is thought to be the clinico-pathological correlation established at autopsy. The long delay which may be present between the onset of the syndrome in question and the time at which autopsy is performed suggests caution when inferring that lesion bilaterality is responsible for a certain symptom. This is especially the case when the patient suffers from a vascular vertebro-basilar artery disease as noted in the chapter on prosopagnosia (Chapter 14). For topographical disorien-

Table 21.1 *Pathological findings in autopsy cases of environmental agnosia (from Landis et al., 1986).*

Source	Autopsy findings
Jackson (1876)	R posterior medial temporal glioma
Förster (1890); Sachs (1895)	Bilateral temporo-occipital infarctions
Wilbrand (1892)	Bilateral temporo-occipital infarctions
Meyer (1900)	Bilateral posteromedial infarctions
Peters (1896)	Bilateral medial occipital and R thalamic infarctions
Touche (1900)	Bilateral occipital infarctions (L larger)
Wendenburg (1909)	R occipital compression by endothelioma
Hemphill and Klein (1948)	R occipital ependymoma
McFie *et al.* (1950)	Large R hemispheric infarction (case 1); choroid plexus papilloma compressing right calcarine region (case 2); large R occipital bronchial metastasis and 3 smaller secondary deposits involving both hemispheres (case 4)
Hecaen and de Ajuriaguerra (1954)	Bilateral parieto-occipital astrocytoma
Gloning *et al.* (1956)	R posterior infarction, including lingual and fusiform guri, lower part of cuneus, spenium and thalamus
Ettlinger *et al.* (1957)	Metastatic tumor of R medial temporal and occipital lobes plus R basal ganglionic infarction
Bornstein and Kidron (1959)	R medial temporo-occipital infarction and
Pevszner *et al.* (1962)	L inferoparietal lobule infarction
Cogan (1979)	R medial temporo-occipital infarction (case 1); R hemisphere glioblastoma (cases 6 and 10)
Vighetto *et al.* (1980)	Large R parietotemporal infarction

tation of types C and D with 'loss of topographical familiarity' (environmental agnosia: Landis *et al.*, 1986; Benson, 1989), a rather clear picture can be derived from the autopsy findings, which are summarized in Table 21.1.

Eight patients had bilateral posterior lesions, and another 8 expanding right-sided neoplasms. Four suffered from infarctions limited to the right hemisphere, 1 of which was a large lesion involving widespread areas anteriorly and posteriorly. The other 3 were posterior cerebral artery occlusions with discrete infarctions of the medial temporal and occipital lobes. Taken together, the cases examined by autopsy suggest that patients suffering from a loss of topographical familiarity often have bilateral posterior hemispheric lesions; nevertheless, a unilateral right-sided posterior medial lesion is evidently sufficient to produce the syndrome of type C topographagnosia.

Neuroimaging and Neurosurgical Findings in Patients Suffering from a Loss of Topographical Familiarity

Until recently, the only localizing information besides that obtained from associated clinical deficits or autopsy reports came from intraoperative findings in patients who had lost topographical familiarity subsequent to the development of circumscribed and well-localizable lesions. For example, the patient reported on by Pommé and Janny (1954) became topographically disoriented following the removal of a right, partly intraventricular peritrigonal glioblastoma. This patient got lost in surroundings with which he had become well acquainted shortly before the operation. He could still draw maps of different locations when actually there, although not from memory. In two of Hécaen *et al.*'s patients (1956) who had undergone operations in which epileptogenic tissue was removed from the right parieto-temporal cortex, topographical disorientation was observed. Temporary loss of topographical memory was found only in the patient reported on by Assal (1969) following the evacuation of a right parieto-temporal haematoma; in the patient reported on by Whitty and Newcombe (1973), who had been operated on almost 40 years earlier because of a large abscess in the right occipito-parietal area, topographical orientation remained disturbed, although this patient had learned to a certain degree to compensate for this impairment. These operation findings, though somewhat crude in terms of precise anatomical location, again suggest the posterior part of the right cerebral hemisphere to be a crucial location with respect to topographical disorientation.

A more precise anatomical localization of lesions is allowed for thanks to modern neuroimaging techniques such as CT or especially MRI. The topographagnosic patient reported on by Hécaen *et al.*, (1980) showed a hypodense lesion near the midline in the right occipital lobe; of the 5 patients with topographical disorientation reported on by Aimard *et al.* (1981), 2 underwent computer tomography. In one case, an old infarction in the right parieto-temporal area was found; in the other, a large right occipito-temporal lesion resulting from cerebral cryptococcosis that extended medially as well as laterally was demonstrated.

The clinical features of our own series of 16 patients suffering from a loss of topographical familiarity (Landis *et al.*, 1986), for whom localization of lesions was made possible by CT, is summarized in Table 21.2. The principle symptom in these 16 patients was an inability to recognize familiar environments. There was no general impairment of intellectual abilities or memory, and spatial orientation was usually achieved by using compensatory verbalizable landmark strategies (cf. p. 416). Although every patient had a visual field disturbance, elementary visual processes were not severely disrupted, and most of the patients could see and accurately describe their environments, i.e. with the exception of four patients they showed no signs of spatial hemineglect or space-related object agnosia. Most could correctly describe familiar environments from memory and could even locate important items on maps. Despite intact primary visual abilities, the patients could not recognize environments with which they had long been familiar; they experienced no sense of topographical familiarity.

Every patient had a demonstrable right posterior medial hemispheric lesion; at least 3 had in addition left-sided lesions. The 11 patients in which brain lesions had been caused by vascular occlusions had typical lesions in the territory of the branches of the right posterior cerebral artery, which led to infarction of the medial temporo-occipital brain areas.

These 16 patients also constitute a representative cross-section in terms of the additional symptoms that accompany loss of topographical familiarity. The most common associated deficits were as follows: prosopagnosia (7 cases), impaired non-verbal learning (6 cases), constructional apraxia deficits (5 cases), alterations in perception of brightness modulation, dressing disturbances, left-sided hemineglect (4 cases each), and visual hallucinations and palinopsia (3 cases each).

Habib and Sirigu (1987) reported 4 more cases of pure topographical disorientation in which CT scans were available. All 4 patients had suffered from strokes of variable extent in the territory of the right posterior cerebral artery. All 4 had left visual field defects, 3 had some constructional deficits; 2 had difficulties with face recognition, 1 in the form of a real prosopagnosia, the other in recognizing photographs of persons (without accessories) fami-

Table 21.2 *Clinical features of patients with loss of environmental familiarity (from Landis et al., 1986).*

Case/age (yr)/sex	Visual field defect	Associated clinical features	Radiological findings
1/54/M	L inferior quadrantanopia	Dressing disturbance, constructional disability, L neglect	R medial occipital infarction
2/58/F	L superior quadrantanopia	L extinction with double simultaneous stimulation, dimness of vision, visual hallucinations, prosopagnosia, absent revisualization, palinopsia	R medial parietal infarction
3/61/M	L homonymous hemianopia	Poor nonverbal learning	R temporo-occipital and R lenticular infarctions
4/51/M	L homonymous hemianopia, R superior quandrantanopia	Transient prosopagnosia, central achromatopsia	Bilateral medial occipital infarctions
5/64/M	L homonymous hemianopia (improved to superior quadrantanopia)	L neglect, transient L arm asterixis, dressing disturbance, unconcern about illness, prosopagnosia	R temporo-occipital infarction
6/33/F	L superior quadrantanopia	Visual hallucinations, visual allesthesia, dimness of vision, absent revisualization, poor nonverbal memory	R temporo-occipital and L medial-occipital infarction
7/46/M	L superior quadrantanopia	Dimness of vision, palinopsia, color-matching difficulties	R temporo-occipital infarction
8/50/M	Stimulus extinction in L visual field with double simultaneous stimulation	Transient prosopagnosia, poor nonverbal learning	R parieto-occipital infarction
9/42/M	L homonymous hemianopia	Visual hallucinations, palinopsia, poor nonverbal memory	R parieto-occipital cystic lesion
10/62/M	L superior quadrantanopia	Transient prosopagnosia, central achromatopsia, poor nonverbal memory, central dazzle	R. parieto-occipital infarction
11/60/F	L homonymous hemianopia	Prosopagnosia, poor non-verbal learning	R temporo-occipital infarction
12/75/M	L homonymous hemianopia	Constructional disturbance, L neglect	R posterior glioblastoma
13/46/M	L homonymous hemianopia	Dressing disturbance, constructional disturbance, difficulty with map reading, L neglect	R parieto-temporo-occipital haematoma
14/55/M	L inferior quadrantanopia	Constructional disturbance	R posterior cerebral infarction
15/58/M	L inferior quadrantanopia	Dressing disturbance, constructional disturbance	R medial occipital and L anterior temporal metastases (undifferentiated adenocarcinoma)
16/26/F	L homonymous hemianopia	Mild prosopagnosia	R medial occipito-temporal infarction

liar to him. One patient had a left-sided hemineglect; an inferior left achromatopsia was found in another.

In each patient, the area below the calcarine fissure was damaged to a more or less extensive degree. This area contains the lingual, fusiform and posterior parahippocampal gyri, known to be the crucial structures in cases of prosopagnosia (cf. Chapter 14). Of particular interest was the second case reported on by Habib and Sirigu (1987), probably the smallest circumscribed lesion ever reported in a case of acute loss of topographic familiarity (Fig. 21.6).

As shown in this figure, the lesion is restricted to the anterior part of the lingual and to the posterior part of the parahippocampal gyri. The common area of damage in all four cases appears to be the region of the posterior right parahippocampal gyrus, posterior to the uncus and anterior to the subsplenial region and its underlying white matter. The right pes hippocampi was spared in all four cases.

Recently, a question about the importance of right temporal lobe structures for topographical orientation was

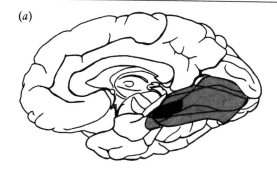

(a)

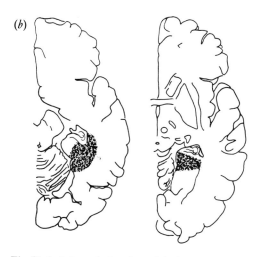

(b)

Fig. 21.6 *Schematic drawings of the lesion found in Patient 2 reported on by Habib and Sirigu (1987), probably the smallest pathologically verified brain lesion to have caused topographagnosia of type C. (a) The lesion is restricted to the right posterior parahippocampal gyrus and to the right anterior lingual gyrus. Outlines of the lesions found in three other patients (grey area) also illustrate that in these cases the right posterior gyrus parahippocampalis was impaired. The lesioned area common to all four patients is drawn in black and corresponds approximately to the lesion of Patient 2. (b) Horizontal sections through the brain of Patient 2. Size of the lesion causing topographagnosia is schematically illustrated (modified from Habib and Sirigu, 1987).*

raised by Beatty *et al.* (1988), who found that topographical memory remained intact in a patient who had undergone a radical right temporal lobectomy in order to remove a large glioblastoma. This finding corroborated our own personal experience with a large number of patients who had been studied after undergoing right amygdala-hippocampectomy for intractable, right tem-

poral lobe seizure disorders. In none of these patients was clinically relevant loss of topographical familiarity observed. This finding suggests that only posterior – and not anterior – 'occipito-limbic' parts of the parahippocampal gyrus and its adjacent structures are of relevance for topographical disorientation of types C and D.

The conclusions about the brain structures involved in topographagnosia (derived from the data on the twenty-four patients who had suffered from loss of topographical familiarity and whose lesions had been confirmed by modern neuroimaging techniques) indicate that the right infero-medial temporo-occipital region, especially the posterior part of the gyrus parahippocampalis, is a crucial area with respect to the symptoms of type C topographagnosia. This conclusion corroborates the autopsy findings mentioned above and is also in accordance with the conclusions advanced by Takahashi *et al.* (1989), who recently described a patient suffering from topographical disorientation and prosopagnosia caused by a right posterior cerebral artery infarction. The cerebral defects were documented by CT scan, MRI scan and positron emission tomography.

Topographical Orientation Disorders and Parietal Lobe Lesions

With the exception of Jackson's early reported case, loss of topographical familiarity, topographical disorientation and topographical amnesia received little attention in early Anglo–American literature. Holmes (1918) and Holmes and Horrax (1919) reported on patients suffering from bilateral parieto–occipital damage accompanied by a profound disorder in space exploration (cf. Chapter 22); these were similar though not identical to the case described by Balint (1909) in which topographical disorientation (type A) was also present. Topographical disorientation in connection with severe disorders of extra-personal space perception represents another type of disorientation impairment, which is discussed in Chapter 22.

Reports presented by Brain (1941), Paterson and Zangwill (1945) and McFie *et al.* (1950) were all part of the revival of behavioural neurological interest in topographical disorientation that took place in the 1940s. Brain (1941) described 8 patients suffering from parietal lobe lesions: in 3 of these, a defect in the visual localization of objects in one visual hemifield was observed. In another 3, subsequent to the occurrence of massive lesions in the right parietal lobe, an inability to follow familiar routes developed; this was caused by the frequently repeated incorrect decision to turn right instead of left, which can be explained by the patient's failure to take into consideration the left half of the external space (cf. Chapter 22). In the last two cases, dressing apraxia was also present. Brain drew attention to the fact that route-finding difficulties as well as difficulties in space perception alone may lead to type A topographic disorientation.

Paterson and Zangwill (1945) extensively studied a patient who had developed topographical disorientation subsequent to receiving a penetrating wound in the right parietal lobe. Elementary visual processes were intact, and he recognized his surroundings as familiar. The authors, who suggested that the syndrome was a specific matching disorder of topographical memory and extra-personal space perception, wrote:

> *In such cases, we are obliged to conclude that despite adequate orientation and perception the patient was unable to bring the perceived material in the proper relation with those experience schemes or memory-dispositions which normally render place-recognition immediate, automatic and correct. This failure, in sharp contrast to the patient's invariably accurate recognition (gnosis) of objects, colours and written symbols, appears to warrant treatment as a specific topographical agnosia.*

In a later paper, McFie *et al.* (1950) reported on 8 cases of patients suffering from profound disturbances in spatial relationship perception; they also had difficulties carrying out constructional tasks under visual control because of right-sided occipito-parietal lesions. Five of these patients also experienced a loss of topographical familiarity, which, according to these authors, should not be considered simply to be a result of unilateral spatial neglect. They emphasized the importance of the right posterior lesion in order to account for topographical agnosia. These cases presumably correspond to either type B or a mixture of type A and B topographical disorientation.

As mentioned above, topographical orientation may be disturbed by the impairment of different mechanisms which are not necessarily related to similar lesions. On the one hand, there appear to be cases of visual disorientation in which an inability to appreciate direction or distance either in one or both visual fields (Holmes, 1918) or in the central field of vision is present, a disturbance which was referred to as '*Ortsblindheit*' by Kleist (1922). Kleist's cases of *Ortsblindheit* would fall into type B topographical disorientation, i.e. the class we have designated as apperceptive topographagnosia. On the other hand, Kleist also reported on cases where spatial perception was relatively intact although specific topographic orientation was disturbed. This disturbance may be interpreted to be a specific topographical agnosia and/or a topographical memory deficit (type C or type D), as in the patient suffering also from prosopagnosia.

Other Cognitive Disabilities Frequently Associated with Topographagnosia

During the last 40 years, a large number of individual cases of topographical disorientation have been published in which either the memory component or the agnosic component has seemed to be relatively more impaired, or in which additional signs and symptoms pointed in either one or the other direction (Pallis, 1955; Macrae and Trolle, 1956; Scotti, 1968; Pomme and Janny, 1954; Gloning *et al.*, 1955; Hécaen *et al.*, 1956; De Renzi and Faglioni, 1962; Hécaen and Angelergues, 1963; Assal, 1969; Whitty and Newcombe, 1973; De Renzi *et al.*, 1977; Whiteley and Warrington, 1978; Vighetto *et al.*, 1980; Hécaen *et al.*, 1980; Fine *et al.*, 1980; for recent reviews see: De Renzi, 1982; Landis *et al.*, 1986; Habib and Sirigu, 1987). Other reports concentrated on describing the association of topographical disorientation with prosopagnosia, central achromatopsia and other visuo-spatial disorders (Hemphill and Klein, 1948; Hécaen and Ajuriaguerra, 1954; Battersby *et al.*, 1956; Ettlinger *et al.*, 1957; Bornstein and Kidron, 1959; Pevzner *et al.*, 1962; Hécaen and Angelergues, 1962; Meadows, 1974; Ross, 1980; Malone *et al.*, 1982).

Of particular interest is the association of loss of environmental topographic orientation with prosopagnosia. Hécaen *et al.* (1952) found 15 such cases of topographical memory disorder in 398 patients suffering from brain damage. Of these 15 patients, 9 suffered from injury to the right hemisphere, 2 to the left; 4 had bilateral damage. In a series of cases published by Hécaen and Angelergues (1963), prosopagnosia was present in 8 of 11 patients suffering from a loss of topographical orientation; the inverse, i.e. topographical disorientation in the presence of prosopagnosia, was recorded in only 8 of 22 prosopagnosic patients, however.

As mentioned above, the symptom of topographical disorientation is not at all homogeneous. It appears in a wide variety of patients having difficulties finding their way, appreciating space and recognizing familiar surroundings, with respect both to the anatomical correlates and to the nature of the underlying functional deficits. Some confusion arose in the literature because the term 'loss of topographical memory' was used not only to designate the patient's inability to recognize the topography of familiar surroundings (which leads to actual topographic disorientation), but also to identify an inability to accurately describe, draw and/or revisualize familiar routes. A comparison of the symptoms described in a patient observed by Pallis (1955) and those of a patient reported on by Macrae and Trolle (1956) suggest that these two abilities may well be dissociable. Although Pallis' patient, who was severely prosopagnosic, lost his way because he was unable to identify places and buildings, he could revisualize in his mind the correct route from one point to another and could also verbally describe this route and trace it on maps. Thus his impairment can be characterized as type C topographical agnosia. Macrae and Trolle's patient, however, could neither describe nor revisualize how to go from one familiar place to another, although he could drive the same way without difficulty, evidently relying on a sequence of local landmarks.

Compensatory Strategies in Topographical Disorientation

Even more striking than compensatory strategies developed by patients with prosopagnosia are those invented by patients suffering from a loss of topographical familiarity. As a consequence, it may be misleading to rely solely on the patients' description of their abilities when asked, for example, to find a certain place, arrive at a certain rendezvous on time, or solve route-finding tests in neuropsychological examinations, in order to determine the presence or absence of environmental familiarity and topographical disorientation.

Few examples have been reported of patients who have to a certain extent recovered from their route-finding difficulties by making increased use of local landmarks, i.e. verbalizable cues such as street names, traffic lights, or the colours and shapes of buildings, etc. (Whitty and Newcombe, 1973; Fine *et al.*, 1980). Probably most clinicians working with patients suffering from topographical disorientation have been struck by the compensatory strategies which may sometimes erroneously be considered to be a sign of complete recovery of a function.

We will try to illustrate this point with some clinical examples. One of Dr D. F. Benson's patients (personal communication) was asked to go to his room just as Dr Benson was preparing to demonstrate topographical disorientation to some visiting neurologists. To the amazement of the visitors, the patient directed his wheel chair fairly quickly along the ward, stopped briskly at the door to the correct room and entered it without hesitation. Having witnessed this obvious demonstration of 'successful' topographical orientation, none of the visiting neurologists could be convinced that this patient had severe topographical disturbances. However, when this patient was later asked how he had achieved this striking performance, he simply responded, 'I know how many doors there are from the end of the hallway to my room, and since all the room doors are open at this time and the room lights can be seen from the hallway, the easiest way to reach my room is to go fast with my wheelchair and

count the lights until I reach the correct number'. It is obvious that this patient used a strategy different from that used by normal subjects in order to orient himself topographically. In a similar manner, we were struck by the remark of a severely topographically disoriented patient who correctly stated that his present location was on a certain floor. When asked how he knew that, he responded, 'Only the first and the fourteenth floor of this hospital have red exit doors.' None of the hospital staff was aware of this – probably because it was not necessary for them to use this information in order to locate themselve topographically.

Patients suffering from topographical disorientation memorize astounding details such as the number of stairs between floors, the number of steps from one location to another, peculiar paintings or inscriptions; as a rule, these details escape the notice of observers who are less dependent on such landmark information in order to orient themselves. It is therefore often more rewarding to ask such patients how they achieve topographical orientation rather than just to look and see if they can orient themselves.

This last point may be illustrated by the case of an unusual patient. This now 73-year-old, right-handed woman (F. H.) has suffered since age 9 from episodes of topographical disorientation lasting from several minutes to one hour. According to family members, although she appeared relatively normal during these periods and could talk, she entered wrong rooms, complained about vertigo, and when left alone, was unable to find her way or sometimes even got lost. The patient described these episodes as follows: 'They start with a funny feeling and suddenly everything looks strange, as if mirror-imaged.' At this stage she could hear other people talk, but had difficulty following the conversation. Sometimes she felt her arms become very long, but, upon measuring them, noticed that their length was, of course, normal, not at all corresponding to the length which she had expected. During these episodes she could not find her way, would enter wrong doors or wrong streets, enter strange houses or even apartments and take streetcars going in the wrong direction. These episodes were usually accompanied by vertigo; subsequent to these episodes, she often also felt nauseated. While initially occurring about twice a month, these episodes soon increased to one a day. At age 40, she underwent for the first time a complete neurological examination including skull X-rays, EEG and pneumoencephalography as well as a lumbar puncture. Neurological examination revealed a mild disturbance of coordination of the left-sided extremities without any other abnormalities (including normal visual fields, which were measured by perimetry). The cerebro-spinal fluid was normal, as was the pneumoencephalogram, but electroencephalographic signs indicating a seizure disorder were present.

Although she had been given a number of anticonvulsants over several years, the frequency of these episodes did not decrease significantly. When she was 58, a complete neurological reevaluation yielded identical results. At age 62, she suffered from an acute onset of severe headaches followed by a progressive left hemiparesis. CT scans, which had in the meantime been developed, revealed an intracerebral right parieto-temporal haematoma. Within one and a half years of observation following this event, the haematoma was completely reabsorbed and she recovered quite well from her hemiparesis. The episodes of topographical disorientation continued, although less frequently. Neuropsychological evaluation before and after the cerebral bleeding indicated the presence of mild figural memory defects and mild constructional disturbances, as well as severe impairment of the body scheme and an inability to learn mazes. In 1981 at the age of 63, she underwent extensive experimental neuropsychological testing in connection with a study of compensation strategies of patients suffering from right posterior cerebral lesions (Christen et al., 1985). Because of the testing, she had to come to our unit several times a week over a period of several weeks. From the description of her episodes, it became apparent that she not only became topographically disoriented, not recognizing the environment, but also did not recognize familiar persons. Having claimed on several occasions to have had one of these episodes while on the way to the unit (which meant that she had to travel for about 40 minutes and change street cars), we wondered how she managed to arrive on time. When specifically asked how she handled this task during such episodes, she initially appeared not to understand what we meant by our questions. Only after the third interview did she finally indicate that her notebook might provide an answer to our queries. This notebook was literally full of hundreds of descriptions of routes covering every possible place the patient had to reach daily. Some of these notes described even the most familiar paths, such as the way leading from the nearby shopping centre to her apartment, as well as others describing the route to her daughter who lived way across the city. One of these descriptions, of course, was how to go to and from our hospital. These notes primarily mentioned landmarks such as tall buildings, names of well-known restaurants or shops, streetcar stations, road names, landmarks such as unusually large window fronts, coloured house walls, and indications such as 'upwards', 'downwards' and 'across the street', as well as the numbers of houses and the numbers or colours of entrances. While usually topographically disorientated patients can readily answer questions about how they deal with their difficulties, we conjecture that the almost lifelong struggle for topographical orientation had rendered the compensatory strategy used by this patient so normal for her that she initially did not even understand the meaning of our questions.

As a final example, we shall describe another simple compensatory strategy used by one of our patients examined in 1987: this 54-year-old owner of a small cheese factory, H. St., suffered from prosopagnosia and topographic disorientation caused by an infarction in the territories of both posterior cerebral arteries. Although he had no difficulties recognizing depth, objects and spatial relations of objects located within the grasping and near–distant action space, he made serious errors in depth perception and distance estimations in the open space of the hospital park and its surroundings. At home he used to go for walks every day after lunch and continued to do so after he had recovered from an acute cerebral incident. He reported that since the cerebral infarction he was no longer able to find his way back to the village or to his home, and as a result regularly got lost on his daily walks in the woods. When asked how he could still take his after-lunch strolls, he smiled and explained his simple surrogate strategy: 'I get lost regularly, but this is no problem. I always take my dog with me and when I want to go home, I just tell my dog "Go home" and the dog guides me along the correct and shortest path.' His relatives reported that Mr St. did not recognize his own home visually, and that he also frequently got lost in his rather large home and in the cheese dairy. They suspected that Mr St. also unconsciously used olfactory signals in order to compensate for his visual topographic disorientation. Although he was not able to recognize his house when sitting in a car with the windows closed, he could recognize it when he had left the car. The patient could not account for this difference.

This report, as well as those of many other patients suffering from type D topographagnosia, indicates that, as a rule, patients are well aware of their defects; anosognosia seems to be rather rare for this type of spatial disorientation, as is the case for prosopagnosia. In addition, the general verbalizable concept of the extra-personal space with its different compartments is not at all affected. Visual orientation is intact in the grasping space, and, in some patients, also in the near–distant action space, i.e. for space compartments within which objects may also be perceived by non-visual cues (cf. p. 415). Since the patients recognize their defect (as in many cases of prosopagnosia), they try to compensate for it by using intelligence and systematic 'detour strategies', which depend on the patient's general intelligence and former learning habits. All these compensatory strategies are possible since these patients possess a general concept of the extra-personal space as a structure. Further investigation is necessary in order to learn more about the different compensatory strategies developed by patients suffering from topographic disorientation.

Neuronal models of topographic disorientation are discussed in chapter 22, where we also present a further discussion of visual neglect and topographic disorientation caused by parietal lobe lesions.

22 Only Half the World: Visual Hemineglect and Related Disorders

Introduction

Hemispatial visual neglect (hemineglect) is an acquired disability. Afflicted individuals can neither respond to nor attend visual stimulus patterns appearing in that part of the extra-personal space contralateral to the side of the brain lesion. In severe cases, hemineglect may also affect the other sense modalities. Visual hemineglect is frequently related to only one side of the attended object, regardless of object location in the extra-personal space. Mild types of visual hemineglect become apparent under competitive stimulation conditions: simultaneous presentation of two visual stimuli located mirror-symmetric to the vertical left–right division of the extra-personal space lead to an 'extinction' of the percept evoked by the stimulus located in the neglected hemispace.

Before we deal with the clinical symptoms and causes of visual hemineglect, we first present some further introductory considerations on space and object perception.

Coordinates, Perceived Constancy and Multimodal Aspects of the Extra-personal Space

The Limited Constancy of Space Perception

Under normal, everyday conditions, man perceives the extra-personal space surrounding him as constant and stable, regardless of his position within this space or of fast (saccadic) or slow (pursuit) gaze movements, which move the image of the extra-personal space across the retina through eye, head or body motion. This extraordinary constancy also holds true even when the head is tilted sidewards, forwards or backwards. Up to a certain limit, the coordinates of the extra-personal space related to the observing subject (the so-called 'egocentric' or 'spatiotopic' coordinates, up–down, left–right or forwards–backwards) are only slightly tilted (Aubert, 1861). When the head is held upside down, as in a headstand, and one simultaneously reads a book held in the normal reading position, what is up and what is down become ambiguous. In other words, the constancy of the perceived coordinates of the extra-personal space has some limits. This is also true for the temporal adjustment of retinal coordinates and egocentric space coordinates. When a subject moves his eyes as fast as possible horizontally to and fro between two targets by means of eye saccades, one perceives an apparent shifting in the extra-personal space ('oscillopsia'; Purkinje, 1825a). The 'recalibration' between retinal ('retinotopic') and egocentric ('spatiotopic') coordinates during and after saccadic eye or gaze movements occurs rather slowly and follows an exponential time function. For large saccades, the time constant is approximately 220 ms (Fig. 22.1; Grüsser et al., 1987). With fast back-and-forth saccades, the recalibration process is not yet finished when the eye movement starts anew. As a result, a doubling of the foveal afterimage occurs when fast, horizontal, back and forth saccades are performed in the dark between two alternating auditory targets (see the caption of Fig. 22.1). Under non-experimental, spontaneous conditions, the fixation period between saccades normally lasts long enough for the spatial recalibration process to be completed, and for object recognition and object localization in spatiotopic coordinates to take place.

We also lose our ability to perceive space constancy when moving above a certain speed through the extra-

(a)

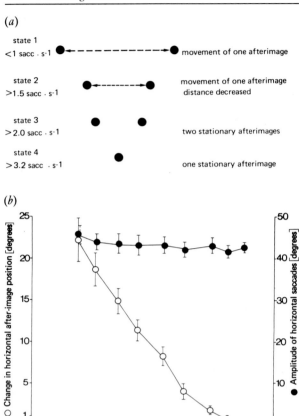

(b)

(c)

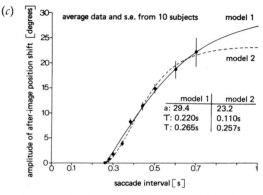

Fig. 22.1 *(a) Illustration of the four stages of afterimage perception during horizontal auditory saccades performed at different rates as indicated. With increasing saccade frequency the perceived distance of horizontal displacement of the foveal afterimages decreases. Above 2 saccades s⁻¹ two stationary afterimages are seen simultaneously, the distance between them decreases with the further increase of saccade frequency. Finally, above 3.2 saccades s⁻¹ one stationary afterimage is seen while the saccadic eye movements are still performed with full amplitude. (b) Relationship between saccade frequency (abscissa), amplitude of horizontal saccades (ordinate, right side, dots) and perceived change in horizontal position of a small foveal afterimage (ordinate, left side, circles). Algebraic mean ± s.e. of data from 10 subjects. Note different scaling of the ordinate for saccade amplitude and afterimage displacement. (c) Change in afterimage position (ordinate) is plotted as a function of saccade interval (abscissa). Model 1 corresponds to a simple exponential function, $f_1(t) = 1 - exp[(T_1 - t)/\tau]$, while for the second model $f_2(t) = [f_1(t)]^2$. (From Grüsser et al., 1987).*

personal space: the parallax movements of the objects located in the extra-personal space, which at a 'natural' speed of locomotion contribute to the percept of spatial depth, gradually transform into perceived visual movement. Our ability to perceive the visual constancy of the extra-personal space is also lost when vestibular stimulation of the semicircular canal receptors occurs above a certain angular acceleration during motion through the extra-personal space. This is especially the case with combined linear and circular acceleration (Coriolis stimulation), which causes severe vertigo. During the state of vertigo, visual space perception and egocentric space coordinates, as well as tactile and motor coordination (with regard to the extra-personal space), are seriously disturbed. In some subjects, a rather small mismatch between visual and vestibular signals is sufficient to cause vertigo. Sensorimotor training during childhood and adolescence affects vertigo thresholds, as the remarkable motor performances of mountaineers, ballet dancers, artistic skaters and acrobats all illustrate.

The perceived coordinates of the extra-personal space

depend not only on vestibular stimuli but also on eye-in-head and head-on-trunk position. The eye-in-head position is partially monitored by efference copy signals derived from gaze motor commands which produce changes in the position of the eye. When normal subjects observe a long-lasting foveal afterimage, shift gaze to the left or right, maintain thereafter gaze position and point towards the afterimage, pointing gain is about 0.6–0.7 when the experiment is performed in total darkness. As soon as background illumination is provided, pointing towards the afterimage (without being able to see the hand) reaches a gain between 0.95 and 1.0 (D. Beier and O.-J. Grüsser, unpublished, 1988), much as when one points to a real spot of light. If the other eye is displaced in the orbit as the subject points towards an afterimage, pointing is not affected. This indicates a rather limited contribution of the extraocular eye muscle mechanoreceptors to the perception of the visual coordinates. Mechanical vibration of one eye seems to have some effect, however, on the perceived position of a target seen with the other eye (Roll and Roll, 1986).

Neck muscle vibration indicates that the contribution of the muscle receptors of the neck muscles to the perception of the egocentric space coordinates is somewhat more effective than that of eye muscle receptors. Lackner and Levine (1979) vibrated the neck muscles in normal human subjects and evoked an illusion of head movement as well as an apparent change in the position of stationary visual targets. Biguer *et al.* (1988) used a small, 0.5-degree red light as a fixation target placed at eye level directly in front of their subjects sitting in an otherwise totally dark room. The subjects were asked to point towards the red spot of light. With unilateral 100-Hz vibration of the left posterior neck muscles by means of a physiotherapy vibrator (estimated vibration amplitude 0.3 mm), the visual target appeared to move towards the right. Although target displacement ceased within 2 to 20 seconds, subjects paradoxically perceived continued target motion without seeing any change in target position. This illusion varied from subject to subject, as did the displacement of pointing, which varied between 0 and approximately 8 degrees. Head movement illusions such as those observed in subjects examined by Lackner and Levine (1979), Lund (1980) and Rossi *et al.* (1985) were not observed in this study. In follow-up experiments, the vibration amplitude was varied between 137 and 431 µm. On average, the apparent shift of the fixation target increased with vibration amplitude; the same was true for the speed of target motion after displacement had ended. These experiments suggest a contribution by the proprioceptive signals in neck muscle receptors to the perception of the egocentric space coordinates.

That the extra-personal space coordinates are perceived independently of our locomotion or gaze movements within that space indicates that a system operates somewhere in the brain that transforms the visual percept from retinotopic to spatiotopic coordinates that are related to our head or body ('ego'), but not to the retinal image. By definition, spatiotopic coordinates are independent of gaze position. The next transformation from spatiotopic to spatial coordinates, the 'allocentric coordinate system', makes the cerebral representation of a certain part of the world (our home, street, city, country, etc.) independent of the actual percept. Our knowledge about the space which we live in is stored mainly in the many more or less coherent mental maps with spatial coordinates. We select one of these mental maps when we evoke a mental image of a certain familiar part of our world, where the imagined position is variable. In pathfinding, for example, the mental map is compared with the perceived space; we decide where to go on the basis of this comparison. We can also find our way, of course, by following the sequence of landmarks stored in the spatiotopic coordinates; this method is rather tedious, however, and frequently space information is not very effective.

Some investigators believed that there was no need for continuous updating between the retinotopic and spatiotopic coordinates during and after gaze movements; instead, they believed that perceptual space constancy is 'assumed' a priori by the central nervous system (MacKay, 1973). We hypothesize, however, that continuous information updating between the retinotopic and spatiotopic coordinates is a *conditio sine qua non* for biologically relevant perception of the extra-personal space. This neuronal operation is also controlled by the vestibular system, which 'sets' the horizontal–vertical coordinates of the extra-personal space by using gravitational information. Signals from other body receptors also play an important role, providing somatosensory information about pressure gradients within the body, pressure on mechanoreceptors found in all those body parts touching the ground, kinaesthetic information from joint, tendon and muscle receptors, and internal feedback signals related to locomotive movements ('efference copy' signals). Furthermore, what is perceived as 'straight ahead' depends on our body scheme as well as on our 'ego space', which is also affected by the sensory modalities just mentioned.

Vection Induced by Visual Movement Stimulation

When we are finding our way under 'normal' conditions, visual signals are more important than those of all the other modalities and determine our direction within the extra-personal space. This visual signal 'dominance' (with respect to the coordinates of the perceived extra-personal space and to the perception of ego movement across that space) can be illustrated by using a modern technical device that was developed to train aircraft pilots: when one sits in the cockpit of a flight (or automobile) simulator, simplified but realistic movie pictures of an artificial visual world created by a computer program are projected onto the 'windows' of the cockpit and change according to the commands given by the pilot (or driver). The illusion of movement through the extra-personal space is nearly perfect. The simple movement signals, as well as the additional movement parallax signals of the simulated extra-personal space, that appear in the windows especially help to perfect the apparent body (or 'aircraft') movement ('vection'). Under these conditions, one easily perceives self-movement in all three dimensions with latencies of less than 250 ms; the perceived body movements depend on the commands given by the pilot. According to the experts who train pilots in such flight simulators, about 70% of what the pilot has learned in a simulator is later used in real flight.

In addition to visual signals, auditory and, under certain conditions, even olfactory signals may contribute to extrapersonal space perception. When one walks in total darkness through a well-known environment (e.g. one's apartment), somatosensory and kinaesthetic information become especially important. For blind people, auditory signals (especially echoes) contribute to extra-personal space perception to a much greater degree than is the case for individuals with normal sight. Although it is much more difficult to induce circular or linear vection by using moving auditory or somatosensory stimuli (as opposed to moving visual stimuli) (Grüsser, 1983), some studies have reported 'arthrokinetic' nystagmus and ego-motion sensations (Brandt *et al.*, 1977).

Global and Local Spatiotopic Coordinates

It seems meaningful to discriminate between global and local coordinates with regard to the perceived coordinates of the extra-personal space (cf. Chapters 6 and 21) surrounding us. The extra-personal space is perceived as a three-dimensional entity, which, at a distance beyond approximately 20 metres, exhibits some non-Euclidean, i.e. non-linear, properties. In addition, for every distinct object and each of its parts within this extra-personal space, there are local coordinates for up–down, left–right and front–behind. The perceived structure of the distinct subcompartments of the extra-personal space depends not only on the global spatiotopic coordinates, but also on the spatial relations between the different objects within that space. Brain lesions affect not only the global, egocentric coordinates of the extra-personal space, but also object perception at the local coordinate level as well. In the latter case, local object shape distortions ('dysmorphopsias') are perceived (Pötzl, 1928).

The Central Vestibular System is Involved in the Transformation of Space Coordinates

The transformation of retinotopic visual signals into spatiotopic signals is a rather complex operation, which is achieved by neuronal networks that are widely spread across the inferior parietal lobe, especially in areas 7a and b in primates and in areas 39 and 40 as well in man. Moreover, all of those regions in the cerebral cortex that integrate visual, vestibular and somatosensory signals (i.e. the vestibular area 2v of the parietal lobe, the parieto–insular vestibular cortex (PIVC) located in the region around the posterior end of the insula, the vestibular area 3aN, the 'neck' region of the somatosensory cortex) are involved in this integration (Grüsser *et al.*, 1982, 1990a, b; Akbarian *et al.*, 1989; Grüsser *et al.*, 1991). Although these cortical structures are about equally strong in the left and right cortical hemispheres in primates, the 'minor' right hemisphere seems to dominate in man for visuo-spatial tasks, especially for those in which spatial perception, goal-

directed attention and visuo–motor interactions are required.

A Short History of the Discovery of Spatial Neglect and Other Visuo-spatial Disorders

Seventeenth and eighteenth century clinicians were aware of visuo-spatial defects caused by brain lesions. Such disturbances were normally mentioned in their textbooks in the chapters dealing with vertigo. For example, Hermann Boerhaave (Leyden, 1668–1738), a leading clinician in his time and head of the famous Leyden School of Medicine, devoted a long chapter ('De vertigine') to the different symptoms and causes of vertigo in his *Praelectiones academicae de morbis nervorum* (pp. 576–641 in the later edition by J. van Eems, 1761). He recognized the correlation between the apparent movement of objects and involuntary eye movements during the state of vertigo and wrote that vertiginous disturbances of perception might be associated with a dimming of vision; he did not however, mention cases of visuo-spatial hemineglect. He also described vertigo as an aura phenomenon preceding epileptic fits. Boerhaave carefully listed the causes of vertigo and believed that these led to a dysfunction of the brain's *sensus communis* (cf. Chapter 2), which was responsible for vertiginous sensations. He also mentioned that mild forms of apoplexias (he called them 'parapoplexias') were frequently associated with vertigo.

In his *Institutiones pathologiae medicinalis* (1757), Boerhaave's prominent pupil Hieronymous David Gaub (Gaubius, 1703–1780) briefly mentioned symptoms of visuo-spatial defects occurring after the formation of brain lesions. He suggested that acute blindness may be caused by cerebral lesions and presented the following list of visuo-spatial disorders as symptoms that may also be caused by cerebral affections: the perception of multiple images for a single object, partition of the images, mutilation or up–down reversal of the image, visual hallucinations and alterations in the location, movement and shape of objects (l.c., p. 383).

This knowledge entered the textbooks on nosology which became quite popular in many European medical schools during the second half of the eighteenth century. For example, G. W. Ploucquet described different causes and symptoms of visual vertigo and mentioned visuospatial dysfunctions (which he called 'allomorpha') in his *System der Nosologie im Umrisse* (1797). As examples of such dysfunctions, he mentioned illusionary changes in the shapes and outlines of objects (phenomena that we refer to today as dysmorphopsias).

Of all the physiologists active during the first half of the nineteenth century, J. E. Purkinje (1787–1869) was the most industrious in trying to investigate the phenomenon of spatial orientation and vertigo experimentally. He did this by performing psychophysical studies on man as well as by studying the effects of experimental brain lesions in animals. Purkinje observed vertigo and eye movements in normal subjects as well as in psychiatric patients, who were rotated for therapeutic reasons in a mechanically driven chair, first described by the British psychiatrist Cox (1804, 1811). Purkinje discriminated between five categories of space vertigo according to aetiology: vertigo caused by different types of motion (movement vertigo), vertigo caused by an electrial potential difference applied between the left and right ear (galvanic vertigo), vertigo caused by general cerebral ischaemia, vertigo caused by the consumption of alcohol or other narcotics, and height vertigo. Purkinje observed that movement vertigo could also be induced by optokinetic stimuli. He discovered that the perceived direction of vertigo is correlated with the rotation of the head in space. This is especially the case when a rotating subject is suddenly stopped and asked to pay attention to the apparent motion that is perceived when the active or passive movement ends and the head is inclined forwards, backwards or sidewards (for details see Grüsser, 1984). Purkinje believed that the three main planes of head rotation constituting the egocentric coordinates of the extra-personal space (pitch, yaw, roll) are sensed and represented by different cerebral structures. On the basis of the symptoms of patients with cerebellar diseases, he assumed that the cerebellum is the site where spatial coordinates and head movements in space are elaborated. Pursuing this idea together with his doctoral student H. C. G. Krauss, he performed a set of lesion experiments on different vertebrates (Krauss, 1824; Purkinje, 1827). These animal experiments were also a reaction to similar experiments performed by the French physiologist P. Flourens (1824). Krauss (1824) provided a detailed description of the comparative studies of the effects of localized cerebellar lesions in dogs, birds (hens, pigeons) and fish performed together with Purkinje:

1. In general, the same lesion effects were found in all species. This convinced Purkinje that they had discovered a general biological law for the cerebral mechanisms involved in space perception and vertigo.

2. Small lesions restricted to the cerebellar surface had no effect or led only to a minor stance instability.

3. Deep lesions in the lateral parts of the cerebellum caused turning movements of the head towards the ipsilateral side, as well as rotation around the long body axis towards the ipsilateral side. These body movements were accompanied by rotatory eye movements, with the slow phase moving towards the side contralateral to the lesion.

4. Deep lesions in the medial part of the cerebellum (saving the brain stem structures) led to retroflection of the head, extension of the anterior limbs and backward bending of the body. Backward rotation and vertical nystagmus were observed in birds; fish also rotated backwards around the pitch axis in the presence of such a lesion.

5. Although lesions in neocortical regions did not produce vertiginous symptoms, they did lead to changes in the 'instinctive behaviour' of the animals.

To our knowledge, this was the first experimentally systematic approach using brain lesions and induced pathological disturbances that tried to find the neuronal substrate representing head movement and the extrapersonal space coordinates. It was also the first experimental search for the pathophysiological basis of vertigo.

A generation after Purkinje, it became evident – again through animal experimentation – that neocortical structures also contribute to visuo–spatial orientation. Ferrier (1886) reported that dogs with lesions in the parietal lobe could no longer orient themselves towards visual stimuli. On the basis of these observations, Ferrier believed that the cerebral centres of vision were located in the parietal lobe. His initial interpretation turned out to be wrong, however (cf. Chapter 2). What Ferrier had actually discovered was the important role played by the parietal lobe in space-directed attention and visuo–motor activity. In expanding upon the studies conducted by Fritsch and Hitzig (1870) on electrical stimulation of the cortex, Ferrier stimulated the posterior part of the parietal lobe and discovered that electrical stimulation of that part of the brain evoked eye movements. This led to a greater understanding of the symptoms of visuo–motor unresponsiveness that appear in an animal after destruction of the parietal lobe regions.

Disturbances in extra-personal space perception caused by brain lesions were reported on by nineteenth century neurologists. For example, Hughlings Jackson (1870) emphasized the idea that the parietal lobe contains multimodal association areas relevant to spatial vision. Without describing the clinical details, he attributed visuo-spatial functions to the right parietal lobe. Interestingly, the first extensive description of symptoms related to parietal lobe lesions was not of a patient with a unilateral defect, but rather of a patient who suffered from bilateral parietal lobe infarctions, which are much rarer (Balint, 1909). This patient's symptoms included general psychic gaze paralysis ('*seelische Blicklähmung*', gaze apraxia) associated with an inability to perform visually directed hand movements within the grasping space ('optic ataxia'), an inability to fixate carefully on a single target, and restriction of the patient's spatially directed attention to the right half of the extra-personal space. Neither primary sensory defects, as indicated by normal visual fields, nor motor palsy were observed. The vestibular reflex eye movements

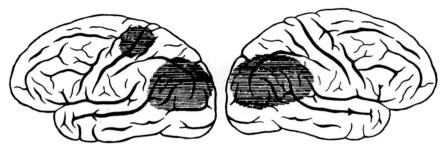

Fig. 22.2 *Schematic illustration of the bilateral brain lesions in Balint's patient (from Balint, 1909).*

(vestibulo–ocular reflexes, VOR) were normal. In the postmortem brain pathology, bilateral posterior parietal lobe lesions were found (Fig. 22.2).

The French ophthalmologist Badal (1888) had earlier described symptoms similar to those observed in Balint's patient, but no brain pathology became available in this case. Badal's patient, a woman suffering from eclampsia, also had other symptoms indicating bilateral posterior cerebral defects (discussed more extensively in Chapter 21). In addition to optical gaze apraxia and optic ataxia, which were revealed by an impaired ability to reach, this patient suffered from topographical disorientation and memory deficits, left–right disorientation, dressing apraxia, constructional apraxia, finger agnosia, alexia and agraphia (cf. also Benton and Meyers, 1956).

A more detailed, systematic investigation of disturbances in space perception and spatial visual orientation was first performed on soldiers suffering from brain wounds received during the First World War (Poppelreuter, 1917; Holmes, 1918; Kleist, 1923, 1934). It became evident in these studies that lesions in the parietal lobe of the right hemisphere lead more frequently to impairment of space perception and spatial orientation than do lesions in the left hemisphere. Poppelreuter, who designed several experimental tests allowing for a semi-quantitative evaluation of extra-personal space perception, was able to demonstrate contralateral hemineglect (as illustrated in Fig. 22.3). Holmes (1918) observed patients suffering from parietal lobe lesions who had extreme difficulty discovering objects in the extra-personal space outside the small regions to which they were actually attending. They could not fixate their gaze and had problems in following a moving target with smooth-pursuit eye movements. The patients studied by Holmes (1918) and Holmes and Horrax (1919) also suffered from a loss of topographical memory. In Holmes's patients, bilateral lesions in the posterior inferior parietal regions and in the gyrus angularis and gyrus circumflexus were either found or assumed.

Holmes and Horrax (1919) performed an extremely meticulous investigation of a soldier with a bilateral gun-

shot wound in the parietal lobe. This study revealed symptoms similar to those described by Balint; moreover, many additional signs of impaired parietal lobe function were observed. The gunshot entered the parieto–occipital region on the right side of the brain and exited through the parietal bone on the left side. From the X-ray localization of the trephine holes, Holmes and Horrax assumed that the inferior parietal region (especially the gyrus angularis) was affected on both sides. After some recovery during the first weeks following the injury, the patient showed the following symptoms:

1. An inferior horizontal hemianopia, which did not affect foveal vision (visual acuity 0.7), indicated a lesion in parts of the visual radiation or area striata on both sides.

2. Although no eye movement palsies were discovered, serious difficulties with spontaneous saccadic exploration of the visual space ('fixing difficulties') were observed. An impairment of convergence and accommodation of the eyes for objects moving towards the patient was also present. These symptoms were quite in contrast to the patient's fast and precise saccadic eye movements in the direction of a finger or any other body part that was touched. Gaze direction towards a source of sound was not impaired. When a single moving visual target appeared in the upper visual field periphery, the patient glanced to the wrong side when intending to fixate this target.

3. In contrast to 'tactile' distance estimation in the grasping space (which was not considered to be disturbed), the ability of the subject to judge the distance of visual objects located either in the grasping space or in the far-distant extra-personal space was extremely impaired.

4. Spatially directed attention was seriously impaired. The patient was also not able to see more than one object at a time (simultaneous agnosia, cf. Chapter 11). He could perceive only one side of a large object when he looked at its centre. This was even true when the two sides of the object were coloured differently. Although he had no object agnosia, only one of two objects presented simultaneously within an otherwise empty field could be recog-

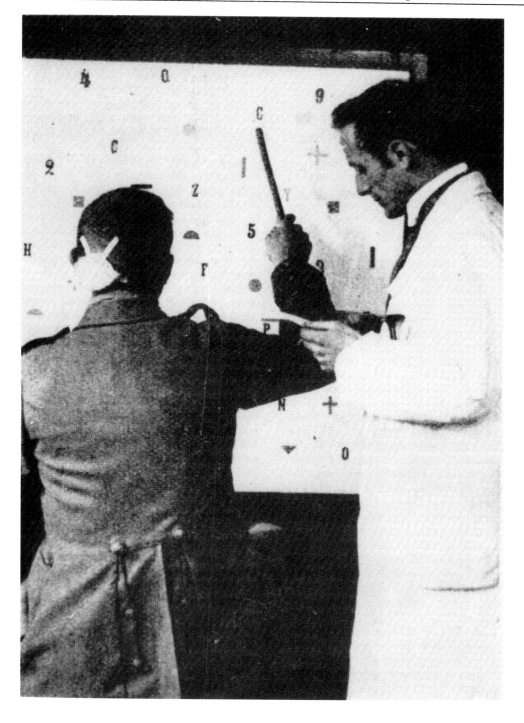

Fig. 22.3 *Poppelreuter examining a brain-lesioned patient in front of a vertical tangent screen on which different numbers, letters and symbols were distributed. The patient had to search for a certain item and point to it with a stick (from Poppelreuter, 1917).*

nized. He had no difficulty recognizing simple geometrical shapes such as circles or squares. When a cross was placed in the centre of a square he had just recognized, however, he only saw the cross and was no longer sure about the square.

5. Spatial localization of objects in the grasping space led to optic ataxia for all objects located outside the restricted field of central vision. Although this was neither a motor problem nor a problem associated with an inability to see details, it was interpreted by Holmes and Horrax as an attentional deficit: 'The essential feature of this inability was to direct his attention to, and the cognizance of, two or more objects that threw the images on the seeing part of the retinae.' Goal-directed hand movements were considerably improved when he took the object into one hand. This was well illustrated by the problems he experienced when eating soup out of a bowl placed on a table. As soon as he was allowed to place the bowl in his hand, he no longer had difficulty directing the spoon.

6. Although visual movement perception was possible for slow movement near the centre of gaze as well as for movement in the visual field periphery, he completely failed to recognize the *direction* of the movement (cf. Chapter 19).

7. A severe defect in the ability to perceive three-dimensionality was referred to by Holmes and Horrax as a loss of 'stereoscopy'. No tests on binocular stereoscopy were performed, however. Evidently the patient's ability to see three-dimensional bodies by evaluating the shading of their surfaces was impaired. The patient could detect only the angles, edges and contours of the object. He explained that he could recognize the objects he saw only because of his ability to detect these features: 'I seem to be able to spot everything that is edged.' His lack of visual depth and distance perception, which included an inability to see more than one object at a time (which prevented him from judging the relative distance between objects), caused serious problems for the patient when he tried to walk around the ward. He bumped into objects located in the near-distant action space as well as into walls. As a consequence, he walked by taking short, slow steps, and held his hands out in front of him 'like a man groping his way through the dark'.

8. The patient suffered from severe topographical disorientation (Chapter 21), lost the ability to describe from memory spatial structures and routes well known to him in the past, and was no longer able to store in memory the spatial relationship of objects he had seen in the grasping space or when walking on the street.

To summarize: visual attention, spatial orientation and the ability to recognize direction were severely disturbed in this patient, who suffered from bilateral, presumably inferior, parietal lobe lesions; in addition, he suffered from topographagnosia and had memory deficits for spatial relations. Although he no longer had the ability to perceive object three-dimensionality, contour perception was preserved. Gaze movements were seriously impaired by the bilateral attentional deficits and the simultaneous agnosia. Holmes and Horrax pointed out the similarity of the symptoms found in their patient to those observed by Pick (1898), Bálint (1909) and van Valkenburg (1908) in patients suffering from parietal lobe lesions in the vascular genesis.

Poppelreuter (1917, 1923) and Kleist (1918, 1923, 1934) reported that unilateral parietal lobe lesions led to a change in the perception and localization of signals originating from the hemispace contralateral to the lesion. Other disturbances in visuo-spatial orientation in the grasping space or in the far-distant extra-personal space were also observed. Scheller and Seidemann (1931) later emphasized disturbances in spatial perception, which they called *optic spatial agnosia* ('optisch-räumliche Agnosie'); these appeared in the presence of a lesion in the left or right side of the parietal lobe. They also reported on a patient suffering from a left-sided hemispatial inattention caused by right parietal lobe lesions. In his investigation of soldiers who had also suffered from parietal lobe lesions received during the Second World War, Brain (1941) discriminated between general visual spatial agnosia and unilateral neglect of the extra-personal space. Spatial hemineglect appears more frequently and more pronounced in the presence of right parietal lobe lesions affecting the left extra-personal space than it does in the presence of left parietal lobe lesions. Brain interpreted the neglect of the contralateral half of the extra-personal space to be an impairment of *spatially related attention*, just as Balint, Holmes and Horrax had explained these defects in their patients. Since Brain's study, contralateral spatial hemineglect has generally been accepted by clinical neurologists as a parietal lobe symptom (Critchley, 1953; Hécaen and Albert, 1978). More recently, however, it has become evident that lesions outside the parietal lobe might also lead to contralateral neglect (p. 460). As a rule, patients suffering from left parietal lobe lesions also have problems with spatial orientation as well as with perceptual coordination of events taking place in the right half of the extra-personal space. Although long-lasting and severe right-sided hemineglect caused by left parietal lobe lesions in right-handers is rare, less severe hemineglect symptoms can also appear, at least transiently, in the presence of left parietal lobe lesions (see below).

The intriguing left–right asymmetry of the cerebral representation of the extra-personal space (presumably of the grasping space as well as of the more distant parts of the extra-personal space) was accepted by most behavioural neurologists after these reports on brain-injured soldiers became available after the Second World War.

This asymmetry is presumably caused by a 'secondary' lateralization: the speech-dominance of the left hemisphere developed during hominid phylogenesis over the last 2 to 3 million years. As a result, the language-related cortical areas expanded at the expense of the spatial functions in the left side of the brain; the right parietal lobe structures had therefore to 'compensate' for the left-hemispheric 'loss' of space-related neuronal operations. Consequently, the hemisphere that is subdominant for language functions became dominant for complex, space-related neuronal operations.

Symptoms of Visual Hemineglect and Other Visuo-spatial Disorders, as Illustrated in the Cases of a Writer and an Artist Suffering from Right Parietal Lobe Lesions

In the following section we describe our own observations of two patients suffering from unilateral posterior parietal lobe lesions. A stroke in the territory of the right middle cerebral artery interrupted a successful career for both of these well-educated patients. One, a well-known poet, was greatly interested in the technical aspects of modern life (Grüsser, 1983). The other was a locally renowned Swiss painter (Schnider *et al.*, 1991).

The Writer

N.N. suffered at the age of 66 from an acute cerebral infarction in the territory of the right middle cerebral artery. Without losing consciousness, he suddenly became hemiplegic on the left side and could no longer orient himself topographically. This acute condition was preceded by repeated attacks of dizziness, disturbances while walking and spatial disorientation. Computer tomography, performed about 3 weeks after the stroke, revealed an extensive lesion in the right parietal lobe, which extended to parts of the white matter below the temporal lobe as well as to the region around the dorsal horn of the lateral ventricle. He had a history of increased alcohol consumption over several years and had suffered at about age 60 from short delirious states. His drinking habits improved thereafter. When one of the authors (O.-J. G.) saw him for the first time 10 days after the stroke, he still suffered from a severe left-sided hemiplegia, a left hemihypaesthesia with relative sparing of the face, a right Horner syndrome, and a left homonymous hemianopia with macular sparing of at least 5 degrees. There were no signs of aphasia, and he could speak fluently without searching for words. Audi-

tory comprehension and the ability to repeat words were both intact. His ability to find synonyms, supra-ordinates or rhymes was also intact, and his verbal short-term memory was normal. A trained ambidextrous left-hander, he had used his right hand to write before the stroke and usually held his cigarette in the left hand. His memory of the past was not impaired and, except for a short period on the day of the stroke, his memory of the recent past was normal. During his first examination after the stroke, he lay in bed and admitted that he could not walk because of 'some problems' with his legs. He was unaware of his left-sided hemiplegia. After more detailed exploration, he reported that he had had some strange experiences on the left side of his body: he noted that his left hand always seemed to mimic the movement of his right hand. In addition, he reported that the left side of his body was 'far away from the self', while the right side of the body was 'intensively near to the self'. He sometimes thought that his left body half had doubled, and that the double lay beside him on the left side of the bed.

He did not spontaneously move his centre of gaze to the left of the midline by means of eye saccades or head movements, and a slight tonic head and eye deviation towards the right side was observed. Smooth-pursuit eye movements (interrupted by saccades) pursuing the investigator's finger or a swinging pendulum stopped at midline position. When asked to move his head to and fro, he moved from the midline position towards the right and then back again to the midline position. When the fixation target was moved towards the right during such horizontal head movements, it could be demonstrated that vestibular–ocular reflex (VOR) and visual pursuit were both possible across a large field of gaze on the right side.

The patient also suffered from extended, left-sided, visual and auditory spatial neglect. When the examiner stood on the left side of the patient's bed, he did not respond to any of the examiner's questions. As the examiner moved into the patient's right extra-personal space, communication became normal once again. When asked to look into the examiner's face as the examiner slowly moved across the patient's right extra-personal space towards the midline, the patient attentively followed him with head and eye movements, regardless of whether or not there was any verbal communication. He stopped pursuing him, however, when the examiner moved into the left side of the patient's extra-personal space. This could not be prevented by talking with the patient, because whenever the examiner 'disappeared' into the neglected hemispace, all conversation immediately stopped: the patient no longer answered even the simplest of questions. When tested from the right extra-personal space, audition was about normal for both ears; whispering could be heard in each ear from a distance of about 4 m.

The subject could correctly name and recognize objects

located in the grasping space and in the near-distant action space, provided that the objects were presented to him directly in front or towards the right side of his grasping space. His ability to perceive the position of two objects relative to one another was impaired within the grasping space, however. Depth perception in the extra-personal space was evidently also affected. Consequently, the patient had some difficulty pointing with his right hand to an object located on the right side of the grasping space. This 'optic ataxia' was caused by problems in estimating the distance and perhaps also the direction of an object with respect to the patient's own body, as well as a possible inability to coordinate hand movements with respect to the object in question. The patient could not point at all to objects located on the left side of the grasping space; when asked to point towards the left, his right hand movements became arbitrary as soon as the hand crossed the midline. The ability to point to parts of his own face (the nose, the left and right eyes or ears, and the chin) with open or closed eyes was not disturbed, although pointing with the right hand to the left hand was arbitrary. He could eat with his right hand, i.e. hand–mouth coordination and fork/spoon–mouth coordination were not seriously affected.

His verbal descriptions of landscapes and objects were fluent. In light of these descriptions, it seems that no spatial neglect of the mental image was present. The patient also correctly described from memory a well-known house and garden in North Germany written about in the novel of another writer. He had visited this house for the last time more than 30 years before. The patient was also able to describe in detail different automobiles as well as the constructional principles of an automobile, boat or aircraft motor. He was a licensed pilot and had gained technical experience during the Second World War as a coastguard boat captain. When asked to describe complex objects such as certain fashionable automobiles from memory, he neglected the left side of the automobile. In other words, although he was familiar with all the parts of an automobile, the transformation of the concept of a certain automobile into a mental image revealed neglect of the left side of his mental image. Although he was not able to draw a face (Fig. 22.4), there were no signs of prosopagnosia; furthermore, his ability to describe different parts of the face verbally was not disturbed.

Although he could read well, when asked to read he ignored about one third or more of each line on the left side of a column. This led to 'spatial dyslexia', which he compensated for by using his imagination; in most cases, this helped him to 'read' a meaningful text that corresponded closely to the actual printed text. His attempts to draw revealed severe constructional apraxia (Fig. 22.6(a–c)), as was the case when he tried to form simple geometrical figures (triangles, squares, crosses, hexagons) by using matches.

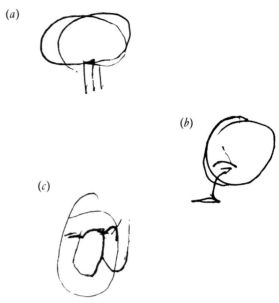

Fig. 22.4 *Drawings from patient N.N. 10 days after a right hemisphere stroke. (a) Drawing of a tree, (b) of a face from memory, (c) copying a schematic face drawn by the examiner (modified from Grüsser, 1983).*

The patient was repeatedly investigated over the next few months. Twenty days after the stroke, the auditory spatial neglect had almost disappeared: he now continued to speak with the investigator even when the latter 'disappeared' into the left half of the patient's extra-personal space; nevertheless, a somewhat reduced attention level was observed. At this point, the patient's contribution to the conversation became intellectually less precise. One gained the impression that when matters of modern German literature were discussed, the patient could respond in his usually brilliant and somewhat malicious manner only when the investigator sat on the right side of the patient's extra-personal space. At between 1 and 6 metres, this 'investigator-directed' attention did not depend on the distance between the patient and the investigator. When asked to write down some autobiographical information, he wrote only on the right side of each page. Even when his hand was moved towards the left border of the page and he was told to write across the whole page, he inevitably shifted to the right third of the page ('spatial dysgraphia', Hécaen and Albert, 1978; Fig. 22.5). This neglect of the left half of the page continued even when the whole page was moved towards the right side of the patient's grasping space. As in the line-bisection task (p. 454), the patient deviated by about one quarter of the page to the right when asked to point to the middle of the page (no errors were made in pointing up or down

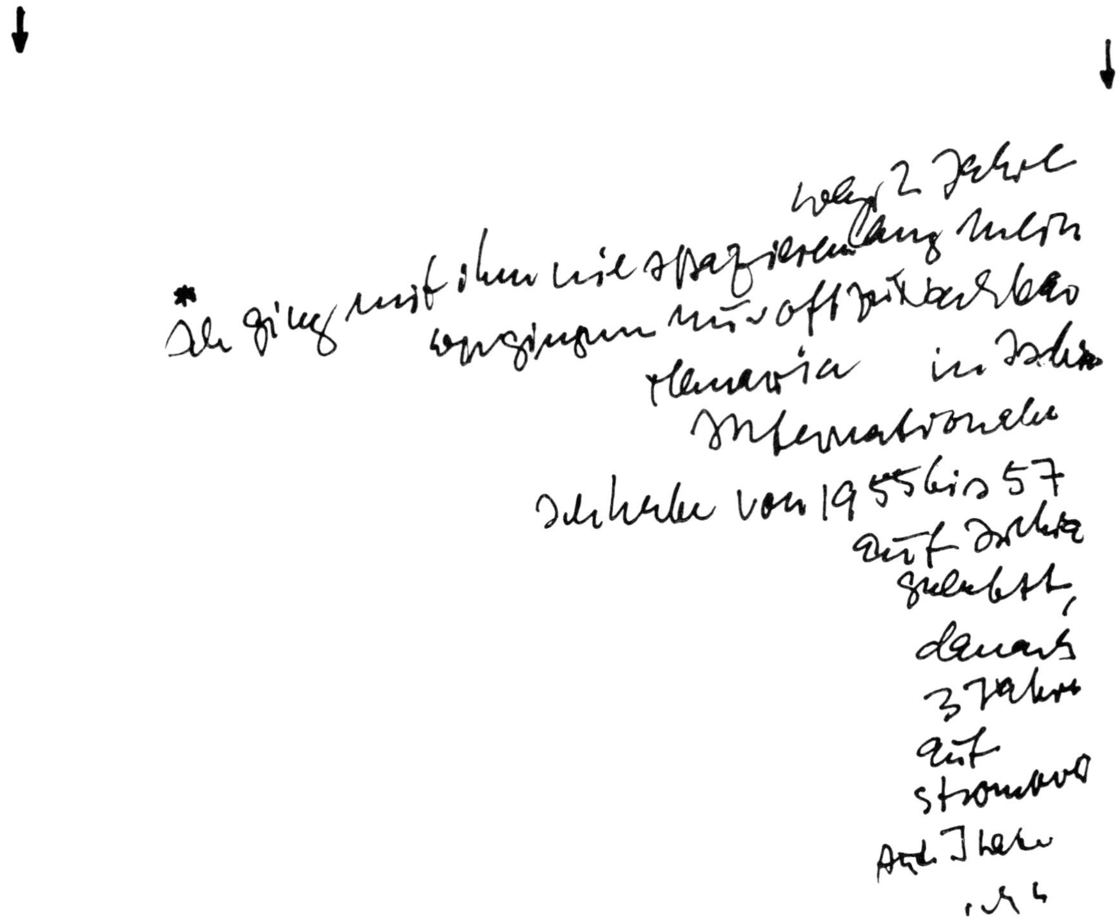

Fig. 22.5 *Patient N.N. wrote a short autobiographical note. He wrote only on the right side of the pages (edges of the page marked by arrows). Before the patient wrote the line marked with the asterisk, his writing right hand was moved towards the left edge of the page by the examiner. He was told to write across the whole page. From the next line on, the patient continued to write only on the right side of the page. This disregard of the left half of the page persisted when the whole page was moved towards the right side of the body. The text contains a few paragraphic errors.*

along the midline position). These pointing errors occurred within the grasping space, regardless of how far away the page was from the patient.

Neglect of the left side of his body and an inability to point correctly with the right hand to different parts of the left half of his body ('autotopagnosia'; Pick, 1907, 1915; Critchley, 1953) continued for several weeks after the stroke. Although left-handed, he was used to writing with his right hand and to holding simultaneously a cigarette in his left hand. Since he was heavily addicted to smoking, he continued to smoke after the stroke, but had serious difficulties when he did not receive help from others. When someone else lit a cigarette for him, he used his right hand to put the cigarette in his mouth; he repeatedly left the cigarette in his mouth and forgot to get rid of the ashes.

When someone suggested that he use the ashtray, he replied, 'But I am using the ashtray.' When asked which hand he had used to move the cigarette from his mouth to the ashtray, he replied, 'With the left hand, of course, as I always do.' Although Figs 22.6(a–f) illustrate the improvement in constructional apraxia that took place during the weeks directly following the stroke, they also indicate that the left side of his drawings was still affected by the neglect. In comparison with his pre-stroke drawing ability, he remained seriously impaired for the rest of his life. His constructional apraxic drawings sometimes showed not only difficulties with the left side of objects, but also with the top and bottom of objects as well (Fig. 22.6(b)).

From about the third week after the stroke, he became

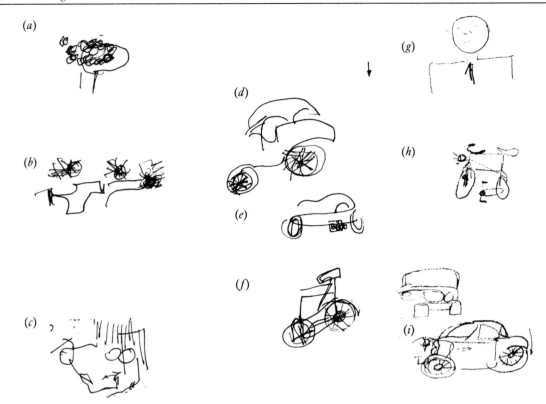

Fig. 22.6 *Patient N.N.: slow recovery of constructional apraxia and left-sided neglect in drawings (see Fig. 22.4) performed 17 days (a–c), 26 days (d–f) and 56 days (g–i) after the stroke. The task was to draw in (a) a tree, (b) a side view of an automobile, (c) a face, (d) a side view of an automobile, (e) a front view of an automobile, (f) a bicycle, (g) a face, (h) a bicycle, (i) an automobile (two attempts) (modified from Grüsser, 1983).*

aware of his left hemiplegia. The 'doubling' experience of his left body side also disappeared. He remained completely anosognosic for his visuo-spatial hemineglect, however. When walking along a straight corridor, and even more so when walking in an open space, he had a strong tendency to wander towards the right side. He had serious difficulties estimating the distances (although not the sizes) of objects located in the far-distant extra-personal space. He could still use perspective and parallax movement to estimate depth. Binocular stereovision was not investigated. When asked to look out of the window and describe the hospital surroundings, he completely neglected everything more than 10 degrees lateral to the midline, even when asked to use his head to look around. He still had trouble turning his head to the left, and voluntary eye saccades rarely went past midline position towards the left. When asked to pursue a moving finger or a swinging pendulum with his eyes, he could now follow the moving target much better than he could during the first examination: in fact, he could even follow it into the

left part of the extra-personal space. When asked to follow the moving target with his head, he was able to move his head almost normally to and fro in both the horizontal and vertical directions.

Upon returning to Berlin after several months of treatment in a rehabilitation centre, the patient had adapted well to walking, despite his left-sided hemiplegia. He moved into a new apartment situated on the ground floor and learned to orient himself without much difficulty in his new environment. He acquired a good topographic memory of his new apartment as well as of other general surroundings. He again became interested in literature and even planned to continue several literary texts that he had begun to write before the stroke. Despite the help of a secretary, he never succeeded in writing a new text, for he had lost all poetic creativity. Over the following years, he neither continued nor finished any old texts, nor did he write any new ones. It is evident from his published texts that descriptions of spatial relations, landscapes, technical conditions, etc., were very important components of his pre-stroke literary style. In contrast to this dramatic reduction in poetic creativity, his critical ability to judge the style and content of modern prose was not at all impaired, and he continued to communicate by telephone or through personal conversation with other writers about professional matters. He also discussed literary and political issues at length with the investigator. Neither his recent verbal memory nor his memory of past biographical literary events was impaired. Slight difficulties that he had memorizing new facts were normal for his age. He could describe vividly from memory landscapes, cities or houses with which he had been familiar prior to the stroke. Because of his high verbal competence, one could not detect any neglect in his descriptions of objects and spaces. The investigator had the impression that he compensated for his spatial neglect by unconsciously putting himself into different positions within the scenery that he recalled from his topographical memory.

In addition to the left-sided hemiplegia, two visuo-spatial defects – the strong left visual hemineglect and the constructional apraxia – did not recover beyond the initial improvements recorded during the first weeks after the stroke. The left homonymous hemianopia showed some improvement, and the macular sparing of the left hemianopia recovered to about 10–12 degrees. In everyday life, his behaviour indicated that he still disregarded the left extra-personal space. For example, to go to the bakery near his home, the patient had to turn right after a short stroll in order to reach his destination, which was located on the right-hand side of the street. After he entered the bakery and bought some rolls, he would leave again to return home. He frequently turned right instead of left, walked to the next street crossing, realized that he had made a mistake, turned around and then walked in the direction of his home, which was now on the left side of his extra-personal space. He regularly passed by the entrance to his house, walked to the next street crossing, realized that he had made another mistake, turned around and walked back. The entrance to his house was now on his right side, and he was able to find it this time. When asked about his not very economic behaviour, he said that it was just his absent-mindedness. Brain (1941a) and De Renzi (1982) had also observed such a pattern of neglect-induced, behaviourally topographical problems, which are usually rare to this extent in the presence of unilateral parietal lobe lesions.

Our patient strongly rejected the examiner's opinion that he was suffering from a left-sided spatial hemineglect and said to him with a smile, 'Your idea that I cannot see the whole space is one of the typical inventions of a scientist.' In his experience, the world and the objects within it were complete. He could even convince an ophthalmologist, who was not familiar with the symptoms of spatial hemineglect, that he had absolutely normal visual perception apart from the remaining left-sided visual field defect.

Hemineglect was present not only for the near-distant and far-distant action spaces, but also for the grasping space as well as for individual objects, even when they were placed on the right side of the grasping space. When eating, he ate only the food placed on the right side of the plate, and then stopped eating. When his friends turned his plate around and he realized that some food was still on the plate, he politely thanked them for their help. Although he responded to large object movements in that part of the left visual field that was still intact, he typically showed all signs of extinction in the neglected half-field when two stimuli were simultaneously moved, one in the right half, the other in the left half of the visual field. An examination of this 'extinction effect' showed that it was strongest when two stimuli were placed symmetrically along the vertical midline. Extinction was weaker when a large stimulus (e.g. the hand of the examiner) was moved on the left side of the grasping space while only a small stimulus (e.g. a finger) was moved on the right side. Single, large, moving objects were perceived in all parts of the extra-personal space.

Even the auditory, left-sided spatial neglect reappeared under competitive situations. During a visit of the examiner and one of the patient's friends, both sat opposite him at a table, one in his left, the other in his right extra-personal space. He repeatedly addressed only the one sitting in his right extra-personal space and ignored the other, even when he posed questions. When the two visitors changed places, this spatial pattern remained,

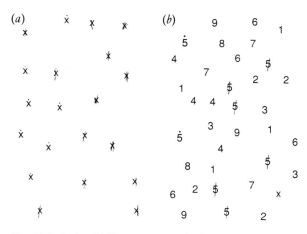

Fig. 22.7 *Patient N.N.: some test results from an investigation 2 years after the stroke which led to a right parietal-lobe lesion. (a) The patient did not cross out all crosses on the page. Those crosses missed are marked with a dot. (b) The patient had to cross out all the number 5s on this page and missed two on the left side (marked with a dot). The pages were about the same size as this page.*

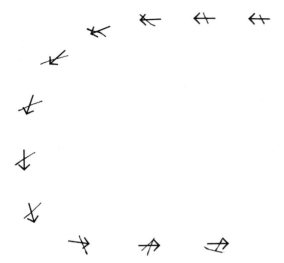

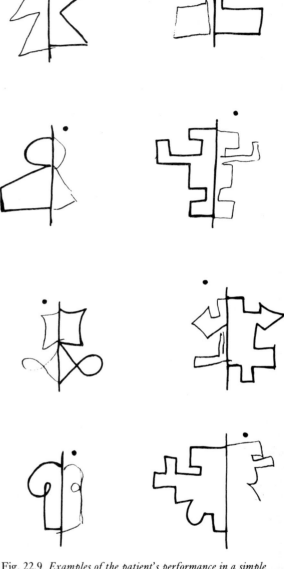

Fig. 22.8 *Patient N.N., examined two years after the stroke. The patient was asked to cross out all arrows. He performed the task correctly, beginning with the right upper arrow. Data from the same day as Figs 22.7 and 22.9. The page was about the same size as this page.*

which indicated that this had nothing to do with the persons visiting him. His left-sided spatial neglect repeatedly caused him problems with cars during strolls. Although he was aware of the near-accidents, he attributed them to the 'rude behaviour of the Berliners'.

Figures 22.7–22.9 show some results obtained approximately two years after the stroke. When he was asked to mark simple symbols such as crosses distributed randomly across the page, he still missed several crosses placed on the left side of the page (Fig. 22.7(a, b)). He did well, however, when asked to follow a set of arrows and to cross out one arrow after the other, and could even follow the arrows towards the left side of the page (Fig. 22.8). Thus he could compensate for the hemineglect by using 'local' directional cues. He could copy simple line drawings mirror-symmetrically along a vertical axis for the simplest figures; he failed in a characteristic manner for more complex ones, however (Fig. 22.9). He still suffered from severe constructional apraxia, and when he wrote spontaneously or on dictation, he used only the right side of the page. When reading newspaper texts, he missed many words in the left quarter of each column, but always filled in these missing words with appropriate substitutes; in this way, he was able to reconstruct a meaningful and syntactically correct text. The neurological and neuropsychological symptoms of N.N. remained stable until his death about 6 years after the stroke. A postmortem examination of the brain was not possible.

The lesion in N.N.'s right hemisphere also evidently

Fig. 22.9 *Examples of the patient's performance in a simple axial symmetry completion test. The halves drawn by the patient are marked by a dot. Simple tasks were performed correctly; with more complex figures the patient showed difficulties owing to constructional apraxia and left-sided hemineglect.*

affected his poetic creativity. We think that this impairment was not a result of his ambidexterity, but rather was related to the right hemisphere's important role in the metaphoric use of language and verbal creativity. N.N.'s

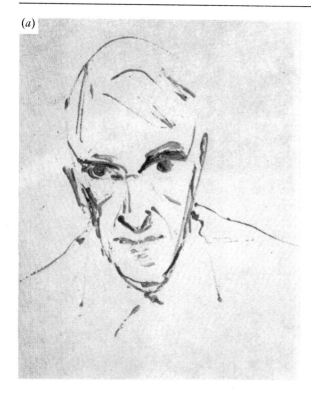

(a)

literary activity before the stroke included many texts related to spatial percepts and technical constructions. It seems probable that his ability to include technical details in his texts was especially impaired by the parietal lesion and by the accompanying 'spatial thought' disorder (Critchley, 1953) – despite the fact that these defects were not immediately apparent when he spoke.

Three German Painters

Right-hemisphere lesions which cause hemispatial neglect are particularly tragic when they occur in a patient whose main artistic skills rely on the individual's visuo-spatial abilities. Jung (1974, 1975) reported on several German painters who suffered from extended right-parietal hemispheric lesions caused by vascular diseases. Two of them were well known, having greatly contributed to the canon of German art during the first decades of the twentieth century. Lovis Corinth (1858–1925) and Anton Räderscheidt (1892–1970) had both suffered from large, right-hemispheric strokes (Corinth in 1911, Räderscheidt in 1967), and both subsequently developed hemispatial neglect. In addition, Corinth had a mild left hemiplegia. Räderscheidt suffered from a left homonymous hemianopia, topographic disorientation and prosopagnosia. After recovering from their acute strokes, both artists con-

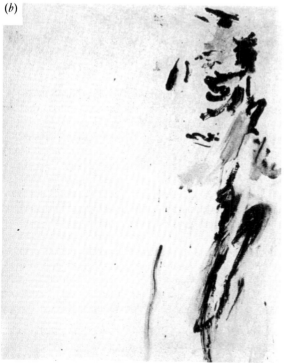

(b)

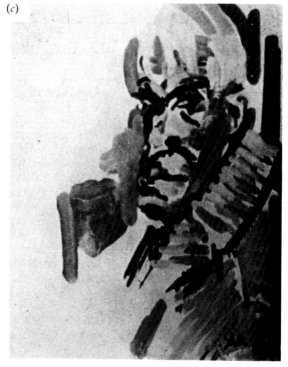

(c)

Fig. 22.10 *Self-portraits by the painter Anton Räderscheidt before (a) and after (b, c) a right parietal lobe lesion (from Jung, 1974).*

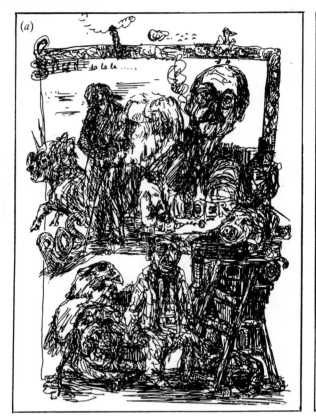

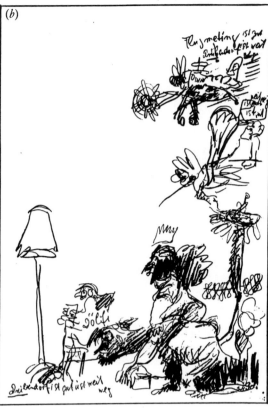

Fig. 22.11 *Drawings by the Swiss painter suffering from a right parietal lobe lesion as described in the text. (a) Drawing before the stroke, (b) drawing after the stroke. Left hemineglect is evident, as well as some changes in drawing style, loss of depth perspective, mild constructional apraxia, and a tendency to write into the drawing.*

tinued to draw and paint. Nine years after his stroke, the precision and details on the left side of one of Corinth's self-portraits were still reduced ('left' related to the observer). An obvious neglect also became evident in Räderscheidt's self-portraits (as illustrated in Fig. 22.10 (Jung, 1974). In addition, marked alterations in the spatial composition of their paintings developed for both painters. This recovered slowly in Corinth's paintings after the stroke but some changes in the vertical/horizontal coordinates of his paintings became noticeable. In an analysis of Räderscheidt's paintings, Gardner (1974, 1982) pointed to the 'fundamental differences in style', which he described as an increase in emotion and as a shift towards 'primitivization'. Jung, who had seen more of Räderscheidt's paintings than Gardner had, observed no significant changes in style.

One of the most famous German painters of the twentieth century, Otto Dix (1891–1969), suffered at age 76 an infarct in the territory of the right medial cerebral artery, which led to left hemiparesis, left partial homonymous hemianopia, hemispatial neglect and mild signs of spatial

agnosia (Baumgartner, personal communication to R. Jung, 1967). Four days after the incident, Dix began to draw again. A left-sided hemineglect became apparent in one of his paintings of a tree. This was demonstrated by Jung (Fig. 13 in Jung, 1974), who compared this drawing with a similiar one made before the stroke. Two weeks after the cerebral infarction, however, no further signs of left-sided neglect were visible in Dix's drawings nor were they in his later lithographs. His drawings and lithographs subsequently became even more vivid and expressive than his pre-stroke style, and are more appreciated today than his work produced during the years immediately prior to the stroke. In contrast to that of Corinth and Räderscheidt, Dix's hemineglect evidently recovered quickly. The change in style and artistic creativity may have been related to introspective reflection about his serious illness.

The Swiss Painter

In the following, we shall describe the impact of a left-sided hemispatial neglect on the artistic performance of a regionally reknowned Swiss painter. This 54-year-old man was admitted to a hospital for a sudden onset of a left-sided sensorimotor hemisyndrome and left hemianopia (Schnider *et al.*, 1991, in preparation). During the first post-stroke days, he experienced visual illusions and hallucinations and perceived a distorted reflection of his own face in the mirror. He misjudged the distances of moving objects and repeatedly saw imaginary snakes moving in a corner of his room. He had used LSD about 15 years prior to the incident; the drug-induced hallucinations had influenced his artistic activity. Since then, he stood in front of his canvases trying to remember the hallucinations he had had when using the drug. It seems that his post-stroke hallucinations were similar to some of these earlier hallucinatory experiences. Despite an initial left hemianopia, no hemispatial neglect was present. The clinical symptoms then changed dramatically: 6 days later he suffered a second stroke, which caused a large right-hemisphere infarction involving the whole territory of the right middle cerebral artery (as shown on a CT scan). After this second incident, he severely neglected the left hemispace and paid attention to examiners only when they addressed him from the right side; in addition, he misplaced visual, auditory and tactile signals originating from the left side into the right hemispace. Like N.N., he also experienced hemispatial neglect for individual objects. This was first realized when the patient complained about not having received the spinach he had so much hoped for at lunch. In fact, he had eaten only the food placed on the right side of the plate. He could not be convinced that the spinach was on the left half of the plate, and was only satisfied when the plate was turned around 180 degrees.

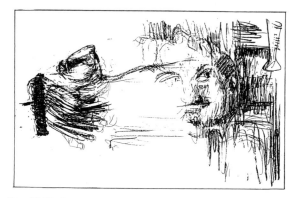

Fig. 22.12 *Drawing by the same patient as Fig. 22.11 at about the same time. 'Local' hemineglect is visible in the drawing of the face on the right side. In addition, the left side of the sheet of paper is dealt with less well. Despite the patient's intention to shade the face on the right side, the apparent depth of the drawing is not very well developed (from Schnider* et al., *in preparation, 1991).*

His hemispatial neglect also became apparent from his performance on cancellation and line bisection tests, as well as in all of his drawings.

Neuropsychological examination showed that there was no aphasia, apraxia or a deficit in his ability to recognize faces, facial expressions, overlapping figures or colours. He had great difficulty, however, in telling the time on analogue watches. His figural and verbal short-term memory was normal, and his visuo-constructive abilities were, surprisingly, still preserved in the right hemispace. He had major problems with symmetries, however, and was virtually unable to make mirror-symmetrical drawings. His visuo-spatial and drawing abilities were tested regularly over a period of 8 months: the left hemispatial neglect was found to fluctuate from day to day. As illustrated in Fig. 22.11 and 22.12, his drawing style changed somewhat after the stroke. Furthermore, he consistently neglected the left side of many figures that he drew, even when the left part of the paper had been brought to his attention. About 3 weeks after the second stroke, visual hallucinations became very rare. The patient experienced auditory hallucinations which usually involved classical music; they were sometimes 'heard' so intensively that he became quite upset. With time, he learned to concentrate on the left side of his extra-personal space, and he made fewer serious errors on the cancellation tests. The patient was transferred to a rehabilitation centre about 6 weeks after the first stroke (without significant improvement of the hemiplegia or hemianopia); he continued to draw there with fluctuating productivity. He sometimes complained of not being able to draw portraits any more. His concentration was also seriously impaired when he drew or painted for more than 10 to 15 minutes. As a sign of this easy exhaustability, he shifted to pencil or charcoal drawings. On certain days, however, he was able to accomplish a great deal. He suffered intermittently from depression, which disturbed his normal life-style to such a degree that he eventually required psychiatric consultation.

Visuo-Spatial Difficulties after Unilateral Impairment of the Left or Right Parietal Lobes

Hemineglect in the Presence of Left Hemisphere Lesions

As already discussed in the preceding sections, extended lesions in the right parietal lobe may lead to pronounced left-sided hemineglect. We interpreted this hemineglect to be a result either of hemi-inattention or of disturbances in space-related perceptual signal processing. As is discussed in greater detail below, we believe that this dichotomy is somewhat artificial, for selective attention plays a role in all space-related visual operations besides simple reflexes. Hemineglect of the right extra-personal space may appear in the presence of lesions in the left parietal lobe. This also is illustrated in another case report below. The idea that hemispatial neglect occurs subsequent to the development of lesions in the language-dominant left hemisphere is rather controversial. It has been claimed that the high rate of hemispatial neglect following the formation of non-dominant, right parietal lesions simply reflects the difficulties involved in examining this phenomenon in the presence of aphasia in left parietal disease, and that the frequency of hemispatial neglect would be the same if one corrected for aphasia. It is common clinical knowledge that hemispatial neglect, especially in regard to severe cases, occurs more frequently after onset of non-dominant parietal diseases. Hécaen (1962) and Hécaen and Angelergue (1963) performed the following statistical study in an attempt to find an answer to this problem: in a sample of 415 patients with brain lesions, they found 59 suffering from hemispatial neglect; 51 had right hemisphere lesions, 4 bilateral and 4 left hemisphere lesions (3 of these last 4 patients were left-handers). This analysis clearly pointed to a right hemisphere dominance with regard to lesion-induced contralateral hemineglect. Gainotti (1968) performed a similar study and reported that in 100 brain-lesioned patients he found 39 with a unilateral spatial neglect, with a 32:7 relation in favour of right hemisphere lesions. This side bias was generally confirmed in later studies (Hécaen, 1972).

Severe hemispatial neglect may be caused by lesions of the left parietal lobe (e.g. Schott *et al.*, 1966; Welman, 1969; Heilman and Watson, 1977; Jeannerod, 1988). This fact will be illustrated in another of our patients, who suffered from a severe global aphasia subsequent to a large left parieto-temporal stroke. In addition to aphasia this patient exhibited all characteristic symptoms of severe hemispatial neglect: he shaved only the left side of his face and ate only the food placed on the left side of his plate, noticing the rest only when the dish was rotated 180 degrees. He failed to copy the right halves of drawings that were presented to him. This example of severe hemineglect in the presence of aphasia certainly is not unique, but in our clinical experience with aphasic patients we have seen only one such case; we have generally found hemineglect in the presence of aphasia to be either mild or transitory in other patients. Some authors did not even observe contralateral hemispatial neglect subsequent to the development of left hemisphere lesions (e.g. Oxbury *et al.*, 1974). While a left-sided neglect resulting from right hemisphere lesions is, as a rule, associated with disturbances in other visuo-spatial operations, visual spatial

defects caused by left hemisphere lesions frequently appear without visual hemispatial neglect. In some tests, the left–right bias in the spatial abilities of patients with right or left hemisphere lesions evidently disappears. In several studies using line bisection tests (Costa *et al.*, 1969; Chain *et al.*, 1979; Colombo *et al.*, 1977), similar 'neglect' frequencies were found in patients with left hemisphere (LH) and right hemisphere (RH) lesions. Evidently, when different tests are applied, the criterion used to determine a diagnosis of 'hemineglect' is changed and rather different statistical numbers for the occurrence of neglect in LH- and RH-lesioned patients result.

Most investigators agree that the neglect found in RH patients is generally more severe than that found in LH patients. In addition, a 'local' object-related hemispatial neglect is less frequently observed in LH patients than in RH patients. Patients suffering from a right-sided hemineglect, but who did not exhibit severe 'local' object-related signs of hemispatial neglect, were able to copy simple symmetrical figures correctly (Colombo *et al.*, 1976).

Dissociation of Spatial Hemineglect Related to the Different Compartments of the Extra-personal Space

As already mentioned in Chapter 21, the extra-personal space may be divided into different compartments. Following Brain (1941), who discerned two space compartments (the 'peripersonal' and the 'extra-personal' spaces), some investigators have explored whether or not brain lesions affect perceptual abilities only in the grasping space or in the extra-personal space as well. The animal experiments discussed in Chapter 6 (Rizzolatti *et al.*, 1983) indicated that in monkeys, lesions in area 8 lead to a reduction in the visual orienting responses related to the far-distant extra-personal space; furthermore, signals related to the grasping space were neglected when area 6 of the prefrontal cortex was destroyed. In many studies of hemispatial neglect in man, this question was not specifically investigated, and the investigators evidently assumed that hemineglect affects all of the compartments in the extra-personal space. Recently, Halligan and Marshall (1991) reported on a 57-year-old, right-handed mechanic who, after a right hemisphere stroke in the territory of the medial cerebral artery, suffered from a severe left hemiparesis and a left inferior quadrantanopia; in addition, he exhibited typical signs of left hemispatial neglect in a behavioural inattention test (Wilson, *et al.*, 1988). The patient was asked to bisect horizontal lines at a distance of 45 cm with a pen and at a distance of 244 cm with a pointing-stick. This 'keen darts player' was also asked to aim darts towards the middle of horizontal lines placed at a distance of 244 cm. These studies, supported by the results of another experiment (division of the horizontal lines into six equal parts), indicated that a severe hemineglect of the grasping space may exist in the absence of hemineglect of the near-distant action space (Chapter 21). This dissociation, which was not found in earlier studies (Pizzamiglio *et al.*, 1989), indicated that within the inferior, posterior parietal lobe, the different compartments of the extra-personal space do indeed seem to have, at least in part, separate representations. It would be rather interesting to repeat this experiment using a glass window with a horizontal line (placed at a distance of approximately 50 cm), and to ask the patient to bisect (by means of a light pointer) this line as well as more distant horizontal lines with the same angular size relative to the observer. Would a similar dissociation also be observed?

Constructional Apraxia

Lesions in the left or right parietal lobes frequently cause constructional apraxia, a symptom that Critchley (1953) considered to be a 'disorder of spatial thought'. Although freehand drawings may be difficult for some normal subjects and are therefore not easily evaluated, constructing simple shapes from matchsticks is a task that all normal subjects should be able to perform. Characteristic differences were observed in patients suffering from left or right parietal lobe lesions; the same differences were observed when patients were asked to copy simple symmetrical drawings or to draw everyday objects from memory. These left/right differences are illustrated by the following description:

> *The patient with a left parietal lesion is moving the matchsticks slowly, perhaps commenting, 'I don't know how to put them', and eventually arriving at a simplified version of the design; while the right parietal patient moves the matchsticks quickly and makes a number of attempts to get the spatial arrangement, but without success.*

(McFie, 1971).

Figure 22.13 illustrates typical results obtained from patients with left and right parietal lesions (McFie and Zangwill, 1960). In several studies, an impaired ability to understand spatial, object-related concepts was found to be more prominent in patients suffering from right parietal lobe lesions than was the case in LH patients (Piercy *et al.*, 1960; Benton and Fogel, 1962; Newcombe, 1969). Nevertheless, other reports indicate that signs of constructional apraxia appear equally severely in RH and LH patients (Dee, 1970; Arena and Gainotti, 1978). Kleist (1912, 1934) believed that constructional apraxia was caused by a defect interrupting both the visual image of the objects as well as the mental programmes that guide the patient's movement as he constructs these objects from simpler parts (two-dimensional objects from sticks or matches, three-dimensional objects from simple building blocks). Because of the different data processing principles that guide the left and right parietal lobes in the construction of simple geometrical figures with matches, the patients' drawings (copying or drawing from memory) also differ for constructional apraxia caused by left or right parietal lobe lesions (McFie and Zangwill, 1960; McFie, 1975).

Tactile Function Disorders

A severe impairment of somatosensory functions in the contralateral body half are observed when a parietal lobe lesion affects both the upper and anterior parietal lobes. If the lesion involves area 5 as well as the upper-posterior parietal lobe areas, contralateral tactile perseveration, polyaesthesia and tactile hallucinations may also develop, depending on the extent of the lesion. These symptoms appear with or without hemianaesthesia. The sensorimotor integration necessary for tactile object recognition might also be impaired, which normally leads to astereognosia. Furthermore, the ability to orient towards one's own body may be lost on the side contralateral to the lesion (hemiasomatognosia). This is described above in the case of patient N.N. Anosognosia for the hemiplegia has been

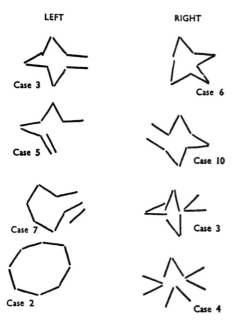

LEFT   RIGHT

Case 3   Case 6

Case 5   Case 10

Case 7   Case 3

Case 2   Case 4

Fig. 22.13 *Attempts to construct a four-pointed star with matchsticks in four patients suffering from left parietal lobe lesions ('left') and four from right parietal lobe lesions ('right'). The cases with right-sided lesions were taken from Ettlinger et al. (1957) (from McFie and Zangwill, 1960, by permission of Macmillan Journals).*

repeatedly reported, as well as the strange but not uncommon phenomenon in which the side of the body contralateral to the lesion is perceived as doubled (p. 439) (cf. Critchley, 1953). Allaesthesia is frequently observed in patients suffering from hemineglect of one body half: when mechanical or painful stimuli are applied to the neglected contralateral side, the subject's attention is directed towards the symmetric part of the body surface ipsilateral to the lesion. This finding indicates that the stimulus is perceived but incorrectly located. Dressing apraxia is a symptom that may appear along with hemineglect in the presence of a right parietal lobe lesion. It indicates an impairment of spatial orientation of the body as well as a breakdown in the planning of coordinated movements related to the body.

Topographic Disorientation

As already described in the preceding chapter, this may appear in RH patients when the lesion extends from the posterior parietal part to the occipital lobe. In comparison with RH patients, topographic disorientation differs characteristically in the presence of LH lesions. General, as opposed to local, familiarity with the extra-personal space is lost, and individual object perception is impaired on the left side in RH patients. In LH patients, however, individual objects are correctly recognized, and the ability to draw is not seriously impaired, provided no hemiplegic symptoms are there. Nevertheless, the relationship between objects and the ability to integrate these objects into a meaningful three-dimensional extra-personal space may be impaired. To illustrate this, we shall describe the case of a patient who suffered from an infarction in the territory of the left cerebral medial artery, which, in addition to other symptoms, led to spatial perceptual difficulties, but not to a pronounced right-sided hemineglect (Grüsser, 1983). This 53-year-old, right-handed woman had a stroke that led to an extended left parieto-temporal lesion: she subsequently suffered from transient spatial and temporal disorientation, a fluent sensory aphasia (Wernicke aphasia), dyslexia and a mild paresis of the right arm and hand. After leaving the hospital, she was unable to use her kitchen appliances and could no longer find her way from her home to different stores. She also had trouble getting dressed: not because of disturbed orientation with regard to her own body, but rather because of an inability to put on her different clothing items in the correct order. During the first months after the incident, she realized that she could no longer use numbers correctly, confused left and right and could not tell the time. She also experienced difficulties when using simple tools such as a hammer or pliers. The ability to eat with a knife, fork and spoon was not impaired, however. Nearly 10 months after the stroke, she reported that she still had great problems in

preparing a meal at home, usually mixing up the order in which she prepared the food. These signs of ideational apraxia slowly improved. Non-automatic handling of objects and instruments in the grasping space was severely disturbed, especially when one object had to be placed relative to another one. The same was true for the operative correlation between the spatial order of objects seen in the grasping space and the motor acts related to these objects. The visuomotor coordination necessary for directly pointing to any object named in the grasping space was not impaired, either on the left or on the right side, or in the case of either hand. She noted her confusion finding her way through her neighbourhood and in the supermarket where she used to shop. She had great trouble understanding the spatial organization of the supermarket and memorizing where dairy products, vegetables, meat, cheese, bread and so forth were located. Despite the serious difficulties finding her way through her neighbourhood, she did not experience a feeling of lost familiarity with the neighbourhood, which is typical for topographic agnosia. She reported having 'forgotten how to get to a certain place, such as a shop or her home', and not being able to integrate the percepts of the different houses or streets which were well known to her into a structural whole. The visuo-constructive disturbances in perceiving a meaningfully structured surrounding recovered to a much lesser extent than did her aphasic disorders. About a year after the incident, all that remained of her aphasia were some paraphasias and some difficulty in finding words. She had no problem guessing distances when looking out the window of the examination room into unfamiliar surroundings, or when performing the same task within the examination room, i.e. within the grasping space or near-distant action space. There were no signs of object agnosia, and the ability to name objects was only minimally disturbed. The problems that she had orienting herself within all compartments of a visually complex extra-personal space were mainly a result of the difficulty she experienced in matching the spatial percept with her spatial memory, or in putting together the details of information about the extra-personal space into a meaningful whole.

Anosognosia

This is frequently associated with left-sided visual hemineglect, as described above in the patient N.N. Dissociations also occur, however. In patients suffering from parieto-temporal right hemisphere lesions, unilateral neglect may become apparent in city traffic situations. For example, one of our patients, a professional singer suffering from a right, temporo-parietal brain lesion (caused by an intracerebral haemorrhage) that led to amusia, left hemiplegia and hemihypaesthesia, discovered this mild hemi-inattention when trying to drive his car again more than a year after the event. He noted that he had extreme difficulties judging what happened on the left side of the extra-personal space, and, as a result, decided to drive no longer.

Somatoparaphrenia

In rare cases, patients with hemispatial neglect and hemiplegia experience illusory phenomena in their paralysed left limbs; in particular, they believe that these limbs are being mechanically interfered with by somebody else. Gerstmann (1942) coined the term somatoparaphrenia for all such paranoid experiences associated with left-sided body parts in patients suffering from right parietal lobe lesions. Observations of this kind have been described repeatedly (e.g. Zingerle, 1913; Kramer, 1917; Pötzl, 1924; Ehrenwald, 1931, 1930; Schilder, 1935; Nielsen, 1937; Weinstein and Kahn, 1950; Nightingale, 1982) and are reviewed in Critchley (1953). We have personally observed somatoparaphrenia twice, once in a patient with a large right parietal glioblastoma and once in a patient who suffered from a right thalamic infarction (Landis, unpublished observations 1981).

The first patient was a 57-year-old locksmith who suffered from Jacksonian seizures, which began in the left arm 1 month prior to an operation for a right parietal glioblastoma. He was treated postoperatively with radiotherapy. He suffered neurologically from a left hemisensory loss and from a mild left hemiparesis that was most pronounced in the left hand. He was readmitted 3 months after the operation because of a regrowth of the tumour, which was indicated by the sudden onset of almost continuous myoclonic jerks in the left arm. The myoclonia disappeared under anticonvulsant therapy. The patient reported that he had episodes at this time of feeling a third, foreign arm on the left side growing within his paretic left forearm, which he considered to be something like a cast. This sensation usually lasted over a period of several minutes. Once this foreign arm had 'reached' his fingers, he had the impression that it inhibited his voluntary hand movements or moved his hand in the wrong, unintended direction. He believed that an unfriendly foreign will, which he ascribed to his wife, controlled this 'third arm'. Such experiences continued for about 2 weeks. The patient died 3 months later; a regrowth of the tumour in the right parietal and temporal lobe as well as in the corpus callosum was found at autopsy. This patient's history of focal seizure disorder suggests that the episodes of somatoparaphrenia were caused by the continuous, deep parieto-temporal epileptic discharges; this is evidently an uncommon cause of somatoparaphrenia.

The second patient, a 62-year-old clerk, suffered from a severe left-sided sensorimotor hemisyndrome and a severe left hemispatial neglect, which developed subsequently into a right thalamic infarction involving the internal capsule. When this patient was shown his own left hand, he considered it to be someone else's hand (usually that of the examining doctor) and refused to believe that it was his own. Hemineglect was clearly tactile and visual in this case. The patient would suddenly complain about other, unspecified enemies who imposed their will on his left arm and hand, supposedly moving them by means of a sophisticated computer program.

Visual Paraphrenia

This patient also displayed a similar paranoic reaction to the neglected part of the visual world. While observing the world or eating, he exhibited classical clinical hemispatial neglect of the left hemispace. A typical neglect of the left side also became apparent in his drawings; this was also the case when he was asked to use his imagination to describe well-known places in his home town (cf. p. 459). When randomly or experimentally confronted with visual, auditory or tactile signals appearing in his left hemispace or affecting the left side of his body, he consistently reacted to these signals; he perceived them, however, in the intact right hemispace (visual allaesthesia). Unlike our patient N.N. described above, this patient could speak with someone located in his left hemispace. Conversation with someone located in his right hemispace was also nearly normal (apart from a reduction in emotional responses, which is frequently observed in patients suffering from right hemisphere lesions). Conversation became distinctly abnormal, however, when the examiner entered the patient's left hemispace. The patient consistently looked towards the right, searching for the source of the voice with which he was talking; he became increasingly irritated and offered paranoic answers to the examiner who had 'disappeared' in the neglected hemispace.

Optic Ataxia

As already mentioned, the patients observed by Pick (1898), Balint (1909) and Holmes and Horrax (1919) all suffered from bilateral parietal lobe lesions. Visually guided hand movements were seriously disturbed in all three patients. This 'optic ataxia' (or visuomotor ataxia) may appear in the absence of the other signs associated with Balint's syndrome (Garcin *et al.*, 1967; De Renzi, 1982), or with only one dominant symptom (Hécaen and Ajuriaguerra, 1954). Bilateral parietal lesions are usually present when the performance with both hands and in both parts of the extra-personal visual space is affected (cf. Table 1 in Rondot, 1989).

Optic ataxia may, however, affect grasping movements in only the left or right half of the grasping space, and possibly in only one hand. In the presence of unilateral right parietal or parieto–occipital lesions, the left half of the grasping space is affected; only the right hand, the left hand or both hands may show signs of optic ataxia, however. This observation led to the hypothesis that the symptoms are caused by different types of lesions: one disturbing the perceptual aspects of object localization in the grasping space, the other the transfer of this information to the brain structures that plan motor intentions. Even a mismatch in the temporal coordination of these two distinct components of goal-directed movements would lead to optic ataxia, especially when delicate finger motions are involved.

A statistical analysis investigating whether optic ataxia more frequently affects the hand ipsilateral or contralateral to the lesion is difficult to perform, since unilateral parietal lobe lesions frequently produce hemiplegic symptoms on the contralateral side. The literature (especially the summary of findings in Table 2 in Rondot, 1989) indicates that a dissociation of optic ataxia is possible regarding either the grasping hand or the side of the space within which visuo-motor grasping is performed (for further discussion see Tzavaras and Masure, 1976; Damasio and Benton, 1979; Heilman et al., 1983; Levine et al., 1978; Vighetto and Perenin, 1981a, b; Jeannerod, 1985; Rondot, 1989).

Tests Used to Evaluate Symptoms of Spatial Hemineglect or Hemi-inattention

Observation of Eye Movements

As a rule, patients suffering from homonymous hemianopia perform less saccades into that half of the field of gaze corresponding to the hemianopic field. Kleist (1934) called this symptom 'gaze asthenia' ('*Blickschwäche*'); it was also described by Poppelreuter (1917) and Pfeifer (1919). Patients with pure hemianopia (without hemineglect) soon adapt and learn to direct gaze movements into the blind hemifield. Consequently, a patient with a unilateral hemianopia is able to read after this adaptation process, during which he learns to direct his gaze towards the blind hemifield. Such an adaptation does not occur in patients with spatial hemineglect. Their random, explorative eye movements remain strongly biased towards the side of the brain lesion, and their centre of gaze usually remains in the 'good' hemispace.

One can record the eye movements of patients by means of DC electrooculography, an eye camera or the infrared reflection technique. This allows for the study of the explorative strategies used by subjects presented with a large, complex visual pattern (e.g. Kömpf and Gmeiner,

1989). With this method, saccades (and head movements) towards the blind hemifield were also found to occur less frequently than towards the normal visual hemifield in hemianopic patients (Karpov et al., 1968; Chedru et al., 1973; Meienberg et al., 1981; Zangemeister et al., 1982). Of course, the better the patients had adapted to the hemianopia, the more they compensated for this bias.

Patients suffering from hemispatial neglect (with or without homonymous hemianopia) behave rather differently. As described above in the case of patient N.N., patients suffering from right posterior parietal lobe lesions do not initially cross the midline with their eyes towards the neglected side and also do not turn the head towards the left. When eye movement recording techniques are not available for a clinical exploration, the following simple tests are recommended: the examiner places 5 to 7 small, white paper dots on his own face and asks the patient to search for these dots (the face should be approximately 40 cm away from the patient). In this way, the examiner can observe explorative eye movements made by the patient; he can simultaneously test whether or not winking with one eye leads to a reflex saccade directed towards the winking eye. In patients suffering from hemineglect, one will, as a rule, easily observe a restriction of saccadic exploration in the attended half of the extra-personal space. One should then ask the patient to point to all the white spots on the examiner's face. One can again observe possible neglect of some of the spots. Finally, one may ask the patient to look at a certain spot on verbal command ('the one on the left cheek', etc.). It again becomes evident that patients suffering from hemineglect are frequently not able, in response to verbal commands, to perform saccades directed towards a given part of their extra-personal space. Testing optokinetic nystagmus (OKN) can be used to identify the patient's difficulties directing the OKN slow phase towards the neglected side. OKN may be evoked at the bedside by using a small, handheld rotating drum (Jung, 1951). Vertical OKN does not show any systematic changes in patients suffering from unilateral spatial hemineglect.

Using DC electrooculography, Girotti et al. (1983) recorded the eye movements of patients suffering from left hemisphere (6) or right hemisphere (16) lesions. Seven of the RH patients had a left-sided hemispatial neglect. The patients were asked to perform fast eye movements towards targets appearing in either predictable or unpredictable positions. In patients suffering from neglect, it was evident that they could not approach a certain target with 1 or 2 saccades, but could with 3 to 7 'hypometric' saccades. Spontaneous, explorative saccades made during inspection of objects and pictures were restricted to the side ipsilateral to the lesion.

Two-dimensional recordings of eye position led to further results regarding changes in eye movement strategies

(a)   (b)

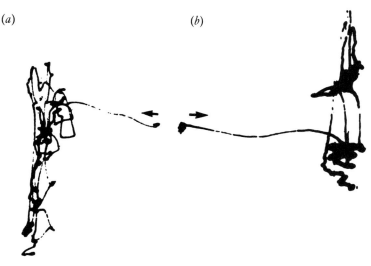

Fig. 22.14 *Two-dimensional recordings of eye position during the exploration of a complex visual pattern. The eye movement started from a central point in the printed visual pattern (marked by arrows). (a) Recordings from a patient suffering from a right-sided spatial hemineglect due to a left parietal-lobe lesion. (b) Recordings from a patient suffering from a left hemispatial neglect due to a right parietal-lobe lesion (modified from Jeannerod, 1987, by permission of the author).*

induced by parietal lobe lesions. Figure 22.14 depicts exploratory eye movements in one patient with a right (a), and in another patient with a left (b), parietal lobe lesion. Gaze trajectories were recorded during free exploration. It is evident that in both cases, the centre of gaze usually remained at the outer range of the part of the picture located ipsilateral to the brain lesion (Jeannerod, 1985). Similar data were reported by Ishiai *et al.*, (1989), who used the line bisection test in order to test the eye movements (recorded with an eye camera) of patients suffering from homonymous hemianopia (with and without spatial hemineglect). Hemianopic patients (without hemineglect) sampled the left and right end of the line with their centre of gaze before bisecting the line; patients suffering from a left hemianopia and a unilateral spatial hemineglect never searched for the end of the line in the left hemianopic field, and consequently made typical errors while performing the line bisection task. When forced to fixate on the left endpoint of the line, however, they recognized their error. This finding suggests interesting conclusions for interpretating performances in the line bisection test. Chain *et al.* (1979) reported that in patients suffering from left parietal lobe lesions the degree of hemineglect increased with the symbolic complexity of the stimuli, while this was not the case for right-hemispheric lesioned patients.

Not only hemispatial neglect caused by parietal lobe lesions but also hemi-inattention caused by other brain lesions (cf. pp. 460–461) led to asymmetric gaze exploration of the extra-personal space. Moser and Kömpf (1990)

described a similar deficit (as shown in Fig. 22.14) related to exploration of the contralateral hemispace in a patient suffering from a right frontal lobe haemorrhage.

Sudden local movement of high-contrast, small stimuli is an effective way in which to evoke goal-oriented saccades, because not only the retino-geniculate cortical but also the retino-tectal visual systems contribute to this elementary visuo-motor response (Chapter 3). When winking does not evoke correctly directed eye saccades during the examination described above, the examiner should put two fingers on the left and right sides of his head, and without saying anything to the patient, move the left or right index finger or both index fingers simultaneously. In normal subjects, this unexpected movement evokes a reflex saccade which can be easily observed. To increase efficiency, the examiner may place a white thimble on the tips of his index fingers. Patients suffering from hemi-inattention either do not respond to the movement of the index finger located in the field of hemineglect, show a delayed and incomplete response, or incorrectly direct their eye movements to the opposite side. As a rule, when both fingers are moved simultaneously, patients suffering from right parietal lobe lesions respond only to the finger moved in the hemispace ipsilateral to the brain lesion. When asked, patients report only having seen the movement within the normal hemispace (extinction phenomenon). Jeannerod (1985) reported that ocular saccades evoked by suddenly illuminated small targets were performed in the correct direction when the target appeared in the hemispace ipsilateral to the parietal lobe lesion. When the spot of light appeared in the neglected region, the saccade was delayed and was often incorrectly directed towards the ipsilateral instead of the contralateral hemispace.

Eye-pursuit movements can easily be studied clinically by using a pendulum, e.g. a plummet suspended on a string, swinging at about 0.5–1 Hz. The patient is asked to follow the swinging pendulum carefully with his eyes. Normally, sinusoidal eye pursuit movements are evoked. In patients with hemineglect, the eye pursuit movements either stop on the midline or continue with a few hypometric saccades into the unattended hemifield. Pursuit movements towards the neglected hemispace are sometimes of the saccadic type, while backward movements towards the normal hemispace are of the smooth-pursuit type. As a rule, when the pendulum is shifted towards the normal part of the extra-personal space, smooth, sinusoidal eye movements are evoked more easily in hemineglect patients, provided that the pendulum does not swing across the midline into the field of hemineglect. The patient is asked not to move his head during these examinations.

Poppelreuter's Visual Exploration Test

Poppelreuter (1917; Fig. 22.3) used a large vertical screen filled with numbers, letters and abstract signs. His subjects were asked to search for a certain letter, number or symbol, and to point with a stick to all these items. Many variants of Poppelreuter's test have been applied and are usually performed using paper and pencil. As a rule, 'visual cancellation', i.e. crossing out a certain type of target, is used in this spatial search test. Patients with a left-sided spatial hemineglect do not see all or many of the targets located on the left side of the screen (Poppelreuter's test) or on a sheet of paper, even when they are able to point correctly to the four corners of the screen or sheet of paper. The following variants of Poppelreuter's test have been applied:

1. All circles or crosses on a sheet of paper have to be crossed out (Fig. 22.7; Bisiach *et al.*, 1979).
2. A certain target letter, number or symbol equally distributed between other letters or symbols serving as camouflage has to be crossed out (Fig. 22.7).
3. Crossing out all or only certain lines (Denny-Brown, 1963; Albert, 1973; Villardita *et al.*, 1983) is used for a quantitative evaluation of unilateral neglect. Short lines of different orientation are drawn on a sheet of paper. The patient has to cross out all lines or only one type of line, determined according to orientation and indicated by a sample line drawn in the centre of the sheet of paper

(Benton *et al.*, 1975; Heilman and Watson, 1978; Vilkki, 1984).

4. One out of three simultaneously presented target words has to be crossed out, whereby the target word is positioned at random on sequentially presented cards (Heilman and Watson, 1978).
5. A modern variant of Poppelreuter's test, which uses more complex items, is the 'searching for animals test' developed by Gainotti *et al.* (1986): black-and-white drawings of 20 animals are placed on a large display board (75 x 50 cm), equally distributed on the right and left sides. Forty different animal figures are then presented on small cards to the patient one at a time; 20 of them are identical to those on the board. The patient is shown one animal at a time and is asked to locate the animal shown to him as quickly as possible on the large board and to decide whether or not it is present. If he is unable to find it then the next item is presented. Great difficulties in finding animals placed on one half of the board were reported for patients suffering from spatial hemineglect.

Line Bisection Test

This is a simple but intriguing test. Lines of different lengths drawn horizontally on sheets of paper or cardboard are presented to the patient, who is asked to bisect the lines and to mark the midsection. Best (1919a) observed that errors in this test corresponded to the perceptual displacement of the visual horizontal directions occurring in patients with parietal lobe lesions. Silberpfennig (1941) demonstrated line bisection difficulties in patients with frontal lobe lesions, which suggested 'frontal lobe neglect'. In normal subjects, Bowers and Heilman (1980) found small errors, which varied somewhat when the bisecting lines were placed in the left, as opposed to the right, grasping space. Bowers *et al.*, (1981), Colombo *et al.*, (1976), Schenkenberg *et al.*, (1980) and Bisiach *et al.* (1983) found the line bisection test to be an easy way in which to diagnose unilateral neglect. Halligan and Marshall (1989), Marshall and Halligan (1989) and Tegnér *et al.*, (1990) investigated how the error, i.e. the deviation of the perceived point of bisection from the actual midpoint, deviates from the 'real' middle as a function of horizontal line length. Their data (presented in Fig. 22.15) indicate that a simple linear relationship between this error and the length of the bisected line seems to be present in only a number of right parietal lobe patients. As mentioned above, Ishiai *et al.*, (1989) recorded the eye movements of their patients as they bisected the lines. Their findings indicate that the incomplete explorative gaze movement strategy is the main reason why errors in line bisection occur. We believe that further studies of this question are necessary.

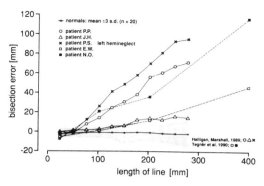

Fig. 22.15 *Results of the line bisection test in different patients suffering from right parietal lobe lesions leading to a left-sided spatial hemineglect. The error E (ordinate) is plotted as a function of the length L of the lines (abscissa), which should bisect. The data on the error E (shifting the bisecting point to the right of the midpoint of the line) are approximated by* $E = aL - c$, *where a and c are constants varying in different patients (data from Halligan and Marshall, 1989; Marshall and Halligan, 1989; Tegnér et al., 1990). Means obtained in normal subjects with standard errors are also displayed.*

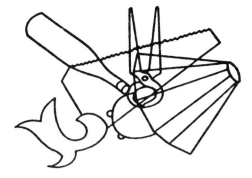

Fig. 22.16 *Poppelreuter investigated visuo-spatial perceptual abilities in brain-lesioned patients, in particular those suffering from occipital or parietal lobe lesions with 'overlapping outline drawings' of several objects. Many of his patients had problems in recognizing the individual objects, while he never found any failure in normal subjects (Poppelreuter, 1917).*

The Overlapping-figures Test

This is another simple test first used by Poppelreuter (1917; Fig. 22.16) to find visuo-spatial difficulties. In this test, simple outline drawings of common objects overlap each other. Poppelreuter wrote that not one normal subject had any trouble whatsoever in correctly recognizing the figures. This test was elaborated upon in Gainotti *et al.*'s study (1989) and was modified in order to maximize errors for patients suffering from unilateral neglect. Recognition of the objects was certainly more difficult because of the overlapping than was the case in the searching-for-animals test mentioned above. Six cards (14 x 21 cm) on which 5 overlapping figures of common objects were drawn were presented to the patients one at a time at a distance of about 40 cm. As Fig. 22.17 illustrates, the complex test pattern was composed of two pairs of overlapping figures and of a fifth figure that overlapped both pairs. The patient was asked to recognize the figures by pointing to identical figures drawn separately on a multiple-choice display presented in one vertical column below the overlapping figures. Patients with right hemisphere lesions made significantly more errors in their attempts to find individual figures on the left side than on the right side of the overlapping figure. This finding indicated local, object-related hemineglect rather than the global difficulties associated with the perception of objects in the hemispace contralateral to the brain lesion. In order to obtain enough data in this test, Gainotti *et al.* used five

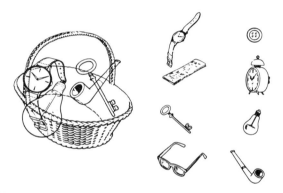

Fig. 22.17 *Modification of the test shown in Fig. 22.16. From the 5 overlapping outline drawings, 2 are placed on the left half and 2 on the right half of the figure. The fifth outline drawing is centred. The patient is asked to point to the corresponding items shown on the right side. In the test these items were placed in a vertical column below the stimulus pattern (from Gainotti et al., 1989).*

other overlapping figures similar to those shown in Fig. 22.17.

Similar to this test are those using hidden figures, such as the tests designed by Gottschaldt (1926) and later used by Thurstone (1944) in a general intelligence test (Fig. 22.18). Teuber *et al.*, (1951) and Teuber and Weinstein (1956) found performances in this test to be about equally impaired in LH and RH patients, but more errors were made by patients suffering from post-Rolandic lesions than by those suffering from pre-Rolandic ones. Orgass *et al.* (1972), Poeck *et al.* (1973) and Pizzamiglio and Carli (1974) found that RH patients made more errors on tests

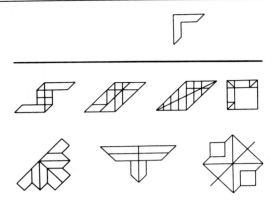

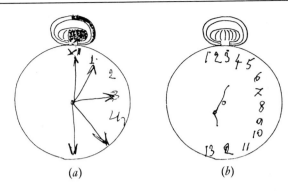

Fig. 22.18 *Example of the hidden-figure test of Gottschaldt (1926/1929) adapted for testing brain-lesioned patients (From Teuber and Weinstein, 1956). Patients are required to search for the simple figure, depicted at the top, which is hidden in all seven complex figures.*

Fig. 22.20 *Drawing of the face of a clock by two patients suffering from right parietal-lobe lesions. The outlines of the figure were given to the patients. They had to fill in the numbers and the hands, setting a certain hour. In both patients the left-sided neglect is evident, but different types of constructional disabilities are visible (from Bisiach et al., 1981, by permission of the authors).*

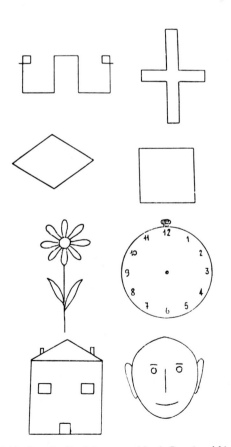

Fig. 22.19 *Standardized figures used by de Renzi and his group in testing the ability of brain-lesioned patients to copy simple shapes and figures (Colombo et al., 1976).*

using embedded figures than did LH patients. Corkin (1979) used this test to demonstrate transient spatial deficits in patients who had undergone unilateral or bilateral cingulotomy for therapeutic reasons.

Copying Simple Drawings and Random Drawings

Patients suffering from right hemisphere parietal lobe lesions are asked to copy a simple drawing; the right half of the copied object is usually drawn with much more detail than the left half. The same is true for drawing from memory (Figs. 22.4, 22.6). Most investigators (e.g. De Renzi, 1982; Colombo *et al.*, 1976) preferred using simple, clearly drawn abstract or concrete figures, such as those shown in Fig. 22.19. An especially interesting item for this task is the face of a clock. In most cases of patients with left or right parietal lobe lesions, this object is drawn oval, and the numbers are squeezed onto the right half of the face by all patients suffering from a left-sided hemispatial neglect. These errors even occur when an empty clockface is presented to the patient and the patient is asked to draw only the hands and numbers (Fig. 22.20).

Axial Symmetry Completion

This is a special drawing task in which patients either have to complete simple, partly completed nonsense figures mirror-symmetrically along a vertical axis, or have to complete simple, meaningful figures drawn only on one side. Patients suffering from left-sided hemineglect sometimes have great difficulties performing this task, especially when the figures are somewhat complicated. Figure 22.9

illustrates examples drawn by the patient N.N. 2 years after his stroke. He was not able to perform this task at all during the first weeks after the stroke. Two years later, when the figure was very simple, he could complete axial symmetric figures on both sides. When he was asked to complete a simple or somewhat complex half-figure drawn on the left side, his own drawings of the right side were considerably smaller, which demonstrated his 'compressed view' of the half-figure left of the vertical axis. He failed to perform the task on both sides for more complex figures. Hemispatial neglect together with constructional apraxia made this task very difficult for him.

Drawing simple, three-dimensional figures such as dice, pyramids or houses becomes an impossible task for many left and right parietal lobe patients. Inevitably, the central perspective required for this task is flattened to two dimensions. This inability to use central perspective cues for drawing has also been observed in professional artists subsequent to a right hemisphere stroke, e.g. in the drawings made by Otto Dix a few days after an RH lesion (Jung, 1974; cf. p. 446). Not only active drawing but also the ability to recognize objects from incomplete drawings (as in Gollin's incomplete pictures; Gollin, 1960) is of course impaired in RH patients. Again, from our experience, RH patients perform especially poorly when asked to detect errors in a drawing in which perceptual three-dimensionality is achieved by using the laws of central perspective.

Keyboard Tapping Task

Using a modified computer keyboard, Chedru (1976) and Gentilini *et al.* (1989) asked patients to tap randomly, but to tap all keys. Not surprisingly, they found that the keys located on the neglected half of the keyboard were tapped less frequently. Since the keyboard gives horizontal and vertical guiding directions, it is perhaps more advisable to use a smaller number of keys (e.g. twelve) arranged in a circle.

Raindrop Test

P. Brugger (Zürich, unpublished 1990) designed a simple test using the screen of a personal computer. The patient is asked to use the computer mouse to place many, equally distributed 'raindrops' onto the PC screen, which should be referred to as a window. Patients suffering from a hemispatial neglect distribute raindrops very unequally, for the most part ignoring the left side of the 'window'.

Looking-out-of-the-window Test

An even simpler test that may be used to discover visual neglect is to ask the patient to look out the window of the examination room (preferably at a park or at a well-

structured part of the city) and to describe what he sees. The number of items described in each of the four quadrants of the extra-personal space are recorded. As a rule, the number of items seen in the non-neglected extra-personal space and the neglected half should differ greatly. In our patient N.N., not a single item on the left side of the extra-personal space was described 3 weeks after the stroke. Two years later, looking at a different view out of the window of another examination room, the ratio of items identified in the right hemispace to those in the left hemispace was about 4:1.

Description of Mental Images

In addition to showing signs of a left-sided spatial hemineglect, patients suffering from right temporo-parieto-occipital lesions also experience impairment of their visual mental representation, as Bisiach and Luzzatti (1978) and Bisiach *et al.* (1981) have emphasized. In order to test this, the examiner should select an area well known to the patient locally. He then asks the patient to imagine this place in his mind's eye while standing at different points. Bisiach and his co-workers chose the Piazza del Duomo in Milan, the city's main square. Characteristic differences were observed when patients were asked to describe the Piazza facing the cathedral and then with their backs to the cathedral, looking towards the square. Under both conditions, RH patients suffering from left hemispatial neglect more or less ignored the left side of the square. This experiment indicates that the spatio-topic memory itself was not impaired, but that the ability to construct the mental image required the use of parietal lobe regions that were asymmetrically impaired. It is possible that the same regions that represent the extra-personal space are therefore also responsible for representing the spatial structure of mental images. After reviewing the literature and reporting on two patients observed by Levine *et al.*, (1985), Farah (1988, 1989) recently came to the same conclusion: the preserved or impaired aspects of visual functions are closely correlated to the preserved or impaired aspects of mental imagery. One of the patients, whose ability to localize objects was impaired, was neither able to describe the location of common landmarks in his neighbourhood, nor to imagine the location of major cities in the Unites States; he had no difficulty with his mental imagination, however, and was able to describe correctly the appearance of different objects, animals or faces. On the contrary, another patient suffering from object agnosia had poor mental imagination abilities for objects, but had no difficulties imagining certain spatial locations.

Poppelreuter (1917) also recommended testing a patient's mental spatial imagination to diagnose visuospatial disturbances. He used much simpler tasks than those used by Bisiach and his co-workers, however. For

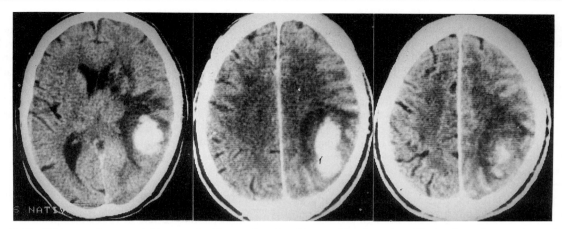

Fig. 22.21 *CT images of an extended intracerebral haemorrhage in a 66-year-old male patient affecting the parieto-temporo-occipital region of the right cerebral hemisphere. The symptoms of this patient are described in the text (case 2 of Landis* et al., *1990).*

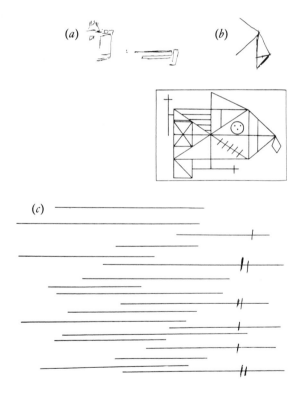

Fig. 22.22 *(a) Drawing of a house by the patient mentioned in Fig. 22.21. (b) Attempt to copy the complex figure of Rey shown below. (c) Line bisection test. The patient attended only to those lines that extended towards the right side of the page. His line bisections demonstrate serious errors. In this patient the error* E *was not systematically related to length of the lines, but depended upon whether the line reached the left 20 per cent of the page. All three tasks (a)–(c) illustrate a severe left-sided hemispatial neglect and (a) and (b) illustrate constructional apraxia.*

example, he asked his patients first to imagine a pentagon and then to imagine how this simple structure changes when a triangle having the same side length as the pentagon is added to each side of the pentagon. He observed that patients suffering from spatio-visual defects performed such mental spatial operations quite poorly; he also noted, however, that some normal subjects too had difficulties performing such a simple task.

One should be cautious when evaluating the findings of Bisiach and his colleagues, however, for even extremely severe hemispatial neglect need not necessarily be accompanied by a hemispatial loss of mental imagination. Landis *et al.*, (1990) observed such a dissociation in a 66-year-old, right-handed patient who suffered from a large parieto-temporo-occipital intracerebral haemorrhage in the right hemisphere (Fig. 22.21), which led to a left homonymous hemianopia, a severe left hemianaesthesia and a mild left hemiplegia. The patient was initially disoriented in time and space, a symptom that disappeared within a few days. This patient's most striking and persistent impairment, however, was his severe left hemispatial neglect (Fig. 22.22(a)). His attempt to draw his own house and garage on the third day after the stroke filled only the very right side and upper angle of the sheet, and the left side of the house was incomplete. This drawing also demonstrated constructional apraxia. Severe hemispatial neglect was also apparent when the patient was asked to copy the complex figure of Rey (Osterrieth, 1944; Fig. 22.22(b)). He continued drawing off the side of the page on the right side, and completely neglected the left half of the page. His performance on a line bisection test also revealed typical deviations (Fig. 22.22(c)). Despite the severe hemispatial neglect, this patient had not lost the visual mental representation of the left hemispace. When tested for mental representation with modified versions of

Bisiach's test, our patient described both sides of a well-known square in Zürich, and correctly described both sides of a road on which he imagined he was driving in both directions. While Bisiach *et al.*'s ingenious test of visual imagination convincingly demonstrated that hemispatial neglect may involve more than just impaired perception of the extra-personal space, this patient demonstrated that even with a relatively intact inner spatial representation, one half of the outer space may be left completely unattended. It is perhaps the coordination between the inner spatial representation and the mapping of the extra-personal space in the brain which provides the crucial differentiating action between these two types of hemispatial neglect.

Another test demonstrating hemispatial impairment of mental imagination was applied by Bisiach *et al.*, (1979). The pattern which the patient was asked to imagine was not seen all at once; rather, it was moved behind a narrow, vertical slit from left to right or from right to left. When the patient was asked to reconstruct the moving object, it became evident that there was neglect of the left side of the mentally constructed object image, as was the case for the perception of real objects completely seen at once. Ogden (1985) reached the same conclusion.

Digit Span

When we are asked to memorize the number 743981504 and are then asked to repeat it, we can perform this task by using either spatial or verbal memory. When we are asked, however, to repeat the memorized number backwards (405 . . .), we have to rely on short-term visual memory, or have to transfer the verbalized number into a mental image. Thus the mental operation required for reading a digit backwards should be particularly impaired in all patients who cannot produce a spatial mental image. Indeed, patients suffering from hemispatial neglect were found to perform this task especially poorly, as compared with normal subjects (Weinberg *et al.*, 1972; Robertson, 1990).

Mental Rotation Tests

In multiple-choice tasks, patients suffering from spatial hemineglect have great difficulty in finding pairs of simple geometrical figures in which one was rotated either in the plane of presentation or in a plane perpendicular to that of presentation. Similarly, finding nonsense figures of different sizes was easier for parietal lobe patients than finding nonsense figures of the same size that were rotated or whose mirror-image was presented (for further discussion see De Renzi, 1982, p. 178ff.).

City Location on Geographic Maps

Hemispatial neglect can also be observed when patients are presented with an unlabelled map of their country and are asked to fill in the positions of the most important cities (McFie *et al.*, 1950; Hécaen *et al.*, 1951). Americans can be asked to fill in the names of the better-known states (Morrow, 1985). Characteristic displacements of cities located on the left (west) or right (east) side of the map have been observed in the presence of left or right hemispatial neglect (Benton *et al.*, 1974). In our opinion, this test clearly indicates that both perception and the patient's conception of spatial relations are disturbed in hemispatial neglect. Marie *et al.* (1922) recognized this inability to develop a concept for topographical relations to be a parietal lobe symptom.

Tachistoscopic Tests

Poppelreuter (1917) wrote that patients with occipito-parietal lesions had considerable problems in correctly recognizing tachistoscopically projected line drawings or photographs of objects. They required much longer projection times than did normal subjects. Tachistoscopic presentation has the advantage of allowing for more precise localization in the left or right hemifield or hemispace. One can, for example, ask how many dots are seen on the flashed targets (1 to 5 dots), or about the orientation of a flashed bar (Warrington and James, 1967; Benton *et al.*, 1978). When asking for line or bar orientation, it seems meaningful to restrict the task to either vertical and horizontal, or to different oblique orientations. Umiltà *et al.* (1974) found visual hemifield differences in normal subjects asked to indicate line orientation. Since horizontal or vertical lines are easy to identify verbally (as opposed to lines of different oblique directions for which no simple verbal descriptions are available), uniform input conditions are present only in those tests where either vertical/horizontal or different oblique line pairs were used for testing.

Not surprisingly, reaction times for tachistoscopically presented stimuli in the left and right visual hemifields were found to be different in patients suffering from left- or right-sided spatial hemineglect. In normal control subjects, spatial cueing improves the response time as well as precision for the perception of stimulus patterns projected into the left or right visual hemifields. The same was found to be true for patients suffering from LH or RH lesions. In general, reaction times for such lateralized tasks increase in the presence of brain lesions. In LH patients this increase was about the same for the left and right visual fields, while in RH patients, this increase was greater in the left than in the right visual field (e.g. Baynes *et al.*, 1986). The spatial cueing paradigm was also used to manipulate visual spatial attention in the study conducted by Petersen *et al.* (1989). The correct visual cue was believed to shift attention towards itself and thereby to facilitate responses, leading in turn to shorter reaction times (as compared with misleading cues). The reaction times for patients suffering from parietal lobe lesions were somewhat impaired for correctly cued targets presented to the side ipsilateral or contralateral to the lesion. A considerable increase in reaction times was found, however, when the cue appeared in the unaffected (ipsilateral) part of the extra-personal space. Interestingly, the performances of patients suffering from temporal and frontal lobe lesions were also affected when tested for the different tasks and reaction times. The increase in response time was much higher in general in the presence of frontal lobe lesions as compared to other neocortical lesions. This was presumably caused by the well-known problems that patients with frontal lobe lesions have when a sudden change in conception with regard to an object is required.

Spatial Hemineglect and Inattention in Patients Suffering from Brain Lesions Located outside the Parietal Lobe

Lesions in the inferior parietal lobe located in the region of the right gyrus circumflexus and gyrus angularis (approximately Brodmann's areas 39 and 40) are the main sites that are found to be impaired in patients exhibiting the symptom of left spatial hemineglect (see the CT scan study by Vallar and Perani, 1986). The posterior parietal lobe regions are part of a complex neuronal network combining perceptual, space-related signals, behavioural intentions leading to a spatial shift of focal attention, and motor programming of goal-directed movements. There are bilateral connections of inferior parietal lobe structures with the frontal and occipital parts of the neocortex, the inferior temporal visual regions, the ventro-lateral thalamus and the pulvinar, the mesencephalic reticular formation, the basal ganglia and the different structures of the limbic system (which includes the gyrus cinguli, phylogenetically the youngest one). In light of these connections, it is not surprising that the symptoms of hemispatial neglect may also appear in the presence of lesions located outside of the parietal lobe; in this case, however, the type of hemineglect seems to be generally somewhat different.

Frontal Lobe Lesions

Frontal lobe lesions, especially when located in the dorsolateral and posterior medial part (including the supple-

mentary motor area, SMA) of the right frontal lobe, cause trimodal (visual, auditory and somatosensory) hemineglect, which is frequently characterized by a general increase in response time to stimuli of these modalities (Silberpfennig, 1941; Gloning, 1965; Heilman and Valenstein, 1972; Damasio *et al.*, 1980, 1985). When the frontal eye fields or the gaze region of the SMA are also damaged, gaze movements towards the contralateral side occur in the presence of hemineglect. Severe reduction in contralateral eye, head and hand movements also occurs when the SMA (located at the mesial surface anterior to the primary motor cortex) is selectively lesioned. Under these conditions, the abolished or reduced responses are, at least in part, certainly caused by an inability to direct 'motor attention' towards the contralateral hemispace.

Goldenberg (1986) described a double-sided neglect in a right-handed woman who suffered from lesions in the anterior two-thirds of the corpus callosum and in the adjacent medial frontal lobe structures. When drawing with her right hand, the patient exhibited a left-sided spatial hemineglect. Her performance on line bisection tests demonstrated a deviation of the left hand towards the left side, and of the right hand towards the right side. Verbal responses to pairs of simple geometrical figures, one tachistoscopically projected to the left, the other to the right hemifield, were restricted to the right hemifield. These findings also support the idea that the attentional components of motor responses, and not elementary, space-related visual perception, are the cause of this type of 'frontal hemineglect'.

Basal Ganglia

This interpretation is perhaps also true for hemineglect reported in the presence of lesions in the basal ganglia, which appears transiently in the visual and auditory domain (Healton *et al.*, 1982; Damasio *et al.*, 1979, 1980; Stein and Volpe, 1983). A severe hemispatial neglect was observed by Ferro and Kertesz (1984) in a patient suffering from a posterior, internal capsule infarction.

Thalamus

From the results of animal experiments, it seems that hemispatial neglect that develops subsequent to damage to the thalamus is mainly caused by lesions in the intrathalamic nuclei or in the nucleus reticularis thalami (Orem *et al.*, 1973; cf. Chapter 4). Watson *et al.* (1981) also emphasized the possible role of the nucleus reticularis thalami in 'thalamic' hemispatial neglect. Almgren *et al.* (1972), Watson and Heilman (1979) and Vilkki (1984) reported considerable contralateral hemineglect in patients who had undergone a right-sided thalamotomy in an effort to treat Parkinson's disease. Left-sided thalamic lesions led to bilateral neglect; the same was true, of course, for bilateral thalamic lesions. One should keep in mind, however, that Parkinson's disease by itself also leads to visual neglect: bilateral and left-sided Parkinson patients have reduced attentiveness for all new objects appearing in the extra-personal space (Villardita *et al.*, 1983). Ogren *et al.* (1984) described unilateral spatial neglect and impairment of unilateral eye movements in a patient suffering from a left pulvinar lesion. A pulvinar 'hemineglect' was also reported by Zihl and von Cramon (1979). These observations may be correlated to the bilateral anatomical projections between the pulvinar and the posterior area 7 found in monkeys (Mesulam *et al.*, 1977; Weber and Yin, 1984; Asanuma *et al.*, 1985; Schmahmann and Pandya, 1990).

Unilateral Cingulectomy

In primates, this leads to hemineglect, hemispatial agnosia and extinction phenomena (stumptail macaques; Watson *et al.*, 1973); frontal lobe lesions also do this (macaques; Latto and Cowey, 1971). As already mentioned above, Corkin (1979) observed transient neglect in psychotic patients who had undergone repeated cingulotomies for therapeutic reasons. Watson *et al.* (1974) also reported on unilateral neglect symptoms caused by lesions in the mesencephalic reticular formation of primates. The direction of the gaze palsy, which of course dominates in the presence of such lesions, depends on the side of the lesion (left–right for the prepontine reticular formation, up–down for the mesencephalic reticular formation; for details see Büttner-Ennever, 1988). To our knowledge, there has been no careful study of brain stem induced gaze palsy leading to signs of hemineglect. Similarly, patients suffering from vertical gaze paralysis in the presence of a Parinaud syndrome correctly report finger movement in all parts of the extra-personal space (unpublished observations, O.-J. Grüsser, 1959).

Alterations in Hemineglect and Hemi-inattention Caused by Vestibular and Optokinetic Stimulation

According to Cappa *et al.* (1987), Silberpfennig (1941) was the first to observe a reduction of hemi-inattention and hemineglect in hemineglect patients after vestibular stimulation. More recently, Rubens (1985) confirmed this observation using caloric vestibular stimulation. He thought that the temporary improvement in the patient's ability to perceive stimuli originating from the neglected part of the extra-personal space was caused by an ocular or gaze motor response directed towards the neglected side. Cappa *et al.* (1987) confirmed Silberpfennig's observations and also reported improvement in their patients' ability to point to distinct parts of the left side of the body. Pizzamiglio *et al.* (unpublished data, mentioned in Pizzamiglio *et al.*, 1990) observed a reduction in hemineglect or hemi-inattention in only some of their patients after vestibular caloric stimulation (iced or warm water applied to one of the external ear canals).

Since it is well known that the afferent and central vestibular system can also be activated by large-field optokinetic stimulation, it seemed worth while to test the effect of horizontal optokinetic stimulation on hemineglect. Long-lasting optokinetic stimulation induces apparent rotation in the direction opposite to the moving field in a stationary patient ('circular vection'; review: Dichgans and Brandt, 1975; Chapter 21). The advantage of optokinetic stimulation (as compared with vestibular stimulation) is the non-adaptive condition: as long as the optokinetic stimulus is rotated and the patient attends to the optokinetic stimuli or, even better, to a stationary target, horizontal vection in the opposite direction is perceived. When a subject is asked under such conditions to point towards the fixation target placed straight ahead at eye level, pointing deviates in the direction of the perceived vection, i.e. in the direction opposite that of the horizontally moving optokinetic field.

Pizzamiglio *et al.* (1990) used the line bisection task to test the effect of optokinetic stimulation on spatial hemineglect. Their patients looked at an 80 x 40 cm acrylic screen placed at a distance of 35 cm from their eyes, with heads rested on a chinrest. Random dots of light appeared on the screen and were either stationary or moved to the right or left at a speed of about 50 cm. s^{-1}, corresponding to about 55 deg. s^{-1}. The subjects were asked to indicate with a stick the point that bisected the luminous strip into two equal segments. As Fig. 22.23 illustrates, errors made in the line bisection task by normal subjects and by RH patients without neglect depended slightly on the speed and direction of movement; in the case of RH patients with hemineglect, errors in line bisection decreased during optokinetic stimulation of the left, neglected field, and increased during optokinetic stimulation of the right, non-neglected field. Thus a displacement of what was considered by the patient to be straight ahead occurred in the direction corresponding to that of the slow phase of optokinetic nystagmus. This observation corresponded to those made by Rubens (1985) and Cappa *et al.* (1987) using vestibular stimulation.

We believe that these findings are consistent with the idea that the network of the parieto-insular vestibular cortex, which normally monitors head-in-space position (Grüsser *et al.*, 1982, 1990a, b), is activated under these

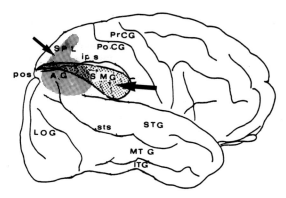

Fig. 22.23 *Schematic representation of the cortical lesions in the patient of Pierrot-Deseilligny* et al. *(1986). The lesion found in the left hemisphere is superposed (small arrow) to the wedge-shaped lesion (large arrow) on the right hemisphere to illustrate the overlapping parts lesioned in both hemispheres. This was the superior anterior part of the angular gyrus (AG) and some cortical structures around the adjacent intraparietal sulcus. On the right side the lesion extended into the supramarginal gyrus (SMG), on the left side into the superior parietal lobule (SPL) (from Pierrot-Deseilligny* et al.*, 1986, modified).*

conditions, and that it shifts the subjective coordinates towards the direction of the slow phase of optokinetic nystagmus. Neurones in this vestibular cortical region are also sensitive to neck receptor input. An obvious horizontal displacement of the fixation point by patients suffering from hemineglect should be expected when vibration is applied on one side of the posterior neck muscles (Biguer *et al.*, 1986, cited by Pizzamiglio *et al.*, 1990).

Bilateral Lesions of the Inferior Parietal Lobule

As illustrated in Fig. 22.2, Bálint's (1909) patient, exhibiting psychic gaze paralysis, optic ataxia and restriction of spatially directed attention, suffered from extended bilateral parieto-occipital lesions. As discussed above, however, the space-related symptoms of the Bálint–Holmes syndrome are most likely caused by lesions of area 39 and 40 located in the inferior parietal lobule (Fig. 2.27). This interpretation is supported by a recent report of Pierrot-Deseilligny *et al.* (1986). They observed a patient suffering from a two-stage infarction of both inferior parietal lobules. The initial left-sided vascular infarct led to a right-sided spatial hemineglect, optic ataxia, impairment of the OKN towards the right side, Gerstmann's syndrome and apraxia of the right hand. The consecutive infarct in the right hemisphere, which occurred 6 weeks

later, utimately led to bilateral visuo-oculomotor disturbances, bilateral visual inattention in the extra-personal space, saccadic dysmetria and major difficulties in performing goal-directed saccades and smooth pursuit eye movements guided by foveal stimuli. Horizontal optokinetic nystagmus was abolished in both directions; vertical OKN was not tested. The patient's ability to perceive visual movement was present for the whole visual field, but his movement perception was reduced in comparison to normals. He was able to perform saccades on command but could not direct his eyes by means of saccades to visual targets appearing within the visual field. His gaze was usually 'frozen' on the initial target. When with a certain degree of effort the patient finally performed a saccade to a visual target, this saccade was as a rule erroneous in direction and always dysmetric in amplitude. Consequently, the reading abilities of the patient were greatly reduced but no real alexia was present. The vestibulo–ocular reflexes were reported as normal. In contrast to Bálint's patient, the bilateral lesions found in this patient were much smaller and affected the superior/anterior part of the angular gyrus and some cortical structures along the intraparietal sulcus region in both hemispheres. On the right hemisphere the lesion extended into the supramarginal gyrus as illustrated in Fig. 22.23. In the left hemisphere a small wedge-shaped part of the superior parietal lobule was also affected.

The observations in this patient allow a more precise restriction of the critical cortical region related to perception of the extra-personal space and the control of attention and eye movements directed towards that space. Unfortunately no detailed distinctions between stimuli related to the different compartments of the extra-personal space were made in this investigation. The observations by Pierrot-Deseilligny clearly suggest that in humans, in addition to area 7, Brodmann's areas 39 and 40 or the access to these areas play a crucial role in the perception of and interaction with the extrapersonal space.

Multilevel Space Representation: a Neuronal Hypothesis

Before discussing the possible neuronal connections providing the basis for perception and cogntion of the environment surrounding us, we will perform a few '*Gedankenexperimente*' to illustrate the problems a neuroscientist faces when he tries to understand the neuronal mechanisms of space perception.

1. Let us assume that an experimental subject is blindfolded and transported for some time with many turns, ups and downs before he is placed in a chair in an experi-

mental room unknown to him. When the blindfold is taken off, he finds himself surrounded by a stationary drum with vertical stripes (Fig. 19.3(a)). When the drum begins to rotate horizontally to the left, the subject will perceive the rotation of the drum and experience simultaneously a stationary 'empty' space outside the rotating drum (about which he knows no details), which seems to form a continuum through the drum with the space surrounding him. The coordinates of the unseen and the seen extra-personal space are the same and are determined by the directions forwards–backwards, left–right and up–down of the subject. Up and down are dependent on the subject's ability to sense the direction of gravitational forces by means of vestibular and somatosensory receptors.

When the drum rotates for a sufficient length of time, the subject begins to experience horizontal circular vection (Fig. 19.1) and perceives the drum rotating to the left and himself rotating simultaneously to the right. Both rotations are perceived as occurring within the extra-personal space, which is experienced as stationary and coherent in the range between the subject and the drum and also outside the drum. As soon as visible objects within the space between the subject and the drum are present, however, they are included in the sensation of circular vection and are seen rotating with the subject. Finally, a third state is reached at which the subject sees the rotating drum as stationary within the extra-personal space and experiences full horizontal vection to the right, whereby the unseen space outside the rotating cylinder now forms a perceptual unity with the cylinder. Both are perceived as stationary when the state of full vection is achieved.

Assuming that the same experiment is performed in a laboratory well-known to the subject, the extra-personal space outside the drum can easily be imagined by the subject during all three experimental conditions mentioned. This known space is also experienced as coherent with the 'empty' space inside the drum, while all visible objects inside the drum are experienced as coherent with the chair on which the subject is sitting. This *Gedankenexperiment*, which we have performed many times as subjects or with other subjects, indicates indeed that under certain conditions circular vection induced by visual movement does not extend beyond the rotating visual pattern into an imagined space outside the cylinder. As soon as one perceives a small part of the space outside the cylinder through a small window in the cylinder, this part is included in circular vection (in this case the rotating pattern is projected to the stationary cylinder wall).

2. Let us now proceed to another *Gedankenexperiment*, which follows the same strategy but in reality would cost much more than the induction of simple horizontal vection as described above. Assume that the subject is transported into a simulated cockpit of an aeroplane and on the

windows of that aeroplane the images of a 3-D visual world are projected in a realistic manner. Whenever these images begin to move as if the aeroplane is rolling along the runway and taking off, within a fraction of a second our subject would perceive 3-D vection of himself and the simulated aeroplane. With adequate visual stimulation he experiences himself and his immediate extra-personal space within the cockpit moving through a landscape, and after 'taking off' our subject can look down to the ground or up to the sky and convince himself that the aeroplane is moving. Some additional realistic auditory and vibratory cues will facilitate this complex 3-D vection. This *Gedankenexperiment* is indeed performed in computer-controlled flight simulators. It also functions when the landscape is artificially generated by computer programs and contains some abstracting simplifications. The near-distant extra-personal coordinates left–right, in front of–behind, and up–down are transferred in this experiment to the perceived space within the cockpit and to the objects seen within that space, while the world outside the cockpit is considered to be stationary and to maintain, as far-distant action space (Fig. 21.1), the coordinates experienced before the 3-D vection began, i.e. the coordinates determined by the gravitational forces.

This experiment teaches us that real gravitational stimuli can be overruled by 3-D visual stimulation inducing complex 3-D vection of the subject, which does not move in space at all. It is not known how large the simulated cockpit must be before this illusion breaks down. During this 3-D vection we can move within the cockpit, gaze from one object to the other, tilt our head and body against an apparent 3-D vection-induced inclination of the cockpit, etc. In simulated complicated flight manoeuvres we even experience a sensation of dizziness. Accordingly, with adequate 3-D visual stimulation all other neuronal signals providing us with information about our position within the extra-personal space may be overruled.

3. When in experiment 2 a well-known landscape appears on the windows of the flight simulator, we orient ouselves immediately within that extra-personal space and can predict what will be seen next, since we match our actual percept with a stored image of a familiar space. What happens when in such a *Gedankenexperiment* space is projected mirror-symmetrically onto the windows of the flight simulator and we experience 3-D vection caused by these moving stimuli, while the familiar space seen is mirror-symmetrical and moving in the 'wrong' direction? What happens when the temporo-spatial sequence of visual images contradicts our stored information about the familiar space? To our knowledge no one has performed this experiment to date, but one can predict some spatial disorientation when the sequence of experienced space contradicts the sequence predicted from spatial memory. One can perform these experiments even better, of course,

in a car simulator and can ask the subject to find his way in the familiar but mirror-symmetrical extra-personal space. We assume that the subject will experience great problems in driving correctly, since matching the mental image of a familiar space with the actual spatial percept will be very difficult.

These three classes of *Gedankenexperiment* illustrate the complexity of neuronal mechanisms a scientist has to consider when trying to explain the neuronal processes controlling normal perception and cognition of the extra-personal space, processes which normally rely not only on visual, but also on vestibular, kinaesthetic, somaesthetic and efference copy signals. The *Gedankenexperimente* also illustrate that the three coordinate systems within which we can describe the experience of extra-personal space, namely the frames of retinotopic, egocentric (spatiotopic) and spatial coordinates, presumably provide only a rather preliminary model by which we may interpret neurophysiological and neuroanatomical data. As the reader can judge for himself, it seems evident that our mental image of a familiar space exists independently of the position from which we view that space with our inner eye, i.e. the mental image of a familiar space is invariant with respect to translation and rotation in an Earth-parallel plane. When we work and move within a familiar space, e.g. our home or place of work, the mental image of that space is transferred to an operational level at which spatiotopic (egocentric) percepts of this space are continuously and unconsciously related to it. We discover this correlation only when the real space has changed. For example when a large piece of furniture is moved to another spot in a familiar room, we immediately note the mismatch between our mental image and the structure of that space. As a rule, we note that change before we realize the type of change made. We think that when man acts within a familiar space this cross-talk between neuronal mechanisms representing the spatial and spatiotopic coordinate systems contributes to the degree of perfection at which we act within that space. With certain restrictions MacKay (1973) seems to be correct in his statement that our brain (and also the brain of other vertebrates) 'assumes' extra-personal space to be constant. In addition to the transformation between the perceived extra-personal space and our mental image of it, a continuous updating and evaluation of visual signals related to the extra-personal space but perceived in retinotopic cordination are necessary. Two different solutions for matching retinotopic and spatiotopic coordinates have been proposed.

Firstly, a map of the visual environment is created in spatiotopic coordinates by means of neuronal operations, as illustrated in the model of Andersen and Zipser described in chapter 6 (Figs. 6.12–6.14). Secondly, instead of this spatial coding the operations related to the extra-personal space are guided by 'vector-coding' (Goldberg

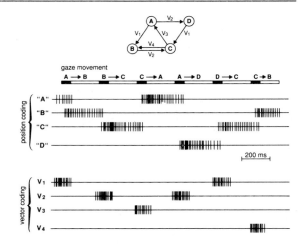

Fig. 22.24.   *Two different modes of neuronal coding of four spatial positions (A, B, C, D) selected for goal-directed movements. With 'spatial position coding' every neurone has a certain gaze field which is modified by the superposed visual receptive field, as illustrated in Fig. 6.13. The whole extra-personal space is represented by neurones having different gaze fields. With 'vector coding' each direction and amplitude of a shift in gaze or attention is represented by a distinct class of neurones operating independently of gaze position and relating their activity to the gaze movement relative to the position of the visual field centre (Figure adapted from Goldberg and Colby, 1987).*

and Colby, 1987). In this model gaze movements are represented by vectors relative to the actual foveal position, and the same is true for hand movements within the grasping space. The principal differences between spatial coding and vector coding are illustrated in Fig. 22.24.

In our opinion one is not forced to decide between the two models of extra-personal space perception, since both principles seem to be realized in certain cortical structures. A spatiotopic representation of the external space is present in some area 7a and 7b neurones, but this spatiotopic mapping seems to differ from the principles guiding the retinotopic mapping of areas V1 or V2 (see below). The coordinates of the spatiotopic maps are adjusted by gravitational signals mediated through the vestibular cortical areas, i.e. through the connections between area PIVC and 7b. The adaptation of spatial perception and motor actions, occurring in subjects wearing reversing prisms, indicates that the cerebral mechanisms of visual-vestibular integration related to extra-personal space perception are highly adaptive even in adults. Furthermore, it seems possible that the fine tuning of extra-personal space perception also depends on vector coding valid for the neuronal networks controlling spatially directed attention, gaze and hand movements. As emphasized by Goldberg and Colby

(1987), for example, vector coding characterizes the relationship between eye movements and frontal eye field neuronal activity. It is probably also valid for the relationship between the activity of prefrontal neuronal structures controlling visually guided grasping movements and the direction and amplitude of the grasping movements.

Perhaps vector coding and spatial coding interact with each other in area 7a and b. This may be illustrated by a simple experiment. As discussed above (Fig. 22.1), oscillopsia occurs – as a breakdown sign of the stability of the extra-personal space perception – when the eyes are moved horizontally or vertically back and forth at a maximum saccade repetition rate (2.5–4 saccades s^{-1}). Oscillopsia is greatly reduced, however, when the saccades are performed between three targets arranged in a triangle, i.e. along a saccade scanning path which requires a spatially preprogrammed commanded structure. In contrast to Goldberg and Colby, we think that vector coding alone is not sufficient to explain perception of the extra-personal space. How could we judge with vector coding, for example, that two objects, moving simultaneously at different places across the extra-personal space, are moving at the same or different speeds or in the same or different directions?

We believe that in Chapters 6, 19, 21 and 22 sufficient evidence is provided to support the hypothesis that at least three main levels of neuronal operations related to the visual perception of the extra-personal space can be assumed (Fig. 21.1). All three levels are in action when man moves through his environment and interacts with the objects of his world.

1. The afferent visual system including the visual cortices V1 and V2 maps the neuronal images of the visual objects into a retinotopic coordinate system and generates from the signals of the two eyes the 'cyclopean retinotopic visual space', within which the spatial relations of the retinal images are preserved. The spatial precision of this retinotopic space decreases with visual acuity, i.e. with the increase in the size of the receptive field with retinal eccentricity, and with the parallel decrease in the number of nerve cells representing a unit area of the binocular visual field in area V1 and V2.

2. The relatively precise retinotopic of area V1 becomes less precise step by step within the hierarchy of peristriate visual cortices: the size of the receptive field diameter increases with the rank of a cortical visual area in the hierarchy of visual cortice (cf. Chapters 4–7). This rule applies for the connections V1-V2-V4-TEO-TE(1–3) and for the movement-sensitive pathway V1-MT-MST-FST. The same is true for the connections of area V1 to area 7a via the different occipito-parietal visual cortices or areas MT and MST (Fig. 6.2).

3. It seems rather probable that within area 7a the extra-personal space is not mapped onto the cortical surface according to simple geometrical spatiotopic rules. If this were the case, one could expect the clinical symptom of neglect to be restricted sometimes to a certain sector of the contralateral hemispace, similar to a scotoma appearing in the visual field when a distinct part of area V1 is lesioned. This has never been observed to our knowledge. Cerebral lesions of the parietal lobe leading to neglect and/or inattention of the contralateral hemispace may be of variable severity, but always affect all parts of the contralateral hemispace. Therefore the spatiotopic representation of the hemispace in areas 7a and b should follow principles other than that of a simple spatiotopic geometry.

4. Since the occipito-parietal visual areas connecting area V1 with area 7a (Fig. 6.2) still exhibit some retinotopic organization, circumscribed lesions within these areas or some of their connections with area 7a will lead to 'local' disturbances in space perception. Indeed dysmorphopsias are observed as clinical symptoms when prestriate cortical regions are impaired.

5. How would the extra-personal visual space be represented within area 7a, leading to a functional spatiotopic organization, without a simple spatiotopic geometry? One could envisage, for example, as in the primary visual cortex, the existence of hypercolumns composed of many neuronal columns in which all nerve cells stand for a distinct direction of space (related to the 'centre' of the extra-personal space straight ahead at eye level) varying from column to column. Within a hypercolumn the individual columns processing data along different directions of the extra-personal space could be arranged either in a circle or side by side along a lattice. All nerve cells within a hypercolumn have receptive fields representing about the same distance from the 'centre' of the extra-personal space'. The whole extra-personal space would then be represented by a set of several hundred such hypercolumns, each one for one of the distances but all of the directions of the contralateral hemispace. It is not necessary for neighbouring hypercolumns to be responsible for similar distances. Neurones located in different hypercolumns but standing for similar distances from the centre of the extrapersonal space and/or similar directions should have close synaptic connection. According to such construction principles, an effective neuronal network is created which operates functionally as a spatiotopic map but at its outputs may also generate 'vector coding' necessary for motor actions related to the extrapersonal space.

6. We still have to discuss how the signal processing within the posterior parietal areas may be related to the different extra-personal space compartments illustrated in Fig. 21.1. Comparing single unit recordings from area 7a and 7b, one gains the impression that area 7a function is related to the perception of the far-distant extra-personal space, while area 7b neuronal activity is involved with action in the grasping space. We believe that during homi-

nid evolution a further differentiation in extra-personal space representation occurred together with the phylogenetic growth of areas 39 and 40 of the hominid brain: while the lateral part of area 7 of the human cortex (Fig. 2.27) is most likely related to the perception of the far-distant extra-personal space, areas 39 and 40 elaborate on object position within the near-distant action space and the grasping space, which in man is the space of tool-making and its implementation. It is within this space compartment that binocular stereodepth perception contributes most to the perceived structure of the extra-personal space. Furthermore, it is the part of the extra-personal space within which object-directed spatial attention plays an essential role in 'focal' amplification of neuronal activity, which depends not only on visual information but also on somatosensory, kinaesthetic and efference copy signals related to the movement directed towards a certain object which is manipulated or worked upon in tool-making or tool usage. Observe how the visual world of a watchmaker or a surgeon 'shrinks' to the object of interest on which he is actually working. Further careful studies in patients suffering from posterior parietal lobe lesions are required to learn more about the different representations of the compartments of the extra-personal space. From more recent clinical observations it is evident, however, that spatial neglect phenomena may indeed be restricted to one of the compartments of the extra-personal space (e.g., Halligan and Marshall, 1991).

7. Finally, the symptoms of type C and type D topographagnosia teach us something about the transfer of parieto-occipital signals related to the perception of the extra-personal space from areas 7, 39 and 40 to limbic structures. Connections appear to exist between the lateral parietal cortex and different structures of the limbic system, especially the gyrus parahippocampalis (Fig. 6.2). Destruction of the gyrus parahippocampalis, particularly in the right hemisphere, abolishes an essential function of spatial orientation, namely the more or less 'automatic' formation of familiarity with the environment. Simultaneously, the transfer between the spatiotopic representations of the perceived space and a mental image of that space stored in spatial memory breaks down in both directions and causes environmental agnosia.

Despite extensive experimental and clinical work on the cerebral mechanisms of spatial representation and topographical orientation, we think that Goldberg's and Colby's (1987) remarks are still applicable and that the 'reader [of this book] must bear in mind, the great, so far unbridged, gap between plausibility and truth in our understanding of spatial vision'.

23 Non-existent Visual Worlds: Afterimages, Illusions, Hallucinations and Related Phenomena

Introduction

In this final chapter, we briefly discuss a large variety of visual sensations that are not at all or only loosely related to the visual stimuli of the extra-personal space. These visual sensations range from the '*Eigengrau*', afterimages, illusionary or delusionary visual percepts, to visual or multimodal hallucinations that are perceived as 'real' objects or events in the extra-personal space. All of these visual perceptions are, of course, caused by corresponding changes in the activity of single neurones in the afferent and/or central visual systems. Microelectrode data, which are available for the more simple visual illusions, demonstrate the close correlation between visual perception and neuronal activity (cf. Fig. 1.1). For complex hallucinatory experiences and the perception of visual sceneries, this correlation is only inferred from more simple observations.

The following text is intended as an introductory review of these sometimes rather strange visual phenomena, which not infrequently occur when local brain lesions or general brain diseases impair the normal function of nerve cell activity in the central visual system. For a detailed description of visual illusions and hallucinations, the reader should consult textbooks on psychiatry or psychopathology, in which further literature on this topic can be found.

The *Eigengrau*

By relaxing in a completely darkened room and attentively observing his visual sensations, the reader can easily make the observations described in this section. In order not to evoke saccadic phosphenes he should avoid large eye saccades (Chapter 10). When sitting in an absolutely dark room, the subject realizes first of all that the extra-personal space does not appear dark black, as one would expect. After a few minutes in such a room, one observes moving light nebulae mixed with very tiny spots of light that rapidly change their luminance levels. Some people observe colours in their *Eigengrau* (Purkinje, 1823, 1825a). In the centre of the visual field, the average brightness of this *Eigengrau* is somewhat different from that of the other parts of the visual field. Depending on the state of adaptation, the region of the visual field centre corresponding to the fovea centralis might appear either somewhat brighter or darker than the background. This difference is a result of the fact that the excitability and the time course of the dark adaptation of the rod-free fovea differs from that of the extrafoveal retina.

The spontaneous sensation of the *Eigengrau* or '*Eigenlicht*' seen in the visual field in total darkness is related to the spontaneous activity of the nerve cells found in the retina and the afferent visual pathway (including area V1). The spontaneous activity of the retinal ganglion cells may be caused in part by thermic isomerization of individual photopigment molecules in the receptor outer segments, which leads to changes in the photoreceptor membrane potential identical to those evoked when a photopigment molecule absorbs a single photon and photoisomerization follows (Chapter 3). Furthermore, both the spontaneous release of transmitter substances at the synaptic contacts between retinal and cerebral visual neurones as well as the Brownian movements of membrane molecules may also contribute to the spontaneous activity of visual neurones. Finally, one should not forget the spontaneous oscillatory processes occurring on the membrane of the dendrites in nerve cells located in the retina or the afferent visual system, which contribute to the variation in spontaneous neuronal activity.

In the cat retina, the average impulse rate (recorded in total darkness) of spontaneous activity of on-centre ganglion cells increases with the duration of dark adaptation, while that of off-centre ganglion cells slightly decreases with duration of dark adaptation (Domberg, 1968). This change in average neuronal activity is presumably also present in the primate retina, where it corresponds to the perceived increase in brightness of the *Eigengrau* with longer dark-adaptation duration. Our interpretation follows a principle already stated in Chapter 1: for elementary visual sensations in the light–dark domain, the perceived brightness or darkness is closely related to the average impulse rate of the on-centre nerve cells and the off-centre nerve cells respectively found in the retina and in the afferent visual system.

Patterns and Scenes Appearing in the *Eigengrau*

Many but not all subjects report that after being in a dark room for a few minutes, they begin to see some visual structures appearing on the *Eigengrau* background. These structures are described either as partially geometric but rather variable and transient, or as simply structured figures usually visible for only a few seconds (Goethe, 1810; Purkinje, 1823, 1825a). The reports sometimes mention short, local flicker sensations that are correlated with the appearance of the above-mentioned structures. Spontaneous movement of the locally appearing geometrical structures, other figures or indistinct spots of light may be observed. Attentive subjects perceive these structures in the dark grey of the extra-personal space, but report that it is difficult to estimate the perceived distance of these phenomena from the observer. It is necessary that the subject maintains accommodation for far distance during such observations; otherwise, accommodation phosphenes, such as those described in Chapter 10, may appear. We believe that the spontaneous illusion of rather fuzzy and short-lasting geometrical figures is caused by a random fluctuation of spontaneous activity in the nerve cells of the primary or secondary visual cortices, whereby the nerve cell activity of the neurones located within a particular orientation column is synchronized. This synchronization spreads to columns of similar orientation preference in the surrounding region. The tendency for self-organization leading to coupled activation of nerve cells in orientation columns of the same orientation is also present in other illusionary visual phenomena, e.g. the

binocular phosphene patterns (Chapter 10). The hypothesis of columnar synchronization of nerve cell activity can also be used to explain the appearance of spatially patterned structures that one perceives when looking at a large, homogenous visual field flickering in a frequency range between 6 and approximately 20 Hz.

A considerable number of subjects perceive more than just fuzzy, geometrical, 'local' patterns in their *Eigengrau*. About 20 per cent report that when they remain for a longer period in total darkness, the *Eigengrau* organizes itself in the foveal region into structures resembling fuzzy human faces or human figures. The faces are rather schematic, as a rule, and do not exhibit any individual expression. They remain small and are visible only for a few seconds. Eye movement may lead to a change in the position of the schematic faces or human figures. The geometrical patterns, human figures or schematic faces seen in the *Eigengrau* appear colourless to the majority of the observers. Some subjects reported the appearance of 'colourful' light nebulae in the *Eigengrau*, however, especially when they became drowsy while staying in a dark room (sleep stage 1; Kuhlo and Lehmann, 1964).

The physiological explanation of these illusionary percepts rests on the same principle used to explain the diffuse *Eigengrau* and the elementary geometrical patterns. As already discussed in Chapters 13 and 14, there are extended occipito-temporal areas in the human brain with neurones that are specialized for the perception of faces, facial expression, human figures and parts of the body. We believe that the illusions of schematic faces and human figures appearing in the *Eigengrau* are somehow related to the changes in the spontaneous activity of these neuronal structures, whereby a kind of 'self-organization' of local activity, in which a large set of cortical columns is coordinated, has to be assumed. This activity presumably spreads from the 'face-specific' temporo-occipital neuronal networks back to the peristriate and even to the striate area, and induces an activation of visual neurons that is presumably related to the subjective perceptions.

From more than 150 questionnaires filled in by medical students asked about their spontaneous visual percepts before falling asleep in total darkness, it seems that the illusionary perception of schematic faces or human figures, as compared with any other meaningful structures, occurs with a much higher frequency during the early state of sleep (sleep phase 1). In addition to observations of the *Eigengrau* and diffuse stationary or moving light nebulae, about 40 per cent of the reports included descriptions of illusionary percepts, such as flashes of light, rudimentary geometric patterns (and movements of these patterns), human faces and figures, and short, indistinct visual scenes. Some reported visual movement illusion accompanied by vestibular sensations.

Afterimages

'Light in the dark' is not only seen as *Eigengrau* or as a phosphene caused by inadequate stimulation of the retina (Chapter 10); it can also appear as the after-effect of a light stimulus. In this case, the visual sensations are called after-images. The reader can easily observe a long-lasting after-image if he fixates for about one minute on a 100-W glowing light bulb located at a distance of about 1 metre in an otherwise dark room, and then closes his eyelids or turns the light off. When he opens his eyes in the dark room, he observes an afterimage of the light bulb which is generally a bright spot having the same shape as the light bulb and which moves with every saccade. When the subject looks at an imaginary point located far away, the afterimage appears to be large. When he looks at his hand in the dark approximately 20 cm in front of his eyes, however, the afterimage seems to shrink in size. When he looks about in the dark room, the afterimage shifts its position. Attentive observers regularly report that their eyes seem to move faster than the afterimage. This effect was used to measure the amount of time needed for the recalibration of retinotopic to spatiotopic coordinates (discussed in Chapter 22). The apparent changes in the position and size of the afterimage indicate that internal feedback mechanisms related to eye saccades and to the neuronal mechanisms of lens accommodation (including concomitant convergence eye movements) interact with the afferent visual signal flow within the central visual system.

When the light is turned off after the subject fixates on a light bulb, the afterimage changes its colour within the next minute. It appears bright yellowish at first, then reddish; it finally becomes darker than the *Eigengrau* for many seconds, may then again appear brighter than the background, and finally disappears after a couple of minutes, depending on the efficiency of illumination. When pressure is exerted on the eyeball for a moment, the afterimage may reappear after having disappeared in the *Eigengrau*. To our knowledge, afterimages were first described in Western literature by Aristotle in his book *On Dreams*:

> *And if, after looking at the sun or some other bright object, we shut our eyes, then, if we watch carefully, an image always appears in the line of sight wherever the eye is directed. It appears first of all in its own proper colour; then it changes to red and then to purple, until it fades to black and disappears* (359b).

Afterimages may last for hours when the stimulus is very bright, i.e. when one fixates on the bright sun for several seconds. Such long-lasting afterimages are accompanied, at least transiently, by degenerative processes in the photoreceptor outer segments; after several days, however, visual acuity may again reach normal values, which indicates regeneration of the photoreceptor outer segments. Sufficiently strong retinal illumination leads, of course, to destruction of the retina that cannot be regenerated, resulting in a corresponding local scotoma.

Long-lasting afterimages are predominantly caused by a change in the primary visual processes related to photopigment molecules, which leads to changes in the membrane potential of photoreceptors in which numerous photopigment molecules are bleached by the strong light stimulus. The changes in the afterimage that occur over a period of time might be caused by the enzymatic resynthesis of unbleached photopigment molecules. A strong light stimulus presumably also leads to rather long-lasting changes in the membrane potential of horizontal cells, and thus has some effect on the neuronal mechanisms responsible for light–dark adaptation within the retina. When one records the activity of single on-centre and off-centre ganglion cells (cat retina), changes in the neuronal activity of the latency class II (X-) on-centre ganglion cells increase or decrease during periods following exposure to a strong, long-lasting light stimulus during which the human observer sees a positive afterimage, i.e. a light sensation brigher than the *Eigengrau* background. As is generally well known, positive and negative afterimages, i.e. sensations where the formerly stimulated part of the visual field becomes brighter or darker than the *Eigengrau* background, follow each other in rather slow periods after a strong retinal stimulation. An increase in activity of latency class II (X-) off-centre retinal ganglion cells is recorded, which corresponds to the negative afterimage period.

A short flash of light ($<$ 10 ms) causes oscillatory light sensations. As illustrated in Fig. 1.8, one perceives a sequence of fast afterimages interrupted by short dark periods. These oscillatory afterimages are especially well observed when a bright light slit is moved across the visual field as the observer fixates on a small target (for reviews see: Fröhlich, 1921a, b, 1922a, b, 1929; Grüsser and Grützner, 1958; Grüsser and Grüsser-Cornehls, 1962). The perceived brightness and duration of the different afterimages following each other in fast succession (Fig. 1.8). The periods of the brightness oscillations of the local afterimage sequences, depend on the stimulus intensity and on the stimulus area. The positive afterimages, i.e. the sensations 'brighter' than the *Eigengrau*, correspond to the activation of on-centre retinal ganglion cells and on-centre nerve cells in the LGN and area V1; the short dark periods in between the afterimages correspond to a periodic activation of off-centre neurones, as illustrated in Fig. 1.8. Like perceived periodic afterimages, the oscillatory activation periods of on-centre and off-centre nerve cells change with stimulus intensity and area (Büttner *et al.*, 1971).

Silent Films without a Cinema: Scenic Visual Illusions (*'phantastische Gesichtserscheinungen'*)

The visual phenomena described in the following section remind us of the perception of faces and human figures that appear when we are falling asleep or are drowsy. In contrast to these spontaneous visual sensations that appear during sleep stage 1, the visual phenomena discussed in the following section exhibit a much wider structural variability: visual sensations that actually appear remain stable over a period of several seconds, and might organize themselves into long-lasting, meaningful visual sceneries. Such visual illusions are seen by about 10 to 15 per cent of normal adult observers, and are more frequently perceived by children and adolescents than by older people (Kroh, 1922; Czycholl, 1985). Johannes Müller (1801–1858), professor of anatomy and physiology at the University of Berlin and one of the leading physiologists of his time, published a book on this topic in 1826, *Über die phantastischen Gesichtserscheinungen. Eine physiologische Untersuchung mit einer physiologischen Urkunde des Aristoteles über den Traum.* Like other scientists of his time who were also interested in visual phenomena (e.g. Alexander von Humboldt, Charles Bell, Jan Evangelista Purkinje), Müller supported the general postulate that all visual percepts are related to simultaneously occurring excitations of certain visual regions of the brain. He referred to the mechanisms of the central nervous system related to vision as the '*Sehsinnsubstanz*' ('substance of visual sensation'), and argued that visual perception can occur only when the *Sehsinnsubstanz* is affected either by signals originating in the retina or by internal excitatory processes. Instead of *Sehsinnsubstanz*, we speak today of the visual areas of the brain. One of Müller's assumptions regarding vision was the idea that the cerebral processes related to vision could be activated by excitation of the retina as well as by mechanisms generated spontaneously or voluntarily in the brain itself. Although Müller thought that the *phantastische Gesichtserscheinungen* ('scenic visual illusions') of his book's title were closely related to dreams, he pointed out that they were certainly not identical with dreams, since they occurred in a wakeful state and were, as a rule, monomodal observations. The content of *phantastische Gesichtserscheinungen* was supposedly only in part modifiable by voluntary intentions. Müller was aware, however, that general psychic relaxation facilitated the appearance of such illusionary perceptions. After he had translated Aristotle's *On Dreams* into German, Müller pointed out that Aristotle had mentioned the *phantastische Gesichtserscheinungen* in this work.

Müller carefully described what he meant by *phantastische Gesichtserscheinungen*. These are illusionary visual perceptions experienced as a sequence of images and not as real events; they are observed not only before falling asleep but also when relaxing in a chair during the daytime with closed eyelids:

At the beginning of the observation, the dark visual field is full of single light spots, light nebulae, moving and changing colours. Soon, circumscribed images of a large variety of objects appear, which are initially seen in a mild shimmer and later on become rather distinct. There is no doubt that these visual perceptions are indeed self-luminant and sometimes also appear coloured. They move, are transmuted and are generated sometimes in the lateral parts of the visual field with such vividness and distinctness not normally seen in these parts of the peripheral visual fields. As soon as the eyes perform the smallest movement, as a rule, the visual illusions disappear .... The [illusionary] perceptions are rarely people with whom one is acquainted; usually strange figures, humans, and animals that I have never seen, illuminated rooms in which I never have been ... There is no connection between these visual phenomena and the experiences of the preceding day. I can see these visual illusions for half an hour before they finally transform into the images of dreams ...

Frequently, these visual images initially appear on a dark visual field, but the visual field may become lighter before the individual images appear, as if the darkness of the visual field were illuminated by an internal, mild daylight which is immediately followed by the structured images ... (Müller, 1826).

Müller pointed out that the illusionary visual images remained stable in space when he gazed across the visual scenery by moving his eyes. There seems to be a distinct difference between the *phantastische Gesichtserscheinungen* and the above-mentioned visual sensations that are observed during the state of falling asleep. Johannes Müller remembered having seen *phantastische Gesichtserscheinungen* as a child, and emphasized that he had always been able to separate these visual perceptions from dreams:

Repeated self-observation enabled me to facilitate making and maintaining illusionary visual percepts. Sleepless nights thus became shorter, for I was able to walk between the illusionary products of my eyes ...

Müller searched through literature for reports of similar visual illusionary perceptions, and quoted famous men, such as Cardano, Spinoza and Goethe, who had observed such phenomena. He repeatedly discussed the relationship between his *phantastische Gesichtserscheinungen* and dream hallucinations, but pointed out that the former were perceived during states of clear consciousness and wakefulness.

The probability that illusionary visual perceptions will appear increases when the observer suffers from fever. Children with high fever especially often report seeing scenic visual hallucinations. The visual scenery may sometimes be accompanied by auditory illusions; the transition from vivid imagery into multimodal hallucinations seems to be rather smooth. The following is a report of complex visual scenes similar to *phantastische Gesichtserscheinungen* that were perceived by a young physician while suffering from high fever:

I was suffering from a serious case of the flu and from inflammation of the tonsils and stayed in bed because of high fever. I observed phenomena that I never perceived before or after this occasion. As soon as I closed my eyelids, I saw colourful visual scenes composed of sequences of images and partly accompanied by sounds and voices. I cannot remember the meaning of what I heard, although I well remember the content of the visual scenes. These were predominantly of men at work on a conveyer belt in a large factory hall. I have never worked under such conditions.

The individual image sequences lasted for only a few seconds and changed rather abruptly into other visual scenes of similar vividness but with different content. I could not make out any meaningful connections between the successive scenes. I observed the whole visual illusion as a sort of modern video-art; I was always aware of the "movie quality" and unrealistic character of the visual scenes that I saw. All the scenes that I saw, however, were not deformed, but appeared in a rather "realistic" fashion. As soon as I opened my eyes, all images and the accompanying auditory noise immediately disappeared and the normal surroundings of the room became clearly visible to me. When I closed my eyelids again, the illusionary visual scenery continued, however, after a delay of about one second. I remember that I remained in this state for about one to two hours. Until today, I have never experienced a similar observation; I believe, however, that I have a good visual imagination, since I can see images of photographs or previously seen scenes very well, and can even look around in these mental pictures ...

One of us (O.-J. G.) found in experiments with this subject that he did indeed possess a very good eidetic ability. After inspecting a painting or any other complex picture by means of saccadic eye movements for about 30 seconds, he could look at a white wall and 'see' the image for about a minute in somewhat faint colours. When asked to describe these eidetic images, he performed saccadic eye movements across the 'projection plane' without perceiving any apparent shift in the projected mental image. He could move his head and body and 'project' the mental image onto another wall of the room, however. It seems rather likely that the ability to see 'eidetic' images ('*subjective optische Anschauungsbilder*'; Urbantschitsch, 1907) is closely related to the ability to see illusionary visual scenes spontaneously.

Johannes Müller's '*phantastische Gesichtserscheinungen*' and related visual phenomena are evidently a result of the self-organizing, spontaneous activity of visual memory mechanisms. One can only speculate about the neurophy-

siological basis of these phenomena: presumably they are produced when the hippocampal and other limbic structures related to visual memory interact closely with the temporal lobe neurones. Since the subject can 'inspect' the perceived visual scenery, as eidetic subjects can gaze about their eidetic after-sensations, the essential mechanisms leading to illusionary visual perception involve the activity of cerebral structures that process the signals in spatiotopic or spatial coordinates and not in retinotopic coordinates (cf. Chapter 22). Thus the primary visual cortex and the higher-order visual association cortices which are still organized in a retinotopic fashion are certainly not the structures that are primarily activated and thereby generate these complex visual scenes. One should not, however, exclude the possibility that 'backward' projections from visual memory areas and spatiotopic organized temporo-parietal association cortices to the visual association cortices in the occipital lobe accompany scenic visual illusions.

To Be or Not to Be: Visual Patterns and Scenes Generated from Meaningless Random Stimuli

A rather fuzzy random structure in part of the visual field might trigger cerebral visual mechanisms, which leads to the perception of figures or scenes. One class of such visual illusions is the pareidolias (Jaspers, 1953), which were well described by Müller (1826). He believed that they were 'creations of the plasticity of the visual phantasy':

During my childhood years, I was frequently fooled by the plasticity of the phantasy .... I remember one such event especially vividly. I gazed out of the living-room window in my parents' home at the house located on the other side of the street. This house had a rather old exterior, and the whitewash on the walls of this house was rather dark in some spots; in other parts, entire chunks had disappeared, and older layers of paint became visible. When I was not allowed to leave the room, I kept myself busy for several hours a day looking through the window at the sooty, decaying walls. I was then able to see several faces in the outlines of the decaying or remaining whitewash, which, when repeatedly observed, took on the appearance of different facial expressions (Müller, 1826).

This description illustrates one of the most frequently occurring illusionary perceptions that takes place when one gazes at unstructured, fuzzy visual patterns: in many subjects, faces or human figures are the most common illusionary percepts. The mechanisms which account for such illusionary visual perceptions are examined in the Rorschach test. The subject is asked to find meaningful visual patterns on the test tables, which contain black or coloured ink-blots having some axial symmetry. These blots are generally just rather fuzzy structures. Some psychologists still believe that characterological judgements can be made based on the illusionary perceptions seen by patients in these ink-blots. Responses, which are called 'interpretations', are categorized according to location (which part of the ink-blot is used) and 'structural determinants' such as colour, shading and inferred movement. In addition, the content of the pareidolias (e.g. faces, human figures, animals, plants, landscapes, etc.) are evaluated (Rorschach, 1942, 1950; Bohm, 1951; Klopfer and Davidson, 1962).

The physician and poet Justinus Kerner (1787–1862) used such ink-blots (*'Kleksographien'*) to inspire his poetic imagination (Fig. 23.1). Leonardo da Vinci also seems to have seen such pareidolic visual percepts, since he recommended to his pupils in his *Book on Painting* to study pareidolias in order to increase their artistic visual phantasy (Ludwig, 1882):

> *I will not hesitate to add to these descriptions a newly discovered method of visual perception, which appears to some people as irrelevant or even ridiculous; nevertheless, this method is very useful in evoking rather variable visual perceptions. This method is nothing other than looking at a wall covered with many spots of variable size or at a stone wall. Whenever you have to invent scenery, you can see scenes on such backgrounds which remind you of different landscapes composed of different types of mountains, rivers, rocks, trees, large planes, valleys and hills. You might see scenes of battles, strange and alien figures in vivid positions with different facial expressions, costumes and innumerable things whose forms you can later draw perfectly . . . .*

Visual illusionary perceptions are also triggered by dynamic random noise, e.g. when one looks at the visual noise of a blank television screen. The most frequent illusionary perceptions reported by subjects under such simple stimulus conditions are faces or small human figures.

Pareidolias and similar illusionary visual sensations are evidently triggered by rather fuzzy and weakly structured visual input signals, which are processed by several neuronal systems tuned to recognize certain orientations or shapes. The 'face-specific' neuronal structures in the temporo–occipital lobe region (as discussed in Chapters 7 and 14) are evidently especially sensitive to such 'noisy' visual input signals; they 'create' illusionary perceptions from these signals.

The activity of the face-specific visual regions is closely related to emotional state, mediated by limbic structures presumably through the gyrus parahippocampalis. Therefore, increased emotionality as well as increased body temperature may lead to misperception of the 'real' visual world. Such experiences also occur with drug use

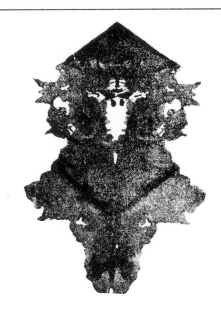

𝕯iese Bilder aus dem Hades,
Alle schwarz und schauerlich,
(Geister sind's, sehr niedern Grades,)
Haben selbst gebildet sich
Ohn' mein Zuthun, mir zum Schrecken,
Einzig nur — aus Tintenflecken.
Habe stets dabei gedacht,
Ueberall wo's schwarz und Nacht

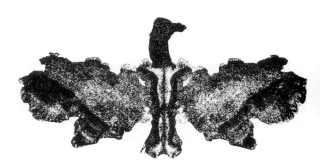

Fig. 23.1 *Two 'kleksographs' that were used by the south German poet and physician Justinus Kerner (1786–1862) as the visual inspiration for short poems (from Kerner, 1890; cf. Grüsser, 1987a).*

(LSD, mescaline, cannabis). The German poet J. W. von Goethe (1749–1832) described just such an experience in his poem '*Der Erlkönig*', perhaps known to some readers through Schubert's song: '*Wer reitet so spät durch Nacht und Wind*'. The feverish child described in this poem experiences severe visual and auditory illusions when riding on a horse with his father across a fen faintly illuminated by moonlight. The illusionary changes in the visual perceptions are facilitated by the fuzzy outlines of the objects seen in scotopic vision. Similarly, subjects who have taken drugs such as those mentioned above report having seen faces in amorphic visual structures; they also perceived unrealistic changes in the facial expressions of others, described as 'paraprosopia' in Chapter 15.

Light Sensations Produced by Inadequate Stimulation of the Retina and the Central Visual System: Phosphenes and Photisms

It is possible to activate the neurones of the retina and the central visual system by means of inadequate stimuli such as mechanical deformation, electrical or magnetic stimuli, drugs, etc. Such stimuli usually produce unstructured or low-level structured light sensations called phosphenes. Phosphenes are non-figural achromatic or coloured light sensations. They are generated within the retina, the afferent visual system or that part of the central visual system which still has a strong retinotopic organization. Phosphenes therefore change their position in the extrapersonal space with eye and gaze movements; they are 'stabilized' within the neuronal representation of the visual field. Similar to phosphenes are photisms, which are evoked by abnormal stimulation of the visual cortical areas beyond area V1. They are characterized by spatially organized structures, i.e. geometric or semi-geometric periods and repetitions. Some patients report having perceived transient geometrical colours appearing in the *Eigengrau* or 'above' the natural visual background. Phosphenes and photisms are described in detail in Chapter 10, and are therefore not discussed again in detail in this short review.

Deep Shadows: Obscurations of the Visual World

When one looks at a homogeneous white background or at the sky and presses both eyes with two fingers from the temporal side with sufficient strength, the visual world changes its appearance within 10 to 15 seconds: it becomes greyish (finally dark grey), and all visual structures disappear. Because of the deformation of the retina, some phosphenes may be present on the dark grey background (Chapter 10). These phosphenes are seen on a darkened background, which obscures all visual input. Eyeball deformation leads to increased intraocular pressure near or even above the blood pressure level, which in turn leads to a transient ischaemia of the retina, because the perfusion pressure, i.e. the difference between the arterial blood pressure and the intraocular pressure, drops to zero. Furthermore, the retina is stretched and the phenomena mentioned in Chapter 10, are evoked.

A decrease in retinal perfusion pressure occurs without eyeball deformation when the arterial blood pressure decreases considerably below normal values. When the difference between the mean arterial blood pressure and the intraocular pressure reaches approximately 40 mmHg, the blood supply to the retina is not sufficient. If blood pressure drops further, one suffers an obscuration of the visual world before one faints. Darkening of the visual field occurs several seconds before fainting, since the perfusion pressure of the brain is higher than the perfusion pressure of the eye, because the venous blood pressure of the brain is below 4 mmHg while the intraocular pressure is normally between 17 and 19 mmHg, regardless of body position. When one carefully observes the obscurations that precede fainting, one realizes that even without eyeball indentation, the obscuration is sometimes accompanied by diffuse light sensations that superpose the darkening of the visual field. One of the authors (O.-J. G.) made such observations experimentally 40 years ago while working as a young student in a factory. After he had painted machine parts located near the ground with a varnish containing vasodilative substances as a solvent, his blood pressure regularly fell to very low levels when he straightened himself into an upright position. In order to prevent himself from fainting, he placed a stool nearby. When sitting on the stool, he could observe the obscurations of his visual field about 15 to 20 times a day. At least half of the obscurations were accompanied by certain local, unstructured illuminations in the darkened field. These observations led to experiments 25 years later in which the activity of single ganglion cells was recorded in anaesthetized cats as the intraocular pressure was slowly raised by means of a cannula located in the anterior eye chamber which was connected to a pressure system (Grehn *et al.*, 1984). In this way, the effect of a decrease in retinal perfusion pressure on retinal ganglion cell activity became measurable. As Fig. 23.2(a) illustrates, the neuronal activity decreased with an increase in intraocular pressure whenever the perfusion pressure was below 40 mmHg. In about 10 per cent of these experiments, transient ischaemic activity was produced in both the on-centre and off-centre ganglion cells before the neuronal response ceased (Fig. 23.2(b)). The recovery period for neuronal activity was approximately proportionate to the duration of total retinal ischaemia. In pentobarbital anaesthesia, the retinal ganglion cells of cats tolerated at least 45 minutes of total ischaemia; after a recovery time of about

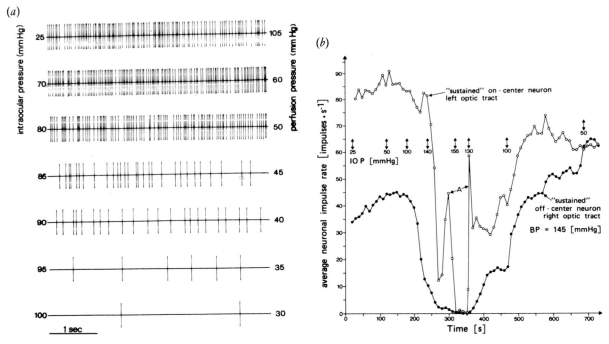

Fig. 23.2 *(a) Recording of an off-centre ganglion cell of the cat retina (pentobarbital anaesthesia). Activity was maintained at different levels of elevated intraocular pressure (left side). Steady illumination of the receptive field and its greater surroundings by a light stimulus of 15 degrees diameter and 35 cd m⁻². The mean arterial blood pressure was 130 mmHg. The perfusion pressure is given on the right side. The intraocular pressure was slowly increased within a period of several minutes. Note the degrees of neuronal activity when the perfusion pressure fell below 50 mmHg. (b) Simultaneous recording of the activity of two retinal ganglion cells (two microelectrodes in the optic tract) of the cat retina (pentobarbital anaesthesia). A step-like change in intraocular pressure was applied, as indicated. The average arterial blood pressure was 145 mmHg. The impulse rates of a latency class II off-centre neurone (dots) and a simultaneously recorded latency class II on-centre neurone (circles) are plotted as a function of time. The two peaks during total retinal ischaemia appearing in the activity of the on-centre retinal ganglion cell are caused by high-frequency activation lasting 2 and 3 seconds respectively. Except for this ischaemic short-time activation present only in the on-centre neurone, the course of activity changes was parallel in the on-centre and off-centre neurone (from Grehn* et al., *1984).*

45 to 60 minutes, their functions appeared to be normal again.

The obscuration of the visual world has probably been experienced by many of those readers who suffer from low blood pressure. There are other types of obscurations of the visual world, however, which are not caused by retinal ischaemia but by direct cerebral dysfunctions. Transient obscurations are reported by patients with papilloedema because of increased intracranial pressure (Gloning *et al.*, 1968). Obscurations resulting from local cerebral ischaemia may be restricted to one half of the visual field; they indicate a temporary insufficiency of blood flow through the posterior cerebral arteries. Bilateral obscurations of the whole visual field may occur because of insufficient blood flow through the vertebral–basilar artery. They are then prodromes of hemianopia or cortical blindness. Obscurations in parts of the visual field are also reported, how-

ever, by patients suffering from temporal, parietal or even frontal lobe lesions. The highest incidence occurs in the presence of occipital lobe lesions. Wieser (1985) observed a patient who reported an 'obscuration of the horizon' during epileptic discharges in the temporal lobe (2 in Fig. 23.3(a)). Gloning *et al.* (1968) reviewed the data of 708 brain-lesioned patients and found 61 with occipital lesions who suffered from obscurations. Only 11 who had lesions not involving occipital regions also reported sudden transient darkenings within the visual field. Several authors (Gruner and Hoff, 1929; Meyerhofer, 1942; Gloning and Hayden, 1953; Gloning *et al.*, 1968) used caloric stimulation of the labyrinths to provoke obscurations or other distortions of vision. Because this stimulation also affects the blood pressure and therefore the cerebral perfusion pressure, this type of experimentally provoked obscured vision cannot simply be attributed to direct neuronal vestibular effects interacting with the responses of nerve cells found in the visual cortex.

Visual Perseveration: Palinopsia

Retinal afterimages have already been described in this chapter. Long-lasting retinal afterimages are mainly caused by changes in the primary photochemical processes and in the connected membrane processes in the photoreceptors. There is a class of visual phenomena which can be considered to consist of 'afterimages' of cerebral origin. Because of pathological changes in the central visual system, the visual images may persist rather distinctly after the visual pattern is removed. A normal correlate of visual persistence is the observation of mental images ('*subjectiv-optische Anschauungsbilder*'; Urbantschitsch, 1907) already mentioned above. Pathological visual persistence or the recurrent appearance of visual images after the stimulus has disappeared is called visual perseveration or palinopsia. As a rule, palinopsia is associated with lesions of the occipital or occipito-temporal visual association areas. Frequently, patients suffering from palinopsia also suffer from temporal lobe epilepsia (cf. Wieser, 1982). Michel and Troost (1980), for example, reported on several patients suffering from palinopsia whose brain lesions could be diagnosed by means of computer tomography. We can illustrate palinopsia with the cases of two patients reported on by Michel and Troost, as follows:

1. A 71-year-old woman was admitted to their neurology department after complaining about 'seeing multiple objects'. Five days before admittance, she suffered from severe vomiting without vertigo or any other ailments. Two days later, she noted that each person she saw had the face of someone she had just seen on television. Some time later, she peeled a banana and then saw for a couple of minutes vivid images of half-peeled bananas on the wall of her living room. She realized that these hallucinations were only images and not real (i.e. were pseudo-hallucinations). Computerized tomography revealed a large area of decreased density in the right occipital lobe, presumably caused by an infarction.

2. Three weeks before admission to the hospital, their second patient suffered from an acute left-sided headache, observed 'blurriness' in the left visual field and 'twirling' object movement. Several minutes after watching television, he saw the features of a face seen on television in the faces of the people present in the room. Computer tomography also revealed changes in the right occipital region, which indicated an infarction of the right occipital lobe. This was later verified by angiography. Figure 14.6 illus-

trates palinopsia in a patient suffering from prosopagnosia. All human faces that she saw were transformed into poodle faces after she had looked for less than a minute at a poodle accompanying a passenger in the tram.

The term *palinopsia* was coined by Pötzl (1954). Other cases of it have been described by Critchley (1951, 1953), Bender (1963), Bender *et al.* (1968), Meadows and Munro (1977), Cleland *et al.* (1981), Cummings *et al.* (1982) and Kömpf *et al.* (1983). Palinopsia is sometimes associated with temporal lobe epilepsy (Robinson and Watt, 1947; Swash, 1979). Palinopsia may also be associated with cerebral polyopia, i.e. multiple, simultaneous percepts of the same object not caused by retinal double images (Bekeny and Peter, 1961; Gloning *et al.*, 1968). In one patient examined by Pötzl (1954), palinopsia was evoked only when the patient gazed upwards. Pötzl therefore assumed that directing the gaze in one critical direction was one of the factors causing palinopsia.

Palinopsia is presumably evoked by maintained neuronal activity in higher-order visual association cortices. One must take into consideration a possible feedback mechanism between area V2 and the higher-order visual cortices, because palinopsia was restricted to rather distinct visual features, such as faces, in some of the cases reported.

Multiplication of Visual Objects: Polyopia

Polyopia is the simultaneous multiple perception of the same object or visual structure. As a rule, polyopia is restricted to foveal vision. Although it may occur at the beginning of a classical migraine attack, it seems otherwise to be a sign of occipital brain lesions. One of the authors (O.-J. G.) observed a patient who had suffered from a closed head trauma during the Second World War. He reported transient obscurations and polyopia restricted to foveal vision.

Mingazzini (1908) was presumably the first to describe polyopia in a patient suffering from a gunshot wound in the occipital lobe. Hoff and Pötzl (1933, 1935b, 1937) confirmed Mingazzini's observation in several patients suffering from polyopia caused by lesions near the occipital pole. Hoff and Pötzl discriminated two types of polyopia: (a) seeing images of about the same size side by side, and (b) 'porroptic polyopia'. In the latter type of polyopia, the multiple images seem to move away from the subject. A third class of polyopia was later described by Gloning *et al.* (1957): 'circular polyopia'. These authors reported on a patient who suffered from transient brain ischaemias resulting from restricted blood supplies through the basilar arteries, which lead to obscurations in the visual field and to a subsequent polyopia in which the patient saw the polyopic images placed in a circle around the fixation target (a lamp on the ceiling). In the 708 brain-lesioned patients screened by Gloning *et al.* (1968), only 10 exhibited the symptom of polyopia; all of them had occipital lesions.

Objects in the Wrong Place: Visual Allaesthesia

While polyopia normally affects only the foveal regions of the visual field, visual allaesthesia is double vision caused by an apparent shift of the visual stimulus to a completely different part of the visual field or extra-personal space. To our knowledge, visual allaesthesia was first described by Beyer (1895), who suffered himself from classical migraines with typical fortification scintillations (cf. Chapter 10). While walking along the street, he once observed his migraine flicker sensations. He suddenly noted that trees and a wall which were actually on the right side of his extra-personal space appeared to him on its left upper part. Evidently he remained aware of where the 'real' walls and trees were located, and realized that the allaesthesia was a pseudohallucination affecting the location of the objects in the extra-personal space. Hermann and Pötzl (1928) wrote a monograph in which they described visual allaesthesia, and pointed out that this rare disorder is generally seen when the parieto-occipital regions are lesioned. As a rule, patients reporting allaesthetic phenomena have experiences similar to Beyer's. They perceive the visual object as shifted from the right to the left half of the extra-personal space. Shifts from the upper to the lower, or from the lower to the upper, half of the extra-personal space are rarely reported (Fuchs and Pötzl, 1917; Bender *et al.*, 1948; Anastosopoulos, 1952). As already discussed in Chapter 22, we assume that visual allaesthesia appears when occipital visual association areas (especially those located on the convexity of the occipital lobe) are impaired. Because of the callosal connections, neuronal structures are activated which represent the mirror-symmetric part of the cortical representation of the visual field or extra-personal space, respectively.

Visual Hallucinations and Pseudohallucinations

While illusionary changes in the visual percept require an external stimulus that activates the afferent visual system,

an external stimulus is not necessary for visual hallucinations. In such hallucinations, the objects or scenes are perceived as realistic events in the extra-personal space. Hallucinatory perceptions are frequently integrated 'harmonically' into the perceptions of the real world; the reports of the patients consist of visual events that an observer can also see, but these visual signals are combined with hallucinated objects or scenes. There are hallucinations that are experienced as dream-like, as unrealistic or as 'images', when the subject is convinced that what he sees is only an illusion. We recommend calling these hallucinatory perceptions 'pseudohallucinations', but are aware that a gradual transition exists between them and hallucinations. The word hallucinations is used frequently in a rather wide sense in the scientific literature, even to denote simple abnormal visual phenomena such as phosphenes and photisms. Since phosphenes, photisms, eidetic imageries, pseudohallucinations and hallucinations are clearly phenomenologically distinct from one another and, in addition, may be connected to abnormal neuronal activity in different parts of the visual brain (see below), we strongly recommend differentiating between these different visual phenomena by using different names. Jaspers (1953) proposed separating pseudohallucinations from hallucinations by the criterion whether or not the visual objects are perceived as images ('*bildhaft*') or as real objects in the extra- personal space ('*leibhaft*'). One has to keep in mind, however, that some patients designate their hallucinations as unreal, even though they perceive 'real' visual objects. The patient then uses his sense of touch in order to determine whether or not a 'seen' object really exists. This is illustrated by the following report of a 60-year-old lady who had been examined by one of us (O.-J. G.). She suffered from multiple metastases of a mammillary carcinoma in the region of the parietal and occipital lobes of both hemispheres:

> It's terrible. I always see a black crow hopping on the little table beside my bed. When I reach towards the crow, I can't feel anything in my hand, but the crow does not disappear. The bird just continues to leap around. This illusion is annoying, but I know that this crow does not really exist and that what I see is therefore caused by my disease.

This type of 'realistic' pseudohallucination is quite different from the animal hallucination frequently reported by patients suffering from an acute, delirious Korsakoff psychosis. These patients report seeing small animals running around the room or even across the bedspread. The animals are perceived as being real, and the strange deformations observed in them are not critically evaluated. A patient suffering from a Korsakoff psychosis reported, for example, that his room was filled with 'numerous small white elephants', which he experienced as being real (G. Baumgartner, personal communication, 1985).

Simple and complex visual hallucinations occur rather

frequently during psychotic states caused by the use of mescaline. With the help of volunteers, Klüver (1928, 1966) and Beringer (1927) performed rather extensive experimental studies on the effect of this drug on the visual sensations. One of Beringer's subjects reported that when he closed his eyes, he perceived bright light which moved; the bright light was supposedly so strong that the subject was convinced that he was sitting in a well-lit room. Evidently, one of the first effects of mescaline is the change in perception of the normal *Eigengrau*. A facilitation in the perception of sceneries and figures (similar to Johannes Müller's '*phantastische Gesichtserscheinungen*') was observed when the mescaline effect increased. Monomodal visual hallucinations also appeared which were so vivid and convincing that the subjects considered them to be real objects or events in the extra-personal space. Similar scenic hallucinations were reported during LSD use (e.g. Leuner, 1962, 1981). Before the advent of modern psychopharmaceuticals, bromide was a frequently used sedative, which, when chronically applied, lead to a considerable increase in plasma bromide levels. In such patients, visual or multimodal scenic hallucinations were observed, often appearing together with delirious changes in consciousness.

Complex visual hallucinations are dominant in the multimodal sceneries perceived by patients suffering from temporal lobe epilepsia or from alcoholic delirium tremens (Korsakoff psychosis). We can use the report of a 36-year-old female patient recorded by one of us (O.-J. G.) more than 30 years ago as an example of visually-dominated multimodal scenic hallucinations associated with this disease. She was admitted to the psychiatric university hospital in Göttingen because of a generalized epileptic seizure. After a short period of reduced consciousness and drowsiness, she reported the following:

I am living in X., a small town in Niedersachsen, where I own a small grocery store. I have always been healthy and have never had any epileptic seizures. I cannot remember any special events that have recently occurred in my life. I work as usual in my grocery store, and have had no special health problems.

After being asked about any special events in the little town, she reported:

About two weeks ago, a television team came to town and began to make a movie about Till Eulenspiegel (ed. note: a medieval German jester). Many artists, jugglers, actors and tightrope walkers assembled in front of my grocery store, which is located in a narrow lane in the medieval part of town. The television scenes were shot in this small lane, and I frequently saw artists and the members of the television team when looking out of a window on the first floor of my home. In order to produce a movie about Till Eulenspiegel's tightrope skills, ropes were attached between the old, half-timbered houses along the lane. The television team also brought along

some well-trained owls and some long-tailed monkeys which were used for the television scenes. As you know, these props really are needed in a movie about Till Eulenspiegel. The owls sat quietly on the shoulders of the actors, who were dressed in "medieval-coloured" clothes, while the long-tailed monkeys ran along the ropes. There were also small groups of street musicians in these scenes, playing music from Till Eulenspiegel's time. Everything happened immediately in front of my grocery store, but I was not hindered in my work, and actually enjoyed the activity of the television team very much . . .

Once, one of the trained long-tailed monkeys was running along one of the ropes and jumped through the window into one of the rooms of my home. When I tried to catch the monkey, I was able to grasp his tail. The tail broke off, and the animal escaped. I held the tail for some time in my hand, however . . .

This patient suffered from severe alcoholic delirium tremens, which was also the cause of the epileptic seizure. This was her first seizure. The entire description of the television team, the actors, the jugglers, Till Eulenspiegel and his owls and long-tailed monkeys, the street musicians, etc., were all part of a continuous hallucinosis caused by an acute Korsakoff psychosis. Typically for this disease, the hallucinations were harmoniously integrated into the perception of real objects, and fitted well into the actual surroundings in which the scenes were 'seen' by the patient. The little medieval lane running through the old district of the town was indeed a highly suitable location for a movie about Till Eulenspiegel. It should be emphasized, however, that not all cases of alcoholic psychosis lead to such pleasant hallucinations. The hallucinations experienced by patients are quite frequently annoying and frightening, and often lead to rather absurd defensive or even aggressive behaviour. Visual hallucinations seem to occur more frequently in endogenic or exogenic psychosis in children than in adults. Eggers (1973) reported on children in the age group between 3 and 9 years who primarily saw animals and figures from fairytales (intoxications and meningoencephalitis cases). Visual hallucinations are also more frequent in schizophrenic children and adolescents than in adults. Again, hallucinations of people or fairytale figures including devils, witches and some animals, are the most common visual hallucinations experienced by schizophrenic children (Eggers, 1973, 1987). In adult schizophrenics it is claimed that in about 50 per cent of the patients visual hallucinations may be lateralized, with a strong dominance in the right visual hemifield (Bracha *et al.*, 1985). The reported percentage of occurrence of visual hallucinations in schizophrenic patients varies considerably. One finds numbers between 5 and 50 per cent in the literature (cf. Spitzer, 1989). In our experience scenic visual hallucinations are very rare in schizophrenia and altogether hallucinations in the auditory domain are at least five times more frequent than visual hallucinations.

Complex visual hallucinations may also appear as symptoms of localized brain lesions caused by infarction, brain tumours or metastases, angiomas, traumatic brain lesions or intracerebral haemorrhages. Gloning *et al.* (1954, 1968) studied 708 patients suffering from brain lesions and found visual hallucinations in 106 of these patients. In 55 patients, they were classified as 'elementary visual hallucinations' (including phosphenes and photisms, as described above). Fifty-one suffered from complex visual hallucinations. In general, 'elementary' visual hallucinations (including phosphenes and photisms) are more frequently observed in patients suffering from occipital lobe lesions (Jackson and Beevor, 1889; Henschen, 1890; Cushing, 1921; Horrax, 1922), while complex scenic hallucinations more often point to a temporal lobe disease. The results of electrical stimulation experiments have confirmed this division: phosphenes, visual illusions and short pseudohallucinatory events are evoked by electrical stimulation of the occipital lobe, while more complex scenes may be evoked by electrical stimulation of the temporal lobe (Penfield and Rasmussen, 1957; Penfield and Pérot, 1963). The localizatory subdivision of phosphenes (stimulation of the afferent visual system and the primary visual cortex), simple hallucinations (stimulation of the retinotopically organized visual association cortices) and complex, scenic hallucinations (stimulation of the temporal lobe visual areas) appears to be neurophysiologically meaningful. It cannot be rigidly applied as a localizatory tool, however, since visual hallucinations can be caused either by a local pathological process leading to hyperexcitation, or by a remote pathological process which interrupts the afferent signal flow to the visual association cortices, which might reach a state of increased activity because of afferent disinhibition (cf. Cogan, 1973). Some clinical reports have emphasized that complex visual hallucinations may be associated with lesions of the afferent visual system (Lhermitte and De Ajuriaguerra, 1936; Weinberger and Grant, 1940; Russell and Whitty, 1955). Since electrical stimulation of the afferent visual system leads only to simple phosphenes in conscious patients, these clinical observations must be considered to be secondary cerebral disinhibitory effects. In addition, the activation of non-visual afferents to the primary visual cortex or to the visual association cortices leads to complex, scenic visual hallucinations. Lesions within the mesencephalic region may lead to a pathological activation of the non-visual input to the central visual system, and thereby evoke a pathological activation of this structure.

The 'peduncular' hallucinations, sometimes (but not necessarily always) appearing in association with delirious states, are caused by pathological processes in the mesencephalic region of the brainstem, which indirectly affect the central visual system. The term 'peduncular hallucinosis' refers to sometimes long-lasting vivid and scenic hallucinations, accompanied frequently by agitation and sleep disturbances. A small number of such patients were described in the literature, and the pathology is usually located in the midbrain (Lhermitte, 1922; van Bogaert, 1924, 1927; Lhermitte *et al.*, 1936; Silverman *et al.*, 1961; Smith *et al.*, 1971; Geller and Bellur, 1987). Also lesions located in the posterior and paramedian thalamus may evoke 'peduncular' hallucinations (e.g. De Morsier, 1938; van Bogaert, 1927; Castaigne *et al.*, 1981; Feinberg and Rapcsak, 1989). Peduncular hallucinations have been considered to be a release phenomenon in conjunction with a lesion of the ascending reticular activating system, as suggested by the concomitant sleep disturbances (Cogan, 1973; Caplan, 1980; Cummings and Miller, 1987). Some evidence exists that peduncular hallucinations are facilitated by reduced visual acuity (Geller and Bellur, 1987; Feinberg and Rapcsak, 1989).

To illustrate the special kind of visual hallucinations or pseudohallucinations present in this syndrome we can describe two of our own patients:

1. S.L., a 61-year-old right-handed man, had suffered from a left thalamic infarct two years prior to the examination. This brain lesion left him with a mild right sensorimotor hemisyndrome. Shortly after the infarction he experienced hallucinatory episodes which have occurred ever since up to several times a day and last between 5 and 20 minutes. He suddenly sees himself surrounded by a number of people who walk around in the room and talk with each other. These people – men, women and children – are German and Italian and unknown to the patient. In every episode new persons appear, speaking Italian or German. The patient never really understands what they say but he can hear them. They may arrive all at once or drop in one after the other, and their presence is not restricted to parts of the visual fields. These people appear like 'normal' men, e.g. they are not transparent, but cover the objects behind them, which is particularly disturbing for the patient when he wants to watch television. The hallucinated men and women are seen in natural colours, but occasionally arms or legs are missing. Initially the patient thought they were real and tried to address them, but they took no notice of him. Nowadays he just watches them acting and performing and is mildly amused by the experience, realizing that none of the persons appearing in such scenes exist at all.

Such episodes may happen while the patient is talking with someone else. To his partner the patient then appears rather absent-minded. The episodes are associated with a mild state of derealization. The patient repeatedly asked himself if what he experiences is real or dream-like. In order to find an answer to this question, he developed a special 'test' as follows: He looked at familiar objects and, realizing that these objects appeared somewhat blurred, took this as a sign that he is hallucinating. During the episodes of peduncular hallucination the patient was unable to recognize letters or numbers in a newspaper. Except for one brief episode with visual metamorphopsias immediately following his stroke, the patient had not experienced other kinds of hallucinatory phenomena and his visual fields were intact.

2. The second patient was a 90-year-old right-handed man with a severely reduced visual acuity known to be of peripheral origin (perhaps retinal degeneration), which could be only partially corrected by glasses. Subsequent to a stroke in the territory of the right posterior cerebral artery 4 months prior to the examination, he suddenly started experiencing visual hallucinations which could last up to 7 or 8 hours daily. Usually he saw tiny men or women at a relatively fixed distance of between 5 and 10 metres in front of him. The men were usually around age 20, the women around 30 and always wearing large hats. They were present in the central part of the extra-personal space and shifted in relation to the patient's eye or head movements. They were always looking at him except when he was walking: then they turned and walked in front of him. The patient had never taken these persons for real – thus his hallucinations belong to the class of pseudohallucinations – but he was disturbed by the fact that the figures covered his real visual surroundings, especially when he was watching television. Their appearance could be brief or last for hours, but on average they were present for several hours a day with interruptions.

In contrast to those of the first patient, these pseudo-hallucinations are purely visual events. The patient sees these figures monocularly as well as with both eyes closed. Viewing the visual hallucinations without glasses, he sees them less clearly and sharply. The figures are coloured and look real, but the body size indicates to him that they are not. They always appear in isolation, i.e. never with a hallucinated background. Although the patient cannot influence these visual delusions voluntarily, they are less frequent when he is talking with someone. They never occur while he is eating and also do not mix with his dreams. The only other visual misperception the patient experienced was an occasional brief distortion of the lower part of the faces of people with whom he was talking. These faces then appeared frightening, like 'horror masks' (cf. paraprosopia, Chapter 15).

As already described in Chapter 9, simple or short complex visual pseudohallucinations may appear within a homonymous visual field defect after the formation of unilateral occipital lesions. These brief, hallucinatory scenes are usually recognized by the patient as not being real, and are experienced like a short movie scene. Engerth *et al.* (1935) reported about patients who saw simple visual hallucinations in the hemianopic visual field. In the first case,

geometric patterns or ornamental schematic faces were perceived; in the second case, letters or more complex visual images were seen for short periods. The latter type of visual pseudohallucinations appeared in this patient only in the evening, while he saw letters only during the daytime (see also Chapter 9).

Complex visual hallucinations appear in patients suffering from cortical blindness caused by bilateral occipital lobe lesions. They are certainly best explained as release phenomena. Gloning *et al.* (1954, 1968) grouped 32 cases of hallucinations and pseudohallucinations from the 51 complex visual hallucinations into the category of unreal, short movie scenes. The remaining 19 patients suffering from complex visual hallucinations experienced vivid, realistic visual scenes that affected perception of the whole extra-personal space. This was not restricted to possibly existing visual field defects. Such scenic visual hallucinations generally appeared when the temporal lobe was affected (in 17 of the 19 cases), and were evidently more frequent when it was the right temporal lobe that was involved than when it was the left. From clinical or EEG data, one must assume that scenic visual hallucinations of this type are predominantly of epileptic origin. This view is advanced in a report published by Penfield and Pérot (1963), who found that electrical stimulation of different parts of the temporal lobe evoked complex visual or multimodal scenic hallucinations in a number of patients suffering from temporal lobe epilepsia. The visual hallucinations evoked by electrical stimulation of the temporal lobe outer surface are primarily reported as short, dream-like events, and not as complex, long-lasting scenes (cf. also Penfield and Rasmussen, 1957). Pötzl (1949b) considered part of the temporal lobe to be the 'visual area of the past' ('*Sehfeld der Vergangenheit*'), and interpreted the dreamy states accompanying the visual perceptions associated with temporal lobe epilepsia as being caused predominantly by abnormal activation in the region of the uncus of the temporal lobe.

Temporal lobe epilepsia is sometimes associated with visual aura phenomena (Janz, 1969). A rather large variety of visual auras have been observed in different patients. Epileptic visual auras can be simple sensations of colour or colourless light nebulae, deformations of the visual percept, the appearance of faces, human figures (frequently seen as multiple objects), or complex, scenic visual hallucinations (Mulder *et al.*, 1957; Palem *et al.*, 1970).

It has been repeatedly reported that epileptic aura phenomena may be related to events experienced just before the first epileptic seizure (Reisner, 1942). Gloning *et al.* (1954) reported on a female patient who suffered from her first epileptic seizure while staying in an air-raid shelter during the Second World War. The aura phenomena that preceded later epileptic seizures consisted of visual and multimodal hallucinations that were related to

Phosphenes
and photisms

Simple-
structured
hallucinations

Kinetopsias
Macropsias
Micropsias

Multimodal
scenic
hallucinations

(Wieser, 1985)

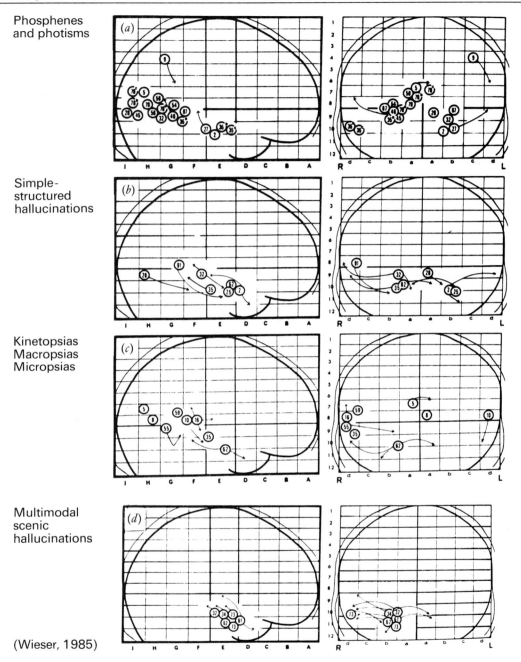

Fig. 23.3 *(a) Projection of the location of intracerebral electrodes onto the lateral surface and onto a coronal cut of the brain. The numbers refer to different patients. Epileptic discharges appearing spontaneously or after a short electrical stimulus train were observed on all marked sites, while the conscious patients reported phosphenes or photisms (chronically implanted intracerebral electrodes). (b) Same as in (a), but the epileptic visual sensations were short, structured images and pseudohallucinations. (c) Same as in (a). The visual sensations were either kinetopsias, macroptic or microptic deformations of objects and persons seen, or visual illusionary transformations of objects in the extra-personal space. (d) Same as in (a). The epileptic discharges on these recording sites were correlated with multimodal complex hallucinations, which together all comprised a complex visual scenery. For further explanation, see the text (from Wieser, 1985, modified).*

the air-raid shelter. Cogan (1973) interpreted episodic, stereotypic hallucinations as ictal attacks, and the continuous variable hallucinations as release phenomena resulting from loss or suppression of the normal visual input.

As repeatedly reported in clinical observations, a correlation between abnormal visual sensations and abnormal activation of the different parts of the visual brain is not easy to establish. Studies involving chronically implanted electrodes in epileptic patients are especially helpful in finding meaningful correlations between abnormal brain function and abnormal visual sensations. Since these electrodes can also be used to stimulate the region of the presumed epileptic foci, pathological visual sensations may be correlated not only with focal epileptic discharges but also with epileptic after-discharges following a short electrical pulse train. Figure 23.3 summarizes several findings obtained in such studies (Wieser, 1982). In Fig. 23.3(a), all sites are schematically projected onto the surface of the right hemisphere and onto a coronal cut through both hemispheres. Epileptic discharges in the electroencephalogram were recorded on these sites during the perception of phosphenes or photisms. The different numbers in Fig. 23.3 refer to the data obtained from different patients. The epileptogenic visual sensations included horizontal stripes, vertical lines, a white ball (like a firework), grey or black moving objects (5), rotating spirals (27), simple

flicker sensation or flashes (28, 32, 45, 59), a white round spot surrounded by a grey ring (35), a snow storm (46), diffuse colour sensations (54, 59), coloured stripes (67) or dots (70), and simple geometrical patterns (78).

In Fig. 23.3(b), pathological epileptogenic visual sensations of elaborated structural complexity (simple visual object hallucinations) were reported: a transformation of objects into 'animal-like humans' (2), a horse stable (28), a rose with many flowers moving in rhythmic movement (32), persons surrounding the subject (35) or vague, imprecisely described scenes (91).

In Fig. 23.3(c), epileptogenic moving fields (kinetopsia), macropsias (5, 8, 16) or micropsias (10, 35, 62), or illusionary transformation of the objects (a small board transformed into a stove, a nurse into a nun wearing a black habit) were reported.

Finally, Fig. 23.3(d) summarizes all recording sites at which epileptic activity was recorded by the electroencephalogram during complex, multimodal, visual scenic hallucinations: a hospital scene experienced during adolescence (32), heautoscopic phenomena (34), hallucinations of persons wellknown during childhood (61), a fast-flowing mountain river (62), persons who change faces and dress, heautoscopy or heautoscopy upon seeing oneself in a mirror (62, 73). Lasting abnormal, multimodal, visually dominated sensations (epileptic dreamy

Table 23.1 *Visual sensations evoked by 'internal' causes. The most probable sites of abnormal excitation and possible lesion sites are listed.*

Visual phenomenon	Sites of abnormal excitation	Possible sites of lesions
Phosphenes	Retina, optic tract, LGN, area V1	Retina, optic tract, LGN, visual radiation
Geometrical pattern or other simple-structured photisms	Areas V2, V3	Visual radiation, area V1
Coloured photisms	Areas V2, V4	Visual radiation, area V1
Abnormal local visual movement sensations	Areas MT, MST, FST	Occipital visual movements association areas, pulvinar
Simple stereotyped shapes, especially human figures, faces, animals	Medio-basal occipito-temporal cortex, RH > LH, gyrus parahippocampalis	Areas V1 and V2, limbic structures
Short visual scenes (pseudohallucinations)	Occipito-temporal lobe	Occipital visual association areas
Complex scenic visual hallucinations	Temporal lobe and limbic connections	Occipital lobe, limbic system
Multimodal scenes, complex hallucinations	Limbic memory areas	Temporal lobe, prefrontal region
Heautoscopy	Limbic areas and vestibular cortex	Temporal lobe

states), which frequently occur in cases of temporal lobe epilepsia (Meyer–Mickeleit, 1953), are, according to Wieser's findings (1982), also associated with high incidence of epileptic activity in the anterior, deep parts of the temporal lobe.

Visual hallucinations may appear during prolonged isolation, in sensory deprivation experiments and in states of somatic exhaustion. Near-death visual or scenic hallucinations belong to this category. Scenic visual hallucinations are experienced by everybody when dreaming. One must assume that dreams are caused by an activation of the limbic and temporal lobe structures during the REM phases of sleep. In many normal subjects, the altered state of consciousness during waking up or falling asleep leads to hypnagogic ('falling asleep') or hypnopomp ('waking up') visual hallucinations or to pseudohallucinations. Hypnopomp hallucinations seem to be associated with narcolepsia, and may be interpreted as recurrent dreams occurring in a state of dissociated consciousness.

In summary, it seems rather probable that all abnormal visual sensations of simple structures (phosphenes, photisms) are caused by a pathological activation within the afferent visual system (including area V1). Pathological processes in these structures can also lead to secondary disinhibitory phenomena in the higher visual association cortices, however. Therefore, complex visual hallucinations may also occur when the afferent visual system is impaired. The direct cause of the visual perception of patterns and simple figures has to be searched for in the pathological activity of the visual association cortices, however. Finally, scenic visual hallucinations and multimodal hallucinations necessarily involve a pathological activation of the occipito-temporal and temporal lobe structures. Whenever long-lasting visual scenes are experienced, one must assume involvement of the visual memory processes related to the limbic structures. Table 23.1 summarizes the findings on abnormal visual sensations as well as the correlation of these sensations with the most probable sites of abnormal excitation and possible sites of lesions which lead to a disinhibition of other cerebral visual structures, causing abnormal activity related to visual sensations having different grades of complexity. Some caution should be exercised in relation to the 'pathological' functions listed in Table 23.1. Extensive comparative psychopathological studies have indicated that the pathognomonic value of the symptom 'visual hallucination' is rather limited. The occasional appearance of short, transient hallucinatory events or dreamy states is so widespread (Parish, 1894) that diagnostic consequences should be deduced only after a thorough neuropsychiatric examination. Furthermore, owing to the increased consumption of hallucinogenic drugs in western society, short visual hallucinations may affect people who have taken drugs weeks or months before ('flashback').

References

Aarkrog, T. (1975). Psychotic and borderline psychotic adolescents: frequency of psychiatric illness and treatment in childhood in 100 consecutive cases. *Acta Psychiatr. Scand.* 52, 58–68

Aarkrog, T., Mortensen, K.V. (1985). Schizophrenia in early adolescence. *Acta Psychiatr. Scand.* 72, 422–429

Aarons, L. (1964). Visual apparent movement research: Review 1935–1955, and bibliography 1955–1963. *Percept. Motor Skills* 18, 239–279

Aarons, L., Goldenberg, L. (1964). Galvanic stimulation of the vestibular system and perception of the vertical. *Perceptual and Motor Skills* 19, 59–66

Aaronson, B., Osmond, H. (eds.) (1971). *Psychedelics: the uses and implications of hallucinogenic drugs.* Hogarth, London

Abadi, R.V., Kulikowski, J.J., Meudell, P. (1981). Visual performance in a case of visual agnosia. In van Hof, M.W., Mohn, G.(eds). *Functional Recovery from Brain Damage. (Developments in Neuroscience 13).* Elsevier/North-Holland, Amsterdam and Oxford, 275–286

Abbot, T.K. (1904). Fresh light on Molyneux's problem. Dr. Ramsey's case. *Mind* (n.s.) 13, 543–554

Abe, T., Nakamura, N., Sugishita, M., Kato, Y., Iwata, M. (1986). Partial disconnection syndrome following penetrating stab wound of the brain. *Eur. Arch. Neurol.* 25, 233–239

Abe, Z. (1951). Influence of adaptation on the strength-frequency curve of human eyes, as determined with electrically produced flickering phosphenes. *Tohoku J. exp. Med.* 54, 37–44

Abelsdorff, G. (1916). Beiderseitiges zentrales Scotom bei im übrigen normalem Gesichtsfelde nach Hinterhauptschuss. *Klin. Monatsblätter für Augenheilkunde* 56, 172

Abraham, F.A., Melamed, E., Lavy, S. (1975). Prognostic value of visual evoked potentials in occipital blindness following basilar artery occlusion. *Appl. Neurophysiol.* 38, 126–135

Abraham, H.D. (1983). Visual phenomenology of LSD flashback. *Arch. Gen. Psychiatry* 40, 884–889

Abrams, R., Redfield, J., Taylor, M.A. (1981). Cognitive dysfunction in schizophrenia, affective disorder and organic brain disease. *Br. J. Psychiatry* 139, 190–194

Ackroyd, C., Humphrey, N.K., Warrington, E.K. (1974). Lasting effects of early blindness. A case study. *Q. J. Exp. Psychol.* 26, 114–124

Acuna, C., Gonzales, F., Dominguez, R. (1983). Sensorimotor unit activity related to intention in the pulvinar of behaving *Cebus apella* monkeys. *Exp. Brain Res.* 52, 411–422

Ad Hoc Committee on Classification of Headache (1962). A classification of headache. *Neurology* 12, 378–380

Adams, A. (1957). Nystagmographische Untersuchungen über den Lidnystagmus und die physiologische Koordination von Lidschlag und rascher Nystagmusphase. *Arch.HNO-Heilk.* 170, 543–558

Adams, G. (1792). *An Essay on Vision briefly explaining the Fabric of the Eye and the Nature of Vision.* Hindmarsh, R., London

Addams, R. (1834). An account of a peculiar optical phaenomenon seen after having looked at a moving body etc. *London and Edinb. Phil. Mag. J. Science*, 3rd series 5, 373–374

Ades, H.W., Raab, D.H. (1949). Effect of preoccipital and temporal decortication on learned visual discrimination in monkeys. *J. Neurophysiol.* 12, 101–108

Adler, A. (1944). Disintegration and restoration of optic recognition in visual agnosia: Analysis of a case. *Arch. Neurol. Psychiat.* 51, 243–259

Adler, A. (1950). Course and outcome of visual agnosia. *J. Nerv. Ment. Dis.* 111, 41–51

Adler, A., Pötzl, O. (1936). Ueber eine eigenartige Reaktion auf Meskalin bei einer Kranken mit doppelseitigen Herden in der Sehsphäre. *Jahrbuch für Psychiatrie* 53, 13

Adler, B., Bock, O., Grüsser, O.-J. (1981). Alpha-stripes: A spatial periodicity appearing in stroboscopically illuminated moving random dot patterns. *Vision Res.* 21, 913–924

Adler, B., Collewijn, H., Curio, G., Grüsser, O.-J., Pause, M., Schreiter U., Weiss, L. (1981). Sigma-movement and Sigma-nystagmus: A new tool to investigate the gaze pursuit system and visual movement perception in man and monkey. *Ann. N.Y. Acad. Sci.* 374, 284–302

Adler, B., Grüsser, O.-J. (1979). Apparent movement and appearance of periodic stripes during eye movements across a stroboscopically illuminated random dot pattern. *Brain Res.* 37, 537–550

Adler, B., Grüsser, O.-J. (1981). Apparent movement perception, eye pursuit movements and optokinetic nystagmus elicited by stroboscopically illumianted stationary periodic stereopatterns. In Fuchs, A.F., Becker, W. (eds.), *Progress in Oculomotor Research*, Elsevier/North-Holland, New York, Amsterdam, Oxford, 577–586

Adler, B., Grüsser, O.-J. (1982). Sigma-movement and optokinetic nystagmus elicited by stroboscopically illuminated stereopatterns. *Exp. Brain Res.* 47, 353–364

Agdogan, C. (1978). *Optics in Albert the Great's 'De sensu et sensato'. An edition, Engl. translation and analysis.* Ph.D. Thesis. University of Wisconsin, Madison

Agdogan, C. (1984). Avicenna and Albert's refutation of the extramission theory of vision. *Islam Studies* 23, 151–157

Aguilar, M.J., Gerbode, F., Hill, J.D. (1971). Neuropathological complications of cardiac surgery. *J. Thorac. Cardiovasc. Surg.* 61, 676–685

Aguilonius, F. (1613). *Opticorum libri VI philosophis iuxta ac mathematicis utiles.* Officina Plantiniana, Antwerpen

Ahlenstiel, H., Kaufmann, R. (1953). Geometrisches Gestalten in optischen Halluzinationen. *Arch. Psychiat. u. Z. ges. Neurol.* 190, 503–529

Ahlenstiel, H., Kaufmann, R. (1962). Über pathologische Illusionen. *Arch. Psychiat. u. Z. ges. Neurol.* 202, 592–605

Ahrens, R. (1954). Beitrag zur Entwicklung des Physiognomie-und Mimikerkennens. *Z. exp. angew. Psychol.* 2, 412–454 and 599–633

Ahrens, R. (1955). Beitrag zur Frage der Prosopagnosie. *Schweiz. Arch. Neurol. Psychiat.* 75, 4–21

Ahrens, R. (1956). Analyse eines Falles von Raumagnosie. Schweiz. Arch. Neurol. Psychiat. 77, 96–122

Aicardi, G., Battaglini, P.P., Galletti, C. (1987). Retinal eye-motion input affects real-motion cell activity in the V3-complex of behaving macaque monkeys. *J. Physiol. (Lond.)* 388, 47P

Aimard, G., Vighetto, A., Confavreux, C., Devic, M. (1981). La désorientation spatiale. *Rev. Neurol. (Paris)* 137, 97–111

Airy, H. (1870). On a distinct form of transient heminopsia. *Proc. Roy. Lond.* 18, 212–229

Airy, H. (1870). On a distinct form of transient hemiopsia. *Philos. Trans. Roy. Soc. Lond.* 160 (1), 247–264

Aizenberg, D., Modai, I. (1985). Autoscopic and drug-induced perceptual disturbances. A case report. *Psychopathology* 18, 237–240

Ajax, E.T. (1964). Acquired dyslexia. *Arch. Neurol.* 11, 66–72

Ajax, E.T. (1967). Dyslexia without agraphia. *Arch. Neurol.* 17, 645–652

Ajax, E.T. (1977). Dyslexia without agraphia: prognostic considerations. *Neurology* 27, 685–688

Ajax, E.T., Schenkenberg, T., Kosteljanetz, M. (1977). Alexia without agraphia and the inferior splenium. *Neurology* 27, 685–688

Ajuriaguerra de, J., Hécaen, H. (1951). La restauration fonctionelle après lobéctomie occipitale. *J. Psychol.* 44, 510–546

Ajuriaguerra, J. de (1954). L'état actuel de la théorie de la Gestalt en psychoneurologie. *Schweizerische Zeitung für Psychologie* 13, 16–53

Akbarian, S., Berndl, K., Grüsser, O.-J., Guldin, W., Pause, M., Schreiter, U. (1988). Responses of single neurons in the parietoinsular vestibular cortex of primates. In Cohen, B., Henn, V. (eds.), *Representation of three-dimensional space in the vestibular, oculomotor, and visual systems. Ann. N.Y. Acad.Sci.* 545, 187–202

Akbarian, S., Guldin, W., Grüsser, O.-J. (1988). The thalamic interconnections of the parieto-insular vestibular region in the Squirrel monkey (Saimiri sciureus). Abstracts of the 11th Annual Meeting of the European Neuroscience Association. Zürich 4–8 Sept. 1988, p. 171

Akelaitis, A.J. (1941). Studies on the corpus callosum. II. The higher visual functions in each homonymous field following complete section of the corpus callosum. *Arch. Neurol. Psychiat.* 45, 788–796

Akelaitis, A.J. (1944). A study of gnosis, praxis and language following section of corpus callosum and anterior commissure. *J. Neurosurg.* 1, 94–101

Akimoto, H., Creutzfeldt, O. (1957). Reaktionen von Neuronen des optischen Cortex nach elektrischer Reizung unspezifischer Thalamuskerne. *Arch. Psychiat. Nervenkr.* 196, 494–519

Alagille, D., Carlier, J.C., Chiva, M., Ziade, R., Ziade, M., Moy, F. (1986). Long-term neuropsychological outcome in children undergoing portal systemic shunts for portal vein obstruction without liver disease. *J. Pediatr. Gastroenterol. Nut.* 5, 861–866

Alajouanine, T. (ed.) (1955). *Les grandes activités du lobe temporal.* Masson et Cie, Paris

Alajouanine, T. (ed.) (1960). *Les grandes activités du lobe occipital.* Masson et Cie, Paris

Alajouanine, T., Lhermitte, F. (1963). Non-verbal communication in aphasia. De Reuch, A., O'Connor, M. (eds.), *Disorder of Language,* Boston

Alajouanine, T., Lhermitte, F., De Ribaucourt-Ducarne,B. (1960). Les alexies agnosiques et aphasiques. In Alajouanine, T. (ed.) *Les grandes activites du lobe occipital,* Masson, Paris, 235–260

Alajouanine, T., Lhermitte, F., Sabouraud, O., De Ribaucourt,

(1953). Agnosie visuelle sans alexie. *Revue Neurol.* 89, 158

Albert, M., Yamadori, A. Gardner, H., Howes, D. (1973). Comprehension in alexia. *Brain* 96, 317–328

Albert, M.L. (1973). A simple test of visual neglect. *Neurology* 23, 658–664

Albert, M.L. (1979). Alexia. In Heilman, K.M., Valenstein, E. (eds.), *Clinical Neuropsychology.* Oxford Press, 59–91

Albert, M.L., Reches, A., Silverberg, R. (1975). Associative visual agnosia without alexia. *Neurology* 25, 322–326

Albert, M.L., Reches, A., Silverberg, R. (1975b). Hemianopic colour blindness. *J. Neurol. Neurosurg. Psychiat.* 38, 546–549

Albert, M.L., Soffer, D., Silverberg, R., Reches, A. (1979). The anatomic basis of visual agnosia. *Neurology* 29, 876–879

Albertotti, J. (1884). Ein automechanisches, selbstregistrierendes Perimeter. *Klin. Monatsbl. f. Augenheilk.* 1884, 465 (quoted after Helmholtz, 1896)

Albertus Magnus (1496, 1506). *Philosophia naturalis.* G. Arrivaenus, Venice/Basel

Albertus Magnus (1880–1899). *De sensu et sensato.* In A. Borgnet (ed.), *Opera Omnia Vol. IX,* Paris, 1–96

Albertus Magnus (1890–1899). *Summae de creaturis.* In: Borgnet, A. (ed.) *Opera Omnia Vol XXXV.* Paris

Albertus Magnus (1916–1921). *De Animalibus, libri XXVI.* 2 Vols. Stadler, H. (ed.), Aschendorff, Münster i.W.

Albertus Magnus (1951). *De Anima.* In Geyer, B. (ed.) *Opera Omnia.* Vol. VII, Part 1 1968, Aschendorff, Münster i.W.

Albertus Magnus (1987). *De Animalibus.* Books 22–26. Engl. Transl. '*Man and the beast*', transl. by J. Scanlan. Medieval and Renaissance Texts and Studies. Center for Medieval and early Renaissance Studies, Binghampton, N.Y.

Albrecht, H., Bielschowsky, A. (1908). Demonstration und Besprechung eines Falles von Seelenblindheit. *Berliner klinische Wochenschrift* 45, 1076

Albright, T.D. (1984a). Direction and orientation selectivity of neurones in visual area MT of the macaque. *J. Neurophysiol.* 52, 1106–1130

Albright, T.D., Desimone, B. (1987). Local precision of visuotopic organization in the middle temporal area (MT) of the macaque. *Exp. Brain Res.* 65, 582–592

Albright, T.D., Desimone, R., Gross, C.G. (1984). Columnar organization of directionally selective cells in visual area MT of the macaque. *J. Neurophysiol.* 51, 16–31

Aldrich, M.S., Alessi, A.G., Beck, R.W., Gilmann, S. (1987). Cortical blindness: Etiology, diagnosis, and prognosis. *Ann. Neurol.* 21, 149–158

Aldrich, M.S., Vanderzant, C., Abou-Khalil, B. et al. (1985). Cortical blindness as an ictal manifestation. *Electroencephalogr. Clin. Neurophysiol.* 61, 37P

Alexander, A. (1867). Ein Fall von hemiopischer Gesichtsfeldbeschränkung. *Klin. Monatsbl. f. Augenhlk.* 5, 88–102

Alexander, G.E. (1982). Functional development of frontal association cortex in monkeys: Behavioral and electrophysiological studies. *Neurosci. Res. Program Bull.* 20, 471–78

Alexander, M.P., Albert, M.L. (1983). The anatomical basis of visual agnosia. In A. Kertesz (ed.), *Localization in neuropsychology.* Academic Press, New York, p. 393–415

Alexander, M.P., Stuss, D.T., Benson, D.F. (1979). Capgras-syndrome: a reduplicative phenomenon. *Neurology* 29, 334–339

Alhazen (1572). *Opticae Thesauros. Alhazeni Arabis libri septem, nuncprimum editi. Eiusdem liber de crepusculis et nubium ascensionibus item Vitellonis Thuringopoloni libri X.,* F.R. Risnerus, Basel

Allard, F., Bryden, M.P. (1979). The effect of concurrent activity on hemispheric asymmetries. *Cortex* 15, 5–17

Allen, I.M. (1930). A clinical study of tumors involving the occipital lobe. *Brain* 53, 194–243

Allen, I.M. (1948). Unilateral visual inattention. *New Zealand Med.*

J. 47, 605–617

Allik, J., Rauk, M., Luuk, A. (1981). Control and sense of eye movements behind closed eyelids. *Perception* 10, 39–51

Allison, R.S., Hurwitz, L.J., White, J.G., Wilmot, T.J. (1969). A follow-up study of a patient with Balint's syndrome. *Neuropsychologia* 7, 319–333

Allman, J. (1977). Evolution of the visual system in the early primates. In Sprague, J.M., Epstein, A.N.(eds.), *Progress in Psychobiology and Physiological Psychology*. Academic Press, New York, p. 1–53

Allman, J., Miezen, F., McGuinness, E. (1985). Direction-and velocity-specific responses from beyond the classical receptive field in the middle temporal visual area (MT). *Perception* 14, 105–126

Allman, J., Miezen, F., McGuinness, E. (1985). Stimulus specific responses from beyond the classical receptive field: neurophysiological mechanisms for local-global comparisons in visual neurons. *Ann. Rev. Neurosci.* 8, 407–430

Allman, J.M. (1977). Evolution of the visual system in the early primates. *Prog. Psychobiol. Physiol. Psychol.* 7, 1–53

Allman, J.M. (1988). The search for area MT in the human brain. In *Proceedings of the European Brain and Behavioral Society Workshop in Segregation of Form and Motion*. Tübingen

Allman, J.M., Baker, J.F., Newsome, W.T., Petersen, S.E. (1981). Visual topography and function: cortical visual areas in the owl monkey. In Woolsey, C.N. (ed.), *Cortical Sensory Organization. Multiple Visual Areas*. Clifton, N.J., Humana, vol. 2, 171–185

Allman, J.M., Kaas, J.H. (1971). A representation of the visual field in the caudal third of the middle temporal gyrus of the owl monkey (Aotus trivirgatus). *Brain Res.* 31, 85–105

Allman, J.M., Kaas, J.H. (1971). Representation of the visual field in striate and adjoining cortex of the owl monkey (Aotus trivirgatus). *Brain Res.* 35, 89–106

Allman, J.M., Kaas, J.H. (1974). The organization of the second visual area (VII) in the owl monkey: A second order transformation of the visual hemifield. *Brain Res.* 76, 247–265

Allman, J.M., Kaas, J.H., Lane, R.H. (1973). The middle temporal visual area (MT) in the bush baby, Galago senegalensis. *Brain Res.* 57, 197–202

Allport, D.A. (1980). Patterns and actions: Cognitive mechanisms are content-specific. In G. Claxton (ed.), *Cognitive psychology: New directions*, Routledge and Kegan Paul, London

Allport, F.H. (1955). *Theories of perception and the concept of structure*. Wiley, New York

Allport, G.W. (1928). The eidetic image and the afterimage. *Am. J. Psychol.* 40, 418–425

Almgren, P.E., Andersson, A.L., Kullberg, G. (1972). Long-term effects of verbally expressed cognition following left and right ventrolateral thalamotomy. *Confin. Neurol.* 34, 162–168

Alouf, I. (1929). Die vergleichende Cytoarchitektonik der Area striata. *J. f. Psychol. Neurol.* (Lpz.) 38, 5

Alpert, M., Martz, M.J. (1977). Cognitive views of schizophrenia in light of recent studies of brain asymmetry, in psychopathology and brain dysfunction. In, Shagass, C., Gershon, S., Friedhoff, A.J. (eds.) Raven Press, New York, 1–12

Alter, I., Rein, S., Toro, A. (1989). A directional bias for studies of laterality. *Neuropsychologia* 27, 251–257

Altmann, S.A., Altmann, J. (1970). *Baboon ecology. African field research*. University of Chicago Press, Chicago

Amassian, V.E., Cracco, R.Q., Maccabee, P.J., Cracco, J.B., Rudell, A., Eberle, L. (1989). Suppression of visual perception by magnetic coil stimulation of human occipital cortex. *EEG Clin. Neurophysiol.* 74, 458–462

Ameli, R., Courchesne, E., Lincoln, A., Kaufman, A.S., Grillon, C. (1988). Visual memory processes in high-functioning individuals with autism. *J. Autism. Dev. Disord.* 18, 601–615

Anastasopoulos, G. (1952). Zur Frage der hemianopischen Hallu-

zinationen, der Orientierungsstörung und der optischen Allästhesie. *Wien. Zschr. Nervenkr.* 6, 34–48

Anastasopoulos, G. K. (1962). Beiträge zu den Halluzinationsproblemen. I. Zur Frage der Entstehung von Herdhalluzinationen. *Psychiat. Neurol. Basel* 143, 233–249

Andersen, J.R. (1976). *Language, memory, and thought*. Lawrence Erlbaum Associates, Hillsdale, NY

Andersen, R.A. (1987). Inferior parietal lobule function in spatial perception and visuomotor integration. In Mountcastle, V.B., Plum, F., Geiger, S.R. (eds.), *Handbook of Physiology. Sect. I. The nervous system* V. Bethesda, MD., American Physiological Soc., p. 483–518

Andersen, R.A. (1988). The neurobiological basis of spatial cognition: role of the parietal lobe. In Stiles-Davis, J., Kritchevsky, M., Bellugi, U. (eds), *Spatial Cognition: Brain Bases and Development*. Univ. of Chicago Press, Chicago, p. 57–80

Andersen, R.A. (1989). Visual and eye movement functions of the posterior parietal cortex. *Ann. Rev. Neurosci.* 12, 2377–2403

Andersen, R.A., Asanuma, C., Cowan, W.M. (1985). Callosal and prefrontal associational projecting cell populations in area 7a of the macaque monkey: a study using retrogradely transported fluorescent dyes. *J. Comp. Neurol.* 232, 443–455

Andersen, R.A., Asanuma, C., Essick, G., Siegel, R.M. (1990). Cortico-cortical connections of anatomically and physiologically defined subdivisions within the inferior parietal lobule. *J. Comp. Neurol.* 296, 65–113

Andersen, R.A., Essick, G.K., Siegel, R.M. (1985). Encoding of spatial location by posterior parietal neurons. *Science* 230, 456–458

Andersen, R.A., Essick, G.K., Siegel, R.M. (1987). Neurons of area 7 activated by both visual stimuli and oculomotor behavior. *Exp. Brain Res.* 67, 316–322

Andersen, R.A., Mountcastle, V.B. (1983). The influence of the angle of gaze upon the excitability of the light-sensitive neurons of the posterior parietal cortex. *J. Neurosci.* 3, 532–548

Andersen, R.A., Siegel, R.M., Essick, G.K., Asanuma, C. (1985). Subdivision of the inferior parietal lobule and dorsal prelunate gyrus of macaque by connectional and functional criteria. *Invest. Ophthalmol. Visual Sci.* 23, 266

Andersen, S. (1985). *Sprachliche Verständlichkeit und Wahrscheinlichkeit*. Brockmeyer, Bochum, 194 p. Quantitative linguistics Vol. 29

Anderson, E., Parkin, A.J. (1985). On the nature of the left visual field advantage for faces. *Cortex* 21, 453–459

Anderson, J.A., Silverstein, J.W., Ritz, S.A., Jones, R.S. (1977). Distinctive features, categorical perception, and probability learning: Some applications of a neural model. *Psychol.Rev.*, 84, 413–447.

Anderson, J.R. (1983). Responses to mirror-image stimulation and assessment of self-recognition in mirror-and peer-reared stumptail macaques. *Quart. J. Exp. Psychol.* 35B, 201–212

Anderson, J.R. (1984a). The development of self-recognition: a review. *Developmental Psychobiology* 17, 35–49

Anderson, J.R. (1984b). Monkeys with mirror: some questions for primate psychology. *Intern. J. Primatology* 5, 81–97

Anderson, M., Semerari, A. (1954). L'eautoscopia negativa. *Il Lavoro Neuropsichiat.* 14, 484–491

Anderson, R.M., Hunt, S.C., van der Stoep, A., Pribram, K.H. (1976). Object permanency and delayed response as spatial context in monkeys with frontal lesions. *Neuropsychologia*, 14, 481–490

Andreassi, J.L., Balinsky, B., Gallichio, J.A., Desimone, J.J., Mellers, B.W. (1976). Hypnotic suggestion of stimulus change and visual cortical evoked potential. *Percept. Mot. Skills* 42, 371–378

Andrews, B.W., Pollen, D.A. (1979). Relationship between spatial frequency selectivity and receptive field profile of simple cells. *J. Physiol. (Lond.)* 287, 163–176.

Anstis, S.M. (1974). A chart demonstrating variations in acuity with retinal position. *Vision Res.* 14, 589–592

Anstis, S.M. (1980). The perception of apparent movement. *Phil. Trans. R. Soc. Lond. B* 290, 153–168

Anton, G. (1895). Über Störungen des Orientierungsvermögens. *Neurol. Centrabl.* 14, 955

Anton, G. (1896). Blindheit nach beiderseitiger Gehirnerkrankung mit Verlust der Orientierung im Raume. *Mittheilungen des Vereins der Ärzte in Steiermark* 33, 41–46

Anton, G. (1898). Ueber Herderkrankungen des Gehirns, welche vom Patienten selbst nicht wahrgenommen werden. *Wiener Klinische Wochenschrift* 11, 227–229

Anton, G. (1899). Beiderseitige Erkrankung der Scheitelgegend des Grosshirnes. *Wiener klinische Wochenschrift* 12, 1193–1199

Anton, G. (1899). Ueber die Selbstwahrnehmung der Herderkrankungen des Gehirns durch den Kranken bei Rindenblindheit und Rindentaubheit. *Arch. f. Psychiat.* 32, 86–127

Anton, G. (1899). Ueber die Selbstwahrnehmungen der Herderkrankungen des Gehirns durch den Kranken bei Rindenblindheit und Rindentaubheit. *Arch. Psychiat. Nervenkr.* 32, 86–127

Aptman, M., Levin, H., Senelick, R.C. (1977). Alexia without agraphia in a left-handed patient with prosopagnosia. *Neurology* 27, 533–537

Arena, R., Gainotti, G. (1978). Constructional apraxia and visuoperceptive disabilities in relation to laterality of cerebral lesions. *Cortex* 14, 463–473

Arieti, S., Bemporad, J.R. (1974). Rare, unclassifiable and collective psychiatric syndromes. In Arieti S. (ed.), *Am. Handbook of Psychiatry 3.* Basic books, New York

Aristoteles (1953). *Über die Sinneswahrnehmung und ihre Gegenstände* ('*De sensu et sensato*'). In Gohlke, P. (ed. and transl.), *Die Lehrschriften* Vol. VI/2: Kleine Schriften zur Seelenkunde, 2nd. ed., Schöningh, Paderborn, p. 22–61

Aristoteles (1970). *Meteorologie.* Werke Vol. VIII, transl. H. Strohm. Wiss. Buchgesellschaft, Darmstadt

Aristotle (1964). *On the soul. Parva naturalia. On breath.* Engl. transl. by W.S. Hett. Loeb Classical Library, Vol. 288. Heinemann, London

Aristotle (1964). *Parva Naturalia: On Dreams.* Text and Translation in: Aristotle Works, Vol. VIII. Harvard University Press, Cambridge, Heinemann, London, p. 348–371

Arlazoroff, A., Carpel, C.L., Zonis, H., Goldenberg, E., Zekler, E. (1984). Incomplete Kluver-Bucy syndrome and fluent aphasia. *Brain Lang.* 23, 300–306

Armaignac, .. (1882). Revue clinique du Sud-Ouest 1882, cited in Charcot, J.M., 1887

Arrigoni, G., DeRenzi, E. (1964). Constructional apraxia and hemispheric locus of lesion. *Cortex* 1, 180–197

Arseni, C., Botez, M.I. (1958). Consideraciones sobre un caso de agnosia de las fisionomias. *Rev. Neuro-Psiquiatria* 21, 583–593

Arseni, C., De Renzi, M. (1965). Consideraciones sobre un caso de agnosia de las fisionomias. *Revista Neuropsiquiatr.* 3, 157–160

Asanuma, C., Andersen, R.A., Cowan, W.M. (1985). The thalamic relations of the caudal inferior parietal lobule and the lateral prefrontal cortex in monkeys: divergent cortical projections from cell clusters in the medial pulvinar nucleus. *J. Comp. Neurol.* 241, 357–381

Aschaffenburg, G. (1927–1929). Handbuch der Psychiatrie. Deuticke, Leipzig

Ashmore, R.J., Snyder, R.T. (1980). Relationship of visual and auditory short-term memory to later reading achievement. *Percept. Mot. Skills* 51, 15–18

Assal, G. (1969). Régression des troubles de la reconnaissance des physionomies et de la memoire topographique chez un malade operé d'un hématome intracérébral parieto-temporal droit. *Rev. Neurol. (Paris)* 121, 184–185

Assal, G., Buttet, J., Jolivet, R. (1979). Aspects ideographiques de l'ecriture: Analyse d'un nouveau type d'agraphie. *La Linguisitque*
14, 79–101

Assal, G., Eisert, H.G., Hecaen, H.E. (1969). Analyse des résultats du test de Farnsworth D15 chez 155 malades atteints de lésions hemisphériques droites ou gauches. *Acta Neurol. Psychiat. Belg.* 69, 705–717

Assal, G., Favre, C., Anderes, J.P. (1984). Non-reconaissance d'animaux familiers chez un paysan. (Nonrecognition of familiar animals by a farmer: Zooagnosia or prosopagnosia for animals). *Rev. Neurol. (Paris)* 140, 580–584

Assal, G., Hadj-Djilani, M. (1976). Une nouvelle observation d'alexie pure sans hemianopsie. *Cortex* 12, 169–174

Assal, G., Regli, F. (1980). Syndrome de disconnexion visuo-verbale et visuo-gesturelle. Aphasie optique et apraxie optique. *Rev. Neurol.* 136, 365–376

Assayama, T. (1914). Über die Aphasie bei Japanern. *Dtsch. Arch. Klin. Med.* 113, 523–529

Atkinson, J., Braddick, O., Braddick, F. (1974). Acuity and contrast sensitivity of infant vision. Nature London 247, 403–404

Atkinson, R.A., Appenzeller, O. (1978): Deer woman. *Headache* 17, 229–232

Attneave, F. (1954). Some informational aspects of visual perception. *Psychol. Rev.* 61, 183–193

Aubert, H. (1857). Beiträge zur Kenntniss des indirecten Sehens II. Ueber die Grenzen der Farbenwahrnehmung auf den seitlichen Theilen der Retina. *Graefes Arch. Ophthalmol.* 3 (2), 38

Aubert, H. (1861). Über eine scheinbare bedeutende Drehung von Objekten bei Neigung des Kopfes nach rechts oder links. *Virchow's Arch. Pathol. Anat. Physiol. klin. Med.* 20, 381–393

Aubert, H. (1865). *Physiologie der Netzhaut.* Morgenstern, Breslau

Aubert, H. (1886). Die Bewegungsempfindung. *Pflügers Arch. ges. Physiol.* 39, 347–370

Aubert, H. (1887). Die Bewegungsempfindung. *Pflügers Arch. ges. Physiol.* 40, 459–480

Aubert, H., Förster, R. (1857). Beiträge zur Kenntniss des indirecten Sehens. I. Untersuchungen über den Raumsinn der Retina. *Graefes Arch. Ophthalmol.* 3(2), 1–37

Auerbach, S.H., Alexander, M.P. (1981). Pure agraphia and unilateral optic ataxia associated with a left superior parietal lobule lesion. *J. Neurol. Neurosurg. Psychiat.* 44, 430

Auersperg, A.P., Sprockhoff, H. (1935). Experimentelle Beiträge zur Frage der Konstanz der Sehdinge und ihrer Fundierung. *Pflügers Arch. ges. Physiol.* 236, 301–320

Augustinus, A. *De genesi ad litteram* (1884). In Migne, J.P. (ed.) *Opera omnia*, Paris

Augustinus, Aurelius (1884). *De spiritu et anima*. In Migne, J.P. (ed.), *Opera omnia, Vol. 6*, Paris

Augustinus, Aurelius (1935). *De trinitate libri XV.* Transl. M. Schmaus, Bibliothek der Kirchenväter, 2. Reihe, Vol. 14, Kösel, München 1935/36

Aulhorn, E., Harms, H., (1972). Visual perimetry. In Jameson, D., Hurvich, L.M. (eds.), *Visual psychophysics. Handbook of sensory physiology.* Vol. VII/4. Springer, Heidelberg, New York, 102–169

Aulhorn, E., Köst, G. (1988). Rauschfeld-Kampimetrie — eine neuartige, perimetrische Untersuchungsweise. *Klin. Monatsbl. Augenheilk.* 192, 284

Aulhorn, E., Köst, G. (1988/89). Noise-field campimetry. In Heijl, A. (ed.), *Perimetry Update Proceedings of the VIIIth International Perimetric Society Meeting.* Kugler & Ghedini Publications, Amsterdam, Berkeley, Milano, 331–336

Averbach, E., Coriell, A.S. (1961). Short-term memory in vision. *Bell. Syst. Techn. J.* 40, 309–328

Avery, G.C., Day, R.H. (1969). Basis of the horizontal-vertical illusion. *J. Exp. Psychol.* 81, 376–380

Avons, S.E., Phillips, W.A. (1980). Visualization and memorization as a function of display time and poststimulus processing time. *J. Exp. Psychol. (Hum. Learn.)* 6, 407–420

Avons, S.E., Phillips, W.A. (1987). Representation of matrix patterns in long-and short-term visual memory. *Acta Psychol. (Amst.)* 65, 227–246

Axenfeld, Th. (1915). Hemianopische Gesichtsfeldstörungen nach Schädelschüssen. *Klin. Monatsbl. Augenheilk.* 55, 126–143

Azam, E.E. (1887). Hypnotisme double conscience et alteration de la personalité. Bailliere, Paris

Baarmann, J. (1882). Ibn al-Haitams Abhandlungen über das Licht. *Zeitschf. f.d.Dtsch. Morgenländische Gesellschaft* 36, 195

Babinski, J. (1914). Contribution a l'étude des troubles mentaux dans l'hemiplegie cerebrale (anosognosie). *Revue Neurologique* 27, 845–847

Babkoff, H., Ben-Uriah, Y. ((1983). Lexical decision time as a function of visual field and stimulus probability. *Cortex* 19, 13–30

Bachevalier, J., Mishkin, M. (1986). Visual recognition impairment follows ventromedial but not dorsolateral prefrontal lesions in monkeys. *Behav. Brain Res.* 20, 249–261

Badal, J. (1888). Contribution ö letude des cécités psychiques. Alexie agraphie, hémianopsie inférieure, trouble du sens d'l'espace. *Arch. d'Ophthalmol.* 140, 97–117

Baddeley, A.D. (1964). Immediate memory and the 'perception' of letter sequences. *J. Exp. Psychol.* 16, 364–367

Baeumker, C. (1928). *Studien und Charakteristiken zur Geschichte der Philosophie, insbesondere des Mittelalters.* Aschendorff, Münster i.W.

Bagshaw, M.H., Benzies, S. (1968). Multiple measures of the orienting reaction and their dissociation after amygdalectomy in monkeys. *Exp. Neurol.* 20, 175–187

Bagshaw, M.H., Mackworth, N.H., Pribram, K.H. (1970b). The effect of inferotemporal cortex ablations on eye movements of monkeys during discrimination training. *Int.J.Neurosci.* 1, 153–158

Bagshaw, M.H., Pribram, K.H. (1953). Cortical organization in gustation (Macaca mulatta). *J. Neurophysiol.* 16, 499–508

Bagshaw, M.H., Pribram, K.H. (1968). Effect of amygdalectomy on stimulus threshold of the monkey. *Exp. Neurol.* 20, 197–202

Bahia, J. (1911). La resensibilisation dans l'hystérie. *Gazette Médicale de Paris*, Juillet 19, 1911, 225–226

Bahrick, H.P., Bahrick, P.O., Wittlinger, R.P. (1975). Fifty years of memory for names and faces: A cross-sectional approach. *J. Exp. Psychol.* 104, 54–57

Bain, A. (1903). *De l'auto-représentation chez les hystériques.* Medical thesis, University of Paris

Baizer, J.S., Robinson, D.L., Dow, B.H. (1977). Visual responses of area 18 neurons in awake, behaving monkey. *J. Neurophysiol.* 40, 1024–1037

Baizer, J.S., Ungerleider, L.G., Desimone, R. (1991). Organization of visual inputs to the inferior temporal and posterior parietal cortex in macaques. *J. Neurosci.* 11, 168–190

Bak, M., Girvin, J.P., Hambrecht, F.T., Kufta, C.V., Loeb, G.E., Schmidt, E.M. (1990). Visual sensations produced by intracortical microstimulationof the human occipital cortex. *Med. and Biol. Eng. and Comput.* 28, 257–259

Bakan, P. (1969). Hypnotizability, laterality of eye-movements and functional brain asymmetry. *Percept. Mot. Skills* 28, 927–932

Baken, B., Putnam, W. (1974). Right-left discrimination and brain lateralization: Sex differences. *Archives of Neurology* 30, 334–335

Baker, C.L., Braddick, O.J. (1984). Eccentricity-dependent scaling of the limits for short-range apparent motion perception. *Vision Res.* 25, 803–812

Baker, C.L. (Jr.), Hess, R.F., Zihl, J. (1991). Residual motion preception in a 'motion-blind' patient, assessed with limited-lifetime random dot stimuli. *J. Neurosci.*, in press

Baker, F.H., Grigg, P., Noorden von, G.K. (1974). Effects of visual deprivation and strabismus on the response of neurons in the visual cortex of the monkey, including studies on the striate and prestriate cortex in the normal animal. *Brain Res.* 66, 185–208

Baker, J.F., Petersen, S.E., Newsome, W.T., Allman, J.M. (1981). Visual response properties of neurons in four extrastriate visual areas of the owl monkey (Aoutus trivirgatus): a quantitative comparison of medial, dorsomedial, dorsolateral and middle temporal areas. *J. Neurophysiol.* 45, 397–416

Baldwin, M. (1970). Neurologic syndroms and hallucinations. In Keup, W. (ed.), *Origin and mechanisms of hallucinations.* Plenum Press, N.Y, London, 3–12

Baley, P., Bonin, G. von (1951). *The isocortex of man.* University of Illinois Press, Urbana Ill.

Baleydier, C., Mauguiere, F. (1980). The duality of the cingulate gyrus in monkey: Neuroanatomical study and functional hypothesis. *Brain* 103, 525–54

Baleydier, C., Mauguiere, F. (1985). Anatomical evidence for medial pulvinar connections with the posterior cingulate cortex, the retrosplenial area, and the posterior parahippocampal gyrus in monkeys. *J. Comp. Neurol.* 232, 219–228

Balint, E. (1987). Memory and consciousness. *Int. J. Psychoanal.* 68, 475–483

Balint, R. (1909). Seelenlähmung des Schauens, optische Ataxie, räumliche Störung der Aufmerksamkeit. *Monatsschr. Psychiat. Neurol.* 25, 51–81

Ballard, D.H. (1986). Cortical connections and parallel processing: structure and function. *Behav. Brain Sci.* 9, 67–90

Baloh, R.W., Yee, R.D., Honrubia, V. (1980). Optokinetic nystagmus and parietal lobe lesions. *Ann. Neurol.* 7, 269–276

Banks, M.S., Geisler, W.S., Bennett, P.J. (1987). The physical limits of grating visibility. *Vision Res.* 27, 1915–1924

Barbas, H. (1988). Anatomic organization of basoventral and mediodorsal visual recipient prefrontal regions in the rhesus monkey. *J. Comp. Neurol.* 276, 313–342

Barbas, H., Mesulam, M.M. (1981). Organization of afferent input to subdivisions of area 8 in the rhesus monkey. *J. Comp. Neurol.* 200, 407–431

Barber, P. (1981). Visual search and number of stimuli reexamined. *Psychol. Bull.* 89, 176–182

Barber, T.X. (1979). Eidetic imagery and the ability to hallucinate at will. *Behav. Brain Sciences* 2, 596

Barbur, L.J., Ruddock, K.H., Waterfield, V.A. (1980). Human visual responses in the absence of the geniculo-calcarine projection. *Brain* 103, 905–928

Barker, A.T., Freeston, I.L., Jalinous, R., Merton, P.A., Morton, H.B. (1985). Magnetic stimulation of the human brain. *J. Physiol. (Lond.)* 369, 3 P

Barker, A.T., Jalinous, R., Freeston, I.L. (1985). Non-invasive magnetic stimulation of the human motor cortex. *Lancet* 1, 1106–1107

Barlow, H.B. (1972). Single units and sensation: a neuron doctrine for perceptual psychology? *Perception* 1, 371–394

Barlow, J.S. (1971). Brain information processing during reading electrophysiological correlates. *Diseases Nerv. Syst.* Vol. 32, p. 668–672

Barnet, A.B., Manson, J.I., Wilner, E. (1970). Acute cerebral blindness in childhood: six cases studied clinically and electrophysiologically. *Neurology* 20, 1147–1156

Barnett, A. (1941). Electrically produced flicker in darkness. *Amer. J. Physiol.* 133, 205–206

Baron, J. (1981). Mechanisms of human facial recognition. *Int. J. Man-Machine Studies* 15, 137–178

Barone, P., Joseph, J.P. (1989). Prefrontal cortex and spatial sequencing in macaque monkey. *Exp. Brain Res.* 78, 447–464

Barrera, M.E., Maurer, D. (1981). The perception of facial expression by three-month-old. *Child Development* 52, 203–206

Barrett, S.E., Rugg, M.D., Perrett, D.I. (1988). Event-related potentials and the matching of familiar and unfamiliar faces. *Neuropsychologia* 26, 105–117

Bartl, G., Benedikt, O. (1974). Rindenblindheit und ihre elektrophysiologische Objektivierung. *Graefes Arch. klin. Ophthalmol.* 192, 255–258

Bartleson, J.D. (1984). Transient and persistent neurological manifestations of migraine. *Stroke* 15, 383–386

Bartlett, J.R., Doty, R.W. (1974). Influence of mesencephalic stimulation on unit activity in striate cortex of squirrel monkeys. *J. Neurophysiol.* 37, 642–652

Bartlett, J.R., Doty, R.W. (1974). Response of units in striate cortex of squirrel monkey to visual and electrical stimuli. *J. Neurophysiol.* 37, 621–641

Bartlett, J.R., Doty, R.W. (1980). An exploration of the ability of macaques to detect microstimulation of striate cortex. *Acta Neurobiol. Exp.* 40, 713–727

Bartlett, J.R., Doty, R.W., Lee, B.B., Negrao, N., Overman, W.H. (1977). Deleterious effects of prolonged electrical excitation of striate cortex in macaques. *Brain Behav. Evol.* 14, 46–66

Bartley, S.H. (1941). *Vision: a study of its basis.* Van Nostrand, New York

Barton, M.I., Goodglass, H., Shai, A. (1965). Differential recognition of tachistoscopically presented English and Hebrew words in right and left visual fields. *Perceptual and Motor Skills* 21, 431–437

Basler, A. (1906). Über das Sehen von Bewegungen. I. Die Wahrnehmung kleinster Bewegungen. *Pflügers Arch. ges. Physiol.* 115, 582–601

Basser, L.S. (1969). The relation of migraine and epilepsy. *Brain* 92, 285–300

Bassili, J.N. (1979). Emotion recognition: the role of facial movement and the relative importance of upper and lower areas of the face. *J. Personality, Soc. Psychol.* 37, 2049–2058

Basso, A., Bisiach, E., Luzzatti, C. (1980). Loss of mental imagery: A case study. *Neuropsychologia* 18, 435–442

Basso, A., Faglioni, P., Spinnler, H. (1976). Non-verbal colour impairment of aphasics. *Neuropsychologia* 14, 183–193

Bastian, H.C. (1898). *A treatise on aphasia and other speech defects.* H.K. Lewis, London

Battersby, W.S., Bender, M.B., Pollack, M., Kahn, R.L. (1956). Unilateral 'spatial' agnosia ('inattention') in patients with cerebral lesions. *Brain* 79, 68–93

Batuev, A.S., Shaefer, V.I., Orlov, A.A. (1985). Comparative characteristics of unit activity in the prefrontal and parietal areas during delayed performance in monkeys. *Behav. Brain Res.* 16, 57–70

Bauer R.M.(1986). The cognitive psychophysiology of prosopagnosia. In Ellis, H.D., Jeeves, M.A., Newcombe, F., Young, A. (eds.), *Aspects of face recognition.* Martinus Nijhoff, Dordrecht, 253–267

Bauer, H. (1911). *Die Psychologie Alhazens auf Grund von Alhazens Optik.* Aschendorff, Münster i.W.

Bauer, R. (1982). A high probability of an orientation shift between layers 4 and 5 in central parts of the cat striate cortex. *Exp. Brain Res.* 48, 245–255

Bauer, R., Dow, B.M., Snyder, A.Z., Vautin, R.G. (1983). Orientation shift between upper and lower layers in monkey visual cortex. *Exp. Brain Res.* 50, 133–145

Bauer, R., Mayr, M., Huber, H.P. (1985). Differences in direction specificity of receptive fields in upper and lower layers of the cat's prestriate area 18. *Neurosci. Letters* 54, 59–63

Bauer, R.M. (1982). Visual hypoemotionality as a symptom of visual-limbic disconnection in man. *Arch. Neurol.* 39, 702–708

Bauer, R.M. (1984). Autonomic recognition of names and faces in prosopagnosia: A neuropsychological application of the Guilty Knowledge Test. *Neuropsychologia* 22, 457–469

Bauer, R.M. (1986). The cognitive psychophysiology of prosopagnosia. In Ellis, H.D., Jeeves, M.A., Newcombe, F., Young, A. (eds.), *Aspects of face processing.* Martinus Nijhoff Publishers, Dordrecht

Bauer, R.M., Rubens, A.B. (1985). Agnosia. In Heilman, K.M., Valenstein, E. (eds.), *Clinical neuropsychology.* Oxford University Press, 2nd. edition, New York, Oxford, 187–241

Bauer, R.M., Trobe, J.D. (1984). Visual memory and perceptual impairments in prosopagnosia. *J. Clin. Neuroophthalmol.* 4, 39–46

Bauer, R.M., Verfaellie, M. (1988). Electrodermal discrimination of familiar but not unfamiliar faces in prosopagnosia. *Brain and Cognition* 8, 240–252

Baumgardt, E., Bujas, Z. (1952). L'influence de la fréquence de stimulation électrique intermittente sur le phosphène liminaire. *Compt. Rend. Soc. de Biol.* 146, 424–

Baumgarten, P. (1878). Hemiopie nach Erkrankung der occipitalen Hirnrinde. *Zentralbl. f. d. Med. Wissensch.* 16, 369

Baumgarten, R. v., Jung, R. (1952). Microelectrode studies on the visual cortex. *Rev. Neurol.* 87, 151–155

Baumgartner, G. (1955). Reaktionen einzelner Neurone im optischen Cortex der Katze nach Lichtblitzen. *Pflügers Arch. ges. Physiol.* 261, 457–469

Baumgartner, G. (1960). Indirekte Grössenbestimmung der rezeptiven Felder der Retina beim Menschen mittels der Hermannschen Gittertäuschung. *Pflügers Arch.* 272, 21–22

Baumgartner, G. (1961). Die Reaktionen der Neurone des zentralen visuellen Systems der Katze im simultanen Helligkeitskontrast. In Jung, R., Kornhuber, H.H. (eds.), *Neurophysiologie und Psychophysik des visuellen Systems.* Springer, Berlin-Göttingen-Heidelberg, 296–311

Baumgartner, G. (1961). Kontrastlichteffekte an retinalen Ganglienzellen: Ableitungen vom Tractus opticus der Katze. In Jung, R., Kornhuber, H.H. (eds.), *Neurophysiologie und Psychophysik des visuellen Systems.* Berlin-Göttingen-Heidelberg, Springer, 45–55

Baumgartner, G. (1961). Neuronale Grundlagen der visuellen Kontrastverschärfung und der Signalübertragung vom Auge zur Hirnrinde. In ed. Nachricht.-techn. Ges. VDE, *Aufnahme und Verarbeitung von Nachrichten durch Organismen.* Hirzel, Stuttgart, 100–108

Baumgartner, G. (1962). Zur Neurophysiologie und Psychophysik des simultanen Helligkeitskontrastes. *Fortschr. Med.* 80, 633–638

Baumgartner, G. (1964). Neuronale Mechanismen des Kontrast-und Bewegungssehens. *Ber. dtsch. Ophthal. Ges.* 66, 111–125

Baumgartner, G. (1977). Neuronal mechanisms of migrainous visual aura. In Rose, C.F. (ed.), *Physiological aspects of clinical neurology.* Blackwell, Oxford, 111–121

Baumgartner, G. (1982). Visuelle Wahrnehmungsstörungen und Halluzinationen bei Epilepsien und anderen Hirnerkrankungen. In Karbowski, K. (ed.), *Halluzinationen bei Epilepsien und ihre Differentialdiagnose*, Huber, Bern, 9–23

Baumgartner, G. (1983). Organization and function of the neocortex. *Neuro-ophthalmology* 3, 1–14

Baumgartner, G. (1983). Psychophysics and central processing. In Ashbury, A.K., McKham, G.M., McDonald W.I. (eds.), Diseases of the nervous system. *Clinical Neurology* II, W.D. Sanders & Co, Philadelphia, W. Heinemann, Medical Books, London, 804–815

Baumgartner, G. (1990). Where do visual signals become a perception? In Eccles, J.C. & Creutzfeldt, O. (eds.), *The principles of design and operation of the brain. Pontificiae Academiae Scientiarum Scripta Varia* 78, 99–114

Baumgartner, G., Brown, J.L., Schulz, A. (1964). Visual motion detection in the cat. *Science* 146, 1070–1071

Baumgartner, G., Brown, J.L., Schulz, A. (1965). Responses of single units of the cat visual system to rectangular stimulus patterns. *J. Neurophysiol.* 28, 1–18

Baumgartner, G., Creutzfeldt, O. (1955). The reaction of cortical neurons upon electrical stimulation of the cerebral cortex. *Electroenceph. clin Neurophysiol.* 7, 662–663

Baumgartner, G., Hakas, P. (1959). Reaktionen einzelner Opticusneurone und corticaler Nervenzellen der Katze im Hell-Dunkel-Grenzfeld (Simultankontrast). *Pflügers Arch. ges. Physiol.* 270, 29

Baumgartner, G., Hakas, P. (1962). Die Neurophysiologie des

simultanen Helligkeitskontrastes. Reziproke Reaktionen antagonistischer Neuronengruppen des visuellen Systems. *Pflüg. Arch. ges. Physiol.* 274, 489–500

Baumgartner, G., Peterhans, E., Heydt, R. von der (1988). Neuronal mechanisms of the first, second and third order contrast in the visual system. In Haken, H. (ed.) *Computational Systems, Natural and Artificial.* Springer, Heidelberg-New York, p. 35–43

Baumgartner, G., von der Heydt, R., Peterhans, E. (1984). Anomalous contours: a tool in studying the neurophysiology of vision. *Exp. Brain Res.* suppl. 9, 413–419

Baxter, D.M., Warrington, E.K. (1983). Neglect dysgraphia. *J. Neurol. Neurosurg. Psychiat.* 46, 1073–1078

Bay, E. (1950). *Agnosie und Funktionswandel. Eine hirnpathologische Studie.* (Monographien aus dem Gesamtgebiete der Neurologie und Psychiatrie Vol. 73) Springer, Berlin

Bay, E. (1951). Über den Begriff der Agnosie. *Nervenarzt* 22, 179–187

Bay, E. (1952a). Analyse eines Falles von Seelenblindheit. *Dtsch. Z. Nervenheilk.* 168, 1–23

Bay, E. (1952b). Der gegenwärtige Stand der Aphasie-Forschung. *Folia Phoniatrica* 4, 9–30

Bay, E. (1953). Disturbances of visual perception and their examination. *Brain* 76, 515–550

Bay, E. (1962). Aphasia and non-verbal disorders of language. *Brain* 85, 411–426

Bay, E. (1965). The concepts of agnosia, apraxia and aphasia after a history of a hundred years. *J. Mt. Sinai Hosp.* 32, 637–650

Bay, E., Lauenstein, O., Cibis, P. (1949). Ein Beitrag zur Frage der Seelenblindheit. Der Fall Schn. von Gelb und Goldstein. *Psychiat. Neurol. Med. Psychol. (Lpz.)* 1, 73–91

Bayley, P., von Bonin, G., Garol, H.W., McCulloch, W.S. (1943). Functional organization of temporal lobe of monkey (Macaca mulatta) and chimpanzee (Pan satyrus). *J. Neurophysiol.* 6, 121–128

Bayley, P.G., von Bonin, G., McCulloch, W. (1950). *The Isocortex of the Chimpanzee.* Univ. of Illinois Press, Urbana

Baylis, G.C., Rolls, E.T. (1987). Responses of neurons in the inferior temporal cortex in short term and serial recognition memory tasks. *Exp. Brain Res.* 65, 614–622

Baylis, G.C., Rolls, E.T., Leonard, C.M. (1985). Selectivity between faces in the responses of a population of neurons in the cortex in the superior temporal sulcus of the monkey. *Brain Res.* 342, 91–102

Baylis, G.C., Rolls, E.T., Leonard, C.M. (1987). Functional subdivisions of the temporal lobe neocortex. *J. Neurosci.* 7, 330–342

Baylor, D.A., Nunn, B.J., Schnapf, J.L. (1987). Spectral sensitivity of cones of the monkey Macaca fascicularis. *J. Physiol. (Lond.)* 390, 145–160

Baynes, K., Holtzman, J.D., Volpe, B.T. (1986). Components of visual attention: alterations in response pattern to visual stimuli following parietal lobe infarction. *Brain* 109, 99–114

Bäumler, Ch. (1925). Über das sogenannte Flimmerskotom. *Dtsch. Z. Nervenheilk.* 83, 11–47

Bear, D.M. (1983). Hemispheric specialization and the neurology of emotion. *Arch. Neurol.* 40, 195–202

Beatty, W.W., MacInnes, W.D., Porphyris, H.S., Troster, A.I., Cermak, L.S. (1988). Preserved topographical memory following right temporal lobectomy. *Brain. Cogn.* 8, 67–76

Beaumont, J.G. (1982). Studies with verbal stimuli. In Beaumont, J.G. (ed.) *Divided visual field studies of cerebral organization.* Academic Press, London, New York, p. 57–86

Beaumont, J.G. (ed.) (1982). *Divided Visual Field Studies of Cerebral Organisation.* Academic Press, London, New York

Beauvois, M.F. (1982). Optic aphasia: A process of interaction between vision and language. *Philos. Trans. Roy. Soc. Lond.* B298, 35–47

Beauvois, M.F., Derouesne, J. (1979). Phonological alexia: three dissociations. *J. Neurol. Neurosurg. Psychiat.* 42, 1115–1124

Beauvois, M.F., Derouesne, J. (1981). Lexical or orthographic agraphia. *Brain* 101, 21–49

Beauvois, M.F., Saillant, B. (1985). Optic aphasia for colours and colour agnosia: a distinction between visual and visuo-verbal impairments in the processing of colours. *Cognitive Neuropsychology* 2, 1–48

Bechterew, W. (1883). Die Funktion der Sehhügel (Thalami optici). Experimentelle Untersuchungen. *Neurol. Centralbl.* 2, 78

Bechterew, W. (1898). *Bewusstsein und Hirnlokalisation.* Weinberg, Georgi, Leipzig

Bechterew, W. (1898). Die Resultate der Untersuchungen mit Reizung von hinteren Partien der Hemisphären und des Frontallappens beim Affen. *Neurol. Centralbl.* 17, 720

Bechterew, W. (1901). Ueber das corticale Sehcentrum. *Monatsschr. Psychiat. Neurol.* 10, 432

Bechterew, W. (1908–1911). Die Funktion der Nervencentra. 3 Vols. Fischer, Jena

Beck, E. (1930). Die Myeloarchitektonik der dorsalen Schläfenlappenrinde beim Menschen. *J. Psychol. Neurol. (Lpz.)* 41, 129

Beck, E. (1937). Sensorische Aphasien. *Z. ges. Neurol. Psychiat.* 158, 193–203

Beck, J., Rosenfeld, A., Ivry, R. (1990). Line segregation. *Spatial Vis.* 4, 75–101

Beck, U., Aschayeri, H., Keller, H. (1978). Prosopagnosie und Farberkennungstörung bei Rückbildung von Rindenblindheit. *Arch. Psychiat. Nervenkr.* 225, 55–66

Becker, A.M. (1952). Über einen Fall von optischer Agnosie. *Wien. Z. Nervenheilk.* 4, 424

Beer, G.J. (1813–1817). *Lehre von den Augenkrankheiten.* 2 Vols. Camesina, Wien

Behr, C. (1909). Zur topischen Diagnose der Hemianopsie. *Graefes Arch. Ophthalmol.* 70, 340–402

Behr, C. (1916). Die homonymen Hemianopsien mit einseitigem Gesichtsfelddefekt im 'reinen temporalen halbmondförmigen Bezirk des binokularen Gesichtsfeldes'. *Klin. Monatsbl. Augenheilk.* 56, 161–172

Behr, C. (1931). Die Erkrankungen der Sehbahn vom Chiasma aufwärts. In Schieck, Brückner (eds.) *Kurzes·Handbuch der Ophthalmologie.* Vol. VI, Springer, Berlin

Behrens, D.S.G. (1733). *Dissertatio de vulnere cerebri non semper et absolute letali.* Frankfurt a.M.

Behrens, F., Collewijn, H., Grüsser, O.-J. (1985). Velocity step responses of the human gaze pursuit system. Experiments with sigma-movement. *Vision Res.* 25, 893–905

Behrens, F., Grüsser, O.-J. (1978). Bewegungswahrnehmung und Augenbewegungen bei Flickerbelichtung unbewegter visueller Muster. In Kommerell, G. (ed.), *Augenbewegungsstörungen.* Bergmann, München, 273–284

Behrens, F., Grüsser, O.-J. (1979). Smooth pursuit eye movements and optokinetic nystagmus elicited by intermittently illuminated stationary patterns. *Exp. Brain Res.* 37, 317–336

Behrens, F., Grüsser, O.-J. (1982). On the additivity of Sigma-and Phi-movement in visual perception and oculomotor control. *Human Neurobiol.* 1, 121–127

Behrens, F., Grüsser, O.-J., Roggenkämper, P. (1989). Open-loop and closed-loop optokinetic nystagmus in Squirrel monkeys. (Saimiri sciureus) and in man. In Allum, J.H.J., Hulliger, M. (eds.), *Progress in brain research,* Vol. 80, Elsevier Science, 183–196

Behrmann, M., Black, S.E., Bub, D. (1990). The evolution of pure alexia: A longitudinal study of recovery. *Brain and Language* 39, 405–427

Beichl, L. (1944). Ueber einen Typus von Scheinbewegungen bei occipitaler Verletzung. *Z. f. d. ges. Neurol. Psychiat.* 177, 486–504

Bekeny, G., Peter, A. (1961). Über Polyopie und Palinopsie. *Psychiat. Neurol. (Basel)* 142, 154–175

Bell, Ch. (1806). *The anatomy and physiology of expressions as con-*

nected with the fine arts. John Murray, London

Bell, Ch. (1811). *Idea of a new anatomy of the brain*. Strahan and Preston, London. Repr. Medical Classics Vol. 1 (1936/1937), p. 105–120

Bell, Ch. (1823). On the motions of the eye in illustration of the uses of the muscles and nerves of the orbit. *Phil. Trans. Roy. Soc. Lond.* 113, 166–186

Belleza, T., Rappaport, M., Hopkins, H.K., Hall, K. (1979). Visual scanning and matching dysfunction in brain-damaged patients with drawing impairment. *Cortex* 15, 19–36

Belyi, B.I. (1988). The role of the right hemisphere in form perception and visual gnosis organization. *Int. J. Neurosci.* 40, 167–180

Ben-Shakhar, G., Gati, I. (1987). Common and distinctive features of verbal and pictorial stimuli as determinants of psychophysiological responsivity. *J. Exp. Psychol. Gen.* Vol. 116, 2, 91–105

Benary, D. (1983). *Polyglossie und ihre Auswirkung auf die optische Differenzierung und das optische Gedächtnis bei Schulkindern*. Univ. Wien, Grund-und Integrativwiss. Fak., Wien, 69 p.

Benary, W. (1922). Studien zur Untersuchung der Intelligenz beim Fall von Seelenblindheit. *Psychol. Forschg.* 2, 209–297

Bender, B.G., Ruddock, K.H. (1974). The characteristics of a visual defect associated with abnormal responses to both colour and luminance. *Vision Res.* 14, 383–393

Bender, D.B. (1981). Retinotopic organization of macaque pulvinar. *J. Neurophysiol.* 46, 672–693

Bender, M., Jung, R. (1948). Abweichung der subjektiven optischen Vertikalen und Horizontalen bei Gesunden und Hirnverletzten. *Arch. Psychiat., Z. Nervenkr od. heilk.* 181, 193–212

Bender, M.B. (1945). Polyopia and monocular diplopia of cerebral origin. *Arch. Neurol.* 59, 323–338

Bender, M.B. (1952). *Disorders in perception*. Charles C. Thomas, Springfield, Ill.

Bender, M.B. (1962). *Neuroophthalmology*. In Baker, A.B. (ed.), *Clinical Neurology* (2nd edn). Hoeber-Harper, New York, 275–347

Bender, M.B. (1984). Dissociated perception of a visual defect. *J. of Nervous and Mental Disease* 172, 364–368

Bender, M.B., Feldman, M. (1965). The so-called 'visual agnosias'. *Proc. 8th. Intern. Cong. Neurol.* 3, 153–156

Bender, M.B., Feldman, M. (1972). The so-called 'visual agnosia'. *Brain* 95, 173–186

Bender, M.B., Feldman, M., Sobin, A.J. (1968). Palinopsia. *Brain* 91, 321–338

Bender, M.B., Furlow, C.T. (1945a). Phenomenon of visual extinction on homonymous fields and psychological principles involved. *Arch. Neurol. Psychiat.* (Chicago) 53, 29–33

Bender, M.B., Furlow, L.T. (1944). Phenomenon of visual extinction and binocular rivalry mechanisms. *Trans. Amer. Neurol. Association* 70, 87–93

Bender, M.B., Furlow, L.T. (1945b). Visual disturbances produced by bilateral lesions of the occipital lobe with central scotomas. *Arch. Neurol. Pychiat.* (Chicago) 53, 165–170

Bender, M.B., Kanzer, M.G. (1939). Dynamics of homonymous hemianopsias and preservation of central vision. *Brain* 62, 404–421

Bender, M.B., Krieger, H.P. (1951). Visual function in perimetrically blind fields. Arch. *Neurol. Psychiat.* (Chicago) 65, 72–79

Bender, M.B., Teuber, H.L. (1946). Phenomena of fluctuation, extinction and completion in visual perception. *Arch. Neurol. Psychiat.* (Chicago) 55, 627–658

Bender, M.B., Teuber, H.L. (1947b). Ring scotoma and tubular fields. Their significance in cases of head-injury. *Arch. Neurol. Psychiat.* (Chicago) 56, 200–226

Bender, M.B., Teuber, H.L. (1948). Spatial organization of visual perception following injury to the brain. *Arch. Neurol. Psychiat.* (Chicago) 58, 721–739 and 59, 39–62

Bender, M.B., Teuber, H.L. (1949). Disturbances in visual perception following cerebral lesions. *J. Psychol.* 28, 223–233

Bender, M.B., Wortis, S.B., Cramer, J. (1948). Organic mental syndrome with phenomena of extinction and allaesthesia. *Arch. Neurol. Psychiat.* 59, 273

Benedict, H. (1830). Augenfunken. In Graefe, C.F. von, Hufeland, C.W., Link, H.F., Rudolphi, K.A., v. Siebold, E. (eds). *Encyclopädisches Wörterbuch der medicinischen Wissenschaften*. Vol. IV. Boike, Berlin, 131–133

Benevento, L.A., Davis, B. (1977). Topographic projections of the prestriate cortex to the pulvinar nuclei in the macaque monkey: an autoradiographic study. *Exp. Brain Res.* 30, 405–424

Benevento, L.A., Fallon, J.H. (1975). The ascending projections of the superior colliculus in the rhesus monkey (*Macaca mulatta*). *J. Comp. Neurol.* 160, 339–362

Benevento, L.A., Miller, J. (1981). Visual responses of single neurons in the caudal lateral pulvinar of the macaque monkey. *J. Neurosci.* 11, 1268–1278

Benevento, L.A., Rezak, M. (1975). Extrageniculate projections to layers VI and I of striate cortex (area 17) in the rhesus monkey (*Macaca mulatta*). *Brain Res.* 96, 51–55

Benevento, L.A., Rezak, M. (1976). The cortical projections of the inferior pulvinar and adjacent lateral pulvinar in the rhesus monkey (*Macaca mulatta*): an autoradiographic study. *Brain Res.* 108, 1–24

Benevento, L.A., Rezak, M., Santos-Anderson, R. (1977). An autoradiographic study of the projections of the pretectum in the rhesus monkey (*Macaca mulatta*): evidence of sonsorimotor links to the thalamus and oculomotor nuclei. *Brain Res.* 127, 197–218

Benevento, L.A., Standage, G.P. (1983). The organization of projections of the retinorecipient and nonretinorecipient nuclei of the pretectal complex and layers of the superior colliculus of the lateral pulvinar and medial pulvinar in the macaque monkey. *J. Comp. Neurol.* 217, 307–336

Benevento, L.A., Yoshida, K. (1981). The afferent and efferent organization of the lateral geniculo-prestriate pathways in the macaque monkey. *J. comp. Neurobiol.* 203, 455–474

Bengtsen, G., Fog, M., Hermann, K. (1941). Zwei Fälle von Atrophia cerebri mit einem speziell psychischen Syndrom (presbyophreniformes Syndrom verbunden mit Agnosie). *Neurol. Psychiat.* 172, 601–607

Benke, T. (1988). Visual agnosia and amnesia from a left unilateral lesion. *Europ. Neurol.* 28, 236–239

Benowitz, L.I., Bear, D.M., Rosenthal, R., Mesulam, M.M., Zaidel, E., Sperry, R.W. (1983). Hemispheric specialization in nonverbal communication. *Cortex* 19, 5–11

Benöhr, R. (1905). Ein Fall von centraler Blindheit. Erweichungsherde in beiden Occipitallappen. Doctoral dissertation, Universität Kiel

Benson, D.F. (1977). The third alexia. *Arch. Neurol.* 34, 327–331

Benson, D.F. (1979). *Aphasia, Alexia, and Agraphia*. Churchill Livingstone, New York

Benson, D.F. (1981). Alexia and the neuroanatomical basis of reading. In Pirozzolo, F.J., Wittrock, M.C. (eds.), *Neuropsychological and cognitive processes in reading*. Academic Press, New York, 69–92

Benson, D.F. (1985). Alexia. In Vinken, P.J., Bruyn, G.W., Klawans, H.L. (eds.), *Handbook of Clinical Neurology* Vol. 4, Elsevier Science Publ., Amsterdam, Chapter 32

Benson, D.F. (1989). Disorders of visual gnosis. In Brown, J.W. (ed.), *Neuropsychology of visual perception*. Erlbaum, Hillsdale, NY, 59–78

Benson, D.F., Greenberg, J.P. (1969). Visual form agnosia. *Arch. of Neurol.* 20, 82–89

Benson, D.F., Barton, M.I. (1970). Disturbances in constructional ability. *Cortex* 6, 19–46

Benson, D.F., Brown, J., Tomlinson, E.B. (1971). Varieties of alexia. Word and letter blindness. *Neurology* 21, 951–957

Benson, D.F., Cummings, J.L., Tsai, S.Y. (1982). Angular gyrus syndrome simulating Alzheimer disease. *Arch. Neurol.* 39, 616–620

Benson, D.F., Davis, R.J., Schnyder, B.D. (1988). Posterior cortical atrophy. *Arch. of Neurol.* 45, 789–793

Benson, D.F., Geschwind, N. (1969). The alexias. In Vinken, P.J., Bruyn, G.W. (eds.) *Handbook of Clinical Neurology*, vol. 4, North Holland Publishing Comp., Amsterdam, 112–140

Benson, D.F., Greenberg, J.P. (1969). Visual form agnosia. *Arch. Neurol.* 20, 82–89

Benson, D.F., Marsden, C.D., Meadows, J. (1974). The amnesic syndrome of posterior cerebral artery occlusion. *Acta Neurol. Scand.* 50, 133–145

Benson, D.F., Segarra, J.(1974). Visual agnosia-prosopagnosia (case report). In Michel, F., Schott, B. (eds.), *Les Syndromes de disconnexion calleuse chez l'homme.* Colloque international de Lyon, 362–370

Benson, D.F., Segarra, J., Albert, M.L. (1974). Visual agnosia-prosopagnosia: A clinicopathologic correlation. *Arch. Neurol.* 30, 307–310

Benson, D.F., Stuss, D.T. (1986). *The frontal lobes.* Raven Pess, New York.

Benson, D.F., Tomlinson, E.B. (1971). Hemiplegic syndrome of the posterior cerebral artery. *Stroke* 2, 559–564

Benton, A. (1979). Visuoperceptual, visuospatial, and visuoconstructive disorders. In K.M. Heilman, E. Valenstein (eds.) *Clinical Neuropsychology*, Oxford University Press, New York, 186–232

Benton, A. (1982). Spatial thinking in neurological patients: historical aspects. In Potegal, M. (ed.) *Spatial Abilities: Development and Physiological Foundations.* Academic Press, London, 253–275

Benton, A. (1984). Hemispheric dominance before Broca. *Neuropsychologia* 22, 807–811

Benton, A. (1985). Facial recognition. In L. Costa, O. Spreen (eds.) *Studies in Neuropsychology. Selected papers of Arthur Benton.* Oxford University Press, New York, 224–235

Benton, A. (1985). Visuoperceptual, visuospatial, and visuoconstructive disorders. In Heilman, K.M., Valenstein, E. (eds.) *Clinical Neuropsychology.* 2nd Ed. Oxford University Press, Oxford, 151–187

Benton, A., Hannay, H.J., Varney, N.R. (1975). Visual perception of line direction in patients with unilateral disease. *Neurology* 25, 907–910

Benton, A., van Allen, M.W. (1972). Prosopagnosia in facial discrimination. *J. Neurol. Sci.* 15, 167–172

Benton, A., van Allen, M.W., Hamsher, K., Levin, H.S. (1975). *Test of facial recognition.* University of Iowa Hospitals, Iowa City

Benton, A.L. (1962). Clinical symptomatology in right and left hemisphere lesions. In Mountcastle, V.B. (ed.), *Interhemispheric Relations and Cerebral Dominance.* John Hopkins Press, Baltimore

Benton, A.L. (1963). *The revised retention test*, 3rd. ed. State University, Iowa

Benton, A.L. (1964). Contributions to aphasia before Broca. *Cortex* 1, 314–327

Benton, A.L. (1965). The problem of cerebral dominance. *The Canad. Psychologist* 6a (no 4), 332–348

Benton, A.L. (1972). The 'minor' hemisphere. *J. Hist. Med. and All. Sci.* 27, 5–14

Benton, A.L. (1975). Visuoperceptive capacity (Benton-Van Allen-Test) In Capt. 6, Baker, A.B. (ed.) *Psychologic Testing*, Clin. Neurol. 1, 10–18, Harper Row, NY, London

Benton, A.L. (1980). The Neuropsychology of Facial Recognition. *Am. Psychologist* 35, 176–186

Benton, A.L., Allen, M.W. van (1972). Prosopagnosia and facial discrimination. *J. Neurol. Sci.* 15, 167–172

Benton, A.L., Eslinger, P.J., Damasio, A.R. (1981). Normative observations on neuropsychological test performances in old age. *J. Clin. Neuropsychol.* 3, 33–42

Benton, A.L., Fogel, M.L. (1962). Three-dimensional constructional praxis: a clinical test. *Arch. Neurol.* (Chicago) 7, 347–354

Benton, A.L., Gordon, M.C. (1971). Correlates of facial recognition. *Trans. Amer. Neurol. Ass.* 96, 146–150

Benton, A.L., Hamsher, K., Varney, N.R., Spreen, O. (1983). Contributions to neuropsychological assessment. Oxford University Press, New York

Benton, A.L., Hannay, H.J., Varney, N.R. (1975). Visual perception of line direction in patients with unilateral brain disease. *Neurology* 25, 907–910

Benton, A.L., Hécaen, H. (1970). Stereoscopic vision in patients with unilateral cerebral disease. *Neurology* 20, 1084–1088

Benton, A.L., Levin, H.S., van Allen, M.W. (1974). Geographic orientation in patients with unilateral cerebral disease. *Neuropsychologia* 12, 183–191

Benton, A.L., Meyers, R. (1956). An early description of the Gerstmann syndrome. *Neurology* 6, 838–842

Benton, A.L., Van Allen, M.W. (1968). Correlates of facial recognition in patients with cerebral disease. *Cortex* 4, 344–358

Benton, A.L., Van Allen, M.W. (1968). Impairment in facial recognition in patients with cerebral disease. *Cortex* 4, 344–358

Benton, A.L., Varney, N.R., Hamsher, K. de S. (1978). Visuospatial judgement. *Arch. Neurol.* 35, 364–367

Benton, H.L., Vogel, M.L. (1962). Three-dimensional constructional praxis: A clinical test. *Arch. Neurol.* 7, 347–354

Benton, S., Levy, I., Swash, M. (1980). Vision in the temporal crescent in occipital infarction. *Brain* 103, 83–97

Berenberg, D., Dorrow, R., Duka, T., Sauerbrey, N. (1988). Benzodiazepine receptor ligands: tools for memory research in clinical pharmacology. *Psychopharmacol. Ser.* 6, 261–274

Berengario da Carpi, J. (1518/1535). *Tractatus de fractura calvae sive cranei.* Nicolinis, Venedig

Berengario da Carpi, J. (1521). *Commentaria cum amplissimis additionibus super anatomia Mundini, una cum textu ejusque in pristino nitorem redacto.* De Benedictis, Bologna

Berent, S. (1977). Functional asymmetry of the human brain in the recognition of faces. *Neuropsychologia* 15, 829–831

Berger, H. (1923). Klinische Beiträge zur Pathologie des Grosshirns. 3. Mitteilung. Herderkrankungen des Occipitallappens. *Arch. Psychiat. Nervenkr.* 69, 569–599

Berger, O. (1885). Zur Lokalisation der corticalen Sehsphäre beim Menschen. *Breslauer ärztliche Zeitung* 7, 1,28,37,51

Bergman, P.S. (1957). Cerebral blindness: an analysis of twelve cases, with special reference to the electroencephalogram and patterns of recovery. *Arch. Neurol. Psychiat.* 78, 568–584

Beringer, K. (1927). *Der Meskalinrausch.* Springer, Berlin

Beringer, K., Stein, J. (1930). Analyse eines Falles von 'reiner' Alexie. *Z. ges. Neurol. Psychiat.* 123, 472–478

Berkeley, G. (1709). *An essay towards a new theory of vision.* Dublin

Berkley, W., Bussey, F.R. (1950). Altitudinal hemianopia: report of 2 cases. *Am. J. Ophthal.* 33, 593–600

Berlin, B., Kay, P. (1969). *Basic color terms: their universality and evolution.* University of California Press, Berkeley

Berlin, E. (1874). Ueber das Accommodationsphosphen. *Graefes Arch. Ophthalmol.* 20, 89–97

Berlucchi, G., Brizzolara, D., Marzi, C.A., Rizzolatti, G., Umilta, C. (1974). Can lateral asymmetries in attention explain interfield differences in visual perception? *Cortex* 10, 177–185

Berlucchi, G., Brizzolara, D., Marzi, C.A., Rizzolatti, G., Umilta, C. (1979). The role of stimulus discriminability and verbal codability in hemispheric specialization for visuospatial tasks. *Neuropsychologia* 17, 195–202

Berlucchi, G., Crea, F., Di Stefano, M., Tassinari, G. (1977). Influence of spatial stimulus-response compatibility on reaction time of ipsilateral and contralateral hand to lateralised light stimuli. *J. exp. Psychol.: Human Percept. Perform.* 3, 505–517

Berlucchi, G., Heron, W., Hyman, R., Rizzolatti, G., Umilta, C. (1971). Simple reaction times of ipsilateral and contralateral hand to lateralised visual stimuli. *Brain* 94, 419–430

Berlucchi, G., Tassinari, G., Marzi, C.A., Di Stefano, M. (1989).

Spatial distribution of the inhibitory effect of peripheral non-informative cues on simple reaction time to non-fixated visual targets. *Neuropsychologia* 27, 201–221

Berndl, K., Cranach, M. von, Grüsser, O.-J. (1986b). Impairment of perception and recognition of faces, mimic expression and gestures in schizophrenic patients. *Eur. Arch. Psychiatr. Neurol. Sci.* 235, 282–291

Berndl, K., Cranach, M. von, Grüsser, O.-J., Kiefer, R.H. (1983). Impairment of recognition of both gestures and miming in schizophrenic patients. *Neurosci. Lett. Suppl.* 14, 27

Berndl, K., Dewitz, W., Grüsser, O.-J., Kiefer, R.H. (1986a). A test movie to study elementary abilities in perception and recognition of mimic and gestural expression. *Eur. Arch. Psychiatr. Neurol. Sci.* 235, 276–281

Berndl, K., Grüsser, O.-J. (1987). Wahrnehmungsstörung bei Schizophrenen. Beeinträchtigung des Erkennens und Wiedererkennens von Gesichtern, Mimik und Gestik bei jugendlichen und erwachsenen Kranken. In Martinius, J. (ed.) *Jugendpsychiatrie. Aktuelle Themen in Diagnostik und Therapie.* MMV Verlag, München, 12–27

Berndl, K., Grüsser, O.-J., Lüdke, M. (1988). Untersuchungen zur Veränderung der Wahrnehmung von Gesichtern, Mimik und Gestik durch schizophrene Patienten. In Oepen, G. (ed.), *Psychiatrie des rechten und linken Gehirns. Neuropsychologische Ansätze zum Verständnis von 'Persönlichkeit', 'Depression' und 'Schizophrenie'.* Deutscher Ärzteverlag, Köln, 93–100

Berndl, K., Grüsser, O.-J., Martin, M., Remschmidt, H. (1986c). Comparative studies on recognition of faces, mimic and gestures in adolescent and middle-aged schizophrenic patients. *Eur. Arch. Psychiatr. Neurol. Sci.* 236, 123–130

Berrini, R., Capitani, E., Sala, S. della, Spinnler, H. (1984). Interaction between lateralization of memory and probe stimulus in the recognition of verbal and spatial visual stimuli. *Neuropsychologia* 22, 517–520

Berson, R.J. (1983). Capgras' syndrome. Amer. J. Psychiat. 140, 969–978

Bertelson, P., Van Haelen, H., Morais, J. (1979). Left hemifield superiority and the extraction of physiognomic invariants. In Steele-Russell, I., Van Hof, M., Berlucci, G. (eds.), *Structure and function of the cerebral commissures.* Macmillan, London

Bertelson, P., Vanhaelen, H. Morais, J. (1979). Left hemifield superiority and the extraction of physiognomic informatin. In Russell S.I., van Hof, M.W., Berlucchi, G. (eds.), *Structure and function of cerebral commissures.* MacMillan, London, 400–410

Berti, A., Papagno, C., Vallar, G. (1986). Balint syndrome: a case of simultanagnosia. *Ital. J. Neurol. Sci.* 7, 261–264

Bertolini, G., Anzola, G.P., Buchtel, H.A., Rizzolatti, G. (1978). Hemispheric differences in the discriminationof the velocity and duration of a simple visual stimulus. *Neuropsychologia* 16, 213–220

Bertulis, A., Guld, C., Lennox-Buchthal, M.A. (1977). Spectral and orientation specificity of single cells in foveal striate cortex of the vervet monkey, *Cercopithecus aethiops. J. Physiol. (Lond.)* 268, 1–20

Besner, D., Coltheart, M. (1979). Ideographic and alphabetic processing in skilled reading of English. *Neuropsychologia* 17, 467–472

Besner, D., Daniels, S., Slade, C. (1982). Ideogram reading and right hemisphere language. *Brit. J. Psychol.* 73, 21–28

Besser, R. (1981). Mediobasale Infarkte der Temporo-Occipital-Region. *Nervenarzt* 52, 167–172

Best, F. (1917). Hemianopsie und Seelenblindheit bei Hirnverletzungen. *Graefes Arch. Ophthalmol.* 93, 49–150

Best, F. (1919a). Über Störungen der optischen Lokalisation bei Verletzungen und Herderkrankungen im Hinterhauptlappen. *Neurol. Cbl. Lpz.* 38, 427–432

Best, F. (1919b). Zur Theorie der Hemianopsie und der höheren Sehzentren. *Graefe's Arch. Ophthalmol.* 100, 1–31

Best, F. (1952). Zur Frage der Seelenblindheit. *Arch. Psychiat.* 188, 511–543

Beyer, E. (1895). Ueber Verlagerungen im Gesichtsfeld bei Flimmerskotom. *Neurol. Zbl.* (Lpz.) 14, 10

Beyn, E.S., Knyazeva, G.R. (1962). The problem of prosopagnosia. *J. Neurol. Neurosurg. Psychiat.* 25, 154–158

Bick, B.A. (1984). The syndrome of intermetamorphosis. *Amer. J. Psychiat.* 141, 588–589

Bidault, E., Luaute, J.P., Tzavaras, A. (1986). Prosopagnosia and the delusional misidentification syndromes. *Bibl. Psychiatr.* 164, 80–91

Biederman, I. (1972). Perceiving real-world scenes. *Science* 177, 77–80

Biederman, I. (1987). Recognition-by-components: A theory of human image understanding. *Psychol. Rev.* 94, 115–147

Biederman, I. (1990). Higher-level vision. In Osherson, D.N., Kosslyn, M., Hollerbach, J.M. (eds.), *Visual cognition and action.* MIT Press, Cambridge, Mass, 41–72

Biederman-Thorson, M., Thorson, J., Lange, G.D. (1971). Apparent movement due to closely spaced sequentially flashed dots in the human peripheral field of vision. *Vision Res.* 11, 889–903

Bigley, G.K., Sharp, F.R. (1983). Reversible alexia without agraphia due to migraine. *Arch. Neurol.* 40, 115

Bignall, K.E., Imbert, M. (1969). Polysensory and cortico-cortical projections to frontal lobe of squirrel and rhesus monkey. *Electroenceph. Clin. Neurophysiol.* 26, 206–15

Biguer, B., Donaldson, M.L., Hein, A., Jeannerod, M. (1988). Neck muscle vibration modifies the representation of visual motion and direction in man. *Brain* 111, 1405–1424

Bihrle, A.M., Bellugi, U., Dells, D., Marks, S. (1989). Seeing either the forest or the trees: dissociation in visuo-spatial processing. *Brain and Cognition* 11, 37–49

Bijl, G.K., Melchior, H.J., Veringa, F. (1980). Recording the visual electrically evoked potential (VEEP). *Electroenceph. Clin. Neurophysiol.* 49, 655–656

Bing, R., Brückner, R. (1954). *Gehirn und Auge. Grundriss der Ophthalmo-Neurologie.* Schwabe, Basel

Bioulac, B., Lamarre, Y. (1979). Activity of postcentral cortical neurons of the monkey during conditioned movements of a deafferented limb. *Brain Res.* 172, 427–437

Birkett, P. (1979). Relationships among handedness, familial handedness, sex and ocular sighting-dominance. *Neuropsychologia* 17, 533–537

Birkmayer, W. (1951). *Hirnverletzungen.* Springer, Wien

Bishop, D.V., Byng, S. (1984). Assessing semantic comprehension: methodological considerations, and a new clinical test. *Cogn. Neuropsychol.* 1, 233–244

Bishop, P.O., Jeremy, D., Lance, J.W. (1953). The optic nerve. Properties of central tract. *J. Physiol.* 121, 415–432

Bishop, P.O., Jeremy, D., McLeod, J.G. (1953). Phenomenon of repetitive firing in lateral geniculate of cat. *J. Neurophysiol.* 16, 437–447

Bishop, P.O., McLeod, J.G. (1954). Nature of potentials associated with synaptic transmission in lateral geniculate of cat. *J. Neurophysiol.* 16, 387–414

Bisiach, E. (1966). Perceptual factors in the pathogenesis of anomia. *Cortex* 2, 90–95

Bisiach, E., Berti, A. (1987). Dyschiria. An attempt at its systemic explanation. In Jeannerod, M. (ed.) *Neurophysiological and neuropsychological aspects of spatial neglect.* North-Holland, Amsterdam, 183–201

Bisiach, E., Berti, A. (1989). Unilateral misrepresentation of distributed information: paradoxes and puzzles. In Brown, J.W. (ed.) *Neuropsychology of visual perception.* Erlbaum, Hillsdale, NJ, 145–165

Bisiach, E., Bulgarelli, C., Sterzi, R., Vallar, G. (1983). Line bisection and cognitive plasticity of unilateral neglect of space. *Brain and Cognition* 2, 32–38

Bisiach, E., Capitani, E. (1976). Cerebral dominance and visual similarity judgements. *Cortex* 12, 347–355

Bisiach, E., Capitani, E., Luzzatti, C., Perani, D. (1981). Brain and conscious representation of outside reality. *Neuropsychologia* 19, 543–551

Bisiach, E., Capitani, E., Porta, E. (1985). Two basic properties of space representation in the brain. *J. Neurol. Neurosurg. Psychiat.* 48, 141–144

Bisiach, E., Capitani, E., Spinnler, H. (1975). Focal hemisphere damage and visuo-perceptural categorization. *J. Neurol. Neurosurg. Psychiat.* 38, 1115–1120

Bisiach, E., Geminiani, G., Berti, A., Rusconi, M.L. (1990). Perceptual and premotor factors of unilateral neglect. *Neurology* 40, 1278–1281

Bisiach, E., Luzzatti, C. (1978). Unilateral neglect of representational space. *Cortex* 14, 129–133

Bisiach, E., Luzzatti, C., Perani, D. (1979). Unilateral neglect, representational schema and consciousness. *Brain* 102, 609–618

Bisiach, E., Perani, D., Vallar, G., Berti, A. (1986). Unilateral neglect: Personal and extrapersonal. *Neuropsychologia* 24, 759–767

Bisiach, E., Vallar, G., Perani, D., Papagno, C., Berti, A. (1986). Unawareness of disease following lesions of the right hemisphere: anosognosia for hemiplegia and anosognosia for hemianopia. *Neuropsychologia* 24 (4), 471–482

Bizzi, E., Schiller, P.H. (1970). Single unit activity in the frontal eye fields of unanesthetized monkeys during eye and head movement. *Exp. Brain Res.* 10, 151–158

Bjerrum, J. (1881). Hemianopsi for far verne. *Dan. Hosp. Tidschr.* 8, 41–49 (quot. after Kölmel, 1988)

Black, S.W., Strub, R.L. (1976). Constructional apraxia in patients with discrete missile wounds of the brain. *Cortex* 12, 212–220

Blackwood, D.H., St. Clair, D.M., Blackburn, I.M., Tyrer, G.M. (1987). Cognitive brain potentials and psychological deficits in Alzheimer's dementia and Korsakoff's amnestic syndrome. *Psychol. Med.* 17, 340–358

Blakemore, C. (1974). Developmental factors in the formation of features extracting neurons. In Schmitt, F.G., Worden, F.G. (eds.), *The neurosciences third study program.* MIT Press, Cambridge, MA., 105–113

Blakemore, C. (1990). Maturation of mechanisms for efficient spatial vision. In Blakemore, C. (ed.), *Vision: Coding and efficiency.* Cambridge Univ. Press, 254–266

Blakemore, C. (1991). Principles of development in the nervous system. (in press)

Blakemore, C. (1991.). Sensitive and vulnerable periods in the development of the visual system (in press)

Blakemore, C., Falconer, M.A. (1967). Long-term effects of anterior temporal lobectomy on certain cognitive functions. *J. Neurol. Neurosurg. Psychiat.* 30, 364–367

Blakemore, C., Garey, L.J., Vital-Durand, F. (1978). The physiological effects of monocular deprivation and their reversal in the monkey's visual cortex. *J. Physiol. (Lond.)* 283, 223–262

Blakemore, C., Molnar, Z. (1990). Factors involved in the establishment of specific interconnections between thalamus and cerebral cortex. Cold Spring Harbor Symposia on Quantitative Biology, Vol. 4

Blakemore, C., Vital-Durand, F., Garey, L.J. (1981). Recovery from monocular deprivation in the monkey. I. Recovery of physiological effects in the visual cortex. *Proc. R. Soc. London Ser. B* 213, 399–423

Blanc-Garin, J. (1984). Perception des visages et reconnaissance de la physionomie dans l'agnosie des visages. *L'année Psychol.* 84, 573–598

Blanc-Garin, J. (1986). Faces and non-faces in prosopagnostic patients. In Ellis, H.D., Jeeves, M.A., Newcombe, F., Young, A. (eds.), *Aspects of face recognition.* Martinus Nijhoff, Dordrecht

Blaney, R.L., Winograd, E. (1978). Developmental differences in children's recognition memory for faces. *Dev. Psychol.* 14, 441–442

Blasdel, G.G., Fitzpatrick, D. (1984). Physiological organization of layer 4 in macaque striate cortex. *J. Neurosci.* 4, 880–895

Blasdel, G.G., Fitzpatrick, D., Lund, J.S. (1983). Physiological and anatomical studies of retinotopic maps in macaque striate cortex. *Invest. Ophthalmol. Vis. Sci.* 24, 266

Blasdel, G.G., Lund, J.S. (1983). Termination of afferent axons in macaque striate cortex. *J. Neurosci.* 3, 1389–1413

Bleuler, E. (1893). Ein Fall von aphasischen Symptomen, Hemianopsie, amnestischer Farbenblindheit und Seelenlähmung. *Arch. Psychiat. Nervenkr.* 25, 32–73

Bleuler, E. (1916). Lehrbuch der Psychiatrie. Springer, Berlin

Bliss, E.L., Clark, L.D. (1962). Visual hallucinations. In West, L.J. (ed.), *Hallucinations.* Grune & Stratton, New York, London, 92–107

Bloch, P. (1980). Bildnis im Mittlalter. Herrscherbild — Grabbild -Stifterbild. In *Bilder vom Menschen in der Kunst des Abendlandes.* Mann, Berlin, 105–141

Bloom, F.E., Lazerson, A., Hofstadter, L. (1985). *Brain, mind and behavior.* Freeman, NY

Blum, B. (1985). Enhancement of visual responses of area 7 neurons by electrical preconditioning stimulation of LP-pulvinar nuclei of the monkey. *Exp. Brain Res.* 59, 434–440

Blum, J.S., Chow, K.L., Pribram, K.H. (1950). A behavioral analysis of the organization of the parieto-temporo-preoccipital cortex. *J. Comp. Neur.* 93, 53–100

Blum, R.A. (1952). Effects of subtotal lesions of frontal granular cortex on delayed reaction in monkeys. *AMA Arch. Neurol. Psychiatry* 67, 375–86

Blundell, E. (1966). Parietal lobe dysfunction in subnormal patients. *J. Ment. Defic. Research* 10, 141–152

Blythe, I.M., Kennard, C., Ruddock, K.H. (1985). Residual function in hemianopia and quadrantanopia. Paper delivered at meeting of European Brain and Behaviour Society, Oxford

Bock, H., Grosshaus, R. (1980). Das Bildnis. Das autonome Portrait seit der Renaissance. In *Bilder vom Menschen in der Kunst des Abendlandes.* Mann, Berlin, 143–196

Bodamer, J. (1947). Die Prosop-Agnosie. (Die Agnosie des Physiognomieerkennens) *Arch. Psychiat. Nervenkr.* 179, 6–54

Bodis-Wollner, I. (1976). Vulnerability of spatial frequency channels in cerebral lesions. *Nature* 261, 309–311

Bodis-Wollner, I. (1977). Recovery from cerebral blindness: evoked potential and psychophysical measurements. *EEG. Clin. Neurophysiol.* 42, 178–184

Bodis-Wollner, I., Atkin, A., Raab, E., Wolkstein, M. (1977). Visual association cortex and vision in man: pattern-evoked occipital potentials in a blind boy. *Science* 198, 629–631

Bodis-Wollner, I., Diamond, S.P. (1976). The measurement of spatial contrast sensitivity in cases of blurred vision associated with cerebral lesions. *Brain* 99, 695–710

Bodis-Wollner, I., Hendley, C.D., Kulikowski, J.J. (1972). Electrophysiological and psychological responses to modulation of contrast of a grating pattern. *Perception* 1, 341–349

Boerhaave, H. (1761). *Praelectiones academicae de morbis nervorum.* van Eems, J. (ed.), Vol. 1, Leyden van der Eyck und de Becker

Bogen, J.E. (1972). Neowiganism. In Smith, W.L. (ed.), *Drugs development and cerebral function.* C.C. Thomas, Springfield, 358–361

Bogen, J.E. (1976). Language function in the short term following cerebral commissurotomy. In Avakian-Whitaker, H., Whitaker, H.A. (eds.), *Current Trends in Neurolinguistics*, Academic Press, New York

Bogen, J.E. (1977). Further discussion on split-brains and hemispheric capabilities. *Br. J. Phil. Sci.* 28, 281–286

Bogen, J.E. (1979). The callosal syndrome. In Heilman, K.M., Valenstein, E. (1979). *Clinical Neuropsychology.* University Press, Oxford, 308–359; 2nd edition 1985, 295–338

Bogen, J.E., Gazzaniga, M.S. (1965). Cerebral commissurotomy in man: minor hemisphere dominance for certain visuospatial functions. *J. Neurosurg.* 23, 394–399

Bogen, J.E., Schultz, D.H., Vogel, P.J. (1988). Completeness of callosotomy shown by magnetic resonance imaging in the long term. *Arch. Neurol.* 45, 1203–1205

Bogousslavsky, J., Miklossy, J., Deruaz, J.P., Assal, G., Regli, F. (1987). Lingual and fusiform gyri in visual processing: a clinicopathologic study of superior altitudinal hemianopia. *J. Neurol. Neurosurg. Psychiat.* 50, 607–614

Bogousslavsky, J., Regli, F. (1986). Pursuit gaze defects in acute and chronic unilateral parieto-occipital lesions. *Europ. Neurol.* 25, 10–18

Bogousslavsky, J., Regli, F., Assal, G. (1986). The syndrome of unilateral tuberothalamic artery territory infacrtion. *Stroke* 17, 434–441

Bogousslavsky, J., Regli, F., Van Melle, G. (1983). Unilateral occipital infarction: evaluation of the risks of developing bilateral loss of vision. *J. Neurol. Neurosurg. Psychiatry* 46, 78–80

Bohm, E. (1951). *Lehrbuch der Rorschach-Diagnostik.* Huber, Bern

Boles, D.B. (1984). Sex in lateralized tachistoscopic word recognition. *Brain and Language* 23, 307–317

Boles, D.B., Eveland, D.C. (1983). Visual and phonetic codes and the process of generation in letter matching. *J. Exp. Psychol (Human Percept).* 9, 657–674

Boller, F., Cole, M., Kim, Y., Mack, J.L., Patawaran, C. (1975). Optic ataxia: clinical-radiological correlations with the EMIscan. *J. Neurol. Neurosurg. Psychiat.* 38, 954–958

Boller, F., De Renzi, E. (1967). Relationship between visual memory defects and hemispheric locus of lesion. *Neurology* 17, 1052–1058

Bolz, J., Gilbert, C.D., Wiesel, T.N. (1989). Pharmacological analysis of cortical circuity. *TINS* Vol. 12, 8, 292–296

Boman, D.K., Hotson, J.R. (1989). Motion perception prominence alters anticipatory slow eye movements. *Exp. Brain Res.* 74, 555–562

Bonhoeffer, K. (1915). Doppelseitige symmetrische Schläfen-und Parietallappenherde als Ursache vollständiger dauernder Worttaubheit bei erhaltener Tonskala, verbunden mit taktiler und optischer Agnosie. *Monatsschr. f. Psychiat. Neurol.* 37, 17–38

Bonhoeffer, K. (1923). Zur Klinik und Lokalisation des Agrammatismus und der Rechts-und Linksdisorientierung. *Monatsschr. Psychiat. Neurol.* 54, 11–42

Bonhoeffer, K. (1924). Die Entwicklung der Anschauungen von der Grosshirnfunktion in den letzten 50 Jahren. *Deutsch. Med. Wochenschr.* 50, 1707–1710

Bonin, G. von, Bailey, P. (1947). *The neocortex of Macaca mulatta.* University of Illinois Press, Urbana, Ill.

Bonnet, C. (1760). *Essai analytique sur les facultés de l'ame.* Philibert, Copenhagen. Reprint Olms, Hildesheim 1973

Bonvicini, G., Pötzl, O. (1907). Einiges über reine 'Wortblindheit'. *Arb. Neurol. Inst. Wien* 15/16, 522–529

Bonvicini, G., Pötzl, O. (1907). Ueber einen Fall von reiner oder subcorticaler Alexia. *Wiener med. Wschr.,* 29

Borelli, G.A. (1680–1682) *De motu animalium.* 2 vols., Bernabo, Rome

Bornstein, B. (1963). Prosopagnosia. In L. Halpern (ed.), *Problems of dynamic neurology.* Studies on the higher functions of the human nervous system. Hadassah Medical Organization, Jerusalem, 283–318

Bornstein, B., Kidron, D.P. (1959). Prosopagnosia. *J. Neurol. Neurosurg. Psychiat.* 22, 124–131

Bornstein, B., Sroka, H., Munitz, H. (1969). Prosopagnosia with animal face agnosia. *Cortex* 5, 164–169

Bornstein, M.H. (1985). Infant into adult: unity to diversity in the development of visual categorization. In J. Mehler, Fox, R. (eds.), *Neonate cognition: beyond the blooming buzzing confusion.* Lawrence Erlbaum Associates, Hillsdale, NJ, 115–138

Bornstein, M.H. (1985). On the development of color naming in young children: data and theory. *Brain and Language* 26, 72–93

Bornstein, M.H., Kessen, W., Weiskopf, S. (1976). Color vision and hue categorization in young human infants. *J. exp. Psychol.: Human perception and performance* 2, 115–129

Borod, J., Caron, H.S., Koff, E.(1981). Asymmetry in positive and negative facial expression: sex differences. *Neuropsychol.* 19, 819–824

Borod, J., Koff, E., Caron, H.S. (1983). Right hemisphere specialisation for the expression and appreciation of emotion: a focus on the face. In Perecman, E. (ed.), *Cognitive processing in the right hemisphere,* Academic Press, New York, 83–109

Borod, J., Koff, E., White,B. (1983). Facial asymmetry in posed and spontaneous expressions of emotion. *Brain and Cognition* 2, 165–175

Borod, J.C., Caron, H.S. (1980). Facedness and emotion related to lateral dominance, sex, and expression type. *Neuropsychologia* 18, 237–241

Borod, J.C., Carper, M., Goodglass, H., Naeser, M. (1984). Aphasic performance on a battery of constructional, visuo-spatial, and quantitative tasks: factorial structure and CT scan localization. *J. Clin. Neuropsychol.* 6, 189–204

Borod, J.C., Koff, E. (1983). Asymmetries in affective facial expression: behavior and anatomy. In Fox, N., Davidson, R. (eds.), *The psychobiology of affective development.* Hilsdale, NJ, Lawrence Erlbaum Associates 293–323

Bosch, G. (1958). Über Phantasiegefährten bei einem hirngeschädigten Kinde. Zugleich ein Beitrag zur Frage des Leiberlebens im Kindesalter. *Nervenarzt* 29, 201–209

Botez, M.I. (1975). Two visual systems in clinical neurology: readaptive role of the primitive system in visual agnosic patients. *Eur. Neurol.* 13, 101–122

Botez, M.I., Olivier, M., Vezina, J.L., Botez, T., Kaufman, B. (1985). Defective revisualization: dissociation between cognitive and imagistic thought, case report and short review of the literature. *Cortex* 21, 375–389

Botez, M.I., Serbanecscu, T., Vernia, I. (1964). Visual static agnosia with special reference to literal agnosic alexia. *Neurology* 14, 1101–1111

Botez, M.I., Serbanescu, T. (1967). Course and outcome of visual static agnosia. *J. Neurol. Sci.* 4, 289–297

Bottini, G., Cappa, S., Geminiani, G., Sterzi, R. (1990). Topographic disorientation — a case report. *Neuropsychologia* 28, 309–312

Boucher, M., Kopp, N., Tomasi, M., Schott, B. (1976). Observation antomo-clinique d'un cas d'alexie sans agraphie. *Rev. Neurol. (Paris)* 132, 656–659

Boucher, M., Michel, F., Tommasi, M., Schott, B. (1974). Alexie sans agraphie (a propos d'un cas anatomique). In Michel, F., Schott, B. (eds.), *Les syndromes de disconnexion calleuse chez l'homme.* Colloque international de Lyon, 371–380

Boudouresques, J., Poncet, M., Cherif, A., Balzamo, M. (1979). L'agnosie des visages: un témoin de la désorganisation fonctionnelle d'un certain type de connaissance des éléments du monde extérieur. *Bulletin de l'Academie Nationale de Médecine* 163, 695–702

Boudouresques, J., Poncet, M., Sebahoun, M., Alicherif, A. (1972). Two cases of alexia without agraphia with disorders of color and image naming. *Bulletin de l'Academie Nationale de Medecine* 44, 297–303

Boulton, J.C., Mullen, K.T. (1990). A case in which colour vision is no longer motion blind. *Clin. Vision Sci.* 5, 175–184

Bouma, H. (1971). Visual recognition of isolated lower-case letters. *Vision Res.* 11, 459–474

Bouma, H. (1973). Visual interference in the parafoveal recognition of initial and final letters of words. *Vision Res.* 13, 767–782

Bouma, H., Voogd, A.H. de (1974). On the control of eye saccades in reading. *Vision Res.* 14, 273–284

Bouman, M.A., Doesschate, J. ten (1969). Adaptation and the electrical excitability of the eye. *Doc. Ophthal.* 26, 240–247

Bouman, M.A., Doesschate, J. ten, Velden, H.A. van der (1951).

Electrical stimulation of the human eye by means of periodical rectangular stimuli. *Doc. Ophthal.* 5–6, 151–167

Bourru, H., Burot, P. (1888). *Variations de la personalité.* Bailliere, Paris

Boussaoud, D., Desimone, R., Ungerleider, L.G. (1991). Visual topography of area TEO in the macaque. *J. Comp. Neurol* 306, 554–575

Boussaoud, D., Ungerleider, L.G., Desimone, R. (1990). Pathways of motion analysis: cortical connections of the medial superior temporal and fundus of the superior temporal visual areas in the macaque. *J. Comp. Neurol.* 296, 462–495

Bower, T.G.R. (1966). The visual world of infants. *Scient. American* 215, 80–92

Bower, T.G.R. (1971). The object in the world of the infant. *Scient. American* 225, 30–44

Bower, T.G.R. (1974). *Development in infancy.* Freeman, San Francisco

Bowers, D., Heilman, K.M. (1976). Material specific hemispherical arousal. *Neuropsychologia* 14, 123–127

Bowers, D., Heilman, K.M. (1980). Psychoneglect: effects of hemispace on tactile line bisection task. *Neuropsychologia* 18, 491–498

Bowers, D., Heilman, K.M. (1984). Dissociation between the processing of affective and non-affective faces: a case study. *J. Clin. Neuropsychol.* 6, 367–379

Bowers, D., Heilman, K.M., Van Den Abell, T. (1981). Hemispacevisual half field (VHF) compatibility. *Neuropsychologia* 19, 757–765

Bowers-Pillsbury, W. (1897). A study of apperception. *Am. J. Psychol.* 8, 315–393

Bowmaker, J.K., Dartnall, H.J.A. (1980). Visual pigments of rods and cones in a human retina. *J. Physiol.* 298, 501–511

Bowmaker, J.K., Dartnall, H.J.A., Mollon, J.D. (1980). Microspectrophotometric demonstration of four classes of photoreceptor in an old world primate, Macaca fascicularis. *J. Physiol.* 298, 131–143

Boycott, B.B., Hopkins, J.M., Sperling, H.G. (1987). Cone connections of the horizontal cells of the rhesus monkey's retina. *Proc. R. Soc.* B229, 345–379

Boyle, R. (1664). Some uncommon observations about vitiated sight. In Birch, T. (ed.), *Robert Boyle, The Works,* vol. V., reprint 1965, Olms, Hildesheim 445–452

Boyle, R. (1664). The experimental history of colours begun, 1st. ed. In *The works of Robert Boyle,* Vol. I London, repr. 1965, Olms, Hildesheim

Boynton, R.M. (1979). *Human color vision.* Holt, Rinehart and Winston, New York, 438 p.

Boynton, R.M. (1988). Color vision. *Ann. Rev. Psychol.* 39, 69–100

Boynton, R.M., Olson, C.X. (1987). Locating basic colors in the OSA space. *Color Res. Appl.* . . . (quoted after Boynton, 1988)

Bötzel, K., Dalbasti, T., Grüsser, O.-J. (1981). Horizontal circular vection and eye movements. *Freiburger Universitätsblätter* 74, 113–117

Bötzel, K., Grüsser, O.-J. (1982). Horizontal and vertical circular vection and eye movements. *Neurosci. Lett. Suppl.* 10, 86–87

Bötzel, K., Grüsser, O.-J. (1987). Potentials evoked by face and nonface stimuli in the human electroencephalogram. *Perception* 16, 239

Bötzel, K., Grüsser, O.-J. (1989). Electric brain potentials evoked by pictures of faces and non-faces: search for 'face-specific' EEG-potentials. *Exp. Brain Res.* 77, 349–360

Bötzel, K., Grüsser, O.-J., Häussler, B., Naumann, A. (1989). The search for face-specific evoked potentials. In Basar, E., Bullock, T.H. (eds), *Brain Dynamics. Progress and Perspectives.* Springer, Berlin, Heidelberg, New York, 449–466

Braak, H. (1977). The pigment architecture of the human occipital lobe. *Anat. Embryol.* 150, 229–250

Braak, J.W.G. ter (1936). Untersuchungen über optokinetischen Nystagmus. *Arch. Neerl. Physiol.* 21, 309–376 English transl. by Collewijn, H. (1981) in *The oculomotor system of the rabbit and its plasticity.* Springer, Berlin

Braak, J.W.G. ter, Schenk, V.W.D., van Vliet, A.G.M. (1971). Visual reactions in a case of long-lasting cortical blindness. *J. Neurol. Neurosurg. Psychiat.* 34, 140–147

Bracha, H.S., Cabrera, F.J. Jr., Karson, C.N., Llewellyn, B.B. (1985). Lateralization of visual hallucinations in chronic Schizophrenia. *Biol. Psychiatry* 20, 1132–1136

Braddick, O.J. (1974). A short-range process in apparent motion. *Vision Res.* 14, 519–527

Braddick, O.J. (1980). Low level and high level processes in apparent motion. *Phil. Trans. R. Soc. Lond.* B. 290, 137–151

Braddick, O.J. (1988). Contours revealed by concealment. *Nature* 333, 803–804

Braddick, O.J., Wattam-Bell, J., Atkinson, J. (1986). Orientation-specific cortical responses develop in early infancy. *Nature (London)* 320, 617–619

Bradley, L., Bryant, P. (1981). Visual memory and phonological skills in reading and spelling backwardness. *Psychol. Res.* 43, 193–199

Bradshaw, G.J., Hicks, R.E., Rose, B. (1979). Lexical discrimination and letter-string identification in the two visual fields. *Brain and Language* 8, 10–18

Bradshaw, J., Gates, A. (1978). Visual field differences in verbal tasks. *Brain and Language* 4, 166–187

Bradshaw, J.L. (1974). Peripherally presented and unreported words may bias the perceived meaning of a centrally fixated homograph. *J. Exp. Psychol.* 103, 1200–1202

Bradshaw, J.L., Bradshaw, J.A. (1988). Notes and discussion. Reading mirror-reversed text: sinistrals really are inferior. *Brain and Language* 33, 189–192

Bradshaw, J.L., Nettleton, N.C. (1983). *Human cerebral asymmetry.* Prentice Hall, Englewood Cliffs, N.J.

Bradshaw, J.L., Nettleton, N.C., Wilson, L.E. (1986). Lateralized recognition of incomplete figures in a prolonged display controlled by eye movements. *Intern. J. Neurosci.* 30, 283–290

Bradshaw, J.L., Sherlock, D. (1982). Bugs and faces in the two visual fields: the analytic/holistic processing dichtomy and task sequencing. *Cortex* 18, 211–226

Bradshaw, J.L., Taylor, M.J., Patterson, K., Nettleton, N.C. (1980). Upright and inverted faces and housefronts, in the two visual fields: a right and a left hemisphere contribution. *J. Clin. Neuropsychol.* 2, 245–257

Bradshaw, J.L., Wallace, G. (1971). Models for the processing and identification of faces. *Percept. Psychophys.* 9, 443–448

Brain, W.R. (1941a). Visual disorientation with special reference to lesions of the right cerebral hemisphere. *Brain* 64, 244–272

Brain, W.R. (1941b). Visual-object agnosia with special reference to the Gestalt theory. *Brain* 64, 43–62

Brain, W.R. (1954). Loss of visualization. *Proc. Roy. Soc. Med.* 47, 288–290

Brain, W.R. (1965). Perception: A Trialogue. *Brain* 88, 697–710

Braitman, J.D. (1984). Activity of neurons in monkey posterior temporal cortex during multidimensional visual discrimination asks. Brain Res. 307, 17–28

Brandeis, D., Horst, A., Lehmann, D. (1987). Topographic effects of attention and subjective figure perception in adaptively segmented ERP map series. In Johnson, R. Jr, Parasuraman R., Rohrbaugh J.W. (ed.), *Current Trends in Event-Related Potential Research* (EEG Supplement 40). Elsevier, Amsterdam, 76–8O

Brandeis, D., Lehmann, D. (1986). Event-related potentials of the brain and cognitive processes: Approaches and applications. *Neuropsychologia* 24, 151–168

Brandeis, D., Lehmann, D. (1989). Segments of ERP map series reveal landscape changes with visual attention and subjective contours. *Electroencephal. clin. Neurophysiol.* 73, 507–519

Brandeis, R., Babkoff, H. (1984). Sorting of hemifield presented temporal and spatial stimuli. *Cortex* 20, 179–192

Brandt, T., Büchele, W., Arnold, F. (1977). Arthrokinetic nystagmus and ego-motion sensation. *Exp. Brain Res.* 30, 331–338

Brandt, T., Dichgans, J., König, E. (1972). Perception of self-rotation (circular vection) induced by optokinetic stimuli. *Pflügers Arch.* 322, R 98

Brandt, T., Dichgans, J., König, E. (1973). Differential effects of central versus peripheral vision in egocentric and exocentric motion perception. *Exp. Brain Res.* 16, 476–491

Brandt, T., Dietrich, M. (1986). Phobischer Attackenschwankschwindel. Ein neues Syndrom. *Münch. med. Wschr.* 128, 247–250

Braun, M. (1988). Die Raumanalysestörung, ein Schlüssel zum Verständnis der Anosognosie beim rechtshirnigen Insult. *Z. Gerontol.* 21, 129–133

Braunstein, M.L. (1976). *Depth perception through motion.* Academic, New York

Bravo, M., Blake, R., Morrison, S. (1988). Cats see subjective contours. *Vision Res.* 28, 861–865

Brazis, P.W., Biller, J., Fine, M. (1981). Central achromatopsia. *Neurology* 31, 920

Bridgeman, B. (1983). Mechanisms of space constancy. In Hein, A., Jeannerod, M. (eds.), *Spatially oriented behavior.* Springer, New York, Berlin, Heidelberg, Tokyo, 263–279

Bridgeman, B., Lewis, S., Heit, G., Nagle, M. (1979). Relation between cognitive and motor-oriented system of visual position perception. *J. Exp. Psychol.: Human Percept. Perform.* 5, 692–700

Bridgeman, B., Staggs, D. (1982). Plasticity in human blindsight. *Vision Res.* 22, 1199–1203

Bridgeman, B., Stark, L. (1979). Omnidirectional increase in threshold for image shifts during saccadic eye movements. *Percept. Psychophysics* 25, 241–243

Brierre de Boimont, A. (1852). *Des hallucinations.* Germer Baillier, Paris

Brierre de Boismont, A. (1953). *Hallucinations or the rational history of apparitions, visions, dreams, ecstasy, magnetism and somnambulism,* transl. from the 2nd French edition. Lindsay and Blakiston, Philadelphia

Brill, N.E. (1882). A case of destructive lesion in the cuneus, accompanied by color-blindness. *Am. J. Neurol. Psychiat.* 1, 356–368

Brindley, G., Merton, P.A. (1960). The absence of position sense in the human eye. *J. Physiol. (Lond.)* 153, 127–130

Brindley, G.S. (1955). The site of electrical excitation of the human eye. *J. Physiol. (Lond.)* 127, 189–200

Brindley, G.S. (1960). *Physiology of the retina and the visual pathway.* Arnold, London

Brindley, G.S. (1962). Beats produced simultaneous stimulation of the human eye with intermittent light and intermittent or alternating current. *J. Physiol. (Lond.)* 164, 157–167

Brindley, G.S. (1970). Sensations produced by electrical stimulation of the occipital poles of the cerebral hemispheres, and their use in constructing visual prostheses. *Ann. Roy. Coll. Surg.* 47, 106–108

Brindley, G.S. (1973). Sensory effects of electrical stimulation of the visual and paravisual cortex in man. In Jung, R. (ed.) *Handbook of Sensory Physiology* Vol. VII/3 Central processing of visual information, Part B, Springer, Berlin, Heidelberg, New York, 583–594

Brindley, G.S. (1982). Effects of electrical stimulation of the visual cortex. *Hum. Neurobiol.* 1, 281–283

Brindley, G.S., Donaldson, P.E.K., Falconer, M.A., Rushton, D.N. (1972). The extent of the region of the occipital cortex that when stimulated gives phosphenes fixed in the visual field. *J. Physiol. (Lond.)* 225, 57–58

Brindley, G.S., Gautier-Smith, P.C., Lewin, W. (1969). Cortical blindness and the functions of the non-geniculate fibres of the optic tracts. *J. Neurol. Neurosurg. Psychiat.* 32, 259–264

Brindley, G.S., Janota, I. (1975). Observations on cortical blindness and on vascular lesions that cause loss of recent memory. *J. Neurol. Neurosurg. Psychiat.* 38, 459–464

Brindley, G.S., Lewin, W.S. (1968). The sensations produced by electrical stimulation of the visual cortex. *J. Physiol. (Lond.)* 196, 479–493

Brissaud, E. (1900). Cecite verbale sans aphasie ni agraphie. Ramolissement cortical de la region Calcarine gauche; degenerescence du Tapetum gauche du Splenum et du Tapetum du cote droit. *Rev. Neurol.* 8, 757

Broadbent, D.E., Broadbent, M.H.P. (1981). Recent effects in visual memory. *J. Exp. Psychol.* 331, 1–15

Broadbent, D.E., Gregory, M. (1968). Visual perception of words differing in letter diagram frequency. *J. Verbal Learning and Verbal Behavior* 7, 569–571

Broadbent, W.H. (1872). Cerebral mechanism of speech and thought. *Med. Chir. Trans.* 55, 145–194

Brodal, P. (1978). Principles of organization of the monkey corticopontine projection. *Brain* 148, 214–218

Broderick, J.P., Swanson, J.W. (1987). Migraine-related strokes. Clinical profile and prognosis in 20 patients. *Arch. Neurol.* 44, 868–879

Brodmann, K. (1905). Beiträge zur histologischen Lokalisation der Grosshirnrinde. Dritte Mitteilung: die Rindenfelder der niederen Affen. *J. Psychol. Neurol. Lpz.* 4, 177–226

Brodmann, K. (1907). Beiträge zur histologischen Lokalisation der Grosshirnrinde. Sechste Mitteilung: die Cortexgliederung des Menschen. *J. Psychol. Neurol. Lpz.* 10, 231–246

Brodmann, K. (1909). *Vergleichende Lokalisationslehre der Grosshirnrinde in ihren Prinzipien dargetellt auf Grund des Zellenbaues.* Barth, Leipzig

Brodmann, K. (1918). Individuelle Variationen der Sehsphäre und ihre Bedeutung für die Klinik der Hinterhauptschüsse. *Allg. Z. Psychiat. (Berlin)* 74, 564–568

Brodmann, K. (1925). *Vergleichende Lokalisationslehre der Grosshirnrinde in ihren Prinzipien dargestellt auf Grund des Zellenbaues.* 2nd. ed. Barth, Leipzig

Brody, B.A., Pribram, K.H. (1978). The role of frontal and parietal cortex in cognitive processing: tests of spatial and sequential functions. *Brain* 101, 607–633

Brokate, A., Grüsser, O.-J., Seeck, M. (1990). Face-responsive components in the visual evoked potential change when the aspect of the faces is varied. In Abstract Book, EBBS Workshop of Cognitive Neuroscience, 24.–29. Mai 1990

Broman, M. (1978). Reaction-time differences between the left and right hemispheres for face and letter discrimination in children and adults. *Cortex* 14, 578–591

Brooks, R.M., Goldstein, A.G. (1963). Recognition by children of inverted photographs of faces. *Child Dev.* 34, 1033–1040

Brosgole, L., Kurucz, J., Plahovinsak, T.J., Gumiela, E. (1981). On the mechanism underlying facial-affective agnosia in senile demented patients. *Intern. J. Neuroscience* 15, 207–215

Brou, P., Sciascia, T.R., Linden, L., Lettvin, J.Y. (1986). The colors of things. *Scient. American* 255, 84–91

Broughton, R.J. (1982). Neurology and dreaming. *Psychiat. J. Univ. Ottava* 7, 101–110

Brouwer, B. (1936). Chiasma, Tractus opticus, Sehstrahlung und Sehrinde. In Bumke, O., Foerster, O. (eds.) *Handbuch der Neurologie*, Vol. VI, 449–532

Brown, J.F. (1931). The visual perception of velocity. *Psychol. Forsch.* 14, 199–232

Brown, J.L. (1961). Orientation to the vertical during water immersion. *Aerospace Medicine* 32, 209–217

Brown, J.W. (1972). *Aphasia, apraxia and agnosia: Clinical and theoretical aspects.* Charles C. Thomas, Springfield, Il.

Brown, J.W. (1983a). Rethinking the right hemisphere. In Perecman, E. (ed.), *Cognitive processing in the right hemisphere.* Academic Press, New York, 41–53

Brown, J.W. (1983b). The microstructure of perception: physiology and patterns of breakdown. *Cognition and Brain Theory* 6, 145–184

Brown, J.W. (1988). *Agnosia and Apraxia: Selected papers of Liepmann, Lange and Pötzl.* Lawrence Erlbaum Associates, Hillsdale NJ

Brown, J.W. (1989). *Neuropsychology of visual perception.* Laurence Erlbaum Associates, Hillsdale NJ

Brown, S., Schäfer, F.R.S. (1888). An investigation into the functions of the occipital and temporal lobes of the monkey's brain. *Philos. Trans. Roy. Soc. Lond.* 179, 303–327

Bruce, A. (1890). On the absence of the corpus callosum in the human brain with a description of a new case. *Brain* 12, 171–190

Bruce, C. (1982). Face recognition by monkeys: Absences of an inversion effect. *Neuropsychologia* 20, 515–521

Bruce, C., Desimone, R., Gross, C.G. (1981). Visual properties of neurons in a polysensory area in superior temporal sulcus of the macaque. *J. Neurophysiol.* 46, 369–384

Bruce, C.J., Goldberg, M.E. (1984). Physiology of the frontal eye fields. *Trends Neurosci.* 7, 436–441

Bruce, C.J., Goldberg, M.E. (1985). Primate frontal eye fields. I. Single neurons discharging before saccades. *J. Neurophysiol.* 53, 603–635

Bruce, C.J., Goldberg, M.E., Bushnell, M.C., Stanton, G.B. (1985). Primate frontal eye fields. II. Physiological and anatomical correlates of electrically evoked eye movements. *J. Neurophysiol.* 54, 714–734

Bruce, V. (1982). Changing faces: visual and nonvisual coding processes in face recognition. *Brit. J. Psychol.* 73, 105–116

Bruce, V. (1983). Recognizing faces. *Phil. Trans. Roy. Soc. Lond. B* 302, 423–436

Bruce, V. (1987). *Recognizing faces.* Erlbaum, London

Bruce, V., Young, A. (1986). Understanding face recognition. *Brit. J. Psychol.* 77, 305–327

Brugger, C. (1980). Blickverhalten und visuelles Gedächtnis. Univ. Wien, Grund-und Integrativwiss., Univ. Wien

Brugger, P. (1979). Doppelgänger und Exkursionshypothese. *Grenzgebiete der Wissenschaft (Innsbruck)* 4, 264–276

Brugger, P., Regard, M., Oelz, O. (1989). Hallucinatory experience in extreme altitude climbers. *J. Clinical and Exp. Neuropsych.* 11, 346–347

Brunn, J.L., Farah, M.J. (in press). The relation between spatial attention and reading. Evidence from the neglect syndrome. *Cognitive Neuropsychology*

Brunner, H., Hoff, H. (1929). Das Nebelsehen bei Labyrinthreizung. *Z. ges. Neurol. Psychiat.* 120, 796

Bruns, L., Stölting, B. (1888). Ein Fall von Alexie mit rechtsseitiger homonymer Hemianopsie ('subcorticale Alexie' Wernicke). Part 1 and 2. *Neurol. Centralbl.* 7, 481–490 and 509–520

Brust, J.C.M. (1980). Music and Language. Musical alexia and agraphia. *Brain* 103, 367–392

Brust, J.C.M., Behrens, M.M. (1977). 'Release hallucinations' as the major symptom of posterior cerebral artery occlusion: A report of 2 cases. *Ann. Neurol.* 2, 432–436

Bruyer, R. (1977). L'agnosie des couleurs. Une brève revue. *Acta Psychiat. Belg.* 77, 309–338

Bruyer, R. (1981). Asymmetry of facial expression in brain-damaged subjects. *Neuropsychologia* 19, 615–624

Bruyer, R. (1981). Perception d'expressions faciales emotionnelles et lesion cerebrale: influence de la netteté du stimulus. *Int. J. Psychol.* 16, 87–94

Bruyer, R. (1986). Foreword: From patchwork to melting pot. In Bruyer, R. (ed.) (1986). *The neuropsychology of face perception and facial expression*, Erlbaum, Hillsdale, N.J., London

Bruyer, R. (1987) (ed.), *The neuropsychology of face perception and facial expression.* Erlbaum, Hillsdale, N.Y. London

Bruyer, R. (1987). Face processing and brain damage: group studies. In Bruyer, R. (ed.), *The neuropsychology of face perception and facial expression*, Erlbaum, Hillsdale, N.J., London, 63–87

Bruyer, R. (1987). *Les méchanismes de reconnaissance des visages.* Press universitaire, Grenoble

Bruyer, R. (1987). Naming faces without recognition. A direct relationship and a new line in the models? *Cahiers de Psychologie Cognitive* 7, 309–313

Bruyer, R., Laterre, C., Seron, X., Feyereisen, P., Strypstein, E., Pierrard, E., Rectem, D. (1983). A case of prosopagnosia with some preserved covert remembrance of familiar faces. *Brain and Cognition* 2, 257–284

Bruyer, R., Rectem, D., Dupuis, M. (1986). Various kinds of face familiarity and a short report on a case of prosopagnosia. *Psychol. Belg.* 26, 221–225

Bryden, M.P. (1965). Tachistoscopic recognition, handedness, and cerebral dominance. *Neuropsychologia* 3, 1–8

Bryden, M.P. (1966). Left-right differences in tachistoscopic recognition: directional scanning or cerebral dominance? *Perceptual and Motor Skills* 23, 1127–1134

Bryden, M.P. (1970). Left-right differences in tachistoscopic recognition as a function of familiarity and pattern orientation. *J. Exp. Psychol.* 84, 120–122

Bryden, M.P. (1976). Response bias and hemispheric differences in dot localization. *Percept. Psychophys.* 19, 23–28

Bryden, M.P., Allard, F. (1976). Visual hemifield differences depend on type face. *Brain Language* 3, 191–200

Bub, D. (1986). Access to the word-form system in letter-by-letter readers. *J. Clin. Exp. Neuropsychol.* 8, 146

Bub, D.N., Black, S., Howell, J. (1989). Word recognition and orthographic context effects in a letter-by-letter reader. *Brain and Language* 36, 357–376

Bub, D.N., Cancelliere, A., Kertesz, A. (1982). The orthographie reading route: evidence for algorithmic grapheme-phoneme conversion in a surface dyslexic. Paper presented at the 20th Annual Meeting of the Academy of Aphasia, New Paltz, N.Y.

Buchtel, H. (1978). Hemispheric differences in discriminative reaction time to facial expressions. *Ital. J. Psychol.* 5, 159–169

Buettner, U.W., Dichgans, J., Grüsser, O.-J. (1982). Efferent motion perception (Sigma-movements) and Sigma-pursuit in neurological patients. In Lennerstrand, G., Zee, D.S., Keller, E.L. (eds.), *Functional basis of ocular motility disorders.* Pergamon Press, Oxford, 359–361

Bulens, C., Meerwaldt, J.D., Van der Wildt, G.J., Keemink, C.J. Spatial contrast sensitivity in unilateral cerebral ischaemic lesions involving the posterior visual pathway. *Brain* 112, 507–520

Bullier, J., Henry, G.H. (1980). Ordinal position and afferent input of neurons in monkey striate cortex. *J. Comp. Neurol.* 193, 913–935

Bullier, J., Kennedy, H. (1983). Projection of the lateral geniculate nucleus onto cortical area V2 in the macaque monkey. *Exp. Brain Res.* 53, 168–172

Burchard, J.M. (1980). *Lehrbuch der systematischen Psychopathologie.* Schattauer, Stuttgart

Burden, V., Bradshaw, J.L., Nettleton, N.C., Wilson, L. (1985). Hand and hemispace effects in tactual tasks in children. *Neuropsychologia* 23, 515–525

Buren, J.M. van, Baldwin, M. (1958). The architecture of the optic radiation in the temporal lobe of man. *Brain* 81, 15–40

Burgmeister, J.J., Tissot, R., Ajuriaguerra, J. (1965). Les hallucinations visuelles des ophthalmopathes. *Neuropsychologia* 3, 9–38

Burkhalter, A., Bernardo, K.L. (1988). Local connections of human visual cortex. *Soc. Neurosci. Abstr.* 14, 601

Burkhalter, A., Felleman, D.J., Newsome, W.T., Van Essen, D.C. (1986). Anatomical and physiological asymmetries related to visual areas V3 and VP in macaque extrastriate cortex. *Vision Res.* 26, 63–80

Burkhalter, A., Van Essen, D.C. (1986). Processing of color, form and disparity information in visual areas VP and V2 of ventral extrastriate cortex in macaque monkey. *J. Neurosci.* 6, 2327–2351

Buschor, E. (1960). *Das Porträt*. Piper, München

Bushnell, M.C., Goldberg, M.E., Robinson, D.L. (1981). Behavioral enhancement of visual responses in monkey cerebral cortex. I. Modulation in posterior parietal cortex related to selective visual attention. *J. Neurophys.* 46, 755–772

Buswell, G.T. (1920). An experimental study of the eye-voice span in reading. Suppl. Educ. Monographies 17

Butler, Th. (1933). Scotoma in migrainous subjects. *Brit. J. Ophthalmol.* 17, 83-

Butter, C.M. (1968). The effect of discrimination training on pattern equivalence in monkeys with inferotemporal and lateral striate lesions. *Neuropsychologia*, 6, 27–40.

Butter, C.M., Evans, J., Kirsch, N., Kewman, D. (1989). Altitudinal neglect following traumatic brain injury: a case report. *Cortex* 25, 135–146

Butter, C.M., Mishkin, M., Rosvold, H.E. (1965). Stimulus generalization in monkeys with inferotemporal and lateral occipital lesions. In Mustofsky, D.J. (ed.), *Stimulus Generalization*. Stanford University Press, Stanford, CA, 119–133

Butters, N., Barton, M., Brody, B.A. (1970). Role of the right parietal lobe in the mediation of cross-modal associations and reversible operations in space. Cortex 6, 174–190

Butters, N., Pandya, D. (1969). Retention of delayed-alternation: effect of selective lesions of *sulcus principalis*. *Science* 165, 1271–1273

Butters, N., Pandya, D., Stein, D., Rosen, J. (1972). A search for the spatial engram within the frontal lobes of monkeys. *Acta Neurobiol. Exp.* 32, 305–29

Button, J., Putman, T. (1962). Visual responses to cortical stimulation in the blind. *J. Iowa med. Soc.* 52, 17–21

Buvat, J.B. (1902). L'auto-représentation organique ou hallucination cinesthésique dans l'hysterie. *Gaz. des hôp.* 133, 1305–1308

Bücherl, B. (1989). Charakterköpfe. In Clair, J., Pichler, C., Pircher, W. (eds.), *Wunderblock. Eine Geschichte der modernen Seele*. Löcker, Wien, 55–67

Bücking, H., Baumgartner, G. (1974). Klinik und Pathophysiologie der initialen neurologischen Symptome bei fokalen Migränen (Migraine ophthalmique, Migraine accompagnée). *Arch. Psychiat. Nervenkr.* 219, 37–52

Bühler, Ch. (1934). Die Reaktionen des Säuglings auf das menschliche Gesicht. *Z. Psychol.* 132, 1–17

Büttner, U., Grüsser, O.-J., Schwanz, E. (1975). The effect of area and intensity on the response of cat retinal ganglion cells to brief light flashes. *Exp. Brain Res.* 23, 259–278

Büttner-Ennever, J. (ed., 1988). Neuroanatomy of the oculomotor system. Reviews of Oculomotor Research, Vol. 2, Elsevier, Amsterdam

Bychowski, Z. (1920). Ueber das Fehlen der Wahrnehmungen der eigenen Blindheit bei zwei Kriegsverletzten. *Neurol. Zbl. Leipzig* 39, 354

Byrne, R.W. (1982). Geographical knowledge and orientation. In Ellis, A.W. (ed.), *Normality and pathology in cognitive functions*. Academic Press, London, 239–264

Cadalbert, A.E. (1990). Qualitative differences in speech from the two sides of the mouth as an indicator of hemispheric motor control: a correlation study between hemibuccal speech and mouth asymmetry during speech. Inaugr. Diss., Univ. Zürich

Caelli, T. (1981). *Visual perception*. Pergamon Press, Oxford

Caelli, T., Hoffman, W.C., Lindman, H. (1978b). Subjective Lorentz transformations and the perception of motion. *J. Opt. Soc. Amer.*, 68, 402–411.

Caelli, T., Hübner, M. (1983). On the efficient two-dimensional energy coding characteristics of spatial vision. *Vision Res.* 23 (10), 1053–1055

Caelli, T., Hübner, M., Rentschler, I. (1985). On the discrimination of micropatterns and textures. *Human Neurobiology* 5, 129–136

Caelli, T., Rentschler, I., Scheidler, W. (1987). Visual pattern recognition in humans. *Biol. Cybernetics* 57, 233–240

Cajal, S.R. (1928). Degeneration and regeneration of the nervous system. Vol. 2, Oxford University Press, London

Callaghan, T.C. (1984). Dimensional interaction of hue and brightness in preattentive field segregation. *Percept. Psychophys.* 36(1), 25–34

Callaghan, T.C. (1989). Interference and dominance in texture segregation: hue, geometric form, and line orientation. *Percept. Psychophys.* 46(1), 299–311

Callaghan, T.C., Lasaga, M.I., Garner, W.R. (1986). Visual texture segregation based on orientation and hue. *Percept. Psychophys.* 39(1), 32–38

Callahan, M.M., Longsdail, S.J., Ron, M.A., Warrington, E.K. (1989). Cognitive impairment in patients with clinically isolated lesions of the type seen in multiple sclerosis. A psychometric and MRI study. *Brain* 112, 361–374

Cambier, J., Elghozi, D., Graveleau, P., Lubetzki, C. (1984). Hemisomatognosie droite et sentiment d'amputation par lesion gauche sous-corticale. Role de la disconnexion calleuse. *Rev. Neurol. (Paris)*. 140, 256–262

Cambier, J., Elghozi, D., Strube, E. (1980). Lesiones du thalamus avec syndrome de l'hemisphere mineur. Discussion du concept de negligence thalamique. *Rev. Neurol.* 136, 105–116

Cambier, J., Graveleau, P., Decroix, J.P., Elghozi, D., Masson, M. (1983). Le syndrome de l'artere choroidienne anterieure. Etude neuropsychologique de 4 cas. *Rev. Neurol. (Paris)* 139, 553–559

Cambier, J., Masson, M., Elghozi, D., Henin, D., Viader, F. (1980). Agnosie visuelle sans hemianopsie droite chez un sujet droitier. *Rev. Neurol (Paris)* 136, 11, 727–740

Caminiti, R., Sbriccoli, A. (1985). The callosal system of the superior parietal lobule in the monkey. *J. Comp. Neurol.* 237, 85–99

Campbell, D.C., Oxbury, J.M. (1976). Recovery from unilateral visuo-spatial neglect? *Cortex* 12, 303–312

Campbell, F.W., Blakemore, C. (1969). On the existence of neurons in the human visual system selectively sensitive to the orientation and size of retinal images. *J. Physiol. (Lond.)* 203, 237–260

Campbell, F.W., Green, D.G. (1965). Optical and retinal factors affecting visual resolution. *J. Physiol.* (London) 181, 576–593

Campbell, F.W., Gubisch, R.W. (1966). Optical quality of the human eye. *J. Physiol.* (London) 186, 558–578

Campbell, F.W., Robson, J.G. (1968). Application of Fourier analysis to the visibility of gratings. *J. Physiol. (Lond.)* 197, 551–566

Campbell, F.W., Robson, J.G., Westheimer, G. (1959). Fluctuations of accommodation under steady viewing conditions. *J. Physiol.* (London) 145, 579–594

Campbell, R. (1978). Asymmetries in interpreting and expressing a posed facial expression. *Cortex* 14, 327–342

Campbell, R. (1986). Asymmetries of facial action: Some facts and fancies of normal face movement. In Bruyer, R. (ed.) *The Neuropsychology of Face Perception and Facial Expression*, Erlbaum, Hillsdale, N.Y., London, 247–267

Campbell, R. (1986). The lateralisation of lipread sounds: a first look. *Brain and Cogn.* 5, 1–21

Campbell, R., Dodd, B. (1980). Hearing by eye. *Quart. J. Exp. Psychol.* 32, 85–99

Campbell, R., Heywood, C.A., Cowey, A., Regard, M., Landis, T. (1990). Sensitivity to eye gaze in prosopagnosic patients and monkeys with superior temporal sulcus ablation. *Neuropsychologia* 28, 1123–1142

Campbell, R., Landis, T., Regard, M. (1986). Face recognition and lipreading. A neurological dissociation. *Brain* 109, 509–521

Campion, J. (1987). Apperceptive agnosia: The specification and description of constructs. In G.W. Humphreys, M.J. Riddoch (eds.), *Visual object processing: A cognitive neuropsychological approach*. London, Lawrence Erlbaum Associates

Campion, J., Latto, R. (1985). Apperceptive agnosia due to carbon monoxide poisoning. An interpretation based on critical band masking from disseminated lesions. *Behav. Brain Res.* 15, 227–240

Campion, J., Latto, R., Smith, Y.M. (1983). Is blindsight an effect of scattered light, spared cortex, and near-threshold vision? *Behavioral and Brain Sci.* 6, 423–486

Campos-Ortega, J.A., Hayhow, W.R. (1972). On the organisation of the visual cortical projection to the pulvinar in macaca mulatta. *Brain, Behav. Evol.* 6, 394–423

Campos-Ortega, J.A., Hayhow, W.R., Clüver, V.P.F. (1970a). A note on the problem of retinal projections to the inferior pulvinar nucleus of primates. *Brain Res.* 22, 126–130

Campos-Ortega, J.A., Hayhow, W.R., Clüver, V.P.F. de (1970b). The descending projections from the cortical visual field of *Macaca mulatta* with particular reference to the question of a cortico-lateral geniculate pathway. *Brain Behav. Evol.* 3, 368–414

Capelle, W. (1953). *Die Vorsokratiker*. 4th ed. Kröner, Stuttgart 1968, 503 p.

Capgras, J., Reboul-Lachaux, J. (1923). Illusion des sosie dans un delire systemise chronique. *Bull. Soc. Clin. Med. Ment.* 2, 6–16

Capitani, E., Scotti, G., Spinnler, H. (1978). Colour imperception in patients with focal excisions of the cerebral hemispheres. *Neuropsychologia* 16, 491–496

Caplan, B. (1985). Stimulus effects in unilateral neglect? *Cortex* 21, 69–80

Caplan, L.R. (1980). 'Top of the basilar' syndrome. *Neurology* 30, 72–79

Caplan, L.R., Hedley-Whyte, T. (1974). Cuing and memory dysfunction in alexia without agraphia: a case report. *Brain* 97, 251–262

Caplan, R., Dodd, B. (1980). Hearing by eye. *Quart. J. Exp. Psychol* 32, 85–99

Cappa, S., Sterzi, R., Vallar, G., Bisiach, E. (1987). Remission of hemineglect and anosognosia during vestibular stimulation. *Neuropsychologia* 25, 775–782

Caramazza, A. (1984). The logic of neuropsychological research and the problem of patient classification in aphasia. *Brain and Language* 21, 9–20

Caramazza, A., Berndt, R.S. (1978). Semantic and syntactic processes in aphasia. A review of the literature. *Psychol. Bull.* 85, 898–918

Carey, S. (1981). The development of face perception. In Davis, G., Ellis, H., Shepherd, J. (eds.), *Perceiving and remembering faces*. Academic Press, London, 9–38

Carey, S., Diamond, R. (1977). From piecemeal to configurational representation of faces. *Science* 195, 312–314

Carey, S., Diamond, R., Woods, B. (1980). Development of face recognition — A maturational component? *Develop. Psychol.* 16, 257–269

Carlow, T.J., Flynn, J.T., Shipley, T. (1976). Color perimetry. *Arch. Ophthalmol.* 94, 1492–1496

Carlson, M., Hubel, D.H., Wiesel, T.N. (1986). Effects of monocular exposure to oriented lines on monkey striate cortex. *Dev. Brain Res.* 5, 71–81

Carmon, A. (1973). Ear asymmetry in perception of emotional nonverbal stimuli. *Acta Psychologica* 37, 351–357

Carmon, A., Gordon, H.W., Bental, E., Harness, B.Z. (1977). Retraining in literal alexia: Substitution of a right hemisphere perceptual strategy for impaired left hemispheric processing. *Bull. L.A. Neurol. Soc.* 42, 41–50

Carmon, A., Nachshon, I., Starinsky, R. (1976). Developmental aspects of visual hemifield differences in the perception of visual material. *Brain Lang.* 3, 463–469

Carpenter, C.R. (1964). *Naturalistic behaviour of nonhuman primates*. Pennsylvania State University Press, University Park

Carpenter, G.C., Tecce, J.J., Stechler, G., Friedman, S. (1970). Dif-

ferential visual behavior to human and humanoid faces in early infancy. *Merrill-Palmer Quarterly* 16, 91–108

Carson, D.H. (1961). Letter constraints within words in printed English. *Kybernetik* 1, 46–54

Casamajor, L. (1913). A case of pure alexia, with localisation confirmed at operation. *Medical Record*, March, 407–409

Casey, T., Ettlinger, G. (1960). The occasional 'independence' of dyslexia and dysgraphia from dysphasia. *J. Neurol. Neurosurg. Psychiat.* 23, 228–236

Cassirer, E. (1944). The concept of group and the theory of perception. *Philos. and Phenomenol. Res.* 5, 1–15

Castaigne, P., Lhermitte, F., Buge, A., Escourelle, R., Hauw, J.J., Lyon-Caen, O. (1981). Paramedian thalamic and midbrain infarcts: clinical and neuropathological study. *Ann. Neurol.* 10, 127–148

Castner, B.M. (1940). Language development. In Gesell, A. et al. (eds.), *The first five years of life*. Harper and Row, New York, Evanston, London

Castro-Caldas, A. (1985). Pure alexia without hemianopia. *Arch. Neurol.* 42, 1035–1036

Castro-Caldas, A., Salgado, V. (1984). Right hemifield alexia without hemianopia. *Arch. Neurol.* 41, 84–87

Cattell, J. McV. (1885). Über die Zeit der Erkennung und Benennung von Schriftzeichen, Bildern und Farben. *Wundt's Philosophische Studien* 2, 635

Cattell, J. McV. (1886). Psychometrische Untersuchungen. *Wundts's Philosophische Studien* 3, 452

Cavada, C., Goldman-Rakic, P.S. (1989). Posterior parietal cortex in rhesus monkey: I. Parcellatation of areas based on distictive limbic and sensory corticocortical connections. *J. Comp. Neurol.* 287, 393–421

Cavada, C., Goldman-Rakic, P.S. (1989). Posterior parietal cortex in rhesus monkey: II. Evidence for segregated corticocortical networks linking sensory and limbic areas with the frontal lobe. *J. Comp. Neurol.* 287, 422–445

Cavanagh, P., Tyler, C.W., Favreau, O. (1984). Perceived velocity of moving chromatic gratings. *J. opt. Soc. Am.* A 1, 893–899

Ceci, S.J. (1982a). Automatic and purposive semantic processing characteristics of normal and language/learning-disabled children. *Developmental Psychology* 19, 427–439

Ceci, S.J. (1982b). Extracting meaning from stimuli: automatic and purposive processing of the language-based learning-disabled. *Topics in Learning and Learning Disabilities* 2, 46–53

Ceci, S.J., Lea, E.E., Ringstrom, M.D. (1980). Coding processes in normal and learning-disabled children: evidence for modality-specific pathways to the cognitive system. *J. Exp. Psychol. (Hum. Learn.)* 6, 785–797

Celesia, G.G., Archer, C.R., Kuroiwa, Y., Goldfader, P.R. (1980). Visual function of the extrageniculo-calcerine system in man. Relationship to cortical blindness. *Arch. Neurol.* 37, 704–706

Chabot, R.J., Petros, Th.V., McCord, G. (1983). Developmental and reading ability differnces in accessing information from semantic memory. *J. Exp. Child Psychol.* 35, 128–142

Chain, F., Leblanc, M., Chedru, F., Lhermitte, F. (1979). Negligence visuelle dans les lesions posterieures de l'hemisphere gauche. *Rev. Neurol.* 135, 105–126

Chalupa, L.M., Coyle, R.S., Lindsley, D.B. (1976). Effect of pulvinar lesions on visual pattern discrimination in monkeys. *J. Neurophysiol.* 39, 354–369

Chamorro, A., Sacco, R.L., Ciercierski, K., Binder, J.R., Tatemichi, T.K., Mohr, J.P. (1990). Visual hemineglect and hemihallucinations in a patient with a subcortical infarction. *Neurology* 40, 1463–1464

Chance, B. (1944). Johannes Müller — a sketch of his life and ophthalmologic works. *Transactions of the American Ophthalmological Society* 42, 230–

Chang, C.H., Damasio, A.R. (1980). Human cerebral asymmetries evaluated by computed tomography. *J. Neurol. Neurosurg. and Psy-*

chiat. 43, 873–878

Chang, H.-T., Kaada, B. (1950). An analysis of primary response of visual cortex to optic nerve stimulation in cat. *J. Neurophysiol.* 13, 305–318

Chapanis, A. (1965). Colour names for colour space. *American Scientist* 53, 327–346

Chapman, C.E., Spidalieri, G., Lamarre, Y. (1984). Discharge properties of area 5 neurones during arm movements triggered by sensory stimuli in the monkey. *Brain Res.* 309, 63–78

Charcot, J.M. (1875). Hemiopie laterale et amblyopie croisèe. *Le Progres Medicale* 3, 481–482

Charcot, J.M. (1876–1880). *Lecon sur les localisations dans les maladies du cerveau. Progres medical.* A. Delahaye, Paris

Charcot, J.M. (1877). *Lectures on the diseases of the nervous system.* Vol. 1 (transl.) The New Sydenham Society, London

Charcot, J.M. (1883). Un cas de suppression brusque et isolé de la vision mentale des signes et des objets (formes et couleurs). *Progr. Med.* 11, 568–571

Charcot, J.M. (1886). Ueber Migraine ophthalmique in der Initialperiode der progressiven Paralyse. In Freud, S. (ed.), *Neue Vorlesungen über die Krankheiten des Nervensystems insbesondere über Hysterie.* Toeplitz & Deuticke, Leipzig, 60–61

Charcot, J.M. (1887). Sur un cas de cécité verbale. In *Lecon sur les maladies du systeme nerveux, vol. III of oeuvres completes de J.M. Charcot,* Delahaye & Lecrosnier, Paris

Charnallet, A., Carbonnel, S., Pellat, J. (1988). Right visual hemiagnosia: a single case report. *Cortex* 24, 347–355

Chasan, B. (1927). Zur Frage der Cytoarchitektonik der Area striata (Rinde vom Calcarinatypus) in ihren Beziehungen zur zentralen optischen Leitung. *Schweizer Arch. f. Neurol. u. Psychiat.* 21, 283–320

Chauffard (1881). Revue de Medicine 1, 393, cited in Charcot, J.M., 1887

Chavis, D.A., Pandya, D.M. (1976). Further observation on corticofrontal connections in the rhesus monkey. *Brain Res.* 117, 369–386

Chedru, F. (1976). Space representation in unilateral spatial neglect. *J. Neurol. Neurosurg. Psychiat.* 39, 1057–1061

Chedru, F., Leblanc, M., Lhermitte, F. (1973). Visual searching in normal and brain-damaged subjects (contribution to the study of unilateral inattention). *Cortex* 9, 94–111

Chen, L. (1968). Talking hand of aphasia stroke patients. *Geriatrics* 23, 145–148

Cheng, M., Outerbridge, J.S. (1975). Optokinetic nystagmus during selective retinal stimulation. *Exp. Brain* 23, 129–139

Cherry, H. (1971). *On human communication.* New York, London

Cheselden, W. (1728). An acount of some observations made by a young gentleman who was born blind, or lost his sight so early, that he had rememberance of ever having seen, and was couch'd between 13 and 14 years of age. *Phil. Trans. Roy. Soc. London* 35, 447

Chevalier-Skolnikoff, S. (1973). Facial expression of emotion in nonhuman primates. In Ekman, P. (ed.), *Darwin and facial expression.* Academic press, N.Y., 11–89

Chisholm, I.H. (1975). Cortical Blindness in cranial arteritis. *Brit. J. Ophthalmol.* 59, 332–333

Chow, K.L. (1950). A retrograde cell degeneration study of the cortical projection field of the pulvinar in the monkey. *J. Comp. Neurol.* 93, 313–340

Chow, K.L. (1951). Effects of partial extirpations of the posterior association cortex on visually mediated behavior in monkeys. *Comp. Psychol. Monogr.* 20, 187–217

Chow, K.L. (1954). Effect of temporal neocortical ablation on visual discrimination learning sets in monkeys. *J. Comp. Physiol. Psychol.* 47, 194–198

Chow, K.L. (1961). Anatomical and electrographical analysis of temporal neocortex in relation to visual discrimination learning in monkey. In Delafresnaye,J.F. (ed.), *Brain Mechanisms and Learn-*

ing. Thomas, Springfield, Ill., 507–525

Chow, K.L. (1961). Changes of brain electropotentials during visual discrimination learning in monkey. *J. Neurophysiol.* 24, 377–390

Christen, L., Landis, T., Regard, M. (1985). Left hemispheric functional compensation in prosopagnosia? A tachistoscopic study with unilaterally lesioned patients. *Hum. Neurobiol.* 4, 9–14

Christman, S. (1989). Perceptual characteristics in visual laterality research. *Brain and Cognition* 11, 238–257

Christodoulou, G.N. (1976). Delusional hyperidentifications of the Fregoli type: organic pathogenetic contributors. *Acta Psychiat. Scand.* 54, 305–314

Christodoulou, G.N. (1977). The syndrome of Capgras. *Brit. J. Psychiat.* 130, 556–564

Christodoulou, G.N. (1978). Course and prognosis of the syndrome of doubles. *J. Nerv. Ment. Dis.* 166, 68–72

Christodoulou, G.N. (ed.) (1986). The delusional misidentification syndromes. Bibl. Psychiat. No. 164. Karger, Basel

Chung, I.H., Grüsser, O.-J., Przybyszewski, A. (1991). Interaction of effects of eyeball deformation and light stimulation in retinal ganglion cells (in preparation)

Chung, T.H., Grüsser, O.-J. Przybyzewski, A. (1990). Interaction of light-stimulation and eyeball deformation on cat retina ganglion cell activity. *European J. Neurosci. suppl.* 3, 341

Chvostek, F. (1892). Beiträge zur Theorie der Hallucinationen. *Jahrbuch für Psychiatrie* 11, 267–289

Cicone, M., Wapner, W., Foldi, N., Zurif, E., Gardner, H. (1979). The relation between gesture and language in aphasic communication. *Brain and Language* 8, 324–349

Ciesielski, K.T., Madden, J.S., Bligh, J.G., Schopflocher, D. (1985). Long-term brain impairment in chronic alcoholics: N2-P3 cognitive potentials in a template-matching memory task. *Alcohol. Alcohol.* 20, 403–408

Clark, C.R., Geffen, G.M., Geffen, L.B. (1989). Catecholamines and the covert orientation of attention in humans. *Neuropsychologia* 27, 131–139

Clark, W.E. Le Gros (1941). Observations on the association fibre system of the visual cortex and the central representation of the retina. *J. Anat.* 75, 225–235

Clarke, E., Dewhurst, K. (1972). *An illustrated history of brain function.* Univ. of Calif. Press, Berkeley, 154 p.

Clarke, E., Dewhurst, K. (1973). *Die Funktionen des Gehirns: Lokalisationstheorien von der Antike bis zur Gegenwart.* Moos, München

Clarke, E., O'Malley, C.D. (1968). *The human brain and spinal cord: a historical study illustrated by writings from antiquity to the twentieth century.* Univ. of Calif. Press, Berkeley,

Clausen, J. (1955). *Visual sensations (phosphenes) produced by AC sinewave stimulation.* Munksgaard, Copenhagen, 101 p.

Clausen, J., Vanderbilt, C. (1957). Visual beats caused by simultaneous electrical and photic stimulation. *Amer. J. Psychol.* 70, 577–585

Cleland, P.G., Saunders, M., Rosser, R. (1981). An unusual case of visual perseveration. *J. Neurol. Neurosurg. Psychiat.* 44, 262–263

Clerk Maxwell, J. (1872). On colour vision. *Proc. Roy. Inst. Great Britain* 6, 260–271

Cobb, S., Lindemann, E. (1943). Symposium on management of Cocoanut Grove Burns at Massachusetts General Hospital: neuropsychiatric observations. *Annals of Surgery* 117, 814–824

Code, C. (1987). *Language, aphasia, and the right hemisphere.* Wiley, Chichester, N.Y.

Cogan, D.G. (1960). Hemianopia and associated symptoms due to parietotemporal lobe lesions. *Am. J. Ophthalmol.* 50, 1056–1066

Cogan, D.G. (1973). Visual hallucinations as release phenomena. *Graefes Arch. klin. Ophthal.* 188, 139–150

Cogan, D.G. (1979). Visuospatial dysgnosia. *Am.J.Ophthal.* 88, 61–68

Cogan, D.G. (1985). Visual disturbances with focal progressive dementing disease. *Am. J. Ophthalmol.* 100, 68–72

Cohen, B., Bodis-Wollner, I. (eds., 1990). *Vision and the brain. The organization of the central visual system.* Raven Press, New York

Cohen, D.N., Salanga, V.D., Hully, W., Steinberg, M.C., Hardy, R.W. (1976). Alexia without agraphia. *Neurology* 26, 455–459

Cohen, G. (1973). Hemispheric differences in serial versus parallel processing. *J. Exp. Psychol.* 97, 349–356

Cohen, L.B., Deloasche, J.S., Pearl, R.A. (1977). An examination of interference effects in infants' memory for faces. *Child Development* 48, 88–96

Cohn, H. (1874). Über Hemiopie bei Hirnleiden. *Klinische Monatsblätter für Augenheilkunde* 12, 203

Cohn, R. (1971). Phantom Vision. *Arch. Neurol.* 25, 468–471

Cohn, R. (1972). Eyeball movements in homonymous hemianopia following simultaneous bitemporal object presentation. *Neurology* 22, 12–14

Cohn, R., Neumann, M.A., Wood, D.H. (1977). Prosopagnosia: a clinicopathological study. *Ann. Neurol.* 1, 177–182

Colby, C.L., Gattass, R., Olson, C.R., Gross, C.G. (1983). Cortical afferents to visual areas in the macaque. *Soc. Neurosci. Abstr.* 9, 152

Colby, C.L., Gattass, R., Olson, C.R., Gross, C.G. (1988). Topographical organization of cortical afferents to extrastriate visual area PO in the macaque: a dual tracer study. *J. Comp. Neurol.* 238, 392–413

Colby, C.L., Miller, E.K. (1986). Eye movement related responses of neurons in superior temporal polysensory area of the macaque. *Neurosci. Abstr.* 12, 1184

Cole, F.J. (1944). *A history of comparative anatomy from Aristotle to the eighteenth century.* MacMillan, London

Cole, M., Perez-Cruet, J. (1964). Prospagnosia. *Neuropsychologia* 2, 237–246

Cole, M., Zangwill, O.L. (1963). Déjö vu in temporal lobe epilepsy. *J. Neurol. Neurosurg. Psychiat.* 26, 37–38

Coles, P.R. (1974). Profile orientation and social distance in portrait paintin. *Perception* 3, 303–308

Collaer, M.L., Evans, J.R. (1982). A measure of short-term visual memory based on the WISC-R coding subtest. *J. Clin. Psychol.* 38, 641–644

Collewijn, H. (1970). An analog model of the rabbit's optokinetic system. *Brain Res.* 36, 71–88

Collewijn, H. (1981). *The oculomotor system of the rabbit and its plasticity.* Springer, Berlin

Collewijn, H., Curio, G., Grüsser, O.-J. (1981). Interaction of vestibulo-ocular reflex and Sigma-optokinetic nystagmus in man. In Fuch, A.F., Becker, W. (eds.), *Progress in oculomotor research.* Elsevier/North-Holland, New York, Amsterdam, Oxford, 567–576

Collewijn, H., Curio, G., Grüsser, O.-J. (1982). Spatially selective visual attention and generation of eye pursuit movements. *Human Neurobiol.* 1, 129–139

Collin, N.D., Conway, A., Latto, R., Marzi, C. (1982). The role of frontal eye fields and superior colliculi in visual search and non-visual search in rhesus monkeys. *Behav. Brain Res.* 4, 177

Colombo, A., De Renzi, E., Faglioni, P. (1976). The occurrence of visual neglect in patients with unilateral cerebral disease. *Cortex* 12, 221–231

Colombo, A., De Renzi, E., Gentilini, M. (1982). The time course of visual hemi-inattention. *Arch. Psychiat. Nervenkrankh.* 231, 539–546

Coltheart, M. (1980). *Deep dyslexia:* a right hemisphere hypothesis. In Coltheart, M., Patterson, K., Marshall, J.C. (eds.), *Deep dyslexia.* Routledge & Kegan Paul, London

Coltheart, M. (1985). Right-hemisphere reading revisited. *Behav. Brain Sci.* 8, 363–365

Coltheart, M., Patterson, K., Marshall, J.C. (1980). Deep dyslexia. Routledge & Kegan Paul, London

Comar, G. (1901). L'auto-représentation de l'organisme chez quelques hystériques. *Rev. Neurol.* 9, 490–495

Comerford, J.P. (1974). Stereopsis with chromatic contours. *Vision Res.* 14, 975–982

Conrad, K. (1947). Über den Begriff der Vorgestalt und seine Bedeutung für die Hirnpathologie. *Nervenarzt* 18, 289

Conrad, K. (1948). Beitrag zum Problem der parietalen Alexie. *Arch. Psychol.* 181, 398–420

Conrad, K. (1948). Über differentiale und integrale Gestaltfunktion und den Begriff der Protopathie. *Nervenarzt* 19, 315–323

Conrad, K. (1953). Über ein eigenartiges Spiegelphantom. Heautoskopische Phänomene als Dauerzustand bei Hypophysentumor. *Nervenarzt* 24, 265–270

Conrad, K. (1979). *Die beginnende Schizophrenie.* Thieme, Stuttgart

Constantinides, C.D. (1954). De l'héautoscopie en général (avec analyse d'un cas). *Ann. Méd.-Psychol.* 112, 336–347

Cook, M. (1978). Eye movement during recognition of faces. In Gruneberg, M.M., Morris, P.E., Sykes, R.N. (eds.), *Practical aspects of memory.* Academic Press, London, New York

Cook, N.D. (1986). *The brain code. Mechanisms of information transfer and the role of the corpus callosum.* Methuen, London and New York

Cooper, L.A., Shepard, R.N. (1973). The time required to prepare for a rotated stimulus. *Memory and Cognition* 1, 246–250

Corballis, M.C. (1988). Recognition of disoriented shapes. *Psychol. Rev.* 95, 115–123

Corballis, M.C. (1989). Laterality and human evolution. *Psychol. Rev.* 96, 492–505

Corballis, M.C., McLaren, R. (1982). Interaction between perceived and imagined rotation. *J. Exp. Psychol.* 8, 215–224

Corballis, M.C., Morgan, M.J. (1978). On the biological basis of human laterality. I. Evidence for a maturational left-right gradient. II. mechnisms of inheritance. *Behav. Brain Sci.* 2, 261–336

Corbett, D., Wise, R.A. (1980). Intracranial self-stimulation in relation to the ascending dopaminergic system of the midbrain: moveable electrode mapping study. *Brain Res.* 185, 1–15

Corbetta, M., Miezin, F.M., Dobmeyer, S., Shulman, G.L., Petersen, S.E. (1990). Attentional modulation of neural processing of shape, color, and velocity in humans. *Science* 248, 1556–1559

Coren, S. (1986). An efferent component in the visual perception of direction and extent. *Psychol. Review* 93, 391–410

Corkin, S. (1965). Tactually-guided maze learning in man: effects of unilateral cortical excisions and bilateral hippocampal lesions. *Neuropsychologia* 3, 339–351

Corkin, S. (1979). Hidden-figures-test performance — Lasting effects of unilateral penetrating head injury and transient effects of bilateral cingulotomy. *Neuropsychologia* 17, 585–605

Corkin, S. (1984). Lasting consequences of bilateral medial temporal lobectomy: Clinical course and experimental findings in HM. *Seminars in Neurology* 4, 249–259

Cornsweet, T.N. (1970). *Visual perception.* Academic Press, New York

Coslett, H.B., Gonzales-Rothi, L.J., Heilman, K.M. (1984). Reading: Selective sparing of closed-class words in Wernicke's aphasia. *Neurology* 34, 1038–1045

Coslett, H.B., Saffran, E.M. (1989). Evidence for preserved reading in 'pure alexia'. *Brain* 112, 327–359

Coslett, H.B., Saffran, E.M. (1989). Preserved object recognition and reading comprehension in optic aphasia. *Brain* 112, 1091–1110

Costa, L.D., Vaughan, H.G. (1962). Performance of patients with lateralised cerebral lesions. I.: Verbal and perceptual tests. *J. Nerv. Ment. Dis.* 134, 162–168

Costa, L.D., Vaughan, H.G., Horwitz, M., Ritter, W. (1969). Patterns of behavioral deficit associated with visual spatial neglect. *Cortex* 5, 242–263

Coughlan, A.K., Hollows, S.E. (1984). Use of memory tests in differentiating organic disorder from depression. *Br. J. Psychiatr.* 145, 164–167

Courbon, P., Fail, G. (1927). Syndrome d'illusion de Fregoli et schizophrenie. *Bull. Soc. Clin. Med. Ment.* 15, 121–125

Courbon, P., Tusques, J. (1932). Illusions d'intermetamorphoses et de charme. *Ann. Med. Psychol. (Paris)* 90, 401–406

Cowey, A. (1964). Projection of the retina onto striate and prestriate cortex in the Squirrel monkey, Saimiri sciureus. *J. Neurophysiol.* 27, 366–393

Cowey, A. (1967). Perimetric study of field defects in monkeys after cortical and retinal ablations. *Quart. J. Psychol.* 19, 232–245

Cowey, A. (1974). Atrophy of retinal ganglion cells after removal of striate cortex in a rhesus monkey. *Perception* 3, 257–260

Cowey, A. (1979). Cortical maps and visual perception. The Grindley Memorial Lecture. *Quart. J. Exp. Psychol.* 31, 1–17

Cowey, A. (1981). Why are there so many visual areas? In Schmitt, F.O., Worden, F.G., Adelman, G., Dennis,, S.G. (eds.), *The Organization of the Cerebral Cortex*. MIT-Press, Cambridge, 395–413

Cowey, A. (1982). Sensory and non-sensory visual disorders in man and monkey. *Philos. Trans. R. Soc. Lond. (Biol.)* 298, 3–13

Cowey, A. (1985). Aspects of cortical organization related to selective attention and selective impairments of visual perception: A tutorial review. In Posner, M.L., Marin, O.S.M. (eds.), *Attention and performance XI*. Hillsdale, Lawrence Erlbaum Ass., 41–62

Cowey, A., Gross, C.G. (1970). Effects of foveal prestriate and inferotemporal lesions on visual discrimination by rhesus monkeys. *Exp. Brain Res.* 11, 128–144

Cowey, A., Porter, J. (1979). Brain damage and global stereopsis. *Proc. Roy. Soc. Lond. B.* 204, 399–407

Cowey, A., Rolls, E.T. (1974). Human cortical magnification factor and its relation to visual acuity. *Exp. Brain Res.* 21, 447–454

Cowey, A., Stoerig, P. (1991). The neurobiology of blindsight. *TINS* 14, 140–145

Cowey, A., Stoerig, P., Perry, V.H. (1989). Transneuronal retrograde degeneration of retinal ganglion cells after damage to striate cortex in macaque monkeys: selective loss of Pö cells. *Neurosci.* Vol. 29, 1, 65–80

Cowey, A., Weiskrantz, L. (1963). A perimetric study of visual field defects in monkeys. *Quart. J. exp. Psychol.* 15, 91–115

Cowey, A., Weiskrantz, L. (1967). A comparison of the effects of inferotemporal and striate cortex lesions on the visual behaviour of rhesus monkeys. *Quart. J. exp. Psychol.* 19, 246–253

Cox, J.M. (1811). Praktische Bemerkungen über geistige Zerrüttung. Transl. J.Ch. Reil. Renger, Halle. English original: London 1804

Cragg, B.G., Ainsworth, A. (1969). The topography of the afferent projections in the circumstriate visual cortex of the monkey studied by the Nauta method. *Vision Res.* 9, 733–747

Crawford, H.J., Allen, S.N. (1983). Enhanced visual memory during hypnosis as mediated by hypnotic responsiveness and cognitive strategies. *J. Exp. Psychol. (Gen)* 112, 662–685

Crawley, A.E. (1911). Doubles. In Hastings, J. (ed.), *Encyclopedia of Religion and Ethics*. Vol. 4. Clark, Edinburgh

Cremonini, W., De Renzi, E., Faglioni, P. (1980). Contrasting performance of right-hemisphere and left-hemisphere patients on short-term and long-term sequential visual memory. *Neuropsychologia* 18, 1–9

Creutzfeldt, O.D. (1956). Reaktionen einzelner Neurone des optischen Cortex nach Reizung unspezifischer Thalamuskerne. Proc. 20th Int. Congr. Physiol., Brussels, p. 387

Creutzfeldt, O.D. (1961). General physiology of cortical neurons and neuronal information in the visual system. In Brazier, M.A.B. (ed.), *Brain and Behavior, Vol. 1*. American Institute of Biological Sciences, Washington, D.C., 299–358

Creutzfeldt, O.D. (1977). Generality of the functional structure of the neocortex. *Naturwissenschaften* 64, 507–517

Creutzfeldt, O.D. (1983). *Cortex-cerebri. Leistung, strukturelle und funktionale Organisation der Hirnrinde*. Springer, Berlin

Creutzfeldt, O.D. (1987). Gibt es eine Mechanik des Denkens?

Forsch. Med. 2, 7–19

Creutzfeldt, O.D. (1988). Cortical mechanisms of eye movements in relation to perception and cognitive processes. In Lüer, G., Lass, U., Shallo-Hoffmann, J. (eds.), *Eye movement research. Physiological and psychological aspects*. Hogreve, Toronto, Zürich, Göttingen, 9–33

Creutzfeldt, O.D.(1979). Repräsentation der visuellen Umwelt im Gehirn. *Verh. Dtsch. Zool. Ges. 1979*, 5–18, Gustav Fischer Verlag, Stuttgart

Creutzfeldt, O.D., Akimoto, H. (1958). Konvergenz und gegenseitige Beeinflussung von Impulsen aus der Retina und den unspezifischen Thalamuskernen an einzelnen Neuronen des optischen Cortex. *Arch. Psychiat. Nervenkr.* 196, 520–538

Creutzfeldt, O.D., Baumgartner, G. (1955). Reactions of neurones in the occipital cortex to electrical stimuli applied to the intralaminar thalamus. *Electroenceph. clin. Neurophysiol.* 7, 664–665

Creutzfeldt, O.D., Grüsser, O.-J. (1959). Beeinflussung der Flimmerreaktion einzelner corticaler Neurone durch elektrische Reize unspezifischer Thalamuskerne. In Bogaert, L. v., Radermecker, J. (eds.), Proc. 1st Int. Congr. Neurol. Sci. Vol. 3, *Electroencephalography, Clinical Neurophysiology and Epilepsy*. Pergamon, London, 349–355

Creutzfeldt, O.D., Kuhnt, U. (1973). Electrophysiology and topographical distribution of visual evoked potentials in animals. In Jung, R. (ed.), *Handbook of sensory physiology. Vol. VII/3B*, Springer, Berlin, 595–646

Creutzfeldt, O.D., Kuhnt, U., Benevento, L.A. (1974). An intracellular analysis of visual cortical neurones to moving stimuli: responses in a co-operative neuronal network. *Exp. Brain Res.* 21, 251–274

Creutzfeldt, O.D., Lange-Malecki, B., Dreyer, E. (1990). Perceived object colour results from a combination of spectral reflectance and chromatic brightness contrast. *J. Opt. Soc. of Am. A.* 7, 1644–1653

Creutzfeldt, O.D., Lee, B.B., Elepfandt, A. (1979). A quantitative study of chromatic organization and receptive fields of cells in the lateral geniculate body of the rhesus monkey. *Exp. Brain Res.* 35, 527–545

Creutzfeldt, O.D., Lee, B.B., Valberg, A. (1986). Colour and brightness signals of parvocellular lateral geniculate neurons. *Exp. Brain Res.* 63, 21–34

Creutzfeldt, O.D., Nothdurft, H.C. (1978). Representation of complex visual stimuli in the brain. *Naturwissenschaften* 65, 307–318

Creutzfeldt, O.D., Weber, H., Tanaka, M., Lee, B.B. (1987). Neuronal representation of spectral and spatial stimulus aspects in foveal and parafoveal area 17 of the awake monkey. *Exp. Brain Res.* 68, 541–564

Crick, F. (1984). The function of the thalamic reticular complex: the searchlight hypothesis. *Proc. Natl. Acad. Sci. USA* 81, 4586–4590

Crick, F.H.C., Asanuma, C. (1986). Certain aspects of the anatomy and physiology of the cerebral cortex. In McClelland, J.L., Rumelhart, D.E.(eds.), *Parallel distributed processing: Explorations in the microstructure of cognition. Vol. II: Psychological and biological models*. MIT Press, Cambridge, MA

Crisco, J.J., Dobbs, J.M., Mulhern, R.K. (1988). Cognitive processing of children with Williams syndrome. *Dev. Med. Child Neurol.* 30, 650–656

Critchley, M. (1933). Neurological aspects of visual and auditory hallucinations. *Brit. Med. J.* 2, 634

Critchley, M. (1939). *The language of gesture*. Arnolds, London

Critchley, M. (1949). Metamorphopsia of central origin. *Trans. Ophthal. Soc. U. K.* 69, 111–121

Critchley, M. (1949). The phenomenon of tactile inattention with special reference to parietal lesions. *Brain* 72, 538–561

Critchley, M. (1949). The problem of awareness or non-awareness of hemianopic field defects. *Transactions Ophthalmol. Soc. UK* 69, 95–109

Critchley, M. (1951). Types of visual perseveration; 'palinopsia' and 'illusory visual spread'. *Brain* 74, 267–299

Critchley, M. (1953/1966). *The parietal lobes.* Hafner, New York

Critchley, M. (1964). The problem of visual agnosia. *J. Neurol. Sci.* 1, 274–290

Critchley, M. (1965). Acquired anomalies of colour perception of central origin. *Brain* 88, 711–724

Critchley, M. (1967). Aphasiological nomenclature and definitions. *Cortex* 3, 3–25

Critchley, M. (1979). *The divine banquet of the brain and other essays.* Raven Press, New York

Critchley, M. (1986). *The citadel of the senses and other essays.* Raven Press, New York

Crockett, D., Bilsker, D., Hurwitz, T., Kozak, J. (1986). Clinical utility of three measures of frontal lobe dysfunction in neuropsychiatric samples. *Int. J. Neurosci.* 32, 895–899

Croog, S.H., Levine, S., Testa, M.A., Brown, B., Bulpitt, C.J., Jenkins, C.D., Klerman, G.L., Williams, G.H. (1986). The effects of antihypertensive therapy on the quality of life. *N. Engl. J. Med.* 314, 1657–1664

Crook, J.M., Lange-Malecki, B., Lee, B.B., Valberg, A. (1988). Visual resolution of macaque retinal ganglion cells. J. Physiol. 396, 205–224

Crook, J.M., Lee, B.B., Tigwell, D.A., Valberg, A. (1987). Thresholds to chromatic spots of cells in the macaque geniculate nucleus as compared to detection sensitivity in man. *J. Physiol.* 392, 193–211

Crowder, R.G. (1972). Visual and auditory memory. In Cavanagh, J.F., Mattingly, I.G. (eds.), *Language by ear and eye. The relationship between speech and reading*, MIT Press, Cambridge, 251–275

Cumming, W.J. (1970). Anatomical findings in a case of alexia without agraphia. *J. Anatomy* 106, 170

Cumming, W.J.K., Hurwitz, L.J., Perl, N.T. (1970). A study of a patient who had alexia without agraphia. *J. Neurol. Neurosurg. Psychiat.* 33, 34–39

Cummings, J.L., Miller, B.L. (1987). Visual hallucinations. Clinical occurrence and use in differential diagnosis. *West. J. Med.* 146, 46–51

Cummings, J.L., Syndulko, K., Goldberg, Z., Treiman, D.M. (1982). Palinopsia reconsidered. *Neurology* 32, 444–447

Curio, G., Grüsser, O.-J. (1985). Visual-vestibular interaction studied with stroboscopically illuminated visual patterns. *Exp. Brain Res.* 58, 294–304

Currie, S., Heathfield, K.W.G., Henson, R.A., Scott, D.F. (1971). Clinical course and prognosis of temporal lobe epilepsy. A survey of 666 patients. *Brain* 94, 173–190

Cusanus, N. (1970). *Compendium.* Tranl. by R. Decker, K. Bormann. Meiner, Hamburg

Cusanus, N. (1971). *De conjecturis. Mutmassungen.* Transl. J. Koch and W. Happ. Meiner, Hamburg

Cusanus, N. (1977). *Der Laie über die Weisheit (Idiota de sapientia).* F. Meiner, Hamburg

Cusanus, N. (1977). *Schrift vom Geist (Liber de mente).* Transl. J. Ritter. In Cassirer, E. (ed.), *Individuum und Kosmos in der Philosophie der Renaissance.* Wiss. Buchges., Darmstadt, 202–300

Cusanus, N. (1982). *Compendium (kurze Darstellung der philosophisch-theologischen Lehre).* Lateinisch-Deutsch. F. Meiner, Hamburg, 110 p.

Cushing, H. (1922). Distortions of the visual fields in cases of brain tumour. The field defects produced by temporal lobe lesions. *Brain* 44, 341–396

Cusick, C.G., Kaas, J.H. (1988). Cortical connections of area 18 and dorsolateral visual cortex in squirrel monkeys. *Vis. Neurosci.* 1, 211–237

Cutting, J. (1981). Judgement of emotional expression in schizophrenics. *Brit. J. Psychiatry* 139, 1–6

Cynader, M.S., Gardner, J.C., Douglas, R.M. (1978). Neural mechanisms underlying stereoscopic depth perception in cat visual cortex. In Cool, S., Smith, E.L. (eds.), *Frontiers in visual science.* Springer, New York

Czermak, I. (1858). Ueber das Accommodationsphosphen. *Graefes Arch. Ophthalmol.* 7, 147–154

Czycholl, D.R. (1985). Die phantastischen Gesichtserscheinungen. Ein Überblick über die Literatur zu dem von Johannes Müller beschriebenen Phänomen und Experimente mit rhythmischer photischer Stimulierung. Lang, Frankfurt a.M.

D'Heilly, Chantemesse (1883). *Progrès médical*, cited in Charcot J.M. (1887)

d'Uzèz, S. (1853). *Essai sur les phosphènes ou anneaux lumineux de la retine.* Masson, Paris

Daffner, K.R., Ahern, G.L., Weintraub, S., Mesulam M.M. (1990). Dissociated neglect behavior following sequential strokes in the right hemisphere. *Ann. Neurol.* 28, 97–101

Dagge, M., Hartje, W. (1985). Influence of contextual complexity on the processing of cartoons by patients with unilateral lesions. *Cortex* 21, 607–616

Dalessio, D.J. (1980). *Wolff's headache and other head pain.* 4th ed., Oxford Univ. Press, New York

Dallenbach, K.M. (1923). Position vs. intensity as a determinant of clearness. *Am. J. Psychol.* 34, 282–286

Dalton, J. (1798). Extraordinary facts relating to the vision of colours: with observations. *Memoirs of the Literary and Philosophical Society of Manchester.* Vol. I, p. 28, Repr. in *Edinbourough Journal of Sciences* 5, 188 (1834)

Damas Mora, J.M.R., Jenner, F.A., Eacott, S.E. (1980). On heautoscopy or the phenomenon of the double: case presentations and review of the literature. *Brit. J. Med. Psychol.* 53, 75–83

Damasio, A.R. (1977). Varieties and significance of the alexias. *Arch. Neurol.* 34, 325–326

Damasio, A.R. (1980). Optic ataxia and apraxia of gaze. *Neurology* 30, 109

Damasio, A.R. (1981). Central achromatopsia. Letter to the editor. *Neurology* 31, 920–921

Damasio, A.R. (1985). Disorders of complex visual processing: Agnosia, achromatopsia, Balint's syndrome, and related difficulties of orientation and construction. In Mesulam, M.M. (ed.), *Principles of behavioral neurology.* F.A. Davis Company, Philadelphia, PA, 259–288

Damasio, A.R. (1990). Category-related recognition defects as a clue to the neural substrates of knowledge. *TINS* 13, 95–98

Damasio, A.R., Benton, A.L. (1979). Impairment of hand movements under visual guidance. *Neurology* 29, 170–178

Damasio, A.R., Chui, H.C., Corbett, J., Kassel, N. (1980). Posterior callosal section in a non-epileptic patient. *J. Neurol. Neurosurg. Psychiat.* 43, 351–356

Damasio, A.R., Damasio, H. (1979). Neglect following damage to frontal lobe or basal ganglia. *Neuropsychologia*

Damasio, A.R., Damasio, H. (1983). Localization of lesions in achromatopsia and prosopagnosia. In Kertesz, A. (ed.), *Localization in neuropsychology.* Academic Press, New York, p. 417–428

Damasio, A.R., Damasio, H. (1983). The anatomic basis of pure alexia and color 'agnosia'. *Neurology* 33, 1573–1583

Damasio, A.R., Damasio, H., Chang, H.C. (1980). Neglect following damage to frontal lobe or basal ganglia. *Neuropsychologia* 18, 123–132

Damasio, A.R., Damasio, H., Tranel, D. (1986). Prosopagnosia: anatomic and physiologic aspects. In H.D. Ellis, M.A. Jeeves, F. Newcombe, A. Young (eds.), *Aspects of face processing*, Martinus Nijhoff, Dordrecht, 268–272

Damasio, A.R., Damasio, H., Van Hoesen, G.W. (1982). Prosopagnosia: anatomic basis and behavioral mechanisms. *Neurology* 32, 331–341

Damasio, A.R., Damasio, J. (1986). The anatomical substrate of prosopagnosia. In Bruyer, R. (ed.) *The neuropsychology of face perception and facial expression*. L. Erlbaum Associates, Hilldale, 31–38

Damasio, A.R., Eslinger, P.J., Damasio, H., Von Hoesen, G.W., Cornell, S. (1985). Multimodal amnesic syndrome following bilateral temporal and basal forebrain damage. *Arch. Neurol.* 42, 252–259

Damasio, A.R., McKee, J., Damasio, H. (1979). Determinants of performance in color anomia. *Brain and Language* 7, 74–85

Damasio, A.R., Yamada, T., Damasio, H., Corbett, J., McKee, J. (1980). Central achromatopsia: behavioral, anatomic and physiologic aspects. *Neurology* 30, 1064–1071

Damasio, H., Damasio, A.R. (1989). *Lesion analysis in neuropsychology*. New York, Oxford, Oxford University Press, 227 p.

Damerow, P., Englund, R.K., Nissen, H.J. (1988). Die Entstehung der Schrift. *Spektrum der Wissenschaft*, February, 74–85

Damerow, P., Englund, R.K., Nissen, H.J. (1988). Die ersten Zahldarstellungen und die Entwicklungen des Zahlbegriffs. *Spektrum der Wissenschaft*, March, 46–55

Danek, A., Bauer, M., Fries, W. (1990). Tracing of neuronal connections in the human brain by magnetic resonance imaging in vivo. *Europ. J. Neuroscience* 2, 112–115

Daniel, P.M., Whitteridge, D. (1961). The representation of the visual field on the cerebral cortex in monkeys. *J. Physiol. (Lond.)* 159, 203–221

Daniels, B. (1932). Über die homonyme Hemianopsie bei Migräne. *Z. f. Augenheilk.* 77, 67–

Dannemiller, J.L. (1989). Computational approaches to color constancy: adaptive and ontogenetic considerations. *Psychol. Review* 96, 255–266

Dannenberg, F.K. (1985). Prosopagnosia: a case study. *Diss. Abstr. Internat.* 45, 2670

Dartnall, H.J.A., Bowmaker, J.K., Mollon, J.D. (1983). Microspectrophotometry of human photoreceptors. In Mollon, J.D., Sharpe, L.T. (eds.), *Colour vision: Physiology and Psychophysics*. Academic Press, New York, 69–80

Darwin, C. (1872). *The expression of emotions in man and animals*. Murray, London, Repr. The University of Chicago Press 1965, Chicago

Darwin, E. (1894/1796). *Zoonomia. Vol. 1, 2*. J. Johnson, London 1794 and 1796. Repr. AMS Press, New York 1974

Daugman, J.G. (1984). Spatial vision channels in the Fourier plane. *Vision Res.* 24, 891–910

Daugman, J.G. (1988a). Complete discrete 2-D Gabor transforms by neural networks for image analysis and compression. *IEEE Transactions on Acoustics, Speech and Signal Processing* 36 (7), 1169–1179

David, M., Hecaen, H., Angelergues, R., Magis, C. (1955). Les tumeurs occipitales. *Neuro-Chirurgie* 1, 85–109/et 177–191

Davidenkov, S.N. (1956a). *Visual agnosias — lecture 8*. State Publishing House of Medical Literature 2

Davidenkov, S.N. (1956b). *Visual agnosias — lecture 9*. State Publishing House of Medical Literature 2

Davidoff, J. (1982). Studies with non-verbal stimuli. In Beaumont, J.G. (ed.), *Divided visual field studies of cerebral organization*. Academic Press, London, New York, p. 29–55

Davidoff, J., Fodor, G. (1989). An annotated translation of Lewandowsky (1908). *Cogn. Neuropsychol.* 6, 165–177

Davidoff, J., Landis, T. (1990). Recognition of unfamiliar faces in prosopagnosia. *Neuropsychologia* 28, 1143–1161

Davidoff, J., Wilson, B. (1985). A case of visual agnosia showing a disorder of pre-semantic visual classification. *Cortex* 21, 121–134

Davidoff, J.B. (1975a). Hemispheric differences in the perception of lightness. *Neuropsychologia* 13, 121–124

Davidoff, J.B. (1976). Hemispheric sensitivity differences in the perception of colour. *Q. J. exp. Psychol.* 28, 387–394

Davidoff, J.B. (1986). The mental representation of faces: spatial and temporal factors. *Percept. Psychophys.* 40, 391–400

Davidoff, J.B.(1986). The specificity of face perception: evidence from psychological investigations. In Bruyer, R. (ed.) *The Neuropsychology of Face Perception and Facial Expression*. Erlbaum, Hillsdale, N.Y., London, 147–166

Davidoff, J.B., Done, D.J. (1984). A longitudinal study of the development of visual field advantage for letter matching. *Neuropsychol.* Vol. 22, p. 311–318

Davidoff, J.B., Donnelly, N. (1990). Object superiority: a comparison of complete and part probes. *Acta Psychologia* 73, 225–243

Davidoff, J.B., Landis, T. (1990). Recognition of unfamiliar faces in prosopagnosia. *Neuropsychologie* 28, 1143–1161

Davidoff, J.B., Ostergaard, A.L. (1984). Colour anomia resulting from weakened short-term colour memory. A case study. *Brain* 107, 415–431

Davidoff, J.B., Troscianko, T., Landis, T., Brugger, P. (1991). Survival of chromatic boundaries in achromatopsia (in preparation).

Davies, G., Ellis, H., Shepherd, J. (1981). *Perceiving and remembering faces*. Academic Press, London

Davis, J.W. (1960). The Molyneux problem. *J. Hist. of Ideas* 21, 392–408

Davis, R., Schmit, V. (1971). Timing the transfer of information between hemispheres in man. *Acta Psychologica* 35, 335–346

Davis, R., Schmit, V. (1973). Visual and verbal coding in the interhemispheric transfer of information. *Acta Psychologica* 37, 229–240

Daw, N.W. (1984). The psychology and physiology of colour vision. *Trends in Neuroscience* 7, 330–335

Day, B.L., Mertens de Noordhout, A., Marsten, C.D., Nakashima, K., Rothwell, J.C., Thompson, P.D. (1987). Temporary interruption of brain processing by an electrical or magnetic cortical shock in man. *J. Physiol. (Lond.)* 390, 197 p.

Day, J. (1979). Visual half-field word recognition as a function of syntactic class and imageability. *Neuropsychologia* 17, 515–519

Day, R.H., Avery, G.C. (1970). Absence of horizontal-vertical illusion in haptic space. *J. Exp. Psychol.* 83, 172–173

Day, R.H., Wade, N.J. (1969). Mechanisms involved in visual orientation constancy. *Psychol. Bull.* 71, 33–42

Day, R.H., Wade, N.J. (1979). Absence of color selectivity in the visual movement aftereffect. *Perception and Psychophysics* Vol. 25 (2), 111–114

De Ajuriaguerra, J., Hecaen, H. (1949). *Le cortex cerebral*. Masson & Cie, Paris, 280–284

De Ajuriaguerra, J., Hecaen, H. (1951). Restauration après lobectomie. *J. Psychol.* 44, 510–546

De Bleser, R., Bayer, J., Luzzatti, C. (1987). Die kognitive Neuropsychologie der Schriftsprache — Ein Überblick mit zwei deutschen Fallbeschreibungen. In Bayer, J. (ed.), *Grammatik und Kognition. Linguistische Berichte Sonderheft* 1, 118–162

De Haan, E.H., Young, A., Newcombe, F. (1987). Faces interfere with name classification in a prosopagnosic patient. *Cortex* 23, 309–316

De Haan, E.H.F., Young, A., Newcombe, F. (1987). Face recognition without awareness. *Cogn. Neuropsych.* 4, 385–415

De Kosky, S.T., Heilman, K.M., Bowers, D., Valenstein, E. (1980). Recognition and discrimination of emotional faces and pictures. *Brain and Language* 9, 206–214

De Massary, J. (1932). L'alexie. *L'Encéphale* 27, 53–78

De Massary, J. (1933). L'alexie. *L'Encéphale* 28, 134–164

De Monasterio, F.M., Gouras, P. (1975). Functional properties of ganglion cells of the rhesus monkey retina. *J. Physiol. (Lond.)* 251, 167–196

De Monasterio, F.M., Gouras, P., Tolhurst, D.J. (1975). Trichromatic colour opponency in ganglion cells of the rhesus monkey retina. *J. Physiol. (Lond.)* 251, 197–216

De Monasterio, F.M., Schein, S.J. (1982). Spectral bandwidths of color oponent cells of geniculocortical pathway of macaque monkeys. *J. Neurophysiol.* 47, 214–224

De Morsier, G. (1938). Les hallucinations visuelles dans les lesions du diencephale (section 2). *Rev. Neuro-Oto-Ophthalmol.* 16, 244–352

De Renzi, E. (1982). *Disorders of space exploration and cognition.* Wiley, New York, Chichester

De Renzi, E. (1982). Memory disorders following focal neocortical damage. *Philos. Trans. R. Soc. Lond. B. Biol. Sci.* 298, 73–83

De Renzi, E. (1985). Disorders of spatial orientation. In Vinken, P.J., Bruyn, G.W., Klawans, H.L. (eds.), *Handbook of Clinical Neurology* 45: Clinical Neuropsychology. Elsevier Science Publishers, Amsterdam, 405–422

De Renzi, E. (1986a). Prosopagnosia in two patients with CT scan evidence of damage confined to the right hemisphere. *Neuropsychologia* 24, 385–389

De Renzi, E. (1986b). Current issues on prosopagnosia. In H.D. Ellis, M.A. Jeeves, F.Newcombe, A. Young (eds.), *Aspects of face processing*, Martinus Nijhoff, Dordrecht

De Renzi, E. (1986c). Slowly progressive visual agnosia or apraxia without dementia. *Cortex* 22, 171–180

De Renzi, E. (1989). Prosopagnosia: A multi-stage, specific disorder? In Young, A.W., Ellis, H.D. (eds.), *Handbook of Research on Face Processing*. Elsevier, North Holland, 27–35

De Renzi, E. Faglioni, P. Scotti, G., Spinnler, H. (1972a). Impairment in associating colour to form, concomitant with aphasia. *Brain* 95, 293–304

De Renzi, E., Bonacini, M.G., Faglioni, P. (1989). Right posterior brain-damaged patients are poor at assessing the age of a face. *Neuropsychologia* 27, 839–848

De Renzi, E., Colombo, A., Faglioni, P., Gibertoni, M. (1982). Conjugate gaze paralysis in stroke patients with unilateral damage. *Arch. Neurol.* (Chicago) 39, 482–486

De Renzi, E., Faglioni, D., Grossi, D., Nichelli, P. (1991). Apperceptive and associative forms of prosopagnosia. *Cortex* 27, 213–221

De Renzi, E., Faglioni, D., Grossi, D., Nichelli, P. (1991). Apperceptive and associative forms of prosopagnosia. *Cortex* 27, 213–221

De Renzi, E., Faglioni, P. (1962). Il disorientamento spaziale da lesione cerebrale. *Sistema Nerv.* 14, 409–436

De Renzi, E., Faglioni, P., Previdi, P. (1977). Spatial memory and hemispheric locus of lesion. *Cortex* 13, 424–433

De Renzi, E., Faglioni, P., Scotti, G. (1970). Hemispheric contribution to the exploration of space through the visual and tactile modality. *Cortex* 6, 191–203

De Renzi, E., Faglioni, P., Scotti, G., Spinnler, H. (1972). Impairment in associating colour to form, concomitant with aphasia. *Brain* 95, 293–304

De Renzi, E., Faglioni, P., Scotti, G., Spinnler, H. (1972b). Impairment of color sorting behavior after hemispheric damage: an experimental study with the Holmgreen skein test. *Cortex* 8, 147-

De Renzi, E., Faglioni, P., Spinnler, H. (1968). The performance of patients with unilateral brain damage on face recognition tasks. *Cortex* 4, 17–34

De Renzi, E., Faglioni, P., Villa, P. (1977). Topographical amnesia. *J. Neurol. Neurosurg. Psychiat.* 40, 498–505

De Renzi, E., Gentilini, M., Barbieri, C. (1989). Auditory neglect. *J. Neurol. Neurosurg. Psychiat.* 52, 613–617

De Renzi, E., Liotti, M., Nichelli, P. (1987). Semantic amnesia with preservation of autobiographic memory: A case report. *Cortex* 23, 575–597

De Renzi, E., Scotti, G., Spinnler, H. (1969). Perceptual and associative disorders of visual recognition: Relationship to the side of the cerebral lesion. *Neurology* 19, 634–642

De Renzi, E., Spinnler, H. (1966). Facial recognition in brain-damaged patients. *Neurology* 16, 143–152

De Renzi, E., Spinnler, H. (1966). Visual recognition in patients with unilateral cerebral disease. *J. Nervous Ment. Disease* 142, 513–525

De Renzi, E., Spinnler, H. (1967). Impaired performance on color tasks in patients with hemisperic damage. *Cortex* 3, 194–216

De Renzi, E., Zambolin, A. Crisi, G. (1987). The pattern of neuropsychological impairment associated with left posterior cerebral artery infarcts. *Brain* 110, 1099–1116

De Valois, K.K., De Valois, R.L., Yund, E.W. (1979). Responses of striate cortex cells to grating and checkerboard patterns. *J. Physiol. (Lond.)* 291, 483–505

De Valois, R.L. (1965). Analysis and coding of color vision in the primate visual system. In Frisch L. (ed.), *Symposia on Quantitative Biology, Vol. 30. Sensory receptors, Cold Spring Harbor*, 567–579

De Valois, R.L. (1973). Central mechanisms of colour vision. In Jung, R. (ed.), *Handbook of Sensory Physiology VII*, Springer, Berlin, Heidelberg, New York (oder in: Central processing of visual information A. Integrative Functions and comparative data, p. 209–253, Springer, Berlin?)

De Valois, R.L., Albrecht, D.G., Thorell, L.G. (1982). Spatial frequency selectivity of cells in macaque visual cortex. *Vision Res.* 22, 545–559

De Valois, R.L., Morgan, H., Snodderly, D.M. (1974). Psychophysical studies of monkey vision: 3. Spatial luminance contrast sensitivity tests of macaque and human observers. *Vision Res.* 14, 75–81

De Valois, R.L., Morgan, H.C., Polson, M.C., Mead, W.R., Hull, E.M. (1974). Psychophysical studies of monkey vision. I. Macaque luminosity and color vision tests. *Vision Res.* 14, 53–67

De Valois, R.L., Thorell, L.G., Albrecht, D.G. (1985). Periodicity of striate-cortex-cell receptive fields. *J. Opt. Soc. Am.* 2, 1115–1123

De Valois, R.L., Yund, E.W., Hepler, N. (1982) The orientation and direction selectivity of cells in macaque visual cortex. *Vision Res.* 22, 531–544

De Weert, C.M.M. (1979). Colour contours and stereopsis. *Vision Res.* 19, 555–564

De Wolfe, A.S., Barrel, R.P., Becker, B.C., Spanner, F.E. (1971). Intellectual deficit in chronic schizophrenia and brain damage. *J. Consult. Clin. Psychol.* 36, 197–204

Debruille, B., Breton, F., Robaey, P., Signoret, J.L., Renault, B. (1989). Cerebral evoked potentials and conscious and unconscious recognition of faces: application to the study of prosopagnosia. *Neurophysiol.Clin.* 19, 393–405

Dee, H.L. (1970). Visuo-constructive and visuo-perceptive deficit in patients with unilateral cerebral lesions. *Neuropsychologia* 8, 305–314

Dee, H.L., Fontenot, D.J. (1973). Cerebral dominance and lateral differences in perception and memory. *Neuropsychologia* 11, 167–173

Dee, H.L., Hannay, H.J. (1973). Asymmetry in perception: Attention versus other determinants. *Acta Psychol.* 37, 241–247

Dejerine, J. (1891). Sur un cas de cécité verbale avec agraphie, suivi d'autopsie. *Mem. Soc. Biol.* 3, 197–201

Dejerine, J. (1892). Contribution a l'étude anatomo-pathologique et clinique des differentes varietés de cécité verbale. *Mem. Soc. Biol.* 4, 61–90

Dejerine, J. (1892). Des differentes varietes de cecite verbale. *Mem. Soc. Biol.* 1892, 1–30

Dejerine, J. (1912). Contribution a l'etude de l'aphasie chez les gauchers. *Rev. Neurol.* 24, 214–226

Dejerine, J. (1914). *Semiologie des affections du systeme nerveux.* Masson, Paris

Dejerine, J., Vialet, N. (1893). Contribution a l'etude de la localisation anatomique de la cécité verbal pure. *C. R. Soc. Biol. (Paris)* 45, 790–795

Delaney, R.C., Rosen, A.J., Mattson, R.H., Novelly, R.A. (1980). Memory function in focal epilepsy: a comparison of non-surgical, unilateral temporal lobe and frontal lobe samples. *Cortex* 16, 103–117

Deleval, J., De Mol, J., Noterman, J. (1983). La perte des images souvenirs. *Acta Neurol. Belg.* 83, 61–79

Delson, E. (ed.) (1965) *Ancestors: the hard evidence*. Liss, New York, 366 p.

Demassary, J. (1932). L'alexie. *Encephale* 27, 134–164

Dembler, J. (1979). Visuelle Entscheidungszeiten und Ratewahrscheinlichkeiten von Wörtern in Abhängigkeit von der Schreibweise (traditionelle Grosschreibung — Kleinschreibung). Inaugural-Dissertation, Physiologisches Institut, Freie Universität Berlin

Denckla, M.B. (1972). Color-naming defects in dyslexic boys. *Cortex* 8, 164–176

Denckla, M.B. (1972). Performance on color tasks in kindergarten children. *Cortex* 8, 177–190

Denckla, M.B., Bowen, F.P. (1973). Dyslexia after left occipito-temporal lobectomy: A case report. *Cortex* 9, 321–328

Denenberg, V.H. (1981). Hemispheric laterality in animals and the effects of early experience. *Behavioral and Brain Sciences* 4, 1–49

Denes, G., Semenza, C., Stoppa, E., Lis, A. (1982). Unilateral spatial neglect and recovery from hemiplegia. *Brain* 105, 543–552

Dennis, M. (1976). Dissociated naming and locating of body parts after left anterior temporal lobe resection: An experimental case study. *Brain and Language* 3, 147–163

Denny-Brown, D. (1963). The physiological basis of perception and speech. In Halpern, L. (ed.), *Problems of dynamic neurology*. Hebrew Univ., Med. Sch. Publ., Jerusalem, p. 30–62

Denny-Brown, D., Banker, B. (1954). Armorphosynthesis from left parietal lesion. *Arch. Neurol. Psychiat.* 71, 302–313

Denny-Brown, D., Chambers, R.A. (1955). Visuo-motor function in the cerebral cortex. *J. Nerv. Ment. Dis.* 121, 288–289

Denny-Brown, D., Chambers, R.A. (1958). The parietal lobe and behavior. *Res. Publ. Assoc. Res. Nerv. Ment. Dis.* 36, 35–117

Denny-Brown, D., Meyer, J.S., Horenstein, S. (1952). The significance of perceptual rivalry resulting from parietal lesions. *Brain* 75, 434–471

Derrington, A.M., Lennie, P. (1982). The influence of temporal frequency and adaptation level on receptive field organization of retinal ganglion cells in cat. *J. Physiol.* 333, 343–366

Derrington, A.M., Lennie, P. (1984). Spatial and temporal contrast sensitivities of neurones in lateral geniculate nucleus of macaque. *J. Physiol.* 357, 219–240

Derwort, A. (1953). Ueber vestibulär induzierte Dysmorphopsien. *Dtsch. Z. Nervenk.* 170, 613

Descartes, R. (1664). *L'homme de René Descartes et un traitté de la formation du foetus*. De la Forge, L. (ed.) Paris: Girard. German transl. (1969) in Rothschuh, K.E. (ed.), *René Descartes 'Über den Menschen' und Beschreibung des menschlichen Körpers*. Schneider, Heidelberg

Descartes, R. (1897–1913). *Dioptrique*. In Adam, C., Tannery P. (eds.) *Oeuvres de Descartes*, Vol. VI, Paris

Desimone, R., Albright, T.D., Gross, C.G., Bruce, C. (1984). Stimulus-selective responses of inferior temporal neurons in the macaque. *J. Neurosci.* 4, 2051–2062

Desimone, R., Fleming, J., Gross, C.G. (1980). Prestriate afferents to inferior temporal cortex: an HRP study. *Brain Res.* 184, 41–55

Desimone, R., Gross, C.G. (1979). Visual areas in the temporal cortex of the macaque. *Brain Res.* 178, 363–380

Desimone, R., Schein, S.J. (1987). Visual properties of neurons in area V4 of the macaque: sensitivity to stimulus from. *J. Neurophysiol.* 57, 835–868

Desimone, R., Schein, S.J., Moran, J., Ungerleider, L.G. (1985). Contour, colour and shape analysis beyond the striate cortex. *Vision Res.* 25, 441–452

Desimone, R., Ungerleider, L.G. (1986). Multiple visual areas in the caudal superior temporal sulcus of the macaque. *J. Comp. Neurol.* 248, 164–189

Desimone, R., Ungerleider, L.G. (1989). Neural mechanisms of visual processing in monkeys. In Boller, F., Grafman, J. (eds.),

Handbook of Neuropsychology. Vol. 2. Elsevier, Amsterdam, New York, Oxford, 267–299

Deuel, R.K., Collins, R.C., Dunlop, N. Caston, T.V. (1979). Recovery from unilateral neglect: Behavioral and functional anatomic correlations in monkeys. *Society of Neuroscience (abstr.)* 5, 624

Deutsch, G. Papanicolaou, A.C., Eisenberg, H.M., Loring, D.W., Levin, H.S. (1986). CBF gradient changes elicited by visual memory tasks. *Neuropsychologia* 24, 283–287

Devinsky, O., Feldman, E., Burrowes, K., Bromfield, E. (1989). Autoscopic phenomena with seizures. *Arch. Neurol.* 46, 1080–1088

Dewdney, D. (1973). A specific distortion of the human facial percept in childhood schizophrenia. *Psychiat. Quart.* 47, 82–94

Dewhurst, K., Pearson, J. (1955). Visual hallucinations of the self in organic disease. *J. Neurol. Neurosurg. Psychiat.* 18, 53–57

DeYoe, E.A., van Essen, D. (1985). Segregation of efferent connections and receptive field properties in visual area V2 of the macaque. *Nature* 317, 58–61

DeYoe, E.A., Van Essen, D.C. (1988). Concurrent processing streams in monkey visual cortex. *Trends Neurosci.* 11, 219–226

Diamond, R., Carey, S. (1977). Developmental changes in the representation of faces. *J. Exp. Child Psychol.* 23, 1–22

Diamond, R., Carey, S. (1986). Why faces are and are not special: An effect of expertise. *J. Exp. Psychol: General* 115, 107–117

Diamond, R., Carey, S., Back, K.J. (1983). Genetic influences on the development of spatial skills during early adolescence. *Cognition* 13, 167–185

Dichgans, J., Brandt, T. (1978). Visual-vestibular interaction: effects on self motion perception and postural control. In Held, R., Leibowitz, H., Teuber, H.L. (eds.), *Handbook of sensory physiology*. 755–804

Dichgans, J., Körner, F., Voigt, K. (1969). Vergleichende Skalierung des afferenten und efferenten Bewegungssehens beim Menschen: Lineare Funktionen mit verschiedener Anstiegssteilheit. *Psychol. Forsch.* 32, 277–295

Dick, M., Ullman, S., Sagi, D. (1987). Parallel and serial processes in motion detection. *Science* 237, 400–402

Dickerson, D.J., Goldfield, E.C. (1981). Development of logical search and visual scanning in children. *Genet. Psychol. Monogr.* 104, 325–337

Dide, M., Botcazo, H. (1902). Amnésie continue, cécité verbale pure, perte du sens topographique, ramollissement double du lobe lingual. *Rev. Neurol.* 10, 676–680

Die, G. van, Collewijn, H. (1982). Optokinetic nystagmus in man: role of central and peripheral retina and occurrence of asymmetries. *Human Neurobiol.* 2, 111–119

Diels, H., Kranz, W. (1951). *Die Fragmente der Vorsokratiker*, Vol. 1, Weidmann, Basel, 504 p.

Dietrich, H. (1962). Capgras' syndrome and Déjö vue. *Fortschr. Neurol. Psychiat.* 30, 617–625

Diller, L., Weinberg, J. (1977). Hemi-inattention in rehabilitation: the evolution of a rational remediation program. In Weinstein, E.A., Friedland, R.P. (eds.), *Advances in Neurology, Vol. 18*. Raven Press, New York, 63–82

DiLollo, V. (1980). Temporal integration in visual memory. *J. Exp. Psychol (Gen.)* 109, 75–97

DiLollo, V., Arnett, J.L., Kruk, R.V. (1982). Age-related changes in rate of visual information processing. *J. Exp. Psychol.* 8, 225–237

Dimond, S., Beaumont, G. (1972). Processing in perceptual integration between and within the cerebral hemispheres. *Br. J. Psychol.* 63, 509–514

Dimond, S.J., Farrington, L., Johnson, P. (1976). Differing emotional response from right and left hemispheres. *Nature* 261, 690–692

Diogenes Laertius (1967). *Leben und Meinungen berühmter Philosophen*. Transl. by O. Appelt, Meiner, Hamburg

Dirks, J., Gibson, E. (1977). Infants' perception of similarity between live people and their photographs. *Child Development* 48, 124–130

Ditchburn, R.W. (1973). *Eye-movements and visual perception.* Clarendon, Oxford

Ditchburn, R.W., Ginsborg, B.L. (1952). Vision with a stabilized retinal image. *Nature* 170, 36–37

Divac, I., Lavail, J.H., Rakic, P., Winston, K.R. (1977). Heterogeneous afferents to the inferior parietal lobule of the rhesus monkey revealed by the retrograde transport method. *Brain Res.* 123, 197–207

Dixon, N.F. (1971). *Subliminal perception: The nature of a controversy.* McGraw-Hill, London

Dixon, N.F. (1981). *Preconscious processing.* Wiley, London

Dobelle, W.H,, Turkel, J., Henderson, D.C., Evans, J.R. (1978). Mapping the projection of the visual field onto visual cortex in man by direct electrical stimulation. *Trans. Am. Soc. Artif. Intern. Organs* 24, 15–17

Dobelle, W.H., Mladejovsky, M.G. (1974). Phosphenes produced by electrical stimulation of human occipital cortex, and their application to the development of a prosthesis for the blind. *J. Physiol.* 243, 553–576

Dobelle, W.H., Mladejovsky, M.G., Evans, J.R., Roberts, T.S., Girvin, J.P. (1976). 'Braille' reading by a blind volunteer by visual cortical stimulation. *Nature* 259, 111–112

Dobelle, W.H., Mladejovsky, M.G., Garvin, J.P. (1974). Artificial vision for the blind: electrical stimulation of visual cortex offers hope for functional prosthesis. *Science* 183, 440–444

Dobelle, W.H., Quest, D.O., Antunes, J.L., Roberts, T.S., Girvin, J.P. (1979). Artificial vision for the blind by electrical stimulation of the visual cortex. *Neurosurgery* 5, 521–527

Dobelle, W.H., Turkel, J., Henderson, D.C., Evans, J.R. (1979). Mapping the representation of visual field by electrical stimulation of human visual cortex. *Am. J. Ophth.* 88, 727–735

Dobson, V., Mayer, D.L., Lee, C.P. (1979). Visual acuity screening of preterm infants. *Invest. Ophthalmol. Vis. Sci.* 19, 1498–1505

Dodd, B. (1979). Lip-reading in infants: Attention to speech presented in-and out-off synchrony. *Cognitive Psychology* 11, 478–484

Dodt, E. (1980). Elektrodiagnostik des visuellen Systems bei krankheitsbedingten und medikamentösen Sehstörungen. AMI-Berichte 2, 73–76

Dodwell, P.C. (1983). Spatial sense of the human infant. In Hein, A., Jeannerod, M. (eds.), *Spatially oriented behavior.* Springer, New York, Berlin, Heidelberg, Tokyo, 197–213

Dodwell, P.C. (1984). Local and global factors in figural synthesis. In Dodwell, P.C., Caelli, T. (eds.) *Figural synthesis,* Lawrence Erlbaum Associates, Hillsdale, 219–248

Dodwell, P.C., Caelli, T. (1984). *Figural synthesis,* Lawrence Erlbaum Associates, Hillsdale,

Doly, M., Isabelle, D.B., Vincent, P., Gaillard, G., Meyniel, G. (1980a). Mechanisms of the formation of X-ray induced phosphenes. I.Electrophysiological investigations. *Radiat. Res.* 82, 93–105

Doly, M., Isabelle, D.B., Vincent, P., Gaillard, G., Meyniel, G. (1980b). Mechanism of the formation of X-ray induced phosphenes. II. Photochemical investigations. *Radiat. Res.* 82, 430–440

Doly, M., Vincent, P., Fourthin, B. et al. (1979). Action des rayons X sur le retine isolée de rat et sur sa rhodopsine. *J. Fr. Biophys. Med. Nuc.* 3/2, 111–117

Domberg, H. (1972). Die Veränderungen der Grösse des receptiven Feldzentrums retinaler on-Zentrum-Neurone der katze bei verschiedener Lichtadaption. FU Berlin, Med. Diss. 1972

Donaldson, I.M. (1985). 'Psychometric' assessment during transient global amnesia. *Cortex* 21, 149–152

Donat, D.C. (1986). Semantic and visual memory after alcohol abuse. *J. Clin. Psychol.* 42, 537–539

Donders, F.C. (1867). Das binoculare Sehen und die Vorstellung von der dritten Dimension. *Grafes Arch. Ophthalmol.* 13, 1

Donders, F.C. (1868). Archiv für Anatomie und Physiologie. 657 ff.

Donders, F.C. (1880). Über Farbenblindheit. *Klin. Monatsbl. f. Augenheilk.* 17, 66

Donders, F.C. (1881). Über Farbensysteme. *Graefes Arch. Ophthalmol.* 27, (I), 155–223

Donini, F. (1939). Su di un caso di aprasia constructiva con grave disorientamento esospaziale e perdita della facolta del riconiscemento della fisionomia della persone. *Note Psichiatre* 68, 469–485

Donnelly, E.F. (1984). Neuropsychological impairment and associated intellectual functions in schizophrenic and other pychiatric patients. *Biol. Psychiat.* 19, 815–824

Doorn, A.J. van, Koenderink, J.J. (1982a).Spatial properties of the visual detectability of moving spatial white noise. *Expl. Brain Res.* 45, 189–195

Doorn, A.J. van, Koenderink, J.J. (1982b). Temporal properties of the visual detectability of moving spatial white noise. *Expl. Brain Res.* 45, 179–182

Doorn, A.J. van, Koenderink, J.J., van de Grind, W.A. (1985). Perception of movement and correlation in stroboscopically presented noise patterns. *Perception* 14, 209–224

Doorn, A.J. van, Koenderink, J.J., van de Grind,W.A. (1984). Limits in spatio-temporal correlation and the perception of visual movement. In Van Doorn et al. (eds.), *Limits in perception.* VNU Science press, 203–234

Dopson, W.G., Beckwith, B.E., Tucker, D.M., Bullard-Bates, P.C. (1984). Asymmetry of facial expression in spontaneous emotion. *Cortex* 20, 243–251

Doty, R.W. (1977). Tonic retinal influences in primates. *Ann. N.Y. Academy Sciences* 290, 139–151

Doty, R.W. (1983). Nongeniculate afferents to striate cortex in macaques. *J. Comp. Neurol.* 218, 159–173

Doty, R.W., Negrao, N. (1972). Forebrain commissures and vision. In Jung, R. (ed.), *Handbook of Sensory Physiology* Vol. 7/3B, Springer, Berlin, 543–582

Doty, R.W., Ringo, J.L., Lewine, J.D. (1988). Forebrain copmissures and visual memory: a new approach. *Behav. Brain Res.* 29, 267–280

Doty, R.W., Wilson, P.D., Bartlett, J.R., Pecci-Saavedra, J. (1973). Mesencephalic control of lateral geniculate nucleus in primates. I. Electrophysiology. *Exp. Brain Res.* 18, 189–203

Dougherty, F.E., Bartlett, E.S., Izard, C.E. (1974). Responses of schizophrenics to expressions of the fundamental emotions. *J. Clin. Psychol.* 30, 243–246

Douglas, R.J., Martin, K.A.C. (1991). Opening the grey box. *Trends Neurosci.* 14, 286–293

Dow, B.M. (1974). Functional classes of cells and their laminar distribution in monkey visual cortex. *J. Neurophysiol.* 37, 927–946

Dow, B.M. (1991). Colour vision. In Dillon, C. (ed.), *Vision and visual dysfunction.* This series Vol. 4, chapter..

Dow, B.M., Baizer, J.S., Robinson, D.L. (1976). Functional organization of area 18 in the rhesus monkey. *Exp. Brain Res. (Suppl)* 1, 412–414

Dow, B.M., Bauer, R. (1984). Retinotopy and orientation columns in the monkey: A new model. *Biol. Cybern.* 49, 189–200

Dow, B.M., Bauer, R., Snyder, A.Z., Vautin, R.G. (1986). Receptive fields and orientation shifts in the foveal striate cortex of the awake macaque monkey. In Edelman, Gall, Cowan, (eds), *Dynamic aspects of neocortical function.* Wiley & Sons, New York

Dow, B.M., Gouras, P. (1973). Color and spatial specificity of single units in rhesus monkey foveal striate cortex. *J. Neurophysiol.* 36, 79–100

Dow, B.M., Snyder, A.Z., Vautin, R.G., Bauer, R. (1981). Magnification factor and receptive field size in foveal striate cortex of the monkey. *Exp. Brain Res.* 44, 213–228

Dow, B.M., Vautin, R.G. (1987). Horizontal segregation of color information in the middle layers of foveal striate cortex. *J. Neurophysiol.* 57, 712–739

Dow, B.M., Yoshioha, T., Vautin, R.G. (1987). Selective suppression of responses of foveal V1, V2 and V4 cells in the macaque during a colour matching task. *Soc. Neurosci. Abstr.* 13, 624

Dowling, J.E. (1987). *The retina: an approachable part of the brain.* Harvard Univ. Press, Cambridge, MA.

Dowling, J.E., Boycott, B.B. (1966). Organization of the primate retina: electron microscopy. *Proc. R. Soc. Lond.* B166, 80–111

Drasdo, N. (1977). The neural representation of visual space. *Nature (Lond.)* 266, 554–556

Dricker, J., Butters, N., Berman, G., Samuels, I., Carey, S. (1978). The recognition and encoding of faces by alcoholic Korsakoff and right hemisphere patients. *Neuropsychologia* 16, 683–695

Dronkers, N.F., Knight, R.T. (1989). Right-sided neglect in a left-hander. *Neuropsychologia* 27, 729–735

Du Prel, C. (1886). *Der Doppelgänger. Sphinx, Monatsschrift der übersinnlichen Weltanschauung,* Vol. 1

Du Prel, C. (1888). *Die monistische Seelenlehre.* Leipzig

Duara, R., Phatak, P.G., Wadia, N.H. (1975). Prosopagnosia and associated disorders. *Neurology India* 23, 149–155

Dubner, R., Zeki, S.M. (1971). Response properties and receptive fields of cells in an anatomically defined region of the superior temporal sulcus in the monkey. *Brain Res.* 35, 528–532

Dubner, R., Zeki, S.M. (1971). Response properties and receptive fields of cells in an anatomically defined region of the superior temporal sulcus in the monkey. *Brain Res.* 35, 528–532

Dubois, M.F.W., Collewijn, H. (1979). Optokinetic reactions in man elicited by localized retinal motion stimuli. *Vision Res.* 19, 1105–1115

Dubois-Charlier, F. (1971). Approche neurolinguistique du probleme de l'alexie pure. *J. Psychol. norm. et pathologique* 1, 39–68

Dubois-Charlier, F. (1972). A propos de l'alexie pure. *Langages* 25, 76–94

Dubois-Charlier, R. (1976). Les analyses neuropsychologiques et neurolinguistiques de l'alexie: 1836–1969. *Langages* 44, 20–62

Dubois-Poulsen, A. (1952). *Le champs visuelle.* Masson, Paris

Ducarne, B., Barbeau, M. (1981). Examen clinique et modes de reeducation des trouble visuels d'orginine cerebral. *Rev. Neurol. (Paris)* 137, 693–707

Duchenne, G. (1862). *Mechanisme de la physiognomie humaine ou analyse electro-physiologique de l'expression des passions.* Paris

Duensing, F. (1952). Beitrag zur Frage der optischen Agnosie. *Arch. Psychiat. Nervenkr.* 188, 131–161

Duensing, F. (1953). Ueber die Wortalexie. *Arch. Psych. Zschr. Neurologie* 191, 163–178

Duensing, F. (1953). Über Alexie mit partiell erhaltenem simultanen Wortlesen. *Arch. Psychiat u. Zeitschr. Neurol.* 191, 179–190

Duensing, F. (1953). Zur Frage der Buchstabenalexie. *Arch. Psychiat. u. Zeitschr. Neurol.* 191, 147–162

Duensing, F. (1954). Zur Frage der optisch-räumlichen Agnosie. *Arch. Psychiat. Nervenkrh.* 192, 185–206

Duffy, R.J. (1981). Three studies of deficits in pantomimic expression and pantomimic recognition in aphasia. *J. Speech Hearing Res.* 24, 70–84

Dufour, H. (1889). Revue de la Suisse romande. Quoted after Wilbrand, H., Saenger, A. (1917). *Die homonymen Hemianopsien.*

Dumont, I., Griggio, A., Dupont, H., Jacquy, J. (1981). A propos d'un cas d'agnosie visuelle avec prosopagnosie et agnosie des coleurs. *Acta Psychiat. Belgica* 81, 25–45

Duncan, E.M., Whitney, P., Kunen, S. (1982). Integration of visual and verbal information in children's memories. *Child. Dev.* 53, 1215–1223

Duncan, J. (1984). Selective attention and the organization of visual information. *Journal of Experimental Psychology: General,* 113, 501–517

Duncan, J., Humphreys, G.W. (1989). Visual search and stimulus similarity. *Psychol. Rev.* 96, 433–458

Duncker, K. (1929). Über induzierte Bewegung. *Psychol. Forsch.* 12,

180–259

Dunn, Th. D. (1895). Double hemiplegia with double hemianopia and loss of geographic center. *Trans. Coll. Physicians Phila.* 3. Ser. 17, 45–55

Dürsteler, M.R., Wurtz, R.H. (1988). Pursuit and optokinetic deficits following chemical lesions of cortical areas MT and MST. *J. Neurophysiol.* 60, 940–965

Dürsteler, M.R., Wurtz, R.H., Newsome, W.T. (1987). Directional pursuit deficits following lesions of the foveal representation within the superior temporal sulcus of the macaque monkey. *J. Neurophysiol.* 57, 1262–1287

Dürsteler, M.R., Wurtz, R.H., Newsome, W.T., Mikimi, A. (1984). Deficits in pursuit eye movements following ibotenic acid lesions of the foveal representation of area MT of macaque monkey. *Soc. Neurosci. Abstr.* 10, 475

Dziurawiec, S., Ellis, H.D. (1986). Neonates' attention to face-like stimuli: A replication of the study by Goren, Sarty and Wu (1975). Quoted in Ellis, Young (1989)

Eagleson, H., Vaughn, G., Knudson, A. (1967). Hand signals for dysphasia. *Arch. phys. Med. Rehab.* 48, 410–414

Eals, M. (1987). Asymmetric processing in perception of apparent movement. *Neuropsychologia* 25, 429–434

Ebbecke, V. (1951). *Johannes Müller, der grosse rheinische Physiologe.* Schmorl & von Seefeld, Hannover

Eccles, J.C. (1986). Do mental events cause neural events analogously to the probability fields of quantum mechanics? *Proc. Roy. Soc. Lond.* 277, 411–428

Ecker, A. (1868). Zur Entwicklungsgeschichte der Furchen und Windungen der Grosshirn-Hemisphären im Foetus des Menschen. *Arch. Anthrop.* 3, 203–223

Ecker, A. (1869). *Die Hirnwindung des Menschen nach eigenen Untersuchungen.* Vieweg, Braunschweig

Eckhorn, R. (1991). Visual cortex: linking of local features into global figures? In Krüger, J. (ed.), *Neuronal cooperativity. Springer Series in Synergetics.* Springer, Berlin, 184

Eckhorn, R., Bauer, R., Jordan, W., Brosch, M., Kruse, W., Munk, M., Reitboeck, H.J. (1988). Coherent oscillations: a mechanism of feature linking in the visual cortex? Multiple electrode and correlation analysis in the cat. *Biol. Cybern.* 60, 121–130

Eckhorn, R., Bauer, R., Reitboeck, H.J. (1989). Discontinuities in visual cortex and possible functional implications: relating cortical structure and function with multi-electrode/correlation techniques. In Basar, E. (ed.), *Springer Series in Brain Dynamics. Vol. 2,* Springer, Berlin, 267–278

Eckhorn, R., Brosch, M., Salem, W., Bauer, R. (1990). Cooperativity between cat area 17 and 18 revealed with signal correlations and HRP. In Elsner, N., Roth, G. (eds.), *Brain, Pereption and Cognition.* Thieme, Stuttgart, New York

Eckhorn, R., Grüsser, O.-J., Kröller, J., Pellnitz, K., Pöpel, B. (1976). Efficiency of different neuronal codes: information transfer calculations for three different neuronal systems. *Biol. Cybern.* 22, 49–60

Eckhorn, R., Reitboeck, H.J. (1989). Stimulus-specific synchronizations in cat visual cortex and their possible role in visual pattern recognition. In Haken, H. (ed.), *Synergetics of Cognition.* Springer Series in Synergetics, 1–14

Eckhorn, R., Reitboeck, H.J., Arndt, M., Dicke, P. (1989). A neural network for feature linking via synchronous activity: results from cat visual cortex and from stimulations. In Cotterill, R.M.J. (ed), *Models of brain function.* Cambridge University Press

Eckhorn, R., Reitboeck, H.J., Arndt, M., Dicke, P. (1989). Feature linking via stimulus-evoked oscillations: experimental results from cat visual cortex and functional implications from a network model. Proc. Int. Joint Confer. Neural Networks, Washington. *IEEE Tab.*

Neural Network Comm., San Diego 1, 723.730

Eckhorn, R., Reitboeck, H.J., Arndt, M., Dicke, P. (1990). Feature linking via synchronization among distributed assemblies: simulations of results from cat visual cortex. *Neural Computation* 2, 293–307

Eckhorn, R., Schanze, T. (1991). Possible neural mechanisms of feature linking in the visual system: stimulus-locked and stimulus-induced synchronizations. In Babloyantz, A. (eds.), *Self-Organization, Emerging Properties and Learning.* Plenum Press

Eckmiller, R., Galley, N., Grüsser, O.-J. (1975). Neurobiologische und nachrichtentechnische Grundlagen des Lesens. In *Lesen und Leben,* Buchhändler Vereinigung GmbH, Frankfurt a.M., 36–81

Eckmiller, R., Grüsser, O.-J. (1972). Electronic stimulation of the velocity function of movement-detecting neurons. In Proceedings of a symposion on: *Cerebral Control of Eye Movements and Perception of Motion in Space* (Freiburg 1971). *Bibl. ophthal.* (Basel) 83, 486–489

Economo, C. von (1927). *Zellaufbau der Grosshirnrinde des Menschen. 10 Vorlesungen.* Springer, Berlin

Economo, C. von (1929). *The Cytoarchitectonics of the human cerebral cortex.* Oxford University Press, London

Economo, C. von (1929). Der Zellaufbau der Grosshirnrinde und die progressive Cerebration. *Erg. Physiol.* 29, 83–128

Economo, C. von, Koskinas, G.W. (1925). *Die Cytoarchitektonik der Hirnrinde des erwachsenen Menschen.* Springer, Wien, Berlin

Edinger, L. (1895). Über die Entwicklung des Rindensehens. *Arch. f. Psychiat.* 27, 950

Efron, R. (1963). Temporal perception, aphasia, déjö vu. *Brain* 86, 403–424

Efron, R. (1968). What is perception? *Boston Studies Philosophy Science* 4, 137–173

Egeth, H., Epstein, J. (1972). Differential specialization of the cerebral hemispheres for the perception of sameness and differences. *Perc. Psychophysics* 12, 218–220

Eggers, C. (1973). *Verlaufsweisen kindlicher und präpuberaler Schizophrenien.* Springer, Berlin, Heidelberg, New York

Eggers, C. (1975). Die akute optische Halluzinose im Kindesalter. Klinische, differentialtypologische, neurophysiologische und entwicklungspsychologische Aspekte. *Fortschr. Neurol. Psychiat. u. Grenzgeb.* 43, 441–470

Eggers, C. (1981). Die Bedeutung limbischer Funktionsstörungen für die Ätiologie kindlicher Schizophrenien. *Fortschr. Neurol. Psychiat.* 49, 101–108

Eggers, C. (1987). Halluzination und Wahn im Kindes-und Jugendalter. In Olbrich, H.M. (ed.), *Halluzination und Wahn.* Springer, Berlin, Heidelberg, N.Y.

Ehrenwald, H. (1930). Über das 'Lesen' mit Umgehung des optischen Wahrnehmungsapparates. Befunde bei einem Fall von reiner Wortblindheit. *Z. ges. Neurol. u. Psychiat.* 123, 204

Ehrenwald, H. (1930). Verändertes Erleben des Körperbildes mit konsekutiver Wahnbildung bei linksseitiger Hemiplegie. *Mschr. Psychiat. Neurol.* 75, 89–97

Ehrenwald, H. (1931). Anosognosie und Depersonaliastion. *Nervenarzt* 4, 681–688

Ehrenwald, H. (1931/32). Störungen der Zeitauffassung, der räumlichen Orientierung, des Zeichnens und des Rechnens bei einem Hirnverletzten. *Z. Neurol. Psychiat.* 132, 518–569

Ehrenwald, J. (1974). Out-of-body-experiences and the denial of death. *J. Nerv. Ment. Dis.* 159, 227–233

Ehrlichman, H., Weiner, S.L., Baker, A.H. (1974). Effects of verbal and spatial questions on initial gaze shift. *Neuropsychologia* 12, 265–277

Eibl-Eibesfeldt, I. (1967). *Grundriss der vergleichenden Verhaltensforschung.* Piper, München

Eibl-Eibesfeldt, I. (1970). *Ethology. The biology of behavior.* Holt, Rinehart, Winston, New York

Eibl-Eibesfeldt, I. (1984). *Die Biologie des menschlichen Verhaltens.*

Grundriss der Humanethologie. Piper, München

Eichmeier, J., Höfer, O., Knoll, M., Meier-Knoll, A. (1974). *Endogene Bildmuster.* Urban und Schwarzenberg, München

Eidelberg, D., Galaburda, A.M. (1984). Inferior parietal lobule: divergent architectonic asymmetries in the human brain. *Arch. Neurol.* 41, 843–852

Eidelberg, E., Schwartz, A.J. (1971). Experimental analysis of the extinction phenomenon in monkeys. *Brain* 94, 91–108

Ekman, P. (1973). Cross-cultural studies of facial expression. In *Darwin and Facial Expression.* Academic Press, New York, London, 169–222

Ekman, P. (1980). Asymmetry in facial expression. *Science* 209, 833–834

Ekman, P. (1989). The argument and evidence about universals in facial expressions of emotions. In Wagner, H., Manstead, A. (eds.), *Handbook of social psychophysiology.* Wiley, Chichester

Ekman, P., Friesen, W.V. (1975). *Unmasking the face.* Prentice-Hall, Englewood Cliffs

Ekman, P., Friesen, W.V. (1976). Measuring facial movement. *J. Environm. Psychol. and Non-Verbal Beh.* 1, 56–75

Ekman, P., Friesen, W.V. (1976). *The pictures of facial affect.* Consulting Psychologists Press, Palo Alto

Ekman, P., Friesen, W.V. (1978). *The facial action coding system.* Englewwod Chiffs, N.J.

Ekman, P., Friesen, W.V., O'Sullivan, M., Chan, A., Diacoyanni-Tarlatzis, I., Heider, K., Krause, R., LeCompte, W.A., Pitcairn, T., Ricci-Bitti, P.E., Scherer, K.R., Tomita, M., Tzavaras, A. (1987). Universal and cultural differences in the judgement of facial expressions of emotion. *J. Personality Soc. Psychol.* 53, 712–717

Ekman, P., Oster, H. (1979). Facial expressions of emotion. *Ann. Rev. Psychol.* 30, 527–554

Ekstrom, R., French, J.W., Harman, H.H. (1976). *Manual for kit of factor-referenced cognitive tests.* Educational Testing Service, Princeton, NY

Elithorn, A. (1955). A preliminary report on a perceptual maze test sensitive to brain damage. *J. Neurol. Neurosurg. Psychiat.* 18, 287–297

Ellen, P., Thinus-Blanc, C. (eds.) (1987). *Cognitive processes and spatial orientation in animal and man.* Vol. II *Neurophysiology and Developmental Aspects.* Nihoff, Dordrecht

Ellenberger, C. (1974). Modern perimetry in neuro-ophthalmic diagnosis. *Arch Neurol.* 30, 193–201

Ellenberger, H.F. (1970). *The discovery of the unconscious. The history and evolution of dynamic psychiatry.* Basic Books, New York

Ellis, H.D. (1975). Recognizing faces. *Br. J. Psychol.* 66, 409–426

Ellis, H.D., Jeeves, M.A., Newcombe, F. Young, A. (1986) (eds.). *Aspects of face processing.* Nijhoff, Dordrecht

Ellis, H.D., Shepherd, J., Bruce, A. (1973). The effects of age and sex upon adolescents' recognition of faces. *J. Genetic Psychol.* 123, 173–174

Ellis, H.D., Shepherd, J., Davies, G.M. (1979). Identification of familiar and unfamiliar faces from internal and external features: Some implications for theories of face recognition. *Perception* 8, 431–439

Ellis, H.D., Shepherd, J.W. (1974). Recognition of abstract and concrete words presented in the left and right visual halffield. *J. exp. Psychol.* 103, 1035–1036

Ellis, H.D., Shepherd, J.W. (1975). Recognition of upright and inverted faces presented in the left and right visual fields. *Cortex* 11, 3–7

Ellis, H.D., Shepherd, J.W., Bruce, A. (1973). The effects of age and sex upon adolescents' recognition of faces. *J. Gen. Psychol.* 123, 173–174

Ellis, H.D., Young, A.W. (1988). *Human cognitive neuropsychology.* Lawrence Erlbaum Associates, Hillsdale, NJ

Ellis, H.D., Young, A.W. (1988). Training in face-processing skills for a child with acquired prosopagnosia. *Developmental Neuropsychol.* 4, 283–294

Ellis, H.D., Young, A.W. (1989). Are faces special? In Young, A.W., Ellis, H.D. (eds.), *Handbook of research on face processing.* North Holland, Amsterdam

Ellis, W., Shepherd, J., Bruce, A. (1973). The effects of age and sex upon adolescents' recognition of faces. *J. Genet. Psychol.* 123, 173–174

Ellis, W.D. (1938). *A sourcebook of Gestalt psychology.* Harcourt Brace, New-York

Endelmann, L. (1912). Über einen Fall von doppelseitiger homonymer Hemianopsie, verbunden mit Alexie und Agraphie nach der Geburt. *Arch. Augenheilk.* 71, 177–188

Engel, A.K., König, P., Gray, C.M., Singer, W. (1990). Synchronization of oscillatory responses: a mechanism for stimulus-dependent assembley formation in cat visual cortex. In Eckmiller, R., Hartmann, G., Hauske, G. (eds.), *Parallel processing in neural systems and computers.* Elsevier, North-Holland, 105–107

Engel, A.K., König, P., Gray, C.M., Singer, W. (1991). Stimulus-dependent neuronal oscillations in cat visual cortex: inter-columnar interaction as determined by cross-correlation analysis. *Eur. J. Neurosci.* (in press)

Engel, F.L. (1971). Visual conspicuity, directed attention and retinal locus. *Vision Res.* 11, 563–576

Engel, F.L. (1974). Visual conspicuity and selective background interference in eccentric vision. *Vision Res.* 14, 459–471

Engel, J.J. (1785). *Ideen zu einer Mimik. 1. Theil.* Mylius, Berlin

Engel, J.J. (1786). *Ideen zu einer Mimik. 2. Theil.* Mylius, Berlin

Engerth, G. (1934). Über isolierte Störungen in der Verwendung der blauen Farben bei parietalen Herderkrankungen. *Z. ges. Neurol. Psychiat.* 149, 723–736

Engerth, G., Hoff, H., Pötzl, O. (1935). Zur Patho-Physiologie der hemianopischen Halluzinationen. *Z. ges. Neurol. Psychiat.* 152, 399–421

Eperon (1884). Hémiachromatopie absolue: avec conservation partielle de la perception lumineuse et de l'acuité visuelle indirecte; dyslexie. Quelques considerations relative ö la localisation des centres visuels corticaux et aux phénomènes mentaux de la lecture. *Arch. Ophthal. Paris* 4, 356–370

Epstein, W. (ed.) (1977). *Stability and constancy in visual perception: mechanisms and processes.* Wiley, New York

Erdmann, B., Dodge, R. (1898). *Psychologische Untersuchungen über das Lesen auf experimenteller Grundlage.* Niemeyer, Halle

Eriksen, B.A., Eriksen, C.W. (1974a). The importance of being first. A tachistoscopic study of the contributions of each letter to the recognition of four letter words. *Perception and Psychophysics* 15, 66–72

Eriksen, B.A., Eriksen, C.W. (1974b). Effects of noise letters upon the identification of a target letter in a non-search task. *Perception and Psychphysics* 16, 143–149

Eriksen, C.W., Spencer, T. (1969). Rate of information processing in visual perception: Some results and methodological considerations. *J. Exp. Psychol. Monographs* 79

Erismann, Th. (1948). *Movie on the effect of inverted vision.* Univ. of Innsbruck

Erismann, Th. (1962). *Experimentelle Psychologie.* De Gruyter, Berlin

Escourolle, R., Hauw, J.J., Gray, F., Henin, D. (1974). Aspects neuropathologiques des lésions du corps calleux. In Michel, F., Schott, B. (eds.), *Les syndromes de disconnexion calleuse chez l' homme.* Colloque international de Lyon

Eskuchen, E. (1911). *Über halbseitige Gesichtsfeldhalluzinationen und halbseitige Sehstörungen.* Inaug. Diss., Heidelberg

Etcoff, N.L. (1984). Selective attention to facial identity and facial emotion. *Neuropsychologia* 22, 281–295

Ettlinger, G. (1956). Sensory deficits in visual agnosia. *J. Neurol. Neurosurg. Psychiat.* 19, 297–308

Ettlinger, G. (1959). Visual discrimination following successive temporal ablations in monkeys. *Brain* 82, 232–250

Ettlinger, G. (1959). Visual discrimination with a single manipulandum following temporal ablations in the monkey. *Quart. J. exp. Psychol.* 11, 164–174

Ettlinger, G. (1977). Parietal cortex in visual orientation. In Rose, F.C. (ed.), *Physiological aspects of clinical neurology.* Blackwell, Oxford, 93–100

Ettlinger, G., Hurwitz, L. (1962). Dyslexia and its associated disturbances. *Neurology* 12, 477–480

Ettlinger, G., Kalsbeck, J.E. (1962). Changes in tactile discrimination and in visual reaching after successive and simultaneous bilateral posterior parietal ablations in the monkey. *J. Neurol. Neurosurg. Psychiat.* 25, 256–268

Ettlinger, G., Warrington, E., Zangwill, O.L. (1957). A further study of visual-spatial agnosia. *Brain* 80, 335–361

Evans, J.R., Gordon, J., Abramov, I., Mladejovsky, M.G., Dobelle, W.H. (1979). Brightness of phosphenes elicited by electrical stimulation of human visual cortex. *Sensory Processes* 3, 82–94

Evarts, E.V. (1962). A neurophysiologic theory of hallucinations. In L.L. West (ed.), *Hallucinations.* Grune, New York

Everitt, B.S., Rushdon, D.N. (1978). A method for plotting the optimum positions of an array of cortical electrical phosphenes. *Biometrics* 34, 399–410

Exner, S. (1875). Über das Sehen von Bewegung und die Theorie des zusammengesetzten Auges. *S.-B. Akad. Wiss. Wien, mat.-nat. Kl.,* Abt. III 72, 156–190

Exner, S. (1881). *Untersuchungen über die Localisation der Functionen in der Grosshirnrinde des Menschen.* Braumüller, Wien

Exner, S. (1894). *Entwurf zu einer physiologischen Erklärung der psychischen Erscheinungen. 1. Theil,* Deuticke, Leipzig, Wien

Exner, S. (1904). Zur Kenntnis des zentralen Sehaktes. *Z. Psychol. Physiol. Sinnesorg.* 36, 194

Eysel, U.Th. (1976). Quantitative studies of intracellular postsynaptic potentials in the lateral geniculate nucleus of the cat with respect to optic tract stimulus response latencies. *Exp. Brain Res.* 25, 469–486

Eysel, U.Th. (1984). Neuronale Mechanismen zur Auffüllung retinaler Skotome. In Herzau, V. (ed.), *Pathohysiologie des Sehens.* Enke, Stuttgart, 10–20

Eysel, U.Th. (1989). Degenerative, regenerative und adaptative Reaktionen auf lokale Schädigungen der Netzhaut. *Fortschr. Ophthalmol.* 86, 604–610

Eysel, U.Th. (1991). Plastizität nach Läsionen im visuellen System. (in preparation for publication)

Eysel, U.Th., Grüsser, O.-J. (1971). Neurophysiological basis of pattern recognition in the cat's visual system. In Grüsser, O.-J., Klinke, R. (eds.), *Zeichenerkennung durch biologische und technische Systeme.* Springer, Berlin-Heidelberg-New York, p. 60–80

Eysel, U.Th., Grüsser, O.-J. (1974). Simultaneous recording of pre-and postsynaptic potentials during degeneration of optic tract fiber input to the cat lateral geniculate nucleus. *Brain Res.* 81, 552–557

Eysel, U.Th., Grüsser, O.-J. (1975). Intracellular postsynaptic potentials of cat lateral geniculate cells and the effects of degeneration of the optic tract terminals. *Brain Res.* 98, 441–455

Eysel, U.Th., Grüsser, O.-J. (1978). Increased transneuronal excitation of the cat lateral geniculate nucleus after acute deafferentation. *Brain Res.* 158, 107–128

Eysel, U.Th., Grüsser, O.-J., Hoffmann, K.-P. (1979). Monocular deprivation and the signal transmission by X-and Y-neurons of the cat lateral geniculate nucleus. *Exp. Brain Res.* 34, 521–539

Eysel, U.Th., Grüsser, O.-J., Pecci Saavedra, J. (1974). Correlation between ultrastructural and electrophysiological signs of degeneration in optic nerve terminals of the cat's lateral geniculate nucleus. *J. neural. Transmission* 35, 337–344

Eysel, U.Th., Grüsser, O.-J., Pecci Saavedra, J. (1974a). Die Signalübertragung durch degenerierende Synapsen nach Unterbrechung des Axoplasmaflusses. Untersuchungen am Corpus geniculatum lateral der Katze. *Bull. Schweiz. Akad. Med. Wiss.* 30, 82–106

Eysel, U.Th., Grüsser, O.-J., Pecci Saavedra, J. (1974b). Signal transmission through degenerating synapses in the lateral geniculate body of the cat. *Brain Res.* 76, 49–70

Eysel, U.Th., Peichl, L., Wässle, H. (1985). Dendritic plasticity in the early postnatal feline retina: quantitative characteristics and sensitive period. *J. Comp. Neurol.* 242, 134–145

Eysel, U.Th., Schmidt-Kastner, R. (1991). Neuronal dysfunction at the border of focal cortical lesions in cat visual cortex. Neuroscience Lett. (in press)

Fabricius ab Aquapendente, H. (1687). *De actione oculorum, pars secunda.* In *Opera omnia anatomica et physiologica.* J.F. Gleditsch, Leipzig

Fagan, J.F. (1972). Infants' recognition memory for faces. *J. Exp. Child Psychol.* 14, 453–476

Fagan, J.F. (1973). Infants' delayed recognition memory and forgetting. *J. Exp. Child Psychol.* 16, 424–450

Fagan, J.F. (1976). Infants' recognition of invariant features of faces. *Child Development* 47, 627–638

Fagan, J.F. (1979). The origins of facial pattern recognition. In Bornstein, M., Kessen, W. (eds.), *Psychological development in infancy: Image to intention.* Erlbaum, Hillsdale, 83–113

Fagan, J.F., Shepherd, P.A. (1979). Infants' perception of face orientation. *Infant Behav. Dev.* 2, 227–324

Faglioni, P., Scotti, G., Spinnler, H. (1971). The performance of brain-damaged patients in spatial localization of visual and tactile stimuli. *Brain* 94, 443–454

Faguet, R.A. (1979). With eyes of the mind. *General Hospital Psychiatry* 1, 311–314

Fairweather, H. (1982). Sex differences: little reason for females to play midfield. In Beaumont, J.G. (ed.), *Divided visual field studies of cerebral organization.* Academic Press, London, New York, 147–194

Falk, F. (1871). *Galen's Lehre vom gesunden und kranken Nervensystem.* Veit & Co., Leipzig

Falkenstein, A. (1936). *Archaische Texte aus Uruk.* Deutsche Forschungsgemeinschaft, Berlin

Fankhauser, F. (1969). Kinetische Perimetrie. *Ophtalmologica* 158, 406–418

Fantz, R.L. (1961). The origin of form perception. *Scient. Amer.* 204, 66–72

Fantz, R.L. (1963). Pattern vision in newborn infants. *Science* 140, 296–297

Fantz, R.L. (1966). Pattern discrimination and selective attention as determinants of perceptual development from birth. In Kidd, A., Revoir, J.L. (eds.), *Perceptual development in children.* International University Press, New York

Fantz, R.L., Fagan, J.F., Miranda, S.R. (1976). Early visual selectivity as a function of pattern variables, previous exposure, age from birth and conception, and expected cognitive deficit. In Cohen, L.B., Salapatek, P. (eds.), *Infant perception: from sensation to cognition. Basic visual processes.* Academic, New York, 249–345

Farah, M.J. (1984). The neural basis of mental imagery: A componential analysis. *Cognition* 18, 245–272

Farah, M.J. (1988). Is visual imagery really visual? Overlooked evidence from neuropsychology. *Psychol. Rev.* 95, 307–317

Farah, M.J. (1989). The neural basis of mental imagery. *TINS* 12, 395–399

Farah, M.J. (1989). The neuropsychology of mental imagery. In Brown, J.W. (ed.), *Neuropsychology of visual perception.* Erlbaum, Hillsdale, 183–202

Farah, M.J. (1990). *Visual agnosia. Disorders of object recognition and what they tell us about normal vision.* MIT Press, Cambridge, Mass.

Farah, M.J. (1991, in press). Patterns of co-occurrence among the associative agnosias: Implications for the nature of visual object representation. *Cognitive Neuropsychology*

Farah, M.J., Gazzaniga, M.S., Holtzman, J.D., Kosslyn, S.M. (1985). A left hemisphere basis for visual mental imagery? *Neuropsychologia* 23, 115–118

Farah, M.J., Hammond, K.H., Mehta, Z., Ratcliff, G. (1989). Category-specificity and modality-specificity in semantic memory. *Neuropsychologia* 27, 193–200

Farah, M.J., Hammond, M., Levine, D.N., Calvanio, R. (1988). Visual and spatial mental imagery: dissociable systems of representation. *Cognitive Psychol.* 20, 439–462

Farah, M.J., Peronnet, F., Gonon, M.A., Giard, M.H. (1988). Electrophysiological evidence for a shared representational medium for visual images and visual percepts. *J. Exp. Psychol: General* 117, 248–257

Farah, M.J., Weisberg, L.L., Monheit, M., Peronnet, F. (1989). Brain activity underlying mental imagery: event-related potentials during mental image generation. *J. Cogn. Neurosci.* 1, 302–316

Farah, M.J., Wong, A.B., Monheit, M.A., Morrow, L.A. (1989). Parietal lobe mechanisms of spatial attention: Modality-specific or supramodal? *Neuropsychologia* 27, 461–470

Farnsworth, D. (1943). The Farnsworth-Munsell 100-hue and dichotomous test for color vision. *J. Opt. Soc. Amer.* 33, 568–678

Faugier-Grimaud, S., Frenois, C., Pernot, F. (1985). Effects of posterior parietal lesions on visually guided movements in monkeys. *Exp. Brain Res.* 59, 125–138

Faugier-Grimaud, S., Frenois, C., Stein, D.G. (1978). Effects of posterior parietal lesions on visually guided behavior in monkeys. *Neuropsychologia* 16, 151–168

Faure-Beaulieu, Jacquet, E. (1924). Alexie pure, reliquat d'agnosie visuelle. *Rev. Neurol.* 2, 495–

Faust, C. (1947). Partielle Seelenblindheit nach Occipitalhirnverletzung mit besonderer Beeinträchtigung des Physiognomieerkennungsvermögens. *Nervenarzt* 18, 294–297

Faust, C. (1948). Über Gestaltzerfall als Symptom des parietookzipitalen Übergangsgebietes bei doppelseitiger Verletzung nach Hirnschuss. *Nervenarzt* 18, 103–115

Faust, C. (1949). Ein Beitrag zur Diagnostik der optischen Agnosie. In Urban, H.J. (ed.), *Festschrift Pötzl.* Universitätsverlag Wagner, Innsbruck, 197–207

Faust, C. (1951). Entwicklung und Abbau optisch-gnostischer Störungen nach traumatischer Hirnschädigung. *Nervenarzt* 22, 176–179

Faust, C. (1955). *Die zerebralen Herdstörungen nach Hinterhauptverletzungen und ihre Beurteilung.* Thieme, Stuttgart

Faust, C. (1956). *Das klinische Bild der Dauerfolgen nach Hirnverletzung.* Thieme, Stuttgart

Fay, T. (1926). Visual hallucinations in organic diseases of the brain. *Arch. Neurol. Psychiat.* 16, 377–379

Fazakas, A. (1928). Über die zentrale und periphere Farbensehschärfe. *Graefes Arch. Ophthalmol.* 120. 555

Fechner, G.T. (1860). *Elemente der Psychophysik.* Vol. 1 and 2. Breitkopf v. Härtel, Leipzig

Fedio, P., Van Buren, J.M. (1975). Memory and perceptual deficits during electrical stimulation in the left and right thalamus and parietal subcortex. *Brain and Language* 2, 78–100

Feilchenfeld, H. (1903). Zur Lageeinschätzung bei seitlichen Kopfneigungen. *Z. Psychol. Physiol. Sinnesorg.* 31, 127–150

Feinberg, I. (1962). A comparison of the visual hallucinations in schizophrenia with those induced by mescaline and LSD–25. In West, L.J. (ed.), *Hallucinations.* Grune & Stratton, New York, p. 64–76

Feinberg, R., Jones, G. (1985). Object reversals after parietal lobe infarction. A case report. *Cortex* 21, 261–271

Feinberg, T.E., Gonzales-Rothi, L.J., Heilman, K.M. (1986). Multimodal agnosia after unilateral left hemisphere lesion. *Neurology* 36, 864–867

Feinberg, T.E., Rifkin, A., Schaffer, C., Walker, E. (1986). Facial discrimination and emotional recognition in schizophrenia and affective disroders. *Arch. Gen. Psychiatry* 43, 276–279

Feinberg, W.M., Rapcsak, S.Z. (1989). 'Peduncular hallucinosis' following paramedian thalamic infarction. *Neurology* 19, 1535–1536

Feinman, S., Entwistle, D.R. (1976). Children's ability to recognize other children's faces. *Child Development* 47, 506–510

Feldman, M., Bender, M.B. (1972). The so-called visual agnosia. *Brain* 95, 173–186

Felleman, D.J., Burkhalter, A., van Essen, D.C. (1987). Visual area PIP: an extrastriate cortical area in the posterior intraparietal sulcus of the macaque monkey. *Soc. Neurosci. Abstr.* 13, 626

Felleman, D.J., DeYoe, E.A., Knierim, J.J., Olavarria, J., van Essen, D.C. van (1988). Compartmental organization of projections from V2 to extrastriate areas V3, V3A, and V4t of macaque monkes. *Invest. Ophthalmol. Visual Sci. Suppl.* 29, 115

Felleman, D.J., Kaas, J.H. (1984). Receptive-field properties of neurons in middle temporal visual area (MT) of owl monkeys. *J. Neurophysiol* 52, 488–513

Felleman, D.J., Knierim, J.J., van Essen, D.C. (1986). Multiple topographic and non-topographic subdivisions of the temporal lobe revealed by the connections of area V4 in macaques. *Soc. Neurosci. Abstr.* 12, 1182

Felleman, D.J., van Essen, D.C. (1983). The connections of area V4 of macaque monkey extrastriate cortex. *Soc. Neurosci. Abstr.* 10, 933

Felleman, D.J., van Essen, D.C. (1987). Receptive field properties of neurons in area V3 of macaque monkey extrastriate cortex. *J. Neurophysiol.* 57, 889–920

Fenstemacher, S.B., Olson, C.R., Gross, C.G. (1984). Afferent connections of macaque visual areas V4 and TEO. *Invest. Ophthalmol. Visual Sci. (Suppl.)* 25, 213

Fentress, J.C., Dotty, R.W. (1971). Effect of tetanization and enucleation upon excitability of visual pathways in squirrel monkeys and cats. *Exp. Neurol.* 30, 535–554

Fenwick, P., Galliano, S., Coate, M.A., Rippere, V., Brown, D. (1985). 'Psychic sensitivity', mystical experience, head injury and brain pathology. *Br. J. Med. Psychol.* 58, 35–44

Fere, Ch. (1898). Hallucinations autoscopiques périodiques. *J. médical de Bruxelles* 3, 101–103

Fere, Ch. (1890). *Les épilepsies et les épileptiques.* (Case 18), Alcan, Paris

Fere, Ch. (1891). Note sur les hallucinations autoscopiques ou spéculaires et sur les hallucinations altruistes. *Compt. Rend. de la Soc. de Biol.* 3, 451–53

Fernandez de Córdoba, E. (1970). Un caso de 'estar en dos' con simultanea (autoscopía en doble sentido). *Actas Lusu-Espanolas de Neurol. y Psiquiat.* 29, 251–254

Fernelius, J. (1542/1607) *Ambiani universa medicinae.* 6th ed. C. Marinius, J. Aubrius, Frankfurt

Ferrero, N. (1952). Leonardo da Vinci: of the eye. *Amer. J. Ophthalmol.* 35, 507–521

Ferrier, D. (1875). Experiments on the brain of monkeys. *Phil. Trans. Roy. Soc. London* 165, 433

Ferrier, D. (1876). *The functions of the brain.* Dawsons, London

Ferrier, D. (1881). Cerebral amblyopia and hemiopia. *Brain* 3, 456–477

Ferrier, D. (1886/1978). *The functions of the brain.* Putnam, London. Reprinted in Robinson, D. (ed.), *Significant contributions to the history of psychology,* Vol. III, Series E.

Ferrier, D. (1888). Schafer on the temporal and occipital lobes. *Brain* 11, 7–30

Ferro, J.M., Kertesz, A. (1984). Posterior internal capsule infarction associated with neglect. *Arch. Neurol.* 41, 422–424

Ferro, J.M., Martins, I.P., Mariano, G.A., Castro Caldas, A. (1983).

CT scan correlates of gesture recognition, *J. Neurol. Neurosurg. Psychiat.* 46, 943–952

Ferro, J.M., Santos, M.E. (1984). Associative visual agnosia: A case study. *Cortex* 20, 121–134

Festinger, L., Sedgwick, H.A., Holtzman, J.D. (1976). Visual perception during smooth pursuit eye movements. *Vision Res.* 16, 1377–1386

Feuchtwanger, E. (1934). Ueber optisch-konstruktive Agnosie (Zugleich ein Beitrag zur Pathologie der optischen Vorstellungstätigkeit). *Z. Neurol. Psychiat.* 151, 49–96

Feyerabend, P. (1975). *Against method. Outline of an anarchistic theory of knowledge.* German transl. H. Vetter (1976): *Wider den Methodenzwang. Skizze einer anarchistischen Erkenntnistheorie.* Suhrkamp, Frankfurt a. M.

Feyereisen, P. (1986). Production and comprehension of emotional facial expressions in brain-damaged subjects. In Bruyer, R.(ed.), *The Neuropsychology of face perception and facial expression,* Erlbaum, Hillsdale, N.J., London, 221–245

Fieandt, K. von (1949). Das phänomenologische Problem von Licht und Schatten. *Acta Psychologica* 6, 337–357

Field, T.M., Woodson, R., Greenberg, R., Cohen, D. (1982). Discrimination and immitation of facial expression by neonates. *Science* 218, 179–181

File, P.E. (1980). Visual memory for colour. *Acta Psychol. (Amst.)* 46, 103–114

Filehne, W. (1922). Über das optische Wahrnehmen von Bewegungen. *Z. Sinnesphysiol.* 53, 134–145

Filimonoff, I.N. (1932). Über die Variabilität der Grosshirnrindenstruktur II. Regio occipitalis beim erwachsenen Menschen. *J. Psychol. Neurol. (Lpz.)* 44, 1–96

Filimonoff, I.N. (1947). A rational subdivision of the cerebral cortex. *Arch. Neurol. and Psychiat.* 58, 296

Fincham, R.W., Nibbelink, D.W., Aschenbrener, C.A. (1975). Alexia with left homonymous hemianopia without agraphia. A case report with autopsy findings. *Neurology* 25, 1164–1168

Fine, E.J., Mellstrom, M., Mani, S.S., Timmins, J. (1980). Spatial disorientation and the Dyke-Davidoff-Masson syndrome. *Cortex* 16, 493–499

Finke, R.A., Freyd, J.J. (1985). Transformations of visual memory induced by implied motions of pattern elements. *J. Exp. Psychol. (Learn Mem Cogn.)* 11, 780–794

Finke, R.A., Freyd, J.J., Shyi, G.C. (1986). Implied velocity and acceleration induce transformations of visual memory. *J. Exp. Psychol (Gen.)* 115, 175–188

Finkelnburg, F.C. (1870). Vortrag bei der Niederrheinischen Gesellschaft in Bonn. Medicinische Section. *Berl.klin.Wschr.* 7, 449–450, 460–461

Finkelstein, D., Grüsser, O.-J. (1965). Frog retina: detection of movement. *Science* 150, 1050–1051

Finkelstein, L.O. (1894). Ueber optische Phänomene bei electrischer Reizung des Sehapparates. *Arch. f. Psychiat.* 26, 867–885

Finlay, D.C., French, J. (1978). Visual field difference in a facial recognition task using signal detection theory. *Neuropsychologia* 16, 103–107

Fiorani, M. Jr., Gattass, R., Rosa, M.G.P., Sousa, A.P.B. (1989). Visual area MT in the Cebus monkey: location visuotopic organization and variability. *J. Comp. Neurol.* 287, 98–118

Fiorentini, A., Berardi, N. (1984). Right hemispheric superiority in the discrimination of spatial phase. *Perception* 13, 695–708

Fiorentini, A., Maffei, L., Sandini, G. (1983). The role of high spatial frequencies in face perception. *Perception* 12, 195–201

Fischer, B., Boch, R. (1981). Enhanced activation of neurons in prelunate cortex before visually guided saccades of trained rhesus monkeys. *Exp. Brain Res.* 44, 129–137

Fischer, B., Poggio, G.F. (1979). Depth sensitivity of binocular cortical neurons of behaving monkeys. *Proc. R. Soc. Lond. B.* 204,

409–414

Fischer, M.H. (1928). Die Regulationsfunktion des menschlichen Labyrinthes und die Zusammenhänge mit verwandten Funktionen. *Erg. Physiol.* 27, 209–379

Fischer, M.H., Kornmüller, A.E. (1930). Egozentrische Lokalisation. I. Optische egozentrische Richtungslokalisation. *Z. Sinnesphysiol.* 61, 87–147

Fischer, M.H., Kornmüller, A.E. (1930). Optokinetisch ausgelöste Bewegungswahrnehmungen und optokinetischer Nystagmus. *J. Psychol. Neurol.* (Lpz.) 41, 273–308

Fischer, R. (1974). A pharmacological and conceptual reevaluation of hallucinations. *Confinia Psychiat.* 17, 143–151

Fitzpatrick, D., Itoh, K., Diamond, I.T. (1983). The laminar organization of the lateral geniculate body and the striate cortex in the squirrel monkey (*Saimiri sciureus*). *J. Neurosci.* 3, 673–702

Fitzpatrick, D., Lund, J.S., Blasdel, G.G. (1985). Intrinsic connections of macaque striate cortex: afferent and efferent connections of lamina 4C. *J. Neurosci.* 5, 3324–3349

Fizgerald, H.P. (1978). Autonomic pupillary reflex of activity during early infancy and its relation to social and nonsocial visual stimuly. *J. Exp. Child Psychology* 6, 470–482

Flandrin, J.M., Jeannerod, M. (1981). Effects of unilateral superior colliculus ablation on oculomotor and vestibulo-ocular responses in the cat. *Exp. Brain Res.* 42, 73–80

Flechsig, P. (1883). *Plan des menschlichen Gehirns.* Veit, Leipzig

Flechsig, P. (1894). Über ein neues Eintheilungsprincip der Grosshirn-Oberfläche. *Neurol. Centralbl.* 13, 674 and 809

Flechsig, P. (1895). Weitere Mittheilungen über die Sinnes-und Associationscentren des menschlichen Gehirns. *Neurol. Centralbl.* 14, 118 and 1177

Flechsig, P. (1927). *Meine myelogenetische Hirnlehre. Mit biographischer Einleitung.* Springer, Berlin

Flechsig, P.E. (1896a). *Gehirn und Seele* (2nd ed.), Velt, Leipzig

Flechsig, P.E. (1896b). *Über die Localisation der geistigen Vorgänge insbesondere der Sinnesempfindungen des Menschen.* Veit, Leipzig

Fleischer, B., Ensinger, T. (1920). Homonym-hemianopische Gesichtsfeldstörungen nach Schädel-spez. Hinterhauptsschüssen. *Klin. Monatsbl. f. Augenheilk.* 65, 181

Fleischman, J.A., Segall, J.D., Judge jr., R.P. (1983). Isolated transient alexia. *Arch. Neurol.* 40, 116

Flesch, J. (1908). Verbale Alexie mit Hemiachromatopsie. *Wiener med. Wochenschr.* 58, 2367

Flin, R.H. (1980). Age effects in children's memory for unfamiliar faces. *Dev. Psychol.* 16, 373–374

Flourens, P. (1846/1978). *Phrenology examined* (Meigs, C.L., trans.). Hogan & Thompson, Philadelphia, PA. Reprinted in Robinson, D.(ed.), *Significant contributions to the history of psychology*, Vol. II, Series E

Flourens, P. (1924). *Recherches éxperimentales sur les propriétés et les fonctions du système nerveux dans les animaux vertébrés.* Crevot, Paris

Flourens, P.J.M. (1824). *Versuche und Untersuchungen über die Eigenschaften und Verrichtungen des Nervensystems bei Thieren mit Rückenwirbeln.* Rein, Leipzig

Flynn, W.R. (1962). Visual hallucinations in sensory deprivation. *Psychiat. Quart.* 36, 55–65

Fodor, J.A. (1980). Methodolocial solipsism as a research strategy for cognitive psychology. *Behav. and Brain Sci.* 3, 63–110

Fodor, J.A. (1983). *The modularity of mind.* MIT Press, Cambridge, M.A.

Foerster, O. (1929). Beiträge zur Pathophysiologie der Sehbahn und der Sehsphäre. *J. Psychol. Neurol. (Lpz.)* 39, 463–485

Foerster, O. (1931). Cerebral cortex in man. *Lancet* 221, 309–312

Foerster, O. (1936). Motorische Felder und Bahnen. Sensible corticale Felder. In Bumke, O., Foerster, O. (eds.), *Handbuch der Neurologie.* Vol. VI, Springer, Berlin, 358–448

Foerster, O., Penfield, W. (1930). Der Narbenzug am und im Gehirn

bei traumatischer Epilepsie in seiner Bedeutung für das Zustandekommen der Anfälle und für die therapeutische Bekämpfung derselben. *Z. ges. Neurol. Psychiat.* 125, 474–572

Foix, C., Hillemand, P. (1925b). Role vraisemblable du splenum dans la pathologenie de l'alexie pure par lesion de la cerebrale posterieure. *Bull. Mem. Soc. Med. Hop. Paris* 41, 393–395

Foix, C., Masson, A. (1923). Le syndrome de l'artère cérébrale postérieure. *Presse Medicale* 32, 361–365

Foix, Ch., Hillemand, P. (1925a). Les syndromes de l'artère cérébrale antérieure. *Encéphale* 20, 209–232

Foote, S.L., Morrison, J.H. (1984). Postnatal development of laminar innervation patterns by monoaminergic fibers in monkey (*Macaca fascicularis*) primary visual cortex. *J. Neurosci.* 4, 2667–2680

Forbes, E.G. (1980). *Tobias Mayer (1723–1762): Pioneer of Enlightened Science in Germany.* Vandenhoeck and Ruprecht, Göttingen

Forsyth, D.M., Chapanis, A. (1958). Counting repeated light flashes as a function of their number, their rate of presentation and retinal location stimulated. *J. Exp. Psychol.* 56, 385–391

Foster, D.H. (1969). The responses of the human visual system to moving spatially-periodic patterns. *Vision Res.* 9, 577–590

Foster, K.H., Gaska, J.P., Nagler, M., Pollen, D.A. (1985). Spatial and temporal frequency selectivity of neurones in visual cortical areas V1 and V2 of the macaque monkey. *J. Physiol. (Lond.)* 365, 331–363

Földes-Papp, K. (1966/1975). *Vom Felsbild zum Alphabet. Die Geschichte der Schrift von ihren frühesten Vorstufen bis zur modernen lateinischen Schreibschrift.* Belser, Stuttgart

Förster, R. (1867). Über Gesichtsfeldmessungen. *Klin. Mbl. Augenheilk.* 5, 293–294

Förster, R. (1890). Ueber Rindenblindheit. *Graefes Arch. Ophthalm.* 36, 94–108

Frank, A. (1987). Facial image and object constancy: a clinical experience and a developmental inference. *Psychoanal. Q.* 56, 477–496

Frank, D.P. (1934). Depersonalisierungserscheinungen bei Hirnerkrankungen. *Z. Neurol. Psychiat.* 149, 563–582

Frederiks, J.A.M. (1969). The agnosias. Disorders of perceptual recognition. In P.J. Vinken, G.W. Bruyn (eds.), *Handbook of Clinical Neurology.* Vol. 4. Holland Publ. Company, Amsterdam

Frederking, U., Glötzner, F., Grüsser, O.-J. (1971). Some cellular aspects of the pathophysiology of epilepsia: responses of single cortical nerve and glial cells during generalized and focal seizures. In Umbach, W. (ed.), Hippokrates Verlag, Stuttgart, 130–148

Freedman, M., Oscar-Berman, M. (1989). Spatial and visual learning deficits in Alzheimer's and Parkinson's disease. *Brain and Cognition* 11, 114–126

Freedman, S.J. (1968). *The neuropsychology of spatially oriented behavior.* Dorsey Press, Homewodd, Ill.

Freeman, R.B. Jr. (1970). A psychophysical metric for visual space perception. *Ergonomics* 13, 73–82

Freud, S. (1891). *On aphasia*, transl. E. Stengl. International Universities Press Inc. (1953), New York

Freud, S. (1891). *Zur Auffassung der Aphasien, eine kritische Studie.* Deuticke, Leipzig, Wien

Freund, C.S. (1889). Ueber optische Aphasie und Seelenblindheit. *Arch. Psychiat. Nervenkr.* 20, 276–297/371–416

Fridrich, J. (1975). Ein Beitrag zur Frage nach den Anfängen des künstlerischen und ästhetischen Sinnes des Urmenschen (Vor-Neanderthal). *Pamatky Archeolocko* 68 (2), 5 (quoted according to Wreschner 1985)

Fried, I., Mateer, C., Ojemann, G., Wohns, R., Fedio, P. (1982). Organization of visuospatial functions in human cortex. Evidence from electrical stimulation. *Brain* 105, 349–371

Friedman, A.P. (1968). Migraine, pathophysiology and pathogenesis. In Finken, P.J., Bruyn, G.W. (eds.), *Handbook of Clinical Neurology*, Vol. V, Elsevier, New York, 38–44

Friedman, A.P. (1972). The headache in history, literature, and legend. *Bulletin of the New York Academy of Medicine* 48 (4), 661–681

Friedman, D.P., Jones, E.G., Burton, H. (1980). Representation pattern in the second somatic sensory area of the monkey cerebral cortex. *J. Comp. Neurol.* 192, 21–41

Friedman, H., Janas, J., Goldman-Rakic, P.S. (1987). Metabolic activity in the thalamus and mammillary bodies of the monkey during spatial memory performance. *Soc. Neurosci. Abstr.* 13, 207

Friedman, R.B., Albert, M.L. (1985). *Alexia*. In Heilmann, K.M, Valenstein, E. (eds.), *Clinical Neuropsychology*. 2nd. ed., Oxford Press, London

Friedman, R.B., Alexander, M.P. (1984). Pictures, images, and pure alexia: A case study. *Cogn. Neuropsychology* 1, 9–23

Friedmann, G. (1970). The judgement of the visual vertical and horizontal with peripheral and central vestibular lesions. *Brain* 93, 313–328

Fries, W. (1981). The projection from the lateral geniculate nucleus to the prestriate cortex of the macaque monkey. *Proc. Roy. Soc. London B* 213, 73–80

Fries, W. (1983). Morphology and distribution of Meynert cells in monkey striate cortex. *Invest. Ophthalmol. Vis. Sci. (Suppl.)* 24, 229

Fries, W. (1984). Cortical projections to the superior colliculus in the macaque monkey: a retrograde study using horseradish peroxidase. *J. Comp. Neurol.* 230, 55–76

Fries, W. (1990). Pontine projection from striate and prestriate visual cortex in the macaque monkey: An anterograde study. *Visual Neurosci.* 4, 205–216

Fries, W., Distel, H. (1983). Large layer VI neurons of monkey striate cortex (Meynert cells) project to the superior colliculus. *Proc. Roy. Soc. Lond.* B219, 53–59

Fries, W., Keizer, K., Kuypers, H.G.J.M. (1985). Large layer VI cells in macaque striate cortex (Meynert cells) project to both superior colliculus and prestriate visual area V5. *Exp. Brain Res.* 58, 613–616

Frith, C.G., Stevens, M., Johnstone, E.C., Owans, D.G.C., Crow, T.J. (1983). Integration of schematic faces and other complex objects in schizophrenia. *J. Nerv. Ment. Dis.* 171, 34–39

Frith, U. (1986). A developmental framework for developmental dyslexia. *Dyslexia* 36, 69–81

Fritsch, G., Hitzig, E. (1870). Über die elektrische Erregbarkeit des Grosshirns. *Arch. Anat. Physiol. wiss. Med.* 37, 300–332

Fröhlich, F.W. (1921). *Grundzüge einer Lehre vom Licht-und Farbsinn*. Gustav Fischer, Jena

Fröhlich, F.W. (1921a). Zur Analyse des Licht-und Farbkontrastes. *Z. Sinnesphysiol.* 52, 89–103

Fröhlich, F.W. (1921b). Untersuchungen über periodische Nachbilder. *Z. Sinnesphysiol.* 52, 60–88

Fröhlich, F.W. (1922a). Über den Einfluss der Hell-und Dunkeladaptation auf den Verlauf der periodischen Nachbilder. *Z. Sinnesphysiol.* 53, 79–107

Fröhlich, F.W. (1922b). Über die Abhängigkeit der periodischen Nachbilder von der Dauer der Belichtung. *Z. Sinnesphysiol.* 53, 108–121

Fröhlich, F.W. (1929). *Die Empfindungszeit*. Gustav Fischer, Jena

Fuchs, A., Pötzl, O. (1917). Beiträge zur Klinik und Anatomie der Schussverletzungen im Bereich der engeren Sehsphäre. *Jahrb. Psychiat. Neurol.* 38, 115

Fuchs, W. (1920). Untersuchungen über das Sehen der Hemianopiker und Hemiamblyopiker. I: Verlagerungserscheinungen. In Gelb, A., Goldstein, K. (eds.), *Psychologische Analysen hirnpathologischer Fälle*. Vol. I. J.A. Barth, Leipzig, 251–353

Fuchs, W. (1920). Untersuchungen über das Sehen der Hemianopiker und Hemiamblyopiker. II: Die totalisierende Gestaltauffassung. In Gelb, A., Goldstein, K. (eds.), *Psychologische Analysen hirnpathologischer Fälle*. Vol. I. J.A. Barth, Leipzig, 419–561

Fuhry, L., Grüsser, O.-J. (1989). Face-responsive components in pattern-induced visual evoked potentials of the Java monkey (Macaca fascicularis). In Elsner, N., Singer, W. (eds.), *Dynamics and Plasticity in Neuronal Systems, Proceedings of the 17th Göttingen Neurobiology Conference*. Thieme, Stuttgart, 380

Fuhry, L., Grüsser, O.-J. (1990). Differences in face-responsive componenets in the visual evoked potentials of Java monkey for human faces and monkey faces. In Elsner, N., Roth, G. (eds.), *Brain-Perception-Cognition. Proceedings of the 18th Göttingen Neurobiology Conference: Gehirn-Wahrnehmung-Kognition*. Thieme, Stuttgart

Fukuzawa, K., Itoh, M., Sasanuma, S., Suzuki, J., Fukusako, Y., Masui, T. (1988). Internal representations and the conceptual operation of color in pure alexia with color naming defects. *Brain and Language* 34, 98–126

Funahashi, S., Bruce, C.J., Goldman-Rakic, P.S. (1986). Perimetry of spatial memory representation in primate prefrontal cortex: evidence for a mnemonic hemianopia. *Soc. Neurosci. Abstr.* 12, 554

Furlow, L.T., Bender, M.B., Teuber, H.L. (1947). *J. Neurosurg.* 4, 380

Fuster, J.M. (1981). Prefrontal cortex in motor control. In Brooks, V.B. (ed.), *Handbook of Physiology. The Nervous System. Motor-Control*. Bethesda, MD., Am. Physiol. Soc., sect. 1, pt. 2, vol. 2, chapt. 25, p. 1149–1178.

Fuster, J.M. (1988). *The prefrontal cortex. Anatomy, Physiology and Neuropsychology of the frontal lobe* (2nd. ed., 1st ed. 1980), Raven Press, NY

Fuster, J.M., Alexander, G.E. (1971). Neuron activity related to short-term memory. *Science* 173, 652–654

Fuster, J.M., Bauer, R.H., Jervey, J.P. (1981). Effects of cooling inferotemporal cortex on performance of visual memory tasks. *Exp. Neurol.* 71, 398–409

Fuster, J.M., Jervey, J.P. (1982). Neuronal firing in the inferotemporal cortex of the monkey in a visual memory task. *J. Neurosci.* 2, 361–375

Gabbard, G.O., Twemlow, S.W., Jones, F.C. (1981). Do 'near-death-experiences' occur only near death? *J. Nerv. and Mental Dis.* 169, 374–377

Gabor, D. (1948). A new microscopic principle. *Nature* 161, 777–778

Gabor, D. (1968). Improved holographic model of temporal recall. *Nature* 217, 1288–1289

Gainotti, G. (1968). Les manifestations de négligence et d'inattention pour l'hémispace. *Cortex* 4, 64–91

Gainotti, G. (1972). Emotional behavior and hemispheric side of lesion. *Cortex* 8, 41–55

Gainotti, G., D'Erme, P., De Bonis, C. (1989). Components of visual attention disrupted in unilateral neglect. In Brown, J.W. (ed.), *Neuropsychology of visual perception*. Erlbaum, Hillsdale; NY, 123–144

Gainotti, G., D'Erme, P., Monteleone, D., Silveri, M.C. (1986). Mechanisms of unilateral spatial neglect in relation to laterality of cerebral lesions. *Brain* 109, 599–612

Gainotti, G., Messerli, P., Tissot, R. (1972). Qualitative analysis of unilateral spatial neglect in relation to laterality of cerebral lesions. *J. Neurol. Neurosurg. Psychiat.* 35, 545–550

Gainotti, G., Tiacci, C. (1970). Patterns of drawing disability in right and left hemispheric patients. *Neuropsychologia* 8, 379–384

Gainotti, G., Tiacci, C. (1971). The relationship between disorders of visual perception and unilateral spatial neglect. *Neuropsychologia* 9, 451–458

Galant, J.S. (1929). Ueber Autohalluzinationen. *Z. Neurol. Psychiat.* 120, 585–586

Galant, J.S. (1935). Ueber selten vorkommende Phänomene bei Dementia-praecox-Kranken. *Psychiat.-Neurol. Wochenschr.* 36, 426–429

Galen, C. (1821–1833). *Opera omnia*. Editionem curavit C.G. Kühn.

20 vols. Cnobloch, Leipzig

Galen, C. (1968). *On the Usefulness of the Parts.* 2 vols. In May, M.T. (ed. and transl.). Ithaca

Galetti, C., Battaglini, P.P. (1989). Gaze-dependent visual neurons in area V3A of monkey prestriate cortex. *J. Neuroscience* 9, 112–125

Galezowski, X. (1868). *Du diagnostic des maledies des yeux per la chromatoscopcie retienienne procede d'une etude sur les lois physices et physiologiques des couleurs.* Bailliere et fils, Paris

Gall, F., Spurzheim, G. (1809). *Recherche sur le systeme nerveux en general et sur selui du cerveau en particulier.* Haussman, Paris

Gallassi, R., Lenzi, P., Stracciari, A., Lorusso, S., Ciardulli, C., Morreale, A., Mussuto, V. (1986). Neuropsychological assessment of mental deterioration: purpose of a brief battery and a probabilistic definition of 'normality' and 'non-normality'. *Acta Psychiatr. Scand.* 74, 62–67

Galletti, C., Battaglini, P.P. (1989). Gaze-dependent visual neurons in area V3A of monkey prestriate cortex. *J. Neurosci.* 9, 1112–1125

Galletti, C., Battaglini, P.P., Aicardi, G. (1988). 'Real-motion' cells in visual area V2 of behaving macaque monkeys. *Exp. Brain Res.* 69, 279–288

Galley, N., Grüsser, O.-J. (1975). Augenbewegungen und Lesen. In Meyer, R., Muth, L., Rüegg, W. (eds.), *Lesen und Leben.* Börsenverband des deutschen Buchhandels, Frankfurt a.M., 65–75

Galli, G. (1965). Prosopagnosie und normale Gesichtswahrnehmung. *Wiener Zeitschr. für Nervenheilk.* 22, 28–37

Gallup, G.G. (1970). Chimpanzees: self-recognition. *Science* 167, 86–87

Gallup, G.G. (1977). Self-recognition in primates. *American Psychologist* 32, 329–338

Gallup, G.G., McClure, M.K., Hill, S.G., Bundy, R.A. (1971). Capacity for self-recognition in differentially reared chimpanzees. *Psychological Records* 21, 69–74

Galper, R.E., Costa, L. (1980). Hemispheric superiority for recognizing faces depends upon how they are learned. *Cortex* 16, 21–38

Galper, R.E., Hochberg, J. (1971). Recognition memory for photographs of faces. *Am. J. Psychol.* 84, 351–354

Galton, F. (1883). *Inquiries into Human Faculty and its Development.* Macmillan, New York

Garcha, H.S., Ettlinger, G. (1980). Tactile discrimination learning in the monkey: the effects of unilateral or bilateral removals of the second somatosensory cortex (area SII). *Cortex* 16, 397–412

Garcin, R., Rondot, P., De Recondo, J. (1967). Ataxie optique localisée aux deux hémichamps visuels homonymes gauches. *Rev. Neurol.* 116, 707–714

Gardner, B.T., Gardner, R.A. (1971). Two-way communication with an infant chimpanzee. In Schrier, A.M., Stollnitz, F. (eds.), *Behavior of nonhuman primates.* Vol. 4. Academic Press, New York, 117–131

Gardner, H. (1974). *The shattered mind.* Lintage Books, New York

Gardner, H. (1982). Artistry following damage to the human brain. In Ellis A.W. (ed.), *Normality and pathology in cognitve functions.* Academic Press, New York, 299–323

Gardner, H., Ling, P.K., Flamm, L., Silverman, J. (1975). Comprehension and appreciation of humorous material following brain damage. *Brain* 98, 399–412

Gardner, H., Zurif, E. (1975). Bee but not Be: Oral reading of single words in aphasia and alexia. *Neuropsychologia* 13, 181–190

Gardner, R.A., Gardner, B.T. (1984). A vocabulary test for chimpanzees. *J. Comp. Psychol.* 98, 381–404

Garland, H., Pearce, J. (1967). Neurological complications of carbon monoxide poisoning. *Quart. J. Medicine,* 36, 445–455

Gassel, M.M. (1969). Occipital lobe syndromes (excluding hemianopia). In Vinken, P.J., Bruyn, G.W. (eds.), *Clinical Neurology, vol. 2.* Amsterdam, North-Holland, 640–679

Gassel, M.M., Williams, D. (1963a). Visual function in patients with homonymous hemianopia. II. Oculomotor mechanisms. *Brain* 86,

1–36

Gassel, M.M., Williams, D. (1963b). Visual function in patients with homonymous hemianopia. III. The completion phenomenon; insight and attitude to the defect; and visual functional efficiency. *Brain* 86, 229–260

Gati, I., Ben-Shakhar, G. (1990). Novelty and significance in orientation and habituation: A feature-matching approach. *J. Exp. Psychol: General* 119, 251–263

Gattass, R., Gross, C.G. (1979). Visual topography of the striate projection zone (MT) in posterior superior temporal sulcus of the macaque. *J. Comp. Neurol.* 46, 621–638

Gattass, R., Gross, C.G., Sandell, J.H. (1981). Visual topography of V2 in the macaque. *J. Comp. Neurol.* 201, 519–540

Gattass, R., Sousa, A.P.B., Gross, C.G. (1988). Visuotopic organization and extent of V3 and V4 of the macaque. *J. Neurosci.* 8, 1831–1845

Gaub, J.D. (1785). *Institutiones pathologiae medicinalis.* Van der Eyck, Leyden

Gaupp, R. (1899). Über corticale Blindheit. *Monatsschr. Psychiat. Neurol.* 5, 28–41

Gaur, A. (1984). *A history of writing.* British Library, London

Gaymard, B., Pierrot-Deseilligny, C., Rivaud, S. (1990). Impairment of sequences of memory-guided saccades after supplementary motor area lesions. *Ann. Neurol.* 28, 622–626

Gazzaniga, M.S. (1970). *The bisected Brain.* Appleton-Century-Crofts, New York

Gazzaniga, M.S., Bogen, J.E., Sperry, R.W. (1962). Some functional effects of sectioning the cerebral commissures in Man. *Proc. nat. Acad. Sci. USA* 48, 1765–1769

Gazzaniga, M.S., Bogen, J.E., Sperry, R.W. (1965). Observations on visual perception after disconnexion of the cerebral hemispheres in man. *Brain* 88, 221–236

Gazzaniga, M.S., Freedman, H. (1973). Observations on visual processes after posterior callosal section. *Neurology* 23, 1126–1130

Gazzaniga, M.S., Hillyard, S.A. (1973). Attention mechanisms following brain bisection. In S. Kornblum (ed.), *Attention and performance IV.* Academic Press, New York, London, 221–238

Gazzaniga, M.S., Le Doux, J.E. (1978). *The integrated mind.* Plenum, New York

Geffen, G., Bradshaw, J.L., Nettleton, N. (1972). Hemispheric asymmetry: verbal and spatial encoding of visual stimuli. *J. Exp. Psychol.* 95, 25–31

Geffen, G., Bradshaw, J.L., Wallace, G. (1971). Interhemispehric effects on reaction time to verbal and nonverbal visual stimuli. *J. exp. Psychol.* 87, 415–422

Geisler, W.S. (1984). Physical limits of acuity and hyperacuity. *J. Opt. Soc. Am. A.* 7, 775–782

Geisler, W.S. (1989). Sequential ideal-observer analysis of visual discriminations. *Psychol. Review* 96, 267–314

Geisler, W.S., Davila, K.D. (1985). Ideal discriminators in spatial vision: two-point stimuli. *J. Opt. Soc. Am. A.* 2, 1483–1497

Geisler, W.S., Hamilton, D.B. (1986). Sampling-theory analysis of spatial vision. *J. Opt. Soc. Am. A.* 3, 62–70

Gelb, A. (1920). Diskussionsbemerkung zu 'Über die durch Kriegsverletzungen bedingten Veränderungen im optischen Zentralapparat'. *Dtsch. Z. Nervenheilk.* 59, 216–225

Gelb, A. (1920). Über den Wegfall der Wahrnehmung von 'Oberflächenfarben'. In Gelb, A., Goldstein, K. (eds.), *Psychologische Analysen hirnpathologischer Fälle.* Vol. I. J.A. Barth, Leipzig, 354–418

Gelb, A. (1921). Über den Wegfall von 'Oberflächenfarben'. *Z. f. Psychol.* 84, 193–257

Gelb, A. (1923). Über eine eigenartige Sehstörung ('Dysmorphopsie') infolge von Gesichtsfeldeinschränkung. Ein Beitrag zur Lehre von den Beziehungen zwischen 'Gesichtsfeld' und 'Sehen'. *Psychologische Forschung* 4, 38–63

Gelb, A. (1926). Die psychologische Bedeutung pathologischer Störungen der Raumwahrnehmung. In Bühler, K. (ed.)., *Bericht über den 9. Kongress für experimentelle Psychologie in München 1925*. Jena, Fischer, 23–80

Gelb, A. (1929). Die 'Farbenkonstanz' der Sehdinge. In Bethe-Bergmann (ed.) *Handbuch der normalen und pathologischen Physiologie* 12, 594–678

Gelb, A., Goldstein, K. (1920). Das 'röhrenförmige Gesichtsfeld' nebst einer Vorrichtung für perimetrische Gesichtsfelduntersuchungen in verschiedenen Entfernungen. In Gelb, A., Goldstein, K. (eds.), *Psychologische Analysen hirnpathologischer Fälle*. Vol. I. J.A. Barth, Leipzig, 143–156

Gelb, A., Goldstein, K. (1920). *Psychologische Analysen hirnpathologischer Fälle*. Barth, Leipzig

Gelb, A., Goldstein, K. (1920). Über den Einfluss des vollständigen Verlustes des optischen Vorstellungsvermögens auf das taktile Erkennen. In Gelb, A., Goldstein, K. (eds.), *Psychologische Analysen hirnpathologischer Fälle*. Vol. I. J.A. Barth, Leipzig, 157–250

Gelb, A., Goldstein, K. (1920). Zur Psychologie des optischen Wahrnehmungs-und Erkennungsvorganges. In Gelb, A., Goldstein, K. (eds.), *Psychologische Analysen hirnpathologischer Fälle*. Vol. I. J.A. Barth, Leipzig, 1–142

Gelb, A., Goldstein, K. (1925). Über Farbennamenamnesie nebst Bemerkungen über das Wesen der amnestischen Aphasie überhaupt und die Beziehung zwischen Sprache und dem Verhalten zur Umwelt. *Psychologische Forschung* 6, 127–186

Gelb, A., Goldstein, K. (1925). Zur Frage nach der gegenseitigen funktionellen Beziehung der geschädigten Sehsphäre bei Hemianopsie (Mikropsie infolge der Vorherrschaft der Vorgänge in der geschädigten Sehsphäre). *Psychologische Forschung* 6, 187

Gelb, I.J. (1952). *A study of writing. The foundation of grammatology*. The University of Chicago Press, Chicago

Gelb, I.J. (1958). *Von der Keilschrift zum Alphabet*. Kohlhammer, Stuttgart

Gellatly, A.R.H. (1980). Perception of an illusory triangle with masked inducing figure. *Perception* 9, 599–602

Geller, T.J., Bellur, S.N. (1987). Peduncular hallucinosis: magnetic resonance imaging confirmation of mesencephalic infaction during life. *Ann. Neurol.* 21, 602–604

Gelpke, Th. (1899). Zur Casuistik der einseitigen homonymen Hemianopsie corticalen Ursprungs, mit eigenartigen Störungen in den sehenden Gesichtsfeldhälften. *Arch. Augenheilk.* 39, 116–126

Gendrin, A.N. (1838). *Traite philosophique de medecine pratique*. 1. Germer Bailliere, Paris

Gennari, F. (1782). *De peculiari structura cerebri nonnullisque eius morbis*. Typographia Regio, Parma

Genner, T. (1947). Das Sehen des eigenen Spiegelbildes als epileptisches Äquivalent. *Wien. Klin. Wschr.* 59, 656–658

Gensicke, P. (1982). Das Capgras-Symptom. *Fortschr. Neurol. Psychiat.* 50, 116–120

Gentilini, M., Barbieri, C., DeRenzi, E., Faglioni, P. (1989). Space exploration with and without the aid of vision in hemisphere-damaged patients. *Cortex* 25, 643–651

Gentilucci, M., Scandolara, C., Pigarev, I.N., Rizzolatti, G. (1983). Visual responses in the postarcuate cortex (area 6) of the monkey that are independent of eye position. *Exp. Brain Res.* 50, 464–468

Georgeson, M.A. (1973). Spatial frequency selectivity of a visual tilt illusion. *Nature* 245, 43–45

Gerlach, J., Krauseneck, P., Liebaldt, G.P. (1977). Rindenblindheit. Klinische, testpsychologische und hirnlokalisatorische Befunde. *Arch. Psychiat. Nervenkr.* 223, 337–350

Gernandt, B., Granit, R. (1947). Single fiber analysis of inhibition and the polarity of the retinal elements. *J. Neurophysiol.* 10, 295–301

Gerrits, H.J.M., Timmerman, G.J.M.E.N. (1969). The filling-in process in patients with retinal scotomata. *Vision Res.* 9, 439–442

Gerrits, H.J.M., Vendrik, A.J.H. (1970). Simultaneous contrast, filling-in process and information processing in man's visual system.

Exp. Brain Res. 11, 411–430

Gerstein, G.L., Gross, C.G., Weinstein, M. (1968). Inferotemporal evoked potentials during discrimination performance by monkeys. *J. Comp. Physiol. Psychol.* 65, 526–528

Gerstenbrand, F., Gloning, I., Weingarten, K. (1956). Störungen der optischen Wahrnehmung bei Hirnstammherden. *Wien Z. Nervenheilk.* 12, 260

Gerstmann, J. (1924). Fingeragnosie. Eine umschriebene Störung der Orientierung am eigenen Körper. *Wien. Klin. Wschr.* 37, 101–102

Gerstmann, J. (1927). Fingeragnosie und isolierte Agraphie — ein neues Syndrom. *Z. ges. Neurol. Psychiat.* 108, 152–177

Gerstmann, J. (1930/1931). Zur Symptomatologie der Hirnläsionen im Übergangsgebiet der unteren Parietal-und mittleren Occipitalwindung. Das Syndrom: Fingeragnosie, Rechts-Links-Störung, Agraphie, Akalkulie. *Nervenarzt* 3, 691–695

Gerstmann, J. (1940). Syndrome of finger agnosia, disorientation for right and left, agraphia and acalculia. Local diagnostic value. *Arch. Neurol. Psychiat.* 44, 398–408

Gerstmann, J. (1942). Problem of imperception of disease and of impaired body territories with organic lesions. *Arch. Neurol. Psychiat.* 48, 890–913

Gerstmann, J. (1957). Some notes on the Gerstmann syndrome. *Neurology* 7, 866–869

Gerstmann, J., Kestenbaum, A. (1930). Monokuläres Doppeltsehen bei cerebralen Erkrankungen I. *Z. s. d. ges. Neurol. u. Psychiat.* 128, 42

Geschwind, N. (1962). The anatomy of acquired disorders of reading. In Money, J. (ed.), *Reading Disability*. John Hopkins Press, Baltimore, 115–129

Geschwind, N. (1965). Disconnexion syndromes in animals and man. Part I and Part II, *Brain* 88, 237–294, 585–645

Geschwind, N. (1974). Le concept de disconnexion: L'histoire d'une idee banale mais importante. In Michel, F., Schott, B. (eds.) *Les syndromes de disconnexion calleuse chez l'homme*. Colloque international de Lyon

Geschwind, N. (1979). Specializations of the human brain. *Scient. Amer.* 241, 158–168

Geschwind, N., Fusillo, M. (1966). Color-naming defects in association with alexia. *Arch. Neurol.* 15, 137–146

Ghent, L. (1956). Perception of overlapping and embedded figures by children of different ages. *Amer. J. Psychol.* 69, 575–587

Giannitrapani, D. (1967). Developing concepts of lateralization of cerebral functions. *Cortex* 3, 353–370

Gibbs, F.A. (1951). Ictal and non-ictal psychiatric disorders in temporal lobe epilepsy. *J. Nerv. Ment. Dis.* 113, 522–528

Gibson, E.J., Pick, A., Osser, H., Hammond, M. (1962). The role of grapheme-phoneme correspondence in the perception of words. *Am. J. Psychol.* 75, 554–570

Gibson, G.A. (1903). Case of right homonymous hemianopia. *Brain* 26, 302

Gibson, J.J. (1954). The visual perception of objective motion and subjective movement. *Psychol. Rev.* 61, 304–314

Gibson, J.J. (1966). *The senses considered as perceptual systems*. Houghton Mifflin, Boston

Gibson, J.J. (1968). What gives rise to the perception of motion. *Psychol. Rev.* 75, 335–346

Gibson, J.J. (1977). On the analysis of change in the optic array in contemporary research in visual space and motion perception. *Scand. J. Psychol.* 18, 161–163

Gibson, J.J. (1979). *The ecological approach to visual perception*. Houghton Mifflin, Boston

Gibson, W.C. (1962). Pioneers of localization of function in the brain. *J. Am. Med. Assoc.* 180, 944–951

Gielen, C.C.A.M., Gisbergen, J.A.M. van, Vendrik, A.J.H. (1982). Reconstruction of cone-sytem contribution to responses of colour-opponent neurones in monkey lateral geniculate. *Biol. Cybern.* 44, 211–221

Gil, R., Pluchon, C., Toullat, G., Michenau, D., Rogez, R., Levevre, J.P. (1985). Disconnexion visuo-verbale (aphasie optique) pour les objets, les images, les couleurs et les visages avec alexie 'abstractive'. *Neuropsychologia* 23, 333–349

Gilbert, C. (1973). Strength of left-handedness and facial recognition ability. *Cortex* 9, 145–151

Gilbert, C. (1977). Non-verbal perceptual abilities in relation to left-handedness and cerebral lateralization. *Neuropsychologia* 15, 779–791

Gilbert, C., Bakan, P. (1973). Visual asymmetry in perception of faces. *Neuropsychologia* 11, 355–362

Gilbert, C.D., Wiesel, T.N. (1989). Columnar specificity of intrinsic horizontal and corticocortical connections in cat visual cortex. *J. Neurosci.* 9, 2432–2442

Giljarowsky, W.A. (1923). Ueber psychische Veränderungen bei Flecktyphus und im Zusammenhang mit demselben. *Z. Psychol., Neurol. Psychiat.* 1, 135–152

Gilliatt, R.W., Pratt, R.T.C. (1952). Disorders of perception and performance in a case of right-sided cerebral thrombosis. *J. Neurol. Neurosurg. Psychiat.* 15, 264–271

Ginsburg, A.P. (1978). *Visual information processing based on spatial filters constrained by biological data.* Wright-Patterson Airbase, Aerospace Medical Research Laboratory Ohio, 78–129

Girotti, F., Casazza, M., Musicco, M., Avanzini, G. (1983). Oculo-motor disorders in cortical lesions in man, the role of unilateral neglect. *Neuropsychologia* 21, 543–553

Girotti, F., Milanese, C., Casazza, M., Allegranza, A., Corridori, F., Avanzini, G. (1982). Oculomotor disturbances in Balint's syndrome: Anatomo-clinical findings and electrooculographic analysis in a case. *Cortex* 18, 603–614

Girvin, J.P., Evans, J.R., Dobelle, W.H., Mladejovsky, M.G., Henderson, D.C., Abramov, I., Gordon, J., Turkel, J. (1979). Electrical stimulation of human visual cortex: the effect of stimulus parameters on phosphene threshold. *Sens. Processes* 3, 66–81

Giuliani, L. (1980). Individuum und Ideal. Antike Bildkunst. In *Bilder vom Menschen in der Kunst des Abendlandes.* Mann, Berlin, 41–86

Glaser, H.S.R. (1971). Differentiation of scribbling in a chimpanzee. *Proc. 3rd. Congr. Primatol.* Zürich. Vol. 3, Karger, Basel, 142–149

Glaser, J.S. (1978). *Neuro-ophthalmology.* Harper and Row, Hagerstown

Glauner, T., Grüsser, O.-J., Ott, B. (1990). Defects in schizophrenic patients related to competent use of script. (in preparation)

Glendenning, K.K., Hall, J.A., Diamond, I.T., Hall, W.C. (1975). The pulvinar nucleus of Galago senegalensis. *J. Comp. Neurol.* 161, 419–458

Glezer, V.D. (1985). Spatial and spatial frequency characteristics of receptive fields of the visual cortex and piecewise Fourier analysis. In, Rose, D., Dobson, V.G. (eds.), *Models of the visual cortex.* Wiley, NY, 265–272

Glezer, V.D., Ivanoff, V.A., Tscherbach, T.A. (1973). Investigation of complex and hypercomplex receptive fields of visual cortex of the cat as spatial frequency filters. *Vision Res.,* 13, 1875–1904

Glickstein, M. (1972). Brain mechanisms in reaction time. *Brain Res.* 40, 33–37

Glickstein, M. (1985). Ferrier's mistake. *TINS* 8, 341–344

Glickstein, M. (1988). The discovery of the visual cortex. *Scientific American* 256 (9), 118–127

Glickstein, M., Cohen, J.L., Dixon, B., Gibson, A., Hollins, M., Labossiere, E., Robinson, F. (1980). Cortico-pontine visual projections in macaque monkeys. *J. Comp. Neurol.* 190, 209–229

Glickstein, M., May, J. (1982). Visual control of movement: the circuits which link visual to motor areas of the brain with special reference to the visual input to the pons and cerebellum. In Neff, W.D.

(ed.), *Contributions to Sensory Physiology.* Academic, New York, vol. 7, 103–145

Glickstein, M., May, J., Mercer, B. (1985). Cortico-pontine projection in the macaque: the distribution of labeled cortical cells after large injections of horseradish peroxidase in the pontine nuclei. *J. Comp. Neurol.* 235, 343–359

Glickstein, M., Rizzolatti, G. (1984). Francesco Gennari and the structure of the cerebral cortex. *Trends in Neuroscience* 7, 464–467

Glickstein, M., Whitteridge, D. (1987). Tatsuji Inouye and the mapping of the visual fields on the human cerebral cortex. *T.I.N.S.* 10, 350–353

Gloning, I., Gloning, K. (1964). Raumzeitliche Transformationen bei Körperschemastörungen. *Neuropsychologia* 2, 221–227

Gloning, I., Gloning, K., Hoff, H. (1954). Über Alexie. *Wien. Z. Nervenheilk.* 10, 149

Gloning, I., Gloning, K., Hoff, H. (1955). Die Störung von Zeit und Raum in der Hirnpathologie. *Wien. Z. Nervenkrh.* 10, 346

Gloning, I., Gloning, K., Hoff, H. (1958). Die Halluzinationen in der Hirnpathologie. *Wien. Z. Nervenhlk.* 14, 289–310

Gloning, I., Gloning, K., Hoff, H. (1961). Die Störungen der optischen Zuwendung. *Wien. Klin. Wschr.* 73, 857

Gloning, I., Gloning, K., Hoff, H. (1967). Über optische Halluzinationen. Eine Studie anhand von 241 Patienten mit autoptisch oder chirurgisch verifizierten Läsionen des Okzipitallappens und seiner Grenzgebiete. *Wien. Z. Nervenkrh.* 25, 1–19

Gloning, I., Gloning, K., Hoff, H. (1968). *Neuropsychological symptoms and syndromes in lesions of the occipital lobe and the adjacent areas.* Gauthier-Villars, Paris

Gloning, I., Gloning, K., Hoff, H., Tschabitscher, H. (1966a). Zur Prosopagnosie. *Neuropsychologia* 4, 113–131

Gloning, I., Gloning, K., Jellinger, K., Quatember, R. (1970). A case of 'prosopagnosia' with necropsy findings. *Neuropsychologia* 8, 199–204

Gloning, I., Gloning, K., Jellinger, K., Tschabitscher, H. (1963). Über einen obduzierten Fall von optischer Körperschemastörung und Heautoskopie. *Neuropsychologia* 1, 217–231

Gloning, I., Gloning, K., Seitelberger, F., Tschabitscher, H. (1955). Ein Fall von reiner Wortblindheit mit Obduktionsbefund. *Wien. Z. Nervenhlk.* 12, 194–215

Gloning, I., Gloning, K., Tschabitscher, H. (1962). Die occipitale Blindheit auf vaskulärer Basis. *Graefes Arch. Ophthalm.* 165, 138–177

Gloning, I., Gloning, K., Weingarten, K. (1954). Ueber optische Halluzinationen. *Wien. Z. Nervenhlk.* 10, 58–66

Gloning, I., Gloning, K., Weingarten, K. (1957). Ueber okzipitale Polyopie. *Wien. Z. Nervenkrh.* 13, 224

Gloning, I., Gloning, K., Weingarten, K., Berner, P. (1955). Über einen Fall mit Alexie der Brailleschrift. *Wien. Z. Nervenkrh.* 10, 260–273

Gloning, I., Tschabitscher, H. (1969). Rückbildung einer corticalen Blindheit. *Wien. Z. Nervenheilk.* 11, 406–407

Gloning, K. (1965). *Die cerebral bedingten Störungen des räumlichen Sehens und des Raumerlebens.* Maudrich Verlag, Wien

Gloning, K., Haub, G., Quatember, R. (1967). Standardisierung einer Untersuchungsmethode der sogenannten 'Prosopagnosie'. *Neuropsychologia* 5, 99–101

Gloning, K., Hayden, R. (1953). Ueber Obnubilationen. *Wien. Z. Nervenheilk.* 14, 289

Gloning, K., Quatember, R. (1966). Methodischer Beitrag zur Untersuchung der Prosopagnosie. *Neuropsychologia* 4, 133–141

Glosser, G., Butters, N., Kaplan, E. (1977). Visuoperceptual processes in brain damaged patients on the digit symbol substitution test. *Intern. J. Neuroscience* 7, 59–66

Gloster, J. (1953). Factors influencing the visual judgement of the vertical direction. *Trans. Ophthal. Soc. U.K* 73, 421–433

Glowic, C., Violon, A. (1981). Un cas de prosopagnosie regressive.

Acta Neurol. Belgica 81, 86–97

Glück, G. (1946). Sui disturbi dello schema corporeo in malati mentali con particolare riguardo all'eautoscopia. Schema corporeo e schema psichico. *Rivista di neurologia (Napoli)* 16, 1–45

Gmelin, E. (1791). *Materialien für die Anthropologie.* Vol. I, Cotta, Tübingen

Gnadt, J.W., Andersen, R.A. (1988). Memory related motor planning activity in posterior parietal cortex of macaque. *Exp. Brain Res.* 70, 216–220

Gnadt, J.W., Anderson, R.A., Blatt, G.J. (1986). Spatial memory and motor planning properties of saccade related activity in the lateral intraparietal area of macaque. *Soc. Neurosci. Abstr.* 12, 458

Gochin, P.M., Miller, E.K., Gross, C.G., Gerstein, G.L. (1991). Functional interactions among neurons in inferior temporal cortex of the awake macaque. *Exp. Brain Res.* 84, 505–516

Godschalk, M., Lemon, R.N., Nijs, H.G.T., Kuypers, H.G.J.M. (1981). Behaviour of neurons in monkey periarcuate and precentral cortex before and during visually guided arm and hand movements. *Exp. Brain Res.* 44, 113–116

Godwin-Austen, R.B. (1965). A case of visual disorientation. *J. Neurol. Neurosurg. Psychiat.* 28, 453–458

Goethe, J.W. v. (1961). *Dichtung und Wahrheit.* In Goethes Werke, Hamburger Ausg. Bd. 9, Hamburg

Goethe, J.W. von (1810). *Zur Farbenlehre. Didaktischer Teil.* Repr. in Goethe, J.W. von (1912), Naturwissenschaftliche Schriften, (K. Goedeke, ed.) Vol 2. Cotta, Stuttgart

Gogol, D. (1874). Aphasie, Apraxie, Agnosie; cited by R. Thiele in Bumke (ed.). *Handb.für Geisteskrankh.* VI. Springer, 1928, Berlin, 243–365

Goldberg, E. (1990). Associative agnosias and the functions of the left hemisphere. *J. Clin. Exp. Neuropsych.* 12, 467–484

Goldberg, E., Gerstman, L.J., Mattis, S., Hughes, J.E., Sirio, C.A., Bilder, R.M. (1982). Selective effects of cholinergic treatment on verbal memory in posttraumatic amnesia. *J. Clin. Neuropsychol.* 4, 219–234

Goldberg, M.E., Bruce, C.J. (1985). Cerebral cortical activity associated with orientationof visual attention in the rhesus monkey. *Vision Res.* 25, 471–481

Goldberg, M.E., Bruce, C.J., Ungerleider, L., Mishkin, M. (1982). Role of the striate cortex in generation of smooth pursuit eye movements (Abstract). *Ann. Neurol.* 12, 113

Goldberg, M.E., Bushnell, M.C. (1981). Behavioral enhancement of visual responses in monkey cerebral cortex. II. Modulation in frontal eye fields specifically related to saccades. *J. Neurophysiol.* 46, 773–787

Goldberg, M.E., Colby, C.L. (1989). The neurophysiology of spatial vision. In Goodglass, H., Damasio, A.R. (eds.), *Handbook of Neuropsychology, Vol. 2.* Elsevier, Amsterdam, N.Y., Oxford, 301–316

Goldberg, M.E., Robinson, D.L. (1977). Visual responses of neurons in monkey inferior parietal lobule: The physiologic substrate of attention and neglect. (Abstr.) *Neurology* 27, 350

Goldberg, M.E., Robinson, D.L. (1980). The significance of enhanced visual responses in posterior parietal cortex. *Behav. Brain Sci.* 3, 503–505

Goldberg, M.E., Wurtz, R.H. (1972). Activity of superior colliculus in behaving monkey. I. Visual receptive fields of single neurons. *J. Neurophysiol.* 35, 542–559

Goldberg, M.E., Wurtz, R.H. (1972). Activity of superior colliculus in behaving monkey. II. Effect of attention on neuronal responses. *J. Neurophysiol.* 35, 560–574

Goldenberg, G. (1986). Neglect in a patient with partial callosal disconnection. *Neuropsychologia* 24, 397–403

Goldenberg, G. (1987). *Neurologische Grundlage bildlicher Vorstellungen.* Springer, Wien, New York

Goldenberg, G. (1989). The ability of patients with brain damage to generate mental visual images. *Brain* 112, 305–325

Goldenberg, G., Mamoli, B., Binder, H. (1985). Die Simultanagnosie als Symptom der Schädigung extrastriärer visueller Rindenfelder: eine Fallstudie. *Nervenarzt* 56, 682–690

Goldiamond, I., Hawkins, W.F. (1958). Vexierversuch: the log-relationship between word-frequency and recognition obtained in the absence of stimulus words. *J. Exp. Psychol.* 56, 457–463

Goldman, P.S., Rosvold, H.E. (1970). Localization of function within the dorsolateral prefrontal cortex of the rhesus monkey. *Exp. Neurol.* 27, 291–304

Goldman-Rakic, P.S. (1984). The frontal lobes: Uncharted provinces of the brain. *Trends in Neuroscience* 7, 425–429

Goldman-Rakic, P.S. (1987). Circuitry of the primate prefrontal cortex and the regulation of behavior by representational memory. *In Mountcastle, V., Blum, F., Geiger, S.R. (eds.), Handbook of Physiology* 5 (Part 1, Ch. 9). Waverly Press, 373–417

Goldman-Rakic, P.S. (1988). Topography of cognition: parallel distributed networks in primate association cortex. *Ann. Rev. Neurosci.* 11, 137–156

Goldstein, A.G. (1965). Learning of inverted and normallly oriented faces in children and adults. *Psychon. Science* 3, 447–448

Goldstein, A.G., Chance, J. (1971). Visual recognition memory for complex configurations. *Percept. Psychophys.* 9, 237–241

Goldstein, A.G., Chance, J.E. (1964). Recogniton of children's faces. *Child Development* 35, 129–136

Goldstein, A.G., Mackenberg, E.G. (1966). Recognition of human faces from isolated facial features: a developmental study. *Psychonomic Science* 6, 149–150

Goldstein, H., Cameron, H. (1952). New method of communication for the aphasic patient. *Ariz. Med.* 8, 17–21

Goldstein, K. (1908). Zur Theorie der Halluzinationen. Studien über normale und pathologische Wahrnehmung. *Arch. f. Psychiat. u. Nervenkr.* 44, 584 and 1036

Goldstein, K. (1923). Über die Abhängigkeit der Bewegungen von optischen Vorgängen. Bewegungsstörungen bei Seelenblinden. *Monatsschr. f.Psychiat. u. Neurol.* 54, 141

Goldstein, K. (1927). Die Lokalisation in der Grosshirnrinde. Nach den Erfahrungen am kranken Menschen. In Bethe, A., Bergmann, G., Embden, G., Ellinger, A. (eds.), *Handbuch der normalen und pathologischen Physiologie.* Vol. X, Spezielle Physiologie des Zentralnervensystems der Wirbeltiere. Springer, Berlin, 600–842

Goldstein, K. (1934). Über monokuläre Doppelbilder. Ihre Entstehung und Bedeutung für die Theorie von der Function des Nervensystems. *Jahrbuch f. Psychiat.* 51, 16

Goldstein, K. (1939). *The Organism.* American Book Publisher, New York

Goldstein, K. (1943). Some remarks on Russell Brain's article concerning visual object-agnosia. *J. Nervous Mental Disease* 98, 148–153

Goldstein, K. (1948). *Language and language disturbances.* Grune & Stratton, N.Y.

Goldstein, K., Gelb, A. (1917/1918). Psychologische Analysen hirnpathologischer Fälle auf Grund von Untersuchungen Hirnverletzter. *Psychol. Forschung,* Vol. 6, 1-

Goldstein, K., Gelb, A. (1918). Psychologische Analysen hirnpathologischer Fälle auf Grund von Untersuchungen Hirnverletzter. I. Abhandlung: Zur Psychologie des optischen Wahrnehmungs-und Erkennungsvorganges. *Z. ges. Neurol. Psychiat.* 41, 1–142

Goldstein, L.H., Canavan, A.G.M., Polkey, C.E. (1989). Cognitive mapping after unilateral temporal lobectomy. *Neuropsychologia* 27, 167–177

Goldstein, M.N., Joynt, R.J., Goldblatt, D. (1971). Word blindness with intact central visual fields. *Neurology* 21, 873–876

Gollin, E.S. (1960). Developmental studies of visual recognition of incomplete objects. *Percept. Mot. Skills* 2, 289–298

Goltz, F. (1892). Über die Verrichtungen des Grosshirns. *Pflüger's Arch. ges. Physiol.* 51, 570–614

Gombrich, E.H. (1984). Maske und Gesicht: die Wahrnehmung physiognomischer Ähnlichkeit im Leben und in der Kunst. In Gombrich, E.H. (ed.), *Bild und Auge*. Klett-Cotta, Stuttgart 105–134

Gomori, A.J., Hawryluk, G.A. (1984). Visual agnosia without alexia. *Neurology* 34, 947–950

Goodale, M.A., Milner, A.D., Jakobson, L.S., Carey, D.P. (1991). A neurological dissociation between perceiving objects and grasping them. *Nature* 349, 154–156

Goodall, J. (1965). Chimpanzees of the Gombe stream reserve. In DeVore, I. (ed), *Primate behavior*. Holt Rinehart, Winston, N.Y., 425–473

Goodall, J. (1986). *The chimpanzees of Gombe. Patterns of behavior*. Belknap, Cambridge, Mass.

Goodglass, H., Barton, M. (1963). Handedness and differential perception of verbal stimuli in left and right visual fields. *Percept. Motor Skills* 17, 851–854

Goodglass, H., Cohen, M.L. (1954). *Disturbance in body-part comprehension in aphasia*. Paper presented at the meeting of the American Psychological Association, Washington D.C.

Goodglass, H., Gleason, J.B., Hyde, M.R. (1970). Some dimensions of auditory language comprehension in aphasia. *J. Speech Hearing Research* 13, 595–606

Goodglass, H., Graves, R., Landis, T. (1980). Le role de l'hemisphere droit dans la lecture. *Rev. Neurol.* 136, 669–673

Goodglass, H., Hyde, M.R., Blumstein, S. (1969). Frequency, picturability, and the availability of nouns in aphasia. *Cortex* 5, 104–119

Goodglass, H., Kaplan, E. (1972). *The assessment of aphasia and related disorders*. Lea and Febiger, Philadelphia, 2nd ed. 1983

Goodglass, H., Kaplan, E., Weintraub, S. (1983). *Boston Naming Test*. Lea and Febiger, Philadelphia

Goodglass, H., Klein, B., Carey, P., Jones, K. (1966). Specific semantic word categories in aphasia. *Cortex* 2, 74–89

Goodglass, H., Wingfield, A., Hyde, M.R., Theurkauf, J.C. (1986). Category specific dissociations in naming and recognition by aphasic patients. *Cortex* 22, 87–102

Goodkin, D.A. (1980). Mechanisms of bromocriptine-induced hallucinations. *New Engl. J. Med.* 302, 1479

Goodwin, D.M. (1989). *Dictionary of Neuropsychology*. Springer, New York

Gordon, H.W., Lee, P.A. (1986). A relationship between gonadotropins and visuospatial function. *Neuropsychologia* 24, 563–576

Goren, C.C., Sarty, M., Wu, R.W.K. (1975). Visual following and pattern discrimination of face-like stimuli by newborn infants. *Pediatrics* 56, 544–549

Gottschaldt, K. (1926). Über den Einfluss der Erfahrung auf die Wahrnehmung von Figuren auf die Sichtbarkeit in umfassenden Konfigurationen. *Psychol. Forsch.* 8, 261–317

Gottschaldt, K. (1929). Vergleichende Untersuchungen über die Wirkung figuraler Einprägung und den Einfluss spezifischer Geschehensverläufe auf die Auffassung optischer Komplexe. *Psychol. Forsch.* 12, 1–87

Gouras, P. (1974). Opponent-colour cells in different layers of foveal striate cortex. *J. Physiol.* 238, 583–602

Gouras, P., Krüger, J. (1979). Responses of cells in foveal visual cortex of the monkey to pure color contrast. *J. Neurophysiol.* 42, I, 850–860

Gouras, P., Padmos, P. (1974). Identification of cone mechanisms in graded responses of foveal striate cortex. *J. Physiol.* 238, 569–581

Gowers, W.R. (1887). *Lectures on the diagnosis of diseases of the brain*. 2nd Edition. J. and A. Churchill, London

Gowers, W.R. (1888). *A manual of diseases of the nervous system*. J. and A. Churchill, London

Gowers, W.R. (1892). *Handbuch der Nervenkrankheiten*. 3 Vols. Cohen, Bonn

Gowers, W.R. (1902). *Epilepsie*. Deuticke, Leipzig

Grabowska, A., Semenza, C., Denes, G., Testa, S. (1989). Impaired grating discrimination following right hemisphere damage. *Neuropsychologia* 27, 259–263

Graefe, A. von (1856). Über die Untersuchung des Gesichtsfeldes bei amblyopischen Affectionen. *Graefes Arch. Ophthalmol.* 2, 258–298

Graefe, A. von (1935). Briefe an F.C. Donders. 1852–1870. *Klin. Monatsblätter f. Augenheilkunde* 95, Beiheft 1

Grafstein, B. (1956a). Mechanism of spreading cortical depression. *J. Neurophysiol.* 19, 154–171

Grafstein, B. (1956b). Locus of propagation of spreading cortical depression. *J. Neurophysiol.* 19, 309–316

Grafstein, B., Forman, D.S. (1980). Intracellular transport in neurons. *Physiol. Rev.* 60, 1167–1283

Graham, C.H. (1965). Perception of movement. In Graham, C.H. (ed.), *Vision and visual perception*. John Wiley & Sons, New York, 575–588

Granit, R. (1947). *Sensory mechanisms of the retina*. Oxford University Press, London

Granit, R. (1948). Neural organization of the retinal elements, as revealed by polarization. *J. Neurophysiol.* 11, 239–251

Granit, R. (1950). The organization of the vertebrate retinal elements. *Erg. Physiol.* 46, 31–70

Gratiolet, P. (1865). *De la physionomie et des mouvements d'expression*. Paris

Graveleau, Ph., Viader, F., Masson, M., Cambier, J. (1986). Négligence thalamique. *Rev. Neurol.* 142, 425–430

Graves, R., Goodglass, H., Landis, T. (1982). Mouth asymmetry during spontaneous speech. *Neuropsychologia* 20, 371–381

Graves, R., Landis, T. (1985). Hemispheric control of speech expression in aphasia: a mouth asymmetry study. *Arch. Neurol.* 42, 249–251

Graves, R., Landis, T. (1990). Asymmetry in mouth opening during different speech tasks. *Intern. J. Psychol.* 25, 179–189

Graves, R., Landis, T., Goodglass, H. (1981). Laterality and sex differences for visual recognition of emotional and non-emotional words. *Neuropsychologia* 19, 95–102

Graves, R., Landis, T., Simpson, C. (1985). On the interpretation of mouth asymmetry. *Neuropsychologia* 23, 121–122

Gray, C.M., Engel, A.K., König, P., Singer, W. (1990). Stimulus-dependent neuronal oscillations in cat visual cortex. I. Receptive field properties and feature dependence. *Eur. J. Neurosci.* (in press)

Gray, C.M., König, P., Engel, A.K., Singer, W. (1989). Oscillatory responses in cat visual cortex exhibit inter-columnar synchronization which reflects global stimulus properties. *Nature* 338, 334–337

Gray, J.H., Fraser, W.L., Lendar, I. (1983). Recognition of emotion from facial expression in mental handicap. *Brit. J. Psychiat.* 142, 566–571

Graybiel, A.M. (1974). Studies on the anatomical organization of posterior association cortex. *J. Neurosci.* 3, 205–214

Green, G.J., Lessell, S. (1977). Acquired cerebral dyschromatopsia. *Arch Ophthalmol.* 95, 121–128

Greenblatt, S.H. (1973). Alexia without agraphia or hemianopia: Anatomical analysis of an autopsied case. *Brain* 96, 307–316

Greenblatt, S.H. (1976). Subangular alexia without agraphia or hemianopia. *Brain and Language* 3, 229–245

Greenblatt, S.H. (1977). Neurosurgery and the anatomy of reading. A practical review. *Neurosurgery* 1, 6–15

Greenblatt, S.H. (1983). Localization of lesions in alexia. In A. Kertesz (ed.), *Localization in Neuropsychology*. Academic Press, New York, 324–356

Gregory, R.L. (1966). *Eye and Brain*. MacGraw-Hill, New York

Gregory, R.L. (1970). *The intelligent eye*. MacGraw-Hill, New York

Gregory, R.L. (1977). Vision with isoluminant colour contrast. 1. A projection technique and observations. *Perception* 6, 113–119

Gregory, R.L., Wallace, J.G. (1963). *Recovery from early blindness: a case study.* Exp. Psychol. Soc. Monogr. Heffer & Sons, London

Grehn, F., Grüsser, O.-J., Stange, D. (1981). The effects of increased intraocular pressure on the response of cat retinal ganglion cells. In Maffei, L. (ed.), *Doc. Ophthal. Proc. Series*, vol. 30, Dr. W. Junk Publishers, The Hague, 31–35

Grehn, F., Grüsser, O.-J., Stange, D. (1984) Effect of short-term intraocular pressure increase on cat retinal ganglion cell activity. *Behav. Brain Res.* 14, 109–121

Greve, K.W., Bauer, R.M. (1989). Implicit learning of faces in prosopagnosia: an application of the mere-exposure paradigm. *J.Clin.Exp.Neuropsychol.* 11, 44

Griesinger, W. (1867). *Die Pathologie und Therapie der psychischen Krankheiten.* Stuttgart. Reprint Bonset, Amsterdam 1964

Griesinger, W. (1868). Über einige epileptoide Zustände. *Arch. Psychiat. Nervenkrh.* 1, 320–333

Grinberg, D.L., Williams, D.R. (1985). Stereopsis with chromatic signals from the blue sensitive mechanism. *Vision Res.* 25, 531–537

Grind, W.A. van de (1988). The possible structure and role of neuronal smart mechanisms in vision. *Cognitive Systems* 2, 163–180

Grind, W.A. van de (1990). Smart mechanisms for the visual evaluation and control of self-motion. In Warren, R., Wertheim A. (eds), *Perception and Control of Self-Motion.* Lawrence Erlbaum Ass., Hillsdale, N.J., 357–398

Grind, W.A. van de, Grüsser, O.-J., (1981). Frequency transfer properties of cat retina horizontal cells. *Vision Res.* 21, 1565–1572

Grind, W.A. van de, Grüsser, O.-J., Lunkenheimer, H.U. (1973). Temporal transfer properties of the afferent visual system. Psychophysical, neurophysiological and theoretical investigations. In Jung, R. (ed.), *Handbook of Sensory Physiology*, Vol. VII/3, Chapter 7, Springer, Berlin, Heidelberg, New York, 431–573

Grind, W.A. van de, Koenderink, J.J., van Doorn, A.J. (1986). The distribution of human motion detector properties in the monocular visual field. *Vision Res.* 26, 797–810

Grind, W.A. van de, Koenderink, J.J., van Doorn, A.J. (1987). Influence of contrast on foveal and peripheral detection of coherent motion in moving random-dot patterns. *J. Optical Soc.of America A* 4, 1643–1652

Grind, W.A. van de, Koenderink, J.J., van Doorn, A.J. (1991). *Viewing —distance invariance of movement detection.* To be subm. June 1991

Grind, W.A. van de, van Doorn, J.A., Koenderink, J.J. (1983). Detection of coherent movement in peripherally viewed random-dot patterns. *J.Optical Soc. of America* 73, 1674–1683

Groenouw, A. (1892). Ueber doppelseitige Hemianopsie centralen Ursprunges. *Arch. Psychiat. Nervenkrh.* 23, 339–366

Gross, C.G. (1972). Visual functions of inferotemporal cortex. In Jung, R. (ed.), *Handbook of Sensory Physiology. Visual Centers in the Brain.* Springer Verlag, Berlin, vol. VII, pt. 3B. p. 451–485

Gross, C.G. (1973). Inferotemporal cortex and vision. In Stellar, E., Sprague, J.M. (eds.), *Progress in Physiological Psychology*, Vol. 5, Academic Press, NY, 77–124

Gross, C.G. (1973). Inferotemporal cortex in vison. *Prog. Psychobiol. Physiol. Psychol.* 5, 77–123

Gross, C.G., Bender, D.B., Gerstein, G.L. (1979). Activity of inferior temporal neurons in behaving monkeys. *Neuropsychologia* 17, 215–229

Gross, C.G., Bender, D.B., Mishkin, M. (1977). Contributions of the corpus callosum and the anterior commissure to the visual activation of inferior temporal neurons. *Brain Res.* 131, 227–239

Gross, C.G., Bender, D.B., Rocha-Miranda, C.E. (1969). Visual receptive fields of neurons in inferotemporal cortex of the monkey. *Science* 166, 1303–1306

Gross, C.G., Bender, D.B., Rocha-Miranda, C.E. (1973). Inferotemporal cortex: A single unit analysis. In: F.O. Schmitt, F.G. Worden (eds.), *The Neurosciences: A Third Study Program.* MIT Press, Cambridge, Mass., 229–238

Gross, C.G., Bruce, C.J., Desimone, R., Fleming, J., Gattass, R. (1981). Cortical visual areas of the temporal lobe: three areas in the macaque. In Woolsey, C.N. (ed.), *Multiple Visual Areas.* Humana, Clifton, N.J., vol. 2, 187–216

Gross, C.G., Cowey, A., Manning, F.J. (1971). Further analysis of visual discrimination deficits following foveal prestriate and inferotemporal lesions in rhesus monkeys. *J. Comp. Physiol. Psychol.* 76, 1–7

Gross, C.G., Desimone, R., Albright, T.D., Schwartz, E.L. (1985). Inferior temporal cortex and pattern recognition. In Chagas, C., Gattas, R., Gross, C. (eds.), *Pattern recognition mechanics. Exp. Brain Res. Suppl.* 11, 179–201

Gross, C.G., Mishkin, M. (1977). The neural basis of stimulus equivalence across retinal translation. In Harnad, S., Doty, R., Jaynes, J., Goldstein, L., Krauthamer, G. (eds.), *Lateralization in the nervous system.* Academic, New York, 109–122

Gross, C.G., Rocha-Miranda, C.E., Bender, D.B. (1972). Visual properties of neurons in infero-temporal cortex of the macaque. *J. Neurophysiol.* 35, 96–111

Gross, C.G., Schiller, P.H., Wells, C., Gerstein, G.L. (1967). Single unit activity in temporal association cortex of the monkey. *J. Neurophysiol.* 30, 833–843

Gross, C.G., Weiskrantz, L. (1964). Some changes in behavior produced by lateral frontal lesions in the macaque. In J.M. Warren, K. Akert, (eds.), *The Frontal Granular Cortex and Behavior.* MacGraw-Hill, New York, 74–101

Gross, M.M. (1972). Hemispheric specialization for processing of visually presented verbal and spatial stimuli. *Percept. Psychophys.* 12, 357–363

Grossberg, S. (1983). The quantized geometry of visual space: the coherent computation of depth, form, lightness. *Behav. Brain Sci.* 6, 625–692

Grossi, D., Fragassi, N.A., Orsini, A., De Falco, F.A., Sepe, O. (1984). Residual reading capability in a patient with alexia without agraphia. *Brain and Language* 23, 337–348

Grotstein, J.S. (1983). The experience of oneself as a double. *Hillside J. Clin. Psychiat.* 5, 259–304

Gruhle, H.W. (1932). Die Psychopathologie. In *Handbuch der Geisteskrankheiten, vol 9, Die Schizophrenie.* Springer, Berlin, 135–210

Gruhle, H.W. (1956). *Verstehende Psychologie (Erlebnislehre).* Thieme, Stuttgart

Gruzelier, J. (1979). Synthesis and critical review of the evidence for hemisphere asymmetries of function in psychopathology. In Gruzelier, J., Flor-Henry, P. (eds.), *Hemisphere Asymmetries of Function in Psychopathology.* Elsevier/North-Holland Biomedical Press, Amsterdam, 647–672

Gruzelier, J., Flor-Henry, P. (eds.) (1979). *Hemisphere Asymmetries of Function in Psychpathology.* Elsevier/North-Holland Biomedical Press, Amsterdam

Gruzelier, J., Hammond, N. (1976). Schizophrenia: a dominant hemisphere temporal-limbic disorder? *Res. Communc. Psychol. Psychiat. Behav.* 1, 33–72

Gruzelier, J.H. (1981). Cerebral laterality and psychopathology: fact and fiction. *Psychological Medicine* 11, 93–108

Grünau, M. von (1978): Form information is necessary for the perception of motion. *Vision Res.* 19, 839–841

Grünau, M.W. (1978). Dissociation and interaction of form and motion information in the human visual system. *Vision Res.* 18, 1485–1489

Grünbaum, A. (1931). Wahrnehmung und Motorik bei der Agnosie. *Arch. Psychiat. Nervenkr.* 95, 725–730

Grünbaum, A.A. (1930). Ueber Apraxie. *Neurol. Zbl. Lpz.* 55, 788

Grünthal, E. (1957). Über phantastische Gesichtserscheinungen bei langdauerndem Augenschluss. *Psychiat. Neurol.* (Basel) 133, 193–206

Grüsser, O.-J. (1957). *Beeinflussung der Flimmerreaktion einzelner corticaler Neurone durch elektrische Reizung unspezifischer Thalamuskerne.* Excerpta med. (Amst.), Intern. Congr. Ser. 11, 148

Grüsser, O.-J. (1960). Mikroelektrodenuntersuchungen zur Konvergenz vestibulärer und retinaler Afferenzen an einzelnen Neruonen des optischen Cortex der Katze. *Pflügers Arch. ges. Physiol.* 270, 227–238

Grüsser, O.-J. (1975). *Einleitung zu 'Neurobiologische und nachrichtentechnische Grundlagen des Lesens' und 'Neurobiologie der visuellen Gestaltwahrnehmung und des Lesens'.* In: *Lesen und Leben.* Buchhändler Vereinigung GmbH, Frankfurt a.M., 36–64

Grüsser, O.-J. (1975). Hirnmechanismen der visuellen Wahrnehmung. In Kurzrock, R. (ed.), *Das menschliche Gehirn.* Colloqium Verlag, Berlin, 21–33

Grüsser, O.-J. (1977). Neurobiologische Grundlagen der Zeichenerkennung. In Posner, R., Reinecke, H.-P. (eds.), *Zeichenprozesse. Semiotische Forschung in den Einzelwissenschaften.* Akademische Verlagsgesellschaft Athenaion, Wiesbaden, 13–45

Grüsser, O.-J. (1979). Cat ganglion cell receptive fields and the role of horizontal cells in their generation. In Schmitt, F.O., Worden, F.G. (eds.), *Neurosciences, fourth study program.* MIT Press, Cambridge Mass, 247–275

Grüsser, O.-J. (1982). Mammalian horizontal cells: spatial and temporal transfer properties. In Drujan, D.D., Laufer, M. (eds.), *The S-potential.* A.R. Liss, New York, 207–233

Grüsser, O.-J. (1982). Space perception and the gazemotor system. *Human Neurobiol.* 1, 73–76

Grüsser, O.-J. (1983). Multimodal structure of the extrapersonal space. In Hein, A., Jeannerod, M. (eds.), *Spatially oriented behavior.* Springer, New York, Berlin, Heidelberg, 327–352

Grüsser, O.-J. (1983). Zeit und Gehirn. Zeitliche Aspekte der Signalverarbeitung in den Sinnesorganen und im Zentralnervensystem. In Peichl, A., Mohler, A. (eds.), *Die Zeit.* Oldenburg-Verlag, 79–132

Grüsser, O.-J. (1984). Face recognition within the reach of neurobiology and beyond it. *Hum. Neurobiol.* 3, 183–190

Grüsser, O.-J. (1984). J.E. Purkyne's contributions to the physiology of the visual, vestibular and the oculomotor system. *Hum. Neurobiol.* 3, 129–144

Grüsser, O.-J. (1986) *Discussion.* In Freund, H.-J., Büttner, U., Cohen, B., Noth, J. (eds.), *Progress in Brain Research 64.* Elsevier Sci. Publ. (Biomedical Div.), 85–86

Grüsser, O.-J. (1986). Interaction of efferent and afferent signals in visual perception. A history of ideas and experimental paradigms. *Acta Psychol.* 63, 3–21

Grüsser, O.-J. (1986). Some recent studies on the quantitative analysis of efference copy mechanisms in visual perception. *Acta Psychol.* 63, 49–62

Grüsser, O.-J. (1986). The effect of gaze motor signals and spatially directed attention on eye movements and visual perception. In Freund, H.-J., Büttner, U., Cohen B., Noth, J. (eds.), *Progress in Brain research 64,* Elsevier Sci. Publ (Biomedical Div.), 391–404

Grüsser, O.-J. (1987a). *Justinus Kerner. 1786–1862. Arzt-Poet-Geisterseher. Nebst Anmerkungen zum Uhland-Kerner-Kreis und zur Medizin-und Geistesgeschichte im Zeitalter der Romantik.* Springer, Berlin, Heidelberg, New York

Grüsser, O.-J. (1987b). Von der Perzeption zur Kognition. Der Beitrag der Neurologie zum Verständnis höherer Hirnfunktionen. *Aus Forschung und Medizin 2,* 47–60

Grüsser, O.-J. (1988). Die phylogenetische Hirnentwicklung und die funktionelle Lateralisation der menschlichen Grosshirnrinde. In Oepen, G. (ed.), *Psychiatrie des rechten und linken Gehirns. Neuropsychologische Ansätze zum Verständnis von 'Persönlichkeit', 'Depression' und 'Schizophrenie'.* Deutsche Ärzte, Köln, 34–50

Grüsser, O.-J. (1988). Funktionelle Lateralisierung des Gehirns. Vom Spurenlesen zum Lesen. *Ärztliche Praxis* 40 oder 60 (11), 249–250

Grüsser, O.-J. (1989). Gehirnvorgänge und bildnerische Kreaktivität. Phylogenetische, historische und individuelle Bedingungen. In Petsche, H. (ed.), *Musik-Gehirn-Spiel: Beiträge zum 4. Herbert von Karajan Symposium in Wien, 24. und 25. Mai 1988 (Herbert von Karajan zum 80. Geburtstag).* Birkhäuser, Basel-Boston-Berlin, 53–90

Grüsser, O.-J. (1989). Quantitative visual psychophysics during the period of European enlightenment. The studies of the astronomer and mathematician Tobias Mayer (1723–1762) on visual acuity and colour perception. *Doc. Ophthalmol.* 71, 93–111

Grüsser, O.-J. (1990). 'Heautognosie' des Gehirns oder Grenzen neurobiologischer Analysen kognitiver Prozese. In Molden, O. (ed.), *Freiheit-Ordnung-Verantwortung.* Europäisches Forum Alpbach 1990, 81–118

Grüsser, O.-J. (1990a). Vom Ort der Seele. Cerebrale Lokalisationstheorien in der Zeit zwischen Albertus Magnus und Paul Broca. *Aus Forschung und Medizin* 5, 75–96

Grüsser, O.-J. (1990b). On the 'Seat of the soul': Cerebral localization theories in mediaevel times and later. In Elsner, N., Roth, G. (eds.), *Brain-Perception-Cognition: proceedings of the 18th Göttingen Neurobiology Conference = Gehirn-Wahrnehmung-Kognition,* Thieme, Stuttgart, New York, 73–81

Grüsser, O.-J. (1991). Impairment of perception and recognition of face, facial expression and gestures in schizophrenic children and adolescents. In Eggers, Ch. (ed.), *Schizophrenia and youth.* Springer, Heidelberg, 100–118

Grüsser, O.-J., Behrens, F. (1988). Open loop optokinetic nystagmus of the Squirrel monkey evoked from a BoTx-immobilized eye. *Soc. Neurosci. Abstr.* 14, 797

Grüsser, O.-J., Creutzfeldt, O. (1957). Eine neurophysiologische Grundlage des Brücke-Bartley-Effektes: Maxima der Impulsfrequenz retinaler und corticaler Neurone bei Flimmerlicht mittlerer Frequenzen. *Pflügers Arch.* 263, 668–681

Grüsser, O.-J., Finkelstein, D., Grüsser-Cornehls, U. (1968). The effect of stimulus velocity on the response of movement-sensitive neurons of the frog's retina. *Pflügers Arch. ges. Physiol.* 300, 49–66

Grüsser, O.-J., Fuhry, L. (1989a). Visual evoked potentials of the Java monkey (Macaca fascicularis) induced by face and non-face stimuli. Abstracts, ENA 12th Annual Meeting/EBBS 21st Annual Meeting, Turin September 1989, 316

Grüsser, O.-J., Fuhry, L. (1989b). Face-responsive components in the temporal lobe visual evoked potentials (EPs) of Java monkeys. *Soc. Neurosci. Abstr.* 15, 120

Grüsser, O.-J., Grüsser-Cornehls, U. (1960). Mikroelektrodenuntersuchungen zur Konvergenz vestibulärer und retinaler Afferenzen an einzelnen Neuronen des optischen Cortex der Katze. *Pflügers Arch.* 270, 227–238

Grüsser, O.-J., Grüsser-Cornehls, U. (1961). Reaktionsmuster einzelner Neurone im Geniculatum laterale und visuellem Cortex der Katze bei Reizung mit optokinetischen Streifenmustern. In Jung, R., Kornhuber, H. (eds.), *Neurophysiologie und Psychophysik des visuellen Systems.* Springer, Berlin-Göttingen-Heidelberg, p. 313–324

Grüsser, O.-J., Grüsser-Cornehls, U. (1962). Periodische Aktivierungsphasen visueller Neurone nach kurzen Lichtreizen verschiedener Dauer. Beziehungen zu den periodischen Nachbildern und dem Charpentier-Intervall. *Pflügers Arch.* 275, 292–311

Grüsser, O.-J., Grüsser-Cornehls, U. (1965). Neurophysiologische Grundlagen des Binocularsehens. *Arch. Psychiat. Nervenkr.* 207, 296–317

Grüsser, O.-J., Grüsser-Cornehls, U. (1968a). Neurophysiologische Grundlagen visueller angeborener Auslösemechanismen beim Frosch. *Z. vergl. Physiol.* 59, 1–24

Grüsser, O.-J., Grüsser-Cornehls, U. (1969). Neurophysiologie des Bewegungssehens. Bewegungsempfindliche und richtungsspezifische Neurone im visuellen System. *Erg. Physiol.* 61, 178–265

Grüsser, O.-J., Grüsser-Cornehls, U. (1972). Interaction of vestibular and visual inputs in the visual system. *Progress in Brain Research* 37, 573–583

Grüsser, O.-J., Grüsser-Cornehls, U. (1973). Neuronal mechanisms of visual movement perception and some psychophysical and behavioural correlations. In Jung, R. (ed.), *Handbook of sensory physiology*, vol.VII/3, Springer, Berlin, Heidelberg, New York, 333–429

Grüsser, O.-J., Grüsser-Cornehls, U. (1973). Physiologie des Sehens. In Schmidt, R.F. (ed.), *Grundriss der Sinnesphysiologie*. Springer, Berlin, Heidelberg, New York

Grüsser, O.-J., Grüsser-Cornehls, U. (1976). Neurophysiology of the anuran visual systems. In Llinas, R., Precht, W. (eds.), *Frog neurobiology*. Springer, Berlin, Heidelberg, 297–385

Grüsser, O.-J., Grüsser-Cornehls, U. (1978). Physiology of vision. In *Fundamentals of sensory physiology*. Springer, New York-Heidelberg-Berlin, 126–179

Grüsser, O.-J., Grüsser-Cornehls, U. (1982). Mother-child holding patterns: A study of Western art. Résumés des Communications; Congrès Internationale de Paléontologie Humaine, 213

Grüsser, O.-J., Grüsser-Cornehls, U., Kusel, R., Przybyszewski, A. (1984). Different responses of cat ganglion cells to ischemia and eyeball deformation. *Soc. Neurosci. Abstr.* 10, 326

Grüsser, O.-J., Grüsser-Cornehls, U., Kusel, R., Przybyszewski, A. (1989). Responses of retinal ganglion cells to eyeball deformation. A neurophysiological basis for pressure phosphenes. *Vision Res.* 29, 181–194

Grüsser, O.-J., Grüsser-Cornehls, U., Müller, J. (1984). Neurophysiologische Grundlagen der Druckphosphene. In Herzau, V. (ed.). *Pathophysiologie des Sehens*. Enke, Stuttgart, 21–37

Grüsser, O.-J., Grüsser-Cornehls, U., Saur, G. (1959). Reaktionen einzelner Neurone im optischen Cortex der Katze nach elektrischer Polarisation des Labyrinths. *Pflügers Arch.* 269, 593–612

Grüsser, O.-J., Grüsser-Cornehls, U., Schreiter, U. (1981). Responses of cat retinal ganglion cells to eyeball deformation. A neurophysiological basis of pressure phosphenes. In Maffei, L. (ed.). *Pathophysiology of the visual system*. Junk, The Hague, 36–52

Grüsser, O.-J., Grützner, A. (1958). Neurophysiologische Grundlagen der periodischen Nachbildphasen nach kurzen Lichtblitzen. *Graefes Arch. Ophthalmol.* 160, 65–93

Grüsser, O.-J., Grützner, A. (1958). Reaktionen einzelner Neurone des optischen Cortex der Katze nach elektrischen Reizserien des Nervus opticus. *Arch. Psychiat. Z. f. d. ges. Neurol.*(Arch. Psychiat. Nervenkr.) 197, 405–432

Grüsser, O.-J., Guldin, W. (1991). *Changes in perceived horizon height during vertical optokinetic stimulation: visual-vestibular interactions.* Abstr. ENA/EBBS-Meeting, Cambridg (in press)

Grüsser, O.-J., Hagner, M. (1990). On the history of deformation phosphenes and the idea of internal light generated in the eye for the purpose of vision. *Doc. Ophthalmol.* 74, 57–85

Grüsser, O.-J., Hagner, M., Przybyszewski, A. (1989). The effect of dark adaptation on the responses of cat retinal ganglion cells to eyeball deformation. *Vision Res.* 29, 1059–1068

Grüsser, O.-J., Hellner, K.A., Grüsser-Cornehls, U. (1962). Die Informationsübertragung im afferenten visuellen System. *Kybernetik* 1, 175–192

Grüsser, O.-J., Kapp, H. (1958). Reaktionen retinaler Neruone nach Lichtblitzen. II. Doppelblitze mit wechselndem Blitzintervall. *Pflügers Arch.* 266, 111–129

Grüsser, O.-J., Kirchoff, N., Naumann, A. (1990). Brain mechanisms for recognition of faces, facial expression, and gestures: neuropsychological and electroencephalographic studies in normals, brain-lesioned patients, and schizophrenics. In Cohen B, Bodis-Wollner I (eds.), *Vision and the Brain*. Raven, New York, 165–193

Grüsser, O.-J., Kirsten, M., Krizic, A., Weiss, L. (1985). The time course of retinal coordinate transformation during and after sac-

cades evoked by auditory stimuli in the dark. *Pflügers Arch.* 403, R67

Grüsser, O.-J., Kirsten, M., Krizic, A., Weiss, L.-R. (1985). The time course of recalibration of retinal spatial values during and after saccades: Comparison of saccades with and without head movements. *Neurosci. Lett. Suppl.* 22, 41

Grüsser, O.-J., Kremer, H. (1986). Face recognition in schizophrenic patients (unpubl.)

Grüsser, O.-J., Krizic, A., Weiss, L.-R. (1987). Afterimage movement during saccades in the dark. *Vision Res.* 27, 215–226

Grüsser, O.-J., Kulikowski, J., Pause, M., Wollensak, J. (1981). Optokinetic nystagmus, Sigma-optokinetic nystagmus and eye pursuit movements elicited by stimulation of an immobilized human eye. *J. Physiol.* 320, 21–22P

Grüsser, O.-J., Kusel, R., Przybyszewski, A. (1984). Cat retinal ganglion cell responses during combined light and electrical sine-wave stimulation of different frequencies. *Perception* 13, A15

Grüsser, O.-J., Kusel, R., Przybyszewski, A. (1984). Interaction of cat ganglion cell responses to sinewave light stimuli (SLS) and sinewave electrical stimuli (SES) of different frequencies. *Neurosci. Lett. Suppl.* 18, S21

Grüsser, O.-J., Naumann, A., Seeck, M. (1990). *Face-responsive components in the visual evoked potential of the human electroencephalogram.* In Abstract Books, EBBS Workshop of Cognitive Neuroscience, 24.–29. Mai 1990

Grüsser, O.-J., Naumann, A., Seeck, M. (1990). Neurophysiological and neuropsychological studies on the perception and recognition of faces and facial expression. In Elsner, N., Roth, G. (eds.), *Brain-Perception-Cognition: Proceedings of the 18th Göttingen Neurobiology Conference*. Thieme, Stuttgart, New York, 83–94

Grüsser, O.-J., Ott, B. (1990). Visual cognitive defects in schizophrenic patients as revealed by a 'pars-pro-toto-test' (in preparation)

Grüsser, O.-J., Pause, M., Schreiter, U. (1979). Three methods to elicit Sigma-optokinetic nystagmus in Java monkeys. *Exp. Brain Res.* 35, 519–526

Grüsser, O.-J., Pause, M., Schreiter, U. (1982). Neuronal responses in the parieto-insular vestibular cortex of alert Java monkeys (Maccaca fascicularis). In Roucoux, A., Crommelinck, M. (eds.), *Physiological and pathological aspects of eye movements*. Dr. W. Junk Publishers, The Hague, Boston, London, 251–270

Grüsser, O.-J., Pause, M., Schreiter, U. (1983). A new vestibular area in the primate cortex. *Soc. Neurosci. Abstr.* Vol. 9, part 1, p. 749

Grüsser, O.-J., Pause, M., Schreiter, U. (1990a). Localization and responses of neurones in the parieto-insular vestibular cortex of awake monkeys (Macaca fascicularis). *J. Physiol. (Lond.)* 430, 537–557

Grüsser, O.-J., Pause, M., Schreiter, U. (1990b). Vestibular neurones in the parieto-insular cortex of monkeys (Macaca fascicularis): Visual and neck receptor responses. *J. Physiol. (Lond.)* 430, 559–583

Grüsser, O.-J., Rabelo, C. (1958). Reaktionen retinaler Neurone nach Lichtblitzen. I. Einzelblitze und Blitzreize wechselnder Frequenz. *Pflügers Arch.* 265, 501–525

Grüsser, O.-J., Reidemeister, Ch. (1959). Flimmerlichtuntersuchungen an der Katzenretina. II. Off-Neurone und Besprechung der Ergebnisse. *Z. Biol.* 3, 254–270

Grüsser, O.-J., Rickmeyer, O. (1981). A simple electronic device to elicit Sigma-movement perception, Sigma-eye movements, Phi-movement perception and Phi-eye movements im man. *J. Pysiol.* 320, 9–10P

Grüsser, O.-J., Saur, G. (1960). Monoculare und binoculare Lichtreizung einzelner Neurone im Geniculatum laterale der Katze. *Plügers Arch. ges. Physiol.* 271, 595–612

Grüsser, O.-J., Selke, T., Zynda, B. (1985). A developmental study of face recognition in children and adolescents. *Human. Neurobiol.* 4, 33–39

Grüsser, O.-J., Selke, Th., Zynda, B. (1988). Cerebral lateralization and some implications for art, aesthetic perception, and artistic creativity. In Rentschler, I., Herzberger, B., Epstein D. (eds.), *Beauty and the brain, biological aspects of aesthetics*. Birkhäuser, Basel, Boston, Berlin, 257–293

Grüsser, O.-J., Weiss, L.-R. (1985). Quantitative models on phylogenetic growth of the hominid brain. In Tobias, Ph.V. (ed.), *Hominid Evolution*. Liss, New York, 457–464

Grüsser-Cornehls, U. (1968). Response of movement-detecting neurons of the frog's retina to moving patterns under stroboscopic illumination. *Pflügers Arch.* 303, 1–13

Grüsser-Cornehls, U., Grüsser, O.-J. (1960). Mikroelektrodenuntersuchungen am Geniculatum laterale der Katze: Nervenzell-und Axonenentladungen nach elektrischer Opticusreizung. *Pflügers Arch.* 271, 50–63

Grützner, A., Grüsser, O.-J., Baumgartner, G. (1958). Reaktionen einzelner Neurone im optischen Cortex der Katze nach elektrischer Reizung des Nervus opticus. *Arch. Psychiat. Z. f. d. ges. Neurol.* 197, 377–404

Grützner, P. (1966). Über erworbene Farbensinnstörungen bei Sehnervenerkrankungen. *Graefes Arch. Ophthalmol.* 169, 366–384

Grützner, P. (1972). Acquired color vision effects. In Jameson, D., Hurvich, L.M. (eds.). *Visual psychophysics. Handbook of Sensory Physiology*. Vol. VII/4. Springer, Berlin, Heidelberg, New York, 643–659

Guard, O., Graule, A., Bellis-Lemerle, F., Giroud, M., Dumas, R. (1985). Le syndrome de disconnexion interhemispherique au cours des gliomes de la partie posterieure du corps calleux. *Encephale* 11, 211–220

Guard, O., Graule, A., Spautz, J.M., Dumas, R. (1981). Anomie fabulante par agnosie visuelle et tactile au cours d'une demence arteriopathique. *Encephale* 7, 275–291

Guard, O., Perenin, M.T., Vighetto, A., Giroud, M., Tommasi, M., Dumas, R. (1984). Syndrome pariétal bilatéral proche d'un syndrome de Balint. *Rev. Neurol.* 140, 358–367

Gueneau de Mussy (1879). Contribution a l'étude pathologique et physiologique de l'amblyopie aphasique. *Rec. Ophtal. (Paris)* 3, 129–142

Guenther, K., Guenther, H. (eds.) (1983). *Schrift, Schreiben, Schriftlichkeit. Arbeiten zur Struktur und Funktion und Entwicklung schriftlicher Sprache*. Niemeyer, Tübingen

Guillery, H. (1905). Weitere Untersuchungen zur Physiologie des Formensinns. *Arch. Augenheilk.* 51, 209

Guillery, H. (1931). Sehschärfe. In Bethe, H. et al. (eds.), *Handbuch der normalen und pathologischen Physiologie* Vol. XII (2)

Guiraud, P. (1955). Langage et communication. *Bull. Soc. Ling. Paris* 50, 119–133

Guiter, H.M., Arapov, V. (1982). *Studies on Zipf's law*. Brockmeyer, Bochum

Guitton, D., Volle, M. (1987). Gaze control in humans: Eye-head coordination during orienting movements to targets within and beyond the oculomotor range. *J. Neurophysiol.* 58, 427–459

Guldin, W., Akbarian, S., Grüsser, O.-J. (1989). The interconnections of the parieto-insular vestibular cortex (PIVC) in the squirrel monkey. *Soc. Neurosci. Abstr.* 15, 519

Guldin, W.O., Grüsser, O.-J. (1987). Single unit responses in the vestibular cortex of squirrel monkeys. *Soc. Neurosci. Abstr.* 13, 1224

Gurewitsch, M. (1933). Weitere Beiträge zur Lehre vom interparietalen Syndrom bei Geisteskrankheiten. *Z. f. Neurol. u. Psychiat.* 146, 126–144

Gutton, D., Buchtel, H.A., Douglas, R.M. (1982). Disturbances of voluntary saccadic eye movement mechanisms following discrete unilateral frontal lobe removals. In Lennerstrand, G., Zee, D.S., Keller, E.L. (eds.), *Functional basis of ocular motility disorders*. Pergamon, Oxford, UK

Gwiazda, J., Brill, S., Mohindra, I., Held, R. (1978). Infant visual acuity and its meridional variation. *Vision Res.* 18, 1557–1564

Gwiazda, J., Brill, S., Mohindra, I., Held, R. (1980). Preferential looking acuity in infants from two to fifty-eight weeks of age. *Am. J. Optom. Physiol. Opt.* 57, 428–432

Gyr, J., Willey, R., Henry, A. (1979). Motor-sensory feedback and geometry of visual space: An attempted replication. *Behav. Brain Sci.* 2, 59–94

Haaxma, R., Kuypers, H. (1974). Role of occipito-frontal cortico-cortical connections in visual guidance of relatively independent hand and finger movement in rhesus monkeys. *Brain Res.* 71, 361–366

Haaxma, R., Kuypers, H.G.J.M. (1975). Intrahemispheric cortical connexions and visual guidance of hand and finger movements in the rhesus monkey. *Brain* 98, 239–260

Haberich, F.J., Fischer, M.H. (1958). Die Bedeutung des Lidschlags für das Sehen beim Umherblicken. *Pflügers Arch. ges. Physiol.* 267, 626–635

Habib, M. (1986). Visual hypoemotionality and prosopagnosia associated with right temporal lobe isolation. *Neuropsychologia* 24, 577–582

Habib, M., Sirigu, A. (1987). Pure topographical disorientation: a definition and anatomical basis. *Cortex* 23, 73–85

Hachinski, V.C., Porchawka, J., Stelle, J.C. (1973). Visual symptoms in the migraine syndrome. *Neurology* 23, 570–579

Hagen, F. (1837). *Die Sinnestäuschungen in Bezug auf Psychologie, Heilkunde und Rechtspflege*. Wigand, Leipzig

Hagen, K.O. von (1941). Two clinical cases of mind blindness (visual agnosia) one due to carbon monoxide poisoning, one due to diffuse degenerative process. *Bull. L.A. Neurol. Soc.* 6, 191–194

Haggard, M.P., Parkinson, A.M. (1971). Stimulus and task factors as determinants of ear advantages. *Quart. J. Exp. Psychol.* 23, 168–177

Hahlweg, K. (1979). Validierung einer Testbatterie zur Erfassung hirnorganischer Schädigungen. *Diagnostica* 25, 229–313

Hahn, E. (1895). Pathologisch-anatomische Untersuchung des Lissauer'schen Falles von Seelenblindheit. *Arbeiten aus der psychiatr. Klinik Breslau* II, 105–119

Haith, M.M. (1980). *Rules that babies look by. The organization of newborn visual activity*. Erlbaum, Hillsdale, N.J.

Haith. M.M., Bergman, T., Moore, M.J. (1977). Eye contact and face scanning in early infancy. *Science* 198, 853–855

Halben, R. (1903). Ein Fall geheilter Wortblindheit mit Persistenz rechtsseitiger Hemianopsie. *Z. Augenheilk.* 10, 487

Hall, K.R.L. (1962): Behaviour of monkeys towards mirror images. *Nature* 196, 1258–1261

Hallett, P.E., Lightstone, A.D. (1976). Saccadic eye movements toward stimuli triggered by prior saccades. *Vision Res.* 16, 99–106

Halligan, P.W., Manning, L., Marshall, J.C. (1990). Individual variation in line bisection: a study of four patients with right hemisphere damage and normal controls. *Neuropsychologia* 28, 1043–1051

Halligan, P.W., Marshall, J.C., Wade, D.T. (1990). Do visual field deficits exacerbate visuo-spatial neglect? *J. Neurol. Neurosurg. Psychiatry* 53, 487–491

Halligan, P.W., Marshall, J.C. (1988). How long is a piece of string? A study of line bisection in a case of visual neglect. *Cortex* 24, 321–328

Halligan, P.W., Marshall, J.C. (1989). Line bisection in visuo-spatial neglect: disproof of a conjecture. *Cortex* 25, 517–521

Halligan, P.W., Marshall, J.C. (1991). Left neglect for near but not far space in man. *Nature* 350, 498–500

Halsband, V., Gruhn, S., Ettlinger, G. (1985). Unilateral spatial neglect and defective performance in one half of space. *Intern. J. Neurosci.* 28, 173–195

Hamanaka, T. (1971a). Ein durch Autopsie verifizierter Fall von Heautoskopie. *Rinsho-Shinkeigaku* 14, 92 (in Japanese, quoted after Hamanaka 1991)

Hamanaka, T. (1971b). Disturbed mirror recognition. *Seishinigaku*,

Tokyo 13, 45–55 (in Japanese, quoted after Hamanaka (1987)

Hamanaka, T. (1987). Justinus Kerners Beitrag zur Psychopathologie des Doppelgängers. Zur Forschungsgeschichte des Doppelgängers und verwandter Phänomene. In Schott, H. (ed.). *Medizin und Romantik. Justinus Kerner als Arzt und Seelenforschung*. Proc. of a Symposion Weinsberg 1986, published in Justinus Kerner Jubiläumsband zum 200. Geburtstag. Weinsberg. Nachrichtenblatt, 376–392

Hamanaka, T., Ikemura, Y. (1968). On the neuropsychology of pure alexia — a case of pure alexia with occipital lobectomy. (in Japanese). *Psychiat. Neurol. Jap.* 70, 689–700

Hampson, E., Kimura, D. (1988). Reciprocal effects of hormonal fluctuations on human motor and perceptual-spatial skills. *Behav. Neurosci.* 102, 456–459

Hamsher, D., Levin, H.S., Benton, A.L. (1979). Facial recognition in patients with focal brain lesions. *Arch. Neurol.* 36, 837–839

Hamsher, K. de. S. (1978). Stereopsis and unilateral brain disease. *Invest. Ophthal. Vis. Sci.* 17, 336–343

Hamsher, K.deS., Levin, H.S., Benton, A.L. (1979). Facial recognition in patients with focal brain lesions. *Arch. Neurol.* 36, 837–839

Han, D.P., Thompson, H.S. (1983). Nomograms for the assessment of Farnsworth-Munsell 100-hue test scores. *Amer. J. Ophthalmol.* 95, 622–625

Hannay, H.J. (1979a). Asymmetry in reception and retention of color. *Brain and Language* 8, 191–201

Hannay, H.J. (1979b). Individual differences and asymmetry effects in memory for unfamiliar faces. *Cortex* 15, 257–267

Hannay, H.J., Dee, H.L., Burns, J.W., Masek, B.S. (1981). Experimental reversal of a left visual field superiority for forms. *Brain and Language* 13, 54–66

Hannay, H.J., Malone, D.R. (1976). Visual field effects and short-term memory for verbal material. *Neuropsycholgia* 14, 203–209

Hannay, H.J., Rogers, J.P. (1979). Individual differences and asymmetry effects in memory for unfamiliar faces. *Cortex* 15, 2

Hansch, E., Pirozzolo, F.J. (1980). Task relevant effects on the assessment of cerebral specialization for facial emotion. *Brain and Language* 10, 51–59

Hansen, R.M., Skavenski, A.A. (1977). Accuracy of eye position information for motor control. *Vision Res.* 17, 919–926

Harcum, E.R., Jones, M.L. (1962). Letter recognition within words flashed right and left of fixation. *Science* 138, 444–445

Hardt, J., Berndt, R.S., Caramazza, A. (1985). Category-specific naming deficit following cerebral infarction. *Nature* 316, 439–440

Hare, E.H. (1966). Personal observations on the spectral marche of migraine. *J. Neurol. Sci.* 3, 259–264

Harlow, H.F., Harlow, M.K. (1962). Social deprivation in monkeys. *Sci. Amer.* 702, 137–146

Harmon, L.D. (1973). The recognition of faces. *Sci. Am.* 229 (5), 71–82

Harms, H. (1969). Die Technik der statischen Perimetrie. *Ophthalmologica* 158, 387–405

Harrington, A. (1985). Nineteenth-century ideas on hemisphere differences and 'duality of mind'. *The Behavioural and Brain Sciences* 8, 617–660

Harrington, D.O. (1981). *The visual fields*. Mosby, St. Louis

Harris, W. (1897). Hemianopia, with special reference to its transient varieties. *Brain* 20, 308–364

Harting, J.K., Casagrande, V.A., Weber, J.E. (1978). The projection of the primate superior colliculus upon the dorsal lateral geniculate nucleus: Autoradiographic analysis of interlaminar distribution of tecto-geniculate axons. *Brain Res.* 150, 593–599

Harting, J.K., Glendenning, K.K., Diamond, I.T., Hall, W.C. (1973). Evolution of the primate visual system: Anterograde degeneration studies of the tecto-pulvinar system. *Am. J. Phys. Anthropol.* 38, 383–392

Harting, J.K., Huerta, M.F., Frankfurter, A.J., Strominger, N.L.,

Royce, G.J. (1980). Ascending pathways from the monkey superior colliculus: an autoradiographic analysis. *J. Comp. Neurol.* 192, 853–882

Hartje, W. (1987). The effect of spatial disorders on arithmetical skills. In Deloche, G., Seron, X. (eds.), *Mathematical disabilities*. Pribaum Publ., Hillsdale, N.J., 121–135

Hartje, W. (1991). Neglect, facial expression and imagery: neuropsychological findings and hypotheses. *Current Opinion in Neurology and Neurosurgery* 4, 104–108

Hartje, W., Ettlinger, G. (1973). Reaching in light and dark after unilateral posterior parietal ablations in the monkey. *Cortex* 9, 346–354

Hartje, W., Hannen, P., Willmes, K. (1986). Effect of visual complexity in tachistoscopic recognition of Kanji and Kana symbols by German subjects. *Neuropsychologia* 24, 297–300

Hartje, W., Schmitz-Gielsdorf, J., Willmes, K. (1984). Corpus callosum — detour of short cut?. Paper pres. at the EBBS Ann. Meeting, Strasbourg, 3.–5. Sep. 1984

Hartmann, F. (1902). *Die Orientierung. Die Physiologie, Psychologie und Pathologie derselben auf biologischen und anatomischen Grundlagen*. F.C.W. Vogel, Leipzig

Hartmann, N. (1912). *Philosophische Grundlagen der Biologie*. Vandenhoeck & Ruprecht, Göttingen

Hartmann, N. (1950). *Philosophie der Natur; Abriss der speziellen Kategorienlehre*. de Gruyter, Berlin

Hartung, J.K., Hall, W.C., Diamond, I.T. (1972). Evolution of the pulvinar. *Brain Behav. Evol.* 6, 424–52

Hasselmo, M.E., Rolls, E.T., Baylis, G.C. (1986b). Selectivity between facial expression in the responses of a population of neurons in the superior temporal sulcus of the monkey. *Neurosci. Lett.* S26, S571

Hasselmo, M.E., Rolls, E.T., Baylis, G.C. (1989). The role of expression and identity in the face-selective responses of neurons in the temporal visual cortex of the monkey. *Behav. Brain Res.* 32, 203–218

Hasselmo, M.E., Rolls, E.T., Baylis, G.C., Nalwa, V. (1989). Object-centered encoding by face selective neurons in the cortex in the superior temporal sulcus of the monkey. *Exp. Brain Res.* 75, 417–429

Hassler, R. (1964). Die zentralen Systeme des Sehens. *Bericht über die 66. Zusammenkunft der Dtsch. Ophthalmolog. Ges. in Heidelberg, 1964*, 229–251

Hassler, R. (1966). Comparative anatomy of the central visual system in day-and night-active primates. In Hassler, R., Stephan, H. (eds.), *Evolution of the forebrain*. Thieme, Stuttgart, 419–434

Hatta, T. (1977a). Recognition of Japanese Kanji in the left and right visual fields. *Neuropsychologia* 15, 685–688

Hatta, T. (1977b). Lateral recognition of abstract and concrete Kanji in Japanese. *Percept. Mot. Skills* 45, 731–734

Hatta, T. (1978). Recognition of Japanese Kanji and Hirakana in the left and right visual fields. *Japanese Psychol. Research* 20, 51–59

Hatta, T. (1981). Differential processing of Kanji and Kana stimuli in Japanese people: some implications from Stroop-test results. *Neuropsychologia* 19, 87–93

Hatta, T. (1983). Visual field differences in semantic comparative judgements with digits and Kanji stimulus materials. *Neuropsychologia* 21, 669–678

Hatta, T., Dimond, S.J. (1980). Comparison of lateral differences for digit and random form recognition in Japanese and Westerners. *J. Exp. Psychol.: Human Percept. Perform.* 6, 368–374

Hatta, T., Honjoh, Y., Mito, H. (1983). Event-related potentials and reaction times as measures of hemispheric differences for physical and semantic Kanji matching. *Cortex* 19, 517–528

Hatta, T., Yamamoto, M., Kawabata, Y. (1984). Functional hemispheric differences in schizophrenia: interhemispheric transfer deficit or selective hemisphere dysfunction? *Biol. Psychiat.* 19, 1027–1035

Hauptmann, A. (1931). Zur Frage der Halluzinationen im hemianopischen Gesichtsfeld. *Z. ges. Neurol. Psychiat.* 131, 90

Hawken, M.J., Parker, A.J., Lund, J.S. (1988). Laminar organization and contrast sensitivity of direction-selective cells in the striate cortex of old world monkey. *J. Neurosci.* 8, 3351–3548

Haxby, J.V., Grady, C.L., Duara, R., Robertson-Tchabo, E.A., Koziarz, B., Cutler, N.R., Rapoport, S.I. (1986). Relation among age, visual memory, and resting cerebral metabolism in 40 healthy men. *Brain Cogn.* 5, 412–427

Hay, D.C., Ellis, H.D. (1981). Asymmetries in facial recognition: evidence for a memory component. *Cortex* 17, 357–368

Hay, D.C., Young, A.W. (1982). The human face. In Ellis, A.W. (ed.), *Normality and pathology in cognitive functions.* Academic Press, London, New York

Hay, W.J., Rickards, A.G., McMenemey, W.H. & Cumings, J.N. (1963). Organic mercury encephalopathy. *J. Neurol. Neurosurg. Psychiat.* 26, 199–202

Häussler, B. (1988). *Visuell evozierte Potentiale bei schematischen Gesichterstimuli.* Doctoral dissertation, F.U. Berlin

Healton, E.B., Navarro, C., Bressman, C., Brust, J.C.M. (1982). Subcortical neglect. *Neurology* 32, 776–778

Hebb, D. O. (1938). The innate organization of visual activity. III. Discrimination of brightness after removal of the striate cortex in the red. *J. Comp. Psychol.* 25, 427–

Hecaen, H. (1962). Clinical symptomatology in right and left hemispheric lesions. In Mountcastle, V.B. (ed.), *Interhemispheric relations and cerebral dominance*, John Hopkins Press, Baltimore, 215–243

Hecaen, H. (1967). Approche sémiotique des troubles du geste. *Langages* 5, 67–83

Hecaen, H. (1967). Aspects des troubles de la lecture (alexies) au cours des lesions cerebrales en foyer. *Word* 23, 265–287

Hecaen, H. (1972). *Introduction ö la neuropsychologie.* Larousse, Paris

Hecaen, H. (1974). Les problèmes des localisation lésionnelles des alexies. *Langages* 44, 111–117

Hecaen, H. (1978). Right hemisphere contribution to language functions. In Buser, P.A., Rougeul-Buser, A. (eds.), *Cerebral correlates of conscious experience.* Elsevier, Amsterdam

Hecaen, H. (1981). The neuropsychology of face recognition. In Davies, G., Ellis, H., Shepherd, J. (eds.), *Perceiving and remembering faces.* Academic Press, London, 39–54

Hecaen, H., Ajuriaguerra de J. (1952). *Méconnaissances et hallucinations corporelles. Intégration et désintégration de la somatognosie.* Masson et Cie., Paris

Hecaen, H., Ajuriaguerra, J. de (1954). Balint's syndrome (psychic paralysis of visual fixation) and its minor forms. *Brain* 77, 373–400

Hecaen, H., Ajuriaguerra, J. de (1956). Agnosie visuelle pour les objets inanimes par lesion unilaterale gauche. *Rev. Neurol. (Paris)* 94, 222–233

Hecaen, H., Ajuriaguerra, J. de, Angelergues, R. (1957). Les troubles de la lecture dans le cadre des modifications des fonctions symboliques. *Psych. Neurol. (Basel)* 134, 97–129

Hecaen, H., Ajuriaguerra, J. de, David, M. (1952). Les deficits fonctionnels apres lobectomie occipitale. *Monatsschr. Psychiatr. Neurol.* 123, 239–291

Hecaen, H., Ajuriaguerra, J. de, Magis, G., Angelergues, R. (1952). Le problème de l'agnosie des physionomies. *Encéphale* 47, 322–355

Hecaen, H., Ajuriaguerra, J. de, Massonet, J. (1951). Les troubles visuo-constructifs par lésion pariéto-occipitale droite. Role des pertubations vestibulaires. *Encéphale* 1, 122–179

Hecaen, H., Ajuriaguerra, J. de, Rouques, L., David, M., Dell, R.B. (1950). Paralysie psychique du regard de Balint au cours de l'évolution d'une leucoencéphalite type Balo. *Rev. Neurol.* 83, 81–104

Hecaen, H., Albert, M.L. (1978). *Human Neuropsychology.* Wiley, New York

Hecaen, H., Angelergues, R. (1962). Agnosia for faces (prosopagnosia). *Arch. Neurol.* 7, 92–100

Hecaen, H., Angelergues, R. (1963). *La cécité psychique.* Masson et Cie., Paris

Hecaen, H., Angelergues, R. (1964). Localization of symptoms in aphasia. In deReuck, A., O'Connor, M. (eds.), *Disorders of Language.* Churchill, London

Hecaen, H., Angelergues, R. (1965). *Neuropsychologie clinique des dysfonctionnement des lobes occipitaux.* Berichte, 8. Intern. Kongress für Neurologie, Vol. 3, Wiener Medizinische Akademie, 29–45

Hecaen, H., Angelergues, R. (1965). *Pathologie du langage.* Larousse, Paris

Hecaen, H., Angelergues, R., Bernhard, C., Chiarelli, J. (1957). Essai de distinction des modalités cliniques de l'agnosie des physiognomies. *Rev. Neurol. (Paris)* 96, 125–144

Hecaen, H., Angelergues, R., Houillier, S. (1961). Les variétés cliniques des acalculies au cours des lésions retrolandiques: approche statistique du problème . *Rev. Neurol.* 105, 85–103

Hecaen, H., Badaraco, J.G. (1956). Séméiologie des hallucinations visuelles en clinique neurologique. *Acta Neurol. Lat.-Am.* 2, 23–57

Hecaen, H., David, M. (1947). Sur certains troubles de la latéralité du regard dans les lésions periétales s'accompagnant de troubles de la somatognosie. *Bull. Soc. Ophtal. (Paris)*, 103–105

Hecaen, H., Goldblum, M.C., Masure, M.C., Ramier, A.M. (1974). Une nouvelle observation d'agnosie d'object. Deficit de l'association ou de la categorisation, spécifique de la modalité visuelle? *Neuropsychologia* 12, 447–464

Hecaen, H., Green, A. (1957). Sur l'héautoscopie. (A propos de quelques cas récents). *Encéphale* 46, 581–594

Hecaen, H., Gruner, J. (1974). Alexie 'pure' avec integrite du corps calleux. In Michel, F., Schott, B. (eds.), *Les Syndromes de Disconnexion calleuse chez l'homme*, Colloque international de Lyon, Hospital Neurologique, Lyon, 347–361

Hecaen, H., Kremin, H. (1975). Neurolinguistic comments on the alexias. In Zülch, K.J., Creutzfeldt, O., Galbraith, G.C. (eds.), *Cerebral Localization.* Springer, Berlin, Heidelberg, NY

Hecaen, H., Kremin, H. (1976). Reading disorders resulting from left hemisphere lesions: aphasic and pure alexias. In Whitaker, H., Whitaker, H.A. (eds.), *Studies in Neurolinguistics.* Academic Press, New York

Hecaen, H., Penfield, W., Bertrand, W., Malmo, R. (1956). The syndrome of apractognosia due to lesions of the minor cerebral hemisphere. *Arch. Neurol. Psychiat.* 75, 400–434

Hecaen, H., Sauguet, J. (1971). Cerebral dominance in left-handed subjects. *Cortex* 7, 19–48

Hecaen, H., Tzavaras, A. (1969). Etude neuropsychologique des troubles de la reconnaissance des visages humaines. *Bull. de Psychologie* 22, 754–762

Hecaen, H., Tzortzis, C., Masure, M.C. (1972). Troubles de l'orientation spatiale dans une épreuve de recherche d'itinéraire lors des lésions corticales unilaterales. *Perception* 1, 325–330

Hecaen, H., Tzortzis, C., Rondot, P. (1980). Loss of topographic memory with learning deficits. *Cortex* 16, 525–542

Hedman, C., Andersen, A.R., Andersson, P.G., Gilhus, N.E., Kangasniemi, P., Olsson, J.E., Strandman, E., Nestvold, K., Olesen, J. (1988). Symptoms of classic migraine attacks: modifications brought about by metoprolol. *Cephalalgia* 8, 279–284

Hedreen, J.C., Yin, T.C.T. (1981). Homotopic and heterotopic callosal afferents of caudal inferior parietal lobule in *Macaca mulatta. J. Comp. Neurol.* 197, 605–621

Hegner, C.A. (1915). Über seltene Formen von hemianopischen Gesichtsfeldstörungen nach Schussverletzungen. *Klin. Monatsbl. f. Augenheilk.* 55, 642–652

Heidenhain, A. (1927). Beitrag zur Kenntnis der Seelenblindheit. *Monatsschr. f. Psychiat. Neurol.* 66, 61–116

Heilbronner, K. (1904). Über Mikropsie und verwandte Zustände.

Dtsch. Z. Nervenheilk. 27, 414–423

Heilbronner, K. (1910). Die aphasischen, apraktischen und agnostischen Störungen. In Lewandowsky, M. (ed.), *Handbuch der Neurologie* I, 982

Heiligtag, F. (1910). Ein Fall von traumatischer Alexie. *Deutsch. med. Wochenschr.* 36, 2147-

Heilman, K.M. (1979). Neglect and related disorders. In Heilman, K.M., Valenstein, E. (eds.), *Clinical neuropsychology*. Oxford University Press, Oxford, New York, 268–307

Heilman, K.M., Bowers, D., Coslett, H.B., Watson, R.T. (1983). Directional hypokinesia in neglect. *Neurology (suppl.2)* 33, 104

Heilman, K.M., Bowers, D., Valenstein, E., Watson, R.T. (1981). A nonvisual test for hemispatial neglect. *Neurology* (abstr., part 2) 83

Heilman, K.M., Bowers, D., Valenstein, E., Watson, R.T. (1986). The right hemisphere: neuropsychological functions. *J. Neurosurg.* 64, 693–704

Heilman, K.M., Bowers, D., Watson, R.T. (1983). Performance on hemispatial pointing task by patients with neglect syndrome. *Neurology* 33, 661–664

Heilman, K.M., Howell, F. (1980). Seizure-induced neglect. *J. Neurol. Neurosurg. Psychiat.* 43, 1035–1040

Heilman, K.M., Musella, L., Watson, R.T. (1977). The EEG in neglect. *Neurology* 23, 437

Heilman, K.M., Odenheimer, G.L., Watson, R.T., Valenstein, E. (1984). Extinction of non-touch. *Neurology* 34, 188 (suppl.)

Heilman, K.M., Pandya, D.N., Geschwind, N. (1970). Trimodal inattention following parietal lobe ablations. *Trans. Amer. Neurol. Ass.* 95, 259–261

Heilman, K.M., Rothi, L., Campanella, D., Wolfson, S. (1979). Wernicke's and global aphasia without alexia. *Arch. Neurol.* 36, 129–133

Heilman, K.M., Safran, A., Geschwind, N. (1971). Closed head trauma and aphasia. *J. Neurol. Neurosurg. Psychiat.* 34, 265–269

Heilman, K.M., Scholes, R., Watson, R.T. (1975). Auditory affective agnosia. *J. Neurol. Neurosurg. Psychiat.* 38, 69–72

Heilman, K.M., Valenstein, E. (1972). Auditory neglect in man. *Arch. Neurol.* 26, 32–35

Heilman, K.M., Valenstein, E. (1972). Frontal lobe neglect in man. *Neurology* 22, 660–664

Heilman, K.M., Valenstein, E. (1979) (eds.). *Clinical neuropsychology*. Oxford Univ. Press, Oxford, New York, 2nd ed. 1989

Heilman, K.M., Valenstein, E. (1979). Mechanisms underlying hemispatial neglect. *Ann. Neurol.* 5, 166–170

Heilman, K.M., Valenstein, E., Watson, R.T. (1983). Localization of neglect. In Kertesz, A. (ed.), *Localization in neuropsychology*. Academic Press, New York, 471–492 (oder 371–392?)

Heilman, K.M., Valenstein, E., Watson, R.T. (1985). The neglect syndrome. In Vinken, P.J., Bruyn, G.W., Klawans, H.L., Frederis, J.A.M.. (eds.), *Handbook of clinical neurology. Vol. 45. Clinical neuropsychology*. Elsevier, Amsterdam, 153–183

Heilman, K.M., Van Den Abell, T. (1979). Right hemispheric dominance for mediating cerebral activation. *Neuropsychologia* 17, 315–321

Heilman, K.M., Van Den Abell, T. (1980). Right hemisphere dominance for attention: the mechanisms underlying hemispheric asymmetries of inattention (neglect). *Neurology* 30, 327–330

Heilman, K.M., Watson, R.T. (1977). The neglect syndrome. A unilateral defect of the orienting response. In Harnard, S., Doty, R.W., Goldstein, L., Jaynes, J., Krauthamer, G. (eds.), *Lateralisation in the nervous system*. Academic Press, New York, 285–302

Heilman, K.M., Watson, R.T. (1977a). Mechanisms underlying the unilateral neglect syndrome. In Weinstein, E.A., Friedland, R.P. (eds.), *Hemi-inattention and hemisphere specialization*. Raven, New York, 93–105

Heilman, K.M., Watson, R.T. (1978). Changes in the symptoms of neglect induced by changes in task strategy. *Arch. Neurol.* 35, 47–49

Heilman, K.M., Watson, R.T., Schulman, H. (1974). A unilateral

memory defect. *J. Neurol. Neurosurg. Psychiat.* 37, 790–793

Heilman, K.M., Watson, R.T., Valenstein, E., Damasio, A.R. (1983). Localization of lesions in neglect. In Kertesz, A. (ed.), *Localization in neuropsychology*. Academic Press, New York, 471–492

Heilman, K.M., Watson, R.T., Valenstein, E., Goldberg, M.E. (1971?). Attention: behavior and neural mechanisms. *Handbook of Physiology*, Chapter 11, 461–481

Hein, A., Diamond, R. (1983). Contribution of eye movement to the representation of space. In Hein, A., Jeannerod, M. (eds.), *Spatially oriented behavior*. Springer, New York, Berlin, Heidelberg, Tokyo, 119–133

Heinrichs, R.W. (1990). Variables associated with Wisconsin card sorting test performacne in neuropsychiatric patients referred for assessment. *Neuropsychiatry, Neuropsychology and Behavioral Neurology* 2, 107–112

Heintel, H. (1965). Heautoskopie bei traumatischer Psychose. Zugleich ein Beitrag zur Phänomenologie der Heautoskopie. *Arch. Psychiat. & Z. ges. Neurol.* 206, 727–735

Heister, G., Landis, T., Regard, M., Schroeder-Heister, P. (1989). Shift of functional cerebral asymmetry during the menstrual cycle. *Neuropsychologia* 27, 871–880

Held, R., Birch, E.E., Gwiazda, J. (1980). Stereoacuity of human infants. *Proc. Natl. Acad. Sci. USA* 77, 5572–5576

Held, R., Rekosh, J. (1963). Motor-sensory feedback and geometry of visual space. *Science* 141, 722–723

Hellige, J.B. (1983). The study of cerebral hemisphere differences: introduction and overview. In Hellige, J.B. (ed.), *Cerebral hemisphere asymmetry*. Praeger, New York

Hellige, J.B., Corwin, W.H., Jonson, J.E. (1984). Effects of perceptual quality on the processing of human faces presented to the left and right cerebral hemispheres. *J. Exp. Psychol.: Hum. Perc. & Perf.* 10, 90–107

Hellige, J.B., Cox, P.J., Litvac, L. (1979). Information processing in the cerebral hemispheres: selective hemispheric activation and capacity limitations. *J. Exp. Psychol.:General* 108, 251–279

Hellige, J.B., Webster, R. (1979). Right hemisphere superiority for initial stages of letter processing. *Neuropsychologia* 17, 653–660

Hellner, K.A., Gauri, K.K. (1982). Über Akkommodationsphosphene. *Fortschr. Ophthalmol.* 79, 169–170

Helmholtz, H. von (1896). *Handbuch der physiologischen Optik*. Voss, Leipzig, 1st ed. 1860

Helmholtz, H. von (1921). *Schriften zur Erkenntnistheorie*. Springer, Berlin

Hemphill, R.E., Klein, R. (1948). Contribution to dressing disability as focal sign and to imperception phenomena. *J. Ment. Sci.* 94, 611–622

Hemsley, D.R. (1982). Cognitive impairment in schizophrenia. In Burton, A. (ed.), *The pathology and psychology of cognition*. Methuan, New York, 169–203

Henderson, D.C., Evans, J.R., Dobelle, W.H. (1979). The relationship between stimulus parameters and phosphene threshold/brightness, during stimulation of human visual cortex. *Trans. Am. Soc. Artif. Intern. Organs* 25, 367–371

Henderson, S.T. (1977). *Daylight and its spectrum*. Wiley, New York

Henderson, V.W. (1982). Impaired hue discrimination in homonymous visual fields. *Arch. Neurol.* 39, 418–419

Henderson, V.W. (1986). Anatomy of posterior pathways in reading: A reassessment. *Brain Lang.* 29, 119–133

Henderson, V.W., Friedman, R.B., Teng, E.L., Weiner, J.M. (1985). Left hemisphere pathways in reading: Inferences from pure alexia without hemianopia. *Neurology* 35, 962–968

Hendricks, I.M., Holliday, I.E., Ruddock, K.H. (1981). A new class of visual defect: spreading inhibition elicited by chromatic light stimuli. *Brain* 104, 813–840

Hendrickson, A.E., Wilson, J.R. (1979). A difference in ^{14}C deoxyglucose audioradiographic patterns in striate cortex between Macaca and Saimiri monkeys following monocular stimulation. *Brain Res.* 170, 353–358

Hendrickson, A.E., Wilson, J.R., Ogren, M.P. (1978). The neuroanatomical organization of pathways between the dorsal lateral geniculate nucleus and visual cortex in old world and new world primates. *J. Comp. Neurol.* 182, 123–136

Henn, V. (1969). Materialien zur Vorgeschichte der Kybernetik. *Studium Generale* 22, 164–190

Henn, V. (1971). The history of cybernetics in the 19th century. In Grüsser, O.-J., Klinke, R. (eds.), *Pattern recognition in biological and technical systems.* Springer, Berlin, 1–7

Henry, W.C. (1854). *Memoirs of the life and scientific researches of John Dalton.* Cavendish Society, London

Henschen, S.E. (1890/1892). *Beiträge zur Pathologie des Gehirns.* Almquist & Wiksell, Uppsala

Henschen, S.E. (1892). *Klinische und anatomische Beiträge zur Pathologie des Gehirns.* Almquist and Wiksell, Uppsala

Henschen, S.E. (1896). *Klinische und anatomische Beiträge zur Anatomie des Gehirns, Teile 1–3,* Almquist & Wiksell, Uppsala

Henschen, S.E. (1909). Über inselförmige Vertretung der Makula in der Sehrindes des Gehirns. *Med. Klinik* 5, 1321

Henschen, S.E. (1910). Die zentralen Sehstörungen. In Lewandowsky, M. (ed.), *Handbuch der Neurologie.* Vol. I, 891–918

Henschen, S.E. (1911). *Klinische und anatomische Beiträge zur Pathologie des Gehirns.* Part IV. Almquist, Wiksell, Uppsala

Henschen, S.E. (1920–1922). *Klinische und anatomische Beiträge zur Pathologie des Gehirns.* Nordiska Bokhandlin, Stockholm

Henschen, S.E. (1923). Vierzigjähriger Kampf um das Sehzentrum und seine Bedeutung für die Hirnforschung. *Z. ges. Neurol. Psychiat.* 87, 505–535

Henschen, S.E. (1925). Über die Lokalisation einseitiger Gesichtshalluzinationen. Kritische Bemerkungen anlässlich Prof. P. Schröders diesbezüglicher Abhandlung. *Arch. f. Psychiat. Nervenkr.* 75, 630–655

Henschen, S.E. (1926). On the function of the right hemisphere of the brain in relation to the left hemisphere in speech, music, and calculation. *Brain* 49, 110–123

Henschen, S.E. (1926a). Zur Anatomie der Sehbahn und des Sehzentrums. *Graefes Arch. Ophthalmol.* 117, 403–418

Henschen, S.E. (1926b). Die Vertretung der beiden Augen in der Sehbahn und in der Sehrinde. I. Die Vertretung der beiden Augen im Corpus geniculatum externum. *Graefes Arch. Ophthalmol.* 117, 419–

Henschen, S.E. (1930). Klinische und anatomische Beiträge zur Pathologie des Gehirns. 8. Teil: Lichtsinn-und Farbensinnzellen im Gehirn. *Dtsch. Z. Nervenheilk.* 112, 146–158

Henschen, S.E. (1930). Lichtsinn-und Farbsinnzellen im Gehirn. *Dtsch. Z. Nervenheilk.* 113, 146 and 305

Herder, J.G. (1772). *Abhandlung über den Ursprung der Sprache.* Voss, Berlin

Hering, E. (1861). *Vom Ortsinne der Netzhaut.* Engelmann, Leipzig

Hering, E. (1872). Zur Lehre vom Lichtsinne. I. Über successive Lichtinduction. *Sitzungsber. Kais. Akad. Wiss. Wien, Math-naturw. Cl. Abth. III,* 66, 5–24

Hering, E. (1874a). Zur Lehre vom Lichtsinne. II. Über simultanen Lichtcontrast. Sitzungsber. *Kais. Akad. Wiss. Wien, Math.-naturw. Cl. Abth. III,* 68, 186–201

Hering, E. (1874b). Zur Lehre vom Lichtsinne. III. Über simultane Lichtinduction und über successiven Contrast. *Sitzungsber. Kais. Akad. Wiss. Wien, Math.-naturw. Cl. Abth. III.* 68, 229–244

Hering, E. (1874c). Zur Lehre vom Lichtsinne. IV. Über die sogenannte Intensität der Lichtempfindung und über die Empfindung des Schwarzen. Sitzungsber. *Kais. Akad. Wiss. Wien, Math.-naturw. Cl. Abth. III.* 69, 85–104

Hering, E. (1874d). Zur Lehre vom Lichtsinne. V. Grundzüge einer Theorie des Lichtsinnes. *Sitzungsber. Kais. Akad. Wiss. Wien,*

Math-naturw. Cl. Abth. III. 69, 179–217

Hering, E. (1875). Zur Lehre vom Lichtsinne VI. Grundzüge einer Theorie des Farbensinnes. *Sitzungsber. Kais. Akad Wiss. Wien, Math.-naturw. Cl. Abth. III.* 70, 169–204

Hering, E. (1879). Der Raumsinn und die Bewegungen des Auges. In Hermann, L. (ed.), *Handbuch der Physiologie.* Vol. 3., 343–601

Hering, E. (1887). Ueber die Theorie des simultanen Contrastes von Helmholtz. I. *Pflügers Arch. ges. Physiol.* 40, 172–191

Hering, E. (1887). Ueber die Theorie des simultanen Contrastes von Helmholtz. II. *Pflügers Arch. ges. Physiol.* 41, 1–29

Hering, E. (1887). Ueber die Theorie des simultanen Contrastes von Helmholtz. III. *Pflügers Arch. ges. Physiol.* 41, 358–367

Hering, E. (1890). Beitrag zur Lehre vom Simultankontrast. *Z. Psychol. und Physiol. der Sinnesorgane.* 1, 18–28

Hering, E. (1891). Untersuchung eines total Farbenblinden. *Pflügers Arch. ges. Physiol.* 49, 563–608

Hering, E. (1903). Ueber die von der Farbenempfindlichkeit unabhängige Aenderung der Weissempfindlichkeit. Nach Versuchen von A. Brückner und E. Hering. *Pflügers Arch. ges. Physiol.* 94, 533–554

Hering, E. (1920). *Grundzüge der Lehre vom Lichtsinn.* Springer, Berlin

Herman, M., Kanade, T. (1986). Incremental reconstruction of 3-D scenes from multiple complex images. *Artificial Intelligence* 30, 289–341

Heron, W. (1957). Perception as a function of retinal locus and attention. *Amer. J. Psychol.* 70, 38–48

Herrmann, G., Pötzl, O. (1926). *Über die Agraphie und ihre lokaldiagnostischen Beziehungen.* Karger, Berlin

Herrmann, G., Pötzl. O. (1928). *Die optische Allaesthesie. Studien zur Psychopathologie der Raumbildung.* S. Karger, Berlin

Hess, C.W., Meienberg, O., Ludin, H.P. (1982). Visual evoked potentials in acute occipital blindness: diagnostic and prognostic value. *J. Neurol.* 227, 193–200

Hess, R.F., Nordby, K. (1986a). Spatial and temporal properties of human rod vision in the achromat. *J. Physiol.* 371, 387–406

Hess, R.F., Nordby, K. (1986b). Spatial and temporal limits of vision in the achromat. *J. Physol.* 371, 365–385

Hess, R.F., Nordby, K., Pointer, J.S. (1987). Regional variation of contrast sensitivity across the retina of the achromat: sensitivity of human rod vision. *J. Physiol.* 388, 101–119

Hess, R.H., Baker, C.L., Jr., Zihl, J. (1989). The 'motion-blind' patient: low-level spatial and temporal filters. *J. Neurosci.* 9, 1628–1640

Hewett, T.D., Ettlinger, G. (1979). Cross-modal performance: The nature of the failure at 'transfer' in non-human primates capable of 'recognition'. *Neuropsychologia* 17, 511–514

Heydt, R. von der (1987). Approaches to visual cortical function. *Rev. Physiol. Biochem. Pharmacol.* 108, 70–150

Heydt, R. von der, Hänny, P., Adorjani, C. (1978). Movement aftereffects in the visual cortex. *Arch. Ital. Biol.* 116, 248–254

Heydt, R. von der, Peterhans, E. (1989). Cortical contour mechanisms and geometrical illusions. In Lam, D.M.K., Gilbert, C.D. (eds.), *Neural mechanisms of visual perception.* Portofolio Publ. Company, The Woodlands, Texas

Heydt, R. von der, Peterhans, E. (1989). Mechanism of contour perception in monkey visual cortex. I. Lines of pattern discontinuity. *J. Neurosci.* 9, 1731–1748

Heydt, R. von der, Peterhans, E., Baumgartner, G. (1984). Illusory contours and cortical neuron responses. *Science* 224, 1260–1261

Heywood, C.A., Cowey, A. (1987). On the role of cortical area V4 in the discrimination of hue and pattern in macaque monkeys. *J. Neurosci.* 7, 2601–2617

Heywood, C.A., Wilson, B., Cowey, A. (1987). A case study of cortical colour 'blindness' with relatively intact achromatic distinction. *J. Neurol. Neurosurg. Psychiat.* 50, 22–29

Heywood, S. (1973). Pursuing stationary dots: smooth eye movements and apparent movement. *Perception* 2, 181–195

Heywood, S., Churcher, J. (1971). Eye movements and the afterimage. I. Tracking the afterimage. *Vision Res.* 11, 1163–1168

Hicks, T.P., Lee, B.B., Vidyasagar, T.R. (1983). The responses of cells in the macaque lateral geniculate nucleus to sinusoidal gratings. *J. Physiol. (Lond.)* 337, 183–200

Hier, D.B., Mohr, J.P. (1977). Incongruous oral and written naming: evidence for a subdivision of the syndrome of Wernicke's aphasia. *Brain and Language* 4, 115–126

Hier, D.B., Moudlock, J., Caplan, L.R. (1983). Behavioral abnormalities after right hemisphere stroke. *Neurology* 33, 337–344

Higier, H. (1894). Über unilaterale Halluzinationen. *Wien. Klinik* 20, 139–170

Higier, H. (1896). Alexia subcorticalis (Wernicke). *St. Petersburger Med. Woch.* 21,

Hikosaka, K., Iwai, E., Saito, H., Tanaka, K. (1988). Polysensory properties of neurons in the anterior bank of the caudal superior temporal sulcus of the macaque monkey. *J. Neurophysiol.* 60, 1615–1637

Hikosaka, O., Sakamoto, M. (1986). Cell activity in monkey caudate nucleus preceding saccadic eye movements. *Exp. Brain Res.* 63, 659–62

Hildreth, E.C. (1984). *The measurement of visual motion.* MIT-Press, Cambridge

Hillebrand, F. (1920). Die Ruhe der Objekte bei Blickbewegungen. *Jahrbuch Psychiat.* 40, 213

Hilliard, R.D. (1973). Hemispheric laterality effects on a facial recognition task in normal subjects. *Cortex* 9, 246–258

Hillyard, S.A. (1985). Electrophysiology of human selective attention. *Trends in Neuroscience* 8, 400–405

Hilz, R., Rentschler, I. (1989). Segregation of color and form. Intact spatial wavelength discrimination in strabismic amblyopia. *Naturwissenschaften* 76, 479–480

Hines, D. (1976). Recognition of verbs, abstract nouns and concrete nouns from the left and right visual half fields. *Neuropsychologia* 14, 211–216

Hines, D. (1984). Position response bias in visual field recognition. *Cortex* 20, 303–306

Hines, D., Jordan-Brown, L., Rossetto Juzwin, K. (1987). Hemispheric visual processing in face recognition. *Brain and Cognition* 6, 91–100

Hines, M. (1929). On cerebral localization. *Physiol. Rev.* 9, 508–517

Hinshelwood, J. (1900). *Letter-, Word-, and Mind-blindness.* H.K. Lewis, London

Hinshelwood, J.(1902). Four cases of word-blindness. *Lancet* 1, 358–358

Hinshelwood, J., Macphail, A. (1904). A case of word blindness with right homonymous hemianopsia. *Brit. med. J.* 2, 1304–1307

Hinton, G.E. (1981). A parallel computation that assigns canonical object-based frames of reference. *Proceedings of the International Joint Conference on Artificial Intelligence,* Vancouver, Canada

Hinton, G.E. (1984). *Distributed Representations.* Carnegie-Mellon, New York, Univ. Press (Tech. Rep. CMU-CS–84–157)

Hinton, G.E., McClelland, J.L., Rumelhart, D.E. (1986). Distributed representations. In D.E. Rumelhart, J.L. McClelland (eds.), *Parallel distributet processing: Explorations in the microstructure of cognition.* MIT Press, Cambridge

Hirata, K., Osaka, R. (1967). Tachistoscopic recognition of Japanese letter materials in left and right visual fields. *Psychologia* 10, 7–18

Hirose, G., Kin, T., Murakami, E. (1977). Alexia without agraphia associated with right occipital lesion. *J. Neurol. Neurosurg. Psychiat.* 40, 225–227

Hirschberg, J. (1887). Die Augenheilkunde bei den Griechen. *Graefes Arch. Ophthalmol.* 33, 47-

Hirschberg, J. (1899). *Geschichte der Augenheilkunde I: Geschichte der Augenheilkunde im Altertum.* In Graefe-Saemisch (ed.), *Handbuch der Augenheilkunde,* Vol. XII/2. Engelmann, Leipzig,

Hirschberg, N. (1932). *Fleckfieber und Nervensystem.* Berlin

Hitch, G.J. , Woodin, M.E., Baker, S. (1989). Visual and phonological components of working memory in children. *Mem. Cognit.* 17, 175–185

Hitzig, E. (1874). *Untersuchungen über das Gehirn: Abhandlungen physiologischen und pathologischen Inhalts.* Hirschwald, Berlin

Hitzig, E. (1903). *Untersuchungen über das Gehirn. Gesammelte Abhandlungen.* Hirschwald, Berlin

Hitzig, E. (1904). *Physiologische und klinische Untersuchungen über das Gehirn.* Hirschwald, Berlin

Hjortsjo, C.H. (1969). *Man's face and mimic language.* Studentlitteratur, Lund

Hochber, J., Galper, R.E. (1974). Attribution of intention as a function of physiognomy. *Mem. Cognit.* 2, 39–42

Hochberg, J. (1968). In the mind's eye. In Haber, R.N. (ed.), *Contemporary theory and research in visual perception.* Holt, Rienhart, Winston, New York, 309–331

Hochberg, J. (1975). On the control of saccades in reading. *Vision Res.* 15, 620-

Hochberg, J., Galper, R.E. (1967). Recognition of faces: I. An exploratory study. *Psychon. Sci.* 9, 619–620

Hoche, A. (1927). *Das träumende Ich.* Fischer, Jena

Hochheimer, W. (1932). Analyse eines 'Seelenblinden' von der Sprache aus. *Psychologische Forschung* 16, 1–69

Hochstein, S., Maunsell, J.H.R. (1985). Dimensional attention effects in the responses of V4 neurons of the macaque monkey. *Soc. Neurosci. Abstr.* 11, 1244

Hoff, H. (1929). Beiträge zur Relation der Sehsphäre und des Vestibularapparates. *Z. f.d. ges. Neurol. u. Psychiat.* 121, 751-

Hoff, H., Gloning, I., Gloning, K. (1954). Über Alexie. *Wien. Z. Nervenheilk.* 10, 149–162

Hoff, H., Gloning, I., Gloning, K. (1962). Das Pötzlsche Syndrom. *Wien. Klin. Wochenschr.* 74, 684–687

Hoff, H., Gloning, I., Gloning, K. (1962). Die zentralen Stöörungen der optischen Wahrnehmung. Part 4. Die reine Wortblindheit, die Ziffern-und Notenblindheit. *Wiener Med. Wochenschr.* 24, 469–473

Hoff, H., Pötzl, O. (1931). Experimentelle Nachbildung von Anosognosie. *Z. Neurol.* 137, 722–734

Hoff, H., Pötzl, O. (1933). Über cerebral bedingte Polyopie und verwandte Erscheinungen. *Jahrbuch f. Psychiat. Neurol.* 50, 35–56

Hoff, H., Pötzl, O. (1935). Über ein neues parieto-occipitales Syndrom. Störungen des Körperschemas. *J. Psychiat.* 52, 173–218

Hoff, H., Pötzl, O. (1935a). Über Störungen des Tiefensehens bei zerebraler Metamorphopsie. *Monatsschr. Psychiat. Neurol.* 90, 305–326

Hoff, H., Pötzl, O. (1935b). Zur diagnostischen Bedeutung der Polyopie bei Tumoren des Okzipitalhirns. *Z. ges. Neurol. Psychiat.* 152, 433–450

Hoff, H., Pötzl, O. (1937). Reine Wortblindheit bei Hirntumor. *Nervenarzt* 10, 385–394

Hoff, H., Pötzl, O. (1937). Über die labyrinthären Beziehungen von Flugsensationen und Flugträumen. *Monatsschr. f. Psychiat. u. Neurol.* 97, 193-

Hoff, H., Pötzl, O. (1937a). Über eine optisch-agnostische Störung des 'Physiognomie-Gedächtnisses'. *Z. Ges. Neurol. Psychiat.* 159, 367–395

Hoff, H., Pötzl, O. (1937b). Über Polyopie und gerichtete hemianoptische Halluzinationen. *Jb. Psychiat.* 54, 55–88

Hoff, H., Pötzl, O. (1938). Anisotropie des Sehraumes bei occipitaler Herderkrankung. *Z. f. Nervenheilk.* 145, 179–217

Hoffman, C., Kagan, S. (1977). Field dependence and facial recognition. *Percept. Mot. Skills* 44, 119–124

Hoffman, W.C. (1966). The Lie algebra of visual perception. *J. Math. Psychol.* 3, 65–98

Hoffman, W.C. (1978). The Lie transformation group approach to visual neuropsychology. In Leeuwenberg, E.L.J., Buffart, H.F.J.M. (eds), *Formal theories of visual perception*, Wiley, New York, 27–66

Hoffmann, K.P. (1983). Control of the optokinetic reflex by the nucleus of the optic tract in the cat. In Hein, A., Jeannerod, M. (eds.), *Spatially oriented behavior*. Springer, New York, Berlin, Heidelberg, Tokyo, 135–153

Hoffmann, K.P., Morrone, C.M., Reuter, J.H. (1980). A comparison of responses of single cells in the LGN and visual cortex to bar and noise stimuli in the cat. *Vision Res.* 20, 771–777

Hofmann, F.B. (1925). *Raumsinn des Auges*. Springer, Berlin

Hojo, K. Willmes, K., Hartje, W. (19..) Tachistoscopic recognition of Kana and Kanji in Japanese subjects. The role of figural complexity in visual field asymmetries (in prepar.)

Hojo, K., Willmes, K., Hartje, W. (1986 unpubl.)...quoted in Hartje et al. 1986

Holden, A.L., Hayes, B.P., Fitzke, F.W. (1987). Retinal magnification factor at the ora terminalis: a structural study of human and animal eyes. *Vision Res.* 27, 1229–1235

Holden, W. A. (1904). A case of mind blindness, unique in that the entire mesial surface of both occipital lobes and both optic radiations were preserved. *Trans. Amer. Ophthal. Soc.* 10, 286-

Holender, D. (1986). Semantic activation without conscious identification in dichotic listening, parafoveal vision, and visual masking. A survey and appraisal. *Behavioral and Brain Sci.* 9, 1–66

Holland, H.C. (1957). The Archimedes spiral. *Nature (Lond.)* 179, 432–433

Holmes, F.B., Lister, W.T. (1916). Disturbance of vision from cerebral lesions with special reference to the cortical representation of the macula. *Brain* 39, 34–73

Holmes, G. (1918a). Disturbances of vision by cerebral lesions. *Brit. J. Ophthalmol.* 2, 353–384

Holmes, G. (1918b). Disturbances of visual orientation. *Brit. J. Ophthalmol.* 2, 449–468 and 506–516

Holmes, G. (1919a). The cortical localization of vision. *Brit. med. J.* 2, 193–199

Holmes, G. (1919b). Disturbances of visual space perception. *Brit. med. J.* 2, 230–233

Holmes, G. (1931). A contribution to the cortical representation of vision. *Brain* 54, 470–479

Holmes, G. (1934). The representation of the mesial sectors of the retinae in the calcarine cortex. *Jahrbücher f. Psychiatrie* 51, 39–47

Holmes, G. (1945). The organization of the visual cortex in man. *Proc. Roy. Soc.(Lond.)* B 132, 348–361

Holmes, G. (1950). Pure word blindness. *Folia Psychiat. Neurol. Neurochir. Neerl.* 53, 279–288

Holmes, G. (1979). *Selected papers of Gordon Holmes*. Ed. by C.G. Phillips. Oxford Univ. Press, Oxford

Holmes, G., Horrax, G. (1919). Disturbances of spatial orientation and visual attention with loss of stereoscopic vision. *Arch. Neurol. Psychiat.* (1965) 1, 385–407

Holmes, G., Lister, W.T. (1916). Disturbances of vision from cerebral lesions, with special reference to the cortical representation of the macula. *Brain* 39, 34–73

Holowinsky, I.Z., Farrelly, J. (1988). Intentional and incidental visual memory as a function of cognitive level and color of the stimulus. *Percept. Mot. Skills* 66, 775–779

Holst, von E., Mittelstaedt, H. (1950). Das Reafferenzprinzip. Wechselwirkungen zwischen Zentralnervensytem und Peripherie. *Naturwissenschaften* 37, 464–476

Holt, E.B. (1903). Eye movement and central anesthesia. *Psychol. Rev. Mon. Suppl.* 4, 3–45

Holtzman, J.D. (1984). Interactions between cortical and subcortical visual areas: evidence from human commissurotomy patients. *Vision Res.* 24, 801–813

Holtzman, J.D., Sedgwick, H.A., Festinger, L. (1978). Interaction of perceptually monitored and unmonitored efferent commands for smooth pursuit eye movements. *Vision Res.* 18, 1545–1555

Holtzman, J.D., Sidtis, J.J., Volpe, B.T., Wilson, D.H., Gazzaniga, M.S. (1981). Dissociation of spatial information for stimulus localization and the control of attention. *Brain* 104, 861–872

Holtzman, R.N.N., Rudel, R.G., Goldensohn, E.S. (1978). Paroxysmal alexia. *Cortex* 14, 592–603

Homa, D., Hayer, B., Schwartz, T. (1976). Perceptibility of schematic face stimuli: evidence for a perceptual Gestalt. *Mem. Cognit.* 4, 176–185

Hooff, J.A.R.A.M. van (1967). The facial display of the catarrhine monkeys and apes. In Morris, D. (ed.), *Primate ethology*. Weidenfeld and Nicolson, London, 7–68

Hooff, J.A.R.A.M. van (1976). The comparison of facial expression in man and higher primates. In Cranach, M. von (ed.), *Methods of inference from animal to human behaviour*. Aldine, Chicago

Hooke, R. (1705). *The posthumous works*. Smith and Wallford, London

Hoppe, I. (1885). Bemerkungen zu Herrn Professor Arndt's Lehre von den Hallucinationen und Illusionen. *Jahrb. f. Psychiatrie* 6, 205–220

Horansky, N. (1936). Kniehöcker und Sehrinde bei einseitiger Opticusatrophie (Einäugigkeit). *Klin. Monatsbl. f. Augenheilk.* 97, 438–443

Horenstein, S., Casey, T.R. (1964). Paropsis associated with hemianopia. *Trans. Amer. neurol. Ass.* 89, 204–206

Horn, L., Helfand, M. (1932). Korrelative Rindenveränderungen im Gehirn einer einseitig Blinden. *Wien. klin. Wochenschr.* 45, 1309

Horowitz, M.J. (1964). The imagery of visual hallucinations. *J. nerv. ment. Dis.* 138, 513–523

Horrax, G. (1923). Visual hallucinations as a cerebral localizing phenomenon, with especial reference to their occurrence in tumors of the temporal lobe. *Arch. Neurol. Psychiat. (Chicago)* 10, 532–547

Horrax, G., Putnam, T.J. (1932). Distortion of the visual fields in cases of brain tumor. The field defects and hallucinations produced by tumors of the occipital lobe. *Brain* 55, 499–523

Horst, L. van der (1932). The psychology of constructive apraxia, psychological views on conception of space. *Psychiat. En. Neurol. Bl.* 36, 661–677

Horst, L. van der (1934). Constructive apraxia. Psychological views on the conception of space. *J. Nerv. Ment. Dis.* 80, 645–650

Horton, J., Hubel, D.H. (1981). Regular patchy distribution of cytochrome oxidase staining in primary visual cortex of macaque monkey. *Nature* 292, 762–764

Horton, J.C., Hedley-Whyte, E.T. (1984). Mapping of cytochrome oxidase patches and ocular dominance columns in human visual cortex. *Phil. Trans. Roy. Soc. London* B 304, 255–272

Hosch, F. (1901). Fall von sogenannter corticaler Hemianopie und Alexie. *Z. Augenheilk.* 5, 5-

Howard, D., Lasaga, M., McAndrews, M. (1980). Semantic activation during memory encoding across the adult life span. *J. Gerontol.* 35, 884–890

Howard, D., McAndrews, M., Lasagna, M. (1980). Automatic and effortful processes in young and old adults: performance on lexical decisions and free recall. Paper repr. at the Ann. Meeting Gerontolog. Soc., San Diego

Howard, I.P. (1982). *Human visual orientation*. Wiley, Chichester, N.Y.

Howells, T.H. (1938). A study of ability to recognize faces. *J. abn. soc. Psychol.* 33, 124–127

Howes, D. (1962). An approach to the quantitative analysis of word blindness. In Money, J. (ed.), *Reading disability*. Johns Hopkins Press, Baltimore

Howes, D., Boller, F. (1975). Simple reaction time: evidence for focal impairment from lesions of the right hemisphere. *Brain* 98, 317–332

Howes, D., Geschwind, N. (1964). Quantitative studies of aphasic language. In Rioch, D.M., Weinstein, E.A. (eds.), *Disorders of com-*

munication. Williams and Wilkins, Baltimore, 229–244

Hoyt, W.F., Kommerell, G. (1973). Der Fundus oculi bei homonymer Hemianopie. *Klin. Monatsbl. Augenheilk.* 162, 456–464

Höber, R. (1934). *Lehrbuch der Physiologie des Menschen.* 7th ed. Springer, Berlin

Hrbek, V. (1984). *Parietal lobes of human cerebral hemispheres.* Statui Pedagogicke Nak Ladatelscvi, Praha

Huang, Y.L., Jones, B. (1980). Naming and discrimination of chinese ideograms presented in the right and left visual fields. *Neuropsychologia* 18, 703–706

Hubel, D.H., Livingstone, M.S. (1981). Regions of poor orientation tuning coincide with patches of cytochrome oxidase staining in monkey striate cortex. *Soc. Neurosci. Abstr.* 7, 357

Hubel, D.H., Livingstone, M.S. (1987). Segregation of form, colour and stereopsis in primate area 18. *J. Neurosci.* 7, 3378–3415

Hubel, D.H., Livingstone, M.S. (1990). Color and contrast sensitivity in the lateral geniculate body and primary visual cortex of the macaque monkey. *J. Neuroscience* 10, 2223–2237

Hubel, D.H., Wiesel, T.N. (1965). Receptive fields and functional architecture in two nonstriate visual areas (18 and 19) of the cat. *J. Neurophysiol.* 28, 229–289

Hubel, D.H., Wiesel, T.N. (1968). Receptive fields and functional architecture of monkey striate cortex. *J. Physiol. (Lond.)* 195, 215–243

Hubel, D.H., Wiesel, T.N. (1972). Laminar and columnar distribution of geniculo-cortical fibers in the macaque monkey. *J. Comp. Neurol.* 146, 421–450

Hubel, D.H., Wiesel, T.N. (1973). A re-examination of stereoscopic mechanisms in area 17 of the cat. *J. Physiol. (Lond.)* 232, 29P–30P

Hubel, D.H., Wiesel, T.N. (1974). Sequence regularity and geometry of orientation columns in the monkey striate cortex. *J. Comp. Neurol.* 158, 267–294

Hubel, D.H., Wiesel, T.N. (1974). Uniformity of monkey striate cortex: A parallel relationship between field size, scatter and magnification factor. *J. Comp. Neurol.* 158, 295–306

Hubel, D.H., Wiesel, T.N. (1977). Functional architecture of macaque monkey visual cortex. *Proc. Roy. Soc. Lond. (Biol.)* 198, 1–59

Hubel, D.H., Wiesel, T.N., LeVay, S. (1977). Plasticity of ocular dominance columns in monkey striate cortex. *Philos. Trans. Roy. Soc. Lond. (Biol.)* 278, 377–409

Huber, W. (1977). Lexikalische Performanz bei Aphasie. In Viethen, H., Bald, W., Sprengel, K. (eds.), *Grammatik und interdisziplinäre Bereiche der Linguistik.* Niemeyer, Tübingen

Huber, W., Poeck, K., Weniger, D., Willmes, K. (1983). *Der Aachener Aphasie-Test.* Hogrefe, Göttingen

Huddart, J. (1777). An account of persons who could not distinguish colours. *Phil. Trans. Roy. Soc. Lond.* 67, 301–302

Huerta, M.F., Krubitzer, L.A., Kaas, J.H. (1986). Frontal eye field as defined by intracortical microstimulation in squirrel monkeys, owl monkeys and macaque monkeys. I. Subcortical connections. *J. Comp. Neurol.* 253, 415–439

Huerta, M.F., Krubitzer, L.A., Kaas, J.H. (1987). Frontal eye field as defined by intracortical microstimulation in squirrel monkeys, owl monkeys and macaque monkeys. II. Cortical connections. *J. Comp. Neurol.* 265, 332–361

Huey, E.B. (1908). *The psychology and pedagogy of reading.* Macmillan, London, reprint MIT Press 1968, Cambridge

Hulme, C., Biggerstaff, A., Moran, G., McKinlay, I. (1982). Visual, kinaesthetic and cross-modal judgements of length by normal and clumsy children. *Dev. Med. Child Neurol.* 24, 461–471

Humphrey, M.E., Zangwill, O.L. (1975). Effects of a right-sided occipito-parietal brain injury in a lefthanded man. *Brain* 75, 312–324

Humphrey, N.K. (1974). Vision in a monkey without striate cortex: a case study. *Perception* 3, 241–255

Humphrey, N.K., Weiskrantz, L. (1967). Vision in monkeys after removal of the striate cortex. *Nature* 215, 595–597

Humphreys, G.W. (1981). On varying the span of visual attention-evidence for 2 modes of spatial attention. *Quart. J. Exp. Psychol.* 331, 17–31

Humphreys, G.W. (1983). Reference frames and shape perception. *Cogn. Psych.* 15, 151–196

Humphreys, G.W., Bruce, V. (1989). *Visual cognition: computational, experimental, and neuropsychological*

Humphreys, G.W., Bruce, W. (1989). *Visual Cognition: Computational, Experimental, and Neuropsychological Perspectives.* Hillsdale NJ: Lawrence Erlbaum Associates

Humphreys, G.W., Bruce, W. (1989). *Visual cognition: computational experimental and neuropsychological perspectives.* Lawrence Erlbaum Ass., London

Humphreys, G.W., Riddoch, M.J. (1984). Routes to object constancy: Implications from neurological impairments of object constancy. *Quart. J. Exp. Psychol.* 36A, 385–415

Humphreys, G.W., Riddoch, M.J. (1985). Author's correction to 'Routes to object constancy'. *Quart. J. Exp. Psychol.* 37A, 493–495

Humphreys, G.W., Riddoch, M.J. (1987). On telling your fruit from your vegetables: a consideration of category-specific deficits after brain damage. *TINS* 10, 145–148

Humphreys, G.W., Riddoch, M.J. (1987). *To see but not to see: a case study of visual agnosia.* Lawrence Erlbaum Associates, Hillsdale, NJ

Humphreys, G.W., Riddoch, M.J. (1987). *Visual object processing: a cognitive neuropsychological approach.* Hillsdale NJ: Lawrence Erlbaum Associates

Humphreys, G.W., Riddoch, M.J. (eds.). *Visual object processing: A cognitive neuropsychological approach.* Lawrence Erlbaum Associates, London

Hun, H. (1887). A clinical study of cerebral localisation illustrated by seven cases. *Am. J. Med. Sci.* 93, 140-

Hurlbert, A., Poggio, T. (1985). Spotlight on attention. *TINS* 8, 309–311

Hurvich, L., Jameson, D. (1957). An opponent-process theory of color vision. *Psychol. Rev.* 64, 384–404

Huxley, A. (1954). *Doors of perception.* Harper, New York

Hylkeena, B.S. (1942a). Fusion frequency with intermittent light under vaious circumstances. *Acta ophthal. (Kbh)* 20, 159–180

Hylkeena, B.S. (1942b). Examination of the visual field by determining the fusion frequency. *Acta ophthal. (Kbh)* 20, 181–193

Hyvärinen, J. (1981). Regional distribution of functions in parietal association area 7 of the monkey. *Brain Res.* 206, 287–303

Hyvärinen, J. (1982a). *The parietal cortex of monkey and man* (Studies of Brain Function 8), Springer, Berlin, Heidelberg, New York

Hyvärinen, J. (1982b). The posterior parietal lobe of the primate brain. *Physiol. Rev.* 62, 1060–1129

Hyvärinen, J., Carlson, S., Hyvärinen, L. (1981a). Early visual deprivation alters modality of neuronal responses in area 19 of monkey cortex. *Neurosc. Lett.* 26, 239–243

Hyvärinen, J., Hyvärinen, L. (1979). Blindness and modification of association cortex by early binocular deprivation in monkeys. *Child* 5, 385–387

Hyvärinen, J., Hyvärinen, L., Carlson, S. (1981b). Effects of binocular deprivation on parietal association cortex in young monkeys. *Doc. Ophthalmol. Proc. Ser.* 30, 177–185

Hyvärinen, J., Hyvärinen, L., Färkkilä, M., Carlson, S., Leinonen, L. (1978). Modification of visual functions of the parietal lobe at early age in monkey. *Med. Biol.* 56, 103–109

Hyvärinen, J., Hyvärinen, L., Linnankovski, I. (1981). Modification of parietal association cortex and functional blindness after binocular deprivation in young monkeys. *Exp. Brain Res.* 42, 1–8

Hyvärinen, J., Lasko, M., Roine, R., Leinonen, L., Sippel, H. (1978). Effects of ethanol on neuronal activity in the parietal association cortex of the alert monkeys. *Brain* 101, 701–715

Hyvärinen, J., Linnankoski, I., Poranen, A., Leinonen, L., Altonen, M. (1978). Use of monkeys as experimental animals: Report of a ten-year experience in a Nordic country. *Ann. Acad. Sic. Fenn. A.V. Medica* 172

Hyvärinen, J., Poranen, A. (1974). Function of the parietal associative area 7 as revealed from cellular discharges in alert monkeys. *Brain* 97, 673–692

Hyvärinen, J., Poranen, A. (1978a). Movement-sensitive and direction and orientation-selective cutaneous receptive fields in the hand area of the post-central gyrus in monkeys. *J. Physiol.* 283. 523–537

Hyvärinen, J., Poranen, A. (1978b). Receptive field integration and submodality convergence in the hand area of the post-central gyrus of the alert monkey. *J. Physiol.* 283, 538–556

Hyvärinen, J., Shelepin, Y. (1979). Distribution of visual and somatic functions in the parietal associative area 7 of the monkey. *Brain Res.* 169, 561–564

Imura, T. (1943). Aphasia: characteristic symptoms in Japanese. *J. Psychiat. Neurol.* 47, 196–218

Indow, T. (1988). Multidimensional studies of Munsell color solid. *Psychol. Reviews* 95, 456–470

Innocenti, G.M. (1981). Growth and reshaping of axons in the establishment of visual callosal connections. *Science* 212, 824–827

Inouye, T. (1909). *Die Sehstörungen bei Schussverletzung der corticalen Sehsphäre, nach Beobachtungen an Verwundeten der letzten japanischen Kriege.* Engelmann, Leipzig

Insausti, R., Amaral, D.G., Cowan, W.M. (1987). The entorhinal cortex of the monkey. II. Cortical afferents. *J. Comp. Neurol.* 264, 356–395

Inui, T. (1988). Properties of human visual memory for block patterns. *Biol. Cybern.* 59, 179–187

Irwin, D.E. (1991). Information integration across saccadic eye movements. *Cognitive Psychology*, (in press)

Irwin, D.E. (1991). Perceiving an integrated visual world. In Meyer, D.E., Kornblum, S. (eds.), *Attention and performance. Vol. XIV: A silver jubilee.* Erlbaum, Hillsdale N.J. (in press)

Irwin, D.E., Brown, J.S., Sun, J.S. (1988). Visual masking and visual integration across saccadic eye movements. *J. exp. Psychol. (General)* 117, 276–287

Irwin, D.E., Yeomans, J.M. (1986). Sensory registration and informational persistence. *J. Exp. Psychol. (Hum. Percept.)* 12, 343–360

Irwin, D.E., Zacks, J.L., Brown, J.S. 1990). Visual memory and the perception of a stable visual environment. *Perception and Psychophys.* 47, 35–46

Iscoe, I., Veldman, D.J. (1963). Perception of an emotional continuum by schizophrenics, normal adults, and children. *J. Clin. Psychol.* 19, 272–276

Isern, R.D. Jr. (1987). Familiy violence and the Kluever-Bucy syndrome. *South Med. J.* 80, 373–377

Ishiai, S., Furukawa, T., Tsukagoshi, H. (1987). Eye-fixation patterns in homonymous hemianopia and unilateral spatial neglect. *Neuropsychologia* 25, 675–679

Ishiai, S., Furukawa, T., Tsukagoshi, H. (1989). Visuospatial processes of line bisection and the mechanisms underlying unilateral spatial neglect. *Brain* 112, 1485–1502

Iverson, S.D. (1973). Visual discrimination deficits associated with posterior inferotemporal lesions in the monkey. *Brain Res.* 62, 89–101

Iwai, E., Mishkin, M. (1968). Two visual foci in the temporal lobe of monkeys. In Yoshii, N., Buchwald, N.A. (eds.), *Neurophysiological basis of learning and behavior.* Osaka UP, Osaka, 1–11

Iwai, E., Mishkin, M. (1969). Further evidence on the locus of the visual area in the temporal lobe of monkeys. *Exp. Neurol.* 25, 585–594

Iwai, E., Yukie, M. (1987). Amygdalofugal and amygdalopetal connections with modality-specific visual cortical areas in macaques (Macaca fuscata, M. mulatta, and M. fascicularis). *J. Comp. Neurol.* 261–362

Iwai, E., Yukie, M., Suyama, H., Shirakawa, S. (1987). Amygdalar connections with middle and inferior temporal gyri of the monkey. *Neurosci. Lett.* 83, 25–29

Iwata, M. (1984). Kanji vs. Kana: Neuropsychological correlations of the Japanese writing system. *Trends in Neuroscience* 7, 290–293

Iwata, M. (1985). Neural mechanisms of reading and writing. Neurogrammatological approach. In Tsukada, Y. (ed.), *Perspectives on Neuroscience: From Molecule to Mind.* University of Tokyo Press, Tokyo, 299–312

Iwata, M. Sugishita, M., Toyokura, Y. (1973). Visual-speech disconnection syndrome of the rigth visual cortex after transection of the splenium of the corpus callosum. *Clin. Neurol.* 13, 308–316

Iwata, M., Sugishita, M., Toyokura, Y. (1981). The Japanese writing system and functional hemispheric specialization. In Katsuki, S., Tsubaki, T., Toyokura, Y. (eds.), *12th World Congress of Neurology.* Excerpta Medica, Amsterdam, 53–62

Iwata, M., Sugishita, M., Toyokura, Y., Yamada, R., Yoshioka, M. (1974). Etude sur le syndrome de disconnexion visuo-linguale après la transection du splenium du corps calleux. *J. Neurol. Sci.* 23, 421–432

Izard, C.E. (1959). Paranoid schizophrenic and normal subjects perceptions of photographs of human faces. *J. Consult. Clin. Psychol.* 23, 119–124

Izard, C.E. (1971). *The face emotion.* Appleton-Century Crofts, New York

Jackson, J.H. (1874). On the nature of the duality of the brain. *Med. Press. Circ.* 17, 19, 41, 63, (reprinted in *Brain* 38, 80–103 (1915))

Jackson, J.H. (1875). Autopsy on a case of hemiopia with hemiplegia and hemianaesthesia. *Lancet* 1, 722

Jackson, J.H. (1876). Case of large cerebral tumour without optic neuritis, and with left hemiplegia and imperception. *Roy. Ophthalm. Hosp. Rep.* 8, London, 434–444. In Selected Writings, vol. 2, Taylor, London 1932, 146–252

Jackson, J.H. (1876). Coloured vision as an 'aura' in epilepsie. *Brit. med. J.* 1, 174

Jackson, J.H. (1878). On the neurology of gestures. *Brain* 1,

Jackson, J.H. (1931/1932). *Selected writings.* 2 vols. Hodder and Stoughton, London

Jackson, J.H., Paton, L. (1909). On some abnormalities of ocular movements. *Lancet* March 27, 900–905

Jacob, H. (1949). *Der Erlebniswandel bei Späterblindeten. Zur Psychopathologie der optischen Wahrnehmung. Abhandlungen zur Psychiatrie, Psychologie, Psychopathologie und Grenzgebieten.* Nölke, Hamburg

Jacobs, L. (1989). Comments on some positive visual phenomena caused by diseases of the brain. In Brown, J.W. (ed.), *Neuropsychology of visual perception,* Erlbaum, Hillsdale, NJ, 165–182

Jacobson, S., Trojanowski, J.Q. (1977). Prefrontal granular cortex of the rhesus monkey. I. Intrahemispheric cortical afferents. *Brain Res.* 132, 209–233

Jaeger, W. (1972). Acquired color vision defects. In Jameson, D., Hurvich, L.M. (eds.), *Visual Psychophysics. Handbook of Sensory Physiology.* Vol. VII/4. Springer, Berlin, Heidelberg, New York, 625–642

Jaeger, W. (1976). *Die Illustrationen von Peter Paul Rubens zum Lehrbuch der Optik des Franciscus Aguilonius 1613.* Brausdruck, Heidelberg

Jaeger, W. (1981). Das Tritanomaloskop. *Ber. Dtsch. Ophthalmol. Ges.* 78, 1017–1030

Jaeger, W., Krastel, H., Braun, S. (1989). Cerebrale Achromatopsie. I. and II. *Klin. Monatsbl. Augenheilk.* 193, 627–634 and 194, 32–36

Jahn, B. (1979). *Die Terminologie der Trugwahrnehmungen von Galen bis Esquirol.*Doctoral dissertation, Freiburg i.Br.

Jakobson, R. (1964). On visual and auditory signs. *Phonetica* 2, 216–220

James, W. (1890). *The principles of psychology.* MacMillan, London

Jameson, D. (1984). Opponent-colours theory in the light of physiological findings. In Ottoson, D., Zeki, S. (eds.) *Central and peripheral mechanisms of colour vision.* Proc. of Internation. Symposium The Wenner-Gren Ctr., Stockholm, MacMillan, London, 83–102

Jameson, D. (1985). Seeing: by art and by design. *Transact. Am. Philosoph. Soc.* 75, 68–78

Jameson, D., Hurvich, L.M. (1989). Essay concerning color constancy. *Ann. Rev. Psychol.* 40, 1–22

Jameson, D., Hurvich, L.M., Varner, D. (1979). Receptoral and postreceptoral visual processes in recovery from chromatic adaptation. *Proc. Natl. Acad. Sci. USA* 76, 3034–3038

Jameson, D., Hurvich, L.M., Varner, D. (1982). Discrimination mechanisms in colour deficient systems. In Verriest, G. (ed.), *Doc. Ophthal. Proc. Ser.* 33, 295–301

Jampel, R.S. (1960). Convergence, divergence, pupillary reactions and accommodation of the eyes from Faradic stimulation of macaque brain. *J. Comp. Neurol.* 115, 371–397

Jantz, H., Behringer, K. (1944). Das Syndrom des Schwebeerlebnisses unmittelbar nach Kopfverletzungen. *Nervenarzt* 17, 197–206

Janz, D. (1969). *Die Epilepsien. Spezielle Pathologie und Therapie.* Thieme, Stuttgart

Jarvik, M.E. (1970). Drugs, hallucinations and memory. In Keup, W. (ed.), *Origin and mechanisms of hallucinations.* Plenum Press, N.Y., London, 277–302

Jason, G.W. (1983). Misreaching in monkeys after combined unilateral occipital lobectomy and splenial transection. *Exp. Neurol.* 81, 114–125

Jason, G.W., Cowey, A., Weiskrantz, L. (1984). Hemispheric asymmetry for a visuo-spatial task in monkeys. *Neuropsychologia* 22, 777–784

Jasper, H.H. (1932). A laboratory study of diagnostic indices of bilateral neuromuscular organisation in stutterers and normal speakers. *Psychol. Monogr.* 43, 72–174

Jaspers, K. (1914). Über leibhafte Bewusstheiten (Bewusstheitstäuschungen), ein psychopathologisches Elementarphänomen. *Z. Pathopsychol.* 2, quoted after Jaspers 1953)

Jaspers, K. (1953). *Allgemeine Psychopathologie.* 6th ed., Springer, Berlin, New York

Jastrow, J.A. (1891). A study of Zöllner's figure and other related illusions. *Amer. J. Psychol.* 4, 381–398

Jeannerod, M. (1971). Espace et regard. In Hecaen, H. (ed.), *Neuropsychologie de la perception visuelle*, Masson et Cie., Paris, 265–279

Jeannerod, M. (1983). How do we direct our actions in space? In Hein, A., Jeannerod, M. (eds.), *Spatially oriented behavior.* Springer, New York, Berlin, Heidelberg, Tokyo, 1–13

Jeannerod, M. (1985). The posterior parietal area as a spatial generator. In Ingle, D.J., Jeannerod, M., Lee, D.N. (eds.), *Brain mechanisms and spatial vision.* Martinus Nijhoff Publishers, Dordrecht, Boston, Lancaster, 278

Jeannerod, M. (1987) (ed.). *Neurophysiological and neuropsychological aspects of spatial neglect.* North Holland, Amsterdam

Jeannerod, M. (1988/1990). Hierarchical model for voluntary goal-directed actions. In Eccles, J., Creutzfeldt, O. (eds.), *The principles of design and operation of the brain.* Pontificiae Academiae Scientiarum Scripta Varia 78, 257–275

Jeannerod, M., Biguer, B. (1987). The directional coding of reaching movements. A visuomotor conception of spatial neglect. In Jeannerod, M. (ed.), *Neurophysiological and neuropsychological aspects of spatial neglect.* Elsevier, North-Holland, 87–113

Jeannerod, M., Biguer, B. (1989). Référence égocentrique et espace

représenté. *Rev. Neurol. (Paris)* 145, 635–639

Jeannerod, M., Gerin, P., Mouret, J. (1965). Influence de l'obscurité et de l'occlusion des paupières sur le controle des mouvements oculaires. *L'Année Psychologique* 65, 309–324

Jeannerod, M., Kennedy, H., Magnin, M. (1979). Corollary discharge: its possible implication in visual and oculomotor interactions. *Neuropsychologia* 17, 241–258

Jeeves, M.A. (1972). Hemisphere differences in response rates to visual stimuli in children. *Psychonom. Sci.* 27, 201–203

Jeeves, M.A. (1984). The historical roots and recurring issues of neurobiological studies of face perception. *Hum. Neurobiol.* 3, 191–196

Jeeves, M.A. (1984). The historical roots and recurring issues of neurobiological studies of face perception. *Human Neurobiol.* 3, 191–196

Jeeves, M.A., Dixon, N.F. (1970). Hemisphere differences in response rates to visual stimuli. *Psychonom. Sci.* 20, 249–251

Jeffreys, D.A., Musselwhite, M.J. (1987). A face-responsive visual evoked potential in man. *J. Physiol. (Lond.)* 390, 36

Jenkner, F.L., Kutschera, E. (1985). Frontal lobe and vision. *Confin. Neurol.* 25, 63–78

Jensen, (1868). Über Doppelwahrnehmungen in der gesunden, wie in der kranken Psyche. *Allgem. Z. f. Psychiat.* 25 (Suppl.), 48–64

Jensen, B.T. (1952). Left-right orientation in profile drawing. *Am. J. Psychol.* 65, 80–83

Jensen, B.T. (1952). Reading habits and left-right orientation in profile drawings by Japanese children. *Am. J. Psychol.* 65, 306–307

Jensen, K., Tfelt-Hansen, P., Lauritzen, M., Olesen, J. (1986). Classic migraine. A prospective recording of symptoms. *Acta Neurol. Scand.* 73, 359–362

Jerusalem, F. (1988). Zur Pathogenese und Therapie der Migräne. *Aktuelle Neurologie* 14, 173–185

Joanette, Y., Brouchon, M., Gauthier, L., Samson, M. (1986). Pointing with left vs right hand in left visual field neglect. *Neuropsychologia* 24, 391–396

Joanette, Y., Goulet, P., Nespoulous, J.L. (1986). Informative content of narrative discourse in right-brain-damaged right-handers. *Brain Lang.* 29, 81–105

Johansson, G. (1971). Studies on visual perception of locomotion. *Perception* 6, 365–376

Johansson, G. (1973). Visual perception of biological motion and a model for its analysis. *Perception and Psychophysics* 14, 201–211

Johansson, G. (1975). Visual motion perception. *Sci. Am.* 232, 76–88

Johansson, T., Fahlgren, H. (1979). Alexia without agraphia: lateral and medial infarction of left occipital lobe. *Neurology* 29, 390–393

Johnston, C.W. (1986). Exploratory eye movements and visual hemineglect. *J. Clin. Exp. Neuropsychol.* 8, 93–101

Johnston, W.A., Dark, V.J. (1986). Selective attention. *Ann. Rev. Psychol.* 47, 43–75

Jolly, F. (1902). Über Flimmerskotom und Migräne. *Berliner Klin. Wochenschr.* 42, 973–976

Jones, A.C. (1969). Influence of mode of stimulus presentation on performance in facial recognition tasks. *Cortex* 5, 291–301

Jones, B. (1979). Lateral asymmetry in testing long-term memory for faces. *Cortex* 15, 183–186

Jones, B. (1979). Sex and visual field effects on accuracy and dicision making when subjects classified male and female faces. *Cortex* 15, 551–560

Jones, B. (1980). Sex and handedness as factors in visual field organization for categorization task. *J. Exp. Psychol. HPP* 6, 494–500

Jones, B., Anuza, T. (1982). Effects of sex, handedness, stimulus and visual field on mental rotation. *Cortex* 18, 501–514

Jones, E.G., Powell, T.P.S. (1969). Morphological variations in the dendritic spines of the neocortex. *J. Cell. Sci.* 5, 509–529

Jones, E.G., Powell, T.P.S. (1970). An anatomical study of converging sensory pathways within the cerebral cortex of the monkey.

Brain 93, 793–820

Jones, G.V., Martin, M. (1985). Deep dyslexia and the right hemisphere hypothesis for semantic paralexia: a reply to Marshall & Patterson. *Neuropsychologia* 23, 685–688

Jones, J.P., Palmer, L.A. (1987). An evaluation of the two-dimensional Gabor filter model of simple receptive fields in cat striate cortex. *J. Neurophysiol.* 58, 1233–1258

Jones-Molfese, V. (1975). Preferences of infants for regular and distorted facial stimuli. *Child Dev.* 46, 1005–1009

Jonides, J. (1979). Left and right visual field superiority for letter classification. *Quart. J. Exp. Psychol.* 31, 423–439

Jordan, D., Baumgartner, G. (1960). Changes of neuronal activity in the primary optic cortex of the cat after elimination of a specific afferent system through pressure schemia of the retina. *Electroenceph. Clin. Neurophysiol.* 12, 258

Jordan, J.R., Geister, W.S., Bovik, A.C. (1990). Color as a source of information in the stereo correspondence process. *Vision Res.* 30, 1955–1970

Jossmann, P. (1929). Zur Psychopathologie der optisch-agnostischen Störungen. *Monatsschr. Psychiat. Neurol.* 72, 81–149

Joynt, R.J., Honch, G.W., Rubin, A.J., Trudell, R.G. (1985). Occipital lobe syndromes. In Vinken, P.J., Bruyn, G.W., Klawans, H.L. (eds.), *Handbook of Clinical Neurology* 45, Clinical Neuropsychology. Elsevier Science Publishers, Amsterdam, 49–62

Judd, T., Gardner, H., Geschwind, N. (1983). Alexia without agraphia in a composer. *Brain* 106, 435–457

Julesz, B. (1971). *Foundation of Cyclopean Perception.* University of Chicago Press, Chicago, Ill.

Julesz, B. (1975). Experiments in the visual perception of texture. *Scientific American* 232, 34–43

Julesz, B. (1981). Textons, the elements of texture discrimination and their interaction. *Nature* 290, 91–97

Julesz, B., Bergen, J.R. (1983). Textons, the fundamental elements in preattentive vision and perception of textures. *Bell Syst. Techn. J.* 62, 1619–1645

Julesz, B., Payne, R.A. (1968). Differences between monocular and binocular stroboscopic movement perception. *Vision Res.* 8, 433–444

Jung, C. (1949). Über eine Nachuntersuchung des Falles Schn. von Goldstein und Gelb. *Psychiatrie, Neurologie und Medizinische Psychologie* 1, 353–362

Jung, R. (1951). Bemerkungen zu Bays Agnosie-Arbeiten. *Nervenarzt* 22, 192–192

Jung, R. (1953). Neuronal discharge. *Electroenceph. clin. Neurophysiol.*, Suppl. 4, 57–71

Jung, R. (1953). Nystagmographie. Zur Physiologie und Pathologie des optisch-vestibulären Systems beim Menschen. In Bergmann, G. von, Frey, W., Schwiegk, H. (eds.), *Handbuch der inneren Medizin*, vol. V/1, Springer, Berlin, Göttingen, Heidelberg, 1325–1379

Jung, R. (1961). Korrelationen von Neuronentätigkeit und Sehen. In Jung, R., Kornhuber, H.H. (eds.), *Neurophysiologie und Psychophysik des visuellen Systems.* Springer, Berlin, Göttingen, Heidelberg, 410–435

Jung, R. (1974). Neuropsychologie und Neurophysiologie des Kontur- und Formsehens in Zeichnung und Malerei. In Wieck, H.H. (ed.), *Psychopathologie musischer Gestaltungen.* Schattauer Verlag, Stuttgart, New York, 27–88

Jung, R. (1975). Compensation of visual neglect of the left side in right hemispheric lesions. In Zülch, K.J., Creutzfeldt, O., Galbraith, C.G. (eds.), *Cerebral localization.* Springer, Berlin, Heidelberg, New York, 302–305

Jung, R. (1979). Translokation kortikaler Migränephosphene bei Augenbewegungen und vestibulären Reizen. *Neuropsychologia* 17, 173–185

Jung, R. (1984). Sensory research in historical perspective: some philosophical foundations of perception. In *Handbook of Physiology*,

Vol. III The nervous system, 1–74

Jung, R., Baumgarten, R. v., Baumgartner, G. (1952). Mikroableitungen von einzelnen Nervenzellen im optischen Cortex der Katze: die lichtaktivierten B-Neurone. *Arch. Psychiat. Nervenkr.* 189, 521–539

Jung, R., Baumgartner, G. (1965). *Neuronenphysiologie der visuellen und paravisuellen Felder.* 3. Intern. Kongress für Neurologie, Wien, Vol. III

Jung, R., Creutzfeldt, O., Grüsser, O.-J. (1957). Die Mikrophysiologie kortikaler Neurone und ihre Bedeutung für die Sinnes-und Hirnfunktionen. *Dtsch. med. Wschr.* 82, 1050–1059

Jung, R., Creutzfeldt, O., Grüsser, O.-J. (1958). The microphysiology of cortical neurones. *Germ. med. Monthly* 3, 269–279

Kaas, J.H. (). *The structural basis for information processing in the primate visual system ....*, 315–340 (keine weiteren Angaben)

Kaas, J.H. (1978). The organization of visual cortex in primates. In Noback, C.R. (ed.), *Sensory Systems of Primates*, Plenum, New York, 151–179

Kaas, J.H. (1989). Changing concepts of visual cortex organization in primates. In Brown, J.W. (ed.), *Neuropsycholgy of visual perception.* Erlbaum, Hillsdale, 3–32

Kaas, J.H., Krubitzer, L.A. (1988). Subdivisions of visuomotor and visual cortex in the frontal lobe of primates: the frontal eye field and the target of the middle temporal area. *Soc. Neurosci. Abstr.* 14, 1123

Kaas, J.H., Krubitzer, L.A., Chino, Y.M., Langston, A.L., Polley, E.H., Blair, N. (1990). Reorganization of retinotopic cortical maps in adult mammals after lesions of the retina. *Science* 248, 229–231

Kaas, J.H., Sur, M., Nelson, R.J., Merzenich, M. (1981). The postcentral somatosensory cortex: multiple representations of the body in primates. In Woolsey, C.N. (ed.), *Cortical Sensory Organization. Multiple Somatic Areas.* Humana, Clifton, N.J. vol. 1, 29–46

Kaeding, F.W. (1898). *Häufigkeitswörterbuch der deutschen Sprache.* Steglitz

Kaess, W.A., Witryol, S.L. (1955). Memory for names and faces: a characteristic of social intelligence? *J. appl. Psychol.* 39, 459–462

Kagan, J., Henker, B.A., Hen-Tov, A.L.J., Lewis, M. (1966). Infants' differential reactions to familiar and distorted faces. *Child Development* 37, 519–532

Kahlbaum, K. (1866). Die Sinnesdelirien. *Allg. Z. Psychiat.* 23, 1–86

Kandel, E.R., Schwartz, J.H. (1985). *Principles of neural science.* Elsevier, New York

Kandinsky, V. (1881). Zur Lehre von den Hallucinationen. *Arch. Psychiat. Nervenkr.* 11, 453–464

Kanizsa, G. (1979). *Organization in vision. Essays on Gestalt perception.* Praeger, New York

Karanth, P. (1981). Pure alexia in a Kanada-English bilingual. *Cortex* 17, 187–198

Karbowski, K. (1982) (ed.). *Halluzinationen bei Epilepsien und ihre Differentialdiagnose.* Huber, Bern, Stuttgart, Wien

Karbowski, K. (1982). Auditive und vestibuläre Halluzinationen epileptischer Genese. In Karbowski, K. (ed.), *Halluzinationen bei Epilepsien und ihre Differentialdiagnose.* Huber, Bern, 24–51

Karlgren, B. (1952). *Sound and Symbol in Chinese.* University Press, Hong Kong. German transl. (1975): Schrift und Sprache der Chinesen. Springer, Berlin, Heidelberg, New York

Karnath, H.O., Hartje, W. (1987). Residual information processing in the neglected visual half-field. *J. Neurol.* 234, 180–184

Karpov, B.A., Meerson, Y.A., Tonkonogii, I.M. (1979). On some peculiarities of the visuomotor system in visual agnosia. *Neuropsychologia* 17, 281–294

Kasanin, J.S. (1946). *Language and Thought in Schizophrenia.* University of California Press, Berkeley

Kasdon, D.L., Jacobson, S. (1978). The thalamic afferents to the inferior parietal lobule of the rhesus monkey. *J. Comp. Neurol.* 177,

685–706

Kase, C.S., Troncoso, J.F., Court, J.E., Tapia, F.J., Mohr, J.P. (1977). Global spatial disorientation. *J. Neurol. Sci.* 34, 267–278

Katz, D. (1911). *Die Erscheinungsweisen der Farben und ihre Beeinflussung durch die individuelle Erfahrung.* J.A. Barth, Leipzig

Katz, D. (1930). *Der Aufbau der Farbenwelt.* J.A. Barth, Leipzig

Katz, D. (1935). *The world of colours.* Kegan Paul, London

Katz, D. (1953). *Studien zur experimentellen Psychologie.* Schwabe, Basel

Katz, D. (1953). Über Zeichnungen von Blinden. In Katz, D. (ed.), *Studien zur experimentellen Psychologie,* Schwabe, Basel, 75–115

Katz, S.E. (1931). Colour preferences in the insane. *J. Abnorm. and Soc. Psychol.* 26, 203–211

Kaufman, L. (1974). *Sight and mind.* Oxford University Press, New York

Kawabata, S., Tagawa, K., Hirata, Y., et al. (1987). A case of alexia with agraphia due to the infarction in the left inferior-posterior temporal lobe. *Rinshou Shinkei* 27, 420–427

Kawahata, N., Nagata, K. (1989). A case of associative visual agnosia: Neuropsychological findings and theoretical considerations. *J. Clin. Exp. Neuropsychol.* 11, 645–664

Kawano, K., Sasaki, M. (1984). Response of neurons in posterior parietal cortex of monkey during visual-vestibular stimulation. II. Optokinetic neurons. *J. Neurophysiol.* 51, 352–360

Kawano, K., Sasaki, M., Yamashita, M. (1980). Vestibular input to visual tracking neurons in the posterior parietal association cortex of the monkey. *Neurosci. Lett.* 17, 55–60

Kawano, K., Sasaki, M., Yamashita, M. (1984). Response properties of neurons in posterior parietal cortex of monkey during visual-vestibular stimulation. I. Visual tracking neurons. *J. Neurophysiol.* 51, 340–351

Kay, M.C., Levin, H.S. (1982). Prosopagnosia. *Americal Journal of Ophthalmology* 94, 75–80

Keen, W.W., Thomson, W. (1871). *Gunshot-wound of the brain, followed by fungus cerebri and recovery with hemiopsia.* Trans. Amer. Ophthal. Soc., 8th Meeting

Kees, H. (1973). *Ägyptische Schrift und Sprache.* Brill, Leiden

Kelly, D.H. (1973). Flicker. In Jameson, D., Hurvich, L.M. (eds.), Visual psychophysics. *Handbook of Sensory Physiol. Vol. VII/4,* Springer, Berlin, 273–302

Kelly, D.H. (1979). Motion and vision. II. Stabilized spatio-temporal threshold surface. *J. opt. Soc. Am.* 69, 1340–1349

Kelly, D.H. (1983). Spatio-temporal variation of chromatic and achromatic contrast thresholds. *J. Opt. Soc. Am.* 73, 742–750

Kemp, D. (1988). Memorial psychophysics for visual area: The effect of retention interval. *Mem. Cognit.* 16, 431–436

Kempe, P., Reimer, Ch. (1976). Halluzinatorische Phänomene bei Reizentzug. *Nervenarzt* 47, 701–707

Kendrick, K.M., Baldwin, B.A. (1987). Cells in temporal cortex of conscious sheep can respond preferentially to faces. *Science* 236, 448–450

Kendrick, K.M., Baldwin, B.A. (1989). Visual responses of sheep temporal cortex cells to moving and stationary human images. *Neurosci. Lett.* 100, 193–197

Kennedy, H., Bullier, J. (1985). A double labeling investigation of the afferent connectivity of cortical areas V1 and V2 of the macaque monkey. *J. Neurosci.* 5, 2815–2830

Kepler, J. (1604). *Ad Vitelloni paralipomena quibus astronomiae pars optica traditur.* Reprint: in Hammer, F. (ed.), J. Kepler, *Gesammelte Werke.* Beck, München

Kepler, J. (1611). *Dioptrice seu demonstratio eorum quae visiu et visibilibus propter conspicilla non ita pridem inventa accidunt.* D. Franc, Ausgustae Vindelicorum. Repr. with an introduction by M. Hoskin, Cambridge Univ. Press., 1962.

Kerner, J. (1824). *Geschichte zweyer Somnambülen nebst einigen anderen Denkwürdigkeiten aus dem Gebiete der magischen Heilkunde und der Psychologie.* Braun, Karlsruhe

Kerner, J. (1829). *Die Seherin von Prevorst. Eröffnungen über das innere Leben des Menschen und über das Hineinragen der Geisterwelt in unsere.* 2 Vols., Cotta, Stuttgart

Kerner, J. (1890). *Kleksographien.* Deutsche Verlagsanstalt, Stuttgart

Kerr, N.H., Voulkes, D. (1981). Right hemispheric mediation of dream visualization: a case study. *Cortex* 17, 603–610

Kerschensteiner, M., Hartje, W., Orgass, B., Poeck, K. (1972). The recognition of simple and complex realistic figures in patients with unilateral brain lesion. *Arch. Psychiat. Nervenkrankh.* 216, 188–200

Kerschensteiner, M., Orgass, B., Poeck, K. (1974). Störungen des visuellen Erkennens nach einseitiger Hirnschädigung. *Nervenarzt* 45, 67–72

Kertesz, A. (1979). Visual agnosia: The dual deficit of recognition. *Cortex* 15, 403–419

Kertesz, A. (1983). Right-hemisphere lesions in constructional apraxia and visuospatial deficit. In Kertesz, A. (ed.), *Localization in neuropsychology.* Academic Press, New York, 455–470

Kertesz, A. (1987). The clinical spectrum and localization of visual agnosia. In G.W. Humphreys, M.J. Riddoch (eds.), *Visual object processing: A cognitive neuropsychological approach.* Lawrence Erlbaum Associates, London

Kertesz, A., Sheppard, A., MacKenzie, R. (1982). Localisation in transcortical sensory aphasia. *Arch. Neurol.* 39, 475–478

Keup, W. (ed.) (1970). *Origin and mechanisms of hallucinations.* Plenum Press, N.Y., London

Kidran, D.P., Bornstein, B. (1959). Prosopagnosia. *J. Neurol. Neurosurg. Psych.* 22, 124–131

Kievet, J., Kuypers, H.G.J.M. (1977). Organization of the thalamocortical connection to the frontal lobe in the rhesus monkey. *Exp. Brain Res.* 29, 299–322

Kikuchi, T. (1987). Temporal characteristics of visual memory. *J. Exp. Psychol.: Hum. Percept* 13, 464–477

Kim, Y., Morrow, L., Passafiume, D., Boller, F. (1984). Visuoperceptual and visuomotor abilities and locus of lesion. *Neuropsychologia* 22, 177–185

Kimura, D. (1961). Cerebral dominance and the perception of verbal stimuli. *Canad. Psychol.* 15, 166–171

Kimura, D. (1966). Dual functional asymmetry of the brain in visual perception. *Neuropsychologia* 4, 275–285

Kimura, D. (1969). Spatial organization in left and right visual fields. *Canad. J. Psychol.* 23, 445–458

Kimura, D., Durnford, M. (1974). Normal studies on the function of the right hemisphere in vision. In Dimond, S.J., Beaumont, J.G: (eds.), *Hemisphere function in the human brain.* Elek Science, London, 25–47

King, M.C. (1981). Effects of non-focal brain dysfunction on visual memory. *J. Clin. Psychol.* 37, 638–643

King-Ellison, P., Jenkins, J.J. (1954). The duration threshold of visual recognition as a function of word-frequency. *Amer. J. Psychol.* 67, 700–703

King-Smith, P.E., Kulikowski, J.J. (1980). Pattern and movement detection in a patient lacking sustained vision. *J. Physiol. (Lond.)* 300,

Kinsbourne, M. (1970). A model for the mechanism of unilateral neglect of space. *Trans. Amer. Neurol. Ass.* 95, 143

Kinsbourne, M. (1972). Eye-head turning indicates cerebral lateralization. *Science* 176, 539–541

Kinsbourne, M. (1973). The control of attention by interaction between the cerebral hemispheres. In Kornblum, S. (ed.) *Attention and performance IV.* Academic Press, New York

Kinsbourne, M. (1974). Direction of gaze and distribution of cerebral thought processes. *Neuropsychologia* 12, 270–281

Kinsbourne, M. (1977). Hemi-neglect and hemispheric rivalry. In Weinstein, E.A., Friedland, R.P. (eds.), *Advances in neurology*, vol. 18. Raven Press, New York

Kinsbourne, M. (1978). *Asymmetrical function of the brain.* London, Cambridge Univ. Press

Kinsbourne, M., Warrington E.K. (1964). Observation on colour agnosia. *J. Neurol. Neurosurg. Psychiat.* 27, 296–299

Kinsbourne, M., Warrington, E.K. (1962). A disorder of simultaneous form perception. *Brain* 85, 461–486

Kinsbourne, M., Warrington, E.K. (1962). Study of finger agnosia. *Brain* 85, 47

Kinsbourne, M., Warrington, E.K. (1962a). A variety of reading disabilities associated with right hemisphere lesions. *J. Neurol. Neurosurg. Psychiat.* 25, 339–344

Kinsbourne, M., Warrington, E.K. (1963). A study of visual perseveration. *J. Neurol. Neurosurg. Psychiat.* 26, 468–475

Kinsbourne, M., Warrington, E.K. (1963). The localizing significance of limited simultaneous form perception. *Brain* 86, 697–702

Kirchhof, J.K.J. (1969a). *Mimische Reaktionen bei Schizophrenie — Einfache Verläufe.* Movie D 949/1968 Inst. Wiss. Film, Göttingen, 3–15

Kirchhof, J.K.J. (1969c). *Mimische Reaktionen bei Schizophrenie. Hebephrene Verläufe.* Movie D 927/1967 Inst. Wiss. Film, Göttingen 3–20

Kirchhof, J.K.J. (1969d). *Mimische Reaktionen bei Schizophrenie Katatonie-Grimassen, Paramimie, Stupor und Angst.* Movie D 906 Inst. Wiss. Film, Göttingen, 3–25

Kirchhof, J.K.J. (1969e). *Mimische Reaktionen bei Schizophrenie. Stereotypien und Defekte.* Movie D 952/1968 Inst. Wiss. Film, Göttingen, 3–20

Kirchhof. J.K.J. (1969b). *Mimische Reaktionen bei Schizophrenie. Paranoide Formen und Paranoia.* Movie D 950/1968 Inst. Wiss. Film, Göttingen, 3–19

Kirshner, H.S., Webb, W.G. (1982). Word and letter reading and the mechnisms of the third alexia. *Arch. Neurol.* 39, 84–87

Kisvarday, Z.F., Cowey, A., Stoerig, P., Somogyi, P. (1991). Direct and indirect retinal input into degenerated dorsal lateral geniculate nucleus after striate cortical removal in monkey: implications for residual vision. Exp. Brain Res. (in press)

Kitterle, F.L., Kaye, K.S. (1985). Hemispheric symmetry in contrast and orientation sensitivity. *Perc. Psychophys.* 37, 391–396

Klee, A. (1975). Perception disorders in migraine. In Pearce, J. (ed.), *Modern topics in migraine.* Heinemann, London, 45–51

Klein, D. (1976). Attentional mechanisms and perceptual asymmetries in tachistoscopic recognition of words and faces. *Neuropsychologia* 14, 55–66

Klein, D., Moscovitch, J., Vigna, C. (1976). Attentional mechanisms and perceptual asymmetries in tachistoscopic recognition of words and faces. *Neuropsychologia* 14, 55–66

Klein, R. (1933). *Über die Funktionen des Parietallappens.*

Klein, R., Ingram, I.M. (1958). Functional disorganization of the left limbs in a tumor of the corpus callosum infiltrating the hemispheres. *J. Mental Sci.* 104, 732–742

Kleist, K. (1912). Der Gang und der gegenwärtige Stand der Apraxieforschung. *Erg. Neurol. Psychiat.* 1, 342–452

Kleist, K. (1918). *Die Gehirnverletzungen in ihrer Bedeutung für die Gehirnlokalisation.* Kriegstagung des Vereins f. Psychiatrie Würzburg

Kleist, K. (1923). Kriegsverletzungen des Gehirns in ihrer Bedeutung für die Hirnlokalisation und Hirnpathologie. In Schjerning, O. (ed.), *Handbuch der ärztlichen Erfahrung im Weltkriege 1914–1818. Vol. 4 Geistes-und Nervenkrankheiten.* Barth, Leipzig

Kleist, K. (1924). *Zur Physiologie und Pathologie der weiteren Sehsphäre (optisch-motorische Störungen, optisch Aufmerksamkeitsstörungen und Beirrungen der absoluten Lokalisation)*

Kleist, K. (1926). Die einzeläugigen Gesichtsfelder und ihre Vertretung in den beiden Lagen der verdoppelten inneren Körnerschicht der Sehrinde. *Klin. Wochenschr.* 5, 3

Kleist, K. (1926). *Gehirnpathologische und gehirnlokalisatorische*

Ergebnisse, vornehmlich aufgrund von Kriegsverletzungen. Festschrift für W. Bechterew

Kleist, K. (1934). *Gehirnpathologie.* Barth, Leipzig

Kleist, K. (1935). Über Form und Ortsblindheit bei Verletzungen des Hinterhautlappens. *Dtsch. Z. Nervenheilk.* 138, 206–214

Kleist, K. (1937). Bericht über die Gehirnpathologie in ihrer Bedeutung für die Neurologie und Psychiatrie. *Z. Ges. Neurol. Psychiat.* 158, 159–193

Klempel, K. (1973). Über Personenverkennung nach dem Muster des sogen. Capgras-Symptoms und verwandte Phänomene. *Psychiatrische Klinik* 6, 17–29

Klengel, H. (1983). *Altbabylonische Texte aus Babylon.* Akademie-Verlag, Berlin

Klicpera, C. (1981). Die Leistungen legasthener Kinder auf einem Zahlen-Symbol-Lerntest. *Z. Kinder-und Jugendpsychiat.* 9, 412–422

Klicpera, C. (1984). Der neuropsychologische Beitrag zur Legasthenieforschung. Eine Übersicht über wichtige Erklärungsmodelle und Befunde. *Fortschr. Neurol. Psychiatr.* 52, 93–103

Klopfer, B., Davidson, H. (1962). *Rorschach technique; an introducing manual.* New York

Klopp, H.W. (1951).Über Umgekehrt-und Verkehrtsehen. *Dtsch. Z. Nervenheilk.* 165, 231–260

Klopp, H.W. (1955). Verkehrtsehen und kurzdauernde Erblindung. *Nervenarzt* 26, 438–441

Klüver, H. (1926). Mescal visions and eidetic vision. *Amer. J. Psychol.* 37, 502

Klüver, H. (1928). *Mescal: the 'divine' plant and its psychological effects.* Kegan Paul, London

Klüver, H. (1941). *Cerebral mechanisms in behavior.* Jeffress, L.A. (ed.). Wiley, New York, 157–199

Klüver, H. (1942). Functional significance of the geniculo-striate system. *Biol. Sympos.* 7, 253–299

Klüver, H. (1942). Mechanisms of hallucinations. In *Studies in personality.* McGraw-Hill, New York, 175–207

Klüver, H. (1951). Visual functions after removal of the occipital lobes. *J. Psychol.* 11, 23

Klüver, H. (1966). *Mescal and mechanisms of hallucinations.* Chicago University Press, Chicago

Klüver, H., Bucy, P.C. (1937). 'Psychic blindness' and other symptoms following bilateral temporal lobectomy in rhesus monkeys. *Amer. J. Physiol.* 119, 352–353

Klüver, H., Bucy, P.C. (1938). An analysis of certain effects of bilateral temporal lobectomy in the rhesus monkey, with special reference to 'psychic blindness'. *J. Psychol.* 5, 33–54

Klüver, H., Bucy, P.C. (1939). Preliminary analysis of functions of the temporal lobes in monkeys. *Arch. Neur. and Psychiat.* 42, 979–1000

Knight, R.A., Elliott, D.S., Freedman, E.G. (1985). Short-term visual memory in schizophrenics. *J. Abnorm. Psychol.* 94, 427–442

Knoll, M. (1967). *Die Welt der inneren Lichterscheinungen.* Rhein, Zürich, Eranos-Jahrbuch 34, 361–397 + 37 Abbildungen.

Kobayashi, S., Mukuno, K., Ishikawa, S., Tasaki, Y. (1985). Hemispheric lateralization of spatial contrast and sensitivity. *Ann. Neurol.* 17, 141–145

Koehler, K., Ebel, H. (1990). Zur Psychopathologie der Personenverkennung — ein multidimensionaler Entwurf. *Fortschr. Neurol. Psychiat.* 58, 310–316

Koehler, P.J., Endtz, L.J., Te Velde, J., Hekster, R.E. (1986). Aware or non-aware. On the significance of awareness for the localization of the lesion responsible for homonymous hemianopia. *J. Neurol. Sci.* 75, 255–262

Koelbing, H. (1973). Kepler und die physiologische Optik. Sein Beitrag und seine Wirkung. In Krafft, F., Meyer, K., Sticker, B. (eds.), *Internationales Kepler-Symposion 1971. Weil der Stadt.* Gerstenberg, Hildesheim, 229–245

Koelbing, H. (1985). *Il Trattato 'De visione' di Girolamo Fabrici d'Acquapendente (Venezia 1600)*. Atti del XXXIII Congresso nazionale della Societa Italiana de Storia della Medicina. La Garangola, Padua, 29–33

Koelbing, H.M. (1988). Zur Geschichte der Farbenlehre. *Klin. Mbl. Augenheilk.* 192, 176–182

Koenderink, J.J. (1984). Geometrical structures determined by the functional order in nervous nets. *Biol. Cybernet.* 50, 43–50

Koenderink, J.J. (1984). The structure of images. *Biol. Cybernet.* 50, 363–370

Koenderink, J.J. (1986). Optic flow. *Vision Res.* 26, 161–180

Koenderink, J.J. (1989). *The brain as a geometry engine. Presentation at the Conference on Domains of Mental Functioning: Attempts at a Synthesis*. ZIF Bielefeld

Koenderink, J.J., van Doorn, A.J. (1978). Visual detection of spatial contrast; influence of location in the visual field, target extent and illuminance level. *Biol. Cybern.* 30, 157–167

Koenderink, J.J., Van Doorn, A.J. (1986). Depth and shape from differential perspective in the presence of bending deformations. *J. Opt. Soc. Amer.* A 3, 242–249

Koenderink, J.J., van Doorn, A.J. (1987). Representation of local geometry in the visual system. *Biol. Cybern.* 55, 367–375

Koenderink, J.J., van Doorn, A.J. (1988). The basic geometry of a vision system. In Trappl, R. (ed.), *Cybernetics and system*. Kluwer Academic Publ., 481–485

Koenderink, J.J., van Doorn, A.J., van de Grind, W.A. (1985). Spatial and temporal parameters of motion detection in the peripheral visual field. *J. Opth. Soc. Am.A* 2, 252–259

Koenderink, J.J., van Doorn, A.J., van de Grind, W.A. (1991). Motion detection at low luminances. *Exp. Brain Res.* (submitted)

Koerner, F. (1972). Optokinetic stimulation of an immobilized eye in the monkey. *Bibl. Ophthalmol.* 82, 298–307

Koerner, F., Schiller, P.H. (1972). The optokinetic response under open and closed loop conditions in the monkey. *Exp. Brain Res.* 14, 318–330

Koffka, K. (1931). Die Wahrnehmung von Bewegung. In Bethe, A. u.a. (eds.), *Handbuch der normalen und pathologischen Physiologie*. Bd. XII/2. Springer, Berlin, 1156–1214

Kohler, I. (1956). Über Aufbau und Wandlungen der Wahrnehmungswelt: insbesondere über bedingte Empfindungen. *Sitzungsbericht Oesterr. Akad. Wiss. Phil.-hist.Kl.* 227, Abh. I. Rohrer, Wien

Kolb, B., Milner, B. (1981). Observations of spontaneous facial expression after cerebral excisions and after intracarotid injection of sodium amytal. *Neuropsychologia* 19, 505–514

Kolb, B., Taylor, L. (1981). Affective behavior in patients with localized cortical excisions: role of lesion side and site. *Science* 214, 89–91

Kolers, P.A. (1969). Clues to a letter's recognition: implications for the design of characters.J. Typograph. Research 3, 145–168

Kolers, P.A. (1970). Three stages of reading. In Levin, H., Williams, J. (eds.), *Basic studies on reading*. Basic Books, NY, London, 90–118

Kolers, P.A. (1972). Experiments in reading. *Scientific Am.* 227, 84–91

Kolers, P.A. (1976). Pattern-analyzing memory. *Science* 191, 1280–1281

Kolers, P.A., Katzman, M.T. (1966). Naming sequentially presented letters and words. *Language and Speech* 9, 84–95

Kolers, P.A., Lewis, C.L. (1972). Bounding of letter sequences and the integration of visually presented words. *Acta Psychol.* 36, 112–124

Kolers, P.A., Perkins, D.N. (1969). Orientation of letters and errors in their recognition. *Percept. Psychophys.* 5, 265–269

Kolers, P.A., Perkins, D.N. (1975). Spatial and ordinal components of form perception and literacy. *Cogn. Psychol.* 7, 228–267

Kolers, P.A., Wolstad, M.E., Bouma, H. (eds.) (1977). *Processing of visible language*. Plenum New York, London

Komatsu, H., Wurtz, R. (1988a). Relation of cortical areas MT and MST to pursuit eye movements. I. Localization and visual properties of neurons. *J. Neurophysiol.* 60, 580–603

Komatsu, H., Wurtz, R. (1988b). Relation of cortical areas MT and MST to pursuit eye movements. III. Interaction with full field visual stimulation. *J. Neurophysiol.* 60, 621–644

Komatsu, H., Wurtz, R.H. (1989). Modulation of pursuit eye movements by stimulation of cortical areas MT and MST. *J. Neurophysiol.* 62, 31–47

Kommerell, G., Täumer, R. (1972). Investigations of the eye tracking system through stabilized retinal images. In Dichgans, J., Bizzi, E. (eds.), *Cerebral control of eye movements and motion perception*. Karger, Basel, 288–297

Konorski, J. (1967). *Integrative activity of the brain*. University of Chicago Press, Chicago

Kornmüller, A.E. (1931). Eine experimentelle Anaesthesie der äusseren Augenmuskeln am Menschen und ihre Auswirkungen. *J. Psychol. Neurol.* (Lpz.) 41, 354–366

Kosky, S.T., Heilman, K.M., Bowers, D., Valenstein, E. (1980). Recognition and discrimination of emotional faces and pictures. *Brain and Language* 9, 206–214

Kosslyn, S.M. (1980). *Image and Mind*. Harvard University Press, Cambridge

Kosslyn, S.M. (1981). The medium and the message in mental imagery: Theory. *Psychol. Rev.* 88, 46–66

Kosslyn, S.M. (1987). Seeing and imagining in the cerebral hemispheres: A computational approach. *Psychol. Rev.* 94, 148–175

Kosslyn, S.M., Flynn, R., Amsterdam, J., Wang, G. (1991). Components of high-level vision: A cognitive neuroscience analysis and accounts of neurological syndromes. *Cognition* (in press)

Kosslyn, S.M., Holtzman, J.D., Farah, M.J., Gazzaniga, M.S. (1985). A computational analysis of mental image generation: evidence from functional dissociations in split-brain patients. *J. Exp. Psychol.* (Gen) 114, 311–341

Köhler, W. (1917). *Intelligenzuntersuchungen an Menschenaffen*. Abh. Preuss. Akad. Wiss. 1917, Physik.-math. Kl. , Nr. 1, 1–223, repr, Springer, Berlin 1966

Köhler, W. (1925). *The mentality of apes*. Routledge and Kegan Paul, London

Köhler, W. (1947). *Gestalt Psychology*. Liveright, New York

Köhler, W., Held, R. (1949). The cortical correlate of pattern vision. *Science*, 110, 414–419.

Köhler, W., Wallach, H. (1944). Figural after effects: An investigation of visual processes. *Proc. Amer. Phil. Soc.* 88, 269–357

Kölmel, H.W. (1982). Visuelle Perseveration. *Nervenarzt* 53, 560–571

Kölmel, H.W. (1983). Photopsien im hemianopen Feld. *Fortschr. Ophthalmol.* 80, 111–112

Kölmel, H.W. (1984). *Visuelle Halluzinationen im hemianopen Feld bei homonymer Hemianopsie*. Springer, Berlin

Kölmel, H.W. (1985). Complex visual hallucinations in the hemianopic field. *J. Neurol. Neurosurg. Psychiat.* 48, 29–38

Kölmel, H.W. (1986). Die Makula bei homonymer Hemianopsie. *Nervenarzt* 57, 439–446

Kölmel, H.W. (1988). Pure homonymous hemiachromatopsia: findings with neuro-ophthalmologic examination and imaging procedures. *Europ. Arch. Psychiat. Neurol. Sci.* 237, 237–243

Kölmel, W. (1988). *Die homonymen Hemianopsien. Klinik und Pathophysiologie zentraler Sehstörungen*. Springer, Berlin

Kömpf, D., Gmeiner, H.J. (1989). Gaze palsy and visual hemineglect in acute hemisphere lesions. *Neuro-Ophthalmology (Amsterdam)* 9, 49–53

Kömpf, D., Piper, H.F., Neundörfer, H.D. (1983). Palinopsie (visuelle Perseveration) und zerebrale Polyopie: klinische Analyse und computertomographische Befunde. *Fortschr. Neurol. Psychiat.*

51, 270–281

Köppen, M. (1893). Ein Fall von urämischer Psychose mit Symptomen der Rindenblindheit. *Charité Annalen* 18, 709–718

Körner, F. (1969). Die Geschwindigkeitsperzeption beim Bewegungssehen. *Ber. dtsch. Ophthal. Ges.* 69, 569–1972

Körner, F., Dichgans, J. (1967). Bewegungswahrnehmung, optokinetischer Nystagmus und retinale Bildwanderung. Der Einfluö visueller Aufmerksamkeit auf zwei Mechanismen des Bewegungssehens. *Graefes Arch. Ophthal.* 174, 34–48

Körner, F., Regli, F., Haynal, A. (1967). Eine durch Farbsinnstörung, Prosopagnosie und Orientierungsstörung charakterisierte visuelle Agnosie. *Arch. Psychiat. u. Z. ges. Neurol.* 209, 1–20

Kraig, R.P., Nicholson, C. (1978). Extracellular ionic variations during spreading depression. *Neurosciences* 3, 1045–1059

Kramer, A.F., Strayer, D.L. (1998). Assessing the development of automatic processing: an application of dual-task and event-related brain potential methodologies. *Biol. Psychol.* 26, 231–267

Kramer, F. (1917). Bulbärapoplexie (Verschluss der Arteria cerebelli posterior inferior) mit Alloästhesie. *Z. ges. Neurol. Psychiat. (Ref.)* 14, 58–60

Krastel, H., Thederan, H., Huber, J. (1985). Zur Systematik des Riddoch-Phänomens. *Klin. Mbl. Augenheilk.* 187, 155–156

Krause, F. (1924). Die Sehbahnen in chirurgischer Beziehung und die faradische Reizung des Sehzentrums. *Klin. Wschr.* 3, 1260–1265

Krause, F., Schum, H. (1931). In Kuttner, H. (ed.), *Neue Deutsche Chirurgie* Vol. 49A,, 3 vols., vol.2: Die epileptischen Erkrankungen. Enke, Stuttgart, 482–486

Krauss, H.C.G. (1824). *De cerebri laesi ad motum voluntarium relatione, certaque vertiginis directione ex certis cerebri regionibus laesis pendente.* Med. Dissertation, Breslau

Krauss, F. (1852). *Nothschrei eines Magnetisch-Vergifteten.* Selbstverlag, Stuttgart

Krauss, F. (1867). *Nothgedrungene Fortsetzung meines Nothschrei gegen meine Vergiftung mit concentrirtem Lebensäther.* Selbstverlag, Stuttgart

Kreindler, A., Ionasescu, Y. (1961). A case of 'pure' word blindness. *J. Neurol. Neurosurg. Psychiat.* 24, 275–280

Kremer-Zech, H. (1987). *Das Wiedererkennen von Gesichtern und Gegenständen durch schizophrene Patienten.* Doctoral dissertation Freie Universität, Berlin

Kremin, H. (1976). L'approche neurolinguistique des alexies: 1969–1976. *Langage* 44, 63–81

Kremin, H. (1976). Les probleme de l'alexie pure. *Langages* 44, 82–110

Kremin, H., Ohlendorf, I. (1988). Einzelwortverarbeitung im Logogen-Modell. Neurolinguistische Evidenzen. *Neurolinguistik* 2, 67–100

Krickl, M., Poser, U., Markowitsch, H.J. (1987). Interactions between damaged brain hemisphere and mode of presentation on the recognition of faces and figures. *Neuropsychologia* 25, 795–805

Kries, J. von (1923). *Allgemeine Sinnesphysiologie.* Vogel, Leipzig

Krill, A.E., Wieland, A.M., Ostfeld, A.M. (1960). The effect of two hallucinogenic agents on human retinal function. *Arch. Ophthal.* 64, 724–733

Kris, E. (1932). Die Charakterköpfe des Franz Xaver Messerschmidt. Versuch einer historischen und physiologischen Deutung. *Jahrbuch der kunsthistorischen Sammlungen in Wien*, NF VI, 169–228

Kris, E. (1977). Ein geisteskranker Bildhauer. In *Die ästhetische Illusion. Phänomene der Kunst aus der Sicht der Psychoanalyse.* Frankfurt a.M.

Kroh, O. (1922). *Subjektive Anschauungsbilder bei Jugendlichen: ein psychologisch-pädagogische Untersuchung.* Vandenhoeck, Göttingen

Kroll, M. (1929). *Die neuropathologischen Syndrome.* Berlin

Kroll, M.B., Stolbun, D. (1933). Was ist konstruktive Apraxie? *Z. ges. Neurol. Psychiat.* 148, 142–158

Kroll, N.E., Ramskov, C.B. (1984). Visual memory as measured by classification and comparison tasks. *J. Exp. Psychol.: Learn. Mem. Cogn.* 10, 395–420

Kroll, N.E., Schepeler, E.M. (1985). Visual priming effects as a measure of short-term visual memory. *Am. J. Psychol.* 98, 449–468

Kruckenburg, M. (1989). *Die Entstehung von Sprache und Schrift.* Dumont, Köln

Krueger, L.E. (1975). The word superiority effect: is its locus visual-spatial or verbal? *Bull. Psychonom. Soc.* 6, 463–468

Krueger, L.E. (1978). A theory of perceptual matching. *Psychol. Rev.* 85, 278–304

Krüger, J., Bach, M. (1982). Independent systems of orientation columns in upper and lower layers of monkey visual cortex. *Neurosci. Lett.* 31, 225–230

Kucera, H., Francis, W.N. (1967). *A computational analysis of present-day American English.* Brown University Press, Providence

Kuhl, P.K., Meltzoff, A.N. (1982). The bimodal perception of speech in infancy. *Science* 218, 1138–1141

Kuhlo, W., Lehmann, D. (1964). Das Einschlaferleben und seine neurophysiologischen Korrelate. *Arch. Psychiat. Nervenkr.* 205, 687–716

Kuhn, M.J., Shekar, P.C. (1990). A comparative study of magnetic resonance imaging and computed tomography in the evaluation of migraine. *Computerized Med. Imag. and Graphics* 14, 148–152

Kulikowski, J.J., Tolhurst, D.J. (1973). Psychophysical evidence for sustained and transient detectors in human vision. *J. Physiol. (Lond.)* 232, 149–162

Kulikowski, J.J., Vidyasagar, T.R. (1986). Space and spatial frequency: analysis and representation in the macaque striate cortex. *Exp. Brain Res.* 64, 5–18

Kumar, N., Verma, A., Maheshwari, M.C., Kumar, B.R. (1986). Prosopagnosia (A report of two cases). *J. Assoc. Physicians of India* 34, 733–735

Kunz, B., Spatz, W.B. (1985). A callosal projection of area 17 upon the border region of area MT in the marmoset monkey, *Callithrix jacchus. J. Comp. Neurol.* 239, 413–419

Kurachi, M., Yamaguchi, N., Inasaka, T., Torii, H. (1979). Recovery from alexia without agraphia: Report of an autopsy. *Cortex*, 15, 297–312

Kurth, W. (1927). *The complete woodcuts of Albrecht Dürer.* W. and G. Foyle, New York, repr. New York, Dover (1963)

Kurucz, J., Feldmar, G. (1979). Prosopo-affective agnosia as a symptom of cerebral organic disease. *J. Amer. Ger. Soc.* 27, 225–230

Kurucz, J., Feldmar, G., Werner, W. (1979). Prosop-affective agnosia associated with chronic organic brain syndrome. *J. Amer. Geriatrics Soc.* 27, 93–95

Kurucz, J., Soni, A., Feldmar, G., Slade, B.R. (1980). Prosopo-affective agnosia and CT findings in patients with cerebral disorders. *J. Amer. Geriatrics Soc.* 28, 475–478

Kussmaul, A. (1877). *Die Störungen der Sprache.* Vogel, Leipzig

Kussmaul, F. (1982). *Ferne Völker, frühe Zeiten. Vol. 1. Afrika, Ozeanien, Amerika.* Bongers, Recklinghausen

Kutzinski (1910). Fall von Rindenblindheit. *Neurologisches Centralblatt* 29, 1324–1326

Kuypers, H.G.J.M., Szwarcbart, M.K., Mishkin, M., Rosvold, H.E. (1965). Occipitotemporal corticocortical connections in the rhesus monkey. *Exp. Neurol.* 11, 245–262

Künzle, H., Akert, K. (1977). Efferent connections of area 8 (frontal eye field) in Macaca fascicularis. A reinvestigation using the autoradiographic technique. *J. Comp. Neurol.* 173, 147–164

Küpfmüller, K. (1954). Die Entropie der deutschen Sprache. *Fernmeldetechnische Zeitschrift* 7, 265–269

Küstermann, K. (1897). Ueber doppelseitige homonyme Hemianopsie und ihre begleitenden Symptome. *Monatschr. Psychiat. Neurol.* 2, 335–352

Lackner, J.R. (1985). Human sensory-motor adaptation to the terrestrial force environment. In Ingle, D.J., Jeannerod, M., Lee, D.N. (eds.), *Brain mechanisms and spatial vision*. Nijhoff, Dordrecht, 175–179

Lackner, J.R. (1988). Some proprioceptive influence on the perceptual representation of body shape and orientation. *Brain* 111, 281–297

Lackner, J.R., Levine, M.S. (1979). Changes in apparent body orientation and sensory localization induced by vibration of postural muscles: vibratory myesthetic illusions. *Aviation, Space and Environmental Medicine* 50, 346–3554

Ladavas, E. (1987). Is the hemispatial deficit produced by right parietal lobe damage associated with retinal or gravitational coordinates? *Brain* 110, 167–180

Ladavas, E., Petronio, A., Umilta, C. (1990). The deployment of visual attention in the intact field of hemineglect patients. *Cortex* 26, 307–317

Laehr, M. (1896). Zur Symptomatologie occipitaler Herderkrankungen. *Charité-Annalen* XXI, 790–814

Laitman, J.T. (1985). Evolution of the hominid upper respiratory tract: the fossile evidence. In Tobias, P.V. (ed.), Hominid evolution. Past, present and future. Liss, New York, 281–286

Laitman, J.T. (1985). Later middle Pleistocene hominids. In Delson, E. (ed.), *Ancestors: the hard evidence*. Liss, New York, 265–267

Laitman, J.T., Crelin, E.S., Conlogue, G.J. (1977). The function of the epiglottis in monkey and man. Yale, *J. Biol. Med.* 50, 43–61

Laitman, J.T., Heimbuch, R.C. (1982). The basicranium of PLIO-Pleistocene hominids as an indicator of their upper respiratory systems. *Am. J. Phys. Anthropol.* 59, 323–331

Laitmann, J.T., Heimbuch, R.C., Crelin, E.S. (1979). The basicranium of fossile hominids as an indicator of their upper respiratory systems. *Am. J. Phys. Anthropol.* 51, 15–24

Lake, D.A., Bryden, M.P. (1976). Handedness and sex differences in hemispheric asymmetry. *Brain and Language* 3, 266–282

Lamansky, H. (1869). Die Bestimmung der Winkelgeschwindigkeit der Augenbewegung. *Pflügers Arch.* 2, 418–422

Lamarre, Y., Spidalieri, G., Chapman, C.E. (1985). Activity of areas 4 and 7 neurons during movements triggered by visual, auditory, and somesthetic stimuli in the monkey: movement-related versus stimulus-related responses. *Exp. Brain Res. Suppl.* 10, 196–210

Lambert, A.J., Beaumont, J.G. (1983). Imageability does not interact with visual field in lateral word recognition with oral report. *Brain and Language* 20, 115–142

LaMettrie, J.O. (1751/1912). L'homme machine, 1751. Engl. tranl. in Bussey, G.C. (ed.), *Man a machine*. Open Court, La Salle, Ill.

Lamontagne, C. (1973). A new experimental paradigm for the investigation of the secondary system of human visual motion perception. *Perception* 2, 167–180

Lamotte, R.H., Acuna, C. (1978). Defects in accuracy of reaching after removal of posterior parietal cortex in monkeys. *Brain Res.* 139, 309–326

Lance, J.W. (1976). Simple formed hallucinations confined to the area of a specific visual field defect. *Brain* 99, 719–734

Land, E. (1977). The retinex theory of color vision. *Scientific Amer.* 237 (Dez.) 108–128

Land, E., McCann, J.J. (1971). Lightness and retinex theory. *J. Opt. Soc. Amer.* 61, 1–11

Land, E.H. (1959a). Color vision and the natural image. Part I. *Proc. Natl. Acad. Sci USA* 45, 115–129

Land, E.H. (1959b). Color vision and the natural image. Part II. *Proc. Natl. Acad. Sci USA* 45, 636–644

Land, E.H. (1986). Recent advances in Retinex theory. *Vision Res.* 26, 7–22

Land, E.H., Hubel, D.H., Livingstone, M.S., Perry, S.H., Burns, M.M. (1983). Colour-generating interactions across the corpus callosum. *Nature* 303, 616–618

Landis, C. (1953). *An annotated bibliography of flicker fusion phenomena*. Armed Forces Nat. Research Council, Ann Arbor

Landis, T. (1987). *Right hemisphere reading: A clinico-experimental approach to the dual brain interaction*. Unpubl. Habil. Schr., University of Zürich

Landis, T. (1988). Die Linke weiss nicht was die Rechte tut: Zur Interaktion der beiden Hirnhälften. *Schweiz. med. Wochenschr.* 118, 1779–1788

Landis, T., Assal, G., Perret, E. (1979). Opposite cerebral hemispheric superiorities for visual associative processing of emotional face and objects. *Nature* 278, 739–740

Landis, T., Buttet, J., Assal, G., Graves, R. (1982). Dissociation of ear preference in monaural word and voice recognition. *Neuropsychologia* 20, 501–504

Landis, T., Cummings, J.L., Benson, D.F. (1980). Le passage de la dominance du langage a l'hemisphere droit: une interpretation de la recuperation tardive lors d'aphasies globale. *Rev. Med. Suisse Romande* 100, 171–177

Landis, T., Cummings, J.L., Benson, D.F., Palmer, E.P. (1986). Loss of topographic familiarity. An environmental agnosia. *Arch. Neurol.* 43, 132–136

Landis, T., Cummings, J.L., Christen, L., Bogen, J.E., Imhof, H. (1986). Are unilateral right posterior cerebral lesions sufficient to cause prosopagnosia? Clinical and radiological findings in six additional patients. *Cortex* 22, 243–252

Landis, T., Graves, R., Benson, F., Hebben, N. (1982). Visual recognition through kinaesthetic mediation. *Psychol. Med.* 12, 515–531

Landis, T., Graves, R., Goodglass, H. (1981). Dissociated verbal awareness of manual performance on two different visual associative tasks: a 'split-brain' phenomenon in normal subjects? *Cortex* 17, 435–440

Landis, T., Graves, R., Goodglass, H. (1982). Aphasic reading and writing: possible evidence for right hemisphere participation. *Cortex* 18, 105–112

Landis, T., Lehmann, D., Mita, T., Skrandies, W. (1984). Evoked potential correlates of figure and ground. *Intern. J. Psychophysiol.* 1, 345–348

Landis, T., Regard, M. (1988). Lateralität und Depression: eine Untersuchung an Patienten mit Insulten im Versorgungsgebiet der A. cerebri posterior. In Oepen, G. (ed.), *Psychiatrie des rechten und linken Gehirns*. Dtsch. Ärzteverlag, Köln

Landis, T., Regard, M. (1988). The right hemisphere's access to lexical meaning: A function of its release from left hemisphere control? In Chiarello, C. (ed.), *Right hemisphere contributions to lexical semantics*. Springer, Heidelberg, 33–47

Landis, T., Regard, M. (1988). Two cases of prosopagnosia and alexia. Part I: Neuropsychological findings. In Bajic, M. (ed.), *Neuron, Brain and Behavior*. Advances in Biosciences. Vol. 70, Pergamon Press, Oxford, 89–95

Landis, T., Regard, M. (1988b). Hemianopsie und Agnosie. *Klin. Mbl. Augenheilk.* 192, 525–528

Landis, T., Regard, M. (1989). Relative interactive hemispheric dominance in reading. In Euler, C.v., Lundberg, I., Lennerstrand, G. (eds.), *Brain and Reading*. Wenner Gren Intern. Symposium Series, Vol. 54, MacMillan, London, 99–115

Landis, T., Regard, M. (1991). Gesichtsfeld-und Wahrnehmungsstörungen bei suprakalkarinen Läsionen. In Gloor, B. (ed.), *Perimetrie mit besonderer Berücksichtigung der automatischen Perimetrie*. 2. Aufl., Enke, Stuttgart

Landis, T., Regard, M., Bliestle, A., Kleihues, P. (1988). Prosopagnosia and agnosia for non-canonical views: An autopsied case. *Brain* 111, 1287–1297

Landis, T., Regard, M., Graves, R., Goodglass, H. (1983). Semantic paralexia: a release of right hemispheric function from left hemispheric control? *Neuropsychologia* 21, 359–364

Landis, T., Regard, M., Serrat, A. (1980). Iconic reading in a case of alexia without agraphia caused by a brain tumor: a tachistoscopic study. *Brain and Language* 11, 45–53

Landis, T., Regard, M., Weniger, D. (1990). Das rechte Hirn. *Schweiz. med. Wochenschr.* 120, 433–439

Landolt, T.E. (1888b). Alexia or word blindness. *Neurol. Cbl.* 7, 605–606

Lane, J.K. (1983). *The Modular Efferent Organization of the Inferior Parietal Lobule and Caudal Principal Sulcus for Their Callosal and Reciprocal Association Projections.* (Dissertation). John Hopkins Univ. Press, Baltimore, MD.

Lange, J. (1936). Agnosien und Apraxien. In O. Bumke, O. Foerster (eds.), *Handbuch der Neurologie*, Springer, Berlin, VI, 807–960

Lange-Malecki, B., Poppinga, J., Creutzfeldt, O.D. (1990). The relative contribution of retinal and cortical mechanisms to simultaneous contrast. *Naturwissenschaften* 77, 394–398

Lannois, M. (1904). A propos des phénomènes d'autoscopie. Un cas de 'vision par la peau'. *Bull. du Lyon médical* 17.7.1904, 161–164

Lansdell, H.C. (1968). Effect of extent of temporal lobe ablations on two lateralised deficits. *Physiol. Behav.* 3, 271–273

Laqueur, L. (1898). Über einen Fall von doppelseitiger homonymer Hemianopsie mit Erhaltung eines minimalen centralen Gesichtsfeldes mit Sectionsbefund. *Versamml. dtsch. ophth. Ges.*, Band 27, 218–229

Larrabee, G.J., Kane, R.L., Schuck, J.R., Francis, D.J. (1985). Construct validity of various memory testing procedures. *J. Clin. Exp. Neuropsychol.* 7, 239–250

Larrabee, G.J., Levin, H.S., Huff, F.J., Kay, M.C., Guinto, F.C. (1985). Visual agnosia contrasted with visual-verbal disconnection. *Neuropsychologia* 23, 1–12

Lasegue, C. (1884). *Etudes médicales.* 2 Vol. Asselin, Paris

Lashley, K.S. (1929). *Brain mechanisms and intelligence.* University Press, Chicago

Lashley, K.S. (1941). Patterns of cerebral integration indicated by the scotomas of migraine. *Arch. Neurol. Psychiat. (Chicago)* 46, 331–339

Lashley, K.S. (1948). The mechanism of vision. XVIII. Effects of destroying the visual 'associative areas' of the monkey. *Genet. Psychol. Monogr.* 37, 107–166

Latto, R. (1978). The effects of bilateral frontal eye-field, posterior parietal or superior collicular lesions on visual search in rhesus monkey. *Brain Res.* 146, 35–50

Latto, R., Cowey, A. (1971). Visual field defects after frontal eye-field lesions in monkeys. *Brain Res.* 30, 1–24

Lauber, H.L., Lewin, B. (1958). Clinical and psychological study of optic hallucinations in the elimination of vision. *Arch. Psychiat. Nervenkr.* 197, 15–31

Laughery, K.R., Alexander, J.F., Lane, A.B. (1971). Recognition of human faces: effects of target exposure time, target position, pose position and type of photograph. *J. Appl. Psychol.* 55, 477–483

Laughery, K.R., Fessler, P.K., Lenorovitz, D.R., Yoblick, D.A. (1974). Time delay and similiarity effects in facial recognition. *J. Appl. Psychol.* 59, 490–496

Lavater, J.C. (1775–1778). *Physiognomische Fragmente zur Beförderung der Menschenkenntnis und Menschenliebe.* Weidmann, Leipzig-Winterthur, 4 vols.

Lawick-Goodall, J. van (1971). *Wilde Schimpansen.* Rowohlt, Hamburg

Lawson, N.C. (1978). Inverted writing in right-and left-handers in relation to lateralization of face recognition. *Cortex* 14, 207–211

Lazar, R.M., Davis,-Lang, D., Sanchez, L. (1984). The formation of visual stimulus equivalences in children. *J. Exp. Anal. Behav.* 41, 251–266

Le Beau, J., Wolinetz, E. (1958). Le phenomene de perseveration visuelle, sa valeur localisatrice pour les lesions occipitales. *Rev. Neurol.* 99, 525–534

Le Beau, J., Wolinetz, E. (1965). *Perseveration visuelle et lobe occipital.*

Vienne, 8. Congres intern. de Neurologie. Pathologie du Lobe Occipital, 201–205

Leao, A.A.P. (1944). Spreading depression of activity in cerebral cortex. *J. Neurophysiol.* 7, 359–390 (oder 391–396?)

Leao, A.A.P. (1947). Further observations on the spreading depression of activity in the cerebral cortex. *J. Neurophysiol.* 10, 409–414

Lebrun, Y., Devreux, F. (1986). L'aphasie optique. *J. Psychologie Normale et Pathologique* 81, 31–40

Lee, B.B., Creutzfeldt, O.D., Elepfandt, A. (1979). The responses of magno-and parvocellular cells of the monkey's lateral geniculate body to moving stimuli. *Exp. Brain Res.* 35, 547–557

Lee, B.B., Valberg, A., Tigwell, D.A., Tryti, J. (1987). An account of responses of spectrally opponent neurons in macaque lateral geniculate nucleus to successive contrast. *Proc. R. Soc. Lond. B.* 230, 293.314

Lee, D.N. (1976). A theory of visual control of braking based on information about time-to-collision. *Perception* 5, 437–457

Leehey, S., Cahn, A. (1979). Lateral asymmetries in the recognition of words, familiar faces and unfamiliar faces. *Neuropsychologia* 17, 619–635

Leehey, S., Carey, S., Diamond, R., Cahn, A. (1978). Upright and inverted faces: the right hemisphere knows the difference. *Cortex* 14, 411–419

Leeuwenberg, E., Boselie, F. (1988). Against the likelihood priciple in visual form perception. *Psychol. Rev.* 95, 485–491

Leff, J.P. (1968). Perceptual phenomena and personality in sensory deprivation. *Brit. J. Psychiat.* 114, 1499–1508

Lehky, S.R., Sejnowski, T.J. (1990). Neural model of stereoacuity and depth interpolation based on a distributed representation of stereo disparity. *J. Neuroscience* 10, 2281–2299

Lehmann, D., Wälchli, P. (1975). Depth perception and location of brain lesions. *J. Neurol.* 209, 157–164

Lehmann, H.E. (1980). Unusual psychiatric disorders. In Kaplan, Freedman, Sedock (eds.), *Comprehensive textbook of psychiatry* Vol. 2, 3rd ed., Williams and Wilkins, Baltimore

Leicester, G., Sidman, M., Stoddard, L.T., Mohr, J.P. (1969). Some determinants of visual neglect. *J. Neurol. Neurosurg. Psychiat.* 32, 580–587

Leichnetz, G.R. (1980). An intrahemispheric columnar projection between two cortical multisensory convergence areas (inferior parietal lobule and prefrontal cortex): an anterograde study in macaque using HRP gel. *Neurosci. Lett.* 18, 119–124

Leinonen, L. (1981). *Functions of posterior temporoparietal cortex in the monkey.* Ph.-Diss. Helsinki.

Leinonen, L., Hyvärinen, J., Nyman, G., Linnankoski, I. (1979). I. Functional properties of neurons in lateral part of associative area 7 in awake monkeys. *Exp. Brain Res.* 34, 299–320

Leinonen, L., Nyman, G. (1979). II. Functional properties of cells in anterolateral part of area 7 associative face area of awake monkeys. *Exp. Brain Res.* 34, 321–333

Leischner, A. (1961). Die autoskopischen Halluzinationen (Heautoskopie). *Fortschr. Neurol. Psychiat.* 29, 550–585

Leischner, R.A. (1957). *Die Störungen der Schriftsprache (Agraphie und Alexie).* G. Thieme, Stuttgart

Lelkins, A.M.M., Koenderink, J.J. (184). Illusory motion in visual displays. *J. opt. Soc. Am.*

Lemaitre, A. (1902). Hallucinations autoscopiques et automatismes divers chez des écoliers. *Arch. de Psychol.* 1, 357–379

Lenneberg, E.H. (1961). Color naming, color recognition, color discrimination: a reappraisal. *Percept. Motor Skills* 12, 275–282

Lenz, G. (1905). Beiträge zur Hemianopsie. *Klin. Monatsbl. Augenheilk.* 43, 263–326

Lenz, G. (1912). Ber. 38. Verh. der ophthalmol. Gesellsch. zu Heidelberg, p. 8

Lenz, G. (1914). Die hirnlokalisatorische Bedeutung der Makulaaussparung im hemianopischen Gesichtsfelde. *Klin. Mbl. Augenheilk.*

53, 30–63

Lenz, G. (1916). Die histologische Lokalisation des Sehzentrums. *Graefe Arch. Klin. Exp. Ophthal.* 91, 254–293

Lenz, G. (1921). Zur Pathologie der cerebralen Sehbahn unter besonderer Berücksichtigung ihrer Ergebnisse für die Anatomie und Physiologie. *Graefes Arch. Ophthalmol.* 72, 1–85 and 72, 179–273

Lenz, G. (1921). Zwei Sektionsfälle mit doppelseitiger zentraler Farbhemianopsie. *Z. ges. Neurol. Psychiat.* 71, 135–186

Lenz, H. (1942). Über frontal bedingte Alexie. *Z. ges. Neurol.* 174, 534–541

Lenz, H. (1944). Raumsinnstörungen bei Hirnverletzungen. *Dtsch. Z. Nervenheilk.* 157, 22–64

Leonard, C.M., Rolls, E.T., Wilson, F.A.W., Baylis, G.C. (1985). Neurons in the amygdala of the monkey with responses selective for faces. *Behav. Brain Res.* 15, 159–176

Leonardo da Vinci (1519/1651). *Trattato della pittura di Lionardo da Vinci.* Langlois, Paris

Leonardo da Vinci (1882). *Das Buch von der Malerei.* Ludwig, H. (ed.) 3 Vols, Wien

Leonardo da Vinci (1952). *Tagebücher und Aufzeichnungen.* Transl. Th. Lücke. P. List, Leipzig

Leonardo da Vinci (1954). *The notebooks of Leonardo da Vinci,* ed. by E. MacCurdy. London. repr. Soc. 2 vols.

Leonardo da Vinci (1979). *Anatomische Zeichnungen aus der Königlichen Bibliothek auf Schloss Windsor.* Hamburger Kunsthalle. Prisma Verlag, Gütersloh

Leonhard, K. (1952). *Reine Agraphie und konstruktive Apraxie als Ausdruck einer Leitungsstörung.*

Leonhard, K. (1957). Aufteilung der endogenen Psychosen. Akademie-Verlag, Berlin

Lepore, F.E. (1986). Visual obscurations: evanescent and elementary. *Sem. Neurol.* 6, 167–175

Leroi-Gourhan, A. (1971). *Prähistorische Kunst. Die Ursprünge der Kunst in Europa.* Herder, Freiburg

Lessell, S., Cohen, M.M. (1979). Phosphenes induced by sound. *Neurology* (NY) 29 (11), 1524–7

Lestienne, F., Whittington, D., Bizzi, E. (1983). Coordination of eye-hand movements in alert monkeys: behavior of eye-related neurons in the brain stem. In Hein, A., Jeannerod, M. (eds.), *Spatially oriented behavior.* Springer, New York, Berlin, Heidelberg, Tokyo, 105–117

Letailleur, M., Morin, J., Le Borgne, Y. (1958). Héautoscopie hétérosexuelle et schizophrénie. Etude d'une observation. *Ann. Méd. Psychol.* 116, 451–461

Lethmate, J., Dücker, G. (1973). Untersuchungen zum Selbsterkennen im Spiegel bei Orang-Utans und einigen anderen Affenarten. *Z. Tierpsychol.* 33, 248–269

Leuner, H. (1960). Über psychopathologische Schlüsselfunktionen in der Modellpsychose. *Med. exp.* 2, 227–232

Leuner, H. (1962). *Die experimentelle Psychose.* Springer, Berlin

Leuner, H. (1968). Ist die Verwendung von LSD-25 für die experimentelle Psychiatrie und in der Psychotherapie heute noch vertretbar? *Nervenarzt* 39, 356–360

Leuner, H. (1981a). *Halluzinogene: Psychische Grenzzustände in Forschung und Psychotherapie.* Huber, Bern

Leuner, H. (1981b). *Katathymes Bilderleben: Grundstufe.* 2nd Ed. Thieme, Stuttgart

Leuret, F. (1834). *Fragments psychologiques sur la folie.* Crochard, Paris

Leuret, F., Gratiolet, P. (1837/1857). *Anatomie comparée des systemes nerveux considérée dans ses rapport avec l'intelligence.* 2 Vols., Bailliere, Paris

LeVay, S., Conolly, M., Houde, J., van Essen, D.C. (1985). The complete pattern of ocular dominance stripes in the striate cortex and visual field of the macaque monkey. *J. Neurosci* 5, 486–501

LeVay, S., Hubel, D.H., Wiesel, T.N. (1975). The pattern of ocular dominance columns in macaque visual cortex revealed by a reduced silver stain. *J. Comp. Neurol.* 159, 559–576

LeVay, S., Wiesel, T.N., Hubel, D.H. (1980). The development of ocular dominance columns in normal and visually deprived monkeys. *J. Comp. Neurol.* 191, 1–51

Levick, Dr. (1866). Abscess of brain. *J. med. Sci. N.5.* 52, 413–414

Levick, R. (1979). Commentary to Wasserman and Kong: *Mental timing. The Behavioral and Brain Sciences* 2, 243–304

Levillain, D., Pouliquen, A., Rogler, M., Samson-Dollfus, D. (1972). Evoked visual potentials in 16 cases of homonymous lateral hemianopsia. Electroclinical study. *Rev. Electroencephalogr. Neurophysiol. Clin.* 2, 299–301

Levin, H.S. (1977). Facial recognition in 'pseudoneurological' patients. *J. Nerv. Ment. Dis.* 164, 135–138

Levin, H.S., Grossman, R.G., Kelly, P.J. (1977). Impairment of facial recognition after closed head injuries of varying severity. *Cortex* 13, 119–130

Levin, H.S., Peters, B.H. (1976). Neuropsychological testing following head injuries: Prosopagnosia without visual field defect. *Diseases of the Nervous System* 37, 68–71

Levine, D.N. (1978). Prosopagnosia and visual object agnosia: A behavioral study. *Brain and Language* 5, 341–365

Levine, D.N., Calvanio, R. (1978). A study of the visual defect in verbal alexia-simultanagnosia. *Brain* 101, 65–81

Levine, D.N., Calvanio, R. (1980). Visual discrimination after lesion of the posterior corpus callosum. *Neurology* 30, 21–30

Levine, D.N., Calvanio, R. (1982). The neurology of reading disorders. In Arbib, M.A., Caplan, D., Marshall, J.C. (eds.), *Neural models of language processes.* Academic Press, NY

Levine, D.N., Calvanio, R. (1989). Prosopagnosia: A defect in visual configural processing. *Brain and Cognition* 10, 149–170

Levine, D.N., Faufman, K.J., Mohr, J.P. (1978). Inaccurate reaching associated with a superior parietal lobe tumor. *Neurology* 28, 556–561

Levine, D.N., Mani, R.B., Calvanio, R. (1988). Pure agraphia and Gerstmann's syndrome as a visuospatial-language dissociation: An experimental case study. *Brain and Lang.* 35, 172–196

Levine, D.N., Warach, J., Farah, M. (1985). Two visual systems in mental imagery: Dissociation of 'what' and 'where' in imagery disorders due to bilateral posterior cerebral lesions. *Neurology* 35, 1010–1018

Levine, M.D. (1985). *Vision in man and machine.* McGraw-Hill, New York

Levy, J. (1974). Psychobiological implications of bilateral asymmetry. In Dimond, S.J., Beaumont, J.G. (eds.), *Hemispheric function in the human brain.* Paul Eleh Ltd, London, 121–183

Levy, J., Heller, W., Banich, N.T., Burton, L.A. (1983). Asymmetry of perception in previewing chimeric faces. *Brain and Cognition* 2, 404–419

Levy, J., Kueck, L. (1986). A right hemispatial field advantage on verbal free-vision task. *Brain and Language* 27, 24–37

Levy, J., Reid, N. (1976). Variations in writing posture and cerebral organization. *Science* 194, 337–339

Levy, J., Trevarthen, C. (1981). Color-matching, color-naming and calor memory in split-brain patients. *Neuropsychologia* 19, 523–541

Levy, J., Trevarthen, C., Sperry, R.W. (1972). Perception of bilateral chimeric figures following hemispheric deconnexion. *Brain* 95, 761–778

Levy, L.H., Orr, T.B., Rosenzweig, S. (1960). Judgments of emotion from facial expressions by college students, mental retardates, and mental hospital patients. *J. Pers.* 28, 342–349

Lewandowsky, M. (1908). Über Abspaltung des Farbensinnes. *Mschr. Psychiat. Neurol.* 23, 488–510

Lewis, M. (1969). Infants' responses to facial stimuli during the first year of life. *Developm. Psychol.* 1, 75–86

Lewis, M. (1969). Infants' responses to facial stimuli during the first year of life. *Develop. Psychol.* 1, 75–86

Lewis, S.W. (1987). Brain imaging in a case of Capgras'syndrome. *Brit. J. Psychiat,* 150, 117–121

Ley, R.G., Bryden, M.P. (1979). Hemispheric differences in processing emotions and faces. *Brain and Language* 7, 127–138

Ley, R.G., Bryden, M.P. (1979). Hemispheric differences in processing emotions and faces. *Brain Lang.* 7, 127–138

Ley, R.G., Strauss, E. (1986). Hemispheric asymmetries in the perception of facial expressions by normals. In Bruyer, R. (ed.), *The Neuropsychology of Face Perception and Facial Expression.* Erlbaum, Hilldsdale, N.Y., London, 269–289

Lezak, M. (1983). *Neuropsychological assessment,* 2nd. ed., Oxford University Press, New York

Lhermitte, F., Beauvois, M.F. (1973). A visual-speech disconnexion syndrome: report of a case with optic aphasia, agnosic alexia and colour agnosia. *Brain* 96, 695–714

Lhermitte, F., Chain, Chedru, F., Penet, C. (1974). Syndrome de deconnexion interhemispherique. Etude des performances visuelles. *Rev. Neurol.* 130, 247–250

Lhermitte, F., Chain, F., Aron, D. (1965). Dix cas d'agnosie des couleurs. Etude comparative avec 10 cas de dyschromatopsies congénitales et acquises d'origine périphérique. *Proc. 8 Congress International de Neurologie,* Wien, 217–221

Lhermitte, F., Chain, F., Aron, D., Leblanc, M., Jouty, O. (1969). Les troubles de la vision des couleurs dans les lésions postérieures du cerveau. *Rev. Neurol.* 121, 5–29

Lhermitte, F., Chain, F., Aron-Rosa, D., Leblanc, M., Souty, O. (1969). Enregistrement des mouvements du regard dans un cas d'agnosie visuelle et dans un cas de desorietation spatiale. *Rev. Neurol. (Paris)* 121, 121–137

Lhermitte, F., Chain, F., Chedru, F. (1975). Syndrome de deconnexion interhemispherique etude: des perfomances visuelle. In Michel, F., Schott, B. (eds.), *Les Syndromes de Disconnexion calleuse chez l'homme,* Colloque International, Lyon

Lhermitte, F., Chain, F., Chedru, F., Penet, C. (1976). A study of visual processes in a case of interhemispheric disconnexion. *J. Neurol. Sci.* 28, 317–330

Lhermitte, F., Chain, F., Escourolle, R., Ducarne, B., Pillon, B. (1972). Etude anatomo-clinique d'un cas de prosopagnosie. *Rev. Neurol. (Paris)* 126, 329–346

Lhermitte, F., Chedru, F., Chain, F. (1973). A propos d'un cas d'agnosie visuelle. *Rev. Neurol.* 128, 301–322

Lhermitte, F., Marteau, R., Serdaru, M., Chedru, F. (1977). Signs of interhemispheric disconnection in Marchiafava-Bignami disease. *Arch. Neurol.* 34, 254

Lhermitte, F., Pillon, B. (1975). La prosopagnosie. Role de l'hemisphere droit dans la perception visuelle. *Rev. Neurol. (Paris)* 131, 791–812

Lhermitte, J. (1922). Syndrome de la calotte pédoncle cérébral. Les troubles psycho-sensorielles dans les lésions du mesencéphale. *Rev. Neurol. (Paris)* 38, 1359–1365

Lhermitte, J. (1934). Les hallucinations visuelles au cours des syndroms pédunculaires. *Ann. Méd.-Psych.* 92, 556–565

Lhermitte, J. (1951a). *Les hallucinations-clinique et physiopathologie.* Doin, Paris

Lhermitte, J. (1951b). Visual hallucinations of the self. *Brit. Med. J.* 3, 431–434

Lhermitte, J., Ajuriaguerra, J. de (1936). Hallucinations visuelles et lesion de l'appareil visuel. *Ann. med. psychol.* 94, 321–351

Lhermitte, J., Ajuriaguerra, J. de (1942). *Psychopathologie de la vision.* Masson et Cie, Paris

Lieber, L. (1976). Lexical decisions in the right and left cerebral hemispheres. *Brain and Language* 3, 443–450

Lieberman, A.R. (1971). The axon reaction: a review of the principal features of perikaryal responses to axon injury. *Int. Rev. Neurobiol.* 14, 49–124

Lieberman, P. (1975). *On the origins of language.* MacMillan, New York

Lieberman, P. (1984). *The biology and evolution of language.* Harvard University Press, Cambridge

Lieberman, P. (1991). *Uniquely human: the evolution of speech, thought and selfless behavior.* Harvard Univ. Press

Liepmann, H. (1900). Das Krankheitsbild der Apraxie. *Monatsschr. Psychiat. Neurol.* 8, 15–44, 102–132, 182–197

Liepmann, H. (1908). Dissolutorische und disjunktive Agnosie. *Neurol. Zentralbl.* 13/14, 608, 664

Liepmann, H. (1908). Über die agnostischen Störungen. *Neurol. Zbl. Lpz.* 27, 1–41, 609–617, 664–675

Lilly, R., Cummings, J.L., Benson, D.S., Frankel, M. (1983). The human Klüver-Bucy syndrome. *Neurology* 33, 1141–1145

Lindberg, D.C. (1976). *Theories of vision from Al-Kindi to Kepler.* The University of Chicago Press, Chicago

Lindemann, E. (1922). Experimentelle Untersuchungen über das Entstehen und Vergehen von Gestalten. *Psychol. Forsch.* 2, 5–60

Linden, M. van der, Seron, X. (1987). A case of dissociation in topographical disorders. The selective break-down of retro-map representation. In Allen, P., Thinus-Blanc, C. (eds.), *Neurobiology of spatial behavior. Vol. II, Neurophysiology and developmental aspects.* Nijhoff, Dordrecht, 173–181

Linden, M. van der, Seron, X., Gillet, J., Predart. S. (1980). Hemineglegence par lesion frontale droite. Apropos des trois observations. *Acta Neurol. Belgica* 80, 298–310

Lindzey, G., Prince, B., Wright, H.K. (1952/53). A study of facial asymmetry. *J. Personality* 21, 68–84

Lippman, C.W. (1951). Hallucinations in migraine. *Am. Psychiat.* 107, 856–858

Lippman, C.W. (1952). Certain hallucinations peculiar to migraine. *J. Nerv. Ment. Dis.* 116, 346–351

Lippman, C.W. (1953). Hallucinations of physical duality in migraine. *J. Neur. Ment. Dis.* 117, 345–350

Lissauer, H. (1890). Ein Fall von Seelenblindheit nebst einem Beitrage zur Theorie derselben. *Arch. Psychiat. Nervenkr.* 21, 222–270

Lissauer, H. (1988). A case of visual agnosia with a contribution to theory. *Cogn. Neuropsychol.* 5, 157–192

Livingstone, M.S., Hubel, D.H. (1984). Anatomy and physiology of a color system in the primate visual cortex. *J. Neurosci.* 4, 309–356

Livingstone, M.S., Hubel, D.H. (1984a). Anatomy and physiology of a colour system in the primate visual cortex. *J. Neurosci.* 4, 309–356

Livingstone, M.S., Hubel, D.H. (1984b). Specificity of intrinsic connections in primate primary visual cortex. *J. Neurosci.* 4, 2830–2835

Livingstone, M.S., Hubel, D.H. (1987a). Connections between layer 4B of area 17 and the thick cytochrome oxidase stripes of area 18 in the squirrel monkey. *J. Neurosci.* 7, 3371–3377

Livingstone, M.S., Hubel, D.H. (1987b). Psychophysical evidence for separate channels for the perception of form, color, movement and depth. *J. Neurosci.* 7, 3416–3468

Livingstone, M.S., Hubel, D.H. (1988). Segregation of form, color, movement, and depth: anatomy, physiology, and perception. *Science* 240, 740–749

Loeb, J. (1885). Die elementaren Störungen einfacher Functionen nach oberflächlicher umschriebener Verletzung des Grosshirns. *Pflüger's Arch. Physiol.* 37, 51–56

Loeb, J. (1886). Beiträge zur Physiologie des Grosshirns. *Pflügers Arch.* 39, 265–346

Loevsund, P., Oberg, P.A., Nilsson, S.E. (1980). Magneto-and electrophosphenes: a comparative study. *Medical Biological Engineering and Computing* 18, 758–764

Loevsund, P., Oberg, P.A., Nilsson, S.E., Reuter, T. (1980). Magnetophosphenes: a quantitative analysis of thresholds. *Medical Biological Engineering and Computing* 18, 326–334

Loewenthal, M., Pevzner, S., Bornstein, M. (1962). Prosopagnosie. *J.*

Neurol. Neurosurg. Psychiat. 25, 336–338

Lohmann, H. (1940). Über die Sichtbarkeitsgrenze und die optische Unterscheidbarkeit sinusförmiger Wechselströme. *Z. Sinnesphysiol.* 69, 27–40

Lokhorst, G.J.C. (1982a). An ancient Greek theory of hemispheric specialization. *Clio Medica* 17, 33–38

Lokhorst, G.J.C. (1982b). The oldest printed text on hemispheric specialization. *Neurology* 32, 762

Long, G.M. (1985). The varieties of visual persistence: Comments on Yeomans and Irwin. *Percept. & Psychophys.* 38, 381–385

Longden, K., Ellis, C., Iversen, S.D. (1976). Hemispheric differences in the discrimination of curvature. *Neuropsychologia* 14, 195–202

Longuet-Higgins, H.C., Prazdny, K. (1980). The interpretation of moving retinal images. *Proc. Roy. Soc. B (London)* 208, 385–397

Loomis, J.M. (1974). Tactile letter recognition under different modes of stimulus presentation. *Perception and Psychophysics* 16, 401–408

Loomis, J.M. (1978). Lateral masking in foveal and eccentric vision. *Vision Res.* 18, 335–338

Loomis, J.M., Apkarian-Stielau, P. (1976). A lateral masking effect in tactile and blurred letter recognition. *Perception and Psychophysics* 20, 221–226

Lorenz, K. (1965). *Über tierisches und menschliches Verhalten.* Vol. I/II. Piper, München

Lovegrove, W. J., Over, R., Broerse, J. (1972). Colour selectivity in motion after-effect *Nature* 338, 334–335

Lowe, D.G. (1987). The viewpoint consistency constraint. *Int. J. Computer Vision* 1, 57–72

Lowe, D.G. (1987). Three-dimensional object recognition from single two-dimensional images. *Artificial Intelligence* 31, 355–395

Löwenfeld, L. (1900). *Somnambulismus und Spiritismus. Grenzfragen des Nerven-und Seelenlebens.* Heft 1, Bergmann, F.J., München

Löwenstein, K., Borchardt, M. (1918). Symptomatologie und electrische Reizung des Nerven bei der Schussverletzung des Hinterhauptlappens. *Dtsch. Z. Nervenheilk.* 58, 264–292

Lu, C., Fender, D.H. (1972). The interaction of color and luminance in stereoscopic vision. *Investigative Ophthalmol. Visiol. Sci.* 11, 482–490

Luce, J. de, Wilder, H.T.. (eds.) (1983). *Language in primates. Perspective and implications.* Springer, Berlin

Luciani, L., Tamburini, A. (1879). Studi clinici: sui centri sensori cortical. *Ann. Univ. di med. et chir.* 247, 293

Luciani. L. (1884). On the sensorial localisations in the cortex cerebri. *Brain* 7, 145–160

Ludwig, H. (ed.) (1882). Leonardo da Vinci, Das Buch *von der Malerei.* (Trattato della pittura 1651). In *Quellenschriften der Kunstgeschichte und Kunsttechnik des Mittelalters und der Renaissance Vol. XVII.* Transl. by H. Ludwig. Braumüller, Wien, (Repr. Osnabrück 1970)

Lueck, C.J., Zeki, S., Friston, K.J., Deiber, M.P., Cope, P., Cunningham, V.J., Lammertsma, A.A., Kennard, C., Farckowiak, R.S.J. (1989). The colour centre in the cerebral cortex of man. *Nature* 340, 386–389

Lueders, H., Lesser, R.P., Hahn, J., Dinner, D.S., Morris, H., Resor, S., Harrison, M. (1986). Basal temporal language area demonstrated by electrical stimulation. *Neurology* 36, 505–510

Luers, Th., Pötzl, O. (1941). Über Verkehrtsehen nach Insult. *Wien. klin. Wschr.* 53, 625

Lufi, D., Cohen, A. (1985). Attentional deficit disorder and short-term visual memory. *J. Clin. Psychol.* 41, 265–267

Luhmann, H.J., Greuel, J.M., Singer, W. (1990). Horizontal interactions in cat striate cortex: II. A current source-density analysis. *Eur. J. Neurosci.* 2, 358–368

Luhmann, H.J., Greuel, J.M., Singer, W. (1990). Horizontal interactions in cat striate cortex: III. Ectopic receptive fields and transient exuberance of tangential interactions. *Eur. J. Neurosci.* 2, 369–377

Luhmann, H.J., Singer, W., Martinez-Millan, L. (1990). Horizontal interactions in cat striate cortex: I. Anatomical substrate and postnatal development. *Eur. J. Neurosci.* 2, 344–357

Lukianowicz, N. (1958). Autoscopic phenomena. *Arch. Psychiat.* 80, 199–220

Lund, J.S. (1973). Organization of neurons in the visual cortex, area 17, of the monkey (*Macaca mulatta*). *J. Comp. Neurol.* 147, 455–496

Lund, J.S., Boothe, R.G. (1975). Interlaminar connections and pyramidal neuron organization in the visual cortex, area 17, of the macaque monkey. *J. Comp. Neurol.* 159, 305–334

Lund, J.S., Boothe, R.G., Lund, R.D. (1977). Development of neurons in the visual cortex (area 17) of the monkey (*Macaca nemestrina*): A Golgi study from fetal day 127 to postnatal maturity. *J. Comp. Neurol.* 176, 149–188

Lund, J.S., Hendrickson, A.E., Ogren, M.P., Tobin, E.A. (1981). Anatomical organization of primate visual cortex area V2. *J. Comp. Neurol.* 202, 19–45

Lund, J.S., Henry, G.H., MacQueen, C.L., Harvey, A.R. (1979). Anatomical organization of the primary visual cortex (area 17) of the cat. A comparison with area 17 of the macaque monkey. *J. Comp. Neurol.* 184, 599–618

Lund, J.S., Lund, R.D., Hendrickson, A.E., Bunt, A.H., Fuchs, A.F. (1975). The origin of efferent pathways from the primary visual cortex, area 17, of the macaque monkey as shown by retrograde transport of horseradish peroxidase. *J. Comp. Neurol.* 164, 287–304

Lund, J.S., Lund, R.D., Hendrickson, A.E., Bunt, A.H., Fuchs, A.F. (1975). The origin of efferent pathways from the primary visual cortex, area 17, of the macaque monkey. *J. Comp. Neurol.* 164, 265–285

Lund, S. (1980). Postural effects of neck muscle vibration in man. *Experientia* 36, 1398

Lungwitz, W. (1937). Zur myeloarchitektonischen Untergliederung der menschlichen Area praeoccipitalis (Area 19, Brodmann). *J. Psychol. Neurol.* 47, 607–688

Lunn, V. (1970). Autoscopic phenomena. *Acta Psychiatrica Scandinavica* 46 (Suppl. 219), 118–125

Lunz, M.A. (1897). Zwei Fälle von corticaler und Seelenblindheit. *Dtsch. Med. Wschr.*, 23, 610–613

Luria, A.R. (1959). Disorders of 'simultaneous perception' in a case of bilateral occipito-parietal brain injury. *Brain* 82, 437–449

Luria, A.R. (1966). *Higher cortical functions in man.* Basic Books, N.Y., 2nd. ed. (1980), Basic Books, N.Y.

Luria, A.R. (1973). *The working brain.* Basic Books, N.Y.

Luria, A.R., Pravdina-Vinarskaya, E.N., Yarbus, A.L. (1963). Disorders of ocular movement in a case of simultanagnosia. *Brain* 86, 219–229

Luria, S.M., McKay, C.L., Ferris, H. (1973). Handedness and adaptation to visual distortions of size and distance. *J. Exp. Psychol.* 100, 263–269

Luria, S.M., Strauss, M.S. (1978). Comparison of eye movements over faces in photographic positives and negatives. *Perception* 7, 349–358

Lüdke, M. (1989). *Störungen des Wahrnehmens und Erkennens mimisch-gestischer Ausdrucksbewegungen bei schizophrenen und nicht-schizophrenen jugendlichen psychiatrischen Patienten. Prüfung eines Kurztestes.* Doctoral dissertation, Freie Universität Berlin

Lüscher, C., Horber, F.F. (1990). Transitory alexia without agraphia in an HIV-positive patient suffering from toxoplasma-encephalitis. A case report. *Europ. Neurol.*

Lyman, R.S., Kwan, S.T., Chao, W.H. (1938). Left occipito-parietal brain tumor with observations on alexia and agraphia in Chinese and English. *Chin. med. J.* 54, 491–516

Lynch, J.C. (1980a). The functional organization of posterior parietal association cortex. *Behav. Brain Sci.* 3, 485–499

Lynch, J.C. (1980b). The role of parieto-occipial association cortex in oculomotor control. *Exp. Brain Res.* 41, A32

Lynch, J.C. (1987). Frontal eye field lesions in monkeys disrupt visual pursuit. *Exp. Brain Res.* 68, 437–441

Lynch, J.C., Acuna, C., Sakata, H., Georgopoulos, A., Mountcastle, V.B. (1973). The parietal association areas and immediate extrapersonal space. Abstr. 3rd. *Ann.. Meet. Soc. Neurosci.* p. 244

Lynch, J.C., Graybiel, A.M., Lobeck, L.J. (1985). The differential projection of two cytoarchitectural subregions of the inferior parietal lobule of macaque upon the deep layers of the superior colliculus. *J. Comp. Neurol.* 235, 241–254

Lynch, J.C., McLaren, J.W. (1982). The contribution of parieto-occipital association cortex to the control of slow eye movements. In Lennerstrand, G., Zee, D.S., Keller, E.L. (eds.), *Functional basis of ocular motility disorders.* Pergamon Press, Oxford, 501–510

Lynch, J.C., McLaren, J.W. (1983). Optokinetic nystagmus deficits following parieto-occipital cortex lesions in monkey. *Exp. Brain Res.* 49, 125–130

Lynch, J.C., Mountcastle, V.B., Talbot, W.H., Yin, T.C.T. (1977). Parietal lobe mechanisms for directed visual attention. *J. Neurophysiol.* 40, 362–389

Lynch, J.C., Yin, T.C.T., Talbot, W.H., Mountcastle, V.B. (1973). Parietal association cortex neurons active during hand and eye tracking of objects in immediate extrapersonal space. *Physiologist* 16, 384

MacCallum, W.A. (1986). The interplay of organic and psychological factors in the delusional misidentification syndromes. *Bibl. Psychiatr.* 164, 92–98

Macchi, G. (1985). Regeneration and plasticity in human CNS: anatomical-clinical approaches. In Bignami, A., Bloom, F.E., Bolis, C.L., Adeloye, M.D. (eds.), *Central nervous system plasticity and repair.* Raven Press, New York, 107–114

Mach, E. (1865). Über die Wirkung der räumlichen Vertheilung des Lichtreizes auf die Netzhaut. *Sitzungsber. Kais. Akad. Wiss., Math.-nat. Cl.* 2, Wien 52, 307–325

Mach, E. (1866a). Über den physiologischen Effect räumlich vertheilter Lichtreize. Sitzungsber. *Kais. Akad. Wiss., Math.-nat. Cl. 2, Wien* 54, 131–144

Mach, E. (1866b). Über die physiologische Wirkung räumlich vertheilter Lichtreize. *Sitzungsber. Kais. Akad. Wiss., Math.-nat. Cl. 2, Wien* 54, 393–408

Mach, E. (1868a). Über die Abhängigkeit der Netzhautstellen von einander. *Vierteljahrschr. f. Psychiat.* 2, 38–51

Mach, E. (1868b). Über die physiologische Wirkung räumlich vertheilter Lichtreize. *Sitzungber. Kais. Akad. Wiss., Math.-nat. Cl. 2,* Wien 57, 11–19

Mach, E. (1886/1906). *Die Analyse der Empfindungen und das Verhältnis des Physischen zum Psychischen.* 4th ed. 1906, Fischer, Jena, English translation (1959): *The Analysis of sensations and the relation of the physical to the psychical.* Dover, New York

Mach, E. (1906). Über den Einfluss räumlich und zeitlich variierender Lichtreize auf die Gesichtswahrnehmung. *Sitzungsber. Kas. Akad. Wiss., Math-nat. Cl. 2, Wien* 115, 623–648

Mack, A., Bachant, J. (1969). Perceived movement of the afterimage during eye movements. *Percept. Psychophys.* 6, 379–384

Mack, J.L., Boller, F. (1977). Associative visual agnosia and its related deficits: the role of the minor hemisphere in assigning meaning to visual perceptions. *Neuropsychologia* 15, 345–349

MacKain, K.S., Studdert-Kennedy, M., Speaker, S., Stern, D. (1983). Infant into modal speech perception is a left hemisphere function. *Science* 290, 1347–1349

MacKay, D.M. (1958). Perceptual stability of stroboscopically lit visual field containing self-luminous objects. *Nature* (Lond.) 181, 501–508

MacKay, D.M. (1969). *Information mechanism and meaning.* MIT Press, Cambridge, MA

MacKay, D.M. (1970). Elevation of visual threshold by displacement of retinal image. *Nature* (Lond.) 225, 90–92

MacKay, D.M. (1973). Visual stability and voluntary eye movements. In Jung, R. (ed.), *Handbook of sensory physiology. Vol. VII 3A. Central processing of visual information. A. Integrative functions and comparative data.* Springer, Berlin, 307–331

MacKay, G. (1888). A discussion on contribution to the study of hemianopsia, with special reference to acquired colour-blindness. *Brit. Med. J.* 2, 1033–1037

MacKay, G., Dunlop, J.C. (1899). The cerebral lesions in a case of complete acquired colour-blindness. *Scott. Med. Surg. J.* 5, 503–512

MacLean, P.D. (1964). Mirror display in the Squirrel monkey, Saimiri sciureus. *Science* 146, 950–952

Macrae, D., Trolle, W. (1956). The defect of function in visual agnosia. *Brain* 79, 94–110

Maeki, N. (1928). Natürliche Bewegungstendenzen der rechten und der linken Hand und ihr Einfluss auf das Zeichnen und den Erkennungsvorgang. *Psychol. Forschung* 10, 1–19

Maffei, L., Fiorentini, A. (1973). The visual cortex as a spatial frequency analyzer. *Vision Res.*, 13, 1255–1267.

Magendi, F. (1834). *Handbuch der Physiologie.* 3rd ed. transl. F. Hensinger. J.F. Bärecke, Eisenach

Magitot, A., Hartmann, A. (1927). La cécité corticale. *Rev. Oto-neuro-oculist.* 5, 81

Magnani, G., Bettoni, L., Mazzucchi, A. (1982). Lesioni atrofiche biocciptali di incerta natura all'origine di una agnosia visiva. *Rivista di Neurologia* 52, 137–148

Magnus, H. (1894). Ein Fall von Rindenblindheit. *Dtsch. Med. Wochenschr.*, Band 20, Thieme, Leipzig/Berlin, 73–76

Magri, R., Mocchetti, E. (1967). Asomatoscopia (autoscopia negativa) parziale in epilettica. *Archivio di Psicologia, Neurologia e Psichiatria* (Milano) 28, 572–585

Mahut, H., Moss, M. (1985). The monkey and the seahorse. Hippocampal ablations in infancy: dissociation of two behavioral functions in the monkey. In Pribram, K., Isaacson, R. (eds.), *The Hippocampus.*

Maki, N. (1978). Psychological analyses of brain damage cases. *J. Biol. Psychol.* 20, 11–21

Malamut, B.L., Saunders, R.C., Mishkin, M. (1984). Monkeys with combined amygdalo-hippocampal lesions succeed in object discrimination learning despite 24-hour intertrial intervals. *Behav. Neurosc.* 98, 759–769

Malis, L., Kruger, L. (1956). Multiple response and excitability of cat's visual cortex. *J. Neurophysiol.* 19, 172–186

Malmo, R.B. (1966). Effects of striate cortex ablation on intensity discrimination and spectral intensity distribution in the rhesus monkey. *Neuropsychologia* 4, 9–26

Malone, D.R., Hannay, H.J. (1978). Hemispheric dominance and normal color memory. *Neuropsychologia* 16, 51–59

Malone, D.R., Morris, H.H., Kay, M.C., Levin, S.H. (1982). Prosopagnosia: A double dissociation between the recognition of familiar and unfamiliar faces. *J. Neurol. Neurosurg. Psychiat.* 45, 820–822

Malpass, R.S., Kravitz, J. (1969). Recognition for faces of own and other race. *J. Personality, Soc. Psychol.* 13, 330–334

Mammucari, A., Caltagirone, C., Ekman, P., Friesen, W., Gianotti, G., Pizzamiglio, L., Zoccolotti, P. (1988). Spontaneous facial expression of emotions in brain-damaged patients. *Cortex* 24, 521–533

Mancuso, R.P., Lawrence, A.F., Hintze, R.W., White, C.T. (1979). Effect of altered central and peripheral visual field stimulation on correct recognition and visual evoked response. *Intern. J. Neurosci.* 9, 113–122

Mandal, M.K., Palchoudhury, S. (1985). Decoding of facial affect in schizophrenia. *Psychol. Rep.* 56, 651–652

Mandelbrot, B. (1953). An informational theory of the statistical structure of language. In Jackson, W. (ed.), *Communication theory.* Butterworths, London

Mandelbrot, B. (1954). Structure formelle des textes et communication. *Word* 10, 1–27

Manis, F.R., Savage, P.L., Morrison, F.J., Horn, C.C., Howell, M.J., Szeszulski, P.A., Holt, L.K. (1987). Paired associate learning in reading-disabled children: evidence for a rule-learning deficiency. *J. Exp. Child Psychol.* 43, 24–40

Marcel, A.J. (1983). Conscious und unconscious perception: Experiments on visual masking and word recognition. *Cognitive Psychology* 15, 197–237

Marcel, T., Rajan, P. (1975). Lateral specialization for recognition of words and faces in good and poor readers. *Neuropsychologia* 13, 489–497

Marchand, L., Ajuriaguerra, J. (1940). Des troubles du schéma corporel. *Ann. Méd.-Psych.* 98, 252–260

Marcie, P., Hecaen, H., Dubois, J., Angelergues, R. (1965). Les troubles de la realisation de la parole au cours des lesions de l'hemisphere droit. *Neuropsychologia* 3, 217–247

Marg, E. (1973). Recording from single cells in the human visual cortex. In Jung, R. (ed.), *Visual centers in the brain. Handbook of Sensory Physiology* Vol. VII/3, *Central processing of visual information*. Springer, Berlin, Heidelberg, New York, 441–449

Marg, E., Adams, J.E. (1970). Evidence for a neurological zoom system in vision from angular changes in some receptive fields of single neurons with changes in fixation distance in the human visual cortex. *Experientia* (Basel) 26, 270–272

Marg, E., Adams, J.E., Rutkin, B. (1968). Receptive fields of cells in the human visual cortex. *Experientia* (Basel) 24, 313–316

Marg, E., Chow, R., Perkins, R.K., Olsen, E.R., Wilson, C.B. (1970). Measurement of unit activity in various systems of the brain postoperatively. *Confinia Neurol.* 32, 53–62

Marg, E., Dierssen, G. (1965). Reported visual percepts from stimulation of the human brain with microelectrodes during therapeutic surgery. *Confin. Neurol.* 26, 57–75

Margolin, D.I. (1984). The neuropsychology of writing and spelling: semantic, phonological, motor, and perceptual processes. *Quart. J. Exp. Psychol.* 36A, 459–489

Mariani, E., Moschini, V., Pastorino, G.C., Rizzi, F., Severgnini, A., Tiengo, M. (1990). Pattern reversal visual evoked potentials (VEP-PR) in migraine subjects with visual aura. *Headache* 30, 435–438

Marie, P. (1922). Questions neurologiques d'actualite. Masson, Paris

Marie, P., Bouttier, H., Bailey, P. (1922). La planotopokinesie. Etude sur les erreurs d'execution de certains mouvements dans leurs rapports avec la representation spatiale. *Rev. Neurol.* 1, 505–512

Marie, P., Chatelin, C. (1915). Les troubles visuels dus aux lesions des voies optiques intra-cerebrales de la sphere visuelle corticale dans les blessures du crane par coup de feu. *Rev. Neurol.* 28, 882

Marie, P., Crouzon, O. (1900). Rammollissement du cuneus et hémianopsie. *Revue Neurol.* 8, 63

Marie, P., Foix, C. (1917). Les aphasies de guerre. *Rev. Neurol.* 2, 53–87

Marin, O.S. (1980). CAT scans of five deep dyslexic patients. In Coltheart, M., Patterson, K., Marshall, J.C. (eds.), *Deep Dyslexia*. Routledge and Kegan Paul, London, 407–411

Mariotte, E. (1668). *Oeuvres.* p. 496–546, quoted after Helmholtz 1896

Markowitsch, H.J., Emmans, D., Irle, E., Streicher, M., Preilowski, B. (1985). Cortical and subcortical afferent connections of the primate's temporal pole: a study of rhesus monkeys, squirrel monkeys and mormosets. *J. Comp. Neurol.* 242, 425–458

Marks, D.F. (1973). Visual imagery differences in the recall of pictures. *Brit. J. Psychol.* 64, 17–24

Marks, R.L., De Vito, T. (1987). Alexia without agraphia and associated disorders. Importance of recognition in the rehabilitation setting. *Arch. Physical Med. Rehabil.* 68, 239–243

Marlowe, W.B., Mancall, E.L., Thomas, J.J. (1975). Complete Klüver-Bucy snydrome in man. *Cortex* 11, 53–59

Marr, D. (1976). Early processing of visual information. *Philos. Trans. Roy. Soc. Lond.* B275, 483–524

Marr, D. (1977). Analysis of occluding contour. *Proc. Roy. Soc. Lond.* B197, 441–475

Marr, D. (1980). Visual information processing: the structure and creation of visual representations. *Phil. Trans. Roy. Soc. Lond.* B290, 199–218

Marr, D. (1982). *Vision: A computational investigation into the human representation and processing of visual information.* Freeman, San Francisco, CA

Marr, D., Hildreth, E. (1980). A theory of edge detection. *Proc. Roy. Soc., Lond.* B207, 187–217

Marr, D., Nishihara, H.K. (1978). Representation and recognition of the spatial organization of three-dimensional shapes. *Proc. Roy. Soc. Lond.* B200, 269–294

Marr, D., Poggio, T., Ullman, S. (1979). Bandpass channels, zero-crossings and early visual processing. *J. opt. Soc. Am.* 69, 914–916

Marrocco, R.T. (1986). The neurobiology of perception. In LeDoux, J.E., Hirst, W. (eds.), *Mind and brain: Dialogues in cognitive neuroscience.* Cambridge University Press, Cambridge, 33–79

Marsh, G.G., Philwin, B. (1987). Unilateral neglect and constructional apraxia in a right-handed artist with a left posterior lesion. *Cortex* 23, 149–155

Marshal, C.R., Maynard, R.M. (1983). Vestibular stimulation for supranuclear gaze palsy. *Arch. Physical Medicine and Rehabilitation* 64, 134–146

Marshall, E., Walker, P. (1987). Visual memory for pictorial stimuli in a serial choice reaction-time task. *Br. J. Psychol.* 78, 213–231

Marshall, J.C., Halligan, P.W. (1988). Blindsight and insight in visuo-spatial neglect. *Nature* 336, 766–767

Marshall, J.C., Halligan, P.W. (1989). Right goes left: an investigation of line bisection in a case of visual neglect. *Cortex* 25, 503–515

Marshall, J.C., Newcombe, F. (1973). Pattern of paralexia. A psycholinguistic approach. *J. Psycholing. Res.* 2, 175–199

Marshall, J.C., Patterson, K.E. (1983). Semantic paralexia and the wrong hemisphere: a note on Landis, Regard, Graves and Goodglass. *Neuropsychologia* 21, 425–427

Marshall, J.C., Patterson, K.E. (1985). Left is still left for semantic paralexias: a reply to Jones and Martin (1985). *Neuropsychologia* 23, 689–690

Marshall, J.F., Turner, B.H., Teitelbaum, P. (1971). Sensory neglect produced by lateral hypothalamic damage. *Science* 174, 523–525

Martin, J.P. (1954). Pure word blindness considered as a disturbance of visual space perception. *Proc. Roy. Soc. Med.* 47, 293–295

Marx, P., Boquet, J., Luce, R., Farbos, J.P. (1970). Spatial agnosia and agnosia of physiogomies, sequelae of cortical blindness. *Bull. Soc. d'Ophthalmol.* Vol. 70,-?

Marzi, C.A., Berlucchi, G. (1977). Right visual field superiority for accuracy of recognition of famous faces in normals. *Neuropsychologia* 15, 751–756 (Titel vergleichen!)

Marzi, C.A., Brizzolara, D., Rizzolatti, G., Umiltö, C., Berlucchi, G. (1974). Left hemisphere superiority for the recognition of well known faces. *Brain Res.* 66, 358–359

Marzi, C.A., Tassinari, G., Agliotti, S., Lutzemberger, L. (1986). Spatial summation across the vertical meridian in hemianopics: a test of blindsight. *Neuropsychologia* 24, 749–758

Marzi, C.A., Tassinari, G., Tressoldi, P.E., Barry, C., Grabowska, A. (1985). Hemispheric asymmetry in face perception tasks of different cognitive requirement. *Human Neurobiol.* 4, 15–20

Mashhour, M. (1964). *Psychophysical relations in the perception of velocity.* Acta Universitatis Stockhomiensis, Stockholm Studies in Psychology, Vol. 3, Almquist & Wiksell, Stockholm,

Maspes, P.E. (1948). Le syndrome experimental chez l'homme de la section du splenium du corps calleux. *Rev. Neurol. (Paris)* 2, 101–113

Massaro, D.W., Taylor, G.A., Venezky, R.L., Jastrzembski, J.E., Lucas, P.A. (1980). *Letter and word perception. Orthographic structure and visual processing in reading.* Amsterdam, North-Holland

Masson, C., Gallet, J.P., Masson, M., Cambier, J. (1988). Epilepsie avec calcifications corticales bilaterales. Discussion d'un deficit post-critique durable. *Rev. Neurol* 144, 499–502

Matelli, M., Olivieri, M.F., Saccani, A., Rizzolatti, G. (1983). Upper visual space neglect and motor deficits after section of the midbrain commissures in the cat. *Behav. Brain Res.* 10, 263-

Mathers, L.H. (1972). The synaptic organization of the cortical projection to the pulvinar of the squirrel monkey. *J. Comp. Neurol.* 146, 43–60

Matin, L. (1972). Eye movements and perceived visual direction. In Jameson, D., Hurvich, L. (eds.), *Handbook of Sensory Physiology. Visual Psychophysics.* Springer-Verlag, Berlin, vol. VII, pt. 4, 331–380

Matin, L., Matin, E., Pearce, D. (1969). Visual perception of direction when voluntary saccades occur. I. Relation of visual direction of a fixation target extinguished before a saccade to a flash presented during the saccade. *Percept. Psychophys.* 5, 65–80

Matin, L., Matin, E., Pola, J. (1970). Visual perception of direction when voluntary saccades occur. II. Relation of visual direction of a fixation target extinguished before a saccade to a subsequent test flash presented before the saccade. *Percept. Psychophys.* 8, 9–14

Matin, L., Pearce, D.G. (1965). Visual perception of direction for stimuli flashed during voluntary saccadic eye movements. *Science N.Y.* 148, 1485–1488

Matin, L., Pearce, D.G., Matin, E., Kibler, G. (1966). Visual perception of direction. Roles of local sign, eye movements and ocular proprioception. *Vision Res.* 6, 453–469

Matin, L., Picoult, E., Stevens, J.K., Edwards, M.W. Jr., Young, D., MacArthur, R. (1982). Oculoparalytic illusion: Visual field dependent spatial mislocations by human partially paralyzed with curare. *Science, N.Y.*, 216, 198–201

Matin, L., Stevens, J.K., Picoult, E. (1983). Perceptual consequence of experimental extraocular muscle paralysis. In Hein, A., Jennerod, M. (eds.), *Spatially oriented behavior.* Springer, New York, 243–262

Matthysse, S., Spring, B.J., Sugarman, J. (1979). *Attention and Information Processing in Schizophrenia.* Pergamon Press, Oxford, New York

Maudsley, H. (1889). The double brain. *Mind* 14, 161–187

Maunsell, J.H.R., Newsome, W.T. (1987). Visual processing in monkey extrastriate cortex. *Ann. Rev. Neurosci.* 10, 363–401

Maunsell, J.H.R., van Essen, D.C. (1983a). Functional properties of neurons in middle temporal visual area of the macaque monkey. I. Selectivity for stimulus direction, speed, and orientation. *J. Neurophysiol.* 49, 1127–1147

Maunsell, J.H.R., van Essen, D.C. (1983b). Functional properties of neurons in middle temporal visual area of the macaque monkey. II. Binocular interactions and sensitivity to binocular disparity. *J. Neurophysiol.* 49, 1148–1167

Maunsell, J.H.R., Van Essen, D.C. (1983c). The connections of the middle temporal visual area (MT) and their relationship to a cortical hierarchy in the macaque monkey. *J. Neurosci.* 3, 2563–2586

Maunsell, J.H.R., van Essen, D.C. (1987). Topographic organization of the middle temporal visual area in the macaque monkey: representational biases and the relationship to callosal connections and myeloarchectonic bounderies. *J. Comp. Neurol.* 266, 535–555

Maurer, B., Salapatek, P. (1976). Development changes in the scanning of faces by young infants. *Child Development* 47, 523–527

Mauthner, L. (1881). *Gehirn und Auge.* Bergmann, Wiesbaden

Maximov, K. (1973). Epilepsie occipitale avec hallucinations héautoscopiques. *Acta neurol. belg.* 73, 320–323

May, J.G., Andersen, R.A. (1986). Different patterns of cortico-pontine projections from separate cortical fields within the inferior parietal lobule and dorsal prelunate gyrus of the macaque. *Exp.*

Brain Res. 63, 265–278

Mayer, L., Dobson, V. (1980). Assessment of vision in young children: a new operant approach yields estimates of acuity. *Invest. Ophthalmol. Vis. Sci.* 19, 566–570

Mayer, T. (1754). Experimente über die Schärfe des Gesichtssinnes. *Göttinger Gelehrte Anzeigen* Nr. 47, 20. Apr.1754, 401–402

Mayer, T. (1755). Experimenta circa visus aciem. *Comment Soc. Reg. Sci. Gottingensis* 1755, 4, 97–112

Mayer, T. (1758). De affinitate colorum (Über die Verwandtschaft der Farben). *Göttinger Gelehrte Anzeigen* Nr. 147, 9. Dez. 1758, 1385–1389

Mayer, T. (1758). *De affinitate colorum commentationes.* In Lichtenberg, G.Ch. 1775: *Tobiae Mayeri, Opera inedita, Vol. 1,* Vandenhoeck, Göttingen

Mayer-Gross, W. (1928). Psychopathologie und Klinik der Trugwahrnehmungen. In Bumke, O. (ed.), *Handbuch der Geisteskrankheiten.* Vol. I. Springer, Berlin

Mayerhofer, J. (1942). Über kombinierte labyrinthäre und occipitale Symptome nach Hinterhauptschuss. *Z. ges. Neurol. Psychiat.* 174, 613

Mayeux, R., Brandt, J., Rosen, J., Benson, D.F. (1980). Interictal memory and language impairment in temporal lobe epilepsy. *Neurology* 30, 120–125

Mays, L.E., Sparks, D.L. (1980). Dissociation of visual and saccade-related responses in superior colliculus neurons. *J. Neurophysiol.* 43, 207–232

Mazzoni, M., Pardossi, L., Cantini, R., Giorgetti, V., Arena, R. (1990). Gerstmann syndrome: a case report. *Cortex* 26, 459–467

Mazzucchi, A., Biber, C. (1983). Is prosopagnosia more frequent in males than in females? *Cortex* 19, 509–516

Mazzucchi, A., Parma, M., Umilta, C., Visintini, D., Zavaroni, G. (1985). Visual attention in patients with unilateral lesional or non-lesional epileptic focus. *Bull. Soc. Ital. Biol. Sper.* 7, 1051–1057

Mazzucchi, A., Posteraro, L., Nuzzi, G., Parma, M. (1985). Unilateral visual agnosia. *Cortex* 21, 309–316

Mazzucchi, A., Visintini, D., Magnani, G., Cattelanie, R., Parma, M. (1985). Hemispheric prevalence changes in partial epileptic patients on perceptual and attentional tasks. *Epilepsia* 26, 379–390

McAllister, D.A., Perri, M.G., Jordan, R.C., Rausher, F.P., Sattin, A. (1987). Effects of ECT given two vs. three times weekly. *Psychiatry Res.* 21, 63–69

McAuley, D.L., Ross-Russel, R.W. (1979). Correlation of CAT scan and visual field defects in vascular lesions of the posterior visual pathways. *J. Neurol. Neurosurg. Psychiat.* 42, 298–311

McCann, J.J., McKee, S., Taylor, T.H. (1976). Quantitative studies in retinex theory. *Vision Res.* 16, 445–458

McCarthy, R.A., Beaumont, J.G. (1983). Analysis of sequential letter matching tasks utilising lateralised tachistoscopic presentation. *Cortex* 19, 79–98

McCarthy, R.A., Warrington, E.K. (1986). Visual associative agnosia: A clinico-anatomical study of a single case. *J. Neurol. Neurosurg. Psychiat.* 49, 1233–1240

McCleary, C., Hirst, W. (1986). Semantic classification in aphasia: A study of basic superordinate and function relations. *Brain and Language* 27, 199–209

McClelland, J.L., Rumelhart, D.E. (1981). An interactive activation model of context effects in letter perception: Part 1. An account of basic findings. *Psychol. Rev.* 88, 375–407

McClelland, J.L., Rumelhart, D.E., Hinton, G.E. (1986). The appeal of parallel distributed processing. In Rumelhart, D.E., McClelland, H.L. (eds.), *Parallel distributed processing: Explorations in the microstructure of cognition.* MIT Press, Cambridge, MA

McConachie, H.R. (1976). Developmental prosopagnosia. A single case report. *Cortex* 12, 76–82

McConkie, G.W., Kerr, P.W., Reddix, M.D., Zola, D. (1988). Eye movement control during reading: I. The location of initial eye fixations on words. *Vision Res.* 28, 1107–1118

McConkie, G.W., Kerr, P.W., Reddix, M.D., Zola, D., Jacobs, A.M. (1989). Eye movement control during reading. II. Frequency of refixating a word. *Percept. Psychophys.* 46, 245–253

McConkie, G.W., Rayner, K. (1975). The span of the effective stimulus during a fixation in reading. *Percept. Psychophysics* 17, 578–586

McConnell, W.B. (1965). The phantom double in pregnancy. *Brit. J. Psychiat.* 111, 67–69

McCormick, G.F., Levine, D.S. (1983). Visual anomia: A unidirectional disconnection. *Neurology* 33, 664–666

McCurdy, H.G. (1949). Experimental notes on the asymmetry of the human face. *J. abn. soc. Psychol.* 44, 553–555

McDaniel, E.D. (1980). Visual memory in the deaf. *Am. Ann. Deaf* 125, 17–20

McFie, J. (1961). The effect of hemispherectomy on intellectual functioning in cases of infantile hemiplegia. *J. Neurol. Neurosurg. Psychiat.* 24, 240–249

McFie, J. (1976). *Assessment of organic intellectual impairment.* Academic Press, London

McFie, J., Piercy, M., Zangwill, O. (1950). Visual-spatial agnosia associated with lesions of the right cerebral hemisphere. *Brain* 73, 167–190

McFie, J., Piercy, M.F. (1952). The relation of laterality of lesion to performance on Weigl's sorting test. *J. ment. Sci.* 98, 299–305

McFie, J., Thompson, J.A. (1972). Picture arrangement: a measure of frontal lobe function? *Brit. J. Psychiat.* 121, 547–552

McFie, J., Zangwill, O.L. (1960). Visual-constructive disabilities associated with lesions of the left cerebral hemisphere. *Brain* 83, 243–260

McGlone, J. (1980). Sex differences in human brain asymmetry: a critical survey. *Behav. Brain Sci.* 3, 215–263

McGlone, J., Davidson, W. (1973). The relation between cerebral speech laterality and spatial ability with special reference to sex and hand preference. *Neuropsychologia* 11, 105–113

McGlone, J., Kertesz, A. (1973). Sex difference in cerebral processing of visuospatial tasks. *Cortex* 9, 313–320

McGurk, H. (1970). The role of object orientation in infant perception. *J. Exp. Child Psychol.* 9, 363–373

McGurk, H. Lewis, M. (1974). Space perception in early infancy: perception within a common auditory visual space? *Science* 186, 649–650

McGurk, H., MacDonald, J. (1976). Hearing lips and seeing voices. *Nature* 264, 746–748

McKee, S.P. (1981). A local mechanism for differential velocity detection. *Vision Res.* 21, 491–500

McKeever, W.F. (1971). Lateral word recognition: effects of unilateral and bilateral presentation, asynchrony of bilateral presentation and forced order of report. *Quart. J. Exp. Psychol.* 23, 410–416

McKeever, W.F., Dixon, M.S. (1981). Right-hemisphere superiority for discriminating memorized from nonmemorized faces: affective imagery, sex, and perceived emotionality effects. *Brain and Language* 12, 246–260

McKeever, W.F., Gill, K.M. (1972). Visual half-field differences in the recognition of bilaterally presented single letters and vertically spelled words. *Perceptual and Motor Skills* 34, 515–518

McKeever, W.F., Huling, M.G. (1971). Lateral dominance in tachistoscopic word recognition performances obtained with simultaneous bilateral input. *Neuropsychologia* 9, 15–20

McLaren, J.W., Lynch, J.C. (1979). Quantitative studies of optokinetic nystagmus in monkeys before and after lesions of parietooccipital association cortex. *Neurosci. Abstr.* 5, 797

McLeod, P., Heywood, C., Driver, J., Zihl, J. (1989). Selective deficit of visual search in moving displays after extrastriate damage. *Nature* 339, 466–467

McLoon, S.C., Santos-Anderson, R., Benevento, L.A. (1975). Some projections of the posterior bank and floor of the superior temporal sulcus in the rhesus monkey. *Neurosci. Abstr.* 64

Meadows, J.C. (1974a). Disturbed perception of colours associated with localized cerebral lesion. *Brain* 97, 615–632

Meadows, J.C. (1974b). The anatomical basis of prosopagnosia. *J. Neurol. Neurosurg. Psychiat.* 37, 489–501

Meadows, J.C., Munro, S.S.F. (1977). Palinopsia. *J. Neurol. Neurosurg. Psychiat.* 40, 5–8

Meerson, Y.A. (1985). Some mechanisms of disturbances of visual gnosis in local brain lesions. *Neurosci. Behav. Physiol.* 15, 69–76

Meeteren, A. von (1974). Calculations on the optical modulation transfer function of the human eye for white light. *Optica Acta* 21, 395–412

Meeteren, A. von, Barlow, H.B. (1981). The statistical efficiency for detecting sinusoidal modulation at average dot density in random figures. *Vision Res.* 21, 765–778

Mehler, J., Bever, T.G., Carey, P. (1967). What we look at when we read. *Perception and Psychophys.* 2, 213–218

Meienberg, O., Harrer, M., Wehren, C. (1986). Oculographic diagnosis of hemineglect in patients with homonymous hemianopia. *J. Neurol.* 233, 97–101

Meienberg, O., Zangemeister, W.H., Rosenberg, M., Hoyt, W.F., Stark, L. (1981). Saccadic eye movement strategies in patients with homonymous hemianopia. *Annals Neurol.* 9, 537–544

Meltzoff, A.N., Moore, M.K. (1977). Imitation of facial and manual gestures by human neonates. *Science* 198, 75–78

Meltzoff, A.N., Moore, M.K. (1983a). Newborn infants imitate adult facial gestures. *Child Dev.* 54, 702–709

Meltzoff, A.N., Moore, M.K. (1983b). The origins of imitation in infancy: paradigm, phenomena and theories. In Lipsitt, L.P., Rovee-Collier, C.K. (eds.), *Advances in infancy research. Vol. 2.* Ablex, Norwood, NJ, 265–301

Meltzoff, A.N., Moore, M.K. (1983c). Methodological issues in studies of imitation: Comments on McKenzie and Over and Koepke et al. *Infant Behav. Dev.* 6, 103–108

Mendez, M.F. (1988). Visuoperceptual function in visual agnosia. *Neurology* 38, 1754–1759

Mendoza, J.E., Thomas, R.K. (1975). Effects of posterior parietal and frontal neocortical lesions in the squirrel monkey. *J. Comp. Physiol. Psychol.* 89, 170–182

Menninger-Lerchenthal, E. (1932). Eine Halluzination Goethes. *Z. f. Neurol. u. Psychiat.* 140, 486–495

Menninger-Lerchenthal, E. (1935). *Das Truggebilde der eigenen Gestalt (Heautoskopie, Doppelgänger).* Karger, Berlin

Menninger-Lerchenthal, E. (1946). *Der eigene Doppelgänger.* Beiheft zur Schweizerischen Zeitschrift für Psychologie und ihre Anwendungen Nr. 11. Huber, Bern

Menninger-Lerchenthal, E. (1961). Heautoskopie. *Wiener Med. Wochenschr.* 111, 745–756

Menzel, E.W. Jr. (1971). Group behavior in young chimpanzees. Responsiveness to cumulative novel changes in a large outdoor enclosure. *J. Comp. Physiol. Psychol.* 74, 46–51

Menzel, E.W., Jr. (1966). Responsiveness to objects in free-ranging Japanese monkeys. *Behaviour* 26, 130–150

Merigan, W.H., Eskin, T.A. (1986). Spatio-temporal vision of macaques with severe loss of Pö ganglion cells. *Vision Res.* 26, 1751–1761

Merrin, E.L., Silberfarb, P.M. (1976). The Capgras phenomenon. *Arch. Gen. Psychiat.* 33, 965–968

Mertens, I., Siegmund, H., Grüsser, O.-J. (1991). Inspection of faces and objects in a visual memory task. *Abstr. Soc. for Neurosci.* (in press)

Merton, P.A., Morton, H.B. (1980a). Electrical stimulation of human motor and visual cortex through the scalp. *J. Physiol.* (Lond.) 305, 9–10

Merton, P.A., Morton, H.B. (1980b). Stimulation of the cerebral cortex in the intact human subject. *Nature* 285, 227

Merzenich, M.M., Kaas, J.H. (1980). Principles of organization of sensory-perceptual systems in mammals. *Prog. Psychobiol. Physiol. Psychol.* 9, 1–42

Mesulam, M.M. (1981). A cortical network for directed attention and unilateral neglect. *Ann. Neurol.* 10, 309–325

Mesulam, M.M. (1985). Attention, confusional states, and neglect. In Mesulam, M.M. (ed.), *Principles of behavioral neurology.* Davis, Philadelphia, 125–168

Mesulam, M.M. (1985). Patterns in behavioral neuroanatomy. In Mesulam, M.M. (ed.), *Principles of behavioral neurology.* Davis, Philadelphia, 1–70

Mesulam, M.M. (ed.). *Principles of behavioral neurology.* Davis, New York

Mesulam, M.M., Mufson, E.J. (1982). Insula of the old world monkey. III. Efferent cortical output and comments on function. *J. Comp. Neurol.* 212, 38–52

Mesulam, M.M., Van Hoesen, G.W., Pandya, D.N., Geschwind, N. (1977). Limbic and sensory connections of the inferior parietal lobule (area PG) in the rhesus monkey: a study with a new method for horseradish peroxidase histochemistry. *Brain Res.* 136, 393–414

Meyendorf, R. (1982). Psychopatho-ophthalmology, gnostic disorders and psychosis in cardiac surgery. Visual disturbances after open heart surgery. *Arch. Psychiatr. Nervenkr.* 232, 119–135

Meyendorf, R., Bender, W., Baumann, E., Athen, D., Ortlieb, S. (1980). Vergleichende Untersuchung zur unilateralen und bilateralen Elektrokrampf-Therapie. Klinische Wirksamkeit und Nebenwirkungen. *Arch. Psychiat. Nervenkrh.* 229, 89–112

Meyer, D., Schvaneveldt, R. (1971). Facilitation in recognizing pairs of words: evidence of a dependence between retrieval operations. *J. Exp. Psychol.* 90, 227–234

Meyer, O. (1900). Ein-und doppelseitige homonyme Hemianopsie mit Orientierungsstörungen. *Monatsschr. Psychiat. Neurol.*, Band VIII, Karger, Berlin, 440–456

Meyer-Eppler, W. (1969). *Grundlagen und Anwendung der Informationstheorie.* 2. Aufl., Springer, Berlin, NY, Heidelberg

Meyer-Gross, W., Stein, J. (1928). Allgemeine Symptomatologie. Pathologie der Wahrnehmung. In Bumke, O. (ed.), *Handbuch der Geisteskrankheiten* allgemeiner Teil, I, 351–507, Springer, Berlin

Meyer-Mickeleit, W.R. (1953). Die Dämmerattacken als charakteristischer Anfallstyp der temporalen Epilepsie (psychomotorische Anfälle, Äquivalente, Automatismen). *Nervenarzt* 24, 331–346

Meyer-Schwickerath, G., Nagun, R. (1951). Über selektive Erregbarkeit verschiedener Netzhautanteile. *Graefes Arch. Ophthalmol.* 151, 693–700

Meyerson, J., Manis, P.B., Miezin, F.M., Allman, J.M. (1977). Magnification in striate cortex and retinal ganglion cell layer of owl monkey. *Science* 198, 855–857

Meynert, T. (1867). Der Bau der Grosshirnrinde und seine örtlichen Verschiedenheiten nebst einem pathologisch anatomischen Corollarium. *Vierteljahresschr. Psychiat.* 1, 198–217

Meynert, T. (1869). Beiträge zur Kenntniss der centralen Projection Sinnesoberflächen. *Sitzungsb. d. Akad. Wissensch. math.-nat. Cl.* 2, Wien 60, 547

Michael, C.R. (1972). Double opponent-color cells in the primate striate cortex. *Physiologist* 15, 216

Michael, C.R. (1973). Opponent-color and opponent-contrast cells in lateral geniculate nucleus of the ground squirrel. *J. Neurophysiol.* 36, 536–550

Michael, C.R. (1978a). Color vision mechanisms in monkey striate cortex: dual-opponent cells with concentric receptive fields. *J. Neurophysiol.* 41, 572–588

Michael, C.R. (1978b). Color vision mechanisms in monkey striate cortex: simple cells with dual opponent-color receptive fields. *J. Neurophysiol.* 41, 1233–1249

Michael, C.R. (1978c). Color-sensitive complex cells in monkey striate cortex. *J. Neurophysiol.* 41, 1250–1266

Michael, C.R. (1979). Color-sensitive hypercomplex cells in monkey striate cortex. *J. Neurophysiol.* 42, 726–744

Michael, C.R. (1985). Laminar segregation of color cells in monkey's striate cortex. *Vision Res.* 25, 415–423

Michea, C.F. (1846). *Du délire des sensations.* Labe, Paris

Michel, D., Laurent, B., Foyatier, N., Blanc, A., Portafaix, M. (1982). Infarctus thalamique paramedian gauche. Etude de la memoire et du langage. *Rev. Neurol. (Paris)* 138, 533–550

Michel, E.M., Troost, B.T. (1980). Palinopsia: cerebral localization with computed tomography. *Neurology* 30, 887–889

Michel, F. (1978). Self-recognition on a TV-screen. In Buser, P.A., Rougoul-Buser, A. (eds.), *Cerebral correlates of conscious experience* North-Holland, Amsterdam, 299–309

Michel, F., Jeannerod, M., Devic, M. (1965). Trouble de l'orientation visuelle dans les trois dimensions de l'espace. *Cortex* 1, 441–466

Michel, F., Perenin, M.T., Sieroff, E. (1986). Prosopagnosie sans hemianaopsie apres lesion unilaterale occipito-temporale droite. *Rev. Neurol. (Paris)* 142, 545–549

Michel, F., Poncet, M., Signoret, J.L. (1989). Les lésions responsables de la prosopagnosie sont-elles toujours bilatérales? *Rev. Neurol. (Paris)* 145, 764–770

Michel, F., Schott, B., Boucher, M., Kopp, N. (1979). Alexie sans agraphie chez un malade ayant un hémisphère gauche deafferente. *Revue Neurol.* 135, 347–364

Michimata, C., Hellige, J.B. (1987). Effects of blurring and stimulus size on the lateralized processing of nonverbal stimuli. *Neuropsychologia* 25, 397–407

Midgley, G.C., Tees, R.C. (1981). Orienting behavior by rats with visual cortical and subcortical lesions. *Exp. Brain Res.* 41, 316–328

Mikami, A., Ito, S., Kubota, A. (1982). Visual response properties of dorsolateral prefrontal neurons during visual fixation task. *J. Neurophysiol.* 47, 593–605

Mikami, A., Nakamura, K. (1988). Behavioral role of stimulus selective neuronal activities in the superior temporal sulcus of macaque monkey. *Neurosci. Abstr.* 14, 10

Mikorey, M. (1952). *Phantome und Doppelgänger.* Lehmann, J.F., München

Miles, C., Madden, C., Jones, D.M. (1989). Cross-modal, auditory-visual Stroop interference: a reply to Cowan and Barron (1987). *Percept. Psychophys.* 45, 77–81

Miles, F.A., Fuller, H.H. (1975). Visual tracking and the primate flocculus. *Science* 189, 1000–1002

Milian, G. (1932). Cécité morphologique. *Bull. de l'Académie de Médecine* 107, 664

Miller, G.A., Bruner, J.S., Postman, L. (1954). Familiarity of letter sequences and tachistoscopic identification. *J. Gen. Psychol.* 50, 129–139

Miller, L. (1985). Cognitive risk-taking after frontal or temporal lobectomy. 1. The synthesis of fragmental visual information. *Neuropsychologia* 23, 359–369

Miller, L., Milner, B. (1985). Cognitive risk-taking after frontal or temporal lobectomy. 2. The synthesis of phonemic and semantic information. *Neuropsychologia* 23, 371–379

Miller, M., Pasik, P., Pasik, T. (1980). Extrageniculate vision in the monkey. VII. Contrast sensitivity functions. *J. Neurophysiol.* 43, 1510–26

Miller, S., Peacock, R. (1982). Evidence for the uniqueness of eidetic imagery. *Percept. Mot. Skills* 55, 1219–1233

Milner, A.D., Dunne, J.J. (1977). Lateralised perception of bilateral chimaeric faces by normal subjects. *Nature* 268, 175–176

Milner, A.D., Heywood, C.A. (1989). A disorder of lightness discrimination in a case of visual form agnosia. *Cortex* 25, 489–494

Milner, A.D., Jeeves, M.A., Silver, P.H., Lines, C.R., Wilson, J. (1985). Reaction times to lateralized visual stimuli in callosal agenesis — stimulus and response factors. *Neuropsychol.* 23, 323–331

Milner, A.D., Perrett, D.I., Johnston, R.S., Benson, P.J., Jordan, T.R., Heeley, D.W., Bettucci, D., Mortara, D., Mutani, R., Terazzi, E., Davidson, D.L.W. (1991). Perception and action in 'visual form agnosia'. *Brain* 114, 405–428

Milner, B. (1958). Psychological defects produced by temporal lobe excision. *Proc. Ass. for Research in Nervous and Mental Disease* 36, 244–257

Milner, B. (1965). Visually-guided maze learning in man: effects of bilateral hippocampal, bilateral frontal, and unilateral cerebral lesion. *Neuropsychologia* 3, 317–338

Milner, B. (1966). Amnesia following operation on the temporal lobes. In Whitty, C.W.M., Zangwill, O.L. (eds.), *Amnesia*. Butterworth, London

Milner, B. (1967). Brain mechanisms suggested by studies of temporal lobes. In Darley, F.L. (ed.), *Brain mechanisms underlying speech and language*. Grune and Stratton, New York

Milner, B. (1968). Visual recognition and recall after right temporal lobe excision in man. *Neuropsychologia* 6, 191–209

Milner, B. (1971). Interhemispheric differences in the localization of psychological processes in man. *Brit. Med. Bull.* 27, 272–277

Milner, B. (1974). Hemispheric specialization: Scope and limits. *Neurosci.* 4, 75–89.

Milner, B. (1979). Complementary functional specializations of the human cerebral hemispheres. *Pontif. Acad. Sci. Scripta Var.* 45, 601–620

Milner, B., Teuber, H.L. (1968). Alteration of perception and memory in man. In Weiskrantz, L.(ed.), *Analysis of behavioral change*. Harper and Row, New York

Milner, P.M. (1958). Note on a possible correspondence between the scotomas of migraine and spreading depression of Leao. *EEG Clin. Neurophysiol.* 10, 705

Mingazzini, G. (1908). Über Symptome infolge von Verletzungen des Occipitallappens durch Geschosse. *Neurol. Zbl.* 27, 1112–1123

Mingolla, E., Todd, J.T. (1986). Perception of solid shape from shading. *Biol. Cybern.* 53, 137–151

Minkowski, M. (1913). Experimentelle Untersuchungen über die Beziehungen der Großhirnrinde und der Netzhaut zu den primären optischen Zentren, besonders zum Corpus geniculatum externum. *Arb. hirnanat. Inst. Zürich* 7, 259–362

Minkowski, M. (1920). Über den Verlauf, die Endigung und die zentrale Repräsentation von gekreuzten Sehnervenfasern bei einigen Säugetieren und beim Menschen. *Schweiz. Arch. Neurol. Psychiat.* 6, 201–252

Minocha, A., Barth, J.T., Herold, D.A., Gideon, D.A., Spyker, D.A. (1986). Modulation of ethanol-induced central nervous system depression by ibuprofen. *Clin. Pharmacol Ther.* 39, 123–127

Mioche, L., Perenin, M.T. (1986). Central and peripheral residual vision in humans with bilateral deprivations amblyopia. *Exp. Brain Res.* 62, 259–272

Miranda, S.B., Fantz, R.L. (1974). Recognition memory in Down's syndrome and normal infants. *Child Development* 45, 651–660

Mishkin, M. (1954). Visual discrimination performance following partial ablations of the temporal lobe: II. Ventral surface vs. hippocampus. *J. Comp. Physiol. Psychol.* 47, 187–193.

Mishkin, M. (1966). Visual mechanisms beyond the striate cortex. In Russell, R. (ed.), *Frontiers of Physiological Psychology*. Academic Press, New York, 93–119

Mishkin, M. (1972). Cortical visual areas and their interaction. In Karczmar, A.G., Eccles, J.C.(eds.), *The brain and human behavior*. Springer-Verlag, Berlin, N.Y., 187–208

Mishkin, M. (1978). Memory in monkeys severely impaired by combined but not by separate removal of amygdala and hippocampus. *Nature* 273, 297–298

Mishkin, M. (1979). Analogous neural models for tactual and visual learning. *Neuropsychologia* 17, 139–151

Mishkin, M. (1982). A memory system in the monkey. *Philos. Trans.*

R. Soc. Lond. B. 298, 85–95

Mishkin, M., Forgays, D.G. (1952). Word-recognition as a function of retinal locus. *J. Exp. Psychol.* 43, 43–48

Mishkin, M., Hall, M. (1955). Discriminations along a size continuum following ablation of the inferior temporal convexity in monkeys. *J. comp. and physiol. Psychol.* 48, 97–101

Mishkin, M., Lewis, M.E., Ungerleider, L.G. (1982). Equivalence of parieto-preoccipital subareas of visuospatial ability in monkeys. *Behav. Brain Res.* 6, 41–55

Mishkin, M., Pribram, K.H. (1954). Visual discrimination performance following partial ablations of the temporal lobe: I. Ventral vs. lateral. *J. comp. and physiol. Psychol.* 47, 14–20

Mishkin, M., Ungerleider, L.G. (1982). Contribution of striate inputs to the visuospatial functions of parieto-preoccipital cortex in monkeys. *Behav. and Brain Res.* 6, 57–77

Mishkin, M., Ungerleider, L.G., Macko, K.A. (1983). Object vision and spatial vision: two cortical pathways. *Trends in Neuroscience* 6, 414–417

Mita, T.H., Dermer, M., Knight, J. (1977). Reversed facial images and the mere-exposure hypothesis. *J. Personality and Social Psychol.* 35, 597–601

Mitchell, D.E., Timney, B. (1984). Postnatal development of function in the mammalian visual system. In Darian-Smith, I., Geiger, S. (eds.), *Handbook of Physiology, Sec.1 The Nervous System.* Am. Physiol. Soc., Bethesda MD, 507–555

Mitzdorf, U. (1985). Current source-density method and application in cat cerebral cortex: investigations of evoked potentials and EEG phenomena. *Physiol. Rev.* 65, 37–100

Mitzdorf, U., Singer, W. (1979). Excitatory synaptic ensemble properties in the visual cortex of the macaque monkey: A current source density analysis of electrically evoked potentials. *J. Comp. Neurol.* 187, 71–84

Miyashita, Y. (1988). Neuronal correlate of visual associative long-term memory in the primate temporal cortex. *Nature* 335, 817–820

Miyashita, Y., Chang, H.S. (1988). Neuronal correlate of pictorial short-term memory in the primate temporal cortex. *Nature* 331, 68–70

Mize, K. (1980). Visual hallucinations following viral encephalitis -a self report. *Neuropsychologia* 18, 193–202

Mochizuki, H., Ohtomo, R. (1988). Pure alexia in Japanese and agraphia without alexia in Kanji. The ability dissociation between reading and writing in Kanji vs. Kana. *Arch. Neurol.* 45, 1157–1159

Moffett, A., Ettlinger, G., Morton, H.B., Piercy, M.F. (1967). Tactile discrimination performance in the monkey: the effect of ablation of various subdivisions of the posterior parietal cortex. *Cortex* 3, 59–96

Mohr, J.P., Leicester, J., Stoddard, L.T., Sidman, M. (1971). Right hemianopia with memory and color deficits in circumscribed left posterior cerebral artery territory infarction. *Neurology* 21, 1104–1111

Mollon, J.D. (1982). Color vision. *Ann. Rev. Psychol.* 33, 41–85

Mollon, J.D. (1989). Uses and origins of primate colour vision. *J. exp. Biol.* 146, 21–38

Mollon, J.D., Newcombe, F., Poldon, P.G., Ratcliff, G. (1980). On the presence of three cone mechanisms in a case of total achromatopsia. In Verriest G. (ed.), *Colour Vision Deficiencies*, Vol. V, chapter 3. Hilger, Bristol, 130–135

Mollon, J.D., Sharpe, L.T. (eds.) (1983). *Colour vision. Physiology and Psychophysics*. Academic Press, London, New York

Monahn, J.S. (1972). Extraretinal feedback and visual localization. *Perc. Psychophys.* 12, 349–353

Monakow, C. von (1885). Experimentelle und pathologisch-anatomische Untersuchungen über die Beziehungen der sogenannten Sehsphäre zu den infracorticalen Opticuszentren und zum N. opticus. *Arch. Psychiat. Nervenkr.* 16, 151–371

Monakow, C. von (1897). *Gehirnpathologie*. A. Hölder, Vienna

Monakow, C. von (1900a). Pathologische und anatomische Mittheilungen über die optischen Centren des Menschen. *Arch. Psychiat. Nervenkr.* 33, 696

Monakow, C. von (1900b). Pathologische und anatomische Mitteilungen über die optischen Centren des Menschen. *Neurologisches Centralblatt* 19, 680–681

Monakow, C. von (1905). *Gehirnpathologie. Vol. 4, Verstopfung der Hirnarterien.* Hölder, Wien

Monakow, C. von (1911). Lokalisation der Hirnfunktionen. *J. Psychol. Neurol.* 17, 185–200

Monakow, C. von (1914). *Die Lokalisation im Grosshirn und der Abbau der Funktion durch corticale Herde.* J.F. Bergmann, Wiesbaden

Money, J., Alexander, D., Walker, H.T. Jr. (1965). *A Standardized Road-map Test of Direction Sense.* The Johns Hopkins Press, Baltimore

Montero, J., Pena, J., Genis, D., et al. (1982). Balint's syndrome. *Acta Neurol. Belg.* 2, 270

Mooney, A.J., Carey, P., Ryan, M., Bofin, P. (1965). Parasagittal parieto-occipital meningioms. *Amer. J. Ophthal.* 59, 197–205

Moran, J., Desimone, R. (1985). Selective attention gates visual processing in extrastriate cortex. *Science* 229, 782–784

Morax, P.V. (1960). La cécité corticale. In Alajouanine, Th. (ed.), *Les grandes activites du lobe occipital.* Masson et Cie, Paris

Morax, V., Moreau, F., Castelain, F. (1919). Les differents types d'alteration de la vision maculaire dans les lesion traumatique occipitales. *Ann Oculist.* 156, 1

Moreland, R.L., Zajonc, R.B. (1977). Is stimulus recognition a necessary condition for the occurence of exposure effects? *J. Pers. Soc. Psychol.* 35, 191–199

Morgagni, G.B. (1719). *Adversaria anatomica omnia.* Padua

Morgagni, G.B. (1719). Epistolae Anatomicae. 16, art. 13

Morgan, M.J. (1977). *Molyneux's question.* Cambridge Univ. Press, Cambridge

Morin, P., Rivrain, Y., Eustache, F., Lambert, J., Courtheoux, P. (1984). Agnosie visuelle et agnosie tactile. *Rev. Neurol.* 140, 271–277

Morita, K., Kaiya, H., Ikeda, T., Namba, M. (1987). Presenile dementia combined with amyotrophy: a review of 34 Japanese cases. *Arch. Gerontol. Geriatr.* 6, 263–277

Morlock, N.L., Mori, K., Ward, A.A. Jr. (1964). A study of single cortical neurons during spreading depression. *J. Neurophysiol.* 27, 1192–1198

Morris, H.H., Lueders, H., Lesser, R.P., Dinner, D.S., Hahn, J. (1984). Transient neuropsychological abnormalities (including Gerstmann's syndrome) during cortical stimulation. *Neurology* 34, 877–883

Morrison, R.L., Tarter, R.E. (1984). Neuropsychological findings relating to Capgras syndrome. *Biological Psychiatry* 19, 1119–1129

Morrone, C.M., Burr, D.C., Maffei, L. (1982). Functional implications of cross-oriented inhibition of cortical visual cells. I. Neurophysiological evidence. *Proc. Roy. Soc. Lond.* B216, 335–354.

Morrow, L.A. (1987). Cerebral lesions and internal spatial representations. In Ellen, P. Thinus-Blanc, C. (eds.), *Neurobiology of Spatial Behaviour II. Neurophysiology and Developmental Aspects.* Dordrecht, Nijhoff, 156–164

Morrow, L.A., Ratcliff, G. (1988). The disengagement of covert attention and the neglect syndrome. *Psychobiology* 3, 16, 261–269

Morrow, L.A., Ratcliff, G., Johnston, S. (1985). Externalizing spatial knowledge in patients with right hemisphere lesions. *Cognitive Neuropsychology* 2, 265–273

Morton, J. (1964). The effects of context upon speed of reading, eye movements and eye-voice span. *Quart. J. Exp. Psychol.* 16, 340–354

Morton, J. (1969). Interaction of information in word recognition. *Psychol. Rev.* 76, 165–178

Morton, J. (1979). Facilitation in word recognition: experiments causing change in the logogen modle. In Kolers, P.A., Wrolstad, M.E., Bouma, H. (eds.), *Processing of visible language Vol. 1.* Plenum Press, New York

Moscovitch, M. (1979). Information processing and the cerebral hemispheres. In Gazzaniga, M.S. (ed.), *Handbook of behavioral neurobiology, Vol. 2, Neuropyschology.* Plenum Press, New York

Moscovitch, M. (1983). Local versus global solutions to problems of hemispheric specialization. *Behav. Brain Sci.* 6, 520–521

Moscovitch, M., Klein, P. (1980). Material specific perceptual interference for visual words and faces: implications for models of capacity limitations, attention and laterality. *J. Exp. Psychol: Hum. Percept. Perform.* 6, 590–604

Moscovitch, M., Olds, J. (1982). Asymmetries in spontaneous facial expressions and their possible relation to hemispheric specialization. *Neuropsychologia* 20, 71–81

Moscovitch, M., Radzins, M. (1987). Backward masking of lateralized faces by noise, pattern and spatial frequency. *Brain and Cognition* 6, 72–90

Moscovitch, M., Scullion, D., Christie, D. (1978). Early versus late stages of processing and their relation to functional hemispheric asymmetries in face recognition. *J. Exp. Psychol.: Hum. Percept. Perform.* 3, 401–416

Moser, A., Kömpf, D. (1990). Unilateral visual exploration deficit in a frontal lobe lesion. *Neuro-ophthalmology* 10, 39–44

Motokawa, K. (1970). *Physiology of color and pattern vision.* Igagu Shoin, Tokyo

Motokawa, K., Ebe, M. (1953). Retinal receptors isolated with AC method and polychromatic theory. *J. opt. Soc. Amer.* 43, 203–209

Motokawa, K., Iwama, K. (1950). Resonance in electrical stimulation of the eye. *Tohoku J. exp. Med.* 53, 201–206

Motter, B.C., Mountcastle, V.B. (1981). The functional properties of the light-sensitive neurons of the posterior parietal cortex studied in waking monkeys: foveal sparing and opponent vector organization. *J. Neurosci.* 1 , 3–26

Motter, B.C., Steinmetz, M.A., Duffy, C.J., Mountcastle, V.B. (1987). Functional properties of parietal visual neurons: mechanisms of directionality along a single axis. *J. Neurosci.* 7, 154–176

Motter, B.C., Steinmetz, M.A., Mountcastle, V.B. (1985). Directional sensitivity of parietal visual neurons to moving stimuli depends upon the extent of the field traversed by the moving stimuli. *Soc. Neurosci. Abstr.* 11, 1011

Mountcastle, V.B. (1976). The world around us: neural command functions for selective attention. *Neurosci. Res. Progr. Bull.* 14, Suppl. 1–47

Mountcastle, V.B. (1978). An organizing principle for cerebral function: the unit module and the distributed system. In Edelman, G.M., Mountcastle, V.B. (eds.), *The mindful brain.* MIT Press, Cambridge, Mass., 7–50

Mountcastle, V.B. (1981). Functional properties of the light sensitive neurons of the posterior parietalcortex and their regulation by state controls: influence on excitability of interested fixation and the angle of gaze. In Pompeiano, O., Ajmone, Marsan C. (eds.), *Brain mechanisms of perceptual awareness and purposeful behavior.* JBRO Monograph Series, Vol. 8. Raven Press, New York, 67–69

Mountcastle, V.B., Andersen, R.A., Motter, B.C. (1981). The influence of attentive fixation upon the excitability of the light-sensitive neurons of the posterior parietal cortex. *J. Neurosci.* 1, 1218–1225

Mountcastle, V.B., Lynch, J.C., Georgopoulos, A., Sakata, H., Acuna, C. (1975). Posterior parietal association cortex of the monkey: command function of operations within extrapersonal space. *J. Neurophysiol.* 38, 871–907

Mountcastle, V.B., Motter, B.C., Steinmetz, M.A., Duffy, C.J. (1984). Looking and seeing: the visual functions of the parietal lobe. In Edelman, G.M., Gall, W.E., Cowan, W.M. (eds.), *Dynamic aspects of neocortical function.* Wiley, New York, 159–194

Mouren, P. Tatossian, A., Trupheme, R., Giudicelli, S., Fresco, R. (1967). L'alexie par deconnection visuo-verbale (Geschwind): A propos d'un cas de cécité verbale pure sans agraphie avec troubles de la denomination des couleurs, des nombres et des images. *Encéphalé*

56, 112–137

Movshon, J.A., Adelson, E.H., Gizzi, M.S., Newsome, W.T. (1985). The analysis of moving visual patterns. *Exp. Brain Res. Suppl.* 11, 117–151

Movshon, J.A., Newsome, W.T. (1984). Functional characteristics of striate cortical neurons projecting to MT in the macaque. *Soc. Neurosci. Abstr.* 10, 933

Movshon, J.A., Thompson, I.D., Tolhurst, D.J. (1978a). Spatial summation in the receptive fields of simple cells in the cat's striate cortex. *J. Physiol. (Lond.)* 283, 53–77

Movshon, J.A., Thompson, I.D., Tolhurst, D.J. (1978b). Receptive field organization of complex cells in the cat's striate cortex. *J. Physiol. (Lond.)* 283, 79–99

Movshon, J.A., Thompson, I.D., Tolhurst, D.J. (1978c). Spatial and temporal contrast sensitivity of neurons in areas 17 and 18 of the cat's visual cortex. *J. Physiol. (Lond.)* 283, 101–120

Moyer, S.B. (1979). Rehabilitation of alexia: a case study. *Cortex* 15, 139–144

Möller, A.R., Burgess, J.E., Sekhar, L.N. (1987). Recording compound action potentials from the optic nerve in man and monkeys. *EEG. Clin. Neurophysiol.* 67, 549–555

Mufson, E.J., Mesulam, M.M. (1982). Insula of the old world monkey. II. Afferent cortical input and comments on the claustrum. *J. Comp. Neurol.* 212, 23–37

Mufson, E.J., Mesulam, M.M. (1984). Thalamic connections of the insula in the rhesus monkey and comments on the paralimbic connectivity of the medial pulvinar nucleus. *J. Comp. Neurol.* 227, 109–120

Mulder, M.E. (1868). Ons oordeel over verticaal, bej neiging van hoofd narr rechts of links. *Arch. Anat. Physiol.* 2, 240–352

Muller, H.J., Findlay, J.M. (1987). Sensitivity and criterion effects in the spatial cuing of visual attention. *Perc. Psychophys.* 42, 383–399

Muller, R.U., Kubie, J.L. (1987). The effects of changes in the environment on the spatial firing of hippocampal complex-spike cells. *J. Neurosci.* 7, 1951–1968

Munk, H. (1878). Weitere Mittheilungen zur Physiologie der Grosshirnrinde. *Arch. Anat. Physiol.* 2, 161–178

Munk, H. (1880). *Über die Sehspären der Grosshirnrinde.* Monatsber. K. Akad. Wiss. Math.-nat. Cl. June 1880, Berlin, reprint, 1–23

Munk, H. (1881). Ueber die Functionen der Grosshirnrinde. Gesammelte Mittheilungen aus den Jahren 1877–1880. Hirschwald, Berlin

Munk, H. (1884). Über die centralen Organe für das Sehen und Hören bei den Wirbelthieren. Sitzungsber. K. Preuss. Akad. Wiss. Berlin 1884, Vol. XXIV, Mai 1884, 1–20

Munk, H. (1890). Sehsphaere und Augenbewegungen. Sitzungsber. K. Preuss. Akad. Wiss. 1890. Vol. III, 1–22

Munk, H. (1890). *Ueber die Functionen der Grosshirnrinde.* Gesammelte Mittheilungen aus den Jahren 1877–1880. Hirschwald, Berlin

Munthe, A. (1931). *Das Buch von San Michele.* Paul List, Leipzig

Muraro, L. (1978). *Giambattista della Porta, mageo scienciato.* Feltrinelli, Milano

Murray, E.A., Mishkin, M. (1983). Severe tactual memory deficits in monkeys after combined removal of the amygdala and hippocampus. *Brain Res.* 270, 340–344

Murray, E.A., Mishkin, M. (1984). Severe tactual as well as visual memory deficits follow combined removal of the amygdala and hippocampus in monkeys. *J. Neurosci.* 4,, 2565–2580

Mustavi, M.J., Fuchs, A.J., Wallman, J. (1984). Smooth-pursuit-related units in the dorsolateral pons of the rhesus macaque. *Soc. Neurosci. Abstr.* 10, 987

Musterle, W., Rössler, O.E. (1986). Computer faces: the human lorenz matrix. *Bio Systems* 19, 61–80

Muzekari, L.H., Bates, M.E. (1977). Judgement of emotion among chronic schizophrenics. *J. Clin. Psychol.* 33, 662–666

Müller, Ch. (1956). *Mikropsie und Makropsie.* S. Karger, Basel, New York

Müller, E. (1971). *Zur Objektivierung des Symptoms 'Personenverkennung'. Eine experimentalpsychologische Untersuchung an psychiatrisch-neurologischen Patientengruppen.* Univ. Wien, Philosphische Fakultät

Müller, F. (1892). Ein Beitrag zur Kenntniss der Seelenblindheit. *Arch. Psychiat. Nervenkr.* 24, 856–871

Müller, G.E. (1916). Über das Aubert'sche Phänomen. *Z. Psychol. Physiol. Sinnesorg.* 49, 109–249

Müller, J. (1826). *Physiologie des Gesichtssinnes.* Coblenz

Müller, J. (1826a). *Ueber die phantastische Gesichtserscheinungen. Eine physiologische Untersuchung mit einer physiologischen Urkunde des Aristoteles über den Traum.* Reprint in Ebbecke, U. (1951) *Johannes Müller der grosse rheinische Physiologe.* Schmorl, von Seelfeld, Hannover

Müller, W., Settgast, J. (1976). *Nofretete — Echnaton.* Catalogue of an exhibition at the Ägyptisches Museum, Berlin

Müller-Beck, H., Albrecht, G. (1987). *Die Anfänge der Kunst vor 30.000 Jahren.* Thieme, Stuttgart

Müller-Erzbach, I. (1951). *Zur Psychologie und Psychopathologie der Doppelgänger-Erscheinungen.* Med.Diss. München

Müller-Karpe, H. (1968). *Das vorgeschichtliche Europa.* Holle, Baden-Baden

Nachmias, J., Sansbury, R.V. (1974). Grating contrast: discrimination may be better than detection. *Vision Res.* 14, 1039–1042

Naegele, J.R., Held, R. (1983). Development of optokinetic nystagmus and effects of abnormal visual experience. In Hein, A., Jeannerod, M. (eds.), *Spatially oriented behavior.* Springer, New York, Berlin, Heidelberg, Tokyo, 155–174

Nagel, W. (1905). *Handbuch der Physiologie des Menschen. Vol. 3. Physiologie der Sinne.* Vieweg, Braunschweig

Nagel, W.A. (1906). Observations on the color-sense of a child. *J. Comp. Neurol. Psychol.* 16, 217–230

Nakada, T., Lee, H., Kwee, I.L., Lerner, A.M. (1984). Epileptic Kluver-Bucy syndrome: case report. *J. Clin. Psychiat.* 45, 87–88

Nakamura, R., Taniguchi, R., Yokochi, F. (1978). Dependence of reaction times on movement patterns in patients with cerebral hemiparesis. *Neuropsychologia* 16, 121–124

Nakamura, R.K., Mishkin, M. (1986). Chronic 'blindness' following lesions of nonvisual cortex in monkey. *Exp. Brain Res.* 63, 173–184

Nakamura, R.K., Schein, S.J., Desimone, R. (1986). Visual responses from cells in striate cortex of monkeys rendered chronically 'blind' by lesions of nonvisual cortex. *Exp. Brain Res.* 63, 185–190

Nakayama, K. (1981). Differential motion hyperacuity under conditions of common image motion. *Vision Res.* 21, 1475–1482

Nakayama, K. (1983). Motion parallax sensitivity and space perception. In Hein, A., Jeannerod, M. (eds.), *Spatially oriented behavior.* Springer, Berlin, 223–243

Nakayama, K. (1985). Biological image motion processing: a review. *Vision Res.* 25, 625–660

Nakayama, K., Loomis, J.M. (1974). Optical velocity patterns, velocity-sensitive neurons, and space perception: a hypothesis. *Perception* 3, 63–80

Nakayama, K., Silverman, G.H. (1984). Temporal and spatial characteristics of the upper displacement limit for motion in random dots. *Vision Res.* 24, 293–299

Nakayama, K., Silverman, G.H. (1985). Detection and discrimination of sinusoidal grating displacements. *J. opt. Soc. Am.* A 2, 267–274

Nakayama, K., Silverman, G.H. (1986). Serial and parallel processing of visual feature conjunctions. *Nature* 320, 264–265

Nardelli, E. Buonanno, F., Coccia, F., Fiaschi, H. Terzian, H., Rizzuto, N. (1982). Prosopagnosia: Report of four cases. *Europ. Neurol.*

21, 289–297

Nashold, B.S. Jr. (1970). Phosphenes resulting from stimulation of the midbrain in man. *Archives of Ophthalmology* NY 84, 433–435

Natale, M., Gur, R.E., Gur, R.C. (1983). Hemispheric asymmetries in processing facial expressions. *Neuropsychologia* 21, 555–566

Natale, M., Gur, R.E., Gur, R.C. (1983). Hemispheric asymmetries in processing emotional expressions. *Neuropsychologia* 21, 555–565

Nathan, P.W. (1946). On simultaneous bilateral stimulation of the body in a lesion of the parietal lobe. *Brain* 69, 325–334

Naudascher, G. (1910). Trois cas d'hallucinations spéculaires. *Ann. Méd.-Psychol.* 68, 284–296

Nauta, W.J.H. (1961). Fiber degeneration following lesions of the amygdaloid complex in the monkey. *J. Anat.* 95, 515–531

Nauta, W.J.H. (1971). The problem of the frontal lobe: A reinterpretation. *J. Psychiat. Res.* 8, 167–187

Navratil, L. (1983). *Die Künstler aus Gugging*. Medusa, Wien

Navratil, L. (1988). *August Walla. Sein Leben und seine Kunst*. Greno, Nördlingen

Neal, L.J. (1978). Encoding and decoding of affective cues in schizophrenic and normal males. *Diss. Abstr. Int.* 39, 6134

Nebes, R. (1971). Handedness and the perception of part-whole relationships. *Cortex* 7, 350–356

Necker, L.A. (1832). Observations on some remarkable optical phenomena seen in Switzerland; and on an optical phenomena which occurs on viewing a figure of crystal or geometrical solid. *London Edinburgh Philos Mag. and J. of Science*, Third Series 1, Nr. 5, 329–337

Neely, J. (1977). Semantic priming and retrieval from lexical memory: roles of inhibitionless spreading activation and limited-capacity attention. *J. Exp. Psychol: Gen.* 106, 226–254

Neisser, U. (1967). *Cognitive Psychology*. Appleton-Century-Crofts, New York

Nelson, D.L., Peebles, J., Pancotto, F. (1970). Phonetic similarity as oposed to information structure as a determinant of word encoding. *J. exp. Psychol.* 86, 117–119

Nelson, R.B., Friedman, D.P., O'Neill, J.B., Mishkin, M., Routtenberg, A. (1987). Gradients of protein kinase C substrate phosphorylation in primate visual system peak in visual memory storage areas. *Brain Res.* 416, 387–392

Nemesius Episcopus Emesenus (1975). De natura hominis. Brill, Leiden

Nemesius of Emesa (1955). The nature of man. In Telfer, W. (ed.), Cyril of Jerusalem and Nemesius of Emesa. Westminster Press, Philadelphia.

Neville, H.J. (1988). Cerebral organization for spatial attention. In Stiles-Davis, J., Kritchevsky, M., Bellugi, U. (eds.), 327–341

Neville, H.J., Lawson, D. (1987). Attention to central and peripheral visual space in a movement detection task: An event-related potential and behavioral study. I. Normal hearing adults. *Brain Res.* 405, 253–267

Newcombe, F. (1969). *Missile wounds of the brain*. Oxford University Press, London

Newcombe, F. (1979). The processing of visual information in prosopagnosia and acquired dyslexia: Functional versus physiological interpretation. In D.J. Oborne, M.M. Gruneberg, J.R. Eiser (eds.), *Research in Psychology and Medicine*. Academic Press, London

Newcombe, F., Ratcliff, G. (1974). Agnosia: A disorder of object recognition. In F. Michel, Schott, B. (eds.), *Les syndromes de disconnexion calleuse chez l'homme*. Colloque International, Lyon

Newcombe, F., Ratcliff, G., Damasio, H. (1987). Dissociable visual and spatial impairments following right posterior cerebral lesions: clinical, neuropsychological and anatomical evidence. *Neuropsychologia* 25, 149–161

Newcombe, F., Russell, W.R. (1969). Dissociated visual perceptual and spatial deficits in focal lesions of the right hemisphere. *J. Neurol. Neurosurg. Psychiat.* 32, 73–81

Newcombe, F., Young, A.W., de Haan, E.H.F. (1989). Prosopagnosia and object agnosia without covert recognition. *Neuropsychologia* 27, 179–191

Newsome, W.T., Britten, K.H., Movshon, J.A., Shadlen, M. (1989). Single neurons and the perception of visual motion. In Lam, D.M.K., Gilbert, C. (eds.), *Neural mechanisms of visual perception*. Proc. of the Retinal Research Foundation Symposium, Vol 2. Portfolio Publishing, The Woodlands, Tx.

Newsome, W.T., Mikami, A., Wurtz, R.H. (1986). Motion selectivity in macaque visual cortex. III. Psychophysics and physiologiy of apparent motion. *J. Neurophysiol.* 55, 1340–1351

Newsome, W.T., Pare, E.B. (1986). MT lesions impair discrimination of direction in a stochastic motion display. *Neurosci. Abstr.* 12, 1183

Newsome, W.T., Pare, E.B. (1988). A selective impairment of motion perception following lesions of the middle temporal visual area (MT). *J. Neurosci.* 8, 2201–2211

Newsome, W.T., Wurtz, R.H. (1981). Response properties of single neurons in the midlle temporal visual area (MT) of alert macaque monkeys. *Soc. Neurosci. Abstr.* 7, 832

Newsome, W.T., Wurtz, R.H., Dürsteler, M.R., Mikami, A. (1985). Deficits in visual motion processing following ibotenic acid lesions of the middle temporal visual area of the macaque monkey. *J. Neurosci* 5, 825–840

Newsome, W.T., Wurtz, R.H., Komatsu, H. (1988). Relation of cortical areas MT and MST to pursuit eye movements. II. Differentiation of retinal from extraretinal inputs. *J. Neurophysiol.* 60, 604–620

Newton, I. (1706). *Opticks or a treatise of the reflections, refractions, inflections and colours of light*. 4th ed. 1730, Repr. Dover, New York, (1952)

Nicholson, C., Philips, J.M., Tobias, C., Kraig, R.P. (1981). Extracellular potassium, calcium and volume profiles during spreading depression. In Sykova, E., Hnik, P., Vyklicky, L. (eds.), *Ion-selective microelectrodes and their use in excitable tissues*, Plenum, New York, 211–223

Nickerson, D. (1981). OSA uniform color scale samples: a unique set. *Color Res. Appl.* 6, 7–33

Nielsen, G.D., Smith, E.E. (1973). Imaginal and verbal representations in short-term recognition of visual forms. *J. Exp. Psychol.* 101, 375–378

Nielsen, J.M. (1937). Unilateral cerebral dominance as related to mind blindness. *Arch. Neurol. Psychiat.* 38, 108–135

Nielsen, J.M. (1939). The unsolved problems in aphasia. Part II: Alexia resulting from a temporal lesion. *Bull. L.A. Neurol. Soc.* 4, 168–183

Nielsen, J.M. (1946). *Agnosia, apraxia and aphasia: Their value in cerebral localization*. Paul Hoeber, New York

Nielsen, J.M., Raney, R.B. (1938). Symptoms following surgical removal of major (left) angular gyrus. *Bull. L.A. Neurol. Soc.* 3, 42–46

Niessl von Mayendorf, E. (1928). Über Seelenblindheit. *Dtsch. Z. Nervenheilk.* 102, 117–119

Niessl von Mayendorf, E. (1935). Zur Lehre von der Seelenblindheit. *Z. ges. Neurol. Psychiat.* 152, 345–382

Nightingale, S. (1982). Somatoparaphrenia: a case report. *Cortex* 18, 463–467

Nilsson, T.H., Nelson, T.M. (1981). Delayed monochromatic hue matches indicate characteristics of visual memory. *J. Exp. Psychol. Hum. Percept.* 7, 141–150

Nissen, H.J. (1977). Aspects of the development of early cylinder seals. In Buccellati, G. (ed.), *Bibliotheca Mesopotamica 6: Seals and Sealing in Ancient Near East* (eds. McGuire Gibson and R.D. Biggs) Undena Publications, Malibu, 15–23

Nissen, H.J. (1988). *The early history of ancient Near East, 9000–2000 B.C.* Chicago

Nissen, H.J., Damerow, P., Englund, R.K. (1990). *Frühe Schrift und Techniken der Wirtschaftsverwaltung im alten Vorderen Orient. Informationsspeicherung und —verarbeitung vor 5000 Jahren.* Franzbecker, Berlin

Noel, G., Meyers, C. (1971). Two cases of visual agnosia with achromatognosia. *Acta Neurol. Belgica* 71, 173–184

Nogrady, H., McConkey, K.M., Perry, C. (1985). Enhancing visual memory: trying hypnosis, trying imagination, and trying again. *J. Abnorm. Psychol.* 94, 195–204

Norden von, G.K., Crawford, M.L.J. (1978). Morphological and physiological changes in the monkey visual system after short time lid closure. *Invest. Ophthalmol.* 17, 762–768

Nothnagel, H. (1879). *Topische Diagnostik der Gehirnkrankheiten.* Berlin

Noton, D., Stark, L. (1971). Scanpaths in eye movements during pattern recognition. *Science* 171, 308–311

Nouet, H. (1923). Hallucinations spéculaires et traumatisme cranien. *Encéphale* 18, 327–329

Novic, J., Luchins, D.J., Perline, R. (1984). Facial affect recognition in schizophrenia. Is there a differential deficit? *Brit. J. Psychiatry* 144, 533–537

Numann, P.J., Torppa, A.J., Blumetti, A.E. (1984). Neuropsychologic deficits associated with primary hyperparathyroidism. *Surgery* 96, 1119–1123

Nyrke, T., Kangasniemiö, P., Lang, A.H. (1990). Transient asymmetries of steady-state visual evoked potentials in classic migraine. *Headache* 30, 133–137

O'Brian, M.D. (1971). Cerebral blood changes in migraine. *Headache* 10, 139–143

O'Connor, N., Hermelin, B. (1973). Short-term memory for the order of pictures and syllables by deaf and hearing children. *Neuropsychologia* 11, 437–442

O'Connor, N., Hermelin, B. (1987). Visual memory and motor programmes: their use by idiot-savant artists and controls. *Br. J. Psychol.* 78, 307–323

O'Keefe, J. (1986). Is consciousness the gateway to the hippocampal cognitive map? A speculative essay on the neural basis of mind. *Brain and Mind* 4, 59–98

O'Keefe, J., Conway, D.H. (1978). Hippocampal place units in the freely moving rat: why they fire where they fire. *Exp. Brain Res.*, 31, 573–590.

O'Keefe, J.B, Nadel, L. (1978). *The hippocampus as a cognitive map.* Clarendon Press, Oxford

Ober, B.A., Stillman, R.C. (1988). Memory in chronic alcoholics: effects of inconsistent versus consistent information. *Addict Behav.* 13, 11–15

Obermaier, H. (1912). *Der Mensch der Vorzeit.* Berlin (quoted after Földes-Papp, 1966)

Ochs, S. (1962). The nature of spreading depression in neuronal networks. *Int. Rev. Neurobiol.* 4, 2–65

Ochs, S. (1982). *Axoplasmic transport and its relation to other nerve functions.* Wiley, New York

Ockleford, E.M., Milner, A.D., Dewar, W., Sneddon, I.A. (1977). Form perception in stumptail macaques follwing posterior parietal and lateral frontal lesions. *Cortex* 13, 361–372

Odom, R.D., Lemond, C.M. (1974). Children's use of component patterns of faces in multidimensional recall problems. *Child Dev.* 45, 527–531

Oelz, O., Largiader, J. (1987). Hallucinations and frostbite on a glacier dome. In Sutton, J.T., Houston, C.S., Coates, G. (eds.), *Hypoxia and cold.* Praeger, New York, 363–365

Ogden, J.A. (1984). Dyslexia in a right-handed patient with a posterior lesion of the right cerebral hemisphere. *Neuropsychologia* 22, 265–280

Ogden, J.A. (1985). Anterior-posterior interhemispheric differences in the loci of lesions producing visual hemineglect. *Brain and Cognition* 4, 59–75

Ogden, J.A. (1985). Contralesional neglect of constructed visual images in right and left brain-damaged patients. *Neuropsychologia* 23, 273–277

Ogden, J.A. (1987). The 'neglected' left hemisphere and its contribution to visuospatial neglect. In Jennerod, M. (ed.), *Neurophysiological and neuropsychological aspects of spatial neglect.* North-Holland, Amsterdam, 251–265

Ogren, M.P., Hendrickson, A.E. (1976). Pathways between striate cortex and subcortical regions in *Macaca mulatta* and *Saimiri sciureus*: evidence for a reciprocal pulvinar connection. *Exp. Neurol.* 53, 780–800

Ogren, M.P., Hendrickson, A.E. (1977). The distribution of pulvinar terminals in visual areas 17 and 18 of the monkey. *Brain Res.* 137, 343–350

Ogren, M.P., Hendrickson, A.E. (1979). The morphology and distribution of striate cortex terminals in the inferior and lateral subdivisions of the Macaca monkey pulvinar. *J. Comp. Neurol.* 188, 179–200

Ogren, M.P., Mateer, C.A., Wyler, A.R. (1984). Alterations in visually related eye movements and following left pulvinar damage in man. *Neuropsychologia* 22, 187–196

Oka, H., Asano, T., Hattori, S., et al. (1985). Pure alexia and alexia with agraphia caused by lesion of the left inferior temporal and fusiform gyri. *Shinkei Naika* 23, 73–76

Oldfield, R.C. (1971). The assessment and analysis of handedness: The Edinburgh inventory. *Neuropsychologia* 9, 97–113

Olesen, J. (1986). The pathophysiology of migraine. In Rose, F.C. (ed.), *Handbook of clinical neurology, Vol. 48,* Elsevier, Amsterdam, 59–83

Olson, R.K., Conners, F.A., Rack, J.P. (1991). Eye movements in dyslexic and normal readers. In Cronley-Dillon, J. (ed.), *Vision and visual dysfunction* (Vol. 13, Stein, J.F. (ed.) (in press))

Olson, R.K., Kliegl, R., Davidson, B.J. (1983). Dyslexic and normal reader's eye movements. *J. Exp. Psychol. (Hum. Percept.)* 9, 816–825

Olszewski, J. (1952). *The Thalamus of the Macaca Mulatta. An Atlas for use in the stereotaxic instrument.* Karger, Basel

Ong, J., Jones, L. Jr. (1982). Memory-for-Designs, intelligence and achievement of educable mentally retared children. *Percept. Mot. Skills* 55, 379–382

Oppenheim, H. (1885). Ueber eine durch eine klinisch bisher nicht verwerthete Untersuchungsmethode ermittelte Form der Sensibilitätsstörung bei einseitigen Erkrankungen des Grosshirns. *Neurol. Centralbl.* 4, 529–533

Optican, L.M., Richmond, B.J. (1987). Temporal encoding of two-dimensional patterns by single units in primate inferior temporal cortex. III. Information theoretic analysis. *J. Neurophysiol.* 57, 162–178

Orbach, J. (1952). Retinal as a factor in the recognition of visually perceived words. *Amer. J. Psychol.* 65, 555–562

Orbach, J. (1967). Differential recognition of Hebrew and English words in right and left visual fields as a function of cerebral dominance and reading habits. *Neuropsychologia* 5, 127–134

Orbaek, P., Lindgren, M. (1988). Prospective clinical and psychometric investigation of patiens with chronic toxic encephalopathy induced by solvents. *Scand J. Work Environ Health* 14, 37–44

Orban, G.A. (1984). *Neuronal operations in the visual cortex.* Studies of Brain Function Vol 11. Springer, Berlin

Orban, G.A. (1991). Quantitative electrophysiology of visual cortical neurons. In Cronly-Dillon, J. (ed.), *Vision and visual dysfunction.* Vol. 4 (Leventhal, A.G. (ed.), chapter 4). Macmillan, London

Orban, G.A., Callens, M. (1977). Influence of movement parameters on area 18 neurones in the cat. *Exp. Brain Res.* 30, 125–140

Orban, G.A., Gulyas, B., Spileers, W. (1988). Influence of moving textured backgrounds on responses of cat area 18 cells to moving bars. In Hicks, T.P., Benedek, G. (eds.), *Progress in Brain Res., Vision within extrageniculo-striate systems*. Vol. 75, 137–145

Orban, G.A., Gulyas, B., Spileers, W., Maes, H. (1987). Responses of cat striate neurons to moving light and dark bars: changes with eccentricity. *J. Opt. Soc. Am. A.*, 4, 1653–1665

Orban, G.A., Gulyas, B., Vogels, R. (1987). Influence of a moving textured background on direction selectivity of cat striate neurons. *J. Neurophysiol.* 57, 1792–1812

Orban, G.A., Hofmann, K.P., Duysens, J. (1985). Velocity selectivity in the cat visual system. I. Responses of LGN cells to moving bar stimuli: a comparison with cortical areas 17 and 18. *J. Neurophysiol* 54, 1026–1049

Orban, G.A., Vandenbussche, E., Sprague, J.M., De Weerd, P. (1988). Stimulus contrast and visual cortical lesions. *Exp. Brain Res.* 72, 191–194

Orem, J., Schlag-Rey, M., Schlag, J. (1973). Unilateral visual neglect and thalamic intralaminar lesions in the cat. *Exp. Neurol.* 40, 784–797

Orenstein, H.B., Hamilton, K.M. (1977). Memory load, critical features and retrieval processes in facial recognition. *Percept. Mot. Skills* 45, 1079–1087

Orenstein, J.B., Meighen, W.B. (1976). Recognition of bilaterally presented words varying in concreteness and frequency: Lateral dominance or sequential processing? *Bull. Psychonomic Society* 7, 179–180

Orgass, B., Kerschensteiner, M. (1975). Die visuellen Agnosien. *Akt. Neurol.* 2, 189–197

Orgass, G., Poeck, K., Kerschensteiner, M., Hartje, W. (1972). Visuo-cognitive performance in patients with unilateral hemipheric lesions. *Z. Neurol.* 202, 177–195

Orgogozo, J.M., Pere, J.J., Strube, E. (1979). Alexie sans agraphie, 'agnosie' des couleurs et atteinte de l'hemichamp visual droit: Un syndrome de l'arterie cerebrale posterieure. *Semaines des Hopitaux de Paris* 55, 1389–1394

Orlov, J.K. (1982a). Dynamik der Häufigkeitsstrukturen. In Guiter, H., Arapov, M.V. (eds.), *Studies on Zipl's law*. Brockmeyer, Bochum, 116–153

Orlov, J.K. (1982b). Ein Modell der Häufigkeitsstruktur des Vokabulars. In Guiter, H., Arapov, M.V. (eds.), *Studies on Zipl's law*. Brockmeyer, Bochum, 154–233

Ormrod, J.E. (1985). Visual memory in a spelling matching task: comparison of good and poor spellers. *Percept. Mot. Skills* 61, 183–188

Ostergaard, A.L., Davidoff, J.B. (1985). Some effects of color and on naming and recognition of objects. *J. Exp. Psychol., Learning, memory and cognition*, 11, 579–587

Osterrieth, P.A. (1944). Le test de copie d'une figure complèxe. *Arch. Psychol.* 30, 206–356

Ott, B., Grüsser, O.-J., Berndl, K. (1989). Visual pattern-completion in normal and schizophrenic subjects. *Soc. Neurosci. Abstr.* 15, 1123

Ottoson, D., Zeki, S. (1984). Central and peripheral mechanisms of colour vision. *Proc. Int. Symposium Wenner-Gren Center.*, Stockholm, Macmillan-Press, London

Overman, W.H. Ormsby, G., Mishkin, M. (1990). Picture recognition vs. picture discrimination learning in monkeys with medial temporal removals. *Exp. Brain Res.* 79, 18–24

Overman, W.H., Doty, R.W. (1978). Hemispheric specialization of facial recognition in man but not in macaque. *Soc. Neurosci. Abstr.* 4, 78

Overman, W.H., Doty, R.W. (1980). Prolonged visual memory in macaques and man. *Neuroscience* 5, 1825–1831

Overman, W.H., Doty, R.W. (1982). Hemispheric specialization displayed by man but not macaques for analysis of faces. *Neuropsychologia* 20, 113–128

Overman, W.H., Ormsby, G. Mishkin. M. (1990). Picture recognition vs. picture discrimination learning in monkeys with medial temporal removals. *Exp. Brain Res.* 79, 18–24

Oxbury, J.M., Campbell, D.C., Oxbury, S.M. (1974). Unilateral spatial neglect and impairments of spatial analysis and visual perception. *Brain* 97, 551–564

Oxbury, J.M., Oxbury, S.M., Humphrey, N.K. (1969). Varieties of colour anomia. *Brain* 92, 847–860

Page, N.G., Bolger, J.P., Sanders, M.D. (1982). Auditory evoked phosphenes in optic nerve disease. *J. Neurol. Neurosurg. Psychiatry* 45, 7–12

Paillard, J. (1982). The contribution of peripheral and central vision to visually guided reaching. In Ingle, D.J., Goodale, M.A., Mansfield, R.J.W. (eds.), *Analysis of human behavior*. Cambridge, MIT-Press, 549–586

Paillard, J. (1987). Cognitive versus sensorimotor encoding of spatial information. In Ellen, P., Thinus-Blanc, C. (eds.), *Cognitive processing and spatial orientation in animal and man*. Martinus Nijhoff, Dordrecht, 43–77

Paillard, J., Amblard, B. (1985). Static versus kinetic visual cues for the processing of spatial relationships. In Ingle, D.J., Jeannerod, M., Lee, D.N. (eds.), *Brain mechanisms and spatial vision*. Martinus Nijhoff, Dordrecht, 299–330

Paillard, J., Brouchon, M. (1974). A proprioceptive contribution to spatial encoding of position cues for balistic movements. *Brain Res.* 71, 273–284

Paillard, J., Hay, L. (1989). Head contribution to visuomotor recalibration after prismatic displacement of the visual field. In Berthoz, A., Graf, W., Vidal, J.P. (eds.), *Abstracts Head-Neck symposium*. Fontainebleau, France

Paillard, J., Jordan, P.L., Brouchon, M. (1981). Visual motion cues in prismatic adaptation: evidence for two separate and additive processes. *Acta Psychologica* 48, 253–270

Paillas, J.E., Cossa, P., Darcourt, G., Naquet, R. (1965). Etude sur l'épilepsie occipitale (ö propos de 36 observations de lésions occipitales verifiées irugicalement). *Proc. 8th Int. Congr. Neurology III* 193

Paivio, A. (1971). *Imagery and verbal processes*. Holt, Rinehart and Wilson, New York

Palem, R.M., Force, L., Esvan, J. (1970). Hallucinations critique épileptique et délire. *Ann. méd.-psychol.* 128, 161–190

Pallis, C.A. (1955). Impaired identification of faces and places with agnosia for colours. *J. Neurol. Neurosurg. Psychiat.* 18, 218–224

Palmer, G. (1777). *Theory of colours and vision*. Leacroft, London.

Palmer, G. (1787). *Theorie de la lumiere, applicable aux arts et principalment a la peinture*. Hardwin et Gattey, Paris

Palmer, J. (1988). Very short-term visual memory for size and shape. *Perc. Psychophys.* 43, 278–286

Palmer, S., Rosch, E., Chase, P. (1981). Canonical perspective and the perception of objects. In J. Long, Baddeley, A. (eds.), *Attention and Performance*, 9. Erlbaum, Hillsdale, 135–151

Palmer, S.E. (1975). The effects of contextual scenes on the identification of objects. *Memory and Cognition* 3, 519–526

Palmer, S.E. (1988). Reference frames in the perception of shape and orientation. In Shepp, B., Ballesteros, S., (eds.), *Object perception: Structure and process*. Lawrence Erlbaum, Hillsdale

Pandya, D. (1974). Interhemispheric connections in primate. In Michel, F., Schott, B. (eds.),. *Les syndromes de disconnexion calleuse chez l'homme*. Colloque international de Lyon, 17–40

Pandya, D.N., Dye, P., Butters, N. (1971). Efferent corticocortical projections of the prefrontal cortex in the rhesus monkey. *Brain Res.* 31, 35–46

Pandya, D.N., Karol, E.A., Heilbron, D. (1971). The topographical distribution of the interhemispheric projections in the corpus callosum of the rhesus monkey. *Brain Res.* 32, 31–43

Pandya, D.N., Kuypers, H.G.J.M. (1969). Cortico-cortical connections in the rhesus monkey. *Brain Res.* 13, 13–36

Pandya, D.N., Seltzer, B. (1982a). Intrinsic connections and architectonics of posterior parietal cortex in the rhesus monkey. *J. Comp. Neurol.* 204, 196–210

Pandya, D.N., Seltzer, B. (1982b). Association areas of the cerebral cortex. *Trends Neurosci.* 5, 386–390

Pandya, D.N., Van Hoesen, G.W., Mesulam, M.M. (1981). Efferent connections of the cingulate gyrus in the rhesus monkey. *Exp. Brain Res.* 42, 319–330

Pandya, D.N., Vignolo, L.A. (1971). Intra-and interhemispheric projections of the precentral, premotor and arcuate areas in the rhesus monkey. *Brain Res.* 26, 217–233

Pandya, D.N., Yeterian, E.H. (1984). Proposed neural circuitry for spatial memory in the primate brain. *Neuropsychologia* 22, 109–122

Panse, F. Shimoyama, T. (1955). Zur Auswirkung aphasischer Störungen im Japanischen. *Arch. Psychiat. Nervenkr.* 193, 131–138

Panse, F.R., Shimoyama, T. (1955). Zur Auswirkung aphasischer Störungen im Japanischen. II. Schreib-und Lesestörungen. *Arch. Psychiat. and Zeitschr. Neurol.* 193, 130–145

Pantle, A. (1974). Motion after-effect magnitude as a measure of the spatio-temporal response properties of direction sensitive analyzers. *Vision Res.* 14, 1229–1236

Pantle, A. (1978). Temporal frequency response characteristics of motion channels measured with three different psychophysical techniques. *Percept. Psychophys.* 24, 285–294

Pantle, A., Sekuler, R. (1969). Contrast response of human visual mechanisms sensitive to orientation and direction of movement. *Vision Res.* 9, 397–406

Pantle, A.J., Sekuler, R.W. (1968). Velocity-sensitive elements in human vision: initial psychophysical evidence. *Vision Res.* 8, 445–450

Papadakis, N. (1974). Subdural hematoma complicated by homonymous hemianopia and alexia. *Surg. Neurol.* 2, 131–132

Papousek, H., Papousek, M. (1974). Mirror image and self-recognition in young human infants: a new method of experimental analysis. *Dev. Psychobiol.* 7, 149–157

Papousek, H., Papousek, M. (1975). Cognitive aspects of preverbal social interaction between human infant and adults. In O'Connor, M. (ed.), *Parent-infant interaction.* Elsevier, Amsterdam, 241–260

Parish, E. (1894). *Ueber die Trugwahrnehmung (Hallucination und Illusion) mit besonderer Berücksichtigung der internationalen Enquete über Wachhallucination bei Gesunden.* Abel, Leipzig

Parish, E. (1897). *Hallucinations and illusions.* Scott, London

Parkhurst, Ch., Feller, R.L. (1982). Who invented the color wheel? *Color, Research and Application* 7, 217–230

Parkinson, D., Rucker, C.W., Craig, W.M. (1952). Visual hallucinations associated with tumors of the occipital lobe. *Arch. Neurol. Psychiat.* 68, 66–68

Parks, T. (1965). Post-retinal visual storage. *Amer. J. Psychol.* 78, 145–147

Parnetti, L., Ciuffetti, G., Signorini, E., Senin, U. (1985). Memory impairment in the elderly: a three-year follow up. *Arch. Gerontol. Geriatr.* 4, 91–100

Parry, C.H. (1825). *Collections from the unpublished writings of C.H. Parry edited by his son. Vol. I.*

Paschinger, E. (1990). *Personal communication.*

Pashler, H., Badgio, P. (1985). Visual attention and stimulus identification. *J. Exp. Psychol.: Human Perc. Perform.* 11, 105–121

Pashler, H., Badgio, P.C. (1987). Attentional issues in the identification of alphanumeric characters. Attention and Performance, Vol. VII: Lawrence Erlbaum Associates, Hillsdale

Pasik, P., Pasik, T. (1964). Oculomotor function in monkeys with lesions of the cerebrum and the superior colliculi. In Bender, M.B. (ed.), *The Oculomotor System.* Hoeber, New York, 40–80

Pasik, P., Pasik, T., Schilder, P. (1969). Extrageniculostriate vision in the monkey: Discrimination of luminous flux-equated figures. *Exp. Neurol.* 23, 421–437

Pasik, T., Pasik, P. (1971). The visual world of monkeys deprived of striate cortex: effective stimulus parameters and the importance of the accesory optic system. In Shipley, T., Dowling, J.E., (eds.), *Visual Processes in Vertebrates* Vision Res. Suppl. 3, Pergamon Press, Oxford, p. 419–435

Pasik, T., Pasik, P. (1980). Extrageniculostriate vision in primates. In Lessell, S., van Dalen, J.T.W., (eds.), *Neuro-ophthalmology Vol. 1.* Elsevier North-Holland, Amsterdam, p. 95–119

Passingham, R.E. (1972). Visual discrimination learning after selective prefrontal ablations in monkeys (*Macaca mulatta*). *Neuropsychologia* 10, 27–39

Pastore, N. (1971). *Selective history of theories of visual perception: 1650–1950.* Oxford Univ. Press, New York

Patat, A., Klein, M.J., Hucher, M., Granier, J. (1988). Acute effects of amitryptiline on human performance and interactions with diazepam. *Eur. J. Clin. Pharmacol.* 35, 585–592

Paterson, A., Zangwill, O.L. (1944). Disorders of visual space perception associated with lesions of the right hemisphere. *Brain* 67, 331–358

Paterson, A., Zangwill, O.L. (1945). A case of topographical disorientation associated with a unilateral cerebral lesion. *Brain* 68, 188–211

Paterson, J.V., Bramwell, E. (1905). Two cases of word blindness. *Med. Press*, 507–508

Patterson, K. (1986). Lexical but nonsemantic spelling? *Cogn. Neuropsychol.* 3, 341–367

Patterson, K., Besner, D. (1984a). Is the right hemisphere literate? *Cogn. Neuropsychol.* 1, 315–341

Patterson, K., Besner, D. (1984b). Reading from the left: a reply to Rubinovics and Moscovitch and to Zaidel and Schweiger. *Cogn. Neuropsychol.* 1, 365–380

Patterson, K., Bradshaw, J.L. (1975). Differential hemispheric mediation of nonverbal visual stimuli. *J. Exp. Psychol: Hum. Perc. Perform.* 1, 246–252

Patterson, K., Kay, J. (1982). Letter-by-letter reading. Psychological description of a neurological syndrome. *Quart. J. exp. Psychol.* 34, 411–441

Patterson, K., Vargha-Khadem F., Polkey, C.E. (1889). Reading with one hemisphere. *Brain* 112, 39–63

Patterson, K.E. (1981). Neuropsychological approaches to a study of reading. *Brit. J. Psychol.* 72, 151–174

Patterson, K.E., Baddeley, A.D. (1977). When face recognition fails. *J. Exp. Psychol: Hum. Learn. Mem.* 3, 406–417

Patterson, K.E., Kay, J. (1982). Letter-by-letter reading: Psychological descriptions of a neurological syndrome. *Quart. J. Exp. Psychol.* 34A, 411–441

Patterson, K.E., Marcel, A.J. (1977). Aphasia, Dyslexia and the phonological coding of written words. *Quart. J. Exp. Psychol.* 29, 307–318

Patterson, K.E., Marshall, J.C., Coltheart, M. (1985). *Surface dyslexia.* Erlbaum, London

Pauletto, D., Toso, V. (1987). Cognitive performance and Parkinson disease: neuropsychological and CT study. *Ital. J. Neurol. Sci.* 8, 121–124

Paulignan, Y., MacKenzie, C., Marteniuk, R., Jeannerod, M. (1991). Selective perturbation of visual input during prehension movements. 1. The effects of changing object position. *Exp. Brain Res.* 83, 502–512

Paulus, W., Zihl, J. (1989). Visual stabilization of posture in a case with selective disturbance of movement vision after bilateral brain damage: Real and apparent motion cues. *Clin. Vis. Sci.* 4, 367–371

Pause, M., Grüsser, O.-J., Schreiter, U. (1980). Sigma-OKN in Java monkeys: Is the apparent motion self-perpetuating by corollary discharge? *Invest. Ophthal. Vis. Sci. Suppl.* 80

Pearce, J. (1975). *Modern topics in migraine.* Heinemann, London

Pearce, J.M.S. (1986). Historical aspects of migraine. *J. Neurol. Neurosurg. Psychiat.* 49, 1097–1103

Pearlman, A.L., Birch, J., Meadows, J.C. (1979). Cerebral color blindness: an acquired defect in hue discrimination. *Ann. Neurol.* 5, 253–261

Pearson, J., Dewhurst, K. (1954). Sur deux cas de phénomènes héautoscopiques consécutifs ö des lésions organiques. *Encéphale* 43, 166–177

Pearson, J., Dewhurst, K. (1955). Visual hallucinations of the self in organic disease. *J. Neur. Neurosurg. Psychiat.* 18, 53–57

Pearson, K.L., Duffy, R.J. (1975). Pantomime recognition in aphasics. *J. Speech and Hearing Res.* 18, 115–132 ?

Pearson, R.C.A., Brodal, P., Powell, T.P.S. (1978). The projection of the thalamus upon the parietal lobe in the monkey. *Brain Res.* 144, 143–148

Pecci Saavedra, J., Vaccarezza, O.L., Reader, T.A., Pasqualini, E. (1970). Synaptic transmission in the degenerating lateral geniculate nucleus: an ultrastructural and electrophysiological study. *Exp. Neurol.* 26, 607–620

Pecci Saavedra, J., Vaccarezza, O.L., Reader, T.A., Pasqualini, E. (1971). Ultrastructural and electrophysiological aspects of denervated synapses in the lateral geniculate nucleus. *Vision Res. (Suppl.)* 3, 229–238

Pedersen, O. (1936). Zur Kenntnis der Symptomatologie der parieto-occipitalen Übergangsregion. *Arch. Psychiat.* 105, 539–549

Peichl, L., Ott, H., Boycott, B.B. (1987). Alpha ganglion cells in mammalian retinae. *Proc. Roy. Soc. Lond. B* 231, 169–197

Pena-Casanova, J., Roig-Rovira, T., Bermudez, A., Tolosa-Sarro, E. (1985). Optic aphasia, optic apraxia and loss of dreaming. *Brain and Language* 26, 63–71

Penfield, W., Jasper, H. (1954). *Epilepsy and the functional anatomy of the human brain.* Churchill, London

Penfield, W., Perrot, P. (1963). The brain's record of auditory and visual experience. A final summary and discussion *Brain* 86, 595–696

Penfield, W., Rasmussen, T. (1952). *The cerebral cortex of man.* Macmillan, New York

Peng, C.Y.Y., Campbell, R. (1988). Different forms of face-knowledge impairment. *Dev. Clin. Exp. Psychol.*(Plenum Press),1–25

Penk, W.E., Brown, A.S., Roberts, W.R., Dolan, M.P., Atkins, H.G., Robinowitz, R. (1981a). Visual memory of black and white male heroin and nonheroin drug users. *J. Abnorm. Psychol.* 90, 486–489

Penk, W.E., Brown, A.S., Roberts, W.R., Dolan, M.P., Atkins, H.G., Robinowitz, R. (1981b). Visual memory of male Hispanic-American heroin addicts. *J. Consult. Clin. Psychol.* 49, 771–772

Pennal, B.E. (1977). Human cerebral asymmetry in color discrimination. *Neuropsychologia* 15, 563–568

Perani, D., Nardocci, N., Broggi, G. (1982). Neglect after right unilateral thalamotomy: a case report. *Ital. J. Neurol. Sci.* 1, 61

Peregrin, J., Pastrnakova, I., Pastrnak, A. (1978). Visual evoked responses to the upper and lower half-field stimulation in a dark-adapted man. *Pflügers Arch.* 376, 81–92

Perenin, M.T. (1978). Visual function within the hemianopic field following early cerebral hemidecortication in man. II. Pattern discrimination. *Neuropsychologia* 16, 697–708

Perenin, M.T., Jeannerod, M. (1975). Residual vision in cortically blind hemifields. *Neuropsychologia* 13, 1–7

Perenin, M.T., Jeannerod, M. (1978). Visual function within the hemianopic field following early cerebral hemidecortication in man. I. Spatial localization. *Neuropsychologia* 16, 1–13

Perenin, M.T., Jeannerod, M., Prablanc, C. (1977). Spatial localization with paralysed eye muscles. *Ophthalmologica* 175, 206–214

Perenin, M.T., Ruel, J., Hécaen, H. (1980). Residual visual capacities

in a case of cortical blindness. *Cortex* 16, 605–612

Perenin, M.T., Vighetto, A. (1983). Optic ataxia: a specific disorder in visuomotor coordination. In Hein, A., Jeannerod, M. (eds.), *Spatially oriented behavior.* Springer, New York, Berlin, Heidelberg, Tokyo, 305–326

Perenin, M.T., Vighetto, A. (1988). Optic ataxia: a specific disruption in visuomotor mechanisms: 1. Different aspects of the deficit in reaching for objects. *Brain* 111, 643–674

Peron, N., Goutner, V. (1944). Alexie pure sans hemianopsie. *Rev. Neurol.* 76, 81–82

Peronnet, F., Farah, M.J. (1989). Mental rotation: an event-related potential study with a validated mental rotation task. *Brain & Cogn.* 9, 279–288

Perrett, D.I., Harries, M., Mistlin, A.J., Chitty, A.J. (1988). Three stages in the classification of body movements by visual neurons. In Barlow, H., Blakemore, C., Weston Smith, M. (eds.), *Images and understanding.* Cambridge Univ. Press

Perrett, D.I., Hietanen, J.K., Oram, M.W., Benson, P.J. (1992). Organization and functions of cells responsive to faces in the temporal cortex. *Proc. Roy. Soc. Lond.* (in press)

Perrett, D.I., Mistlin, A.J., Chitty, A.J. (1987). Visual neurones responsive to faces. *Trends in Neuroscience* 10, 358–363

Perrett, D.I., Rolls, E.T., Caan, W. (1982). Visual neurones responsive to faces in the monkey temporal cortex. *Exp. Brain Res.* 47, 329–342

Perrett, D.I., Smith, P.A.J., Mistlin, A.J., Chitty, A.J., Head, A.S., Potter, D.D., Broennimann, L.R., Milner, A.D., Jeeves, M.A. (1985a). Visual analysis of body movements by neurones in the temporal cortex of the macaque monkey: a preliminary report. *Behav. Brain Res.* 16, 153–170

Perrett, D.I., Smith, P.A.J., Potter, D.B., Mistlin, A.J., Head, A.S., Milner, A.D., Jeeves, M.A. (1984). Neurones responsive to faces in the temporal cortex: studies of functional organization, sensitivity to identity and relation to perception. *Hum. Neurobiol.* 3, 197–208

Perrett, D.I., Smith, P.A.J., Potter, D.D., Mistlin, A.J., Head, A.S., Milner, A.D., Jeeves, M.A. (1985b). Visual cells in the temporal cortex sensitive to face view and gaze direction. *Proc. Roy. Soc. Lond. (Biol.)* 223, 293–317

Perry, V.H., Cowey, A. (1981). The morphological correlates of X- and Y-like retinal ganglion cells in the retina of monkeys. *Exp. Brain Res.* 43, 226–228

Perry, V.H., Cowey, A. (1985). Retinal ganglion cells that project to the superior colliculus and pretectum in the macaque monkey. *Neuroscience* 12, 1125–1137

Perry, V.H., Cowey, A. (1988). The ganglion cell and cone distributions in monkey's retina: implications for central magnification factors. *Vision Res.* 25, 1795–1810

Perry, V.H., Oehler, R., Cowey, A. (1984). Retinal ganglion cells that project to the dorsal lateral geniculate nucleus in the macaque monkey. *Neuroscience* 12, 1101–1123

Perry, V.H., Silveira, L.C.L. (1988). Functional lamination in the ganglion cell layer of the macaque's retina. *Neuroscience* 25, 217–224

Peterhans, E., von der Heydt, R. (1987). The role of end-stopped receptive fields in contour perception. In Elsner, N., Creutzfeldt, O. (eds.), *New Frontiers in Brain Research.* Proc of the 15th Göttingen Neurobiology Conf. Thieme, Stuttgart

Peterhans, E., von der Heydt, R. (1988). Anomalous contour responses and effects of common motion in V2 of the alert monkey. A correlation with the anatomical cytochrome oxidase pattern. Abstract of ENA, Suppl. *Europ. J. Neurosci.* 98, 356

Peterhans, E., von der Heydt, R. (1989). Mechanisms of contour perception in monkey visual cortex. II. Contours bridging gaps. *J. Neurosci.* 9, 1749–1763

Peterhans, E., von der Heydt, R. (1991). Elements of form perception in monkey prestriate cortex. In Gorea, A., Fregnac, Y., Kapoula, Z., Findlay, J. (eds.), *Representations of vision. Trends and tacit assump-*

tions in vision research. Cambridge Univ. Press, Cambridge, 111–124

Peterhans, E., von der Heydt, R. (1991). Subjective colours bridging the gap between psychophysics and physiology. *Trends in Neurosciences* 14, 112–119

Peterhans, E., von der Heydt, R., Baumgartner, G. (1986). Neuronal responses to illusory contours stimuli reveal stages of visual cortical processing. In Pettigrew, J.D., Sanderson, K.J., Levick, W.R. (eds.), *Visual neuroscience.* Cambridge Univ. Press, 343–351

Peters, A. (1896). Ueber die Beziehungen zwischen Orientierungsstörungen und ein-und doppelseitiger Hemianopsie. *Arch. Augenheilk.* 32, 175–187

Peters, A. (1908). Kongenitale Wortblindheit. *Münchner med. Wochenschr.*

Petersen, S.E., Fox, P.T., Snyder, A.Z., Raichle, M.E. (1990). Activation of extrastriate and frontal cortical areas by visual words and word-like stimuli. *Science* 249, 1041–1044

Petersen, S.E., Miezin, F.M., Allman, J.M. (1988). Transient and sustained responses in four extrastriate visual areas in the owl monkey. *Exp. Brain Res.* 70, 55–60

Petersen, S.E., Morris, J.D., Robinson, D.L. (1984). Modulation of attentional behavior by injection of GABA-related drugs into the pulvinar of macaque. *Soc. Neurosci. Abstr.* 10, 475

Petersen, S.E., Robinson, D.L., Currie, J.N. (1989). Influences of lesions of parietal cortex on visual spatial attention in humans. *Exp. Brain Res.* 76, 267–280

Petersen, S.E., Robinson, D.L., Keys, W. (1982). A physiological comparison of the lateral pulvinar and area 7 in the behaving macaque. *Soc. Neurosci. Abstr.* 8, 681

Petersen, S.E., Robinson, D.L., Keys, W. (1985). Pulvinar nuclei of the behaving rhesus monkey: visual responses and their modulation. *J. Neurophysiol.* 54, 867–886

Peterson, N.L., Kirshner, H.S. (1981). Gestural impairment and gestural ability in aphasia. *Brain and Language* 14, 333–348

Peterzell, D.H. (1990). History of human cerebral hemispheric research. (iIn preparation)

Peterzell, D.H. (1991). On the non-relation between spatial frequency and cerebral hemispheric competence. Brain & Cognition (in press)...

Peterzell, D.H., Harvey, L.O. Jr, Hardyck C.D. (1989). Spatial frequencies and the cerebral hemispheres: contrast sensitivity, visible persistence, and letter classification. *Percept. Psychophys.* 46, 443–455

Petit-Dutaillis, D., Chavany, J.A., Fenelon, F. (1949). Disparation des phenomenes agnosiques apres amputation du lobe occipital gauche chez un droitier opere d'un meningiome du pressoir. *Rev. Neurol. (Paris)* 81, 424–427

Petras, J.M. (1971). Connections of the parietal lobe. *J. Psychiat. Res.* 8, 189–201

Petrides, M., Iversen, S.D. (1979). Restricted posterior parietal lesions in the rhesus monkey and performance on visuospatial tasks. *Brain Res.* 161, 63–77

Petrides, M., Pandya, D.N. (1984). Projections to the frontal cortex from the posterior parietal region in the rhesus monkey. *J. Comp. Neurol.* 228, 105–116

Petry, S., Meyer, G.E. (1987). *The perception of illusory contours.* Springer, Berlin

Pevzner, S., Bornstein, B., Loewenthal, M. (1962). Prosopagnosia. *J. Neurol. Neurosurg. Psychiat.* 25, 336–338

Pfaff, C.H. (1795). *Ueber thierische Electricität und Reizbarkeit. Ein Beytrag zu den neuesten Entdeckungen über diese Gegenstände.* Crusius. London

Pfeifer, R.A. (1919). Die Störungen des optischen Suchaktes bei Hirnverletzten. *Dtsch. Z. Nervenheilk.* 64, 140–152

Pfloeger, A. (1965). Seelenblindheit bei Röhrensehen? Dtsch. Z. *Nervenheilk.* 187, 485–490

Philips, W.A., Christie, D.F.M. (1977). Components of visual memory. *Quart. J. Exp. Psychol.* 29, 117–133

Phillips, C.G., Zeki, S., Barlow, H.G. (1984). Localizations of functions in the cerebral cortex. Past, present, future. *Brain* 107, 327–361

Pichler, E. (1943). Ueber Störungen des Raum-und Zeiterlebens bei Verletzungen des Hinterhauptlappens. *Z. ges. Neurol. Psychiat.* 176, 434–464

Pichler, E. (1957). Über Verkehrtsehen als Grosshirnsymptom. *Wien. klin. Wschr.* 69, 625–630

Pick, A. (1898). *Beiträge zur Pathologie und pathologischen Anatomie des Centralnervensystems.* Karger, Berlin

Pick, A. (1903). Clinical studies. III. On reduplicative paramnesia. *Brain* 26, 260–267

Pick, A. (1904). The localizing diagnostic significance of so-called hemianopic hallucinations, with remarks on temporal scintillating scotomata. *Am.J.Med.Sci.* 127, 82–92

Pick, A. (1907). *Zur Symptomatologie des atrophischen Hinterhauptslappens.* Karger, Berlin

Pick, A. (1915). Zur Pathologie des Bewusstseins vom eigenen Körper. Ein Beitrag aus der Kriegsmedizin. *Neurologisches Zentralblatt* 34 257–265

Pick, A. (1916). Kritische Bemerkungen zur Lehre von der Farbenbenennung bei Aphasischen. *Z. ges. Neurol. Psychiat.* 32, 310–325

Piderit, Th. (1858). *Grundsätze der Mimik und Physiognomik.* Vieweg, Braunschweig

Piderit, Th. (1867). *Wissenschaftliches System der Mimik und Physiognomik.* Meyers, Detmold

Pierce, J. (1960). Some sources of artifact in studies of the tachistoscopic perception of words. *J. Exp. Psychol.* 66, 363–370

Piercy, M., Hecaen, H., Ajuriaguerra, J. (1960). Constructional apraxia associated with unilateral cerebral lesions — left and right-sided cases compared. *Brain* 83, 225–242

Pierrot-Deseilligny, C., Gray, F., Brunet, P. (1986). Infarcts of both inferior parietal lobules with impairment of visually guided eye movements, peripheral visual inattention and optic ataxia. *Brain* 109, 81–97

Pierrot-Deseilligny, C., Rivaud, S., Gaymard, B., Agid, Y. (1990). Cortical control of memory-guided saccades in man. *Exp. Brain Res.* in press

Pillon, B. (1981). Négligence de l'hémi-espace gauche dans des épreuves visuo-constructives (influence de la complexité spatiale et de la méthode de compensation). *Neuropsychologia* 19, 317–320

Pillon, B. (1981). Troubles visuo-constructifs et méthodes de compensation: résultats de 85 patients atteints de lésions cérébrales. *Neuropsychologia* 19, 375–383

Pillon, B., Bakchine, S., Lhermitte, F. (1987). Alexia without agraphia in a left-handed patient with a right occipital lesion. *Arch. Neurol.* 44, 1257–1262

Pillon, B., Signoret, J.L., Lhermitte, F. (1981). Agnosie visuelle associative: Role de l'hemisphere gauche dans la perception visuelle. *Rev. Neurol. (Paris)* 137, 831–842

Pillsbury, W.B. (1987). A study in apperception. *Am. J. Psychol.* 8, 315–393

Pilowsky, I., Bassett, D. (1980). Schizophrenia and the response to facial emotions. *Compr. Psychiatry.* 21, 236–244

Pilowsky, I., Thornton, M., Stokes, B.B. (1986). Towards the quantification of facial expressions with the use of a mathematical model of the face. In Ellis, H.D. Jeeves, M.A., Newcombe, F., Young, A. (eds.), *Aspects of face processing.* Nijhoff, Dordrecht, 340–348

Pinker, S. (1985). Visual cognition: An introduction. In S. Pinker (ed.), *Visual cognition.* MIT Press, Cambridge

Pirozzolo, F.J., Kerr, K.L., Obrzut, J.E., Morley, G.K., Haxby, J.V., Lundgren, S. (1981). Neurolinguistic analysis of the language abilities of a patient with a 'double disconnection syndrome': a case of subangular alexia in the presence of mixed transcortical aphasia. *J.*

Neurol. Neurosurg. Psychiat. 44, 152–155

Pirozzolo, F.J., Rayner, K. (1980). Handedness, hemispheric specialization and saccadic eye movement latencies. *Neuropsychologia* 18, 225–229

Pishkin, V. (1966). Perceptual judgment of schizophrenics and normals as a function of social cues and symbolic stimuli. *J. Clin. Psychol.* 22, 3–10

Pitblado, C. (1979). Visual field differences in perception of the vertical with and without a visible frame of reference. *Neuropsychologia* 17, 381–392

Pittenger, J.B., Shaw, R.E. (1975). Aging faces as visco-elastic events: implications for a theory of nonrigid shape perception. *J. Exp. Psychol.* 1, 374–382

Pizzamiglio, L., Cappa, S., Valler, G., Zoccolotti, P., Bottini, G., Ciurli, P., Guariglia, C., Antonucci, G. (1989). Visual neglect for far and near extra-personal space in humans. *Cortex* 25, 471–477

Pizzamiglio, L., Carli, R. (1974). Visual, tactile and acoustic embedded figure tests in patients with unilateral brain damage. *Cortex* 10, 238–246

Pizzamiglio, L., Frasca, R., Guariglia, C., Incoccia, C., Antonucci, G. (1990). Effect of optokinectic stimulation in patients with visual neglect. *Cortex* 26, 535–540

Pizzamiglio, L., Zoccolotti, P. (1981). Sex and cognitive influence on visual hemifield superiority for face and letter recognition. *Cortex* 17, 215–226

Plant, G.T., Wilkins, A.J. (1988). Preserved movement sensitivity following occipital lobe damage: a case report of spatio-temporal contrast sensitivity in the Riddoch phenomenon. *Clin. Vis. Sci.* 2, 321–329

Plateau, J. (1872). Sur la mesure des sensations physique, et sur la loi qui lie l'intensité de ces sensations ö l'intensité de la cause excitante. *Bull. de L'Acad. Roy. Belg.* 33, 376–388

Plateau, J. (1873). Über die Messung physischer Empfindungen und das Gesetz, welches die Stärke dieser Empfindungen mit der Stärke der erregenden Ursache verknüpft. *Poggendorfs Ann. der Physik und Chemie*, 5th series, 30, 465–476

Plater, F. (1583). *De corporis humani structura et usu*. Froben, Basel

Platon. (1969). *Timaios*. In Loewenthal, E. (ed.), *Sämtliche Werke* Vol. III, Hegner, Köln, Olten, 93–191

Ploog, D. (1979). Soziobiologie der Primaten. In Kisker, K.P., Meyer, J.E., Müller, C., Strömgren, E. (eds.), *Psychiatrie der Gegenwart. Vol. I, 2*, Springer, Berlin, 380–544

Ploucquet, W.G. (1797). *System der Nosologie im Umrisse*. Heerbrandt, Tübingen

Podros, L.Z., Wyke, M.A., Waters, J.M. (1981). Vision and kinesthesis in spatial short-term memory. *Percept. Mot. Skills* 53, 459–466

Poeck, K. (1969). Pathophysiology of emotional disorders associated with brain damage. In Vinken, P.J., Bruyn, G.W. (eds.), *Handbook of Clinical Neurology Vol. 3, Disorders of higher nervous activity*. Willey, North Holland, Amsterdam, 343–367

Poeck, K. (1975). Neuropsychologische Symptome ohne eigenständige Bedeutung. *Akt. Neurol.* 2, 199–208

Poeck, K. (1984). Neuropsychological demonstration of splenial interhemispheric disconnection in a case of optic anomia. *Neuropsychologia* 22, 707–713

Poeck, K. (1989) (ed.). *Klinische Neuropsychologie*. 2nd. ed. Thieme, Stuttgart

Poeck, K., Kerschensteiner, M., Hartje, W., Orgass, B. (1973). Impairment in visual recognition of geometric figures in patients with circumscribed retrorolandic brain lesions. *Neuropsychologia* 11, 311–317

Poeck, K., Stachowiak, F.J. (1975). Farbbenennungsstörungen bei aphasischen und nicht-aphasischen Hirnkranken. *J. Neurol.* 209, 95–102

Poffenberger, A.T. (1912). Reaction time to retinal stimulation with special reference to the time lost in conduction through nerve centers. *Archs. Psychol.* 23, 1–73

Poggio, G.F. (1972). Spatial properties of neurons in striate cortex of unanaesthetized macaque monkey. *Invest. Opthalmol. Vis. Sci.* 11, 368–377

Poggio, G.F., Baker, F.H., Mansfield, R.J.W., Sillito, A., Grigg, P. (1975). Spatial and chromatic properties of neurons subserving foveal and parafoveal vision in rhesus monkeys. *Brain Res.* 100, 25–59

Poggio, G.F., Doty Jr., R.W., Talbot, W.H. (1977). Foveal striate cortex of behaving monkey: single-neuron responses to square-wave gratings during fixation of gaze. *J. Neurophysiol.* 40, 1369–1391

Poggio, G.F., Fischer, B. (1977). Binocular interaction and depth sensitivity in striate and prestriate cortex of behaving rhesus monkey. *J. Neurophysiol.* 40, 1392–1405

Poggio, G.F., Gonzales, F., Krause, F. (1988). Stereoscopic mechanisms in monkey visual cortex: binocular correlation and disparity selectivity. *J. Neurosci.* 8, 4531–4550

Poggio, G.F., Talbot, W.H. (1981). Mechanisms of static and dynamic stereopsis in foveal cortex of the rhesus monkey. *J. Physiol. (Lond.)* 315, 469–492

Pohl, W. (1973). Dissociation of spatial discrimination deficits following frontal and parietal lesions in monkeys. *J. Comp. Physiol. Psychol.* 82, 227–239

Poizner, H., Kaplan, E., Bellugi, U., Padden, C.A. (1984). Visual-spatial processing in deaf brain-damaged signers. *Brain and Cognition* 3, 281–306

Pokorny, J., Shevell, S.,K., Smith, V.G. (1991). Colour appearance and colour constancy. In Cronly-Dillon, J.(ed.), *Vision and visual dysfunction Vol. 6, Gouras, P. (ed.), Chapter 4*

Pola, J., Wyatt, H. (1980). Target position and velocity: the stimuli for pursuit eye movements. *Vision Res.* 20, 523–534

Polich, J. (1984). Hemispheric patterns in visual search. *Brain and Cognition* 3, 128–139

Pollen, D.A. (1977). Responses of single neurons to electrical stimulation of the surface of the visual cortex. *Brain, Behav. Evol.* 14, 67–86

Pollen, D.A., Feldon, S.E. (1979). Spatial periodicities of periodic complex cells in the visual cortex cluster at one-half octave intervals. *Invest. Ophthal. and Visual Sci.* 18 (4), 429–434

Pollen, D.A., Lee, J.R., Taylor, J.H. (1971). How does the striate cortex begin reconstruction of the visual world? *Science* 173, 74–77

Pollen, D.A., Taylor, J.H. (1974). The striate cortex and the spatial analysis of visual space. In Schmitt, F.O., Worden, F.G. (eds.), *The Neurosciences Third Study Program*. The MIT Press, Cambridge, MA, 239–247

Polyak, S. (1957). *The vertebrate visual system. Its origin, structure and function and its manifestations in disease with an analysis of its role in the life of animals and in the origin of man.* H. Klüver (ed.) University of Chicago Press, Chicago

Polyak, S.L. (1941). *The retina*. Univ. of Chicago Press, Chicago

Pomme, A., Janny, P. (1954). Trouble de la mémoire topographique consécutif ö une intervention sur l'hémisphère non dominant. *Rev. Neurol.* 91, 307–308

Pontius, A.A. (1975). Developmental phases in visual recognition of the human face pattern exemplified by the 'smiling response'. *Experimentia* 31, 126–129

Popoff, N. (1927). Zur Kenntnis der Grösse der Area striate und Methodik ihrer Ausmessung. *J. Psychol. Neurol.* 34, 238–242

Poppelreuter, W. (1917). *Die psychischen Schädigungen durch Kopfschuss im Kriege 1914/16. Mit besonderer Berücksichtigung der pathopsychologischen, pädagogischen, gewerblichen und sozialen Beziehungen. Vol. 1, Die Störungen der niederen und höheren Sehleistungen durch Verletzungen des Okzipitalhirns*. Voss, Leipzig

Poppelreuter, W. (1917). Die Störungen des Lesens und Schreibens bei zerebral Sehgestörten. In *Die psychischen Schädigungen durch Kopfschuss im Kriege* 1, 256–270

Poppelreuter, W. (1923). Zur Psychologie und Pathologie der optischen Wahrnehmung. *Z. ges. Neurol. Psychiat.* 83, 26–152

Porta, G. della (1586). *De humana physiognomia.*

Porter, P.B. (1954). Another puzzle picture. *Amer. J. Psychol.* 67, 550–551

Posner, M.I. (1980). Orienting of attention. The 7th. Sir Frederic Bartlett Lecture. *Quart. J. Exp. Psychol.* 32, 3–25

Posner, M.I., Boies, S.J., Eichelmann, W.H., Taylor, R.L. (1969). Retention of visual and name codes of single letters. *J. Exp. Psychol. Monographs* 79

Posner, M.I., Cohen, Y. (1984). Components of visual orienting. In Bouma, H., Bowhuis, D. (eds.), *Attention and performance.* Erlbaum Ass., Hillsdale, NJ, 531–556

Posner, M.I., Cohen, Y., Rafal, R.D. (1982). Neural system control of spatial orienting. *Philos. Trans. Roy. Soc. Lond.* 298, 187–198

Posner, M.I., Snyder, C.R.R., Davidson, B.J. (1980). Attention and the detection of signals. *J. Exp. Psychol.* 109, 160–174

Posner, M.I., Walker, J.A., Friedrich, F.J., Rafal, R.D. (1984). Effects of parietal lobe injury on covert orienting of visual attention. *J. Neurosci.* 4, 1863–1874

Potegal, M. (1982). *Spatial abilities: development and psychological foundations.* Academic Press, New York

Potter, M.C., Faulconer, B.A. (1975). Time to understand pictures and words. *Nature* 253, 437–438

Pouliquen, A., Levillain, D., Gray, F., Samson-Dollfus, D., Rogler, M. (1974). 4 cas anatomocliniques d'hemianopsies laterales homonymes etudies a l'aide des potentiels evoques. *Rev. Otoneuroophthalmol.* 46, 133–136

Pöppel, E. (1973). Fortification illusion during an attack of ophthalmic migraine. *Naturwissenschaften* 60, 554–555

Pöppel, E. (1985). Bridging a neuronal gap. Perceptual completion across a cortical scotoma is dependent on stimulus motion. *Naturwissenschaften* 72, 599

Pöppel, E. (1986). Long-range colour-generating interactions across the retina. *Nature* 320, 523–525

Pöppel, E., Brinkmann, R., Cramon, D. von, Singer, W. (1978). Association and dissociation of visual functions in a case of bilateral occipital lobe infarction. *Arch. Psychiat. Nervenkr.* 225, 1–21

Pöppel, E., Cramon, D. von, Backmund, H. (1975). Eccentricity-specific dissociation of visual functions in patients with lesions of the central visual pathways. *Nature* 256, 489–490

Pöppel, E., Held, R., Frost, D. (1973). Residual visual function after brain wounds involving the central visual pathways in man. *Nature Lond.* 243, 295–296

Pöppel, E., Held, R., Frost, D. (1973). Residual visual function after brain wounds involving the central visual pathways in man. *Nature* 243, 295–296

Pöppel, E., Richards, W. (1974). Light sensitivity in cortical scotomata contralateral to small islands of blindness. *Exp. Brain Res.* 21, 125–130

Pöppel, E., Stoerig, P. (1986). Eccentricity-dependent residual target detection in visual field defects. *Exp. Brain Res.* 64, 469–475

Pöppel, E., Stoerig, P., Logothetis, N., Fries, W., Boergen, K.-P., Oertel, W., Zihl, J. (1987). Plasticity and rigidity in the representation of the human visual field. *Exp. Brain Res.* 68, 445–448

Pötzl, O. (1917). Experimentell erregte Traumbilder in ihren Beziehungen zum indirekten Sehen. I. *Z. ges. Neurol. Psychiat.* 37, 278–349

Pötzl, O. (1918). Bemerkungen über den Augenmassfehler der Hemianopiker. *Wien. klin. Wschr.* 31, 1149–1152

Pötzl, O. (1919). Über die Rückbildung einer Wortblindheit. *Z. ges. Neurol. Psychiat.* 52, 251

Pötzl, O. (1919). Vergleichende Betrachtung mehrerer Herderkrankungen in der Sehsphäre. *Jahrbücher f. Psych.* 39, 402–447

Pötzl, O. (1924). Ueber Störungen der Selbstwahrnehmung bei linksseitiger Hemiplegie. *Z. ges. Neurol. Psychiat.* 93, 117–168

Pötzl, O. (1927). Zur Kausuistik der Wortblindheit-Notenblindheit.

Mschr. Psychiat. Neurol. 66, 1–12

Pötzl, O. (1928). *Die Aphasielehre vom Standpunkte der klinischen Psychiatrie. Erster Band: Die optisch-agnostischen Störungen.* In Aschaffenburg, G. (ed.), *Handbuch der Psychiatrie.* F. Deuticke, Leipzig, Wien

Pötzl, O. (1933). Polyopie und gnostische Störung. *Jahrb. Psychiat. Neurol.* 50, 57

Pötzl, O. (1933). Über einige Beziehungen der traumhaften epileptischen Aura. *Wien. med. Wschr.* 87 (17), 465–468

Pötzl, O. (1949a). Ueber einige zentrale Probleme des Farbensehens. *Wiener Klin. Wochenschr.* 61, 706

Pötzl, O. (1949b). Zur Pathophysiologie des Uncus Syndroms und der traumhaften Aura. *Mschr. Psychiat. Neurol.* 117, 153

Pötzl, O. (1951). Ueber Verkehrtsehen. *Z. ges. Neurol. Psychiat.* 176, 780

Pötzl, O. (1952/53). Zur Agnosie des Physiognomiegedächtnisses. *Wien. Z. Nervenheilk.* 6, 335–354

Pötzl, O. (1954). Über Palinopsie (und deren Beziehung zu Eigenleistungen occipitaler Rindenfelder). *Wien. Z. Nervenheilk.* 8, 161–186

Pötzl, O. (1958). *Über die Beziehungen des Grosshirns zur Farbenwelt (abgeleitet aus hirnpathologischen Befunden).* W. Maudrich, Wien

Pötzl, O., Redlich, E. (1911). Demonstration eines Falles von bilateraler Affektion beider Occipitallappen. *Wiener Klin. Wochenschr.* 24, 517–518

Preilowski, B. (1975). Facial self-recognition after separate right and left hemisphere stimulation in two patients with complete cerebral commissurotomy. *Exp. Brain Res.* 23, Suppl. 165

Preilowski, B. (1979). Consciousness after complete surgical section of the forebrain in man. In Steele Russell, I., van Hof, M.W., Berlucchi, E. (eds.), *Structure and function of cerebral commissures.* The Macmillan Press, London, 411–420

Premack, A.J., Premack, D. (1972). Teaching language to an ape. *Sci. Amer.* 227(4), 92–99

Premack, D. (1971). On the assessment of language competence in the chimpanzee. In Schrier, A.M., Stollnitz, F. (eds.), *Behavior of nonhuman primates, Vol. 4.* Academic Press, New York, 185–228

Premack, D. (1975). Putting a face together. Chimpanzees and children reconstruct and transform disassembled figures. *Science* 188, 228–236

Premack, D. (1976). *Intelligence in ape and man.* Hillsdale, NJ, Earlbaum

Premack, D. (1976). *Language and intelligence in ape and man.* Erlbaum, Hillsdale, N.J. (s.o.? Titel?)

Prendes, J.L. (1978). Transient cortical blindness following vertebral angiography. *Headache* 18, 222–224

Preobrashensky, P. (1902). Zur Lehre von der subcorticalen Alexie und ähnlichen Störungen. *Neurol. Centralbl. Lpz.* 21, 734–736

Prevec, F.H. (1990). Functional specialization in the lower and upper visual fields in humans: Its ecological origins and neurophysiological implications. *Behav. and Brain Sciences* (in press)

Pribram, K.H. (1967). Neurophysiology and learning. I. Memory and organization of attention. In Lindsley, D.B., Lumsdaine, A.A. (eds.), *Brain Function. Vol. 4: Brain function and learning.* Univ. Calif. Press, Berkeley

Pribram, K.H. (1975). Toward a holonomic theory of perception. In Ertel, S., Kemmler, L., Stadler, M. (eds.), *Gestalttheorie in der modernen Psychologie* Erich Wengenroth, Köln, 161–184

Pribram, K.H. (1982b). Localization and distribution of function in the brain. In Orbach, J. (ed.), *Neuropsychology after Lashley.* Erlbaum, 273–296

Pribram, K.H., Bagshaw, M.H. (1953). Further analysis of temporal lobe syndrome utilizing fronto-temporal ablation. *J. Comp. Neurol.* 99, 347–375

Pribram, K.H., Blehart, S.R., Spinelli, D.N. (1966). Effects on visual discrimination of crosshatching and undercutting the inferotemporal cortex of monkey. *J. Comp. and Physiol. Psychol.*, 62, 358–364

Pribram, K.H., Carlton, E.H. (1986). Holonomic brain theory in imaging and object perception. *Acta Psychol.*, 63, 175–210

Pribram, K.H., McGuiness, D. (1975). Arousal, activation and effort in the control of attention. *Psychol. Rev.* 182, 116–149

Pribram, K.H., Reitz, S., McNeil, M., Spevack, A.A. (1979). The effect of amygdalectomy on orienting and classical conditioning in monkeys. *Pavlovian J.* 14 (4), 203–217

Pribram, K.H., Spinelli, D.N., Reitz, S.L. (1969). Effects of radical disconnexions of occipital and temporal cortex on visual behaviour of monkeys. *Brain*, 92, 301–312

Prince, M. (1906). *The dissociation of a personality.* Longman's Green and Co., New York, London

Prinzhorn, H. (1922/1968). *Bildnerei der Geisteskranken. Ein Beitrag zur Psychologie und Psychopathologie der Gestaltung.* Springer, Berlin Heidelberg New York

Prior, M., McCorriston, M. (1983). Acquired and developmental spelling dyslexia. *Brain Lang.* 20, 263–285

Probst, M. (1901). Ueber einen Fall vollständiger Rindenblindheit und vollständiger Amusie. *Mschr. Psychiat. Neurol.* 9, 5–21

Prohovnik, I., Risberg, J., Hagstadius, S., Maximilian, V. (1981). Cortical activity during unilateral tactile stimulation: a regional cerebral blood flow study. Meet. Int. Neuropsychol. Soc., Atlanta, Georgia, Febr. 1981

Proudfoot, R.E. (1983). Hemiretinal differences in face recognition: Accuracy versus reaction time. *Brain and Cognition* 2, 25–31

Przybyszewski, A., Chung, H.T., Grüsser, O.-J. (1990). Interaction of light stimulation and eyeball deformation in the cat retina. In Elsner, N., Roth, G. (eds.), *Brain — Perception — Cognition.* Proc. 18th Göttingen Neurobiology Conference, Thieme, Stuttgart, p. 222

Purdy, J.E., Olmstead, K.M. (1984). New estimate for storage time in sensory memory. *Percept. Mot. Skills* 59, 683–686

Purkinje, J.E. (1819/1823). *Beyträge zur Kenntniss des Sehens in subjectiver Hinsicht.* Calve, Prag

Purkinje, J.E. (1825a). *Beobachtungen und Versuche zur Physiologie der Sinne. II. Neue Beyträge zur Kenntniss des Sehens in subjectiver Hinsicht.* Reimer, Berlin

Purkinje, J.E. (1825b). Über die Scheinbewegungen, welche im subjectiven Umfange des Gesichtssinnes vorkommen. *Bull. der naturwissenschaftlichen Sektion der Schlesischen Gesellschaft* 4, 9–10

Purkinje, J.E. (1827). Über die physiologische Bedeutung des Schwindels und die Beziehung desselben zu den neuesten Versuchen über die Hirnfunctionen. *Magazin ges. Heilkunde* 23, 284–310

Purkinje, J. (1837/1838). Neueste Untersuchungen aus der Nerven- und Hirnanatomie. Bericht über die Versammlung deutscher Naturforscher und Ärzte. Prag 1837 (ed. Sternberg, K., Kromholz, J.V.), Haase, Prag, 177–181

Purtscher, (1900). Ueber die Einwirkung von Leuchtgas-Vergiftung auf das Seh-Organ. *Centralbl. prakt. Augenheilk.*, Jahrgang 24, 225–232

Putnam, T.J. (1926). Studies on the central visual system. IV. The details of the organization of the geniculostriate system in man. *Archs. Neurol. Psychiat. Lond.* 16, 683–707

Putnam, T.J., Liebman, S. (1942). Cortical representation of the macula lutea. *Arch. Ophthal.* 28, 415–443

Pylyshyn, Z.W. (1981). The imagery debate: analogue media versus tacite knowledge. *Psychol. Rev.* 87, 16–45

Pylyshyn, Z.W. (1984). *Computation and cognition.* MIT Press, Cambridge, MA

Quaglino, A. (1867). Emiplegia sinistra con amaurosi-Guarigione-Perdita totale della percezione dei colori e della memoria della configurazione degli oggetti. *Giornale d'oftalmologia italiane* 10, 106–117

Quensel, F. (1927). Ein Fall von rechtsseitiger Hemianopsie mit Alexie und zentral bedingtem monokulärem Doppeltsehen. *Mschr. Psychiat. Neurol.* 65, 173–207

Quensel, F. (1931). Die Alexie. In Schieck, F., Brückner, A. (eds.), *Kurzes Handbuch der Ophthalmologie*, Springer, Berlin, 324–475

Quensel, F. (1931). Die Erkrankungen der höheren optischen Zentren. In Schieck, F., Brückner, A. (eds), *Kurzes Handbuch der Ophthalmologie 6.* Springer-Verlag, Berlin, 324–475

Rabbitt, P., Cumming, G., Vyas, S. (1979). Modulation of selective attention by sequential effects in visual search tasks. *Quart. J. Exp. Psychol.* 31, 305–317

Rabbitt, P., Vyas, S. (1979). Memory and data-driven control of selective attention in continuous tasks. *Can. J. Psychol/Rev. Canad. Psychol.* 33, 71–87

Rabelo, C., Grüsser, O.-J. (1961). Die Abhängigkeit der subjektiven Helligkeit intermittierender Lichtreize von der Flimmerfrequenz (Brücke-Effekt, 'brightness-enhancement'): Untersuchungen bei verschiedener Leuchtdichte und Feldgrösse. *Psychol. Forsch.* 26, 299–312

Rachewiltz, B. de (1966). *An introduction to Egyptian art.* Spring Books, London

Radil, T., Radilová, I., Bohdanecky, Z., Bozkov. V. (1985). Psychophysiology of unconscious and conscious phenomena during visual perception. In Klix, F., Näätänen, R., Zimmer, K. (eds.), *Psychophysiological approaches to human information processing.* Elsevier, North Holland Amsterdam, 97–127

Rafal, R., Smith, J., Krantz, J., Cohen, J., Brennan, C. (1990). Extrageniculate vision in hemianopic humans: saccade inhibition by signals in the blind field. *Science* 250, 118–121

Rafal, R.D., Posner, M.I. (1987). Deficits in human visual spatial attention following thalamic lesions. *Proc. Natl. Acad. Sci. USA* 85, 7349–7353

Raizada, V.N., Raizada, I.N. (1972). Visual agnosia. *Neurology India* 20, 181–182

Rakic, P. (1977). Prenatal development of the visual system in rhesus monkey. *Philos. Trans. R. Soc. Lond. B Biol. Sci* 278, 245

Rakic, P. (1979). Genesis of visual connections in the rhesus monkey. In Freeman, R.D. (ed.), *Developmental neurobiology of vision.* Plenum Publ., New York, 249–260

Ramon y Cajal, S. (1894). *Die Retina der Wirbelthiere.* Bergmann, Wiesbaden

Ranschburg, P., Schill, E. (1932). Über Alexie und Agnosie. *Z. Neurol.* 139, 192–240

Rapaczynski, W., Ehrlichman, H. (1979). Opposite visual hemifield superiorities in face recognition as a function of cognitive style. *Neuropsychologia* 17, 645–652

Rapoport, A. (1982). Zipf's law re-visited. In Guiter, H., Arapov, M.V. (eds.), *Studies on Zipf's law.* Brockmeyer, Bochum, 1–28

Raskin, N.R. (1980/1988). *Headache.* Churchill Livingstone, New York

Ratcliff, G. (1979). Spatial thought, mental rotation and the right cerebral hemisphere. *Neuropsychologia* 17, 49–54

Ratcliff, G. (1987). Spatial cognition in man: the evidence from cerebral lesions. In Ellen, P., Thinus-Blanc, C. (eds.), *Neurophysiology and Developmental Aspects* Vol. II. Martinus Nijhoff Publ., Dordrecht-Boston-Lancaster, 78–90

Ratcliff, G., Davies-Jones, G.A.B. (1972). Defective visual localization in focal brain wounds. *Brain* 95, 46–60

Ratcliff, G., Newcombe, F. (1973). Spatial orientation in man: effects of left, right and bilateral posterior cerebral lesions. *J. Neurol., Neurosurg. and Psychiat.* 36, 448–454

Ratcliff, G., Newcombe, F. (1982). Object recognition: Some deductions from the clinical evidence. In A.W. Ellis (ed.), *Normality and pathology in cognitive functions.* Academic Press, New York, 147–171

Ratcliff, G., Ridley, R.M., Ettlinger, G. (1977). Spatial disorientation in the monkey. *Cortex* 13, 62–65

Ratcliff, G., Ross, J.E. (1981). Visual perception and perceptual disorder. *Br. Med. Bull.* 37, 181–186

Ratliff, F. (1965). *Mach bands: quantitative studies on neural networks in the retina.* Holden-Day, San Francisco, London, Amsterdam

Raybourn, M.S. (1983). The effects of direct-current magnetic field on turtle retinas in vitro. *Science* 220, 715–717

Rayner, K. (1979). Eye guidance in reading: fixation locations with words. *Perception* 8, 21–30

Rayner, K., Bertera, J.H. (1979). Reading without a fovea. *Science* 206, 468–469

Rayner, K., McConkie, G.W. (1976). What guides a reader's eye movements? *Vison Res.* 16, 829–837

Reda, G.C., Anderson, M. (1953). L'eautoscopia. *Rivista di Neurologia* 23, 26–42

Redican, W.K. (1975). Facial expressions in non-human primates. In Rosenblum, L.A. (ed.), *Primate behavior: developments in field and laboratory research.* Vol. 4. Academic Press, New York

Redlich, E. (1895). Ueber die sogenannte subcorticale Alexie. *Jb. Psychiat. Neurol.* 13, 1–60

Redlich, E., Bonvicini, G. (1911). Weitere klinische und anatomische Mitteilungen über das Fehlen der Wahrnehmung der eigenen Blindheit bei Hirnkrankheiten. *Neurol. Centralblatt,* 30. Jg., Veit, Leipzig, 227–238 u. 301–309

Redlich, E., Bonvicini, G. (1907). Über mangelnde Wahrnehmung (Autoanaesthesie) der Blindheit bei cerebralen Erkrankungen. *Neurol. Zbl.* 26, 945–951

Redlich, E., Bonvicini, G. (1909). Über das Fehlen der Wahrnehmung der eigenen Blindheit bei Hirnerkrankungen. *Jb. Psychiat. Neurol.* 29, 1–133

Redlich, E., Bonvicini, G. (1911). Weitere klinische und anatomische Mitteilungen über das Fehlen der Wahrnehmung der eigenen Blindheit bei Hirnkrankheiten. *Dtsch. Z. Nervenheilkunde* 41, 121

Redlich, F., Dorsay, J.F. (1945). Denial of blindness by patients with cerebral disease. *Arch. Neurol. Psychiat.* 53, 407

Reed, J.L. (1970). Schizophrenic thoughts disorder: A review and hypothesis. *Comp. Psychiat.* 11, 403–432

Reeves, A. (1986). Attention and the order of items in short-term visual memory. *Psychol. Res.* 48, 239–250

Reeves, A., Sperling, G. (1986). Attention gating in short-term visual memory. *Psychol. Rev.* 93, 180–206

Regal, D.M., Boothe, R., Teller, D.Y., Sackett, G.P. (1976). Visual acuity and visual responsiveness in dark-reared monkeys (Macaca nemestrina). *Vision Res.* 16, 523–530

Regan, D., Beverley, K.I. (1983). Visual fields for frontal plane motion and changing size. *Vision Res.* 23, 673–676

Regan, D., Beverley, K.I. (1984). Figure-ground segregation by motion contrast and by luminance contrast. *J. opt. Soc. Am.* 1, 433–442

Regard, M., Landis, T. (1984). Experimentally induced semantic paralexias in normals: a property of the right hemisphere. *Cortex* 20, 263–270

Regard, M., Landis, T. (1986). Affective and cognitive decisions on faces in normals. In Ellis, H.D., Jeeves, M.A., Newcombe, F., Young, A. (eds.), *Aspects of face processing.* Martinus Nijhoff, Dordrecht, 363–369

Regard, M., Landis, T. (1988). Beauty may differ in each half of the eye of the beholder. In Rentschler, I., Herzberger, B., Epstein, D. (eds.), *Beauty and Brain,* Birkhäuser, Basel, 243–257

Regard, M., Landis, T. (1988). Persönlichkeit und Lateralität. In Oepen, G. (ed.), *Psychiatrie des rechten und linken Gehirns.* Dtscher Ärzte-Verlag, Köln, 225–231

Regard, M., Landis, T., Graves, R. (1985). Dissociated hemispheric superiorities for reading stenography versus print. *Neuropsychologia* 23, 431–435

Regard, M., Landis, T., Hess, K. (1985). Preserved stenography reading in a patient with pure alexia. *Arch. Neurol.* 42, 400–402

Regard, M., Landis, T., Wieser, H.G., Hailemariam, S. (1985). Functional inhibition and release: unilateral tachistoscopic performance and stereoencephalographic activity in a case with left limbic status epilepticus. *Neuropsychologia* 23, 575–581

Reichardt, M. (1918). *Allgemeine und spezielle Psychiatrie.* Vol. 2, 2nd ed., Fischer, Jena

Reichardt, W. (1961). Autocorrelation, a principle for the evaluation of sensory information by the central nervous system. In Rosenblith, W.A. (ed.), *Sensory Communication.* MIT Press, Cambridge, Mass., 303–317

Reichel, F.D. , Todd, J.T. (1990). Perceived depth inversion of smoothly curved surfaces due to image orientation. *J. exp. Psychol: Human Perception Performance* 16, 653–644

Reicher, G.M. (1969). Perceptual recognition as a function of meaningfulness of stimulus material. *J. Exp. Psychol.* 81, 275–280

Reidemeister, C., Grüsser, O.-J. (1959). Flimmerlichtuntersuchungen an der Katzenretina. I. On-Neurone und on-off Neurone. *Z. Biol.* 111, 241–253

Reil, J.C. (1803). *Rhapsodieen über die Anwendung der psychischen Curmethode auf Geisteszerrüttungen.* Halle 1803, reprint Bonset, Amsterdam 1968,

Reinhard, C. (1887a). Zur Frage der Hirnlocalisation mit besonderer Berücksichtigung der cerebralen Sehstörungen. *Arch. Psychiat.* 18, 240–258

Reinhard, C. (1887b). Zur Frage der Hirnlocalisation mit besonderer Berücksichtigung der cerebralen Sehstörungen. *Arch. Psychiat.* 18, 449–486

Reinhard, C. (1986). Zur Frage der Hirnlocalisation mit besonderer Brücksichtigung der cerebralen Sehstörungen. *Arch. Psychiat.* 17, 717–756

Reisch, G. (1517). *Margerita philosophica.* Frobenius, Basel

Reisner, H. (1942). Über situationsbedingte Erlebnisse in der epileptischen Aura. *Nervenarzt* 16, 317–322

Reitz, S.L., Pribram K.H. (1969). Some subcortical connections of the inferotemporal gyrus of monkey. *Exp. Neurol.* 26, 632–645

Remschmidt, H., Schmidt, L. (eds) (1981). *Neuropsychologie des Kindesalters.* Enke, Stuttgart

Renault, B., Signoret, J.L., Debruille, B., Breton, F., Bolgert, F. (1989). Brain potentials reveal covert facial recognition in prosopagnosia. *Neuropsychologia* 27, 905–912

Rentschler, I., Baumgartner, G., Campbell, F.W., Lehmann, D. (1982). Analysis and restitution of visual function in a case of cerebral ambyopia. *Human Neurobiol.* 1, 9–16

Rentschler, I., Christen, L., Christen, S., Landis, T. (1986). Features versus spatial phase in a tachistoscopic laterality experiment. *Percept. & Psychophysics* 39, 205–209

Rentschler, I., Encke, W., Landis, T., Treutwein, B. (1991). Local and global components of global visual perception. *Percept. & Psychophysics,* in press

Rentschler, I., Hübner, M., Caelli, T. (1988). On the discrimination of compound Gabor signals and textures. *Vision Res.* 28, 279–291

Reuter-Lorenz, P. (1981). Differential contribution of the two cerebral hemispheres to the perception of happy and sad faces. *Neuropsychologia* 19, 609–613

Rey, A. (1964). *L'examen clinique en psychologie.* Presses Universitaires de France, Paris

Reynolds, D.M., Jeeves, M.A. (1978). A developmental study of hemisphere specialization for recognition of faces in normal subjects. *Cortex* 14, 511–520

Rezak, M., Benevento, L.A. (1979). A comparison of the organization of the projections of the dorsal lateral geniculate nucleus, the inferior pulvinar and adjacent lateral pulvinar to primary visual cortex (area 17) in the macaque monkey. *Brain Res.* 167, 19–40

Rhodes, G. (1985). Perceptual asymmetries in face recognition. *Brain and Cognition* 4, 197–218

Richards, J.S. (1980). Visual memory in left hemiplegia: a clinical evaluation of verbally mediated theories of visual memory. *Percept. Mot. Skills* 51, 13–14

Richards, W. (1968). Spatial remapping in the primate visual system. *Kybernetik* 4, 146–156

Richards, W. (1970). Stereopsis and stereoblindness. *Exp. Brain Res.* 10, 380–388

Richards, W. (1971). Anomalous sterescopic depth perception. *J. opt. Soc. Am.* 61, 410–414

Richards, W. (1971). Motion detection in man and other animals. *Brain Behav. Evol.* 4, 162–181

Richards, W. (1971). The fortification illusion of migraine. *Scient. Am.* 224, 89–96

Richards, W.A. (1975). Maps and migraines. *J. Opt. Soc. Am.* 65, 1185A

Richardson, J.T.E. (1975). Further evidence on the effect of word imageability in dyslexia. *Quart. J. Exp. Psychol.* 27, 445–449

Richardson, J.T.E. (1975). Imagery, concreteness and lexical complexity. *Quart. J. exp. Psychol.* 27, 211–223

Richardson, J.T.E. (1975). The effect of word imageability in acquired dyslexia. *Neuropsychologia* 13, 281–287

Richmond, B.J., Optican, L.M. (1987). Temporal encoding of two-dimensional patterns by single units in primate inferior temporal cortex. II. Quantification of response waveform. *J. Neurophysiol.* 57, 147–161

Richmond, B.J., Optican, L.M., Podell, M., Spitzer, H. (1987). Temporal encoding of two-dimensional patterns by single units in primate inferior temporal cortex. I. Response characteristics. *J. Neurophysiol.* 57, 132–146

Richmond, B.J., Sato, T. (1982). Visual responses of inferior temporal neurons are modified by attention to different stimulus dimensions. *Soc. Neurosci. Abstr.* 8, 812

Richmond, B.J., Wurtz, R.H., Sato, T. (1983). Visual responses of inferior temporal neurons in the awake monkey. *J. Neurophysiol.* 50, 1415–1432

Riddoch, G. (1917). Dissociation of visual perceptions due to occipital injuries, with especial reference to appreciation of movement. *Brain* 40, 15–57

Riddoch, G. (1935). Visual disorientation in homonymous half-fields. *Brain* 58, 376–382

Riddoch, M.J., Humphreys, G.W. (1983). The effect of cuing on unilateral neglect. *Neuropsychologia* 21, 589–599

Riddoch, M.J., Humphreys, G.W. (1987a). A case of integrative visual agnosia. *Brain* 110, 1431–1462

Riddoch, M.J., Humphreys, G.W. (1987b). Visual object processing in optic aphasia: a case of semantic access agnosia. *Cogn. Neuropsychol.* 4, 131–185

Riddoch, M.J., Humphreys, G.W. (1989). Finding the way around topographical impairments. In Brown, J.W. (ed.), *Neuropsychology of visual perception*. Erlbaum, Hillsdale, 79–104

Ridley, R.M., Baker, H.F., Murray, T.K. (1988). Basal nucleus lesions in monkeys: recognition memory impairment or visual agnosia? *Psychopharmacology (Berlin)* 95, 289–290

Riege, W.H., Kelly, K., Klane, L.T. (1981). Age and error differences on Memory-for-Designs. *Percept. Mot. Skills* 52, 507–513

Riege, W.H., Klane, L.T., Metter, E.J., Hanson, W.R. (1982). Decision speed and bias after unilateral stroke. *Cortex* 18, 345–355

Riegel, K.F., Riegel, R.M. (1961). Prediction of word-recognition thresholds on the basis of stimulus parameters. *Language and Speech* 4, 157–?

Rieger, C. (1909). Über Apparate in dem Hirn. *Arbeiten der Psychiatrischen Klinik zu Würzburg*, Heft 5, 176–197, Fischer, Jena

Riese, W. (1947). The early history of aphasia. *Bull. Hist. Med.* 21, 322–334

Riese, W., Hoff, E.C. (1950). A history of the doctrine of cerebral localization: sources, anticipations and basic reasoning. *J. Hist. Med.* 5, 50–71

Riklan, M., Levita, E. (1970). Psychological studies of thalamic lesions in humans. *J. Nerv. Ment. Dis.* 150, 251–265

Ringo, J.L. (1988). Seemingly discrepant data from hippocampectomized macaques are reconciled by detectability analysis. *Behav. Neurosci* 102, 173–177

Rinn, W.E. (1984). The neuropsychology of facial expression: a review of the neurological and psychological mechanisms for producing facial expressions. *Psychol. Bull.* 95, 52–77

Risos, A. (1965). Die visuelle Wahrnehmung während des optokinetischen Nystagmus des Menschen. *Pflügers Arch. ges. Physiol.* 283, R 63

Ritter, I.W. (1802). *Beyträge zu nähern Kenntniss des Galvanismus und der Resultate seyner Untersuchung*. Frommann, Jena

Ritter, I.W. (1805). Neue Versuche und Bemerkungen über den Galvanismus. *Gilbert's Annalen* 19, 6–8

Rixecker, H., Hartje, W. (1980). Kimura's recurring-figures-test: a normative study. *J. clin. Psychol.* 36, 465–567

Rizzo, M., Corbett, J.C., Thompson, H.S., Damasio, A.R. (1986). Spatial contrast sensitivity in facial recognition. *Neurology* 36, 1254–1256

Rizzo, M., Hurtig, R. (1987). Looking but not seeing: Attention, perception, and eye movements in simultanagnosia. *Neurology* 37, 1642–1648

Rizzo, M., Hurtig, R., Damasio, A.R. (1987). The role of scanpaths in facial recognition and learning. *Ann. Neurol.* 22, 41–45

Rizzolatti, G., Buchtel, H.A. (1977). Hemispheric superiority in reaction time to faces: a sex difference. *Cortex* 13, 300–305

Rizzolatti, G., Camarda, R. (1987). Neural circuits for spatial attention and unilateral neglect. In Jeannerod, M. (ed.), *Neurophysiological and neuropsychological aspects of spatial neglect*. Elsevier, Amsterdam, p. 289–313

Rizzolatti, G., Gallese, V. (1988). Mechanisms and theories in spatial neglect. In Boller, F., Grafman, J. (eds.), *Handbook of Neuropsychology*. Elsevier, Amsterdam, p. 223–246

Rizzolatti, G., Gentilucci, M., Fogassi, L., Luppino, G., Matelli, M., Ponzoni, M.S. (1987). Neurons related to goal-directed motor act in inferior area 6 of macaque monkey. *Exp. Brain Res.* 67, 220–224

Rizzolatti, G., Matelli, M., Pavesi, G. (1983). Deficits in attention and movement following the removal of postarcuate (area 6) and prearcuate (area 8) cortex in macaque monkeys. *Brain* 106, 655–673

Rizzolatti, G., Scandolara, C., Gentilucci, M., Camarda, R. (1981). Response properties and behavioral modulation of 'mouth' neurons of the postarcuate cortex (area 6) in macaque monkeys. *Brain Res.* 255, 421–424

Rizzolatti, G., Scandolara, C., Matelli, M., Gentilucci, M. (1981a). Afferent properties of periarcuate neurons in macaque monkeys. I. Somatosensory responses. *Behav. Brain Res.* 2, 125–146

Rizzolatti, G., Scandolara, C., Matelli, M., Gentilucci, M. (1981b). Afferent properties of periarcuate neurons in macaque monkeys. II. Visual responses. *Behavioural Brain Res.* 2, 147–163

Rizzolatti, G., Umilta, C., Berlucchi, G. (1971). Opposite superiorities of the right and left cerebral hemispheres in discriminative reaction time to physiognomical and alphabetical material. *Brain* 94, 431–442

Rizzolatti, G., Umilta, C.A., Berlucchi, G. (1970). Dimonstratione di differenze firzionali fra gli emisferi cerebrali dell'vomo normale per mezzo della tecnica dei tempi di reazione. *Arch. Fisiol.* 68, 96–97

Rizzuto, N. (1982). Prosopagnosia: report of four cases. *Europ. Neurol.* 21, 289–297

Robertson, I. (1989). Anomalies in the laterality of omissions in unilateral left visual neglect: implications for an attentional theory of neglect. *Neuropsychologia* 27, 157–165

Robertson, I.H. (1990). Digit span and visual neglect: a puzzling relationship. *Neuropsychologia* 28, 217–222

Robinson, C.J., Burton, H. (1980). Organization of somatosensory receptive fields in cortical areas 7b, retroinsular postauditory and granular insula of *M. fascicularis. J. Comp. Neurol.* 192, 69–92

Robinson, C.J., Burton, H. (1980). Somatic submodality distribution within the second somatosensory (SII), 7b, retroinsular, postauditory, and granular insular cortical areas of *M. fascicularis. J. Comp. Neurol.* 192, 93–108

Robinson, D.A. (1975). Oculomotor control signals. In Lennerstrand, G., Bach-y-Rita, P. (eds.), *Basic Mechanisms of Ocular Motility and Their Clinical Implications.* Pergamon, Oxford, 337–374

Robinson, D.L., Goldberg, M.E., Stanton, G.B. (1978). Parietal association cortex in the primate: sensory mechanisms and behavioral modulations. *J. Neurophysiol.* 41, 910–932

Robinson, D.L., Morris, J.D., Petersen, S.E. (1984). Cued visual behavior and the pulvinar of the awake macaque (Abstract). *Invest. Ophthalmol. Visual Sci.* 25, S33

Robinson, P.K., Watt, A.C. (1947). Hallucinations of remembered scenes as an epileptic aura. *Brain* 20, 440–448

Robinson, T.W., Vanderwolf, C.H., Pappas, B.A. (1977). Are the dorsal noradrenergic bundle projections from the locus coeruleus important for neocortical or hippocampal activation? *Brain Res.* 8, 75–98

Robson, J.G. (1975). Receptive fields: Neural representation of the spatial and intensive attributes of the visual image. In Carterette, E.C. (ed.), *Handbook of Perception*, Vol. V, *Seeing.* Academic Press, NY, 81–116

Rocha-Miranda, C.E., Bender, D.B., Gross, C.G., Mishkin, M. (1975). Visual activation of neurons in inferotemporal cortex depends on striate cortex and forebrain commissures. *J. Neurophysiol.* 38, 475–491

Rockland, K.S., Pandya, D.N. (1979). Laminar origins and terminations of cortical connections of the occipital lobe in the rhesus monkey. *Brain Res.* 179, 3–20

Rockland, K.S., Pandya, D.N. (1981). Cortical connections of the occipital lobe in the rhesus monkey: interconnections between areas 17, 18, 19 and the superior temporal sulcus. *Brain Res.* 212, 249–270

Rockland, K.S., Virga, A. (1990). Organization of individual cortical axons projecting from area V1 (area17) to V2 (area 18) in the macaque monkey. *Visual Neurosci.* 4, 11–28

Rodel, M. (1989). *Unterschiedliche Struktur-und Verarbeitungsprinzipien von Sprachzusammenhängen in den beiden Hirnhemisphären.* Doctoral dissertation, University Zürich

Rodel, M., Landis, T., Regard, M. (1989). Hemispheric dissociation in semantic relation. *J. Clin. Exp. Neuropsychol.* 11, 70

Rodieck, R.W. (1973). *The vertebrate retina: principles of structure and function.* Freeman, San Francisco

Rodieck, R.W., Binmoeller, K.F., Dineen, J. (1985). Parasol and midget ganglion cells of the human retina. *J. Comp. Neurol.* 233, 115–132

Rodieck, R.W., Brening, R.K. (1983). Retinal ganglion cells: properties, types, genera, pathways and trans-species comparisons. *Brain Behav. Evol.* 23, 121–164

Rodman, H.R., Albright, T.D. (1987). Coding of visual stimulus velocity in area MT of the macaque. *Vision Res.* 27, 2035–2048

Roellgen, D. (1985). *Agraphia.* In Heilman, K.M., Valenstein, E. (eds.), *Clinical Neuropsychology.* 2nd ed. Oxford Press, London

Roheim, G. (1916). Spiegelzauber. *Imago* 5, 63–120

Rohr, M. (1923). Auswahl aus der Behandlung des Horopters bei Franciscus Aguilonius um 1613. *Z. ophthalm. Optik* 11, 41

Roland, P.E. (1982). Cortical regulation of selective attention in man. A regional cerebral blood flow study. *J. Neurophysiol.* 48, 1059–1078

Roland, P.E., Friberg, L. (1985). Localization of cortical areas activated by thinking. *J. Neurophysiol.* 53, 1219–43

Roll, J.P., Gilhodes, J., Roll, R., Velay, J.L. (1990). Contribution of skeletal and extraocular proprioception to kinaesthetic representation. In Jeannerod, M. (ed.), *Attention and performance XIII*, Erlbaum, Hillsdale, 549–566

Roll, J.P., Roll, R. (1986a). Kinesthetic and motor effects of extraocular muscle vibration in man. In O'Regan, J.K., Lévy-Schoen, A. (eds.), *Eye movement, from physiology to cognition.* Elsevier, North-Holland, Amsterdam, 57–68

Roll, R., Roll, J.P. (1986b). Perceptual and motor effects induced by extraocular muscle vibration in man. *Neurosci. Lett. Suppl.* 26, S330

Rolls, E.T. (1981). Responses of amygdaloid neurons in the primate. In Ben-Ari, Y. (ed.), *Amygdaloid Complex.* Elsevier, Amsterdam, 383–393

Rolls, E.T. (1984). Neurons in the cortex of the temporal lobe and in the amygdala of the monkey with responses selective for faces. *Hum. Neurobiol.* 3, 209–222

Rolls, E.T. (1985). Neuronal activity in relation to the recognition of stimuli in the primate. In Chagas, C., Gattas, A., Gross, C. (eds.), *Pattern recognition mechanisms.* Springer-Verlag, Berlin, 203–213

Rolls, E.T. (1990) A theory of emotion, and its application to understanding the neural basis of emotion. *Cognition and Emotion* 4, 161–190

Rolls, E.T. (1992). Face processing mechanisms within and beyond the temporal cortical visual areas. *Proc. Roy. Soc. Lond.* (in press)

Rolls, E.T., Baylis, G.C. (1986). Size and contrast have only small effects on the responses to faces of neurons in the cortex of the superior temporal sulcus of the monkey. *Exp. Brain Res.* 65, 38–48

Rolls, E.T., Baylis, G.C., Hasselmo, M.E. (1987). The responses of neurons in the cortex in the superior temporal sulcus of the monkey to band-pass spatial farequency filtered faces. *Vision Res.* 27, 311–326

Rolls, E.T., Baylis, G.C., Hasselmo, M.E., Nalwa, V. (1989). The effect of learning on the face-selective responses of neurons in the cortex in the superior temporal sulcus of the monkey. *Exp. Brain Res.* 76, 153–164

Rolls, E.T., Baylis, G.C., Leonard, C.M. (1985). Role of low and high spatial frequencies in the face-selective responses of neurons in the cortex in the superior temporal sulcus in the monkey. *Vision Res.* 25, 1021–1035

Rolls, E.T., Cowey, A. (1970). Topography of the retina and striate cortex and its relationship to visual acuity in rhesus monkeys and squirrel monkeys. *Exp. Brain Res.* 10, 298–310

Rolls, E.T., Perrett, D., Thorpe, S.J., Puerto, A., Roper-Hall, A., Maddison, S. (1979). Responses of neurons in area 7 of the parietal cortex to objects of different significance. *Brain Res.* 169, 194–198

Rolls, E.T., Sanghera, M.K., Roper-Hall, A. (1979). The latency of activation of neurones in the lateral hypothalamus and substantia innominata during feeding in the monkey. *Brain Res.* 164, 121–135

Rolls, E.T., Treves, A. (1990). The relative advantages of sparse versus distributed encoding for associative neuronal networks in the brain. *Network* 1, 407–421

Rondot, P. (1975). Visuomotor disconnexion. Optical ataxia. *Brain and Nerve (Tokyo)* 27, 933–940

Rondot, P. (1989). Visuomotor ataxia. In Brown, J.W. (ed.), *Neuropsycholgy of visual perception.* Erlbaum, Hillsdale, 105–119

Rondot, P., de Recondo, J., Ribadeau Dumas, J.L. (1977). Visuomotor ataxia. *Brain* 100, 355–376

Rondot, P., Tzavaras, A. (1969). La prosopagnosie après vingt années d'études cliniques et neuropsychologiques. *J. Psychol. norm. path.* 2, 133–165

Rondot, P., Tzavaras, A., Garcin, R. (1967). Sur un cas de prosopagnosie persistant depuis quinze années. *Rev. Neurol. (Paris)* 117, 424–428

Rorschach, H. (1958). *Psychodiagnostik, Methodik und Ergebnis eines wahrnehmungsdiagnosti. Experiments.* 6th ed. Huber, Bern, 302 p.

Rosa, M.G.P., Sousa, A.P.B., Gattass, R. (1988). Representation of the visual field in the second visual area in the Cebus monkey. *J. Comp. Neurol.* 275, 326–345

Rosati, G., De Bastiani, P., Gilli, P., Paolino, E. (1980). Oral aluminum and neuropsychological functioning. A study of dialysis patients receiving aluminum hydroxide gels. *J. Neurol.* 223, 251–257

Rosch, E., Mervis, C.B., Gray, W., Johnson, D., Boyes-Braem, P. (1976). Basic objects in natural categories. *Cogn. Psychol.* 8, 382–439

Rose, D. (1983). An investigation into hemisphere differences in adaptation to contrast. *Perception & Psychophysics* 34, 89–95

Rose, J.E. (1949). The cellular structure of the auditory region of the cat. *J. Comp. Neurol.* 91, 409–440

Rosenberger, P.B. (1974). Discriminative aspects of visual hemi-inattention. *Neurology.* 24, 17–23

Rosenfeld, S.A., van Hoesen, G.W. (1979). Face recognition in the rhesus monkey. *Neuropsychologia* 17, 503–509

Rosenstein, L.M., Rawkin, J.G. (1929). Zur Psychopathologie der Gewebevergiftungen. *Z. Neurol.Psychiat.* 122, 1–22

Rosenthal, R., Bigelow, L.B. (1972). Quantitative brain measurements in chronic schizophrenia. *Br. J. Psychiat.* 121, 259–264

Ross, E.D. (1980). Sensory-specific and fractional disorders of recent memory in man: I. Isolated loss of visual recent memory. *Arch. Neurol.* 37, 193–200

Ross, E.D. (1980). The anatomic basis of visual agnosia. *Neurology* 30, 109–110

Ross, E.D. (1981). The aprosodias. Functional-anatomic organisation of the affective components of language in the right hemisphere. *Arch. Neurol.* 38, 561–569

Ross, H.E., Ross G.M. (1976). Did Ptolemy understand the moon illusion? *Perception* 5, 377–385

Rossi, A., Rossi, B., Santarcangelo, E. (1985). Influence of neck vibration on lower limb extensor muscles in man. *Arch. Ital. Biol.* 123, 241–253

Rossi, A., Stratta, P., D'Albenzio, L., Tartaro, A., Schiazza, G., di Michele, V., Bolino, F., Casacchia, M. (1990). *Biol. Psychiat.* 27, 61–68

Rossi, O. (1912). Regenerative Vorgänge im Nervus opticus. *J. Psychol. Neurol.* 19, 160–186

Roth, B. (1976). Narcolepsy and hypersomnia: review and classification of 642 personally observed cases. *Schweiz. Arch. Neurol. Psychiat.* 119, 31–41

Rothi, L.J.G., Goldstein, L.P., Teas, E., Schoenfeld, D., Moss, S., Ochipa, C. (1985). Treatment of alexia without agraphia: a case report. *J. Clin. and Exp. Neuropsychol.* 7, 607

Rothi, L.J.G., Mack, L., Heilman, K.M. (1986). Pantomime agnosia. *J. Neurol. Neurosurg. Psychiat.* 49, 451–454

Rousseaux, M., Cabaret, M., Lesoin, F., Devos, P., Dubois, F., Petit, H. (1986). Bilan de l'amnesie des infarctus thalamiques restreints, 6 cas. *Cortex* 22, 213–228

Rouzaud, M. Ribadeau, J.L., Degiovanni, E. Larmande, P., Ployet, M.J., Laffont, F. (1978). Troubles associatifs visuels (agnosie et syndrome de dysconnexion); atteinte auditive d'origine ischemique. *Rev. Otoneuroophthalmologique* 50, 365–382

Rovamo, J. (1978). Receptive field density of retinal ganglion cells and cortical magnification factor in man. *Med. Biol.* 56, 97–102

Rovamo, J., Virsu, V. (1979). An estimation and application of the human cortical magnification factor. *Exp. Brain Res.* 37, 1–20

Rovet, J., Netley, C. (1981). Turner syndrome in a pair of dizygotic twins: a single case study. *Behav. Genet.* 11, 65–72

Rozanski, J. (1952). Peduncular hallucinosis following vertebral angiography. *Neurology* 2, 341–349

Röhler, R. (1962). Die Abbildungseigenschaften der Augenmedien. *Vision Res.* 2, 391–429

Röhler, R., Miller, U., Aberl, M. (1969). Zur Messung der Modulationsübertragungfunktion des lebenden menschlichen Auges im reflektierten Licht (Measurement of the modulation transfer function of the eye by means of reflected light.). *Vision Res.* 9, 407–428

Rubens, A.B. (1979). Agnosia. In Heilman, K.M., Valenstein, E. (eds.), *Clinical Neuropsychology*. University Press, Oxford, 233–267

Rubens, A.B. (1985). Caloric stimulation and unilateral visual neglect. *Neurology* 35, 1019–1024

Rubens, A.B., Benson, D.F. (1971). Associative visual agnosia. *Arch. Neurol.* 24, 305–315

Rubin, E. (1921). *Visuell wahrgenommene Figuren*. Gyldendals, Copenhagen

Rubin, M.L., Walls, G.L. (1969). *Fundamentals of visual science*. Thomas, Springfield, Ill.

Rubin, W. (1984). *Primitivism in 20th century art: affinity of the Tribal and the Modern*. 2 Vols. Museum of Modern Art, New York

Ruddock, K.H. (1978). Evidence concerning the functional organisation of human vison derived from experiments with anomalous subjects. *Photobiology Bull.* 1, 6–14

Ruddock, K.H., Waterfield, V.A. (1978). Selective loss of function associated with a central visual defect. *Neurosci. Letters* 8, 93–98

Rudel, R.G., Teuber, H.L. (1971). Pattern recognition within and across sensory modalities in normal and brain-injured children. *Neuropsychologia* 9, 389–399

Ruff, R.L., Volpe, B.T. (1981). Environmental reduplication associated with right frontal and parietal lobe injury. *J. Neurol. Neurosurg. Psychiat.* 44, 382–386

Rumbaugh, D.M. (ed.) (1977) *Language learning by a chimpanzee. The Lana Project.* Academic Press, New York

Rumbaugh, D.M., Glasersfeld, E. von, Warner, H., Pisani, P., Gill, T.V. (1974). Lana (chimpanzee) learning language: a progress report. *Brain and Language* 1, 205–212

Rumelhart, D.E., Siple, P. (1974). Process of recognizing tachistoscopically presented words. *Psychological Review* 81, 99–113

Runge, Ph. O. (1810). *Die Farbenkugel*. Hamburg. repr. Stuttgart: Verlag Freies Geistesleben (1959)

Rushton, D.N., Brindley, G.S. (1977). Short-and long-term stability of cortical electrical phosphenes. In Rose, F.C. (ed.), *Physiological aspects of clinical neurology*. Blackwell, Oxford, 123–153

Rushton, D.N., Brindley, G.S. (1978). Properties of cortical electrical phosphenes. In Cool, S.J., Smith, E.L. (eds.), *Frontiers in Visual Science*. Springer, New York, 574–593

Russel, W.R., Whitty, C.W.M. (1955). Studies in traumatic epilepsy, III. Visual fits. *J. Neurol. Neurosurg. Psychiat.* 18, 79–96

Russell, I.S. (1982). Some observations on the problem of recovery of function following brain damage. *Hum. Neurobiol.* 1, 68–72

Russo, M., Vignolo, L.A. (1967). Visual figure-ground discrimination in patients with unilateral cerebral disease. *Cortex* 3, 113–127

Sabelaish, S., Hilmi, G. (1976). Ocular manifestations of mercury poisoning. *Bull. World Health Org.* 53 (suppl.), 83–86

Sachs, H. (1893). *Vorträge über Bau und Tätigkeit des Grosshirns*. Preuss & Jünger, Breslau

Sachs, H. (1895). Das Gehirn des Förster'schen 'Rindenblinden'. *Arb. Psychiatr. Klin. Breslau* 2, 53–127

Sackheim, H.A., Greenberg, M.S., Weiman, A.L., Gur, R.C., Hungerbuhler, J.P., Geschwind, N. (1982). Hemispheric asymmetry in the expression of positive and negative emotions. *Arch. Neurol.* 39, 210–218

Sackheim, H.A., Gur, R.C. (1978). Lateral asymmetry in intensity of emotional expression. *Neuropsychologia* 16, 473–481

Sackheim, H.A., Gur, R.C. (1982). Facial asymmetry and the communication of emotion. In Cacioppo, J.G., Petty, R.E. (eds.), *Social Psychophysiology*. Guilford, New York

Sackheim, H.A., Gur, R.C., Saucy, M.C. (1978). Emotions are expressed more strongly on the left side of the face. *Science* 202, 434–435

Sacks, O. (1985). *Migraine*. Duckworth, London

Sacks, O. (1985). *The man who mistook his wife for a hat*. Summit Books, New York

Sacks, O., Wasserman, R. (1987). The case of the colorblind painter. New York, *Review of Books* 34, 25–34

Sacks, O.,Wasserman, R.L., Zeki, S., Siegel, R.M. (1988). Sudden color-blindness of cerebral origin. *Soc. Neurosci. Abstr.* 14, 1251

Sadeh, M., Goldhammer, Y., Kuritsky, A. (1983). Postictal blindness in adults. *J. Neurol. Neurosurg. Psychiat.* 46, 566–569

Saenger, A. (1918). Über die durch die Kriegsverletzungen bedingten Veränderungen im optischen Zentralapparat. *Dtsch. Z. f. Nervenheilk.* 59, 192–228

Saenger, A. (1919). Ein Fall von dauernder zerebraler Erblindung nach Hinterhauptverletzung. *Zbl. Neurol. Psychiat.* 38, 210

Saffran, E.M. (1980). Reading in deep dyslexia is not ideographic. *Neuropsychologia* 18, 219–223

Saffran, E.M., Bogyo, L.C., Schwartz, M.F., Marin, O.S.M. (1980). Does deep dyslexia reflect right-hemisphere reading. In Coltheart, M., Patterson, K., Marshall, J.C. (eds.), *Deep dyslexia*. Routledge & Kegan Paul, London, 381–406

Saffran, E.M., Marin, O.S.M. (1977). Reading without phonology: Evidence from aphasia. *Quart. J. Exp. Psychol.* 29, 515–525

Safran, A.B., Kline, L.B., Glaser, J.S., Daroff, R.B. (1981). Television-induced formed hallucinations and cerebral diplopia. *Br. J. Ophthalmol.* 65, 707–711

Saito, H., Yukio, M., Tanaka, K., Hikosaka, K., Fukada, Y., Iwai, E. (1986). Integration of direction signals of image motion in the superior temporal sulcus of the macaque monkey. *J. Neurosci.* 6, 145–157

Sakata, H., Shibutani, H., Ito, Y., Tsurugai, K. (1986). Parietal cortical neurons responding to rotary movement of visual stimuli in space. *Exp. Brain Res.* 61, 658–663

Sakata, H., Shibutani, H., Kawano, K. (1978). Parietal neurons with dual sensitivity to real and induced movements of visual stimuli. *Neurosci Lett.* 9, 165–169

Sakata, H., Shibutani, H., Kawano, K. (1980). Spatial properties of visual fixation neurons in posterior parietal association cortex of the monkey. *J. Neurophysiol.* 43, 1654–1672

Sakata, H., Shibutani, H., Kawano, K. (1983). Functional properties of visual tracking neurons in posterior parietal association cortex of the monkey. *J. Neurophysiol.* 49, 1364–1380

Sakata, H., Shibutani, H., Kawano, K., Harrington, T.L. (1985). Neural mechanisms of space vision in the parietal association cortex in the monkey. *Vision Res.* 25, 453–464

Sakata, H., Takaoka, Y., Kawarasaki, A., Shibutani, H. (1973). Somatosensory properties of neurons in the superior parietal cortex (area 5) of the rhesus monkey. *Brain Res.* 64, 85–102

Sakitt, B., Barlow, H.B. (1982). A model for the economic cortical encoding of the visual image. *Biol. Cybernetics* 43, 97–108

Salama, A. (1981). The autoscopic phenomenon: case report and review of literature. *Canad. J. Psychiat.* 26, 475–476

Salmon, J.H. (1968). Transient postictal hemianopia. *Arch. Ophthalmol.* 29, 523–525

Salzen, E.A., Kostek, E.A., Beavan, D.J. (1985). The perception of action versus feeling in facial expression. In Ellis, H.D. (ed.), *NATO-Buch.* 326–339

Samelsohn, J. (1881). Zur Frage des Farbensinncentrums. *Centralblatt med. Wiss.* 29, 850–853

Samuels, I., Butters, N., Gooodglass, H. (1971). Visual memory defects following cortical-limbic lesions: effect of field of presentation. *Physiol. Behav.* 6, 447–452

Sandell, J.H., Schiller, P.H. (1982). Effects of cooling area 18 on striate cortex cells in the squirrel monkey. *J. Neurophysiol.* 48, 38–48

Sandras, N.K. (1968). *Prehistoric art in Europe*. Penguin Books, London, p. 350

Sands, S.F., Lincoln, E.E., Wright, A.A. (1982). Pictorial similarity judgements and the organization of visual memory in the rhesus monkey. *J. Exp. Psychol. (Gen.)* 111, 369–389

Sands, S.F., Wright, A.A. (1982). Monkey and humand pictoral memory scanning. *Science* 216, 1333–1334

Sanford, A.J., Garrod, S.C. (1981). *Understanding written language*. Wiley, Chichester, New York, Brisbane, Toronto

Sanford, H.S., Bair, H.L. (1939). Visual disturbances associated with tumors of the temporal lobe. *Arch. Neurol. Psychiat.* 42, 21–43

Sanger-Brown,H., Schafer, E.A. (1888). An investigation into the functions of the occipital and temporal lobes of the monkey's brain. *Philos. Trans. Roy. Soc. Lond.* 179, 303–327

Saper, C.B., Plum, F. (1985). Disorders of consciousness. In Frederiks, J.A.M. (ed.), *Handbook of Clinical Neurology. Clinical Neuropsychology*. Elsevier, Amsterdam, vol. 1, 107–128

Sasanuma, S. (1975). Kana and Kanji processing in Japanese aphasics. *Brain and Language* 2, 369–383

Sasanuma, S. (1980). Acquired dyslexia in Japanese: clinical features and underlying mechanisms. In Coltheart, M., Patterson, K., Marshall, J.C. (eds.), *Deep dyslexia*. Routledge and Kegan Paul, London, 48–90

Sasanuma, S. (1985). Surface dyslexia and dysgraphia. How are they manifested in Japanese? In Patterson, K.E., Marshall, J.C., Coltheart, M., *Surface Dyslexia. Neuropsychological and Cognitive Studies of Phonological Reading*. Erlbaum, London

Sasanuma, S., Fujimura, O. (1971). Selective impairment of phonetic and non-phonetic transcription of words in Japanese aphasic patients: Kana vs. Kanji in visual recognition and writing. *Cortex 7*, 1–18

Sasanuma, S., Fujimura, O. (1972). An analysis of writing errors in Japanese aphasic patients: Kanji versus Kana words. *Cortex 8*, 265–282

Sasanuma, S., Fujimura, O. (1974). Kanji versus Kana processing in alexia with transient agraphia: a case report. *Cortex 10*, 88–97

Sasanuma, S., Itoh, M., Kobayashi, Y., Mori, K. (1980). The nature of the task-stimulus interaction in the tachistoscopic recognition of Kana and Kanji word. *Brain and Language* 9, 298–306

Sasanuma, S., Itoh, M., Mori, K., Kobayashi, Y. (1977). Tachistoscopic recognition of Kana and Kanji words. *Neuropsychologia* 15, 547–553

Sasanuma, S., Monoi, H. (1975). The syndrome of Gogi (word-meaning) aphasia. Selective impairment of kanji processing. *Neurology* 25, 627–632

Sato, T. (1988). Effects of attention and stimulus interaction on visual responses of inferior temporal neurons in macaque. *J. Neurophysiol.* 60, 344–364

Savage-Rumbaugh, E.S. (1986). *Ape language: from conditioned responses to symbols*. Columbia University Press, New York

Savage-Rumbaugh, E.S., McDonald, K., Sevcik, R.A., Hopkins, W.D., Rubert, E. (1986). Spontaneous symbol acquisition and communicative use by pygmy chimpanzees (Pan paniscus). *J. Exp. Psychol.* 115, 211–235

Savage-Rumbaugh, E.S., Rumbaugh, D.M., McDonald, K. (1985). Language learning in two species of apes. *Neurosci. Biobehav. Rev.* 9, 653–665

Savage-Rumbaugh, E.S., Wilkerson, B.J. (1978). Socio-sexual behavior in *Pan paniscus* and *Pan troglodytes*: A comparative study. *J. Human Evol.* 7, 327–344

Savage-Rumbaugh, S., Rumbaugh, D.M., McDonald, K. (1985). Language learning in two species of apes. *Neurosci. Biobehav. Rev.* 9, 653–665

Säring, B., Prosiegel, M., Cramon von, D. (1988). Zum Problem der Anosognosie und Anosodiaphorie bei hirngeschädigten Patienten. *Nervenarzt* 59, 129–137

Scapinello, K.I., Yarmey, A.D. (1970). The role of familiarity and orientation in immediate and delayed recognition of pictorial stimuli. *Psychonom. Sci.* 21, 329–330

Scarone, S., Strambi, L.F., Cazzullo, C.L. (1981). Effects of two dosages of chlordesmethyldiazepam on mnestic information processes in normal subjects. *Clin. Ther.* 4, 184–191

Scarpatetti, A., Ketz, E., Jung, W. (1983). Zentralbedingte Achromatopsie. *Klin. Mbl. Augenheilk.* 183, 132–135

Schaefer, K.P. (1970). Unit analysis and electrical stimulation in the optic tectum of rabbits and cats. *Brain Behav. Evol.* 3, 222–240

Schafer, E.A. (1888). On the functions of the temporal and occipital lobes: a reply to Dr. Ferrier. *Brain* 11, 145–165

Schaternikoff, J. (1902). Über den Einfluss der Adaptation auf die Erscheinung des Flimmerns. *Z. Sinnesphysiol.* 29, 241–263

Scheidler, W., Landis, T., Rentschler, I., Regard, M., Encke, W., Baumgartner, G. (in press). A pattern recognition approach to visual agnosia. *Clin. Vis. Sci.*

Schein, S.J. (1988). Anatomy of macaque fovea and spatial densities of neurons in foveal representation. *J. comp. Neurol.* 269, 479–505

Schein, S.J., Desimone, R. (1990). Spectral properties of V4 neurons in the macaque. *J. Neurosci.* 10, 3369–3389

Schein, S.J., Marrocco, R.T., De Monasterio, F.M. (1982). Is there a high concentration of color-selective cells in area V4 of monkey visual cortex? *J. Neurophysiol.* 47, 193–213

Scheiner, C. (1619/1648). *Oculus: Hoc es: Fundamentum opticum.* Agricola, Innsbruck

Scheller, H. (1951). Über das Wesen und die Abgrenzung optisch-agnostischer Störungen. *Nervenarzt* 22, 187–190

Scheller, H. (1966). Benennen und Erkennen. Klinischer und anatomischer Bericht ueber einen Fall von optischer Aphasie, Alexie und optischer Agnosie. *Nervenarzt* 37, 93–96

Scheller, H., Seidemann, H. (1931). Zur Frage der optisch-räumlichen Agnosie (zugleich ein Beitrag zur Dyslexie). *Mschr. Psychiat. Neurol.* 81, 97–188

Schenkenberg, T., Bradford, D.C., Ajax, E.T. (1980). Line bisection and unilateral visual neglect in patients with neurologic impairment. *Neurology* 30, 509–517

Schilder, P. (1914). *Selbstbewusstsein und Persönlichkeitsbewusstsein. Eine psychopathologische Studie. Monographien aus dem Gesamtgebiete der Neurologie und Psychiatrie* 9. Julius Springer, Berlin

Schilder, P. (1923). *Das Körperschema.* Springer, Berlin

Schilder, P. (1931). Fingeragnosie, Fingerapraxie, Fingeraphasie. *Nervenarzt* 4, 625–???

Schilder, P. (1935). *The image and appearance of the human body.* Kegan Paul, Trench, Trubner, London

Schilder, P., Isakower, O. (1928). Optisch-räumliche Agnosie und Agraphie. *Z. ges. Neurol. Psychiat.* 113, 102–142

Schilder, P., Pasik, P., Pasik, T. (1972). Extrageniculate vision in the monkey. III. Circle vs. triangle and 'red vs. green' discrimination. *Exp. Brain Res.* 14, 436–48

Schilder, P., Pasik, P., Pasik, P. (1971). Extrageniculate vision in the monkey. II.Demonstration of brightness discrimination. *Brain Res.* 32, 383–98

Schiller, P.H. (1966). Developmental study of color-word interference. *J. Exp. Psychol.* 72, 105–108

Schiller, P.H., Finlay, B.L., Volman, S.F. (1976). Quantitative studies of single cell properties in monkey striate cortex. I. Spatiotemporal organization of receptive fields. *J. Neurophysiol.* 39, 1288–1319

Schiller, P.H., Finlay, B.L., Volman, S.F. (1976a). Quantitative studies of single-cell properties in monkey striate cortex. III. Spatial frequency. *J. Neurophysiol.* 39, 1334–1351

Schiller, P.H., Malpeli, J.G. (1977). The effect of striate cortex cooling on area 18 cells in the monkey. *Brain Res.* 126, 366–369

Schiller, P.H., Malpeli, J.G. (1978). Functional specificity of lateral geniculate nucleus laminae of the rhesus monkey. *J. Neurophysiol.* 41, 788–797

Schiller, P.H., Stryker, M. (1972). Single-unit recording and stimulation in superior colliculus of the alert rhesus monkey. *J. Neurophysiol.* 35, 915–924

Schiller, P.H., Treue, S.D., Conway, J.L. (1980). Deficits in eye movements following frontal eye-field and superior colliculus ablations. *J. Neurophysiol.* 44, 1175–1189

Schilling, T.B., König, P. (1990). Coherency detection by coupled oscillatory responses – synchronizing connections in neural oscillator layers. In Eckmiller, R., Hartmann, G., Hauske, G. (eds.), *Parallel processing in neural systems and computers.* Elsevier, North Holland, 139–142

Schlag, J., Schlag-Rey, M. (1983). Interface of visual input and oculomotor command for directing the gaze on target. In Hein, A., Jeannerod, M. (eds.), *Spatially oriented behavior.* Springer, New York, Berlin, Heidelberg, Tokyo, 87–103

Schlag-Rey, M., Schlag, J. (1980). Eye movement neurons in the thalamus of monkey. *Invest. Ophthal. Vis. Sci. ARVO Suppl.* 176

Schlag-Rey, M., Schlag, J. (1984). Visuomotor functions of central thalamus in monkey. I. Unit activity related to spontaneous eye movements. *J. Neurophysiol.* 51, 1149–1174

Schlanger, B.B., Schlanger, P., Gerstman, L.J. (1976). The perception of emotionally toned sentences by right-hemisphere-damaged and aphasic subjects. *Brain and Language* 3, 396–403

Schlesinger, B. (1928). Zur Auffassung der optischen und konstruktiven Apraxie. *Z. ges. Neurol. Psychiat.* 117, 649–697

Schliephake, H. (1874). Beyträge zur Kenntniss der Einwirkung des galvanischen Stromes auf das menschliche Auge. Wirkung der Santonin-Vergiftung auf den Einfluö des galvanischen Stromes. *Pflügers Arch.* 8, 565

Schmahmann, J.D., Pandya, D.N. (1990). Anatomical investigation of projections from thalamus to posterior cortex in the rhesus monkey: a WGA-HRP and fluorescent tracer study. *J. Comp. Neurol.* 295, 299–326

Schmandt-Besserat, D. (1977). An archaic recording system and the origin of writing. *Syro-Mesopotamian Studies* 1, 31–70

Schmandt-Besserat, D. (1988). Tokens at Uruk. *Baghdader Mitteilungen. Deutsches Archäologisches Institut* 19, 1–176

Schmeing, K. (1937). *Das zweite Gesicht in Niederdeutschland, Wesen und Wahrheitsgehalt.* Barth, Leipzig

Schmeing, K. (1943). *Zur Geschichte des zweiten Gesichts.* Oldenburg

Schmitt, B. (1948). L'héautoscopie. *Cahiers de psychiatrie* 2, 21–26

Schmitz-Gielsdorf, J., Willmes, K., Vondenhoff, C., Hartje, W. (1988). Effects of spatial arrangement of letter pairs in a name-matching task with unilateral and bilateral hemifield stimulation. *Neuropsychologia* 26, 591–602

Schmuller, J. (1979). Hemispheric asymmetry for alphabetic identification: scaling analyses. *Brain and Language* 8, 263–274

Schneider, K. (1959). *Klinische Psychopathologie.* 5. Aufl. Thieme, Stuttgart

Schnider, A., Landis, Th., Regard, M. (1991). Balint's syndrome in subactue HIV-encephalitis. *J. Neurol Neurosurg. Psychiat* 54,

Schnider, A., Regard, M., Landis, Th. (1991). Neglect in an artist: space perception disrupted but style preserved. (in preparation)

Schnider, A., Vaney, C. (1989). Neglekt — das oft vernachlässigte Syndrom der Vernachlässigung. *Schweiz. med. Wschr.* 119, 1583–1590

Schober, H. (1948). Erworbene Farbenblindheit nach Schädeltrauma. *Graefes Arch. Ophthal.* 148, 93–100

Schober, H., Rentschler, I. (1966). *Das Bild als Schein der Wirklichkeit.* Moos, München

Schoeler, H., Uhthoff, W. (1884). *Beiträge zur Pathologie des Sehnerven und der Netzhaut bei Allgemeinerkrankungen.* Berlin

Schoenen, J., Jamart, B., Delwaide, P.-J. (1987). Electroencephalographich mapping in migraine during the critical and intercritical periods. *Rev. Electroencephalogr. Neurophysiol. Clin.* Vol. 17(3)

Schoonbart, L., Cardyn-Oomen, E., Todts, H. (eds.) (1989). *James Ensor Exhibition catalogue.* Kunsthalle der Hypo-Kulturstiftung München, Hirmer, München

Schott, B., Jeannerod, M., Zahin, M.A. (1966). L'agnosie spatiale unilaterale: perturbation en secteur des mechanisms d'exploration et de fixation du regard. *J. de Medicine de Lyon* 47, 169–195

Schöne, H. (1964). The role of gravity in human spatial orientation. *Aerospace Medicine* 35, 764–772

Schöne, H. (1983). Orientierungskonzepte: Geschichtliches und Aktuelles. *Naturwissenschaften* 70, 342–348

Schreber, D.P. (1903). *Denkwürdigkeiten einer Nervenkranken.* Reprint in Heiligenthal, P., Volk, R. (eds.) (1973), *Bürgerliche Wahnwelt um 1900.* Focus, Wiesbaden, 1–246

Schröder, P. (1925). Über Gesichtshalluzinationen bei organischen Hirnleiden. *Arch. Psychiat. Nervenkr.* 75, 630–655

Schubert, G.H. (1814). *Die Symbolik des Traumes.* Reprint Lambert-Schneider, Heidelberg

Schubert, G.H. (1818). Ansichten von der Nachtseite der Naturwissenschaften. Arnold, Dresden

Schulhoff, C., Goodglass, H. (1969). Dichotic listening, side of brain injury and cerebral dominance. *Neuropsychologia* 7, 149–160

Schultze, M. (1866). Zur Anatomie und Physiologie der Retina. *Arch. mikrosk. Anat.* 2, 175–286

Schultze, M. (1866). *Zur Anatomie und Physiologie der Retina.* Cohen, Bonn

Schultze, M. (1867). Bemerkungen über Bau und Entwicklung der Retina. *Arch. mikrosk. Anat.* 3, 371–382

Schultze, M.I.S. (1872). *Sehorgan. I. Die Retina.* In Stricker, H. (ed.), *Handbuch der Lehre von den Geweben.* Vol. 2. Engelmann, Leipzig

Schumann, M. (1943). Sich-selbst-Sehen in einer zyklothymen Depression. *Nervenarzt* 16, 518–521

Schuster, P. (1909). Beitrag zur Kenntnis der Alexie und verwandter Störungen. *Mschr. Psychiat. Neurol.* 25 (Ergänzungsband), 349–378 und 389–424

Schuster, P., Taterha, H. (1920). Zur Klinik und Seelenblindheit. *Dtsch. Z. Nervenheilk.* 102, 112–122

Schuster, P., Taterka, H. (1926). Beitrag zur Anatomie und Klinik der reinen Worttaubheit. *Z. Neurol. Psychiat.* 105, 498–538

Schvaneveldt, R., Meyer, D. (1973). Retrieval and comparison processes in semantic memory. In Kornblum, S. (ed.), *Attention and performance.* Vol. 4. Academic Press, New York

Schwartz, A.S., Eidelberg, E. (1968). 'Extinction' to bilateral simultaneous stimulation in the monkey. *Neurology (Minneap.)* 18, 61–68

Schwartz, B.D., Winstead, D.K. (1982). Visual processing deficits in acute and chronic schizophrenics. *Biol. Psychiatry* 17, 1377–1387

Schwartz, D. (1982). Care of the acutely ill older adult. Part 1. Catastrophic illness: how it feels. *Geriatr. Nurs. (N.Y.)* 3, 302–306

Schwartz, E.L., Desimone, R., Albright, T.D., Gross, C.G. (1983). Shape recognition and inferior temporal neurons. *Proc. Nat. Acad. Sci.* 80, 5776–5778

Schwartz, J.H. (1979). Axonal transport: components, mechanisms and specificity. *Ann. Rev. Neurosci.* 2, 467–504

Schwartz, M., Smith, M.L. (1980). Visual asymmetries with chimeric faces. *Neuropsychologia* 18, 103–106

Schwartz, M.F., Marin, O.S.M., Saffran, E.M. (1979). Dissociation of language function in dementia: a case study. *Brain and Lang.* 7, 277–306

Schwartz, M.F., Saffran, E.M., Marin, O.S.M. (1980). Fractionating the reading process in dementia: Evidence for word-specific print-to-sound associations. In M. Coltheart, K.E. Patterson, J.C. Marshall (eds.), *Deep dyslexia.* Routledge and Kegan Paul, London

Schwartz, M.L., Goldman-Rakic, P.S. (1982). Single cortical neurones have axon collaterals to ipsilateral cortex in fetal and adult primates. *Nature* 299, 154–155

Schwartz, M.L., Goldman-Rakic, P.S. (1984). Callosal and intrahemispheric connectivity of the prefrontal association cortex in rhesus monkey: relation between intraparietal and principal sulcal cortex. *J. Comp. Neurol.* 226, 403–420

Schwartz, O. (1889). Ueber die Wirkung des constanten Stromes auf das normale Auge. *Arch. Psychiat. Nervenkr.* 21, 500

Schwartzbaum, J.S., Pribram, K.H. (1960). The effects of amygdalectomy in monkeys on transposition along a brightness continuum. *J. Comp. Physiol. Psychol.* 53, 396–399

Schwartzkroin, P.A., Cowey, A., Gross, C.G. (1969). A test of an 'efferent model' of the function of inferotemporal cortex in visual discrimination. *EEG. Clin. Neuropyhsiol.* 27, 594–600

Schwarz, F. (1940). Über die Reizung des Sehorgans durch niederfrequente elektrische Schwingungen. *Z. Sinnesphysiol.* 69, 92–118

Schwarz, F. (1944). Über die elektrische Reizbarkeit des Auges bei Hell-und Dunkeladaptation. *Pflügers Arch. Ges. Physiol.* 248, 76–86

Scotti, G. (1968). La perdita della memoria topografica: descrizione di un caso. *Sistema Nerv.* 20, 352–361

Scotti, G., Spinnler, H. (1970). Colour imperception in unilateral hemisphere-damaged patients. *J. Neurol. Neurosurg. Psychiat.* 33, 22–28

Scoville, W.B., Milner, B. (1957). Loss of recent memory after bilateral hippocampal lesions. *J. Neurol. Neurosurg. Psychiatr.* 20, 11–21

Seal, J., Commenges, D. (1985). A quantitative analysis of stimulus- and movement-related responses in the posterior parietal cortex of the monkey. *Exp. Brain Res.* 58, 144–153

Seal, J., Gross, C., Bioulac, B. (1982). Activity of neurons in area 5 during a simple arm movement in monkeys before and after deafferentation of the trained limb. *Brain Res.* 250, 229–243

Seal, J., Gross, C., Doudet, D., Bioulac, B. (1983). Instruction-related changes of neuronal activity in area 5 during a simple forearm movement in the monkey. *Neurosci. Lett.* 36, 145–150

Seamon, J.G., Gazzaniga, M. (1973). Coding strategies and cerebral laterality effects. *Cogn. Psychol.* 3, 552–631

Sedgwick, H.A., Festinger, L. (1976). Eye movements, efference, and visual perception. In Monty, R.A., Senders, J.W. (eds.), *Eye Movements and Psychological Processes.* Halsted, New York, 221–230

Seeck, M., Fuhry, L., Grüsser, O.-J. (1990). Item-related visual evoked potentials in the human EEG when human faces, animal faces, objects with 'physiognomic' components and 'neutral' objects served as stimuli. Abstracts Book, EBBS Workshop of Cognitive Neuroscience, 24.–29. Mai 1990, p. 88

Seeck, M., Grüsser, O.-J. (1991). Category-responsive components in visual evoked potentials. Photographs of faces, persons, tools and flowers as stimuli (submited).

Seeck, M., Naumann, A., Grüsser, O.-J. (1989). *Visual evoked potentials to silhouettes of human figures and other patterns.* Abstracts, ENA 12th Annual Meeting/EBBS 21st Annual Meeting, Turin, September 1989, p. 316

Segalowitz, S.J., Stewart, C. (1979). Left and right lateralization for letter matching: strategy and sex differences. *Neuropsychologia* 17, 521–525

Seggern, H. von (1881). Achromatopsie bei homonymer Hemianopsie mit voller Sehschärfe. *Klin. Monatsbl. Augenheilk.* 71, 101–104

Seguin, E.G. (1886). A contribution of the pathology of hemianopsis of central origin (cortex-hemianopsia). *J. nerv. ment. Dis.* 13, 1–38

Seidler, W., Grüsser, O.-J., Seeck, M. (1990). Visual evoked potentials in the human electroencephalogram to faces and selected parts of the face. In: Abstracts Book, EBBS Workshop of Cognitive Neuroscience, 24.–29. Mai 1990, p. 90

Seidman, L.J. (1983). Schizophrenia and brain dysfunction: an integration of recent neurodiagnostic findings. *Psychological Bulletin* 94, 195–238

Sekuler, R.W., Ganz, L. (1963). After-effects of seen motion with a stabilized retinal image. *Science* 139, 419–420

Selke, T. (1987). *Der Einfluss des Lebensalters auf die Fähigkeit von Kindern und Jugendlichen, Gesichter wiederzuerkennen.* Doctoral Dissertation. Freie Universität, Berlin

Seltzer, B., Pandya, D.N. (1976). Some cortical projections of the parahippocampal area in the rhesus monkey. *Exp. Neurol.* 50, 146–160

Seltzer, B., Pandya, D.N. (1978). Afferent cortical connections and architectonics of the superior temporal sulcus and surrounding cortex in the rhesus monkey. *Brain Res.* 149, 1–24

Seltzer, B., Pandya, D.N. (1980). Converging visual and somatic sensory cortical input to the intraparietal sulcus of the rhesus monkey. *Brain Res.* 192, 339–351

Seltzer, B., Pandya, D.N. (1984). Further observations on parieto-temporal connections in the rhesus monkey. *Exp. Brain Res.* 55, 301–312

Seltzer, B., Pandya, D.N. (1986). Posterior parietal projections to the intraparietal sulcus of the rhesus monkey. *Exp. Brain Res.* 62, 459–69

Seltzer, B., Van Hoesen, G.W. (1979). A direct inferior parietal lobule projection to the presubiculum in the rhesus monkey. *Brain Res.* 179, 157–161

Semmes, J. Weinstein, S., Ghent, L., Teuber, H.L. (1963). Correlates of impaired orientation in personal and extrapersonal space. *Brain* 86, 747–772

Senden, M. von (1932). *Raum-und Gestaltauffassung bei operierten Blindgeborenen vor und nach der Operation.* Barth, Leipzig (Engl. transl.: *Space and sight.* Free Press, Glencoe, Ill. (1960)

Sengoku, A., Kawai, I., Ohashi, H., Fujinawa, A. (1981). Paroxysmal autoscopy. *Seishinigaku* (Tokio) 23, 239–243 (quoted after Hamanaka, 1991)

Seppaelaeinen, A.M., Lindstroem, K., Martelin, T. (1980). Neurophysiological and psychological picture of solvent poisoning. *Am. J. Ind. Med.* 1, 31–42

Sereno, M.I., Allman, J.M. (1991). Cortical visual areas in mammals. In Cronly-Dillon, J. (ed.), *Vision and visual dysfunction.* Vol. 4 *The neural basis of visaul function.* ed. by Leventhal, A.G., chapter 7, MacMillan, London

Sergent, J. (1982). The cerebral balance of power: confrontation or cooperation. *J. Exp. Psych.: Human Perception and Performance* 8, 253–272

Sergent, J. (1983). Role of input in visual hemispheric asymmetries. *Psych. Bull.* 93, 481–512

Sergent, J. (1984a). An investigation into component and configural processes underlying face perception. *Brit. J. Psychol.* 75, 221–242

Sergent, J. (1984b). Configural processing of faces in the left and the right cerebral hemispheres. *J. Exp. Psychol.: Hum. Perc. Perf.* 10, 554–572

Sergent, J. (1984c). Inferences from unilateral brain damage about normal hemispheric functions in visual pattern recogniton. *Psychol. Bull.* 96, 99–115

Sergent, J. (1986). Methodological constrains on neuropsychological studies of face perception in normals. In Bruyer, R. (ed.), *The neuropsychology of face perception and facial expression.* Erlbaum, Hillsdale, N.J., 91–124

Sergent, J. (1989). Image generation and processing of generated images in the cerebral hemispheres. *J.Exp.Psychol.: Hum. Perc. Perform.* 15, 170–178

Sergent, J. (1990). The Neuropsychology of Visual Image Generation: Data, Method, and Theory. *Brain and Cogn.* 13, 98–129

Sergent, J. Corbalis, M.C. (1989). Categorization of disoriented faces in the cerebral hemispheres of normal and commissurotomized subjects. *J. Exp. Psychol: Human Perception and Performance A* 15, 701–710

Sergent, J., Bindra, D. (1981). Differential hemispheric processing of faces: methodological considerations and reinterpretation. *Psych. Bull.* 89, 541–554

Sergent, J., Corballis, M.C. (1990). Generation of multipart images in the disconnected cerebral hemispheres. *Bull. Psychonom. Soc.* 28, 309–311

Sergent, J., Hellige, J.B. (1986). Role of input factors in visual field asymmetries. *Brain and Cognition* 5, 174–199

Sergent, J., Poncet, M. (1990). From covert to overt recognition of faces in a prosopagnosic patient. *Brain* 113, 989–1004

Sergent, J., Switkes, E. (1984). Differential hemispheric sensitivity to spatial-frequency components of visual patterns. *Soc. Neurosci.*

Abstr. 10, 317

Sergent, J., Villemure, J.G. (1989). Prosopagnosia in a right hemispherectomized patient. *Brain* 112, 975–995

Seron, X., Van der Kaa, M.A., Remitz, A. (1979). Pantomime interpretation and aphasia. *Neuropsychologia* 17, 661–668

Serre d'Uzes, H. A. (1853). *Essai sur les phosphenes ou anneaux lumineux de la retine.* Lib. Victor Masson, Paris.

Sethe, K. (1939). *Vom Bilde zum Buchstaben. Die Entstehungsgeschichte der Schrift.* Reprint: Olms, Hildesheim

Severin, H.G. (1980). Bildnisse zwischen Antike und Mittelalter. In *Bilder vom Menschen in der Kunst des Abendlandes.* Mann, Berlin, 87–104

Sextus Empiricus (1936). *Against the physicists. Against the Ethicists. Transl. from the Greek by R.G. Bury.* Heinemann, London

Sextus Empiricus (1968–1985). *Grundriss der pyrrhonischen Skepsis. Einleitung und aus den Altgriechischen übersetzt von H. Hossenfelder.* Frankfurt, Suhrkamp

Shahrokhi, F., Hoagland, V.A., Randt, C.T. (1980). Retention of visual discrimination learning reinforced by brain stimulation in mice. *Neurosci. Lett.* 20, 109–113

Shallice, T. (1982). Specific impairments in planning. *Philos. Trans. R. Soc. London Ser. B* 298, 199–209

Shallice, T. (1988). *From neuropsychology to mental structure.* Cambridge University Press, New York

Shallice, T., Safran, E. (1986). Lexical processing in the absence of explicit word identification: evidence from a letter-by-letter reader. *Cogn. Neuropsychol.* 3, 429–458

Shallice, T., Warrington, E.K. (1975). Word recognition in a phonemic dyslexix patient. *Q. J. Exp. Psychol.* 27, 187–199

Shallice, T., Warrington, E.K. (1980). Single and multiple component central dyslexic syndromes. In Coltheart, M., Patterson, K., Marshall, J.C. (eds.), *Deep dyslexia.* Routledge and Kegan Paul, London

Shallice, T., Warrington, E.K., McCarthy, R. (1983). Reading without semantics. *Quart. J. Exp. Psychol.* 35A, 111–138

Shannon, C.E. (1951). Prediction and entropy of printed English. *Bell System Technical Journal* 30, 50–64

Shannon, C.E., Weaver, W. (1949/1964). *The mathematical theory of communications.* The University of Illinois Press, Urbana, IL, 125 p.

Shapley, R. (1990). Visual sensitivity and parallel retinocortical channels. *Ann. Rev. Psychol.* 41, 635–658

Shapley, R., Kaplan, E., Soodak, R. (1981). Spatial summation and contrast sensitivity of X and Y cells in the lateral geniculate nucleus of the macaque. *Nature* 292, 543–545

Shapley, R., Lennie, P. (1985). Spatial frequency analysis in the visual system. *Amer. Rev. Neurosci.* 8, 547–583

Sharpe, J.A., Johnston, J.L. (1989). Ocular motor paresis versus apraxia. *Ann. Neurol.* 25, 209

Shaw, M.L. (1984). Division of attention between spatial locations: A fundamental difference between detection of letters and detection of luminance increments. In H. Bouma, D.G. Brouwhuis (eds.), *Attention and performance* X. Lawrence Erlbaum Associates, Hillsdale, 109–121

Sheils, D. (1978). A cross-cultural study of beliefs in out-of-the-body experiences, waking and sleeping. *J. Society for Psychical Research* 49, 697–741

Shelton, P.A., Bowers, D., Heilman, K.M. (1990). Peripersonal and vertical neglect. *Brain* 113, 191–205

Shepard, R.N. (1978). The mental image. *Americ. Psychol.* 33, 125–137

Shepard, R.N. (1987b). Toward a universal law of generalization for psychological science. *Science*, 237, 1317–1323

Shepard, R.N. (1988). The role of transformations in spatial cognition. In Stiles-David, J., Kritchevsdy, M., Bellugi, U. (eds.), *Spatial cognition: Brain bases and development.* Lawrence Erlbaum Associates, Hillsdale, NY, 81–110

Shepard, R.N., Metzler, J. (1971). Mental rotation of three-dimensional objects. *Science* 171, 701–703

Shepherd, J.W., Deregowski, J.B., Ellis, H.D. (1974). A cross-cultural study of recognition memory for faces. *Int. J. Psychol.* 9, 205–212

Shepherd, J.W., Ellis, H.D. (1986). The effect of attractiveness on recognition memory for faces. *Am. J. Psychol.* 86, 627–633

Sheppard, J.I. (1968). *Human color perception. A critical study of the experimental foundation.* Elsevier, New York, 192 p.

Sherman, P.D. (1982). *Colour vision in the nineteenth century.* Hilger, Bristol

Sherman, S.M., Wilson, J.R., Kass, J.H., Webb, S.V. (1976). X-and Y-cells in the dorsal lateral geniculate nucleus of the owl monkey (*Aotus trivirgatus*). *Science* 192, 474–477

Sherrington, C.S. (1898). Further note on the sensory nerves of muscles. *Proc. Roy. Soc.* 62, 120–121

Shibutani, H., Sakata, H., Hyvärinen, J. (1984). Saccade and blinking evoked by microstimulation of the posterior parietal association cortex of the monkey. *Exp. Brain Res.* 55, 1–8

Shiffrin, R.M., Gardner, G.T. (1982). Visual processing capacity and attentional control. *J. Exp. Psychol.* 93, 72–83

Shiota, J., Kawamura, M., Isono, O. (1986). Alexia with agraphia produce by a localized infarction in the inferior posterior region of the left temporal lobe (in Jap.). *Nou Shinkei* 38, 1051–1055

Shiota, J., Sugita, K., Kikushima, S., Maki, T., Takeuchi, T. (1989). A case of multiple sclerosis with pure alexia. *Nou Shinkei* 41, 961–964

Shipkin, P,M., Gray, B.S., Daroff, R.B., Glaser, J.S. (1981). Alexia without agraphia in a right-handed patient with a left field defect and diffuse cerebral atrophy. *Neuro-ophthalmology* 2, 123

Shipley, T. (1964). Quantitative psychophysical methods applied to the neuropsychiatric examination of the visual agnosias. *Neuropsychologia* 2, 145–152

Shipp, S., Zeki, S. (1985). Segregation of pathways leading from area V2 to areas V4 and V5 of macaque monkey visual cortex. *Nature* 315, 322–325

Shipp, S., Zeki, S. (1989). The organization of connections between areas V5 and V1 in macaque monkey visual cortex. *Eur. J. Neurosci.* 1, 309–332

Shipp, S., Zeki, S. (1989). The organization of connections between areas V5 and V2 in macaque monkey visual cortex. *Eur. J. Neurosci.* 1, 333–354

Shuttleworth, E.C., Syring, V., Allen, N. (1982). Further observations on the nature of prosopagnosia. *Brain and Cognition* 1, 302–332

Sidtis, J.J., Volpe, B.T., Holtzman, J.D., Wilson, D.H., Gazzaniga, M.S. (1981). Cognitive interaction after staged callosal section: evidence for transfer of semantic activation. *Science* 212, 344–346

Siegel, R.E. (1970). *Galen on Sense perception. His doctrines, observations and experiments on vision, hearing, smell, taste, touch and pain, and their historical sources.* Karger, Basel

Siegel, R.K., West, L.J. (eds.) (1975). *Hallucinations: behavior, experience and theory.* Wiley, New York

Siegel, R.M., Andersen, R.A., Essick, G.K., Asanuma, C. (1985). The functional and anatomical subdivision of the inferior parietal lobule. *Soc. Neurosci. Abstr.* 11, 1012

Siegel, R.M., Anderson, R.A. (1986). Motion perceptual deficits following ibotenic acid lesions of the middle temporal area (MT) in the behaving rhesus monkey. *Soc. Neurosci. Abstr.* 12, 1183

Siegel, R.M., Anderson, R.A. (1988). Perception of three-dimensional structure from two-dimensional visual motion in monkey and man. *Nature* 331, 259–261

Siemerling, E. (1890). Ein Fall von sogenannter Seelenblindheit nebst anderweitigen cerebralen Symptomen. *Arch. Psychiat. Nervenkr.* 21, 284–299

Silberpfennig, J. (1941). Contributions to the problem of eye movements. III. Disturbances of ocular movements with pseudohemianopia in frontal lobe tumors. *Confin. Neurol.* 4, 1–13

Sillito, A.M., Kemp, J.A., Milson, J.A., Berardi, N. (1980). A reevaluation of the mechanism underlying simple cell orientation selectivity. *Brain Res.* 194, 517–520

Silva, P.S. (1965). Alucinacoes autoscopicas na epilepsia temporal: o fator emocional em nossa vida psiquica. *Revista Brasileira de Medicina* 22, 746–747

Silverman, S.M., Bergman, P.S., Bender, M.B. (1961). The dynamics of transient cerebral blindness. *Arch. Neurol.* 4, 333–348

Silverstein, A., Krieger, H.P. (1960). Neurologic complications of cardiac surgery. *Arch. Neurol.* 3, 601–605

Simon, M. (ed.) (1906). *Sieben Bücher Anatomie des Galen.* Leipzig

Simpson, J.I. (1984). The accessory optic system. *Ann. Rev. Neurosci.* 7, 13–41

Simpson, K.H., Smith, R.J., Davies, L.F. (1987). Comparison of the effects of atropine and glycopyrrolate on cognitive function following general anaesthesia. *Br. J. Anaest.* 59, 966–969

Singer, I. (1958). *The Spinoza of market street.* Farrar, Strauss and Giroux, New York

Singer, W. (1973). The effect of mesencephalic reticular stimulation on intracellular potential of cat lateral geniculate. *Brain Res.* 61, 55–68

Singer, W. (1989). Search for coherence: A basic principle of cortical self-organization. *Concepts in Neurosci.* 1 (1), 1–25.

Siqueira, E.B. (1965). The temporo-pulvinar connections in the rhesus monkey. *Arch. Neurol.* 13, 321–330

Siqueira, E.B. (1971). The cortical connections of the nucleus pulvinaris of the dorsal thalamus in rhesus monkey. *Int. J. Neurol.* 8, 139–154

Sirk, H. (1956). *Mathematik für Naturwissenschaftler und Chemiker.* Steinkopf, Dresden, Leipzig

Sittig, O. (1921). Störungen im Verhalten gegenüber Farben bei Aphasischen. *Monatsschr. Psychiat. Neurol.* 49, 63–68, 169–187

Sivadon, P. (1937). Phénomènes autoscopiques au cours de la grippe. *Ann. méd.-psych.* 95, 215–220

Sivak, M., Hill, C.S., Olson, P.L. (1984). Computerized video tasks as training techniques for driving-related perceptual deficits of persons with brain damage: a pilot evaluation. *Int. J. Rehabil. Res.* 7, 389–398

Skavenski, A.A. (1972). Inflow as a source of extraretinal eye position information. *Vision Res.* 12, 221–229

Skavenski, A.A., Hansen, R.M. (1978). Role of eye position information in visual space perception. In Senders, J.W., Fisher, D.F., Monty, R.A. (eds.), *Eye Movements and the Higher Psychological Functions.* Halsted, New York, 15–34

Skinner, B.F. (1965). *Science and human behavior.* Macmillan, New York

Skworzoff, K. (1931). Doppelgänger-Halluzinationen bei Kranken mit Funktionsstörungen des Labyrinths. *Z. ges.Neurol. Psychiat.* 133, 762–766

Skwotzoff (1881). *De la cécité des mots.* Thèse, Paris (cited in Charcot J.M. 1887)

Slater, A., Morison, V., Rose, D. (1982). Visual memory at birth. *Br. J. Psychol.* 73, 519–525

Sloan, L.L. (1971). The Tübinger perimeter of Harms and Aulhorn. *Arch. Ophthalmol.* 86, 612–622

Small, M. (1983). Asymmetrically evoked potentials in response to face stimuli. *Cortex* 19, 441–450

Small, M. (1988). Visual evoked potentials in a patient with prosopganosia. *Electroencephalogr. Clin. Neurophysiol.* 71, 10–16

Smith, A.D., Winograd, E. (1978). Adult age differences in remembering faces. *Dev. Psychol.* 14, 443–444

Smith, J.L. (1962). Homonymous hemianopia. A review of hundred cases. *Am. J. Ophthal.* 54, 616–622

Smith, J.L., Cogan, D.G. (1959). Optokinetic nystagmus: a test for parietal lobe lesion. A study of 31 anatomically verified cases. *Am. J. Ophthalmol.* 48, 187–193

Smith, J.L., Cross, S.A. (1983). Occipital lobe infarction after open heart surgery. *J. Clin. Neuroophthalmol.* 3, 23–30

Smith, K.V., Smith, W.M. (1962). *Perception and motion.* Saunders, Philadelphia, London, 341 p.

Smith, L.M. (1987). The encoding and recall of spatial location after right hippocampal lesions in man. In Ellen, P., Thinus-Blanc, C. (eds.), *Neurobiology of Spatial Behaviour II. Neurophysiology and Developmental Aspects.* Dordrecht, Nijhoff, 165–172

Smith, M.L., Milner, B. (1981). The role of the right hippocampus in the recall of spatial location. *Neuropsychologia* 19, 781–793

Smith, R.A., Gelles, D.B., Vanderhaeghen, J.J. (1971). Subcortical visual hallucinations. *Cortex* 7, 162–168

Smith, S., Holmes, G. (1916). A case of bilateral motor apraxia with disturbance of visual orientation. *Brit. Med. J.* 1, 437–441

Smythe, F.S. (1934). The second assault. In *Everest 1933.* Hodder and Stoughton, London, 164

Smythies, J.R. (1959a). The stroboscopic patterns: I. The dark phase. *Brit. J. Psychol.* 50, 106

Smythies, J.R. (1959b). The stroboscopic patterns: II. The phenomenology of the bright phase and afterimages. *Brit. J. Psychol.* 50, 305

Smythies, J.R. (1960). The stroboscopic patterns: III. Further experiments and discussion. *Brit. J. Psychol.* 51, 247

Snell, L. (1860). Die Personenverkennung als Symptom der Geistesstörung. *Allg. Z. Psychiat.* 17, 545–554

Snodderly, D.M., Kurtz, D. (1985). Eye position during fixation tasks: comparison of macaque and human. *Vision Res.* 25, 83–98

Sobotka, S., Pizlo, Z., Budohoska, W. (1984). Hemispheric differences in evoked potentials to pictures of faces in the left and right visual fields. *EEG Clin. Neurophysiol.* 59, 441–453

Solbrig, K.A.V. (1864). Bemerkung zu J. Jessens Vortrag 'Über doppeltes Bewusstsein'. *Allg. Z. Psychiat.* 22, 412

Sollier, P. (1901). Perte de la vision spéculaire. *Ann. Méd.-Psychol.* 1901, 87

Sollier, P. (1902). Les hallucinations autoscopiques. *Bull. de l'institut psychol.* 1902, 39–55

Sollier, P. (1903). *Les phénomènes d'autoscopie.* Alcan, Paris

Sollier, P. (1908). Quelques cas d'autoscopie. *J. de psychologie normale et pathologique* 5, 160–165

Solomon, A.P. (1932). Acalculia, other agnosias and multiple neuritis following carbon monoxide poiseming. *Med. Clin. North Am.* 16, 531–538

Solomon, R.L., Postman, L. (1952). Frequency of usage as a determinant of recognition thresholds for words. *J. Exp. Psychol.* 43, 195–201

Solomon, S., Hotchkiss, E., Saravay, S.M., Bayer, C., Ramsey, P., Blum, R.S. (1983). Impairment of memory function by antihypertensive medication. *Arch. Gen. Psychiat.* 40, 1109–1112

Souques, A. (1907). Un cas d'alexie ou cécité verbale dite pure suivie d'autopsie. *Bull. Soc. méd. des Hop.* 24, 213–218

Soury, J. (1895/96). The occipital lobe and mental vision. *Revue Philosophique,* Paris, Jan., Febr., Dec. 1895, Febr., March 1896. Review in *Brain* 19, 432–458 (1896)

Spalding, J.M.K. (1952a). Wounds of the visual pathway. Part I: The visual radiation. *J. Neurol. Neurosurg. Psychiat.* 15, 99–109

Spalding, J.M.K. (1952b). Wounds of the visual pathway. Part II: The striate cortex. *J. Neurol.Neurosurg. Psychiat.* 15, 169–183

Sparks, D.L., Mays, L.E. (1983). Role of monkey superior colliculus in the spatial localization of saccade targets. In Hein, A., Jeannerod, M. (eds.), *Spatially oriented behavior.* Springer, New York, Berlin, Heidelberg, Tokyo, 63–85

Sparks, R., Geschwind, N. (1968). Dichotic listening in man after section of the neocortical commissures. *Cortex* 4, 3–16

Sparr, S.A., Milton, J., Drislane, F.W., Nagagopal, V. (1991). A historic case of visual agnosia revisited after 4O Years. *Brain* 114,

789–800

Spatz, W.B. (1977). Topographically organized reciprocal connections between areas 17 and MT (visual area of superior sulcus) in the marmoset Callithrix jacchus. *Exp. Brain Res.* 27, 559–572

Spatz, W.B., Tigges, J. (1972). Experimental-anatomical studies on the 'middle temporal visual area (MT)' in primates. *J. Comp. Neurol.* 146, 451–464

Spatz, W.B., Tigges, J., Tigges, M. (1970). Subcortical projections, cortical associations and some intrinsic intralaminar connections of the striate cortex in the squirrel monkey (*Saimiri*). *J. Comp. Neurol.* 140, 155–174

Spehlmann, R. Gross, R.A., Ho, S.U. et al. (1977). Visual evoked potentials and postmortem findings in a case of cortical blindness. *Ann. Neurol.* 2, 531–534

Spehlmann, R., Gross, R.A., Ho, S.U., Leestma, J.E., Norcross. K.A. (1977). Visual evoked responses and postmortem findings in a case of cortical blindess. *Trans. Am. Neurol. Assoc.* 102, 157–159

Sperry, R.W. (1950). Neural basis of the spontaneous optokinetic response produced by visual inversion. *J. comp. Physiol. Psychol.* 43, 482–489

Sperry, R.W. (1980). Mind-brain interaction: Mentalism, yes; Dualism, no. *Neurosci.* 5, 195–206

Sperry, R.W., Gazzaniga, M.S. (1967). Language following surgical disconnection of the hemispheres. In Millikan, C.H., Darley, F.L. (eds.), *Brain mechanisms underlying speech and language.* Grune and Stratton, New York

Sperry, R.W., Gazzaniga, M.S., Bogen, J.E. (1969). Interhemispheric relationships: The neocortical commissures; syndromes of hemisphere disconnection. In Vinken, P.J., Bruyn, G.W. (eds.), *Handbook of clinical neurology,* Vol. 4. North Holland, Amsterdam, 273–290

Sperry, R.W., Zaidel, E., Zaidel, D. (1979). Self recognition and social awareness in the disconnected minor hemisphere. *Neuropsychologia* 17, 153–166

Spinelli, D.N., Pribram, K.H. (1966). Changes in visual recovery functions produced by temporal lobe stimulation. *EEG Clin. Neurophysiol.* 20, 44–49

Spitz, R.A., (1969). *Vom Säugling zum Kleinkind.* 2nd ed. Klett, Stuttgart

Spitz, R.A., Wolf, K.M. (1946). The smiling response: a contribution to the ontogenesis of social relations. *Genet. Psychol. Mongr.* 34, 57–125

Spitzer, H., Desimone, R., Moran, J. (1988). Increased attention enhances both behavioral and neuronal performance. *Science* 240, 338–340

Spitzer, M. (1988). *Halluzinationen.* Springer, Heidelberg, Berlin

Spoerri, E., Glaesemer, J. (eds.) (1976). *Adolph Wölfli. Catalogue of an exhibition.* 2nd ed. Basler Druck-und Verlagsanstalt, Basel

Sprague, J.M. (1966). Interaction of cortex and superior colliculus in mediation of visually guided behavior in the cat. *Science* 153, 1544–1547

Sprague, J.M., Chambers, W.W., Stellar, E. (1961). Attentive affective and adaptive behavior in the cat. *Science* 133, 165–173

Sprague, J.M., Levy, J.D., Berlucchi, C. (1977). Visual cortical areas mediating from discrimination in the cat. *J. Comp. Neurol.* 172, 441–488

Sprague, J.M., Meikle, T.H. (1965). The role of the superior colliculus in visually guided behavior. *Exp. Neurol.* 11, 115–146

Spreen, O., Benton, A.L., Van Allen, M.W. (1966). Dissociation of visual and tactile naming in amnesic aphasia. *Neurology* 16, 807–814

Springer, S.P., Deutsch, G. (1981/1989). *Left brain, right brain.* Freeman, San Francisco

Squire, L.R. (1987). *Memory and Brain.* Oxford University Press, New York

Srebro, R. (1985a). Localization of visually evoked cortical activity in humans. *J. Physiol. (Lond.)* 360, 233–246

Srebro, R. (1985b). Localization of cortical activity associated with visual recognition in humans. *J. Physiol. (Lond.)* 360, 247–259

Sroka, H., Solsi, P., Bornstein, B. (1973). Alexia without agraphia with complete recovery. *Confin. Neurol.* 35, 167–176

St. John, R.C. (1981). Lateral asymmetry in face perception. *Can.J. Psychol.* 35, 213–223

Stachowiak, F.J., Poeck, K. (1976). Functional disconnection in pure alexia and color naming deficit demonstrated by deblocking methods. *Brain and Language* 3, 135–143

Staller, J., Buchanan, D., Singer, M., Lappin, J., Webb, W. (1978). Alexia without agraphia: an experimental case study. *Brain Lang.* 5, 378–387

Stamm, J.S., Pribram, K.H. (1961). Effects of epileptogenic lesions of inferotemporal cortex on learning and retention in monkeys. *J. Comp. Physiol. Psychol.* 54, 614–618

Standage, G.P., Benevento, L.A. (1983). The organization of connections between the pulvinar and visual area MT in the macaque monkey. *Brain Res.* 262, 288–294

Stanton, G.B., Cruce, W.L.R., Goldberg, M.E., Robinson, D.L. (1977). Some ipsilateral projections to areas PF and PG of the inferior parietal lobule in monkeys. *Neurosci. Lett.* 6, 243–250

Stark, L., Bridgeman, B. (1983). Role of corollary discharge in space constancy. *Percept. Psychophys.* 34, 371–380

Staudenmaier, L. (1912). *Die Magie als experimentelle Naturwissenschaft.* Leipzig

Staufenberg, W. von (1914). Über Seelenblindheit (opt. Agnosie). Nebst Bemerkungen zur Anatomie der Sehstrahlung. In Monokow, C.V. (ed.), *Arbeiten aus dem hirnanatomischen Institut in Zürich.* Vol. 8. Bergmann, Wiesbaden, 1–212

Staufenberg, W. von (1918). Klinische und anatomische Beiträge zur Kenntnis der aphasischen, agnostischen und apraktischen Symptome. *Z. ges. Neurol. Psychiat.* 39, 71–212

Steffan, Ph. (1881). Beitrag zur Pathologie des Farbensinnes. *Graefes Arch. Ophthalmol.* 27, 1–24

Stein, D.G., Rosen, J.J., Butters, N. (eds.) (1974). *Plasticity and recovery of function in the central nervous system.* Academic Press, New York, S. Francisco, London

Stein, J. (1928). Pathologie der Wahrnehmung. In Bumke, O. (ed.), *Handbuch für Geisteskrankheiten I.* Springer-Verlag, Berlin

Stein, J.F. (1978). The effect of parietal lobe cooling on manipulative behaviour in the conscious monkey. In Gordon, G. (ed.), *Active Touch — The Mechanism of Recognition of Objects by Manipulation. A Multidisciplinary Approach.* Pergamon, Oxford, UK, 79–90

Stein, J.F. (1989). Representation of egocentric space in the posterior parietal cortex. *Quart. J. Exp. Physiol.* 74, 583–606

Stein, S., Volpe, B.T. (1983). Classical 'parietal' neglect syndrome after subcortical right frontal lobe infarction. *Neurology* 33, 797–799

Steinbach, M.J. (1967). Pursuing the perceptual rather than the retinal stimulus. *Vision Res.* 16, 1371–1376

Steinbach, M.J., Smith, D.R. (1981). Spatial localization after strabismus surgery: Evidence for inflow. *Science, N.Y.* 213, 1407–1409

Steinbuch, J.G. (1811). *Beytrag zur Physiologie der Sinne.* Schrag, Nürnberg

Steinitz, K. (1958). *Leonardo da Vinci's trattato della pittura. A bibliography 1651–1956.* Kopenhagen

Steklis, H.D., Raleigh, N.J. (eds.) (1979). *Neurobiology of Social Communication in Primates,* Academic Press, New York, London

Stender, S. (1987). Gedanken zur Nutzung des Tempo-und Merkfähigkeitstest (TME) von Roether in der Alkoholikerbetreuung. *Psychiatr. Neurol. Med. Psychol. (Leipz.)* 39, 744–747

Stengel, E. (1948). The syndrome of visual alexia with colour agnosia. *J. Mental Sciences* 94, 46–58

Stenon, N. (1910). *Opera philosophica.* Maar, V. (ed.), Vol. 1: *Life and work of Nicolaus Steno.* Vol. 2: *Discours sur l'anatomie du cerveau.* Munsgaard, Kopenhagen

Stensaas, S.S., Eddington, E.E.., Dobelle, W.H. (1974). The top-

ography and variability of the primary visual cortex in man. *J. Neurosurg.* 40, 747–755

Sterling, T.D. (1971). *Visual prosthesis: the interdisciplinary dialogue.* Academic Press, New York

Stern, B., Stern, J.M. (1985). The Rey-Osterieth complex as a diagnostic measure of neuropsychological outcome of brain injury. *Scand. J. Rehab. Med. Suppl.* 12, 31–35

Stern, K., McNaughton, D. (1945). Capgras-syndrome. *Psychiatric Quarterly* 19, 139–163

Sternberg, S. (1967). Two operations in character recognition: Some evidence from reaction-time measurements. *Perception and Psychophysics* 2, 45–53

Stevens, K.A. (1983). Evidence relating subjective contours and interpretations involving interposition. *Perception* 12, 491–500

Stiles, W.S. (1978). *Mechanisms of colour vision.* Academic Press, London, New York, San Francisco, 298 p.

Stockert, F.G. von (1934). Das Gerstmann'sche Syndrom der Fingeragnosie mit besonderer Berücksichtigung der Sprach-und Schreibstörungen. *Monatsschrift für Psychiatrie* 88, 121-???

Stoerig, P. (1987). Chromaticity and achromaticity. *Brain* 110, 869–886

Stoerig, P., Cowey, A. (1989). Residual target detection as a function of stimulus size. *Brain* 112, 1123–1139

Stoerig, P., Cowey, A. (1989). Wavelength sensitivity in blindsight. *Nature* 342, 916–918

Stoerig, P., Hübner, M., Pöppel, E. (1985). Signal detection analysis of residual vision in a field defect due to a post-geniculate lesion. *Neuropsychologia* 23, 589–599

Stoerig, P., Pöppel, E. (1986). Eccentricity-dependent residual target detection in visual field defects. *Exp. Brain Res.* 64, 469–475

Stoffregen, T.A., Riccio, G.E. (1988). An ecological theory of orientation and the vestibular system. *Psychol. Rev.* 95, 3–14

Stollreiter-Butzon, L. (1950). Zur Frage der Prosop-Agnosie. *Arch. Psychiat. Z. Neurol.* 184, 1–27

Stone, J. (1983). *Parallel processing in the visual system.* Plenum, NY

Stoper, A.E. (1967). *Vision during pursuit movement: The role of oculomotor information.* Ph.D. Thesis. Brandeis University

Stoper, A.E. (1973). Apparent motion of stimuli presented stroboscopically during pursuit movement of the eye. *Percept. Psychophys.* 13, 201–211

Storch, E. (1903). Zwei Fälle von reiner Alexie. *Monatsschr. Psychiat. Neurol.* 13, 499–531

Straschill, M., Hoffmann, K.P. (1969). Response characteristics of movement-detecting neurons in pretectal region of the cat. *Exp. Neurol.* 25, 165–176

Straschill, M., Schick, F. (1974). Neuronal activity during eye movements in a visual association area of cat cerebral cortex. *Exp. Brain Res.* 19, 467–477

Stratton, G. (1896). Some preliminary experiments on vision without inversion of the retinal image. *Psychol. Rev.* 3, 611–617

Stratton, G. (1897a). Upright vision and the retinal image. *Psychol. Rev.* 4, 182–187

Stratton, G. (1897b). Vision without inversion of the retinal image. *Psychol. Rev.* 4, 341–360, 463–481

Stratton, G.M. (1917). *Theophrastus and the Greek physiological Psychology before Aristotle.* Allen and Unwin, London, Reprint: Bonset, Amsterdam 1964

Strauss, E., Kaplan, E. (1980). Lateralized asymmetries in self-perception. *Cortex* 16, 289–293

Strauss, E., Moscovitch, M. (1981). Perception of facial expressions. *Brain and Language* 13, 308–332

Strauss, E., Wada, J., Kosaka, B. (1983). Spontaneous facial expressions occurring on the onset of focal seizure activity. *Arch. Neurol.* 40, 545–547

Strauss, H. (1924). Über konstruktive Apraxie. *Monatsschr. Psychiat. Neurol.* 56, 65–124

Street, R.F. (1931). *A Gestalt completion test.* Teachers College, Columbia University, New York

Streitfeld, B., Wilson, M. (1986). The ABC's of categorical perception. *Cognitive Psychol.* 18, 432–451

Striano, S., Grossi, D., Chiacchio, and Fels, A. (1981). Bilateral lesion of the occipital lobes. *Acta Neurologica (Napoli)* 26, 690–694

Studdert-Kennedy, M. (1983). On learning to speak. *Human Neurobiol.* 2, 191–195

Sturm, W., Reul, J., Willmes, K. (1989). Is there a generalized right hemisphere dominance for mediating cerebral activation? Evidence from a choice reaction experiment with lateralizedsimple warning stimuli. *Neuropsychologia* 27, 747–751

Stuss, D.T., Benson, D.F. (1983). Frontal lobe lesions and behavior. In Kertesz, A. (ed.), *Localization in neuropsychology.* Academic Press, New York, 429–454

Suberi, M., Mc Keever, W.F. (1977). Differential right hemispheric memory storage of emotional and non-emotional faces. *Neuropsychologia* 15, 757–768

Sugishita, M., Ettlinger, G., Ridley, R.M. (1979). Disturbance of cage-finding in the monkey. *Cortex* 14, 431–438

Sugishita, M., Iwata, M., Toyokura, Y., Yoshioka, M., Yamada, R. (1978). Reading of ideograms and phonograms in Japanese patients after partial commissurotomy. *Neuropsychologia* 16, 417–426

Sugishita, M., Iwata, M., Yamada, R., Yoshioka, M., Toyokura, Y. (1973). Disconnection syndrome in patients with partially split brain. Excerpta Medica. Intern. Congress Series 293, 65

Sugishita, M., Yoshioka, M., Kawamura, M. (1986). Recovery from hemialexia. *Brain Lang.* 29, 106–118

Sutter, A., Beck, J., Graham, N. (1989). Contrast and spatial variables in texture segregation: testing a simple spatial-frequency channels model. *Percept. & Psychophys.* 46, 312–332

Suzuki, D.A., Keller, E.L. (1984). Visual signals in the dorsolateral pontine nucleus of the alert monkey: their relationship to smooth-pursuit eye movements. *Exp. Brain Res.* 53, 473–478

Suzuki, D.A., May, J., Keller, E.L. (1984). Smooth pursuit eye movement deficits with pharmacological lesions in monkey dorsolateral pontine nucleus. *Soc. Neurosci. Abstr.* 10, 58

Swammerdam, J. (1737/1738). *Biblia naturae.* 2 vols. Boerhaave, H. (ed.). Severinus, Amsterdam

Swanson, H.L. (1984). Semantic and visual memory codes in learning disabled readers. *J. Exp. Child Psychol.* 37, 124–140

Swanzy, H.R. (1883). Case of hemiachromatopsia. *Trans. Ophthalmol. Soc. United Kingdom* 3, 185–189

Swash, M. (1979). Visual perseveration in temporal lobe epilepsy. *J. Neurol. Neurosurg. Psychiat.* 42, 569–571

Swerdloff, M.A., Zieker, A.B., Krohel, G.B. (1981). Movement phosphenes in optic neuritis. *J. Clin. Neuro-Ophthalmol.* 1, 279–282

Symonds, C., Mackenzie, L. (1957). Bilateral loss of vision from cerebral infarction. *Brain* 80, 415–455

Synolds, D.L., Pronko, N.H. (1949). An exploratory study of color perception of children. *J. Gen. Psychol.* 74, 17–21

Szatmari, A. (1938). Ueber optische Sinnestäuschungen als epileptisches Aequivalent bei traumatischer Schädigung des Hinterhauptlappens. *Arch. f. Psychiat. Nervenkh.* 107, 290–299

Szentagothai, J. (1973). Neuronal and synaptic architecture of the lateral geniculate nucleus. In *Handbook of Sensory Physiology,* Vol.VII, Springer, Berlin, 141–176

Szentagothai, J. (1985). Functional anatomy of the visual centers as cues for pattern recognition concepts. In Chagas, D., Gattas, R., Gross, C., (eds.), *Pattern recognition mechanisms* Springer-Verlag, Berlin, 39–52

Szentagothai, J., Hamori, J., Tömböl, T. (1966). Degeneration and electron microscope analysis of the synaptic glomeruli in lateral geniculate body. *Exp. Brain Res.* 2, 283–301

Takahashi, N., Kawamura, M., Hirayama, K., Tagawa, K. (1989). Non-verbal facial and topographic visual object agnosia — a problem of familiarity in prosopagnosia and topographic disorientation. *No-To-Shinkei* 41, 703–710

Takahashi, R., Mori, H., Yoshino, T. (1956). Charges in electrical excitability of the human eye for sinusoidal alternating currents, caused by illumination with white and monochromic lights. *Nichiganshi (Jap.)* 60, 727–734

Talalla, A., Bullara, L., Pudenz, R. (1974). Electrical stimulation of the human visual cortex: preliminary report. *Can. J. Neurol. Sci.* 1, 236–238

Talbot, S.A., Marshall, W.H. (1941). Physiological studies of neuronal mechanisms of visual localization and discrimination. *Amer. J. Ophthalmol.* 24, 1255–1263

Tanaka, K., Fukada, Y., Saito, H.A. (1989). Underlying mechanisms of the response specificity of expansion-contraction and rotation cells in the dorsal part of the medial superior temporal area of the macaque monkey. *J. Neurophysiol.* 62, 642–656

Tanaka, K., Hikosaka, K., Saito, H., Yukie, M., Fukada, Y., Iwai, E. (1986). Analysis of local and wide-field movements in the superior temporal visual areas of the macaque monkey. *J. Neurosci.* 6, 134–144

Tanaka, K., Saito, H.A. (1989). Analysis of motion of the visual field by direction, expansion-contraction, and rotation cells clustered in the dorsal part of the medial superior temporal area of the macaque monkey. *J. Neurophysiol.* 62, 626–641

Tanaka, M., Lee, B.B., Creutzfeldt, O.D. (1983). Spectral tuning and contour representation in area 17 of the awake monkey. In Mollon, J.D., Sharpe, L.T. (eds.), *Colour vision: physiology and psychophysics.* Academic Press, London, 269–276

Tanaka, M., Lindsley, E., Lausmann, S., Creutzfeldt, O.D. (1990). Afferent connections of the prelunate visual association cortex (areas V4 and DP). *Anat. Embryol.* 181, 19–30

Tanaka, M., Weber, H., Creutzfeldt, O.D. (1986). Visual properties and spatial distribution of neurones in the visual association area on the prelunate gyrus of the awake monkey. *Exp. Brain Res.* 63, 11–37

Tapley, S.M., Bryden, M.P. (1983). Handwriting position and hemispheric asymmetry in right-handers. *Neuropsychologia* 21, 129–138

Tasker, R.R., Organ, L.W., Hwrylyshyn, P. (1980). Visual phenomena evoked by electrical stimulation of the human brainstem. *Appl. Neurophysiol.* 43, 89–95

Taylor, A., Warrington, E.K. (1971). Visual agnosia: A single case report. *Cortex* 7, 152–161

Taylor, A., Warrington, E.K. (1973). Visual discrimination in patients with localized cerebral lesions. *Cortex* 9, 82–93

Taylor, E.A. (1966). The fundamental reading skill. As related to eye movement photography and visual anomalies. Springfield, Illinois

Taylor, J. (1727). *An account of the mechanism of the eye.* Norwich

Taylor, J. (1738). *Le mechanisme ou le nouveau traite de l'anatomie du globe de l'oeil avec l'usage de see differentes partis, et de celles qui lui sont contigues.* Paris 1738

Taylor, J. (1743). *An impartial enquiry into the seat of the immediate organ of sight.* London

Taylor, J. (1750). *Mechanismus oder Neue Abhandlung von der künstlichen Zusammensetzung des Menschlichen Auges.* Stoks Erben and Schilling, Frankfurt a.M.

Taylor, M.A., Abrams, R. (1984). Cognitive impairment in schizophrenia. *Am. J. Psychiatry* 141, 196–201

Tegner, R. (1990). Through the looking glass. *J. Clin. Exp. Neuropsych. (Abstract)* 12, 408

Tegner, R., Levander, M., Caneman, G. (1990). Apparent right neglect in patients with left visual neglect. *Cortex* 26, 455–458

Teller, D.Y., Regal, D.M., Videen, T.O., Pulos, E. (1978). Development of visual acuity in infant monkeys (Macaca nemestrina) during the early postnatal weeks. *Vision Res.* 18, 561–566

Tello, F. (1907). La regeneration dans les voies optiques. *Trav. Lab.*

Rech. Biol. Univ. Madr. 5, 237–248

Temple, C.M. (1987). *The alexias.* In Beech, J.R., Colley, A.M. (eds.), *Cognitive approaches to reading.* Chapter 11, John Wiley & Sons, New York, 271–295

Tenenbaum, J.M., Barrow, H.G. (1976). Experiments in interpretation-guided segmentation. *Stanford Research Institute Technical Note* 123

Terrace, H.S. (1959). The effect of retinal locus and attention on the perception of words. *J. Exp. Psychol.* 58, 382–389

Terraces, H.S., Petitto, L.A., Sanders, R.J., Bever, T.G. (1979). Can an ape create a sentence? *Science* 206, 891–900

Tetens, J.N. (1796). *Über den Ursprung der Sprache und der Schrift.* Reprint 1966: Akademie-Verlag, Berlin

Teuber, H.L. (1960). *Perception.* Chapter 65. In Field, J., Magoun, H.W., Hall, U.E. (eds.), *Handbook of Physiology Section I.* Am. Physiol. Society, Washington, 1593–1668

Teuber, H.L. (1962). Effects of brain wounds implicating right or left hemispheres in man. In Mountcastle, V.B. (ed.), *Interhemispheric relations and cerebral dominance.* John Hopkins Press, Baltimore, 131–157

Teuber, H.L. (1963). Space perception and its disturbances after brain injury in man. *Neuropsychologia* 1, 47–57

Teuber, H.L. (1965). Postscript: Some needed revisions of the classical views of agnosia. I. Tactile thresholds and shape discrimination. *Neuropsychologia* 3, 371–378

Teuber, H.L. (1965). Somatosensory disorders due to cortical lesions. Preface: disorders of higher tactile and visual functions. Postscript: some needed revisions of the classical views of agnosia. *Neuropsychologia* 3, 287–294

Teuber, H.L. (1968). Alteration of perception and memory in man. In L. Weiskrantz (ed.), *Analysis of behavioral change.* Harper and Row, New York

Teuber, H.L., Battersby, W.S., Bender, M.B. (1949). Changes in visual searching performance following cerebral lesions. *Amer. J. Physiol.* 159, 592

Teuber, H.L., Battersby, W.S., Bender, M.B. (1951). Performance of complex visual tasks after cerebral lesions. *J. Nerv. ment. Dis.* 114, 413–429

Teuber, H.L., Battersby, W.S., Bender, M.B. (1960). *Visual field defects after penetrating missile wounds of the brain.* Harvard Univ. Press, Cambridge

Teuber, H.L., Weinstein, S. (1956). Ability to discover hidden figures after cerebral lesions. *Arch. Neurol. Psychiat.* 76, 369–379

Thase, M.E., Liss, L., Smeltzer, D., Maloon, J. (1982). Clinical evaluation of dementia in Down's syndrome: a preliminary report. *J. Ment. Defic. Res.* 26, 239–244

Thase, M.E., Tigner, R., Smeltzer, D.J., Liss, L. (1984). Age-related neuropsychological deficits in Down's syndrome. *Biol. Psychiatry* 19, 571–585

Theios, J., Amrhein, P.C. (1989). Theoretical analysis of the cognitive processing of lexical and pictorial stimuli: Reading, naming, and visual and conceptual comparisons. *Psychol. Rev.* 96, 5–24

Theophrastus of Eresos (1917). *On the senses.* Translated from the Greek; in Stratton, G.M. (ed.), *Theophrastus and the Greek physiological psychology before Aristotle.* Reprint Bonset, E.J., Amsterdam 1964

Thomas, H., Molfese, V.J. (1977). Infants and I scales: Inferring change from the ordinal stimulus selections of infant for configural stimuli. *J. Exp. Child Psychol.* 23, 329–339

Thomas, J.L. (1985). Visual memory: adult age differences in map recall and learning strategies. *Exp. Aging Res.* 11, 93–97

Thompson, C. (1982). Anwesenheit: Psychopathology and clinical associations. *Br. J. Psychiat.* 141, 628–630

Thompson, J.K. (1983). Visual field, exposure duration, and sex as factors in the perception of emotional facial expressions. *Cortex* 19, 293–308

Thorndike, E.L., Lorge, I. (1944). *The teachers' work book of 30.000 words.* Columbia University, New York Teachers College, Columbia University

Thornton, M., Pilowsky, I. (1982). Facial expression can be modelled mathematically. *Brit. J. Psychiat.* 140, 61–63

Tiberghien, G., Clerc, I. (1986). The cognitive locus of prosopagnosia. In R. Bruyer (ed.), *The neuropsychology of face perception and facial expression.* Laurence Erlbaum, Hillsdale

Tigges, J., Spatz, W.B., Tigges, M. (1973a). Reciprocal point-to-point connections between parastriate and striate cortex in the squirrel monkey (*Saimiri*). *J. Comp. Neurol.* 148, 481–490

Tigges, J., Tigges, M., Perrachio, A.A. (1977). Complementary laminar terminations of afferents to area 17 originating in area 18 and in the lateral geniculate nucleus in squirrel monkey (*Saimiri*). *J. Comp. Neurol.* 176, 87–100

Tilgner, R.D. (1978). Einfluss von Rotation auf die Erkennung von Buchstaben. In Schüle, W. (ed.), *Wahrnehmungspsychologie, aktuelle experimentelle Beiträge.* Fachbuchhandlung für Psychologie, Frankfurt, 92–105

Tilgner, R.D., Hauske, G. (1980). Untersuchungen zur Rotationsinvarianz bei der Erkennung von Buchstaben. *Z. exp. angew. Psychol.* 27, 147–462

Tinker, M.A. (1958). Recent studies of eye movements in reading. *Psychol. Bull.* 55, 215–231

Tinker, M.A., Patterson, D.G. (1955). The effect of typographical variations upon eye movements in reading. *J. Educ. Res.* 49, 171–184

Tinker, M.A., Patterson, D.G. (1963). Influence of simultaneous variation in size of type, width of line and leading for newspaper type. *J. Appl. Psychol.* 47, 380–382

Tobias, P.V. (1971). *The brain in hominid evolution.* Columbia University Press, New York

Tobias, P.V. (1979). *The evolution of the human brain, intellect and spirit.* University of Adelaide, Information Office, Adelaide

Tobias, P.V. (ed.) (1985). *Hominid evolution. Past, present and future.* Liss, New York

Todd, J. (1955). The syndrome of Alice in Wonderland. *Canad. Med. Association J.* 73, 701–704

Todd, J. (1962). The significance of the Doppelgänger (hallucinatory double) in folk-lore and neuropsychiatry. *Practitioner* 188, 377–382

Todd, J., Dewhurst, K. (1957). The double — its psychopathology and psychophysiology. *J. Nerv. Ment. Dis.* 122, 47–54

Todd, J.T. (1982). Visual information about rigid and nonrigid motion: a geometric analysis. *J. Exp. Psychol.* 8, 238–252

Todd, J.T. (1984). The perception of three-dimensional structure from rigid and nonrigid motion. *Percept. Psychophys.* 36, 97–103

Todd, J.T., Akerstrom, R.A. (1987). Perception of three-dimensional form from patterns of optical texture. *J. Exp. Psychol.: Human Perc. Perf.* 13, 242–255

Todd, J.T., Reichel, F.D. (1989). Ordinal structure in the visual perception and cognition of smoothly curved surfaces. *Psychol. Review* 96, 643–657

Todd, J.T., Reichel, F.D. (1990). Visual perception of smoothly curved surfaces from double-projected contour patterns. *J. Exp. Psychol.* 16, 665–674

Tomkins, S.S. (1962). *Affect, imagery and consciousness.* Vol. 1 *The positive affects.* Vol. 2. *The negative affects.* Tavistock-Springer, New York, London

Tomlinson-Keasey, C. (1979). A task analysis of hemispheric functioning. *Neuropsychologia* 17, 345–351

Tomlinson-Keasey, C., Brewer, A., Huffman, K. (1983). The importance of being first: an analysis of tachistoscopic presentations of words. *Cortex* 19, 309–325

Tonkonogy, J. (1988). Microsaccades and vision. *Neurology* 38, 664–665

Tootell, R.B.H., Hamilton, S.L. (1989). Functional anatomy of the second visual area (V2) in the macaque. *J. Neurosci.* 9, 2620–2644

Tootell, R.B.H., Hamilton, S.L., Silverman, M.S. (1985). Topography of cytochrome oxidase activity in owl monkey cortex. *J. Neurosci.* 5, 2786–2800

Tootell, R.B.H., Hamilton, S.L., Silverman, M.S., Switkes, E. (1988). Functional anatomy of macaque striate cortex. I. Ocular dominance, binocular interactions, and baseline conditions. *J. Neurosci.* 8, 1500–1530

Tootell, R.B.H., Hamilton, S.L., Switkes, E. (1988). Functional anatomy of macaque striate cortex. IV. Contrast and magno-parvo streams. *J. Neurosci.* 8, 1594–1609

Tootell, R.B.H., Silverman, M.S., DeValois, R.L. (1981). Spatial frequency columns in primary visual cortex. *Science* 214, 813–815

Tootell, R.B.H., Silverman, M.S., DeValois, R.L., Jacobs, G.H. (1983). Functional organization of the second cortical visual area in primates. *Science* 220, 737–739

Tootell, R.B.H., Silverman, M.S., Hamilton, S.L., DeValois, R.L., Switkes, E. (1988). Functional anatomy of macaque striate cortex. III. Color. *J. Neurosci.* 8, 1569–1593

Tootell, R.B.H., Switkes, E., Silverman, M.S., Hamilton, S.L. (1988). Functional anatomy of macaque striate cortex. II. Retinotopic organization. *J. Neurosci.* 8, 1531–1568

Torii, H., Enokida, H. (1979). Alexia without agraphia: Its seminological features in Japanese language (in Jap.). *Shinkei Naika* 10, 413–419

Torjussen, T. (1978). Visual processing in cortically blind hemifields. *Neuropsychologia* 16, 15–21

Torre, M. della (1776). *Nuove osservazioni microscopiche.* Napoli

Touche, R. (1900). Cécité cérébrale. — Perte du sens topographique autopsié. *Ann. d'Occulist.* 124, 212–220

Towle, V.L., Brigell, M., Spire, J.P. (1989). Hemi-field pattern visual evoked potentials: a comparison of display and analysis techniques. *Brain Topogr.* 1 (4), 263–270

Tranel, D., Damasio, A.R. (1985). Knowledge without awareness: an autonomic index of facial recognition by prosopagnosics. *Science* 228, 1453–1454

Tranel, D., Damasio, A.R. (1988). Non-conscious face recognition in patients with face agnosia. *Behav. Brain Res.* 30, 235–249

Tranel, D., Damasio, A.R., Damasio H. (1988). Intact recognition of facial expression, gender, and age in patients with impaired recognition of face identity. *Neurology* 38, 690–696

Traquair, H.M. (1927). *An introduction to clinical perimetry.* Mosby, St. Louis

Travis, D., Thompson, P. (1989). Spatio-temporal contrast sensitivity and colour vision in multiple sclerosis. *Brain* 112, 283–301

Treisman, A. (1982). Perceptual grouping and attention in visual search for features and for objects. *J. exp. Psych.: Human perception and performance* 8, 194–214

Treisman, A., Souther, J. (1985). Search asymmetry: a diagnostic for preattentive processing of separable features. *J. exp. Psych.: General* 114, 285–310

Treisman, A.M. (1969). Strategies and models of selective attention. *Psychol. Rev.* 76, 282–299

Treisman, A.M., Gelade, G. (1980). A feature-integration theory of attention. *Cognitive Psychol.* 12, 97–136

Treisman, A.M., Riley, J.G.A. (1969). Is selective attention selective perception or selective response? A further test. *J. Exp. Psych.* 79, 27–34

Treisman, A.M., Schmidt, H. (1982). Illusionary conjunctions in the perception of objects. *Cognitive Psychol.* 14, 107–141

Treitel, T. (1879). Ueber den Werth der Gesichtsfeldmessung mit Pigmenten für die Auffassung der Krankheiten des nervösen Sehapparates. *Graefes Arch. Ophthalmol.* 25, Abt. II, 29–51, Abt. III, 47–110

Trelles, J.O., Boggiano, L., Donayre, J. (1962). Sobre un caso de heautoscopia. *Revista de Neuro-Psiquiatria* 25, 265–280

Trendelenburg, W. (1961). *Der Gesichtssinn.* Springer, Berlin, Göttingen, Heidelberg

Trescher, J.H., Ford, F.R. (1937). Colloid cyst of the third ventricle. *Arch. Neurol. Psychiat.* 37, 959–973

Trevarthen, C. (1968). Two mechanisms of vision in priamtes. *Psychologische Forschung.* 31, 299–337

Trevarthen, C. (1970). Experimental evidence for a brain-stem contribution to visual perception in man. *Brain, Behaviour and Evolution* 3, 338–352

Trevarthen, C. (1985). Facial expressions of emotion in mother-infant interaction. *Human Neurobiol.* 4, 21–32

Trevarthen, C.B., Kinsbourne, M. (1972). *Perceptual completion of words and figures by commissurotomy patients.* Cited in Levy, Trevarthen and Sperry (1972)

Trobe, J.D., Lorber, M.L., Schletzinger, N.S. (1973). Isolated homonymous hemianopsia. A review of 104 cases. *Arch. Ophthalm.* 89, 377–381

Trobe, J.R., Bauer, R.M. (1986). Seeing but not recognizing. *Surv.Ophthalmol.* 30, 328–36

Trojanowski, J.Q., Jacobson, S. (1974). Medial pulvinar afferents to frontal eye fields in rhesus monkey demonstrated by horseradish peroxidase. *Brain Res.* 80, 395–411

Trojanowski, J.Q., Jacobson, S. (1975). Peroxidase labeled subcortical afferents to pulvinar in rhesus monkey. *Brain Res.* 97, 144–150

Trojanowski, J.Q., Jacobson, S. (1976). Areal and laminar distribution of some pulvinar cortical efferents in rhesus monkey. *J. Comp. Neurol.* 169, 371–392

Troxler, D. (1804). Über das Verschwinden gegebener Gegenstände innerhalb unseres Gesichtskreises. In Himly, K., Schmidt, J.A. (eds.), *Ophthalmische Bibliothek* Vol. 2, Fromann, Jena, 51–53

Tsao, Y.C., Feustel, T., Soseos, C. (1979). Stroop interference in the left and right visual fields. *Brain and Language* 8, 367–371

Tschermak, A. von (1930). *Optischer Raumsinn und Augenbewegungen.* In Bethe, H., Bergmann, G.. von, etc. (eds.), *Handbuch der normalen und pathologischen Physiologie.* Vol 12, 834

Tucker, D.M. (1976). Sex differences in hemispheric specialization for synthetic visuospatial functions. *Neuropsychologia* 14, 447–454

Tucker, G., Harrow, M., Detre, T., Hoffman, B. (1969). Perceptual experiences in schizophrenic and non-schizophrenic patients. *Arch. Gen. Psychiat.* 20, 159–166

Tulving, E. (1983). *Elements of episodic memory.* Clarendon Press, Oxford

Tulving, E., Gold, C. (1963). Stimulus information and contextual information as determinants of tachistoscopic recognition of words. *J.Exp. Psychol.* 66, 319–327

Turgman, J., Goldhammer, Y., Braham, J. (1979). Alexia without agraphia due to brain tumor: A reversible syndrome. *Ann. Neurol.* 6, 265–268

Turkewitz, G., Ross, O. (1983). Changes in visual field advantages for facial recognition: The development of a general processing strategy. *Cortex* 19, 179–185

Tusa, R.J., Ungerleider, L.G. (1987). The inferior longitudinal fasciculus: A reexamination in humans and monkeys. *Ann. Neurol* 18, 583–591

Tyler, Ch. (1978). Some new entoptic phenomena. *Vision Res.* 18, 1633–1639

Tyler, H.R. (1968). Abnormalities of perception with defective eye movements (Balint's syndrome). *Cortex* 4, 154–171

Tyler, H.R. (1969). Defective stimulus explorations in aphasic patients. *Neurology* 19, 105–112

Tymms, R. (1982). The history of the syndrome of Capgras. In Rose, F.C., Bynum, W.F. (eds.), *Historical Aspects of the Neurosciences.* Raven, New York

Tzavaras, A., Hecaen, H., Le Bras, H. (1970). Le problème de la specificité du deficit de la reconnaissance du visage humain lors des lesion hémisphèrique unilaterales. *Neuropsychologia* 8, 403–416

Tzavaras, A., Hécaen, H., Le Bras, H. (1971). Troubles de la reconnaissance du visage humain et lateralisation hemispherique lesionnelle chez les sujets gauchers. *Neuropsychologia* 9, 475–477

Tzavaras, A., Masure, M.C. (1976). Aspects différents de l'ataxie optique selon la latéralisation hémisphérique de la lésion. *Lyon Médical* 236, 673–683

Tzavaras, A., Merienne, L., Masure, M.C. (1973). Prosopagnosie, amnesie et troubles du langage par lesion temporale gauche chez un sujet Gaucher. *L'Encéphale* 62, 382–394

Tzeng, O.J.L., Hung, D.L., Cotton, B., Wang, W.S.Y. (1979). Visual lateralization effect in reading Chinese characters. *Nature* 282, 499–501

Uexküll, J. von (1920). *Theoretische Biologie.* (2nd. ed. 1928) Springer, Berlin

Uhthoff, W. (1899). Beiträge zu den Gesichtstäuschungen (Halluzinationen, Illusionen etc.) bei Erkrankung des Sehorgans. *Mtschr. Psychiat. Neurol.* 4, 241–264

Uhthoff, W. (1915). Beiträge zu den hemianopischen Gesichtsfeldstörungen nach Schädelschüssen, besonders solcher im Bereich des Hinterhauptes. *Monatsbl. Augenheilk.* 55, 104–125

Ullman, S. (1979). *The interpretation of visual motion.* MIT-Press, Cambridge

Ullman, S. (1986). Artificial intelligence and the brain. Computational structure of visual system. *Ann. Rev. Neurosci.* 9, 1–26

Ulrich, G. (1977). Das Syndrom der akustischen Agnosie. Fallbericht und der Versuch einer neuropsychologischen Qualifizierung. *Archiv Psychiat. Nervenkrh.* 224, 221–233

Umilta, C., Bagnara, S., Simion, F. (1978). Laterality effects for simple and complex geometrical figures and nonsense patterns. *Neuropsychologia* 16, 43–49

Umilta, C., Rizzolatti, G., Marzi, C.A., Zamboni, G., Franzini, C. Camarda, R., Berlucchi, G. (1974). Hemispheric differences in the discrimination of line orientation. *Neuropsychologia* 12, 165–174

Ungerleider, L.G. (1985). The corticocortical pathways for object recognition and spatial perception. In Chagas, C., Gattass, R., Gross, C.G. (eds.), *Pattern Recognition Mechanisms.* Vatican City, Pontificia Scientiarum Academia, 21–38

Ungerleider, L.G., Brody, B.A. (1977). Extrapersonal spatial orientation: the role of posterior parietal, anterior frontal, and inferotemporal cortex. *Exp. Neurol.* 56, 265–280

Ungerleider, L.G., Christensen, C.A. (1977). Pulvinar lesions in monkeys produce abnormal eye movements during visual discrimination training. *Brain Res.* 136, 189–196

Ungerleider, L.G., Christensen, C.A. (1979). Pulvinar lesions in monkeys produce abnormal scanning of a complex visual array. *Neuropsychologia* 17, 493–501

Ungerleider, L.G., Desimone, R. (1986a). Projections to the superior temporal sulcus from the central and peripheral representations of V1 and V2. *J. Comp. Neurol.* 248, 147–163

Ungerleider, L.G., Desimone, R. (1986b). Cortical projections of visual area MT in the macaque. *J. Comp. Neurol.* 248, 190–222

Ungerleider, L.G., Desimone, R., Galkin, T.W., Mishkin, M. (1984). Subcortical projections of area MT in the macaque. *J. Comp. Neurol.* 223, 368–386

Ungerleider, L.G., Galkin, T.W., Mishkin, M. (1983). Visuotopic organization of projections from striate cortex to inferior and lateral pulvinar in rhesus monkey. *J. Comp. Neurol.* 217, 137–157

Ungerleider, L.G., Ganz, L., Pribram, K.H. (1977). Size constancy in Rhesus monkeys: Effects of pulvinar, prestriate and inferotemporal lesions. *Exp. Brain Res.* 27, 251–269

Ungerleider, L.G., Gattass, R., Sousa, A.F.B., Mishkin, M. (1983). Projections of area V2 in the macaque. *Soc. Neurosci. Abstr.* 9, 152

Ungerleider, L.G., Mishkin, M. (1979). The striate projection zone in the superior temporal sulcus of Macaca mulatta: location and topographic organization. *J. Comp. Neurol.* 188, 347–366

Ungerleider, L.G., Mishkin, M. (1982). Two cortical visual systems. In Ingle, D.J., Mansfield, R.J.W., Goodale, M.S. (eds.), *The Analysis of Visual Behavior.* MIT Press, Cambridge, Mass., 549–586

Ungerleider, L.G., Pribram, K.H. (1977). Inferotemporal versus combined pulvinar-prestriate lesions in the rhesus monkey: effects on color, object and pattern discrimination. *Neuropsychologia* 15, 481–498

Ungerstedt, U. (1971). Striatal dopamine release after amphetamine or nerve degeneration revealed by rotational behavior. *Acta Physiol. Scand (suppl. 367)* 82, 49–68

Ungerstedt, U. (1974) Brain dopamine neurones and behavior. In Schmidt, F.O., Woren, F.G. (eds.), *The Neuroscience. Vol. 3.* Cambridge Mass, MIT Press, 695–703

Ungerstedt, U. (1981). Stereotaxic mapping of the monoamine pathway in the rat brain. *Acta Physiol. Scand. (suppl. 367)* 82, 1–48

Urban, H. (1937). Zur Physiologie der Occipitalregion des Menschen. *Z. ges. Neurol. Psychiat.* 158, 257–261

Urbantschitsch, F. (1907). *Über subjective optische Anschauungsbilder.* Wien

Vaegan and Taylor, D. (1980). Critical period for deprivation amblyopia in children. *Trans. Ophthalmol. Soc. UK* 99, 432–439

Vaina, L.M. (1988b). Effects of right parietal lobe lesions on visual motion analysis in humans. *J. Opt. Soc. Amer.* (Suppl). 29, 434

Vaina, L.M. (1989). Selective deficits of visual motion interpretation in patients with right occipito-parietal lesions. *Biol. Cyb.* 61, 1–13

Vaina, L.M. (1989). Selective impairment of visual motion interpretation following lesions of the right occipito-parietal area in humans. *Biol. Cyb.* 61, 347–359

Vaina, L.M., Lemay, M., Bienfang, D.C., Choi, A.Y., Nakayama, K. (1990). Intact 'biological motion' and 'structure from motion' perception in a patient with impaired motion mechanisms: a case study. *Visual Neurosci.* 5, 353–369

Vaina, L.M., LeMay, M., Choi, A., Kemper, T., Bienfang, D. (1989). Visual motion analysis with impaired speed perception: psychophysical and anatomical studies in humans. *Soc. Neurosci. Abstr.* 15, 1256

Vaina, L.M., LeMay, M., Naili, S., Amarillio, P., Bienfang, D., Montgomery, C. (1988). Deficits of visual motion analysis after posterior right hemisphere lesions. *Soc. Neurosci. Abstr.* 14, 485

Valberg, A., Lee, B.B., Tigwell, D.A., Creutzfeldt, O.D. (1985). A simultaneous contrast effect of steady remote surrounds on responses of cells in macaque lateral geniculate nucleus. *Exp. Brain Res.* 58, 604–608

Valberg, A., Seim, T., Lee, B.B., Tryti, J. (1986). Reconstruction of equidistant color space from responses of visual neurones of macaques. *J. Opt. Soc. Am. A* 3, 1726–1734

Valenstein, E., Heilman, K.M. (1978). Apraxic agraphia with neglect induced paragraphia. *Arch. Neurol.* 36, 506–508

Valenstein, E., Heilman, K.M. (1981). Unilateral hypokinesia and motor extinction. *Neurology* 31, 445–448

Valenstein, E., Van Den Abell, T., Tankle, R., Heilman, K.M. (1980). Apomorphine-induced turning after recovery from neglect induced by cortical lesions. *Neurology* 30, 358 (abstr.)

Valenstein, E., Van Den Abell, T., Watson, R.T., Heilman, K.M. (1982). Nonsensory neglect from parietotemporal lesions in monkeys. *Neurology* 32, 1198–1201

Valentin, G. (1844). *Lehrbuch der Physiologie des Menschen.* Vieweg, Braunschweig

Valkenburg, C.T. van (1908). Zur Kenntnis der gestörten Tiefenwahrnehmung. *Dtsch. Z.f. Nervenheilk.* 34, 322–337

Vallar, G., Perani, D. (1986). The anatomy of unilateral neglect after right-hemisphere stroke lesions. A clinical/CT-scan correlation study in man. *Neuropsychologia* 24, 609–622

Vallar, G., Perani, D. (1987). The anatomy of spatial neglect in humans. In Jeannerod, M. (ed.), *Neurophysiological and neuropsychological aspects of spatial neglect*. North-Holland, Amsterdam, 235–258

Valverde, F. (1968). Structural changes in the area striata of the mouse after enucleation. *Exp. Brain Res.* 5, 274–292

Valverde, F. (1991). The organization of the striate cortex. In Cronly-Dillon (ed.), *Vision and Visual Dysfunction*. Vol. 4. Chapter 4. Macmillan, London

Valvo, A. (1971). *Sight restoration after long-term blindness*. Am. Found. for the Blind, New York

Van Allen, M.W., Benton, A.L. (1972). Prosopagnosia and facial discrimination. *J. Neurol. Sci.* 15, 167–172

Van Bogaert, L. (1924). Syndrome inferieur du noyau rouge, troubles psycho-sensoriels d'origine mesocephalique. *Rev. Neurol. (Paris)* 40, 417–423

Van Bogaert, L. (1927). L'hallucinose pédoncolaire. *Rev. Neurol.* 43, 608–617

Van Buren, J.M. (1963). *The retinal ganglion cell layer*. Thomas, Springfield, III.

Van Buren, J.M., Baldwin, M. (1958). The architecture of the optic radiation in the temporal lobe of man. *Brain* 81, 15–40

Van Essen, D.C. (1979). Visual areas of the mammalian cerebral cortex. *Ann. Rev. Neurosci.* 2, 227–263

Van Essen, D.C. (1985). Functional organization of primate visual cortex. In Peters, A., Jones, E.C. (eds.), *The cerebral cortex, Vol. 3 Visual Cortex*. Plenum, New York

Van Essen, D.C., Felleman, D.J., De Yoe, E.A., Olavarria, J., Knierim, J. (1991). Cold Spring Harbor Symposion on Quantitative Biology. Vol. 55 (in press, quoted after Douglas and Martin, 1991)

Van Essen, D.C., Maunsell, J.H.R. (1980). Two-dimensional maps of the cerebral cortex. *J. Comp. Neurol.* 191, 255–281

Van Essen, D.C., Maunsell, J.H.R. (1983). Hierarchical organization and functional streams in the visual cortex. *Trends Neurosci.* 6, 370–375

Van Essen, D.C., Maunsell, J.H.R., Bixby, J.L. (1981). The middle temporal visual area in the macaque: myeloarchitecture, connections, functional properties and topographic organization. *J. Comp. Neurol.* 199, 293–326

Van Essen, D.C., Newsome, W.T., Bixby, J.L. (1982). The pattern of interhemispheric connections and its relationship to extrastriate visual areas in macaque monkey. *J. Neurosci.* 2, 265–283

Van Essen, D.C., Newsome, W.T., Maunsell, J.H.R. (1984). The visual representation in striate cortex of macaque monkey: asymmetries, anisotropies and individual variability. *Vision Res.* 24, 429–448

Van Essen, D.C., Newsome, W.T., Maunsell, J.H.R., Bixby, J.L. (1986). The projections from striate cortex (V1) to areas V2 and V3 in the macaque monkey. Asymmetries, areal bounderies, and patchy connections. *J. Comp. Neurol.* 244, 451–480

Van Essen, D.C., Zeki, S.M. (1978). The topographic organization of rhesus monkey prestriate cortex. *J. Physiol. (Lond.)* 277, 193–226

Van Lancker, D.R., Canter, G.J. (1982). Impairment of voice and face recognition in patients with hemispheric damage. Brain Cogn. 1, 185–195

Van Santen, J.P.H., Jonides, J. (1978). A replication of the face-superiority effect. *Bull. Psychonom. Soc.* 12, 378-

Van Wagenen, W.P., Bornstein, B. (1973). Surgical division of commissural pathways in the corpus callosum. *Arch. Neurol. Psychiat.* 44, 740–759

Varin, D. (1971). Fenomeni di contrasto diffusione chromatica dell' organizzazione spaziale dell campo percettivo. *Rev. di Psychol.* 65, 101–128

Varner, D., Jameson, D., Hurvich, L.M. (1984). Temporal sensitivities related to color theory. *J. opt. Soc. Amer. A*, 1, 474–481

Varney, N.R. (1978). Linguistic correlates of pantomime recognition in aphasic patients. *J. Neurol. Neurosurg. Psychiat.* 41, 564–568

Varney, N.R., Digre, K. (1983). Color 'amnesia' without aphasia.

Cortex 19, 545–550

Varnhagen, C.K., Das, J.P., Varnhagen, S. (1987). Auditory and visual memory span: cognitive processing by TMR individuals with Down syndrome or other etiologies. *Am. J. Ment. Defic.* 91, 398–405

Vater, A., Heinicke, J.Ch. (1723). *Dissertatio inauguralis medica qua visus vitia duo rarissima, alterum duplicati, alterum dimidiati, physiologice et pathologice considerata*. Dr. med. dissertation. Univ. of Wittenberg, Vidua Gerdesia, Wittenberg

Vaughan, H.G. (Jr.), Gross, C.G. (1969). Cortical responses to light in unanaesthetized monkeys and their alteration by visual system lesions. *Exp. Brain Res.* 8, 19–36

Ventre, J., Faugier-Grimaud, S. (1986). Effects of posterior parietal cortex lesions (area 7) on VOR in monkeys. *Exp. Brain Res.* 62, 654–658

Ventre, J., Flandrin, J.M., Jeannerod, M. (1984). In search for the egocentric reference. A neurophysiological hypothesis. *Neuropsychologia* 22, 797–806

Veraart, C., De Volder, A.G., Wanet-Defalque, M.C., Bol, A., Michel, Ch., Goffinet, A.M. (1990). Glucose utilization in human visual cortex is abnormally elevated in blindness of early onset but decreased in blindness of late onset. *Brain Res.* 510, 115–121

Veringa, F. (1964). Electro-optical stimulation of the human retina as a research technique. Doc. *Ophthal.* 18, 72–82

Veringa, F., Roelofs, J. (1966). Electro-optical interaction in the retina. *Nature* 211, 321–322

Verleger, R. (1988). Event-related potentials and cognition: A critique of the context updating hypothesis and an alternative interpretation of P3. *Behav. and Brain Sci.* 11, 343–427

Vermeire, B.A., Erdmann, A.L., Hamilton, C.R. (1983). Laterality in monkeys for discriminating facial expression and identity. *Soc. Neurosci. Abstr.* 9, 651

Veroff, A.E. (1978). A structural determinant of hemispheric processing of pictorial material. *Brain and Language* 5, 139–148

Verrey, D. (1888). Hemiachromatopsie droite absolue. Conservation partielle de la perception lumineuse et des formes. Ancient kyste hemorrhagique de la partie inferieure du lobe occipitale gauche. *Arch. Ophthalmol. (Paris)* 8, 289–300

Verriest, G. (ed.) (1973). *Colour vision deficiencies II*. Karger, Basel

Verriest, G. (ed.) (1975). *Colour vision deficiencies III*. Karger, Basel

Verriest, G. (ed.) (1979). *Colour vision deficiencies*. Hilger, Bristol

Vesalius, A. (1543). *De humani corporis fabrica, libri septem*. J. Oporinus, Basel

Vialet, N. (1893). Les centres cerebraux de la vision et l'appareil nerveux visuel intra-cerebral. Faculte de Medecine de Paris, Paris

Victor, J.D. (1988). Evaluation of poor performance and asymmetry in the Farnsworth-Munsell 100-hue-test. *Invest. Ophthal. Visual Sci.* 29, 476–481

Victor, J.D., Maiese, K., Shapley, R., Sidtis, J., Gazzaniga, M.S. (1989). Acquired central dyschromatopsia: analysis of a case with preservation of color discrimination. *Clin. Vision Sci.* 4, 183–196

Vighetto, A., Aimard, G., Confavreux, C., Devic, M. (1980). Une observation anatomo-clinique de fabulation (ou délire) topographique. *Cortex* 16, 501–507

Vighetto, A., Henry, E., Garde, P., Aimard, G. (1985). Le delire spatial: une manifestation des lesions de l'hemisphere mineur. *Rev. Neurol. (Paris)* 141, 476–481

Vighetto, A., Perenin, M.T. (1981a). Ataxie optique: analyse des responses oculaires et manuelles dans une tache de pointage vers une cible visuelle. *Rev. Neurol.* 137, 357–372

Vighetto, A., Perenin, M.T. (1981b). Pure agraphia and unilateral optic ataxia associated with a left superior parietal lobule lesion. *J. Neurol. Neurosurg. Psychiat.* 44, 430

Vilkki, J. (1984). Visual hemi-inattention after ventrolateral thalamotomy. *Neuropsychologia* 22, 399–408

Vilkki, J., Laitinen, L.V. (1974). Differential effects of left and right ventrolateral thalamotomy on receptive and expressive verbal performances and face-matching. *Neuropsychologia* 12, 11–19

Vilkki, J., Laitinen, L.V. (1976). Effects of pulvinotomy and ventro-lateral thalamotomy on some cognitive functions. *Neuropsychologia* 14, 67–78

Villardita, C., Smirni, P., Zappala, G. (1983). Visual neglect in Parkinson's disease. *Arch. Neurol.* 40, 737–739

Vincent, C., David, M., Puech, P. (1930). Sur l'alexie. Production du phenomene a la suite de l'extirpation de la corne occipitale du ventricule laterale gauche. *Rev. Neurol.* 1, 262–272

Vincent, F.M., Sadowsky, C.H., Saunders, R.L., Reeves, A.G. (1977). Alexia without agraphia, hemianopia or color-naming defect. A disconnection syndrome. *Neurology* 27, 689–691 (abstract: *Neurology* 26, 354–355 (1976))

Virsu, V., Lee, B.B., Creuzfeldt, O.D. (1987). Mesopic spectral responses and the Purkinje shift of macaque lateral geniculate nucleus cells. *Vision Res.* 27, 191–200

Virsu, V., Rovamo, J. (1979). Visual resolution, contrast sensitivity and the cortical magnification factor. *Exp. Brain Res.* 37, 475–494

Vizioli, R., Liberati, F. (1964). L'autoscopia epilettica. *Acta neurol. (Napoli)* 19, 866–873

Vizioli, R., Severini, P. (1955). Epilessia e autoscopia. *Riv. Neurol.* 25, 491–493

Vliegen, J., Koch, H.R. (1974). Die klinische Bedeutung der homonymen Hemianopsie. *Nervenarzt* 45, 449–457

Vogel, R.F. (1974). The Capgras-syndrome and its psychopathology. *Amer. J. Psychiat.* 131,922–924

Vogt, B.A., Pandya, D.N. (1978). Cortico-cortical connections of somatic sensory cortex (area 3, 1 and 2) in the rhesus monkey. *J. Comp. Neurol.* 177, 179–192

Vogt, B.A., Rosene, D.L., Pandya, D.N. (1979). Thalamic and cortical afferents differentiate anterior from posterior cingulate cortex in the monkey. *Science* 204, 205–207

Vogt, C., Vogt, O. (1919). Allgemeine Ergebnisse unserer Hirnforschung. *J. Psychol. Neurol. Lpz.* 25, 273–462

Vogt, C., Vogt, O. (1919). Allgemeine Ergebnisse unserer Hirnforschung. Vierte Mitteilung. Die physiologische Bedeutung der architektonischen Rindenfelderung auf Grund neuer Rindenreizungen. *J. Neurol. Psychol. Lpz.* 25, 399–462

Vogt, C., Vogt, O. (1926). Die vergleichend-architektonische und die vergleichend-reizphysiologische Felderung der Grosshirnrinde unter besonderer Berücksichtigung der menschlichen. *Naturwissenschaften* 14, 1190–1194

Volpe, B.T., Ledoux, J.E., Gazzaniga, M.S. (1979). Information processing of visual stimuli in an 'extinguished' field. *Nature* 282, 722–724

Vorster, O. (1893). Ueber einen Fall von doppelseitiger Hemianopsie mit Seelenblindheit, Photopsien und Gesichtstäuschungen. *Allg. Z. Psychiat. u. psychisch-gerichtl. Med.* 49, 227–249

Vrechia, C.I., Cremene, V., Popescu, P. (1948). Hemianopsie avec chromoagnosie. *Rev. Neurol. (Paris)* 80, 70

Wade, N.J. (1968). Visual orientation during and after lateral head, body and trunk tilts. *Perception and Psychophysics* 3, 215–219

Wagman, I.H. (1964). Eye movements induced by electric stimulation of cerebrum in monkeys and their relationship to bodily movement. In Bender, M.B. (ed.), *Oculo-motor system.* Hoeber, New York, 18–39

Wagner, W. (1932). Über Raumstörungen. *Monatschr. Psychiat. Neurol.* 84, 281–307

Wagner, W. (1937). Scheitellappensymptome und das Lokalisationsprinzip. *Z. Neurol.* 157, 169

Wagner, W. (1943). Anosognosie, Zeitrafferphänomen und Uhrzeitagnosie als Symptome der Störungen im rechten Parieto-occipitallappen. *Nervenarzt* 16, 49

Wagor, E., Lin, C.S., Kaas, J.H. (1975). Some cortical projections of

the dorsomedial visual area (DM) of association cortex in the owl monkey, *Aotus trivirgatus*. *J. Comp. Neurol.* 163, 227–250

Walker, E. (1981). Emotion recognition in disturbed and normal children: a research note. *J. Child Psychol. Psychiatry* 22, 263–269

Walker, E., Ceci, S.J. (1985). Semantic priming effects for stimuli presented to the right and left visual field. *Brain and Language* 25, 144–159

Walker, E., Marwit, S.J., Emory, E. (1980). A cross-sectional study of emotion recognition in schizophrenics. *J. abnorm. Psychol.* 89, 428–436

Walker, E., Mcguire, M., Bettes, B. (1984). Recognition and identification of facial stimuli by schizophrenics and patients with affective disorders. *Brit. J. Clin. Psychol.* 23, 37–44

Walker, P. (1979). Short-term visual memory — importance of the spatial and temporal separation of successive stimuli. *Quart. J. exp. Psychol.* 30, 665–680

Walker, P., Marshall, E. (1982). Visual memory and stimulus repetition effects. *J. Exp. Psychol. (Gen.)* 111, 348–368

Walker, R.Y. (1933). The eye movements of good readers. *Psychol. Monog.* 44, 95–117

Walker-Smith, G.J., Gale, A.G., Findlay, J.M. (1977). Eye-movement strategies involved in face perception. *Perception* 6, 313–326

Wallach, H., O'Connell, D.N. (1953). The kinetic depth effect. *J. Exp. Psych.* 45, 205–217

Walls, G.L. (1951). The problem of visual direction. I. The history to 1900. *J. Optom. Physiol. Opt.* 28, 55–83

Walls, G.L. (1956). The G. Palmer Story. *J. Hist. Med. allied Sci.* 11, 66–96

Walls, G.L. (1963). *The vertebrate eye and its adaptive radiation.* Hafner, New York, London

Walsh, F.B., Hoyt, W.F. (1969a). *Clinical Neuro-Ophthalmology*, 3rd. ed. Vol. 1–3. Williams & Wilkins, Baltimore

Walsh, F.B., Hoyt, W.F. (1969b). The visual sensory system. In Vinken, P.J., Bruyn, G.W. (eds.), *Handbook of clinical neurology* Vol. 2. North —Holland, Amsterdam

Walsh, T.J. (1972). *Neuroophthalmology. Clinical signs and symptoms.* Lea and Febiger, Philadelphia

Walter, W.G. (1973). Human frontal lobe function in sensory-motor association. In Pribram, K.H., Luria, A.R. (eds.), *Psychophysiology of the Frontal Lobes.* Academic Press, New York, 109–122

Wang, P.L. (1980). Interaction between handedness and cerebral functional dominance. *Int. J. Neurosci.* 11, 35–40

Wapner, W., Hamby, S., Gardner, H. (1981). The role of the right hemisphere in the apprehension of complex linguistic materials. *Brain and Language* 14, 15–33

Wapner, W., Judd, T., Gardner, H. (1978). Visual agnosia in an artist. *Cortex* 14, 343–364

Ward, R., Morgan, M. (1978). Perceptual effects of pursuit eye movements in the absence of a target. *Nature* 274, 158–159

Warner, S.J. (1949). The colour preferences of psychiatric groups. *Psychol. Monogr* ...., 301-...

Warrington, E.K. (1962). The completion of visual forms across hemianopic field defects. *J. Neurol. Neurosurg. Psychiatry* 25, 208–217

Warrington, E.K. (1975). The selective impairment of semantic memory. *Quart. J. Exp. Psychol* 27, 635–657

Warrington, E.K. (1981). Concrete word dyslexia. *Brit. J. Psychol.* 72, 175–196

Warrington, E.K. (1982). Neuropsychological studies of object recognition. *Philos. Trans. Roy. Soc. London* B298, 15–33

Warrington, E.K. (1985). Agnosia: The impairment of object recognition. In P.J. Vinken, G.W. Bruyn, H.L. Klawans (eds.), *Handbook of clinical neurology* 45. Chapter 23, Elsevier, Amsterdam

Warrington, E.K., Baddeley, A.D. (1974). Amnesia and memory for visual location. *Neuropsychologia* 12, 257–263

Warrington, E.K., James, M. (1967). An experimental investigation of facial recognition in patients with unilateral cerebral lesions. *Cortex* 3, 317–326

Warrington, E.K., James, M. (1967). Disorders of visual perception in patients with localised cerebral lesions. *Neuropsychologia* 5, 253–266

Warrington, E.K., James, M. (1967). Tachistoscopic number estimation in patients with unilateral cerebral lesions. *J. Neurol. Neurosurg. Psychiat.* 30, 468–474

Warrington, E.K., James, M. (1986). Visual object recognition in patients with right-hemisphere lesions: axes or features. *Perception* 15, 355–366

Warrington, E.K., James, M. (1988). Visual apperceptive agnosia: a clinico-anatomical study of three cases. *Cortex* 24, 13–32

Warrington, E.K., James, M., Kinsbourne, M. (1966). Drawing disability in relation to laterality of cerebral lesion. *Brain* 89, 53–82

Warrington, E.K., McCarthy, R. (1983). Category specific access to dysphasia. *Brain* 106, 859–878

Warrington, E.K., McCarthy, R. (1987). Categories of knowledge: Further fractionation and an attempted integration. *Brain* 110, 1273–1296

Warrington, E.K., Rabin, P. (1971). Visual span of apprehension in patients with unilateral cerebral lesions. *Q. J. Exp. Psychol.* 23, 423–431

Warrington, E.K., Shallice, T. (1979). Semantic access dyslexia. *Brain* 102, 43–63

Warrington, E.K., Shallice, T. (1980). Word-form dyslexia. *Brain* 103, 99–112

Warrington, E.K., Shallice, T. (1984). Category specific semantic impairments. *Brain* 107, 829–854

Warrington, E.K., Taylor, A.M. (1973a). Immediate memory for faces: Long-or short-term memory? *Quart. J. Exp. Psychol.* 25, 316–322

Warrington, E.K., Taylor, A.M. (1973b). The contribution of the right parietal lobe to object recogniton. *Cortex* 9, 152–164

Warrington, E.K., Taylor, A.M. (1978). Two categorical stages of object recognition. *Perception* 7, 695–705

Warrington, E.K., Zangwill, O.L. (1957). A study of dyslexia. *J. Neurol. Neurosurg. Psychiat.* 20, 208–215

Wasserman, G.S. (1978). *Color vision: an historical introduction.* Wiley, New York

Watanabe, S. (1985). *Pattern recognition. Human and mechanical.* John Wiley, New York

Watson, A.B., Ahumanda, A.J., Jr. (1985). A model of human visual motion sensing. *J. Opt. Soc. Amer.* A2, 322–342

Watson, B.U., Sullivan, P.M., Moeller, M.P., Jensen, J.K. (1982). Nonverbal intelligence and English language ability in deaf children. *J. Speech Hear. Disord.* 47, 199–204

Watson, J.S., Hayes, L.A., Vietze, P., Becker, J. (1979). Discriminative infant smiling to orientations of talking faces of mother and stranger. *J. Exp. Child Psychol.* 28, 92–99

Watson, R.T., Andriola, M., Heilman, K.M. (1977). The EEG neglect. *J. Neurol. Sci.* 34, 343–348

Watson, R.T., Heilman, K.M. (1979). Thalamic neglect. *Neurology* 29, 690–694

Watson, R.T., Heilman, K.M., Cauthen, J.C., King, F.A. (1973). Neglect after cingulectomy. *Neurology* 23, 1003–1007

Watson, R.T., Heilman, K.M., Miller, B.D., King, F.A. (1974). Neglect after mesencephalic reticular formation lesions. *Neurology* 24, 294–298

Watson, R.T., Miller, B., Heilman, K.M. (1977). Evoked potential in neglect. *Arch. Neurol.* 34, 224–227

Watson, R.T., Miller, B.D., Heilman, K.M. (1978). Nonsensory neglect. *Ann. Neurol.* 3, 505–508

Watson, R.T., Valenstein, E., Heilman, K.M. (1981). Thalamic neglect: possible role of the medial thalamus and nucleus reticularis

thalami in behavior. *Arch. Neurol.* 38, 501–507

Watt, R.J. (1984). Further evidence concerning the analysis of curvature in human foveal vision. *Vision Res.* 24, 251–253

Watt, R.J. (1988). *Visual processing: Computational, psychophysical and cognitive research.* Lawrence Erlbaum Associates, Hove

Wayland, S., Taplin, J.E. (1985). Feature-processing deficits following brain injury. I. Overselectivity in recognition memory for compound stimuli. *Brain Cognition* 4, 338–355

Wayland, S., Taplin, J.E. (1985). Feature-processing deficits following brain injury. II. Classification learning, categorical decision making, and feature production. *Brain Cognition* 4, 356–376

Weale, R. (1988). Leonardo on the eye. *Doc. Ophthalmol.* 68, 19–34

Weale, R.A. (1982). *Focus on vision.* Harvard University Press, Cambridge, Mass.

Weber, J.T., Huerta, M.F., Kaas, J.H., Harting, J.K. (1983). The projections of the lateral geniculate nucleus of the squirrel monkey: Studies in the interlaminar zones and the S-layers. *J. Comp. Neurol.* 213, 135–145

Weber, W.C., Jung, R.(1940). Über die epileptische Aura. *Z. Neurol. Psychiat.* 170, 211–265

Webster, M.J., Ungerleider, L.G., Bachevalier, J. (1991). Connections of inferior temporal areas TE and TEO with medial temporal-lobe structures in infant and adult monkeys. *J. Neurosci.* 11, 1095–1116

Wechsler, A.F. (1972). Transient left hemialexia. *Neurology* 22, 628–633

Wechsler, A.F. (1973). The effect of organic brain disease on recall of emotionally charged versus neutral narrative texts. *Neurology* 23, 130–135

Wechsler, A.F. (1977). Dissociative alexia. *Arch. Neurol.* 34, 257

Wechsler, A.F., Weinstein, E.A., Antin, S.P. (1972). Alexia without agraphia. *Bull. Los Angeles Neurol. Soc.* 37, 1–11

Wechsler, D. (1945). A standardized memory scale for clinical use. *J. Psychol.* 19, 87–95

Wechsler, D. (1955). *Wechsler adult intelligence scale, manual.* Psychological Corporation, New York

Wechsler, D. (1981). *WAIS-R Manual.* Psychological Corporation, New York

Wechsler, I.S. (1933). Partial cortical blindness with preservation of color vision. *Arch. Ophthal.* 9, 957–965

Weeler, D.D. (1970). Processes in word recognition. *Cognitive Psychology* 1, 59–85

Weigl, E. (1941). On the psychology of the so-called processes of abstraction. *J. Abn. Soc. Psychol.* 36, 3–33

Weigl, E. (1964). Some critical remarks concerning the problem of so-called simultanagnosia. *Neuropsychologia* 2, 189–207

Weigl, E. (1968). On the problem of cortical syndromes. Experimental studies. In Simmel, M.L. (ed.), *The reach of mind: essays in memory of Kurt Goldstein.* Springer, New York, 143–159

Weigl, E. (1974). Neuropsychological experiments on transcoding between spoken und written language structures. *Brain Lang.* 1, 227–240

Weigl, E. (1981). Personal communication.

Weigl, E., Bierwisch, M. (1976). Neuropsychologie et neurolinguistique. Themes de recherche commune. *Langages* 44, 4–19

Weigl, E., Milhailescu, L., Sewastopol, N., Lander, J. (1967). Zur Psychologie und Pathologie des Bilderkennens. *Z. f. Psychol.* 173, 45–76

Weinberger, D.R., Berman, K.F., Chase, N. (1988). Mesocortical dopaminergic function and human cognition. In Kalivas, P.W., Nemeroff, C.B. (eds.), *The mesocorticolimbic dopamine system.* New York Academy of Sciences, New York, 330–334

Weinberger, L.M., Grant, F.C. (1941). Visual hallucinations and their neuro-optical correlates. *Arch. Ophthal.* 23, 166–199

Weiner, I.B. (1970). Perceptual functioning in schizophrenia: implications for the study of perceptual processes. *Ann. N.Y. Acad. Sci.*

169, 718–730

Weinstein, E.A., Friedland, R.P. (eds.) (1977). Hemi-inattention and hemispheric specialization. *Advances in Neurology* 18, New York, Raven Press

Weinstein, E.A., Kahn, R.L. (1950). The syndrome of anosognosia, *Arch. Neurol. Psychiat.* 64, 772–791

Weinstein, E.A., Kahn, R.L. (1955). Denial of illness. Ch.T. Thomas, Springfield, Ill.

Weintraub, S., Mesulam, M.M. (1989). Neglect: hemispheric specialization, behavioral components and anatomical correlates. In Boller, F., Gratman, J., *Handbook of Neurophysiology*, Vol. 2 (Goodglass, H., Damasio, A.R., eds.), Elsevier, Amsterdam, 357–374

Weisenburg, T.S., McBride, K.L. (1935/1964). *Aphasia*. Hafner Publishing Co., New York

Weiskrantz, L. (1963). Contour discrimination in a young monkey with striate cortex ablation. *Neuropsychologia* 1, 145–164

Weiskrantz, L. (1972). Behavioural analysis of the monkey's visual nervous system. *Proc. Roy. Soc. London B* 182, 427–455

Weiskrantz, L. (1974). The interaction between occipital and temporal cortex in vision: An overview. In F.O. Schmitt, F.G. Worden (eds.), *The Neurosciences: A Third Study Program*. MIT-Press, Cambridge, Mass., 189–204

Weiskrantz, L. (1977). Trying to bridge some neuropsychological gaps between monkey and man. *Brit. J. Psychol.* 68, 431–445

Weiskrantz, L. (1978). Some aspects of visual capacity in monkey and man following striate cortex lesion. *Arch. Ital. Biol.* 116, 318–23

Weiskrantz, L. (1980). Varieties of residual experience. *Quart. J. exp. Psychol.* 32, 365–86

Weiskrantz, L. (1982). A follow-up study of blindsight. Paper presented at the Fifth INS European Conference, Deauville, France, June 16–18

Weiskrantz, L. (1986). *Blindsight: A case study and implications.* Oxford University Press, Oxford

Weiskrantz, L., Cowey, A. (1963). Striate cortex lesions and visual acuity of the rhesus monkey. *J. comp. physiol. Psychol.* 56, 225–32

Weiskrantz, L., Cowey, A. (1967). A comparison of the effects of striate cortex and retinal lesions on visual acuity in the monkey. *Science* 155, 104–106

Weiskrantz, L., Cowey, A. (1970). Filling in the scotoma: A study of residual vision after striate cortex lesions in monkeys. In Stellar, E., Sprague, J.M. (eds.), *Progress in physiological psychology.* Vol. 3, Academic Press, NY, 237–260

Weiskrantz, L., Cowey, A., Passingham, C. (1977). Spatial responses to brief stimuli by monkeys with striate cortex ablations. *Brain* 100, 655–670

Weiskrantz, L., Warrington, E.K, Sanders, M.D., Marshall, J. (1974). Visual capacity in the hemianopic field following a restricted occipital ablation. *Brain* 97, 709–728

Weisstein, N., Harris, C.S. (1974). Visual detection of line segments: An object superiority effect. *Science* 196, 752–755

Weizsäcker, V. von (1928). Pathophysiologie der Sensibilität. *Dtsch. Z. Nervenhk.* 101, 184–211

Welch, K., Stuteville, P. (1958). Experimental production of neglect in monkeys. *Brain* 81, 341–347

Welch, R.B., Goldstein, G. (1972). Prism adaptation and brain damage. *Neuropsychologia* 10, 387–394

Weller, R.E., Kaas, J.H. (1983). Retinotopic patterns of connections of area 17 with visual areas V-II and MT in macaque monkeys. *J. Comp. Neurol.* 220, 253–279

Weller, R.E., Kaas, J.H. (1985). Cortical projections of the dorsolateral visual area in owl monkeys: the prestriate relay to inferior temporal cortex. *J. Comp. Neurol.* 234, 35–59

Weller, R.E., Kaas, J.H. (1987). Subdivisions and connections of inferior temporal cortex in owl monkeys. *J. Comp. Neurol.* 256, 137–172

Weller, R.E., Wall, J.T., Kaas, J.H. (1984). Cortical connections of

the middle temporal visual area (MT) and the superior temporal cortex in owl monkeys. *J. Comp. Neurol.* 228, 81–104

Welman, A.J. (1969). Right-sided unilateral visual spatial agnosia, asomatognosia and anosognosia with left hemisphere lesions. *Brain* 92, 571–580

Wendenburg, K. (1909). Ein Tumor des rechten Hinterhauptlappens mit ungewöhnlichen klinischen Begleiterscheinungen. *Monatsschr. Psychiatr. Neurol.* 25, 428–440

Werner, A. (1990). Studies on colour constancy in man using a 'Checkerboard-Mondrian'. Unpublished manuscript, F.U. Berlin, Neurobiol. Sect.

Werner, J.S., Peterzell, D.H., Scheetz, A.J. (1989). Light, vision, and aging. *Optometry and Vision Sci.* 67, 214–229

Werner, J.S., Walraven, J. (1962). Effect of chromatic adaptation on the achromatic locus: the role of contrast, luminance and background color. *Vision Res.* 22, 929–943

Wernicke, C. (1874). *Der aphasische Symptomencomplex.* Franck & Weigert, Breslau

Wernicke, C. (1881). *Lehrbuch der Gehirnkrankheiten.* Th. Fischer, Kassel und Berlin

Wernicke, C. (1903). Ein Fall von isolierter Agraphie. *Mschr. Psychiat. Neurol.* 13, 1–24

Werth, R. (1983). 'Blindsight': some conceptual considerations. *Beh. Brain Sci.* 6. 467–468

Werth, R., Pöppel, E. (1988). Compression and lateral shift of mental coordinate systems in a line bisection task. *Neuropsychologia* 26, 741–745

Wertheim, T. (1894). Über die indirekte Sehschärfe. *Z. Psychol. Physiol. Sinnesorg.* 7, 172–189

Wertheimer, G. (1912). Experimentelle Studien über das Sehen von Bewegungen. *Z. Psychol.* 61, 161–265

West, L.J. (ed.) (1962). *Hallucinations.* Grune & Stratton, New York

Westheimer, G. (1981). Visual hyperacuity. In Ottoson, D. (ed.), *Progress in sensory physiology* 1. Springer-Verlag, Berlin, 1–30

Westheimer, G. (1982). The spatial grain of the perifoveal visual field. *Vision Res.* 22, 157–162

Westheimer, G., Campbell, F.W. (1962). Light distribution in the image formed by the living human eye. *J. Optical Soc. America* 52, 1040–1045

Westheimer, G., Hauske, G. (1975). Temporal and spatial interference with vernier acuity. *Vision Res.* 15, 1137–1141

Westheimer, G., McKee, S.P. (1977a). Integration regions for visual hyperacuity. *Vision Res.* 17, 89–93

Westheimer, G., McKee, S.P. (1977b). Spatial configurations for visual hyperacuity. *Vision Res.* 17, 941–947

Weston, M.J., Whitlock, F.A. (1971). The Capgras-syndrome following head injury. *Brit. J. Psychiat.* 119, 25–31

Westphal, K. (1881). Zur Frage von Lokalisation der unilateralen Convulsionen und Hemianopsie bedingten Hirnerkrankunge. *Charité-Annalen* 6, 342–365

Weymouth, F.B. (1958). Visual sensory units and the minimal angle of resolution. *Amer. J. Ophthal.* 46, 102–113

Weymouth, F.W., Hines, D.C., Acres, L.H., Raaf, J.E., Wheeler, M.C. (1928). Visual acuity within the area centralis and its relation to eye movements and fixation. *Amer. J. Ophthalmol.* 11, 947–960

Whelan, T.B., Schteingart, D.E., Starkman, M.N., Smith, A. (1980). Neuropsychological deficits in Cushing's syndrome. *J. Nerv. Ment. Dis.* 168, 753–757

White, M.J. (1969). Laterality differences in perception: a review. *Psychol. Bull.* 72, 387–405

White, N.J. (1980). Complex visual hallucinations in partial blindness due to eye disease. *Brit. J. Psychiat.* 136, 284–286

Whitehouse, P.J. (1981). Imagery and verbal encoding in left and right hemisphere damaged patients. *Brain and Language* 14, 315–332

Whiteley, A.M., Warrington, E.K. (1977). Prosopagnosia: A clinical, psychological, and anatomical study of three patients. *J. Neurol. Neurosurg. Psychiat.* 40, 395–430

Whiteley, A.M., Warrington, E.K. (1978). Selective impairment of topographical memory: a single case study. *J. Neurol. Neurosurg. & Psychiat.* 41, 575–578

Whitlock, D.G., Nauta, W.J. (1956). Subcortical projections from the temporal neocortex in Macaca Mulatta. *J. Comp. Neurol.* 106, 183–212

Whitty, C.W.M., Newcombe, F. (1973). R.C. Oldfield's study of visual and topographic disturbances in a right occipito-parietal lesion of 30 years duration. *Neuropsychologia* 11, 471–475

Wicker, I. (1930). Ein eigenartiger Fall von räumlicher Orientierungsstörung. *Mschr. f. Psychiat. Neurol.* 77, 310,317

Wiedemann, E. (1910). Zu Ibn Al Haitams Optik. *Arch. Gesch. Naturw. u. Technik* 3, 1–153

Wiedemann, E. (1913). Ibn Sinas Anschauung vom Sehvorgang. *Arch. Gesch. Naturw. u. Technik* 4, 239–241

Wiesel, T.N., Hubel, D.H. (1966). Spatial and chromatic interactions in the lateral geniculate body of the rhesus monkey. *J. Neurophysiol.* 29, 1115–1156

Wieser, H.G. (1982). Zur Frage der lokalisatorischen Bedeutung epileptischer Halluzinationen. In Karbowski, K. (ed.), *Halluzinationen bei Epilepsie und ihre Differentialdiagnose.* Huber, Bern, 67–92

Wieser, H.G., Valavanis, A., Roos, A., Isler, P., Renella, R.R. (1989). 'Selective' and 'superselective' temporal lobe amytal tests: I. Neuroradiological, neuroanatomical and electrical data. *Adv. Epileptology* 17, 20–27

Wigan, A.L. (1844). *A new view of insanity: the duality of the mind.* Longman, Brown, Green and Longmans, London. Reprinted by J. Simon, Malibu 1985

Wilbrand, H. (1881). *Über Hemianopsie und ihr Verhältnis zur topischen Diagnose der Gehirnkrankheiten.* Hirschwald, Berlin

Wilbrand, H. (1884). *Ophthalmiatrische Beiträge zur Diagnostik der Gehirn-Krankheiten.* Bergmann, Wiesbaden

Wilbrand, H. (1887). *Die Seelenblindheit als Herderscheinung und ihre Beziehungen zur homonymen Hemianopsie.* J.F. Bergmann, Wiesbaden

Wilbrand, H. (1892). Ein Fall von Seelenblindheit und Hemianopsie mit Sectionsbefund. *Dtsch. Z. Nervenheilk.* 2, 361–387

Wilbrand, H., Saenger, A. (1917). Die homonyme Hemianopsie nebst ihren Beziehungen zu den anderen cerebralen Herderscheinungen. In Wilbrand, H., Saenger, A. (eds.), *Die Neurologie des Auges. Ein Handbuch für Nerven-und Augenärzte.* Vol. 7. Bergmann, Wiesbaden

Wilbrand, H., Saenger, A. (1918). Die Verletzungen der Sehbahnen des Gehirns mit besonderer Berücksichtigung der Kriegsverletzungen. Bergmann, Wiesbaden

Wilcox, J.A. (1986). The anatomical basis of misidentification. *Bibl. Psychiatr.* 164, 59–67

Wilder, J. (1928). Über Schief-und Verkehrtsehen. *Dtsch. Z. Nervenheilk.* 104, 222–256

Wilkins, A.J., Andermann, F., Ives, J. (1975). Stripes, complex cells and seizures. An attempt to determine the locus and nature of the trigger mechanism in pattern-sensitive epilepsy. *Brain* 98, 365–380

Wilkins, A.J., Binnie, C.D., Darby, C.E. (1980). Visually-induced seizures. *Progr. in Neurobiol.* 15, 85–118

Williams, D. (1956). Emotions reflected in epileptic experiences. *Brain* 79, 29–67

Williams, D., Gassel, M.M. (1962). Visual function in patients with homonymous hemianopia. Part I: The visual fields. *Brain* 85, 175–250

Williams, D., Phillips, G., Sekuler, R. (1986). Hysteresis in the perception of motion direction as evidence for neural cooperativity. *Nature* 324, 253–255

Williams, M. (1970). *Brain damage and the mind.* Penguin Books, Baltimore

Williams, R.A., Essock, E.A. (1986). Areas of spatial interaction for a hyperacuity stimulus. *Vision Res.* 26, 349–360

Williams, R.W., Herrup, K. (1988). The control of neuron number. *Ann. Rev. Neurosci.* 11, 423–453

Willis, Th. (1664/1672). *Cerebri anatome.* London

Willis, Th. (1672/1676). *De anima brutorum, exercitationes duae, prior physiologica, altera pathologica.* De Tournes, Genf

Willis, Th. (1681/1720). *Opera omnia.* Huguetan, Leyden and Malachinus, Venedig

Wilson, A.E., Harper, D.W. (1977). The locus of maximum weighting within attentive fields: An empirical investigation. *Quart. J. Exp. Psychol.* 29, 97–106

Wilson, B., Cockburn, J., Halligan, P.W. (1987). Behavioural inattention test. Thames Valley Test Company, Titchfield

Wilson, C.C. (1972). Spatial factors and the behavior of non-human primates. *Folia Primatol.* 18, 226–275

Wilson, C.L., Babb, T.L., Halgren, E., Crandall, P.H. (1983). Visual receptive fields and response properties of neurons in human temporal lobe and visual pathways. *Brain* 106, 473–502

Wilson, J.T., Wiedmann, K.D., Philips, W.A., Brooks, D.N. (1988). Visual event perception in alcoholics. *J. Clin. Exp. Neuropsychol.* 10, 222–234

Wilson, M. (1957). Effects of circumscribed cortical lesions upon somesthetic and visual discrimination in the monkey. *J. Comp. Physiol. Psychol.*, 50, 630–635.

Wilson, M., Debauche, B.A. (1981). Inferotemporal cortex and categorical perception of visual stimuli by monkeys. *Neuropsychologia* 19, 29–41

Wilson, M., Stamm, J.S., Pribram, K.H. (1960). Deficits in roughness discrimination after posterior parietal lesions in monkeys. *J. Comp. Physiol. Psychol.* 53, 535–539

Winner, E. (1979). Do chimpanzees recognize photographs as representations of objects? *Neuropsychologia* 17, 413–420

Winnick, W.A., Daniel, S.A. (1970). Two kinds of response priming in tachistoscopic recognition. *J. exp. Psychol.* 84, 74–81

Winograd, E. (1976). Recognition memory for faces following nine different judgements. *Bull. Psychon. Soc.* 8, 419–421

Winterstein, H. (1932). *Schlaf und Traum.* Springer, Berlin

Wisniewski, K.E., Dalton, A.J., McLachlan, C., Wen, G.Y., Wisniewski, H.M. (1985). Alzheimer's disease in Down's syndrome: clinicopathologic studies. *Neurology* 35, 957–961

Wispé, L.G., Drambarean, N.C. (1953). Physiological need, word frequency, and visual duration thresholds. *J. exp. Psychol.* 46, 25–31

Witelson, S.F. (1976). Sex and the single hemisphere: specialization of the right hemisphere for spatial processing. *Science* 193, 425–427

Witt, E.D., Ryan, C. Hsu, L.K. (1985). Learning deficits in adolescents with anorexia nervosa. *J. Nerv. Ment. Dis.* 173, 182–184

Wohlgemuth, A. (1911). On the aftereffect of seen movement. *Br. J. Psychol. Monogr. Suppl.*

Wolf, M.E., Goodale, M.A. (1987). Oral asymmetries during verbal and non-verbal movements of the mouth. *Neuropsychologia* 25, 375–396

Wolff, Ch. (1725/1980). *Vernünftige Gedancken vom Gebrauche der Theile in Menschen, Thieren und Pflantzen, den Liebhabern der Wahrheit mitgetheilet,* 1725. Renger, Frankfurt/Leipzig. Repr. in *Gesammelte Werke* 1. Abt.: *Deutsche Schriften,* Vol. 8, G. Olms, Hildesheim

Wolff, W. (1933/1934). The experimental study of forms of expression. *Charcater and Personality* 2, 168–176

Wollaston, W.H. (1824). On semi-decussation of optic nerves. *Philos. Trans. Roy. Soc. Lond.* 114, 222

Wolpert, I. (1924). Die Simultanagnosie — Störung der Gesamtauffassung. *Z. ges. Neurol. Psychiat.* 93, 397–415

Wolpert, I. (1925). Zur Psychologie der agnostischen Störungen. *Dtsch. Z. Nervenheilk.* 83, 340–344

Wolpert, I. (1930). Über das Wesen der literalen Alexie. *Mschr. Psychiat. Neurol.* 75, 207–266

Wong-Riley, M.D.T. (1977). Connections between the pulvinar nucleus and the prestriate cortex in the squirrel monkey as revealed by peroxidase histochemistry and autoradiography. *Brain Res.* 134, 249–267

Wong-Riley, M.D.T. (1978). Reciprocal connections between striate and prestriate cortex in squirrel monkey as demonstrated by combined peroxidase histochemistry and autoradiography. *Brain Res.* 147, 159–164

Wong-Riley, M.D.T. (1979). Changes in the visual system of monocularly sutured or enucleated cats demonstrable with cytochrome oxidase histochemistry. *Brain Res.* 171, 11–28

Wong-Riley, M.D.T. (1979). Columnar cortico-cortical interconnections within the visual system of the squirrel and macaque monkeys. *Brain Res.* 162, 201–217

Woods, B.T., Pöppel, E. (1974). Effect of print size on reading time in a patient with verbal alexia. *Neuropsychologia* 12, 31–41

Wreschner, E.E. (1985). Evidence and interpretation of red ochre in the early prehistoric sequences. In Tobias, Ph.V. (ed.), *Hominid evolution. Past, present and future.* Liss, New York, 387–394

Wundt, W. (1893). *Grundzüge der physiologischen Psychologie.* Vol. I and II, 4th ed. Engelmann, Leipzig

Wundt, W. (1894). Über psychische Kausalität und das Princip des psychophysischen Parallelismus. *Philosophische Studien* 10, 1–124

Wundt, W. (1904/1911). *Vorlesung über die Menschen-und Tierseele.* Voss, Hamburg, Leipzig

Wurtz, R.H. (1969). Response of striate cortex neurons to stimuli during rapid eye movements in the monkey. *J. Neurophysiol.* 32, 975–986

Wurtz, R.H. (1969). Visual receptive fields of striate cortex neurons in awake monkeys. *J. Neurophysiol.* 32, 727–742

Wurtz, R.H., Goldberg, M.E. (1972). Activity of superior colliculus in behaving monkeys. III. Cells discharging before eye movements. *J. Neurophysiol.* 35, 575–586

Wurtz, R.H., Goldberg, M.E., Robinson, D.L. (1982). Brain mechanisms of visual attention. *Sci. Am.* 246, 124–135

Wurtz, R.H., Mohler, C.W. (1976). Enhancement of visual responses in monkey striate cortex and frontal eye fields. *J. Neurophysiol.* 39, 766–772

Wurtz, R.H., Mohler, C.W. (1976). Organization of monkey superior colliculus: enhanced visual response of superficial layer cells. *J. Neurophysiol.* 39, 745–765

Wurtz, R.H., Newsome, W.T. (1985). Divergent signals encoded by neurons in extrastriate areas MT and MST during smooth pursuit eye movements. *Soc. Neurosci. Abstr.* 11, 1246 (124?)

Wurtz, R.H., Richmond, B.J., Newsome, W.T. (1984). Modulation of cortical visual processing by attention, perception and movement. In Edelman, G., Gall, W.E., Cowan, W.M. (eds.), *Dynamic aspects of neocortical function.* Wiley, New York

Wydler, A., Perret, E. (1978). Neuropsychologische Erfassung der Steropsis bei hirngeschädigten Patienten. *Nervenarzt* 49, 366–369

Wygotski, L.S. (1934/1974). *Denken und Sprechen.* 1. ed. Moskau 1934. German edition: Frankfurt

Wyke, M., Holgate, D. (1973). Colour-naming defects in dysphasic patients. A qualitative analysis. *Neuropsychologia* 11, 451–461

Wyler, F., Graves, R., Landis, T. (1987). Cognitive task influence on relative hemispheric motor control: Mouth asymmetry and lateral eye movements. *J. Clin. Exp. Neuropsychol.* 9, 105–116

Wyszecki, G., Stiles, W.S. (1982). *Color Science* (2nd. ed.) J. Wiley and Sons, New York

Yamada, M. (1966). Five natural troops of Japanese monkeys in Shodoshima Island. I. Distribution of social organization. *Primates* 7,

Yamadori, A. (1975). Ideogram reading in alexia. *Brain* 98, 231–238

Yamadori, A. (1980). Right unilateral dyscopia of letters in alexia without agraphia. *Neurology* 30, 991–994

Yamadori, A. (1982). Alexia with agraphia and angular gyrus (in Jap.). *Shitsugoshou Kenkyu* 2, 41–47

Yamadori, A., Albert, M.L. (1973). Word category aphasia. *Cortex* 9, 112–115

Yamadori, A., Motumura, N., Endo, M., et al. (1985). Category-specific alexia and a neuropsychological model of reading. *Shitsugoshou Kenkyu* 5, 23–27

Yamadori, A., Osumi, S., Masuhara, S., et al. (1977). Preservation of singing in Brocas' aphasia. *J. Neurol. Neurosurg. Psychat.* 40, 221–224

Yamane, S., Kaji, S., Kawano, K. (1988). What facial features activate face neurons in infereotemporal cortex of the monkey. *Exp. Brain Res.* 73, 209–214

Yamane, S., Komatsu, H., Kaji, S., Kawano, K. (1990). Neural activity in the cortex of monkeys during a face discrimination task. In Iwai, E. (ed.), *Vision, memory and temporal lobe.* Elsevier, New York, 89–100

Yandell, L., Elias, J.W. (1983). Left hemispheric advantage for a visuospatial-dichaptic matching task. *Cortex* 19, 69–77

Yarbus, A.L. (1967). *Eye movements and vision.* Transl. by B. Haigh. Plenum Press, New York

Yarmey, A.D. (1970). The effects of mnemonic instructions on paired associates recognition memory for faces or names. *Canad. J. behav. Sci.* 2, 181–190

Yarmey, A.D. (1974). Proactive interference in short-term retention of human faces. *Can. J. Psychol.* 28, 333–338

Yarmey, A.D. (1979). Through the looking glass: sex differences in memory for self-facial poses. *J. Res. Personality* 13, 450–459

Yates, A.J. (1966). Data-processing levels and thought disorder in schizophrenia. *Aust. J. Psychol.* 18, 103–129

Yeterian, E.H., Pandya, D.N. (1985). Corticothalamic connections of the posterior parietal cortex in the rhesus monkey. *J. Comp. Neurol.* 237, 408–426

Yin, R.K. (1969). Looking at upside-down faces. *J. exp. Psychol.* 81, 141–145

Yin, R.K. (1970). Face recognition by brain-injured patients: a dissociable ability? *Neuropsychologia* 8, 395–402

Yin, R.K. (1970). Face recognition: a special process? Unpubl.doc. diss., MIT Cambridge

Yin, R.K. (1978). Face perception: a review of experiments with infants, normal adults, and brain-injured persons. In Held, R., Leibowith, H.W., Teuber, H.L. (eds.), *Handbook of sensory physiology. Vol. VIII: Perception.* Berlin, 593–605

Yin, T.C.T., Mountcastle, V.B. (1977). Visual input to the visuomotor mechanisms of the monkey's parietal lobe. *Science* 197, 1381–1383

Yin, T.C.T., Mountcastle, V.B. (1978). Mechanisms of neural integration in the parietal lobe for visual attention. *Federation Proc.* 37, 2251–2257

Young, A.W. (1984). Right cerebral hemisphere superiority for recognizing the internal and external features of famous faces. *Brit. J. Psychol.* 75, 161–169

Young, A.W. (1987). Finding the mind's construction in the face. *Cognitive Neuropsychology* 4, 45–53

Young, A.W. (1988). Functional organization of visual recognition. In L. Weiskrantz (ed.), *Thought without language.* Oxford University Press, Oxford

Young, A.W., Bion, P.J. (1980). Absence of any developmental trend in right hemisphere superiority for face recognition. *Cortex* 16, 213–220

Young, A.W., Bion, P.J. (1981). Accuracy of naming laterally presented known faces by children and adults. *Cortex* 17, 97–106

Young, A.W., Bion, P.J. (1983). The nature of the sex difference in right hemisphere superiority for face recognition. *Cortex* 19,

215–226

Young, A.W., De Haan, E.H.F. (1988). Boundaries of covert recognition in prosopagnosia. *Cognitive Neuropsychology* 5, 317–336

Young, A.W., de Haan, E.H.F., Newcombe, F., Hay, D.C. (1990). Facial neglect. *Neuropsychologia* 28, 391–415

Young, A.W., Ellis, A.W. (1981). Asymmetry of cerebral hemispheric function in normal and poor readers. *Psychol. Bull./Amer. Psychol. Ass. Wash.* 89, 183–190

Young, A.W., Ellis, H.D. (1976). An experimental investigation of developmental differences in ability to recognize faces presented to the left and right cerebral hemispheres. *Neuropsychologia* 14, 495–498

Young, A.W., Ellis, H.D. (1989). Childhood prosopagnosia. *Brain Cogn.* 9, 16–47

Young, A.W., Ellis, H.D. (1989). *Handbook of research on face processing.* Elsevier, North Holland

Young, A.W., Hay, D.C., McWeeney, K.H. (1985). Right cerebral hemisphere superiority for constructing facial representations. *Neuropsychologia* 23, 195–202

Young, A.W., Hellawell, D., De Haan, E.H. (1988). Cross-domain semantic priming in normal subjects and a prosopagnosic patient. *Q. J. Exp. Psychol.* 40, 661–580

Young, A.W., Ratcliff, G. (1983). Visuospatial abilities of the right hemisphere. In A.W. Young (ed.), *Functions of the right cerebral hemisphere*, Academic Press, London, 1–32

Young, R.S., Fishman, G.A. (1980). Loss of colour vision and Stiles' II1 mechanism in a patient with cerebral infarction. *J. Opt. Soc. Amer.* 70, 1301–1305

Young, R.S., Fishman, G.A., Chen, F. (1980). Traumatically acquired color vision defect. *Investigative Ophthal. Vis.Sci.* 19, 545–549

Young, T. (1802). On the theory of light and colours. *Phil. Trans. Roy. Soc. London* 92, 12–48

Yuille, A.L., Ullman, S. (1990). Computational theories of low-level vision. In Osherson, D.N., Kosslyn, M., Hollerbach, J.M., *Visual cognition and action*. MIT-Press, Cambridge, Mass, 5–39

Yukie, M., Iwai, E. (1981). Direct projection from the dorsal lateral geniculate nucleus to the prestriate cortex in macaque monkeys. *J. comp. Neurobiol.* 201, 81–97

Yves, J., Goulet, P., Ska, B., Nespulous, J.L. (1986). Informative content of narrative discourse in right-brain-damaged right-handers. *Brain & Lang.* 29, 81–105

Zabel, L., Bouma, H., Legein, Ch.P. (1978). Visual recognition by dyslectic children. A comparison of monocular and binocular reading and word recognition. *IPO Ann. Progr. Rep.* 13, 68–73

Zachary Jacobson, J., Dodwell, P.C. (1979). Saccadic eye movements during reading. *Brain Lang.* 8, 303–314

Zador, J. (1930). Meskalinwirkung bei Störungen des optischen Systems. *Z. Neurol.* 127, 30–107

Zaidel, E. (1978). Lexical organization in the right hemisphere. In Buser, P., Rougeul-Buser, A. (eds.), *Cerebral Correlates of Conscious Experience*. INSERM Symposium No 6. Elsevier North-Holland, Amsterdam & Oxford, 177–197

Zaidel, E. (1985). Language in the right hemisphere. In D.F. Benson, E. Zaidel (eds.), *The dual brain*. The Guilford Press, New York, 205–231

Zaidel, E., Peters, A.M. (1981). Phonologic encoding and ideographic reading by the disconnected right hemisphere: two case studies. *Brain Lang.* 14, 205–234

Zangemeister, W.H., Meienberg, O., Stark, L., Hoyt, W.F. (1982). Eye-head coordination in homonymous hemianopia. *J.Neurol.* 226, 243–254

Zangwill, O.L. (1964). The current status of cerebral dominance. In The Brain and Disorders of Communication. *Res. Publ. Assoc. Nerv.*

Ment. Dis. 42, 103–118

Zangwill, O.L., Blakemore, C. (1972). Dyslexia: reversal of eye movements during reading. *Neuropsychol.* 10, 371–373

Zangwill, O.L., Wyke, M.A. (1990). Hughlings Jackson on the recognition of places, persons, and objects. In Trevarthen, C. (ed.), *Brain circuits and functions of the mind. Essays in honor of Roger W. Sperry.* Cambridge University Press, Cambridge, 281–292

Zarith, S.H., Kahn, R.L. (1974). Impairment and adaptation in chronic disabilities: Spatial inattention. *J. Nervous Mental Dis.* 159, 63–72

Zazzo, R. (1948). Images du corps et conscience de soi. Enfance, 29–43, quoted after Bruyer, 1986

Zazzo, R. (1979). Des enfants, des singes et des chiens, devant le miroir. *Rev. Psychol. Appl.* 29, 235–246

Zeal, A.A., Rhoton, A.L. (1978). Microsurgical anatomy of the posterior cerebral artery. *J. Neurosurg.* 48, 534–559

Zee, D.S., Yamazaki, A., Butler, P.H., Gücer, G. (1981). Effects of ablation of flocculus and paraflocculus on eye movements in primate. *J. Neurophysiol.* 46, 878–899

Zeitler, J. (1900). Tachistoskopische Versuche über das Lesen. *Wundt's Philosophische Studien* 16, 380–463

Zeki, S. (1988). Anatomical guides to the functional organization of the visual cortex. In Rakic, P., Singer, W. (eds.), *Neurobiology of neocortex.* Wiley, New York, 241–251

Zeki, S., Shipp, S. (1989). Modular connections between areas V2 and V4 of macaque monkey visual cortex. *Eur. J. Neurosci.* 1, 494–506

Zeki, S.M. (1969). Representation of central visual fields in prestriate cortex of monkey. *Brain Res.* 14, 271–291

Zeki, S.M. (1970). Interhemispheric connections of prestriate cortex of monkey. *Brain Res.* 19, 63–75

Zeki, S.M. (1971). Convergent input from the striate cortex (area 17) to the cortex of the superior temporal sulcus in the rhesus monkey. *Brain Res.* 28, 338–340

Zeki, S.M. (1971b). Cortical projections from two prestriate areas in the monkey. *Brain Res.* 34, 19–35

Zeki, S.M. (1973a). Colour coding in rhesus monkey prestriate cortex. *Brain Res.* 53, 422–427

Zeki, S.M. (1973b). Comparison of the cortical degeneration in the visual regions of the temporal lobe of the monkey following section of the anterior commissure and the splenium. *J. Comp. Neurol.* 148, 167–176

Zeki, S.M. (1974a). Functional organization of a visual area in the posterior bank of the superior temporal sulcus of the rhesus monkey. *J. Physiol. (Lond.)* 236, 549–573

Zeki, S.M. (1974b). Cells responding to changing image size and disparity in the cortex of the rhesus monkey. *J. Physiol. (Lond.)* 242, 827–841

Zeki, S.M. (1975). The functional organization of projections from striate to prestriate visual cortex in the rhesus monkey. *Cold Spring Harbor Symp. Quant. Biol.* 40, 591–600

Zeki, S.M. (1977). Colour coding in the superior temporal sulcus of rhesus monkey visual cortex. *Proc. R. Soc. London Ser. B* 197, 195–223

Zeki, S.M. (1978). Functional specialisation in the visual cortex of the rhesus monkey. *Nature* 274, 423–428

Zeki, S.M. (1978). The cortical projections of foveal striate cortex in the rhesus monkey. *J. Physiol. (Lond.)* 277, 227–244

Zeki, S.M. (1978). The third visual complex of rhesus monkey prestriate cortex. *J. Physiol. (Lond.)* 277, 245–272

Zeki, S.M. (1978). Uniformity and diversity of structure and function in rhesus monkey prestriate visual cortex. *J. Physiol. (Lond.)* 277, 273–290

Zeki, S.M. (1979). Zu Brodmanns Area 18 und Area 19. *Exp. Brain Res.* 36, 195–197

Zeki, S.M. (1980). A direct projection from area V1 to area V3A of rhesus monkey visual cortex. *Proc. Roy. Soc. Lond. B* 207, 499–506

Zeki, S.M. (1980). The representation of colours in the cerebral cortex. *Nature*, 284, 412–418

Zeki, S.M. (1983a). Colour coding in the cerebral cortex: The reaction of cells in monkey visual cortex to wavelengths and colours. *Neurosci.* 9, 741–765

Zeki, S.M. (1983b). Colour coding in the cerebral cortex: The responses of wavelength-selective and colour-coded cells in monkey visual cortex to changes in wavelength composition. *Neuroscience* 9, 767–781

Zeki, S.M. (1984). Colour coding in the superior temporal sulcus of Rhesus monkey visual cortex. *Proc. R. Soc. Med. (Lond.) B* 197, 555–562

Zeki, S.M. (1990a). A century of cerebral achromatopsia. *Brain* 113, 1721–1777

Zeki, S.M. (1990b). The form vision of achromatopsic patients. *The Brain*, LV Cold Spring Harbor Symposium on Quantitative Biology, May 30–Jun 6, p. 16

Zeki, S.M. (1991). Cerebral akinetopsia (visual motion blindness). *Brain* 114, 811–824

Zeki, S.M., Watson, J.D.G., Lueck, C.J., Friston, K.J., Kennard, C., Frackowiak, R.S.J. (1991). A direct demonstration of functional specialization in human visual cortex. *J. Neurosci.* 11, 641–649

Zelenkova, T.P. (1984). Evoked potentials of posterior association areas of the cortex during discrimination and recognition of human portraits. *Human Physiology* 9, 83–89

Zemanek, H. (1959). *Elementare Informationstheorie*. Oldenbourg, Wien, München

Zenkov, L.R., Fishman, M.N., Melnichuk, P.V., Losev, N.I. (1974). Visual evoked potentials in persons with visual pathway disorders (in Russisch). *Zh. VYSSH. Nerv. Deiat.* 24, 2142–2148

Ziehl, H. (1895). Ueber einen Fall von Alexie mit Farbenhemiopie. *Neurologisches Centralblatt* 14, 892–893

Zihl, J. (1980). 'Blindsight': improvement of visually guided eye movements by systematic practice in patients with cerebral blindness. *Neuropsychologia* 18, 71–77

Zihl, J. (1981). Recovery of visual functions in patients with cerebral blindness effect of specific practice with saccadic localization. *Exp. Brain Res.* 44, 159–169

Zihl, J. (1988). Homonyme Hemianopsie und ihre Rehabilitation. *Klin. Mbl. Augenheilk.* 192, 555–558

Zihl, J. (1989). Cerebral disturbances of elementary visual functions. In Brown, J.W. (ed.), *Neuropsychology of visual perception*. Erlbaum, Hillsdale, NY, 35–58

Zihl, J., Cramon, D. von (1979). Restitution of visual function in patients with cerebral blindness. *J. Neurol. Neurosurg. Psychiat.* 42, 312–322

Zihl, J., Cramon, D. von (1979). The contribution of the 'second' visual system to directed visual attention in man. *Brain* 102, 835–856

Zihl, J., Cramon, D. von (1980). Colour anomia restricted to the left visual hemifield after splenial disconnexion. *J. Neurol. Neurosurg. Psychiat.* 43, 719–724

Zihl, J., Cramon, D. von (1980). Registration of light stimuli in the cortically blind hemifield and its effect on localization. *Behav. Brain Res.* 1, 287–298

Zihl, J., Cramon, D. von (1985). Visual field recovery from scotoma in patients with postgeniculate damage: a review of 55 cases. *Brain* 108, 335–365

Zihl, J., Cramon, D. von (1986). Amblyopie nach Hirnschädigung. *Z. prakt. Augenheilkd.* 7, 283–286

Zihl, J., Cramon, D. von (1986). *Zerebrale Sehstörungen*. Kohlhammer, Stuttgart

Zihl, J., Cramon, D. von, Brinkmann, R., Backmund, H. (1977). *Nervenarzt* 48, 219–224

Zihl, J., Cramon, D. von, Mai, N. (1983). Selective disturbance of movement vision after bilateral brain damage. *Brain* 106, 313–340

Zihl, J., Cramon, D. von, Mai, N., Schmid, Ch. (1991). Disturbance of movement vision after bilateral posterior brain damage: further evidence and follow up observations. Submitted to *Brain*

Zihl, J., Cramon, D. von, Pöppel, E. (1978). Sensorische Rehabilitation bei Patienten mit postchiasmalen Sehstörungen. *Nervenarzt* 49, 101–111

Zihl, J., Krischer, C., Meissen, R. (1984). Die heminanopische Lesestörung und ihre Behandlung. *Nervenarzt* 55, 317–323

Zihl, J., Pöppel, E., Cramon, D. von (1977). Diurnal variation of visual field size in patients with postretinal lesions. *Exp. Brain Res.* 27, 245–249

Zihl, J., Roth, W., Kerkhoff, G., Heywood, C.A. (1988). The influence of homonymous visual field disorders on colour sorting performance in the FM 100-hue-test. *Neuropsychologia* 26, 869–876

Zihl, J., Tretter, F., Singer, W. (1980). Phasic electrodermal responses after visual stimulation in the cortically blind hemifield. *Beh. Brain Res.* 1, 197–203

Zihl, J., Tretter, F., Singer, W., Pöppel, E. (1978). Vegetative Reaktionen nach optischer Reizung im blinden Gesichtsfeld eines Patienten mit einer Okzipitallappenläsion. *Med. Psychol.* 3, 241–242

Zihl, J., Werth, R. (1984a). Contributions to the study of 'blindsight' — I. Can stray light account for saccadic localization in patients with postgeniculate damage? *Neuropsychologia* 22, 1–11

Zihl, J., Werth, R. (1984b). Contributions to the study of 'blindsight' — II. The role of specific practice for saccadic localization in patients with postgeniculate visual field defects. *Neuropsychologia* 22, 13–22

Zihlman, A. (1984). Body build and tissue composition in *Pan paniscus* and *Pan troglodytes*, with comparisons to other hominoids. In Sussman, R. (ed.), *The pygmy chimpanzee: evolutionary biology and behavior*. Plenum Press, New York

Zihlman, A., Cronin, J.E., Cramer, D.L., Sarich, V.M. (1978). Pygmy chimpanzee as a possible prototype for the common ancestor of humans, chimpanzees, and gorillas. *Nature* 275, 744–746

Zillig, G. (1947). Psychopathologische Untersuchungen bei Hirnverletzten. Störungen der Wahrnehmung des Aussenraumes und des Körperschemas bei biparietaler Verletzung. Der Fall B.U. *Dtsch. Z. Nervenheilk.* 158, 224

Zimmer, D.E. (1989). Migräne. *Zeit-Magazin* Nr.19, 74–84

Zingerle, H. (1913). Über Störungen der Wahrnehmung des eigenen Körpers bei organischen Gehirnerkrankungen. *Mschr. Psychiat. Neurol.* 34, 13–36

Zipf, G.K. (1935). *The psycho-biology of language*. Boston

Zipf, G.K. (1949). *Human behavior and the principle of least effort*. Maddison-Wesley, Cambridge, Mass.

Zipser, D., Andersen, R.A. (1988). A back-propagation programmed network that simulates the response properties of a subset of posterior parietal neurones. *Nature* 331, 679–684

Zola-Morgan, S., Kritchevsky, M. (1988). Spatial cognition in adults. In Stiles-Davis, J., Kritchevsky, M., Bellugi, U. (eds.), *Spatial cognition*. Brain Bases and Development. Hillsdale, N.J., Erlbaum, 415–21

Zollinger, H. (1973). Zusammenhänge zwischen Farbenbenennung und Biologie des Farbensehens beim Menschen. *Vjschr. Naturf. Ges. Zürich* 118, 227–255

Zollinger, H. (1984). Why just turquoise? Remarks on the evolution of color terms. *Psychol. Res.* 46, 403–409

Zollinger, H. (1988). Biological aspects of color naming. In Rentschler, J., Herzberger, B., Epstein, D. (eds.), *Beauty and the brain*. Birkhäuser, Basel, 149–164

Zrenner, C. (1985). Theories of pineal function from classical antiquity to 1900: a history. *Pineal Res. Review* 3, 1–40

Zrenner, E. (1983). *Neurophysiological aspects of color vision in primates*. Springer, Berlin

Zuckermann, M. (1969). Hallucinations, reported sensations and images. In Zubeck, J.P. (ed.), *Sensory deprivation: fifteen years of research*. Appleton-Centry-Crofts, New York

Zumbroich, T.J., Blakemore, C., Price, D.J. (1988). Stimulus selectivity and its postnatal development in the cat's suprasylvian visual cortex. In Hicks, T.P., Benedek, G. (eds.), *Progress in Brain Research, Vol. 75,* 211–230. Elesevier Publ.

Zusne, L. (1970): *Visual perception of form.* Academic Press, New York,

Zutt, J. (1953). 'Ausser-sich-sein' und 'Auf sich selbst zurückblicken' als Ausnahmezustand. *Nervenarzt* 24, 24–30

Zynda, B. (1984). *Über das Wiedererkennen von Gesichtern.* Doctoral Diss. Freie Universität, Berlin

Index